# PEDIATRIC BURNS

# PEDIATRIC BURNS

Edited By

BRADLEY J. PHILLIPS, MD

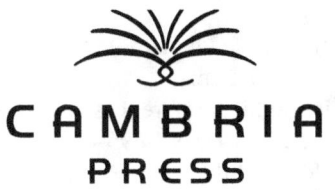

CAMBRIA PRESS

Amherst, New York

Editor: Bradley J. Phillips, M.D.
Director, Burn Program
Director, Surgical Critical Care
Associate Director, Trauma Surgery
Swedish Medical Center: Level 1 Trauma—Adult & Pediatric Injury

Phillips Surgical, PC: from tragedy … Hope!
Burn-Trauma-ICU & Emergency Surgery
499 E. Hampden Rd: Suite 380
Englewood, CO 80113
Office: 303-788-5300
Fax: 303-788-5363
Email: bjpmd2@aol.com

Requests for permission should be directed to:
permissions@cambriapress.com, or mailed to:
Cambria Press
100 Corporate Parkway, Suite 128
Amherst, NY 14226

Paperback ISBN: 978-1-60497-850-6

The Library of Congress has cataloged the earlier, hardcover edition as follows:

Library of Congress Cataloging-in-Publication Data

Pediatric burns / edited by Bradley Phillips.
p. ; cm.
Includes bibliographical references and index.
ISBN 978-1-60497-696-0
1. Burns and scalds in children. I. Phillips, Bradley.
[DNLM: 1. Burns. 2. Adolescent. 3. Child. 4. Infant. WO 704 P371 2010]

RD96.4.P42 2010
617.1'10083—dc22

2010006665

*To my parents*

# TABLE OF CONTENTS

# ACKNOWLEDGMENTS

I would like to deeply thank and acknowledge Dr. Ronald Hunt and Dr. Richard Dennis; their guidance helped a young student learn the art of medicine.

Throughout my career, I have had many teachers and mentors—three who stand out in terms of my burn experience are Dr. David Herndon, Dr. David Greenhalgh, and, of course, Dr. Robert Sheridan.

I owe each of these gentlemen more than they realize and I hope that this book will be accepted as some small form of payment. All of us that treat injured children are motivated by these physicians, day in and day out.

This book exists because of the work of many: the authors, the reviewers, and the publishing staff. I want to especially thank each of the chapter authors—in our busy, hectic world they have taken the time to help put this textbook together. I would also like to thank Ms. Amy Halm for all of her time and dedication to this project.

With the dynamic support of Cambria Press, Inc. this book is now in your hands and I will ask of you one favor:

to help us create
hope from tragedy…

we shall not warmly nor gently embrace
the manifestations of burn injury

for she is the devil's haunt
she is the invading crusader
she is the omnipresent masquerade

and as such, we must strike at her very heart
we must attack her cascading armies and drive them to the gates of hell
we must stand and defend the very weak—lifting them up in loving arms

we are tasked to keep guard—a constant vigil -
every minute, every hour, every day
until the battle is won

these deeds, at all costs, I say
for the price of failure is death

so let us not pause in doubt or fear
let us push forward into the darkness
and hunt for her hidden truths

if our work is just,
our acts are bold,
our efforts are courageous,
then we shall overcome

we shall
and we must

# INTRODUCTION

The practice of pediatric burns is a dynamic and ever evolving field. Many aspects of care are unique to this patient population and the delivery of care is a challenge even for the most experienced medical team.

It is in this framework that we have composed *Pediatric Burns:* a comprehensive guide for the diagnosis, treatment and follow up of the burned child from Time Zero through Long-term Rehabilitation. Mindful of the complexities of burn injuries themselves, with the many divergent causes, as well as, the social and psychological harm associated with severe burn wounds, we have endeavored to create this text for the medical professional involved in attaining the most positive outcome possible for the patient and his or her family.

## THE STUDY OF PEDIATRIC BURNS: TEXTBOOK AND RELATED LEARNING MATERIAL

This project describes the most advanced practices in use throughout the world in every type of burn wound category, providing clear descriptions of treatment methods from every discipline's perspective. Contributors represent practitioners from a wide variety of backgrounds, locations and cultures, all with a common goal: to ensure the healthiest and most highly functioning young burn survivors possible.

## THE REALITY AND SEVERITY OF THE PEDIATRIC BURN

In the United States alone, burns are the third leading cause of death among children 0 to 14 years of age. In addition, each year greater than 125,000 children suffer serious burn injuries, with a disturbing percentage of those through abuse. Yet the number of specialized burn centers in the U.S. is not near enough to be in proximity or even accessible to the majority of these patients. The situation is even worse in most other regions of the world. Therefore, it is critical that we reach as many caregivers as possible with the information contained in these pages, as treatment of burn injuries has undergone dramatic changes over time in every area, from surgical procedures to respiratory and fluid resuscitation and even nourishment and metabolic support. The ability to recognize and react appropriately to pediatric injury can greatly affect the outcome and prognosis, up to and including the patient's future quality of life.

## THE NEED FOR SPECIALIZATION

A seriously burned child requires an immediate, unique and complex order of care from a myriad of disciplines if survival and full functional recovery are to be achieved. When we remember that serious burn injuries are trauma cases first, a comprehensive understanding of these injuries is called for. First responders who can recognize, assess, and take rapid and correct actions in a serious burn case can greatly impact patient survivability until handoff to the ER and surgical team.

This project is an important resource for medical students interested in pursuing a specialty of pediatrics or burns, as well as current practitioners or those in the study of family practice, emergency medicine, surgery and critical care. Surgical and critical care nurses and allied health professionals in respiratory, physical and occupational therapy, psychology and social work will benefit from learning about the comprehensive nature of treatment of the burn-injured child. Clinic and hospital administrators will have a greater appreciation of the specialized equipment and expertise required to deliver optimal care to this most vulnerable patient population after reading this book.

## FROM TRAGEDY....HOPE

*Pediatric Burns* is a multi-authored volume that is solely dedicated to providing a comprehensive roadmap to caregivers involved in treating and rehabilitating a child with a serious burn injury. It is my hope that this work will have a profound effect on the lives of young burn survivors and their families.

–Bradley J. Phillips

# PEDIATRIC BURNS

# CHAPTER ONE

# HISTORICAL PERSPECTIVE AND THE DEVELOPMENT OF MODERN BURN CARE

LEOPOLDO C. CANCIO, MD, FACS COLONEL, MEDICAL CORPS, US ARMY,
US ARMY INSTITUTE OF SURGICAL RESEARCH

BASIL A. PRUITT JR, MD, FACS CLINICAL PROFESSOR OF SURGERY,
UNIVERSITY OF TEXAS HEALTH SCIENCES CENTER AT SAN ANTONIO

## INTRODUCTION

Before WWII and the creation of specialized units for the care of thermally injured patients, deep burns in excess of 30% were almost invariably fatal[1]; the pathophysiology of death following thermal injury was misunderstood, and effective options for resuscitation, wound care, and surgical closure did not exist. What conditions made possible the extraordinary revolution of the last 60 years? Answering this question is important in order to continue to progress in addressing the unsolved problems in burn care and to make our most lifesaving advances available to the rest of the world.

## ORGANIZATIONAL LANDMARKS

Of the various innovations which led to the marked reduction in postburn mortality of the last 60 years, no technology or surgical technique has been more important than the burn center concept itself, which involves the institutional commitment to excellence in research, teaching, and clinical care. Several landmarks in the history of the burn center are provided in the Table. The first burn hospital was established in 1843 by James Syme in Edinburgh, who felt that mixing burn and other surgical patients would represent "the highest degree of culpable recklessness." Subsequently, space was created in a former workshop. Five years later, however, the burn patients were transferred in order to accommodate an increased number of patients from railway and other accidents.[2]

## The World Wars and Fire Disasters

Subsequent developments in burn care, as in trauma care generally, were clearly given impetus by the world wars and civilian fire disasters.[3-5] In 1916, Sir Harold Gillies, who is recognized as the founder of modern plastic surgery, returned from service in France during WWI to establish the first plastic and oral-maxillofacial surgery service in the United Kingdom, treating combat casualties, including burn patients, at Cambridge Military Hospital, Aldershot. Gillies proceeded to develop forward-deployed units during WWII to care for patients with burns and other injuries meriting plastic surgical attention.[6] His cousin, Archibald McIndoe, became consultant in plastic surgery to the Air Ministry and established a burn hospital at East Grinstead during the Battle of Britain in 1940. One of McIndoe's most important contributions was his recognition of the need for a social support system for burn survivors, which was provided for these airmen not only by their own "Guinea Pig Club," but also by hospital staff and local townspeople. McIndoe condemned the use of tannic acid for topical wound care, defined the need for early rehabilitation, and developed techniques for facial reconstruction based on experience with 600 patients with severe facial burns.[7,8] He later recalled his state of mind upon embarking on this uncharted path: "A good, competent surgeon, experienced, yes…but when I looked at a burned boy for the first time and saw I must replace his eyelids, God came down my right arm."[9]

Even though no dedicated burn unit was employed for the care of US combat casualties during WWII, that conflict nonetheless accelerated the development of burn care in the United States, just as in England. The Japanese attack on Pearl Harbor generated several hundred burn casualties,[10] propelled the United States into war, and was followed in January 1942 by a National Research Council symposium on burns, with the initiation of several research programs in burn care. Two such federally funded programs were in place at the Massachusetts General Hospital (MGH) (in burn and complex wound infections and in the physiology of burns) when, on November 28, 1942, a fire at the Cocoanut Grove nightclub in Boston killed 492 of approximately 1000 occupants.[11] One hundred fourteen patients arrived at MGH within a 2-hour period, of whom 39 survived to be admitted to a special casualty ward which remained open till December 13. The hospital course of these 39 patients was carefully documented, and although MGH did not establish a permanent burn unit at the time, these observations (which ranged from fluid resuscitation and management of inhalation injury to social work and rehabilitation) formed a foundation for subsequent research.[12]

Dr Chester Keefer, who supervised the US national program to evaluate penicillin, released enough of the new drug to Dr Champ Lyons, a young surgeon at Massachusetts General Hospital, to treat 13 of the 39 burn patients.[13] Dr Lyons authored the microbiology chapter in the Cocoanut Grove

burns monograph, in which he remarked on the benign nature of the burn wounds of patients who received penicillin.[14] In the spring of 1943, Dr Lyons became a major in the US Army's Surgical Consultants and began a study of penicillin in the treatment of soldiers with complicated orthopedic injuries at the Bushnell General Hospital in Brigham, Utah.[15] In June 1943, a second clinical unit to study penicillin was established at Halloran General Hospital on Staten Island, New York. Dr Lyons was placed in charge of the Wound Unit's study of penicillin, in the course of which 209 combat casualties were treated with the new drug. After completing the studies at Halloran General Hospital, Lyons was reassigned to the Surgical Consultants Division, a new addition to the Army Medical Department. He served as surgical infections and wound management consultant in the Mediterranean theater of operations, where he continued to refine methods of penicillin usage.[15]

In 1947, the Wound Unit was relocated from Staten Island to Fort Sam Houston, Texas, and renamed the Surgical Research Unit (SRU).[16] In this unit, patients with infected burns and other infected wounds were treated on a special ward at Brooke General Hospital.[17] Two years later (1949), due to growing concerns about the possibility of nuclear war with the Soviet Union and recognition (based on experience in Japan) that such a war could generate thousands of burn survivors, the SRU established the nation's second burn unit and refocused its research effort from the evaluation and use of antibiotics to the treatment of burns.[18]

## Organization of the Burn Unit

The organization and subsequent development of the SRU was one of the US Army's most important contributions to burn care. Under a single commander and within a small organization separate from the host military, hospital surgeons, physicians, basic scientists, therapists, nurses, enlisted medics, and support personnel were brought together. The members of this prototypical multidisciplinary burn team had one objective: to improve patient outcomes by conducting integrated basic and clinical research. That is, they sought to take problems from the clinic to the laboratory, where models of injury were developed and the solutions were then transferred back to the clinic and applied to patient care. Along with a growing number of civilian burn units, the SRU (later the US Army Institute of Surgical Research, USAISR) made numerous contributions, several of which are discussed later. Also critical for improving care in the United States was the unit's commitment to training surgeons, many of whom became directors of civilian burn centers.[19-21] Finally, designation of the unit as a single destination for all US military burn casualties, as well as for civilians in the region, provided a constant and sufficient number of patients during both war and peace.

Another major factor in the development of burn care in the United States was the decision on July 4, 1962, by the Shriners Hospitals for Crippled Children to privately fund the construction and operation of 3 pediatric burn units. The center in Galveston, Texas, opened in 1963 under Dr Curtis Artz as chief of staff; the unit in Cincinnati, Ohio, in 1964 under Dr Bruce Macmillan; and the unit in Boston, Massachusetts in 1964 under Dr Oliver Cope. Other dedicated facilities were constructed from through 196in the late 1960s. Similar to the USAISR, they became centers of excellence in care, teaching, and research.[22-24]

The period of most rapid growth in the number of burn units in the United States occurred during the decade 1970-1979, in which the number of units tripled.[23] One hundred fifty units were open in 1979, with a mean of 11 beds each. By 2007, the number of units had decreased to 125, but there was a slight increase in the mean number of beds, to 14. Currently, this translates to a ratio of 1 burn unit per 2.5 million people in the United States.[25] Possible future trends involve a further decrease in the number of burn units, with a concomitant increase in the number of beds per burn unit and increased regionalization of care.[26]

## National and International Burn Associations

The exponential growth in the number of burn professionals led to a series of National Burn Seminars (1959-1967), followed by creation of the American Burn Association (ABA) in 1968. A noteworthy aspect of the ABA has been its inclusion of representatives of all specialties involved in the care of burn patients, that is, all members of the multidisciplinary team. Abroad, similar national (eg, British Burn Association, 1968) and international (eg, International Society for Burn Injuries, 1965; European Burns Association, 1981)[27,28] organizations were formed.

In addition to sponsoring an annual meeting for burn care professionals, the ABA has played an increasing role in carrying out several functions of national importance. These functions have included education, disaster planning, promulgation of standards, and collection of data. Educational efforts include publication of the *Journal of Burn Care and Research* and sponsorship of the Advanced Burn Life Support course (formerly managed by the Nebraska Burn Institute). The ABA supports research primarily via its newly formed Multicenter Trials Group, which, since 2001, has contributed several publications to the field.[29,30] The organization represents its members before Congress, for example, by advocating safe sleepwear for children, fire-safe cigarettes, appropriate payment for burn care services,

and timely qualification of burn survivors for Social Security disability.

With respect to disaster planning, the USAISR and the ABA collaborated during Gulf War I in 1991 and then again during Operation Iraqi Freedom in 2003 to determine, on a daily basis, the number of available beds at burn centers across the country in case of a mass casualty event.[31,32] The relevance of this system to civilian disaster planning led to its continuation by the ABA along with the US Department of Health and Human Services. Disasters such as the World Trade Center attacks in 2001[33] and the Station nightclub fire of 2003[34] further highlighted the need for regional and national burn disaster plans. The ABA has made such planning a priority, as have several regional burn organizations.[35-37] The ABA publishes a continuing series of clinical practice guidelines to address various issues in burn care.[38] The organization's verification committee, which began work in 1992, plays an indispensable role in both promulgating a standard of care for burn center operation as well as providing burn centers with individualized guidance to assist them in achieving that standard.[25,39] Finally, the National Burn Repository, which began collecting data in 1991, provides data for research and enables the setting of performance benchmarks.[40]

## MILESTONES IN RESEARCH AND CLINICAL CARE

The creation of specialized centers dedicated to integrated clinical and laboratory research in burns and to excellence in clinical care and teaching made possible a series of changes in patient management which markedly reduced postburn mortality.

## Fluid Resuscitation

The first milestone was an understanding of the pathophysiology of burn shock and the development of fluid resuscitation formulae. In the early 20th century, it was commonly believed that early postburn deaths were caused by "toxemia." According to this view, the eschar released a toxic substance or substances into the circulation, which caused death. Topical treatment of the burn wound was directed at "tanning" the eschar in an effort to prevent the release of this toxin (see following). The toxemia theory also inspired the rebirth of therapeutic bleeding in the form of partial exchange transfusion:

> Should a patient be admitted after the toxaemia has developed...we have practiced exsanguination transfusion. In the adult we have made no attempt to

completely exsanguinate the patient, and in the child we have removed about 20 c.c. per lb. body weight.[41]

Fluid resuscitation, by contrast, was rarely practiced before WWII. In 1945 the Medical Research Council of the United Kingdom reviewed 1200 admissions from 1937 through 1941 to the Glasgow Royal Infirmary and discovered that one-half of deaths occurred within the first 24 hours and 72 percent within 3 days. Only 4 patients received intravenous plasma or serum.[7] Similarly, Artz and Fox found that the "majority" of burn patients in this era died from inadequate or inappropriate fluid replacement.[18]

Three developments formed the foundation for the method of burn resuscitation used today. First, Underhill, writing in 1930 about his experiences following the Rialto Theatre fire in New Haven, Connecticut, of 1921, argued that the toxemia theory was "an obstruction." Rather, anhydremia, or loss of water from the blood, magnified "the circulatory deficiency" (ie, shock). "The thick, sticky blood… finds great difficulty in passing through the capillaries…the tissues in general suffer from inadequate oxygenation… the heart pumps only a portion of its normal volume." Tissue damage and inflammation caused increased capillary permeability and loss of plasma-like fluid. This was manifested by an increase in hemoglobin, which could also be used as an index of resuscitation. Therapy should consist of intravenous, oral, subcutaneous, and/or rectal infusions of saline solutions, at a rate not to exceed 1.5 liters per hour.[42]

Second, Blalock in 1931 demonstrated that thermal injury in unresuscitated dogs caused loss of over half of the total plasma volume as interstitial edema fluid. He concluded that "fluid loss probably is the initiating factor in the decline of blood pressure"—not toxemia. He also revealed the protein content of edema fluid to be almost as high as that of blood. Interestingly, he did not (at that time) propose that these fluid losses be replaced, but incorrectly speculated that tannic acid and other escharotics might effect a reduction in fluid loss rates.[43]

The third major contribution was the demonstration that plasma, now available in sufficient quantities for clinical use, could be used to resuscitate burn patients when guided by burn-size-based formulae to estimate plasma dose. Use of plasma for burn resuscitation was described by several authors after 1939[44-46]; consistent with Underhill's recommendations, complex formulae based on frequent determinations of the hematocrit or hemoglobin were used to adjust the infusion rate. Mass production of plasma was begun by the Blood for Britain program under Dr Charles Drew et al. in August 1940.[47] As a consequence, plasma was used in the treatment of the approximately 300 thermally injured casualties admitted to the US Naval Hospital Pearl Harbor following the Japanese attack.[10] At the National Research Council meeting of January 7, 1942, chaired by I. S. Ravdin, Harkins proposed for far-forward military use (where laboratory facilities for calculation of the hematocrit were not available) the first formula for resuscitation based on burn size, known as the first aid formula. Fifty ml of plasma were to be given per percent total body surface area burned (TBSA), "in divided doses."[46,48] Later, he defined a more rapid initial rate of infusion—one-third of the estimated volume given in the first 2 hours, one-third in the next 4 hours, and one-third in the next 6 hours.[49] It should be noted that this volume is considerably less than would be recommended by later formulae. After the Cocoanut Grove fire, Cope and Rhinelander reported giving plasma to all but 10 of the 39 patients admitted to MGH. In a fortuitous modification of the NRC formula,

[f]or each 10 percent of the body surface involved, it was planned to give 500 cc. in the first 24 hours. Because the plasma delivered by the Blood Bank during the first 36 hours was diluted with an equal volume of physiologic saline solution, the patient was to receive 1000 cc. for each 10 per cent burned. The plasma dosage was modified subsequently on the basis of repeated hematocrit and serum protein determinations.[50]

In Cope and Moore's follow-up paper of 1947, a further refinement called the surface area formula is described: 75 ml of plasma and 75 ml of isotonic crystalloid solution per TBSA, with one-half given over the first 8 hours and one-half over the second 16 hours. The urine output was to be used as the primary index of resuscitation.[51] Subsequent refinements of this basic concept included the following:

- Evans formula: incorporation of body weight; colloid 1 ml/kg/TBSA and crystalloid 1 ml/TBSA[52]
- Brooke formula: decrease in colloid content to 0.5 ml/kg/TBSA, with crystalloid 1.5 ml/kg/TBSA; replacement of plasma with 5% albumin due to risk of hepatitis[53]
- Parkland formula: elimination of colloid; increase in crystalloid to 4 ml/kg/TBSA[54]
- Modified Brooke formula: elimination of colloid during first 24 hours; crystalloid 2 ml/kg/TBSA[55]

The net effect of this effort was the virtual elimination of postburn renal failure during the early 1950s and a reduction in burn shock as the cause of postburn death by approximately 13%. Currently, the hazards of over-resuscitation (extremity and abdominal compartment syndromes, airway and pulmonary edema, progression of wound depth)[56] mandate a continued search for an approach to resuscitation which reduces the rate of edema formation.

## The Burn Wound: Topical Treatment

In 1954, Liedberg and colleagues at the SRU noted that effective fluid resuscitation now kept many patients with greater than 50% TBSA burns alive past the 2-day mark, only to succumb later. Whereas previous authors had attributed these delayed deaths to "toxemia" or "exhaustion," the presence of positive blood cultures, particularly in patients with large full-thickness burns, pointed at bacteremia of burn wound origin as the cause of death. This hypothesis was confirmed in the animal model of invasive pseudomonal burn wound infection developed by Walker and Mason.[57,58] At that time, however, no effective topical therapy had been identified.[59]

Early descriptions of treatment of wounds are found in ancient Egyptian papyri. Several agents are recommended for the topical treatment of burns in the Ebers papyrus (1550 BC), ranging from boiled, ground goat dung in fermenting yeast, to copper filings and honey, to rubbing a frog warmed in oil on the wound.[60] Hippocrates (460-377 BC), whose influence permeated Western medicine for more than 5 centuries, mentioned several topical agents for the treatment of burns and seemed to favor old hog seam (lard) mixed with any or all of several other agents such as wax, bitumen and resin, and wine. Topical treatment was little changed in the 9th and 10th centuries, when Rhazes (850-932), the most famous Arabian physician of that time, proposed treating burns more gently by application of cold water or egg yolk in attar of roses. He is also credited with being the first to write about the use of animal gut for ligatures in operations. In the next century, Avicenna (Ibn Sina, 980-1037) is said to have recommended ice water for the treatment of burns. That treatment achieved no popularity in ancient times, but has elicited renewed interest in recent years.[61]

The application of various topical agents to the burn wound was continued by surgeons throughout the Middle Ages and Renaissance, with the stature of the physician, rather than data, determining the force of the recommendation. Ambroise Paré (1510-1590) is credited with a comparative trial showing that treatment with mashed onion and salt improved the healing of burns compared to an unspecified "control" substance. William Clowes and Richard Wiseman, the leading British surgeons of the 16th and 17th centuries, respectively, were also proponents of the onion treatment of fresh burns, as was Fabricius Hildanus in Germany.[61,62] A less irritating agent, carron oil, a 50/50 mixture of lime water and linseed oil, was widely used in topical dressings in the 18th and 19th centuries.[61]

The topical application of silver nitrate was initially, in concentrated form (*lapis infernalis*), used to remove granulation tissue from slow-healing burns and to produce a crust on the surface of fresh burns. Silver at that concentration caused severe pain in partial-thickness injuries and could, by itself, cause tissue necrosis. Johann Nepomuk Rust (1775-1840), a surgeon in the Prussian army, was an early advocate of dilute silver nitrate solution (0.2%) for the immediate treatment of burn wounds.[63] Unfortunately, a single application of the dilute solution of silver nitrate could not affect long-term control of microbial proliferation. Consequently, that use of silver nitrate did not win general acceptance.

In the colonial years of the United Sates, American physicians commonly traveled to Europe and England to "complete" their medical education. Consequently, burn care mirrored that practiced in Europe. In 1684, Dr Stafford of London gave Governor John Winthrop of Plymouth Colony a detailed recipe for the preparation of an ointment containing "rine of Eelder, Ssambucus, Ssempervive, and Mmosse" boiled in oil, to which was added barrow's grease (lard from castrated male hogs). At the end of the 18th century, Mr John Vinal of Boston reported the beneficial effects of electricity on his burned thumb, and near the midpoint of the 19th century, Dr Samuel W. Francis described his invention of a glass glove which was used for continuous lime water irrigation of burns on extremities. In the very next year, Dr George Derby of Boston reported on the use of finely powdered dry earth for the successful treatment of burns of the leg and feet.[64]

Throughout the remainder of the 19th century and during the early years of the 20th century, topical therapy of burn wounds changed little, with a wide variety of agents preferred by individual surgeons, without evidence of clinical effectiveness. In 1925, E. C. Davidson described the topical application of tannic acid to bind toxins and coagulate damaged tissue. The tannic acid treatment achieved transient popularity, but findings such as liver damage, impaired distal circulation (when used on the hands), and failure to reduce plasma losses, to prevent subeschar infection, or to improve patient survival led to its abandonment by the early 1940s.[22] The triple-dye treatment (gentian violet, acriflavine, and brilliant green) of Aldrich had similarly transient popularity due to a lack of effect on patient outcome.[22]

With the development of antimicrobial agents such as sulfonamides and other antibiotics in the 1930s and 1940s, it was only a matter of time until effective topical burn wound chemotherapy was developed. Initial trials of penicillin cream by Leonard Colebrook at the Birmingham Accident Hospital Burns Unit were frustrated by the rapid development of microbial resistance, and an early trial of sulfadiazine by Fraser Gurd in Canada was foiled by its low solubility and renal toxicity.[64] In the mid-1960s, Sulfamylon® (mafenide acetate) burn cream was developed by Moncrief and colleagues at the US Army Institute of Surgical Research, at the same time as the effectiveness of 0.5% silver nitrate soaks in controlling burn wound infection was confirmed by Moyer and Monafo.[65-68] Silver sulfadiazine was subsequently developed by Dr Charles Fox to combine the advantages of a sulfonamide and the silver ion, while minimizing the complications of both.[69] Those three agents, along with the recently developed silver-impregnated fabrics,[70] are the most commonly employed chemotherapeutic antimicrobials used in modern burn wound care. Effective topical therapy resulted in a dramatic reduction in invasive gram-negative burn wound infection (burn wound sepsis) as a cause of death (from 59% to 10% of deaths), and in postburn mortality.[65]

## The Burn Wound: Surgical Treatment

Originally, the surgical treatment of burn wounds, if performed, was limited to contracture release and reconstruction after the wound had healed by scar formation. In patients with larger wounds or burns of functional areas, this was wholly unsatisfactory. The creation of burn units committed to care for these patients led to the development of more effective techniques for wound closure. Artz noted that one should "wait until natural sequestration has occurred and a good granulating barrier has formed beneath the eschar…After removing the eschar…skin grafting should be performed as soon as the granulating surface is properly prepared."[71] Debridement to the point of bleeding or pain during daily immersion hydrotherapy (Hubbard tanks) was used to facilitate separation of the eschar.[72] Then, cadaver cutaneous allografts (homografts) were often used to prepare the granulating wound bed for autografting.[73]

In patients with larger (>50% TBSA) burns and in the absence of topical antimicrobials, this cautious approach did not prevent death from invasive burn wound infection, leading some to propose a more radical solution: primary excision of the burn wound. Surgeons at the SRU suggested that a "heroic" practice of early excision, starting postburn day 4, should be considered for patients with large burns. This would reduce the "large pabulum" of dead tissue available for microbial proliferation, while immediate coverage with a combination of autograft and cadaver allograft would further protect the wound.[59] Several authors during the 1950s and 1960s demonstrated the feasibility of this approach, but without an improvement in mortality.[74]

In 1968, Janzekovic described the technique of tangential primary excision of the burn wound with immediate grafting; operating in postwar Yugoslavia, she recalled

that "a barber's razor sharpened on a strap was the pearl among our instruments."[75,76] In a retrospective study, Tompkins et al. reported an improvement in mortality attributed to excision over the course of 1974 through 1984.[77] McManus and colleagues compared patients with burn size >30% TBSA who underwent excision with those who did not from 1983 through 1985. Unfortunately, an improvement in mortality could not be attributed to excision due to the presence of preexisting organ failure precluding surgery in many unexcised patients. However, only 6 of the 93 patients (6.5%) who died in this study had invasive bacterial burn wound infection, whereas 54 of the 93 (58%) developed pneumonia—indicating a shift from wound to nonwound infections.[78]

In McManus' study, excision was performed a mean of 13.5 days postburn. By contrast, Herndon et al. at Galveston implemented a method of excision within 48 to 72 hours of admission, which relied on widely meshed (4:1) autograft covered by allograft. In a small study of children from 1977 through 1981, these authors noted a decrease in length of stay, but not in mortality with this technique.[79] From 1982 through 1985, adults were randomized to undergo early excision versus excision after eschar separation 3 weeks later. Young adults without inhalation injury and with burns >30% TBSA showed an improvement in mortality.[80] A recent meta-analysis found a decrease in mortality but an increase in blood use in early excision patients without inhalation injury.[81]

Despite the limitations of prior studies, early excision is performed today in most US burn centers; however, controversy remains about the definition of "early" and the feasibility of performing radical, total excision during one operation, especially in adults. For patients with the largest wounds and limited donor sites, new methods of temporary and permanent closure have been sought. Burke and Yannas developed the first successful dermal regeneration template (Integra®), composed of a dermal analog (collagen and chondroitin-6-sulfate) and a temporary epidermal analog (Silastic).[82] Cultured epidermal autografts provide material for wound closure for patients with the most extensive burns, although the cost is high and final take rates are variable.[83,84] The ultimate goal of an off-the-shelf bilaminar product for permanent wound closure, with a take rate similar to that of cutaneous autografts, has not yet been achieved.

## Inhalation Injury

Improvements in fluid resuscitation and wound care refocused attention on inhalation injury. Although the term "acute respiratory distress syndrome" (ARDS) was first applied to post-traumatic pulmonary failure in 1967,[85] direct injury to the lung parenchyma by inhalation of toxic gases such as chlorine and phosgene was recognized during WWI. This injury featured "pulmonary oedema, rupture of the pulmonary alveoli and concentration of the blood, with increased viscosity and a tendency to thrombosis." Treatment included oxygen and (for patients with deep cyanosis) venesection of as much as 400 ml of blood.[86]

The potential of indoor fire disasters to cause rapid, early death by asphyxia or inhalation injury was demonstrated by the Cleveland Clinic fire of 1929. This fire, started by ignition of highly flammable X-ray film, claimed 125 lives. Most of the deaths have been attributed to inhalation of carbon monoxide, hydrogen cyanide, and nitrogen oxides.[87] Those caring for the Cocoanut Grove victims were aware of that earlier experience and noted that the majority of patients arriving at MGH who did not survive to admission had elevated carbon monoxide levels. A sense of the situation can be gleaned from this description: "The first clue to the high incidence of pulmonary burns was afforded by the number who died within the first few minutes after reaching the hospital. They were very cyanotic, comatose or restless, and had severe upper respiratory damage."[88] From this description, it appears likely that some patients died with airway obstruction. In the patients surviving to admission, these authors provided a classic description of smoke inhalation injury. Severe upper respiratory and laryngeal edema mandated "radical therapy" in 5 patients, namely endotracheal intubation followed by immediate tracheotomy. Oxygen was provided via tent or transtracheal catheter. Those surviving this initial phase developed diffuse bronchiolitis, bronchial plugging, and alveolar collapse.[88]

Further improvements in the care of patients with inhalation injury required the development of positive-pressure mechanical ventilators. In the course of thoracic trauma research in North Africa during WWII, Brewer, Burbank, and colleagues of the Second Auxiliary Surgical Group (with the support of theater consultant surgeon Colonel Churchill) delivered oxygen via mask along with an intermittent, hand-operated positive airway pressure device to casualties with "wet lung of trauma."[89,90] Dr Forrest Bird, V. R. Bennett, and J. Emerson built mechanical positive-pressure ventilators towards the end of WWII, all inspired by technology developed during the war to deliver oxygen to pilots flying at high altitudes.[91] The availability of these and similar machines, as well as the Scandinavian polio epidemic of 1952, spurred the creation of intensive care units (ICUs).[92] At the USAISR and several other centers, burn ICUs were located within the burn unit under the direction of surgeons who ensured continuity of care and clinical research.

Once accurate diagnosis of inhalation injury by bronchoscopy and xenon-133 lung scanning became available, it became apparent that these patients were at increased risk of pneumonia and death.[93] Large animal models were developed and the pathophysiology of the injury was defined.[94] Unlike ARDS as a result of mechanical trauma or alveolar injury due to inhalation of chemical warfare agents, smoke inhalation injury was found to damage the small airways, with resultant ventilation-perfusion mismatch, bronchiolar obstruction, and pneumonia.[95,96] This injury process featured activation of the inflammatory cascade, which in animal models was amenable to modulation by various anti-inflammatory agents. However, the most effective interventions to date are those directly aimed at maintaining small airway patency and avoiding injurious forms of mechanical ventilation. These include use of high-frequency percussive ventilation with the Volumetric Diffusive Respiration (VDR-4®) ventilator developed by Bird and delivery of heparin by nebulization.[97,98]

## Metabolism and Nutrition

Bradford Cannon described the nutritional management of survivors of the Cocoanut Grove fire: "All patients were given a high protein and high vitamin diet...it was necessary to feed [one patient] by stomach tube with supplemental daily intravenous amogen, glucose, and vitamins."[99] But it soon became apparent that survivors of major thermal injury evidenced a hypermetabolic, hypercatabolic state which continued at least until wounds were closed and often resulted in severe loss of lean body mass. Cope and colleagues reported measurements of metabolic rate up to 180% of normal in the early postburn period and recognized a relationship between wound size and metabolic rate.[100] Wilmore and colleagues identified the role of catecholamines as mediators of the postburn hypermetabolic state.[101] They further documented that the burn patient is internally warm and not externally cold, and that hypermetabolism is wound-directed, as evidenced by elevated blood flow to the burn wound.[102-104] Consequently, the metabolic needs of the burn patient should be met rather than suppressed.

Earlier (1971), Wilmore et al. demonstrated the feasibility of providing massive amounts of calories by a combination of intravenous and enteral alimentation.[105] Curreri published the first burn-specific formula for estimating caloric requirements: calories/day = 25(wt in kg) + 40(TBSA).[106] However, the provision of adequate calories and nitrogen failed to arrest hypermetabolism and reduced, but did not eliminate, erosion of lean body mass in these patients. Three approaches have recently been taken to address this problem: the use of anabolic steroids such as oxandrolone,[29] the use of propranolol,[107] and the use of insulin,[108] insulin-like growth factor,[109] or human growth hormone.[110]

## Rehabilitation

As postburn mortality decreased, the problems encountered by burn survivors, particularly those with deep and extensive injuries, became paramount.[111] The scientific study of the occupational, physical, and psychosocial rehabilitation of the thermally injured patient is a relatively young field. The Cocoanut Grove monograph briefly states that 6 patients with dorsal hand burns who had been splinted in extension were referred to the Physical Therapy Department after completion of surface healing.[112] In the 1950s, Moncrief began rehabilitation soon after admission and resumed it 8 to 10 days after skin grafting.[113,114] The advent of heat-malleable plastic (thermoplastic) material made it possible to fabricate increasingly complex and effective positioning devices.[115] This was followed by the introduction of pressure to treat hypertrophic scars and the development of customized pressure garments.[116] Others reduced or eliminated the delay between skin grafting and ambulation, without deleterious effects on graft take.[117,118] In brief, burn rehabilitation is no longer viewed as a "phase" which begins after completion of wound healing, but as a highly specialized process which must begin immediately upon patient admission and often continues for 24 or more months. A recent review noted a need for more research in this area, to include prevention and management of hypertrophic scarring and contractures, pain management, post-traumatic stress disorder, affective disorders, and body-image problems.[119]

## Conclusion

The 1910 edition of the *Encyclopedia Britannica* stated that death "almost invariably" results when one-third or more of the TBSA is burned.[1] For young adults, the 20th century in the West featured an extraordinary diminution in the lethal-area 50% (LA50—that burn size which is lethal for 50% of a given cohort of patients), from 43% TBSA in 1945 through 1957 to 82% in 1987 through 1991.[21] At the Galveston Shriners' Burn Center, the mortality rate in children with 96-100% TBSA burns during 1982 through 1996 was only 69%. This led the authors to conclude that "prompt intravenous access and resuscitation, aggressive operative therapy, and the avoidance of sepsis and organ failure by meticulous critical care should enable any child with almost any burn size to live." At that hospital[120] and others providing comprehensive long-term psychosocial and physical rehabilitation,[121] follow-up data indicate that

young survivors of massive thermal injury can experience reasonably well-adjusted lives. No one intervention was solely responsible for these improvements; rather, it is the combined effects of fluid resuscitation, wound care, infection control, inhalation injury management, nutritional support, and aggressive rehabilitation. All these interventions, however, were directed in a coordinated fashion at correcting what Burke called "the fundamental defects of burn injury—the destruction of skin and its immediate physiologic effects."[1] This revolution has been possible only because of integrated clinical and laboratory research, carried out by multidisciplinary teams in specialized centers supported by generous public and private funding. New challenges remain—in maintaining and expanding adequate numbers of fully trained nurses, therapists, and physicians,[122] in caring for the most severely injured, in facilitating their return to a successful role in society, and in translating the most effective of these advances to that large portion of the world which has not yet adopted them.

## Key Points

- Civilian fire disasters and military conflicts focused attention on the burn problem and motivated the creation of a new type of specialized care facility: the burn unit. The success of these units depends on multidisciplinary teams engaged in closely integrated laboratory and translational research and evidence-based clinical care.
- Postburn shock is primarily caused by loss of fluid similar to plasma from the blood into the interstitium (edema formation). Fluid resuscitation formulae were developed based on the recognition that these losses are proportional to burn size.
- Before the development of effective topical antimicrobials, invasive gram-negative burn wound infection was the leading cause of postburn death. The commonly used topical agents are mafenide acetate or some form of the silver cation (silver sulfadiazine, silver-impregnated dressings).
- Early excision and grafting of deep partial and full-thickness burn wounds has become the standard of care for burn patients.
- Inhalation injury increases postburn mortality. Effective therapies include not only gentle mechanical ventilation, but also those which maintain small airway patency.
- Thermal injury causes hypermetabolism and hypercatabolism, which persist to some degree

long after the wound is closed. Caloric requirements are roughly proportional to the burn size.

- Effective rehabilitation must begin immediately upon admission and must be directed at minimizing disability from hypertrophic scarring, contracture, and deconditioning.
- Particularly in children and young adults, striking improvements in postburn survival call into question the notion of futile care and refocus attention on long-term psychosocial rehabilitation.

## ACKNOWLEDGMENTS

The authors gratefully acknowledge the support of Ms Gerri Trumbo, USAISR librarian.

## TABLE 1. Organizational landmarks in the history of modern burn care.

**1843:** Syme establishes first burn hospital in Edinburgh[2]

**1884:** Burn patients admitted to a special ward at the Glasgow Royal Infirmary[7]

**1915:** Sir Harold Gillies sets up the first plastics and oral-maxillofacial unit in the United Kingdom at Cambridge Military Hospital, Aldershot[6]

**1940:** During the Battle of Britain, Archibald McIndoe inaugurates a Royal Air Force burn unit at East Grinstead[7]

**1941:** Japanese attack on Pearl Harbor marks entry of United States into WWII and tests US military burn care capabilities[10]

**1942:** US National Research Council holds national meeting, establishes research program in burns[51]

**1942:** Fire disaster at the Cocoanut Grove nightclub in Boston leads to documentation of several aspects of burn pathophysiology and treatment[12]

**1944:** Colebrook establishes a burn unit with Medical Research Council support at the Birmingham Accident Hospital[123,124]

**1947:** Evans establishes the first burn unit in the United States in Richmond, Virginia

**1949:** US Army Surgical Research Unit (SRU) establishes the US Army Burn Center at Fort Sam Houston, Texas

**1951:** SRU begins aeromedical evacuation of critically ill burn patients[125,126]

**1953:** Dobrkovsky founds the burn unit in Prague[123]

**1962:** Shriners Hospitals set up three burn units for children in the United States[22]

**1959–1967:** National burn seminars are held in the United States[127]

**1965:** International Society for Burn Injuries is founded[27]

**1968:** British Burn Association and American Burn Association (ABA) are founded

**1974:** *Burns Including Thermal Injury* (later, *Burns*) begins publication

**1980:** *Journal of Burn Care and Rehabilitation* (later, *Journal of Burn Care and Research*) begins publication

**1991:** ABA and American College of Surgeons Committee on Trauma begin verification of US burn centers

**1991:** ABA creates the National Burn Repository database

**2003:** US Army Institute of Surgical Research and ABA reinstitute a national burn-bed reporting system developed during Operation Desert Storm to support combat operations in Iraq and other crises[32]

## REFERENCES

**1.** Burke JF. Burn treatment's evolution in the 20th century. *J Am Coll Surg.* 2005; **200:** 152–153.

**2.** Wallace AF. Recent advances in the treatment of burns—1843–1858. *Br J Plast Surg.* 1987; **40:** 193–200.

**3.** Pruitt BA Jr. Combat casualty care and surgical progress. *Ann Surg.* 2006; **243:** 715–729.

**4.** Eldad A. "Out of the strong came forth sweetness": on the contribution of military conflicts to the development of burn treatment in Israel. *J Burn Care Rehabil.* 1998; **19:** 470–479.

**5.** Eldad A. Notes on the contribution of wars and conflicts to medical achievements. *Burns.* 1998; **23:** 523.

**6.** Mills SMH. Burns down under: lessons lost, lessons learned. *J Burn Care Rehabil.* 2005; **26:** 43–52.

**7.** Jackson D. Thirty years of burn treatment in Britain—where now? *Injury.* 1978; **10:** 40–45.

**8.** Jackson DM. Burns: McIndoe's contribution and subsequent advances. *Ann R Coll Surg Engl.* 1979; **61:** 335–340.

**9.** Mayhew ER. *The Reconstruction of Warriors.* London: Greenhill Books; 2004.

**10.** Anonymous (Administrative History Section, Administrative Division, Bureau of Medicine and Surgery Pearl Harbor navy medical activities. In: *The United States Navy Medical Department at War, 1941–1945.* Vol. 1, parts 1-2. Washington, DC: The Bureau of Medicine and Surgery; 1946.

**11.** Saffle JR. The 1942 fire at Boston's Cocoanut Grove nightclub. *Am J Surg.* 1993; **166:** 581–591.

12. Aub JC, Beecher HK, Cannon B, et al. *Management of the Cocoanut Grove Burns at the Massachusetts General Hospital.* Philadelphia: JB Lippincott; 1943.

13. Dalton ML. Champ Lyons: an incomplete life. *Ann Surg.* 2003; **237:** 694–703.

14. Lyons C. Problems of infection and chemotherapy. In: Aub JC, Beecher HK, Cannon B, et al., eds. *Management of the Cocoanut Grove Burns at the Massachusetts General Hospital.* Philadelphia: JB Lippincott; 1943: 94–102.

15. Neushul P. Fighting research: army participation in the clinical testing and mass production of penicillin during the Second World War. In: Cooter R, Harrison M, Sturdy S, eds. *War, Medicine and Modernity.* Gloucestershire: Sutton Publishing Ltd; 1998: 208–211.

16. McAllister SE, Pulaski EJ. A technic for dressing septic wounds. *Am J Nurs.* 1947; **47:** 396–398.

17. Anonymous.—Annual Report of Brooke General Hospital, Brooke Army Medical Center, Fort Sam Houston, Texas for Calendar Year 1947, p. 44.

18. Artz CP. Burns in my lifetime. *J Trauma.* 1969; **9:** 827–833.

19. Heimbach DM. We can see so far because… *J Burn Care Rehabil.* 1988; **9:** 340–346.

20. Pruitt BA Jr. The integration of clinical care and laboratory research. A model for medical progress. *Arch Surg.* 1995; **130:** 461–471.

21. Pruitt BA Jr. Centennial changes in surgical care and research. *Ann Surg.* 2000; **232:** 287-301.

22. Artz CP. History of burns. In: Artz CP, Moncrief JA, Pruitt BA Jr, eds. *Burns: A Team Approach.* Philadelphia: WB Saunders; 1979: 3–16.

23. Dimick AR, Brigham PA, Sheehy EM. The development of burn centers in North America. *J Burn Care Rehabil.* 1993; **14:** 284–299.

24. McCollough NC III. The evolution of Shriners Hospitals for Children in North America. *Clin Orthop.* 2000; **374:** 187–194.

25. Brigham PA, Dimick AR. The evolution of burn care facilities in the United States. *J Burn Care Res.* 2008; **29:** 248–256.

26. Warden GD, Heimbach D. Regionalization of burn care—a concept whose time has come. *J Burn Care Rehabil.* 2003; **24:** 173–174.

27. Pruitt BA Jr. The development of the International Society for Burn Injuries and progress in burn care: the whole is greater than the sum of its parts. *Burns.* 1999; **25:** 683–696.

28. Königová R. History of burn medicine. *Acta Chir Plast.* 2004; **46:** 37–38.

29. Wolf SE, Edelman LS, Kemalyan N, et al. Effects of oxandrolone on outcome measures in the severely burned: a multicenter prospective randomized double-blind trial. *J Burn Care Res.* 2006; **27:** 131–139.

30. Palmieri TL, Caruso DM, Foster KN, et al. Effect of blood transfusion on outcome after major burn injury: a multicenter study. *Crit Care Med.* 2006; **34:** 1602–1607.

31. Shirani KZ, Becker WK, Rue LW, Mason AD Jr, Pruitt BA Jr. Burn care during Operation Desert Storm. *US Army Med Dep J.* 1992; PB 8-92-1/2: 37–39.

32. Barillo DJ, Jordan MH, Jocz RJ, Nye D, Cancio LC, Holcomb JB. Tracking the daily availability of burn beds for national emergencies. *J Burn Care Rehabil.* 2005; **26:** 174–182.

33. Yurt RW, Bessey PQ, Bauer GJ, et al. A regional burn center's response to a disaster: September 11, 2001, and the days beyond. *J Burn Care Rehabil.* 2005; **26:** 117–124.

34. Harrington DT, Biffl WL, Cioffi WG. The Station nightclub fire. *J Burn Care Rehabil.* 2005; **26:** 141–143.

35. Barillo DJ, Dimick AR, Cairns BA, Hardin WD, Acker JE III, Peck MD. The Southern Region burn disaster plan. *J Burn Care Res.* 2006; **27:** 589–595.

36. Yurt RW, Lazar EJ, Leahy NE, et al. Burn disaster planning: an urban region's approach. *J Burn Care Res.* 2008; **29:** 158–165.

37. ABA Board of Trustees, Committee on Organization and Delivery of Burn Care Disaster management and the ABA plan. *J Burn Care Rehabil.* 2005; **26:** 102–106.

38. Gibran NS; Committee on Organization and Delivery of Burn Care of the ABA. Practice guidelines for burn care, 2006. *J Burn Care Res.* 2006; **27:** 437–438.

39. American Burn Association; American College of Surgeons. Guidelines for the operation of burn centers. *J Burn Care Res.* 2007; **28:** 134–141.

40. Latenser BA, Miller SF, Bessey PQ, et al. National Burn Repository 2006: a ten-year review. *J Burn Care Res.* 2007; **28:** 635–658.

41. Ravdin IS, Ferguson LK. The early treatment of superficial burns. *Ann Surg.* 1924: 439–456.

42. Underhill FP. The significance of anhydremia in extensive superficial burns. *JAMA.* 1930; **95:** 852–857.

43. Blalock A. Experimental shock. VII. The importance of the local loss of fluid in the production of the low blood pressure after burns. *Arch Surg.* 1931; **22:** 610–616.

44. Black DAK. Treatment of burn shock with plasma and serum. *Br Med J.* 1940; **2:** 693–697.

45. Elkington JR, Wolff WA, Lee WE. Plasma transfusion in the treatment of the fluid shift in severe burns. *Ann Surg.* 1940; **112:** 150–157.

46. Harkins HN, Lam CR, Romence H. Plasma therapy in severe burns. *Surg Gynecol Obstet.* 1942; **75:** 410–420.

47. Kendrick DB. *Blood Program in World War II.* Washington, DC: Office of the Surgeon General, Department of the Army; 1964.

48. Harkins HN. The general treatment of the patient with a severe burn. In: Harkins HN. *Burns, Shock Wound Healing and Vascular Injuries.* Philadelphia: WB Saunders; 1943: 3–26.

49. Harkins HN. The present status of the problem of thermal burns. *Physiol Rev.* 1945; **25**: 531–572.

50. Cope O, Rhinelander FW. The problem of burn shock complicated by pulmonary damage. In: Aub JC, Beecher HK, Cannon B, et al., eds. *Management of the Cocoanut Grove Burns at the Massachusetts General Hospital.* Philadelphia: JB Lippincott; 1943: 115–128.

51. Cope O, Moore FD. The redistribution of body water and the fluid therapy of the burned patient. *Ann Surg.* 1947; **126**: 1010–1045.

52. Evans EI, Purnell OJ, Robinett PW, Batchelor A, Martin M. Fluid and electrolyte requirements in severe burns. *Ann Surg.* 1952; **135**: 804–817.

53. Reiss E, Stirman JA, Artz CP, Davis JH, Amspacher WH. Fluid and electrolyte balance in burns. *JAMA.* 1953; **152**: 1309–1313.

54. Baxter CR, Shires T. Physiological response to crystalloid resuscitation of severe burns. *Ann N Y Acad Sci.* 1968; **150**: 874–894.

55. Pruitt BA Jr, Mason AD Jr, Moncrief JA. Hemodynamic changes in the early postburn patient: the influence of fluid administration and of a vasodilator (hydralazine). *J Trauma.* 1971; **11**: 36–46.

56. Pruitt BA Jr. Protection from excessive resuscitation: "pushing the pendulum back". *J Trauma.* 2000; **49**: 567–568.

57. Teplitz C, Davis D, Mason AD Jr, Moncrief JA. Pseudomonas burn wound sepsis. I.Pathogenesis of experimental pseudomonas burn wound sepsis. *J Surg Res.* 1964; **4**: 200–216.

58. Walker HL, Mason AD Jr, Raulston GL. Surface infection with Pseudomonas aeruginosa. *Ann Surg.* 1964; **160**: 297–305.

59. Liedberg NC, Reiss E, Artz CP. Infection in burns. III. Septicemia, a common cause of death. *Surg Gynecol Obstet.* 1954; **99**: 151–158.

60. Rutkow IM. Ancient civilizations. In: Rutkow IM. *Surgery: An Illustrated History.* St. Louis, MO: Mosby; 1993: 12–13.

61. Klasen HK. Introduction. In: Klasen HK. *History of Burns.* Rotterdam: Erasmus Publishing; 2004: 13–20.

62. Haeger K. *The Illustrated History of Surgery.* London: Harold Starke; 1989: 122–127.

63. Klasen HK. The use of silver in the treatment of burns. In: Klasen HK. *History of Burns.* Rotterdam: Erasmus Publishing; 2004: 483–518.

64. Pruitt BA Jr. Multidisciplinary care and research for burn injury: 1976 presidential address, American Burn Association meeting. *J Trauma.* 1977; **17**: 263–269.

65. Pruitt BA Jr, O'Neill JA Jr, Moncrief JA, Lindberg RB. Successful control of burn-wound sepsis. *JAMA.* 1968; **203**: 1054–1056.

66. Lindberg RB, Moncrief JA, Mason AD Jr. Control of experimental and clinical burn wound sepsis by topical application of Sulfamylon compounds. *Ann N Y Acad Sci.* 1968; **150**: 950–960.

67. Moyer CA, Brentano L, Gravens DL, Margraf HW, Monafo WW Jr. Treatment of large burns with 0.5% silver nitrate solution. *Arch Surg.* 1965; **90**: 812–867.

68. Bondoc CC, Morris PJ, Wee T, Burke JF. The metabolic effects of 0.5 per cent $AgNO_3$ in the treatment of major burns in children. *J Pediatr Surg.* 1967; **2**: 22–28.

69. Fox CL Jr. Silver sulfadiazine—a new topical therapy for pseudomonas in burns. Therapy of pseudomonas infection in burns. *Arch Surg.* 1968; **96**: 184–188.

70. Tredget EE, Shankowsky HA, Groeneveld A, Burrell R. A matched-pair, randomized study evaluating the efficacy and safety of Acticoat silver-coated dressing for the treatment of burn wounds. *J Burn Care Rehabil.* 1998; **19**: 531–537.

71. Artz CP, Soroff HS. Modern concepts in the treatment of burns. *JAMA.* 1955; **159**: 411–417.

72. Dobbs ER. Burn therapy of years ago. *J Burn Care Rehabil.* 1999; **20**: 62–66.

73. Jackson D. A clinical study of the use of skin homografts for burns. *Br J Plastic Surg.* 1954; **7**: 26–43.

74. Jackson D, Topley E, Cason JS, Lowbury EJL. Primary excision and grafting of large burns. *Ann Surg.* 1960; **152**: 167–189.

75. Janzekovic Z. A new concept in the early excision and immediate grafting of burns. *J Trauma.* 1970; **10**: 1103–1108.

76. Janzekovic Z. Once upon a time…how West discovered East. *J Plast Reconstr Aesthetic Surg.* 2008; **61**: 240–244.

77. Tompkins RG, Burke JF, Schoenfeld DA, et al. Prompt eschar excision: a treatment system contributing to reduced burn mortality. A statistical evaluation of burn care at the Massachusetts General Hospital (1974–1984). *Ann Surg.* 1986; **204**: 272–281.

78. McManus WF, Mason AD Jr, Pruitt BA Jr. Excision of the burn wound in patients with large burns. *Arch Surg.* 1989; **124**: 718–720.

79. Herndon DN, Parks DH. Comparison of serial debridement and autografting and early massive excision with cadaver skin overlay in the treatment of large burns in children. *J Trauma.* 1986; **26**: 149–152.

80. Herndon DN, Barrow RE, Rutan RL, Rutan TC, Desai MH, Abston S. A comparison of conservative versus early excision. Therapies in severely burned patients. *Ann Surg.* 1989; **209**: 547–552.

81. Ong YS, Samuel M, Song C. Meta-analysis of early excision of burns. *Burns.* 2006; **32**: 145–150.

82. Burke JF, Yannas IV, Quinby WC Jr, Bondoc CC, Jung WK. Successful use of a physiologically acceptable artificial skin in the treatment of extensive burn injury. *Ann Surg.* 1981; **194**: 413–428.

83. Gallico GG III, O'Connor NE, Compton CC, Kehinde O, Green H. Permanent coverage of large burn wounds with autologous cultured human epithelium. *N Engl J Med.* 1984; **311**: 448–451.

84. Rue LW III, Cioffi WG, McManus WF, Pruitt BA Jr. Wound closure and outcome in extensively burned patients treated with cultured autologous keratinocytes. *J Trauma.* 1993; **34**: 662–667.

85. Ashbaugh DG, Bigelow DB, Petty TL, Levine BE. Acute respiratory distress in adults. *Lancet.* 1967; **2**: 319–323.

86. *The Medical Manual of Chemical Warfare*. London: His Majesty's Stationery Office; 1941.

87. Gregory KL, Malinoski VF, Sharp CR. Cleveland Clinic Fire Survivorship Study, 1929–1965. *Arch Environ Health*. 1969; **18**: 508–515.

88. Aub JC, Pittman H, Brues AM. The pulmonary complications: a clinical description. In: Aub JC, Beecher HK, Cannon B, et al., eds. *Management of the Cocoanut Grove Burns at the Massachusetts General Hospital*. Philadelphia: JB Lippincott; 1943: 34–40.

89. Brewer LA, Burbank B, Samson PC, Schiff CA. The "wet lung" in war casualties. *Ann Surg*. 1946; **123**: 343–362.

90. Brewer LA III. A historical account of the "wet lung of trauma" and the introduction of intermittent positive-pressure oxygen therapy in World War II. *Ann Thorac Surg*. 1981; **31**: 386–393.

91. Morris MJ. Acute respiratory distress syndrome in combat casualties: military medicine and advances in mechanical ventilation. *Mil Med*. 2006; **171**: 1039–1044.

92. Rosengart MR. Critical care medicine: landmarks and legends. *Surg Clin North Am*. 2006; **86**: 1305–1321.

93. Shirani KZ, Pruitt BA Jr, Mason AD Jr. The influence of inhalation injury and pneumonia on burn mortality. *Ann Surg*. 1987; **205**: 82–87.

94. Shimazu T, Yukioka T, Hubbard GB, Langlinais PC, Mason AD Jr, Pruitt BA Jr. A dose-responsive model of smoke inhalation injury. Severity-related alteration in cardiopulmonary function. *Ann Surg*. 1987; **206**: 89–98.

95. Shimazu T, Yukioka T, Ikeuchi H, Mason AD Jr, Wagner PD, Pruitt BA Jr. Ventilation-perfusion alterations after smoke inhalation injury in an ovine model. *J Appl Physiol*. 1996; **81**: 2250–2259.

96. Cancio LC, Batchinsky AI, Dubick MA, et al. Inhalation injury: pathophysiology and clinical care. Proceedings of a symposium conducted at the Trauma Institute of San Antonio, San Antonio, TX, USA on 28 March 2006. *Burns*. 2007; **33**: 681–692.

97. Cioffi WG Jr, Rue LW III, Graves TA, McManus WF, Mason AD Jr, Pruitt BA Jr. Prophylactic use of high-frequency percussive ventilation in patients with inhalation injury. *Ann Surg*. 1991; **213**: 575–582.

98. Desai MH, Mlcak R, Richardson J, Nichols R, Herndon DN. Reduction in mortality in pediatric patients with inhalation injury with aerosolized heparin/N-acetylcystine therapy. *J Burn Care Rehabil*. 1998; **19**: 210–212.

99. Cannon B. Procedures in rehabilitation of the severely burned. In: Aub JC, Beecher HK, Cannon B, et al., eds. *Management of the Cocoanut Grove Burns at the Massachusetts General Hospital*. Philadelphia: JB Lippincott; 1943: 103–110.

100. Cope O, Nardi GL, Quijano M, Rovit RL, Stanbury JB, Wight A. Metabolic rate and thyroid function following acute thermal trauma in man. *Ann Surg*. 1953; **137**: 165–174.

101. Wilmore DW, Long JM, Mason AD Jr, Skreen RW, Pruitt BA Jr. Catecholamines: mediators of the hypermetabolic response to thermal injury. *Ann Surg*. 1974; **180**: 653–669.

102. Wilmore DW, Mason AD Jr, Johnson DW, Pruitt BA Jr. Effect of ambient temperature on heat production and heat loss in burn patients. *J Appl Physiol*. 1975; **38**: 593–597.

103. Aulick LH, Wilmore DW, Mason AD Jr, Pruitt BA Jr. Influence of the burn wound on peripheral circulation in thermally injured patients. *Am J Physiol*. 1977; **233**: H520–H526.

104. Wilmore DW, Aulick LH, Mason AD, Pruitt BA Jr. Influence of the burn wound on local and systemic responses to injury. *Ann Surg*. 1977; **186**: 444–458.

105. Wilmore DW, Curreri PW, Spitzer KW, Spitzer ME, Pruitt BA Jr. Supranormal dietary intake in thermally injured hypermetabolic patients. *Surg Gynecol Obstet*. 1971; **132**: 881–886.

106. Curreri PW, Richmond D, Marvin J, Baxter CR. Dietary requirements of patients with major burns. *J Am Diet Assoc*. 1974; **65**: 415–417.

107. Herndon DN, Hart DW, Wolf SE, Chinkes DL, Wolfe RR. Reversal of catabolism by beta-blockade after severe burns. *N Engl J Med*. 2001; **345**: 1223–1229.

108. Sakurai Y, Aarsland A, Herndon DN, et al. Stimulation of muscle protein synthesis by long-term insulin infusion in severely burned patients. *Ann Surg*. 1995; **222**: 283–297.

109. Cioffi WG, Gore DC, Rue LW III, et al. Insulin-like growth factor-1 lowers protein oxidation in patients with thermal injury. *Ann Surg*. 1994; **220**: 310–319.

110. Herndon DN, Hawkins HK, Nguyen TT, Pierre E, Cox R, Barrow RE. Characterization of growth hormone enhanced donor site healing in patients with large cutaneous burns. *Ann Surg*. 1995; **221**: 649–659.

111. Pereira C, Murphy K, Herndon D. Outcome measures in burn care. Is mortality dead? *Burns*. 2004; **30**: 761–771.

112. Watkins AL. A note on physical therapy. In: Aub JC, Beecher HK, Cannon B, et al., eds. *Management of the Cocoanut Grove Burns at the Massachusetts General Hospital*. Philadelphia: JB Lippincott; 1943: 111–114.

113. Moncrief JA. Complications of burns. *Ann Surg*. 1958; **147**: 443–475.

114. Moncrief JA. Third degree burns of the dorsum of the hand. *Am J Surg*. 1958; **96**: 535–544.

115. Willis B. The use of Orthoplast isoprene splints in the treatment of the acutely burned child: preliminary report. *Am J Occup Ther*. 1969; **23**: 57–61.

116. Larson DL, Abston S, Evans EB, Dobrkovsky M, Linares HA. Techniques for decreasing scar formation and contractures in the burned patient. *J Trauma*. 1971; **11**: 807–823.

117. Schmitt MA, French L, Kalil ET. How soon is safe? Ambulation of the patient with burns after lower-extremity skin grafting. *J Burn Care Rehabil*. 1991; **12**: 33–37.

118. Burnsworth B, Krob MJ, Langer-Schnepp M. Immediate ambulation of patients with lower-extremity grafts. *J Burn Care Rehabil*. 1992; **13**: 89–92.

119. Esselman PC, Magyar-Russell G, Fauerbach JA. Burn rehabilitation: state of the science. *Am J Phys Med Rehabil*. 2006; **85**: 383–413.

**120.** Wolf SE, Rose JK, Desai MH, Mileski JP, Barrow RE, Herndon DN. Mortality determinants in massive pediatric burns. An analysis of 103 children with > or = 80% TBSA burns (> or = 70% full-thickness). *Ann Surg.* 1997; **225:** 554–569.

**121.** Sheridan RL, Hinson MI, Liang MH, et al. Long-term outcome of children surviving massive burns. *JAMA.* 2000; **283:** 69–73.

**122.** Gamelli RL. Who will follow? *J Burn Care Res.* 2006; **27:** 1–7.

**123.** Artz CP. Historical aspects of burn management. *Surg Clin North Am.* 1970; **50:** 1193–1200.

**124.** Lawrence JC. Some aspects of burns and burns research at Birmingham Accident Hospital 1944–93: A. B. Wallace Memorial Lecture, 1994. *Burns.* 1995; **21:** 403–413.

**125.** Maxwell E. *Memorandum from Director of Professional Services, Office of the Surgeon General of the Air Force, Headquarters, U.S. Air Force.* Washington, DC: US Air Force; November 27, 1951.

**126.** Cancio LC, Pruitt BA Jr. Management of mass casualty burn disasters. *Int J Disaster Med.* 2004; **2:** 114–129.

**127.** Baxter CR. Before the American Burn Association. *J Burn Care Rehabil.* 1993; **14:** 228–229.

# Principles of Pediatric Burn Injury

Alice Leung, MD,

and

Bradley J. Phillips, MD

## Outline

## Introduction

Over 250,000 children suffer from burn injuries each year, accounting for one-third of all burns in the United States.[1] Thirty thousand of these patients sustain injuries that require admission to a hospital.[2] In the last 25 years, pediatric mortality has decreased through improved resuscitation and aggressive operative treatment. However, burn injuries are still the fifth leading cause of death in pediatric patients and are estimated to cost society $2.3 billion each year.[3,4]

Burn injuries are ubiquitous, affecting every age, class, and ethnicity. Toddlers are most at risk for injury, as their newly gained mobility and ability to explore their environment outpace their cognitive development and sense of danger.[5] In all age groups, males are 50% to 100% more likely to be burned than females. The majority of pediatric burns are scald injuries, followed by flame injuries. Chemical and electrical injuries occur less frequently; these burns tend to be small, involving less than 10% of the body. One of the greatest dangers in caring for pediatric burn patients is underestimation of the severity of the injury, both by physicians and by families. The presence of an inhalation injury in children younger than 4 years is associated with a poor prognosis. Even small burns in the absence of inhalation in infants have been known to be fatal.[6] Although death from burn injury can result from burn shock in the immediate postinjury period, it is more commonly due to septic complications such as pneumonia, respiratory distress syndrome, and multisystem organ failure.[7] The best outcome for patients with large burns is achieved by referral to the multidisciplinary setting of specialized burn centers. The first line of care is often given by emergency medical services, pediatricians, and emergency department physicians. It is essential that patients be properly triaged for care. Smaller burns should be treated as outpatients, while referral of more significant injuries to multidisciplinary burn centers is necessary to optimize patient care. In order to treat patients effectively, all health care providers should have a general understanding of burn physiology and care.

## PATHOPHYSIOLOGY

The skin is the largest organ in the human body, providing structural support, immunity, and regulation of heat and water loss.[3] It is comprised of 3 layers: epidermis, dermis, and subcutaneous tissue. The epidermis is comprised of avascular sheets of keratinocytes. The basal layer of the epithelium continues to replicate as the superficial layers are constantly exfoliated. The epidermis acts as a mechanical barrier to infection by preventing invasion of bacteria. The dermis is more physiologically active and can be divided into 2 layers. The papillary dermis interdigitates with the epidermis, supplying the avascular layer with nutrients and oxygen. The reticular dermis is rich in collagen and elastin, giving skin its strength and elasticity.[8] This strong reticular layer is embedded with hair follicles, nerves, sebaceous glands, and sweat glands.

Once a thermal injury is sustained, it can be separated into 3 zones: (1) the zone of coagulation, (2) the zone of stasis, and (3) the zone of hyperemia.

The zone of coagulation is characterized by severe injury with irreversible damage. This area of devitalized tissue is surrounded by the zone of stasis, which sustains lesser injury but demonstrates significant inflammation and impaired vasculature. The outermost zone of hyperemia exhibits vasodilation and increased blood flow. Injury to this area is reversible and typically resolves in 7 to 10 days.[8,9] The boundaries of these zones are dynamic and affected by management. The zone of coagulation may continue to expand in the setting of impaired blood supply. These wounds are at risk of deepening in the setting of hypovolemia, hypotension, catecholamine-induced vasoconstriction, and infection. The best-case scenario is for the zone of coagulation to remain stable while the zone of hyperemia ingresses, replacing the zone of stasis.[8] Appropriate fluid resuscitation in the first 24 to 48 hours is the best means of avoiding worsening of wounds.[3]

Determining the extent of damage in a burn injury is based on the depth and the total body surface area involved. The actual thickness of skin will vary between different patients and different sites of the body. Therefore, wound depth is described relative to the layer of skin injured rather than as a numeric measurement. Knowing the remaining

layer of uninjured skin provides insight on the wound's ability to spontaneously heal versus the need for surgical intervention. Many tools have been developed in recent years to help assess the depth of injury, including dyes, laser Doppler, and thermography.[3,10] However, these methods are expensive and often not readily accessible in the daily care of patients. The depth of a wound remains primarily a clinical diagnosis, taking into account the physical examination and mechanism of injury. The preferred nomenclature divides the depth of burn injury into 4 classes: (1) superficial, (2) superficial partial thickness, (3) deep partial thickness, and (4) full thickness.

A superficial burn involves only the epidermis and is characterized by erythema and edema in the absence of blistering and desquamation. Superficial burns heal spontaneously in days and are commonly seen in sunburns.

Both superficial partial-thickness and deep partial-thickness burns involve the entire epidermis and a portion of the dermis.[1] These wounds are commonly seen in scald and flash burns.[1] Superficial partial-thickness injuries are contained within the papillary dermis, while deep partial-thickness injuries extend into the reticular dermis. Both wounds are characterized by pain and fluid-filled blisters. Debridement of superficial partial-thickness wounds will expose moist, pink tissue which blanches with pressure. These wounds will reepithelialize from retained epithelial islands and dermal appendages. They can be expected to heal within 7 to 28 days with minimal scarring.[1] Deep partial-thickness injuries destroy the epithelial interstices of the papillary dermis along with a greater proportion of the vasculature. The surface of these wounds will appear drier and will be slower to blanch with digital pressure on exam. If uncomplicated by infection, deep partial-thickness wounds can spontaneously heal in 3 to 8 weeks from the wound edges and remnant dermal appendages.[1,3] The protracted course of healing renders these deeper wounds prone to complications, such as hypertrophy and pigment changes.[3,11]

The epidermis and dermis are completely destroyed in full-thickness injuries. These burns will not heal spontaneously due to destruction of dermal appendages. Full-thickness burns are leathery, insensate, and fail to blanch, corresponding to destruction of elastin fibers, nerve endings, and vasculature of the dermis.[1] Full-thickness burns are seen in flame, grease, and solid contact injuries. They are associated with multiple complications, such as acute renal failure, hyperkalemia, rhabdomyolysis, myoglobinuria, and compartment syndrome.[8]

The other major factor in defining the extent of damage is determining the total body surface area (TBSA) involved. Calculation of the TBSA includes all partial-thickness and full-thickness burns, with the exclusion of superficial injuries.[11] Due to the highly variable body proportions in the pediatric population, the commonly used "rule of nines" in adult burn management is not applicable without significant modification. An alternative method to estimate the area involved, referred to as the "rule of palms," uses the patient's hand as an internal control. The surface area of one side of the patient's hand, including the fingers, is equal to 1% of the TBSA. This palm estimate is particularly useful with injuries that present with a splattered or blotchy distribution. A more precise calculation of the TBSA involves the use of an age-appropriate Lund-Browder chart (Table 1).[1] In particular, emergency medical services and the emergency department may find the modified "rule of nines" and the palm estimate very helpful. In these circumstances, the TBSA is used for triage purposes and serves only as a marker of the extent of injury. Upon admission to a burn center or intensive care setting, the TBSA will influence initial resuscitation and management until the Lund-Browder chart is utilized for a more accurate assessment.[8]

## BURN MANAGEMENT

History should be obtained from the patient, the patient's caregivers, and the responding emergency medical services, if applicable. The mechanism of injury as well as the temperature of the agent and duration of contact should be determined. The surrounding circumstances should be documented very carefully, as up to 20% of pediatric burns are a result of negligence or abuse.[12] Health care providers should be alert and aware of the warning signs of abuse, such as an inconsistent or changing history, an unexplained delay in seeking medical attention, and treatment being sought by an unrelated adult (Table 2).[8]

## Triage

### Outpatient Care

Outpatient care of a pediatric burn is preferable whenever possible. Management of smaller burns (TBSA less than 10%) in the normal home environment provides a less traumatic as well as a more cost-effective means of providing care, to the benefit of both the patient and society. In order to permit outpatient care, the patient must be able to maintain oral nutrition and hydration, and the family must be able to manage appropriate wound care.[1] The caregiver should be reliable and should demonstrate wound care competence prior to discharge.[9] Daily care involves washing the wound with a mild detergent in warm water and providing gentle debridement with a wet washcloth. A thin layer of topical antimicrobials, such as silvadene or bacitracin, should be applied to the affected area in order to maintain a

moist environment conducive to wound healing and to help with pain control. The wound can then be covered with a nonadherent dry dressing. The patient's pain should be sufficiently controlled with oral medications to permit dressing changes and regular use of the affected areas. In addition to patient education, physical therapy should be considered, particularly if the injury crosses a joint.[2]

### Inpatient Care

The American Burn Association has recommended guidelines for admission or transfer to a burn center. All children with a burn greater than 10% TBSA or with involvement of an area of functional importance should be immediately admitted for care.[11] Other cutaneous injuries requiring admission, which may be more significant than initially appreciated, are chemical and electrical burns and the presence of inhalation injury. Pediatric patients initially treated in a facility without qualified caregivers should be transferred to a burn center specializing in pediatric care. The child may require intubation prior to transportation and should be covered in dry, sterile sheets to maintain body temperature.[12]

### Pre-hospital Preparation

In preparing for the patient's arrival, the room should be warmed to 31.5°C ± 0.7°C and equipped with warming blankets.[12] The materials necessary for airway management and intravenous access should be readily available, as well as large volumes of warm intravenous fluids. All personnel should be gowned, gloved, and masked to protect themselves and the patient.[8]

Burn management can be divided into 3 phases (Figure 1): (1) emergent, (2) acute, and (3) rehabilitation and reintegration.

### Emergent

The goal of the emergent phase in pediatric burn management is to stop the injury process and stabilize the patient. Health care providers should follow the pediatric advanced life support and advanced trauma life support protocols, attending to the patient's airway, breathing, and circulation. Adequate fluid resuscitation and maintenance of core body temperature are also very important throughout the management of a pediatric burn.

### Airway—Upper Airway Injury

Airway obstruction occurs with injury to the soft tissues of the head, face, and neck, including the upper airway. The upper airway is defined as the oropharynx above the glottis and is typically injured from direct heat to the mucosa. This injury responds with formation of edema within 45 to 60 minutes. Patients with inhalation injury may initially present with a patent airway but can rapidly deteriorate within 12 to 24 hours of injury as edema peaks from aggressive fluid resuscitation. Some warning signs of exposure to high heat include singed nasal hairs and facial burns.[1] Common signs of a compromised airway include progressive hoarseness, stridor or inspiratory grunting, and increased respiratory rate and work of breathing. Providers should continue to monitor the patient's airway throughout the emergent phase, with a low threshold for intubation in burn patients. Upon any sign of a deteriorating airway, an endotracheal tube should be placed, as delay in securing the airway can lead to a difficult and potentially dangerous emergent intubation. Edema can be minimized by elevating the head of the bed 20° to 30° and typically resolves in 2 to 3 days[12]; thus, tracheostomy is typically not required.[1]

Particular care must be taken to properly secure the endotracheal tube once placement is confirmed. Failure to secure the tube may be disastrous due to the difficulty of reintubation in the setting of massive edema. The tube may be secured carefully with umbilical tape, but the surrounding skin must be monitored regularly for signs of pressure necrosis.[1]

## Breathing—Lower Airway Injury

Lower airway inhalation injuries (defined as injury below the glottis, including the lung parenchyma) greatly increase the severity of the burn. Lower airway injuries are the result of smoke inhalation, usually within an enclosed space, such as a house fire. The inhalation of smoke results in exposure of the terminal bronchioalveolar tree to chemical irritants. With the notable exception of steam injuries, lower airway injuries are not a result of direct thermal injury, since the upper airway dissipates the energy prior to exposure to the lower airway.[8] Pediatric patients become disoriented easily and may hide rather than making an attempt to escape from an enclosed space.[13] Young children in particular are at high risk of inhalation injury due to relative immobility and lack of situational awareness.[7]

The diagnosis of lower airway injury in pediatric patients is typically clinical. Visualization of subglottic structures via bronchoscopy requires an internal diameter of at least 8.0 mm and can be technically demanding in small children. Any patient who presents with a history of being involved in an enclosed space fire, loss of consciousness, or change in mental status should be presumed to have some degree of inhalation injury and closely monitored. These injuries may occur in the absence of cutaneous damage and may present with dyspnea, rales and rhonchi, and carbonaceous sputum.[8]

These signs and symptoms typically develop within 24 to 48 hours of the initial insult.[1]

The treatment of lower airway injuries is mainly supportive.[14] Bronchodilators may be useful in treating bronchospasm caused by aerosolized irritants. Mechanical ventilation with positive end expiratory pressure may be necessary in the event of a declining respiratory status. Permissive hypercapnia is allowed in patients with inhalation injury as long as the pH remains above 7.20.[12] Meticulous pulmonary toilet plays an important role, particularly in younger children, where the small diameter of pediatric endotracheal tubes can result in an increased risk of obstruction by secretions as well as wound exudates and topical wound care agents.[1]

Systemic poisoning caused by inhaled toxins, frequently carbon monoxide and cyanide, is also very common. Carbon monoxide poisoning is the leading cause of death at the scene of a fire.[8] This toxin binds over 200 times more efficiently to hemoglobin than oxygen does, thereby impairing oxygen uptake and delivery to tissues.[13] Patients can present with headaches, dizziness, nausea, and seizures. A high clinical suspicion is required based on the history and mechanism of injury. Pulse oxymetry will be unreliable in carbon monoxide poisoning, as hemoglobin will be detected in its bound form. Treatment with high-flow oxygen via a nonrebreather mask is initiated while blood carboxyhemoglobin levels are measured to confirm the diagnosis. Treatment is continued until carboxyhemaglobin is less than 10% total hemoglobin.[8]

Cyanide poisoning is associated with incomplete combustion of nitrogenous materials such as silks and polyesters.[15] The severity of poisoning is directly related to the extent of smoke exposure and results in metabolic acidosis. Patients with cyanide poisoning present with nonspecific symptoms such as nausea, tachypnea, and changes in mentation. Unfortunately, treatment is limited and the patient is notably unresponsive to supplemental oxygen.[3] There is no available widespread testing method, and patients are typically diagnosed postmortem.[8]

## Circulation

Predictable hemodynamic changes occur following severe burn injury. The patient exhibits an elevated cardiac output and decreased total peripheral resistance, making assessment of intravascular volume difficult.[12] Intravenous access is very important in patient management. In large burns, 2 large-bore peripheral IVs are required.[1] Obtaining access may be difficult secondary to distribution of the burn, edema, and reluctance to penetrate burned skin. Though not ideal, access may be obtained through areas of burn injury, followed by venous cut-downs and intraosseous access.

Once acquired, lines should be secured by sutures, as exudative fluid will not permit adhesive tapes and edema will render wraps impractical.[1]

## Fluids

Though the skin's gross appearance may be deceptively intact, burn injuries have 5 to 10 times the evaporative loss of normal skin. In smaller burns, patients are able to maintain hydration with oral fluids or with a combination of oral fluids supplemented with low volumes of intravenous fluids.[3] Patients with burns involving greater than 15% TBSA have substantial exudative and evaporative fluid loss and require intravenous fluid resuscitation.[8] Different factors, such as electrical or chemical injury, may lead to higher than expected fluid requirements. Inhalation injury is known to increase resuscitation requirements by up to 50%.[8] Large burn injuries will cause systemic physiologic changes which exacerbate intravascular loss. Inflammatory mediators are released from the wound and lead to significant capillary leak. Fluid is able to escape the intravascular space and migrate into the interstitium. Capillary permeability peaks 18 hours following injury, and maximum edema is observed at 48 hours.[9] The use of colloid as resuscitation fluid is controversial and generally not recommended in the first 24 hours. Extravasation of colloid during the initial resuscitation period is thought to prolong edema secondary to capillary leak. Instead, colloid use in resuscitation should be reserved for persistent hypotension or to possibly prevent overresuscitation in patients who manifest a less than ideal response to crystalloids.[3] Beyond the first 24 hours, colloid may be given regularly in order to supplement the disproportionate protein loss observed in pediatric patients.

Initial resuscitation may be calculated based on a number of formulae, such as the Parkland formula and the Galveston formula (Figure 2).[16]

In addition to the resuscitation volume, maintenance fluids must be added and will constitute a greater proportion of the fluid delivered to patients relative to adults.[1] The goal of resuscitation is adequate end organ perfusion, which can be evaluated by a combination of clinical and laboratory findings. A Foley catheter, rather than diapers or urine bags, should be placed to more accurately monitor hourly urine output in order to evaluate fluid resuscitation. Appropriate goals are 1 cc to 1.5 cc urine/hour in children and 1.5 cc to 2.0 cc urine/hour in infants. In the event that urine output does not respond to resuscitation after substantial amounts of crystalloid fluids, such as lactated Ringers solution, a transesophageal echo or pulmonary artery catheter may be invaluable to determine intravascular fluid status. Resuscitation efforts can be evaluated based on vital signs, peripheral temperature, capillary refill, and level of mentation.

Lab values such as hematocrit, base deficit, central venous pressure, and lactate levels may be helpful in evaluating tissue perfusion and should be monitored regularly throughout the emergent phase.

Although certain injuries will require more fluid than calculated by the resuscitation formula, health care providers must be cognizant of possible overresuscitation. Complications of excessive resuscitation include pulmonary edema, electrolyte imbalances, and prolific third spacing. Electrolyte imbalance is commonly seen in conjunction with the massive cellular damage of a significant burn injury. Specifically, hyponatremia can occur, while hypovolemia and the generous use of albumin may lead to hyperkalemia. Large fluctuations of sodium in the pediatric population can lead to seizures, cerebral edema, herniation, and central pontine myelinosis,[3,12,17] which are all associated with increased mortality. Such significant electrolyte fluctuations may be prevented by close monitoring. Continued third spacing of excess fluid from overresuscitation can result in abdominal compartment syndrome. This complication should be considered when bladder pressure, acting as a marker for abdominal pressure, exceeds 30 mmHg (thus overcoming capillary filling pressures).[18] Abdominal compartment syndrome may be relieved by reducing intravenous fluids or by performing a paracentesis or decompressive laparotomy. Diuretics are inappropriate in the setting of acute burns.

Infants and small children younger than 2 years and with a weight less than 20 kg require the addition of glucose to their resuscitative fluids since they have sparse glycogen stores and are susceptible to hypoglycemia.[1,12,18] Their glucose should be monitored hourly during the initial resuscitation period and replaced as necessary.

## Temperature

Temperature dysregulation is a hallmark of burn injury, with a tendency towards hypothermia. A subnormal body temperature should be minimized, as it leads to coagulation dysfunction and is associated with increased mortality. The use of warm intravenous fluids, particularly during resuscitation, when large volumes are used, can help maintain core body temperature.[1] The ambient temperature in the intensive care setting and operating room should be kept warm in order to decrease radiant heat loss through large, hyperemic burns.[8]

## Secondary Assessment

Though the temptation is to immediately address a burn injury, a systemic head-to-toe evaluation should be performed. Any potentially life-threatening injury should be addressed before wound management is initiated.

Head and Neurological—A change in mental status or loss of consciousness is an indication for a head CT scan in order to evaluate for accompanying intracranial trauma. Other causes to be considered include intoxication, hypoxia, hypotension, and inhalation injury.

Eyes and Ears—In the event of facial involvement, an ophthalmology consultation should be obtained early, as a delayed evaluation will be difficult with advancing facial edema. A fluorescein exam to evaluate the cornea is helpful to evaluate for subtle eye injuries. External ear burns should be debrided and treated with mafenide acetate to prevent suppurative chondritis.

Chest—The patient's ability to ventilate should be reevaluated during the secondary survey, particularly with a deep, circumferential injury. Full-thickness burns will result in an inelastic eschar which restricts the chest wall's ability to rise with inspiration. Signs of respiratory distress and elevated peak airway pressures will be seen with decreased chest compliance. An escharotomy, in which incisions through the eschar to healthy tissue are made along the flanks and below the costal margins, allows the anterior chest wall to dissociate from the posterior chest wall and abdomen.[19] This results in relieving the constriction and improving the patient's respiratory status.

Extremities—Deep circumferential burns to the limbs may cause a complication similar to that described above. The leathery eschar constricts the underlying soft tissue as subcutaneous structures proceed to swell with aggressive fluid resuscitation and systemic inflammation. This constriction results in an increase in compartment pressure. When the pressure exceeds 25 mmHg to 30 mmHg, capillary filling pressure is overcome and tissue becomes hypoperfused. This hypoperfusion can lead to limb ischemia, functional disability, and amputation.[3] The injured limb should be kept at the level of the heart to maintain optimal mean arterial pressure while limiting dependent pooling.[12] Early findings of compartment syndrome include pain on stretching, a tense limb, palpable pulses, brisk capillary refill, and paresthesia.[19] Once the syndrome develops, treatment via escharotomy to release constriction is indicated.[3] Warm ischemia leads to soft tissue death within 2 to 3 hours, allowing escharotomies to be performed in the controlled environment of an operating room. The incision should be performed with electrocautery to minimize blood loss and should follow the proceeding guidelines: avoid named nerves, preserve longitudinal veins, and avoid crossing joints in straight lines to minimize future contractures.[19]

Abdomen—The patient should be evaluated for associated injuries, particularly in the setting of excess fluid requirements and rapidly decreasing hematocrit levels. Abdominal fluid and pressure should be monitored in efforts to avoid massive overresuscitation. With sympathetic activity decreasing splanchnic flow, the patient should be initiated on H2 antagonist prophylaxis to prevent Curling's ulcers of the gastroduodenum. Since burn patients are also prone to swallowing air and gastric dilation, a nasogastric tube should be placed to decompress the stomach during the emergent phase.[12]

## Tetanus

As open wounds, burn injuries are vulnerable to tetanus infection.[8] If the patient's immune status is unknown, he or she should receive active immunization with injection of tetanus toxoid. If the patient is not immunized, passive immunization in the form of antitetanus immunoglobulin should be administered in addition to tetanus toxoid.[20]

## Acute Phase

The goal of the acute phase is to cover the wound in order to decrease water vapor loss, prevent desiccation, and aid in pain control and bacterial inhibition.[20] Complications seen during this period include wound infection, sepsis, pulmonary insufficiency, and multisystem organ failure.[2]

Pain control throughout this phase is very important in order to minimize trauma and additional stress. Dose-appropriate intravenous morphine, oral acetaminophen, and acetaminophen with codeine are commonly used in pediatric burn management. Similar to other pediatric medications, these analgesics should be dosed by weight.[21]

Morphine IV: 0.1-0.2 mg/kg/dose Q2-4 hr PRN (**max. dose:** 15 mg/dose).
Oxycodone PO: 0.05-0.15 mg/kg/dose Q4-6 hr PRN (**max. dose:** 5 mg/dose).
Acetaminophen PO: 10-15 mg/kg/dose Q4-6 hr PRN (**max. dose:** 90 mg/kg/24 hr).

Extended-release oxycodone can help with pain control in older children. Conscious sedation with the use of ketamine is helpful during procedures such as extensive dressing changes.[9]

Intact blisters of partial-thickness wounds are managed by using firm, sweeping motions with warm saline-soaked gauze to unroof and debride them. The wounds are then treated with topical antimicrobials and covered with dry, nonadherent dressings. Bacitracin is commonly used and has coverage against some gram-positive bacteria. Its primary function is to maintain a moist environment conducive to healing. Silvadene is an agent which has a broader spectrum of antimicrobial coverage, including gram-positive and gram-negative bacteria and fungi. However, as an opaque white cream, Silvadene renders wound assessment more difficult between dressing changes. The most common adverse drug reaction of Silvadene is self-limited leukocytosis, but other potential complications include anaphylaxis and kernicturus. Its use should be avoided in patients with known sulfa allergies and children younger than 2 years. Mafenide acetate, a carbonic anhydrase inhibitor with good penetration of devitalized tissue and cartilage, is commonly used on the tip of the nose and ears. It covers a broad range of gram-positive and gram-negative bacteria, pseudomonas, and some anaerobes. Broader use of mafenide acetate in pediatrics is generally limited due to pain associated with its application.[3]

With the increased antibiotic resistance seen with hospital-acquired infections, the choice of topical antimicrobials for wound management is becoming increasingly important. The provider must choose a regimen which meets the patient's tolerance of dressing changes and appropriately covers the specific pathogens identified.[22]

## Operative Management

Early excision and grafting of burn wounds is a key component in the management of burns. Epinephrine (0.5 µg/ml) is used as tumescence during excision and helps control blood loss. The use of epinephrine decreases typical blood loss of 3.5% to 5% total blood volume per percent of TBSA excised by up to 80%.[17] Excision within 48 hours of injury has been shown to be effective in improving care and decreasing mortality.[17,23] In addition, patients display decreased risk of infection, decreased antibiotic requirements, and improved long-term outcomes, such as reduced hypertrophic scarring. Patients are also able to leave the hospital earlier, and the cost of care as a whole is minimized.[23]

There are many options for coverage once the wound is excised, including autograft, allograft, xenograft, and a number of synthetic coverings. The standard of care for definitive coverage is autograft in the form of split-thickness skin graft (STSG). The grafts are harvested from an unburned area using a pneumatic-powered dermatome at a thickness of 0.010 inch to 0.012 inch. The scalp is a good harvest site in children because of its ability to reepithelialize very quickly. Repeated harvesting of donor sites for wound coverage may be allowed as necessary once healing occurs. STSGs are typically meshed 1:1 or 2:1 in order to protect wounds. Besides permitting drainage of fluid from the wound bed to maximize graft viability, meshing also allows for the possibility of graft expansion. STSGs may be placed as sheets over cosmetically or functionally important areas such as the face and hands. Sheet grafts are pie-holed using a knife in order to allow drainage of exudates during the immediate postoperative period. Meshing at ratios greater than 1:1 permits the graft to cover a larger area. Ratios of up to 3:1 and 4:1 are commonly used for coverage of large wounds. Greater ratios are uncommon secondary to fragility of the grafts and the greater distance epithelial cells must migrate to facilitate full wound coverage. Even with substantial meshing, there may be insufficient uninjured skin available for full burn coverage. These patients benefit from cultured epithelial autografts to aid in definitive coverage. Within the first few days of care, a healthy sample of the patient's skin is taken and sent for cell culture. The cultured epithelial cells are then applied to the patient's excised wounds. Some surgeons use the cultured epithelial cells in conjunction with STSG meshed with large expansion ratios, such as 8:1, to encourage reepithelialization of the mesh interstices. Cultured epithelial autografts are capable of organizing into epidermal structures within weeks and allow for coverage of extensive open wounds.[24] Allograft and xenograft may be used as temporary biologic dressings for excised burns. These wound coverings act as physical barriers to infection, limit fluid loss, and decrease the inflammatory response.[25] Temporary coverage of the wound is capable of promoting dermal regeneration of the wound bed in preparation for definitive coverage with autograft. Even though these biologic dressings are chemically treated to reduce immunogenicity, they will still be rejected within days to weeks.[26]

Alternative nonimmunogenic synthetic dressings, such as Biobrane and Integra, have been developed in recent years. Biobrane is a porous mesh of nylon filaments embedded with type I collagen which is covered with a layer of silicone. The collagen fibers adhere to the wound bed and allow for improved migration of epithelial cells. The pores allow leakage of exudates and reciprocal passage of topical antimicrobials down to the wound. Integra is another synthetic bilayer commonly used in the coverage of complex burn wounds. The chondroitin sulfate layer serves as a dermal regeneration template and is protected by a silastic membrane. Once the Integra becomes vascularized, the superficial silastic layer is removed and replaced with a thin STSG.[26]

## Sepsis

With the loss of an important barrier for infection, burn patients are at high risk of developing infection and sepsis. The use of elevated temperature as a marker for sepsis is unreliable in pediatric burn patients since these children are often febrile in the absence of infection secondary to the release of inflammatory mediators.[20] A heightened suspicion of sepsis is warranted if the patient becomes toxic, hypotensive, thrombocytopenic, leukocytic, or experiences a change in mental status.[27] In the context of these signs and symptoms, the patient's wound should be examined and a pan-culture, including blood, sputum, and urine, should be obtained. Quantitative cultures of the wound are useful to differentiate infection from colonization. Broad-spectrum antibiotic coverage should be started immediately and continued until culture sensitivities can further direct treatment. If no infection is found, then antibiotics may be stopped after 48 to 72 hours to avoid overuse of broad-spectrum antibiotics. Preventative protocols, such as the scheduled rotation of central venous catheters, also help to reduce the prevalence of sepsis.[20]

## Antibiotics/Antifungals

There is no role for systemic antibiotic prophylaxis in burn care. Antibiotics should only be initiated to treat known or suspected infections and continued as directed by culture sensitivities.[12] Prudent, sensitivity-driven antibiotic use is important in limiting antibiotic resistance in a population very prone to sepsis and infection. Fungal wound infections are very common in large burns and typically occur at day 16 following injury.[28] Because these infections are associated with a very high mortality rate, oral prophylaxis with antifungal agents is appropriate and has been shown to decrease the incidence of fungal infections.[29]

## Nutrition and Metabolism

Patients with large burns experience a hypercatabolic state over an extended period, well beyond their initial injury.[30] This state is characterized by increased insulin resistance, gluconeogenesis, and protein catabolism.[3] In injuries involving greater than 40% TBSA, a patient's resting energy expenditure is 150% to 200% higher than normal.[31] In these large burns, patients can lose up to 25% of their preburn body weight by the third week following their injury.[32] The effects of hypercatabolism include loss of lean body mass and growth delay for up to 2 years.[25] As bone mineral density is chronically lower in children with severe burns, these patients have an increased lifelong risk of osteoporosis. The goal of nutrition and metabolism in the acute phase is to maintain preadmission weight, which may be difficult to assess initially due to fluctuations in fluid status. Laboratory findings are also unreliable in the acute phase and cannot be used in the evaluation of nutritional status. Hypoalbuminemia is expected acutely as the liver shifts production in favor of acute phase reactants such as C-reactive protein.[33] Early excision of injured tissue helps to decrease catabolism, presumably by removing a major source of inflammatory mediators. Early initiation of nutrition is an important component in counteracting catabolism.[34] Delays in initiating nutritional support have been shown to exacerbate catabolism, impair wound healing, and increase the risk of infection.[8] Therefore, a nasogastric tube should be placed early

in order to begin a high caloric diet with carbohydrates as the main source of calories. Early enteral feeding has also been shown to maintain the gut barrier, prevent gut atrophy, and potentially decrease enterogenic infections. Care should be taken to avoid overfeeding, which can lead to hepatic dysfunction, hyperglycemia, and increased carbon dioxide production. When initiating enteral feedings in the acute phase, patients should be monitored for hypotension, splanchnic hypoperfusion, and intestinal necrosis.[30]

Therapy, in addition to nutrition, can help to attenuate lean body mass loss. While aerobic exercise is effective for older children in maintaining lean body mass, muscle strength, and power, it has limited use in infants and toddlers.[31] Anabolic agents have also been shown to benefit pediatric burn patients. Oxandrolone given orally twice daily at a dose of 0.1 mg/kg will increase protein synthesis and decrease loss of lean body mass. Insulin supplementation can help overcome burn-induced insulin resistance. When titrated between 400 mU/ml and 900 mU/ml to control blood glucose levels for 7 days, patients demonstrate improved healing time and increased muscle protein synthesis.[31]

Catabolism-blocking agents can also be useful in these patients. Propanolol, a beta blocker, can attenuate the stress-induced hypermetabolism. When titrated to decrease the patient's baseline heart rate by 20% for several weeks, beta blockade is able to decrease excess thermogenesis, tachycardia, cardiac work, and superphysiologic resting energy expenditure.[35]

## Rehabilitation and Reintegration

Improved resuscitation, along with early excision and grafting, permits most pediatric patients to survive deep burns. Currently, even a child with a large burn of up to 60% TBSA may be expected to survive with appropriate care in a specialized burn center.[36] With more severely burned children surviving their injuries, the focus has shifted to improving their quality of life.[37] The morbidity of these burns is significant and includes common complications such as scarring, contraction, and weakness from loss of muscle. The ultimate goal of this phase is to facilitate psychological and functional recovery, and is best accomplished in the multidisciplinary setting of a specialized burn center.

## Hypertrophic Scarring

Hypertrophic scarring is a common complication of burns and occurs most often in deep dermal burns that are left to heal spontaneously over a protracted period of greater than 3 weeks.[1] Hypertrophic areas have an exaggerated inflammatory response which stimulates excess growth of collagen fibers. These scars typically form in areas of high elasticity and tension, such as the lower face, anterior chest, and submental triangle.[2] The formation of these scars peaks at 3 to 6 months. The course of each scar will vary, but most will partially resolve in 12 to 18 months as the scar matures, becoming softer and flatter with decreased hyperemia.[7] Hypertrophy is also associated with significant pruritus, which can be difficult to treat and very distressing to the patient. The first line of therapy for pruritus includes oral antihistamines and emollient creams.[38]

Keloid scars are another complication, with a similar appearance to hypertrophic scarring. However, they continue to expand beyond the original borders of the injury and occur more often in darker-pigmented patients.[2]

The treatment of hypertrophic and keloid scars begins conservatively with the application of pressure garments. These garments apply 24 mmHg of pressure to the scar and help remodel collagen fibers.[2] Patients who are at risk of developing scars or who show early signs of hypertrophy should be fitted for these garments as soon as wounds are closed and the majority of edema has resolved. In order to be effective, the garments must be worn 23 hours each day for months.[39] The greatest challenge in using these garments in pediatric care is compliance, particularly in adolescents. If the garments produce insufficient results, steroid injections may also be helpful. Steroid therapy requires many injections spaced 1 cm apart with 1 mg triamcinolone/site. This treatment can be effective but may lead to hypopigmentation, atrophy, telangiectasia, and recurrence of scarring.[2] Scars which are unresponsive to conservative treatment and cause a functional deficit or undue stress to the patient are referred to a reconstructive surgeon for management. Multiple options exist, including dermabrasion and release of tension using transposition flaps such as Z-plasties.

## Contracture

Contractures occur when hypertrophic scarring develops across joints.[36] This predisposition of hypertrophy in areas of tension is worsened by the tendency of patients to assume a flexed position in order to help alleviate pain. Over time, the scar matures and effectively tethers the joint as it becomes thicker and tighter.[2] If left immobile, the underlying muscles and tendons become shortened with subsequent capsular contraction.[12] The best treatment for contractures is to continue range-of-motion exercises. Occupational and physical therapy should follow the patient to ensure appropriate use of the area and recommend exercises to help regain range of motion. Pediatric burns in areas of functional importance should be closely followed to monitor for contractures. Since the scar does not grow or stretch proportionately as the child develops, there is the potential for contractures to

occur even years after the burn.[2] Early treatment of these contractures focuses on prevention with use of pressure garments and splinting. In patients who may have developed mild to moderate contractures, serial splinting can be effective. With severe contractures or those unresponsive to splinting, contracture release may be planned by a burn or reconstructive surgeon.[2]

## Heterotopic Ossification

Heterotopic ossification is an uncommon complication of burns where normal bone forms ectopically in soft tissue via calcium deposition. This dilemma occurs most commonly following deep burns of the elbow, followed by the shoulder, hip, knee, and forearm. The patient will present with pain, edema, and decreased range of motion of the affected joint.[40] Diagnosis is confirmed radiographically. Because conservative treatment is unlikely to help resolve this complication, surgical intervention is often necessary once ossification begins to limit function and activities of daily living.

## Leukoderma

Hypopigmentation, or leukoderma, is a very common sequela of burn injury, particularly in patients with darker skin pigmentation. This complication has no functional deficit, but may need to be addressed for psychological or cosmetic reasons. Treatment can be provided by a plastic and reconstructive surgeon who may restore more normative pigmentation through dermabrasion and regrafting of the affected area.[2]

## Psychological

Severe burns can remove a child from a normal home and school environment for weeks to months.[36] Regardless of the size of the burn injury, the severity is not directly correlated with the psychological impact of the injury.[36] Therefore, consultation with a child-life specialist is very important with every pediatric burn in helping to normalize the patient's care. The ability of the family to cope and the presence of other psychological issues are better predictors of the impact of injury, particularly in young children. Care must be taken to minimize additional trauma during management of the burn by suitable pain and anxiety control.

Providers should also be aware of the possibility of post-traumatic stress disorder in pediatric burn patients. During this phase of burn management, health care providers should inquire about hypervigilance, nightmares, and chronic fearfulness.[2] Early referral to a counselor is helpful in managing this disorder. The development of acute stress and post-traumatic stress disorder is strongly associated with the actions of caregivers and their projection onto their charges.[41] Depending on the patient's age and stage of development, family counseling may be an appropriate option as well.

## Follow-Up

Patients suffering from burns have a better prognosis when consistent, long-term follow-up and early integration occurs.[6] A multidisciplinary team can help provide physical and occupational therapy, scar management, reconstructive surgery, and family support.[32] A significant burn is often a life-changing event for the patient as well as for his or her family. Health care providers must involve family in their children's management as early as possible since a functional family and early reintegration are key components of a good prognosis.[42] Severe burns are no longer synonymous with a poor quality of life, and it is our responsibility to make it a priority to help return these children to normal, meaningful, and productive lives.

## KEY POINTS

- Determination of the extent of burn injury is based on depth and total body surface area (TBSA) involvement.
- Extent of the burn injury is based on the temperature and duration of contact with the offending agent.
- Burn management should always begin with PALS and ATLS protocols, along with specific management of fluid resuscitation and temperature maintenance.
- Early excision and grafting is imperative in optimizing patient outcomes from significant burns.
- Physical therapy with early range of motion and exercise will improve long-term outcome.
- Continued follow-up for years with the patient and his or her family with a multidisciplinary burn center improves long-term rehabilitation and reintegration.

TABLE 1

**The Lund and Browder Chart, Calculating the Percent Total Body Surface Area Involved in Burn Injury**

| | | Newborn | 1 Year Old | 5 Years Old | 10 Years Old | 15 Years Old |
|---|---|---|---|---|---|---|
| Head | Anterior | 9.5 | 8.5 | 6.5 | 5.5 | 4.5 |
| | Posterior | 9.5 | 8.5 | 6.5 | 5.5 | 4.5 |
| Neck | Anterior | 1 | 1 | 1 | 1 | 1 |
| | Posterior | 1 | 1 | 1 | 1 | 1 |
| Chest | Anterior | 13 | 13 | 13 | 13 | 13 |
| | Posterior | 13 | 13 | 13 | 13 | 13 |
| Right: Upper Arm | Anterior | 2 | 2 | 2 | 2 | 2 |
| | Posterior | 2 | 2 | 2 | 2 | 2 |
| Left: Upper Arm | Anterior | 2 | 2 | 2 | 2 | 2 |
| | Posterior | 2 | 2 | 2 | 2 | 2 |
| Right: Forearm | Anterior | 1.5 | 1.5 | 1.5 | 1.5 | 1.5 |
| | Posterior | 1.5 | 1.5 | 1.5 | 1.5 | 1.5 |
| Left: Forearm | Anterior | 1.5 | 1.5 | 1.5 | 1.5 | 1.5 |
| | Posterior | 1.5 | 1.5 | 1.5 | 1.5 | 1.5 |
| Right: Hand | Anterior | 1.25 | 1.25 | 1.25 | 1.25 | 1.25 |
| | Posterior | 1.25 | 1.25 | 1.25 | 1.25 | 1.25 |

*continued on next page*

TABLE 1 (continued)

|  |  | Newborn | 1 Year Old | 5 Years Old | 10 Years Old | 15 Years Old |
|---|---|---|---|---|---|---|
| Left: Hand | Anterior | 1.25 | 1.25 | 1.25 | 1.25 | 1.25 |
|  | Posterior | 1.25 | 1.25 | 1.25 | 1.25 | 1.25 |
| Perineum |  | 1 | 1 | 1 | 1 | 1 |
| Right: Buttock |  | 2.5 | 2.5 | 2.5 | 2.5 | 2.5 |
| Left: Buttock |  | 2.5 | 2.5 | 2.5 | 2.5 | 2.5 |
| Right: Thigh | Anterior | 2.75 | 3.25 | 4 | 4.5 | 4.5 |
|  | Posterior | 2.75 | 3.25 | 4 | 4.5 | 4.5 |
| Left: Thigh | Anterior | 2.75 | 3.25 | 4 | 4.5 | 4.5 |
|  | Posterior | 2.75 | 3.25 | 4 | 4.5 | 4.5 |
| Right: Calf | Anterior | 2.5 | 2.5 | 2.75 | 3 | 3.25 |
|  | Posterior | 2.5 | 2.5 | 2.75 | 3 | 3.25 |
| Left: Calf | Anterior | 2.5 | 2.5 | 2.75 | 3 | 3.25 |
|  | Posterior | 2.5 | 2.5 | 2.75 | 3 | 3.25 |
| Right: Foot | Anterior | 1.75 | 1.75 | 1.75 | 1.75 | 1.75 |
|  | Posterior | 1.75 | 1.75 | 1.75 | 1.75 | 1.75 |
| Left: Foot | Anterior | 1.75 | 1.75 | 1.75 | 1.75 | 1.75 |
|  | Posterior | 1.75 | 1.75 | 1.75 | 1.75 | 1.75 |
|  | SUM - TBSA |  |  |  |  |  |

TABLE 2

**Common signs of child abuse in pediatric
patients sustaining thermal injury.**

**Signs of Child Abuse**

- Delay in seeking medical treatment
- Changing reports of how injury was sustained
- Injury inconsistent with reported mechanism
- Clean line of demarcation in injury
- Injury to buttocks, ankles, wrist, palms, soles
- Other injuries present (fractures, bruises, healed burns)
- Multiple hospitalizations

FIGURE 1

**The phases of thermal injury care, consisting of preparatory, emergent, acute, and rehabilitation and reintegration.**

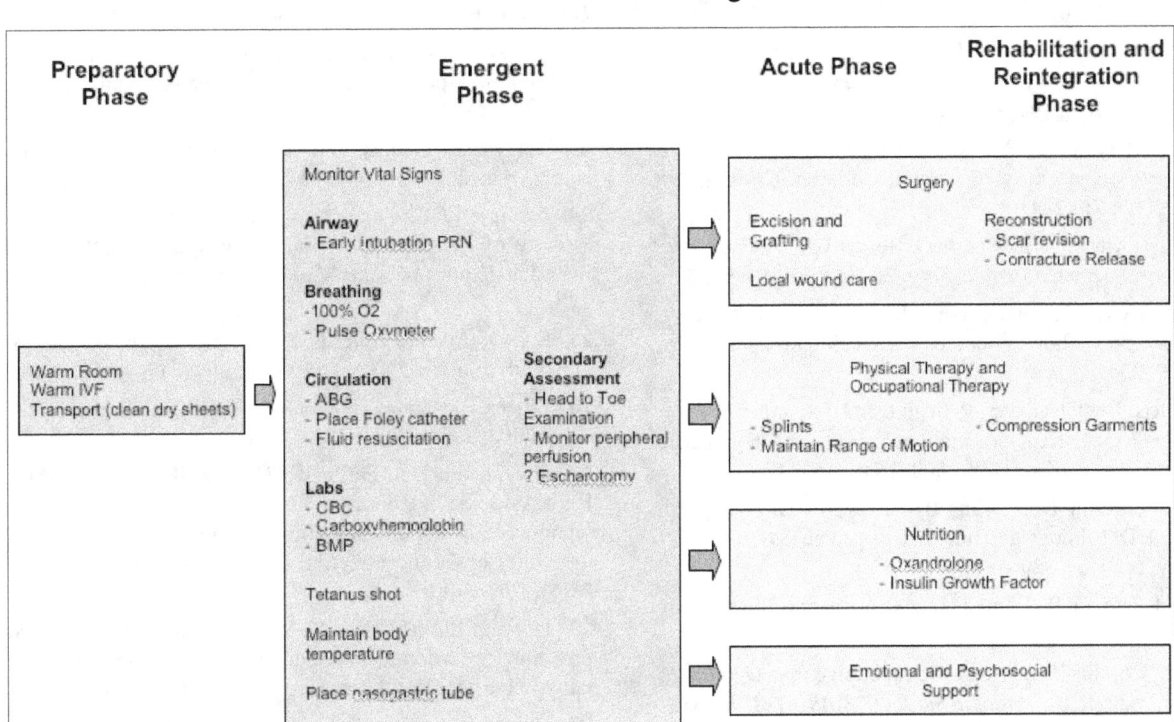

FIGURE 2

**The Parkland formula and the Galveston formula, calculating the amount of fluid required for resuscitation.**

# Parkland formula:
### 4cc/kg/percent TBSA burned
Initial 8 hrs: 1/2 of the fluid administered
Following 16 hrs: Remaining 1/2 fluid administered

# Galveston formula:

Initial 24 hrs: **5000 cc LR/m2 TBSA burned + 2000 cc LR/m2 BSA** (D5W for total BSA component in children > 2 years old is recommended)
Initial 8 hrs: 1/2 of the fluid administered
Following 16 hrs: Remaining 1/2 fluid administered

Following 24 hours: **3750 cc/m2 TBSA burned + 1500 cc LR/m2 BSA**

# REFERENCES

1. Purdue G, Hunt JL, Burris AM. Pediatric burn care. *Clin Pediatr Emerg Med.* 2002; **3**: 76–82.

2. Davoodi P, Fernandez JM, O SJ. Postburn sequelae in the pediatric patient: clinical presentation and treatment options. *J Craniofac Surg.* 2008; **19**(4): 1047–1052.

3. Duffy BJ, McLaughlin PM, Eichelberger MR. Assessment, triage, and early management of burns in children. *Clin Pediatr Emerg Med.* 2006; **7**: 82–93.

4. Corpron CA, Martin AE, Roberts G, Besner GE. The pediatric burn unit: a profit center. *J Pediatr Surg.* 2004; **39**: 961–963.

5. Tse T, Poon CHY, Tse KH, Tsui TK, Ayyappan T, Burd A. Paediatric burn prevention: an epidemiological approach. *Burns.* 2006; **32**: 229–234.

6. Sheridan RL, Remensnyder JP, Schnitzer JJ, Schulz JT, Ryan CM, Tompkins RG. Current expectations for survival in pediatric burns. *Arch Pediatr Adolesc Med.* 2000; **154**: 245–249.

7. Morrow SE, Smith DL, Cairns BA, Howell PD, Nakayama DK, Peterson HD. Etiology and outcome of pediatric burns. *J Pediatr Surg.* 1996; **31**(3): 320–333.

8. Duncan RT, Dunn KW. Immediate management of burns. *Surgery.* 2006; **24**(1): 9–14.

9. Pizano LR, Corallo JP, Davies J. Nonoperative management of pediatric burn injuries. *J Craniofac Surg.* 2008; **19**(4): 877–881.

10. Monstrey S, Hoeksema H, Verbelen J, Pirayesh A, Blondeel P. Assessment of burn depth and burn wound healing potential. *Burns.* 2008; **34**(6): 761–769.

11. O'Brien SP, Billmire DA. Prevention and management of outpatient pediatric burns. *J Craniofac Surg.* 2008; **19**(4): 1034–1039.

12. Sheridan RL. Burns. *Crit Care Med.* 2002; **30**(11)(suppl): S500–S514.

13. Heimbach DM, Warckerle JF. Inhalation injuries. *Ann Emerg Med.* 1988; **17**(12): 1316–1320.

14. Sheridan RL. Burn care: results of technical and organizational progress. *JAMA.* 2003; **190**(6): 719–722.

15. Geller RJ, Barthold C, Saiers JA, Hall AH. Pediatric cyanide poisoning: causes, manifestations, management, and unmet needs. *Pediatrics.* 2006; **118**(5): 2146–2158.

16. Barret JP, Desai MH, Herndon DN. Survival in paediatric burns involving 100% total body surface area. *Ann Burns Fire Disasters.* 1999; **12**(3): 139–142.

17. Young AE. The management of severe burns in children. *Curr Paediatr.* 2004; **14**: 202–207.

18. Schulman CI, King DR. Pediatric fluid resuscitation after thermal injury. *J Craniofac Surg.* 2008; **19**(4): 910–912.

19. Burd A, Noronha FV, Ahmen K, et al. Decompression not escharotomy in acute burns. *Burns.* 2006; **32**(3): 284–292.

20. Sheridan RL. Sepsis in pediatric burn patients. *Pediatr Crit Care Med.* 2005; **6**(3)(suppl): S112–S119.

21. Custer EJW, Rau, RE. Johns Hopkins Hospital. *The Harriet Lane Handbook.* 18th ed. Philadelphia: Elsevier Mosby, 2009.

22. Patel PP, Vasquez SA, Granick MS, Rhee ST. Topical antimicrobials in pediatric burn wound management. *J Craniofac Surg.* 2008; **19**(4): 913–933.

23. Mandal A. Quality and cost-effectiveness—effects in burn care. *Burns.* 2007; **33**: 414–417.

24. Compton CC. Current concepts in pediatric burn care: the biology of cultured epithelial autografts: an eight-year study in pediatric burn patients. *Eur J Pediatr Surg.* 1992; **2**(4): 216–222.

25. Stal D, Cole P, Hollier L. Nonoperative management of complex burn injuries. *J Craniofac Surg.* 2008; **19**(4): 1016–1019.

26. Lineen E, Namias N. Biologic dressing in burns. *J Craniofac Surg.* 2008; **19**(4): 923–928.

27. Greenhalgh DG, Saffle JR, Holmes JH IV, et al.; American Burn Association Consensus Conference on Burn Sepsis and Infection Group. American Burn Association consensus conference to define sepsis and infection in burns. *J Burn Care Res.* 2007; **28**(6): 776–790.

28. Horvath EE, Murray CK, Vaughen GM, et al. Fungal wound infection (not colonization) is independently associated with mortality in burn patients. *Ann Surg.* 2007; **245**(6): 978–985.

29. Desai MH, Abston S. Candida infection in massively burned patients. *J Trauma.* 1981; **21**(3): 237–239.

30. Schulman CI, Ivascu FA. Nutritional and metabolic consequences in the pediatric burn patient. *J Craniofac Surg.* 2008; **19**(4): 891–894.

31. Przkora R, Herndon DN, Jeschke MG. The factor age and the recovery of severely burned children. *Burns.* 2008; **34**: 41–44.

32. Herndon DN, Tompkins RG. Support of the metabolic response to burn injury. *Lancet.* 2004; **363**(9424): 1895–1902.

33. Fuhrman MP. The albumin-nutrition connection: separating myth from fact. *Nutrition.* 2002; **18**(2): 199–200.

34. Przkora R, Barrow RE, Jeschke MG, et al. Body composition changes with time in pediatric burn patients. *J Trauma.* 2006; **60**: 968–971.

35. Herndon DN, Hart DW, Wolf SE, Chinkes DL, Wolfe RR. Reversal of catabolism by beta-blockade after severe burns. *N Engl J Med.* 2001; **345**(17): 1223–1229.

36. Esselman PC. Burn rehabilitation: an overview. *Arch Phys Med Rehabil.* 2007; **88**(12)(suppl 2): S3–S6.

37. Sheridan RL, Hinson MI, Liang MH. Long-term outcome of children surviving massive burns. *JAMA.* 2000; **283**(1): 69–73.

38. Brooks JP, Malic CC, Judkins KC. Scratching the surface—managing the itch associated with burns: a review of current knowledge. *Burns.* 2008; **34**(6): 751–760.

39. Anzarut A, Olson J, Singh P, Rowe BH, Tredget EE. The effectiveness of pressure garment therapy for the prevention of abnormal scarring after burn injury: a meta-analysis. *J Plast Reconstr Aesthet Surg*. 2009 Jan; **62**(1): 77–84.

40. Hunt JL, Arnoldo BD, Kowalske K, Helm P, Purdue GF. Heterotopic ossification revisited: a 21-year surgical experience. *J Burn Care Res*. 2006; **27**(4): 535–540.

41. Stoddard FJ, Saxe G, Ronfeldt H, et al. Acute stress symptoms in young children with burns. *J Am Acad Child Psychiatry*. 2006; **45**(1): 87–93.

42. Druery M, Brown TLH, Muller M. Long term functional outcomes and quality of life following severe burn injury. *Burns*. 2005; **31**: 692–695.

# CHAPTER THREE

# EPIDEMIOLOGY AND ECONOMICS OF PEDIATRIC BURNS

BRUCE CHUNG, MD, STEVEN A. KAHN, MD,
UNIVERSITY OF ROCHESTER SCHOOL OF MEDICINE,
ROCHESTER, NY DEPARTMENT OF SURGERY DIVISION OF BURN,
ACUTE CARE, AND TRAUMA SURGERY
AND
CHRISTOPHER W. LENTZ, MD, FACS, FCCM,
UNIVERSITY OF NEW MEXICO HEALTH SCIENCES CENTER
DEPARTMENT OF SURGERY, DIVISION OF GENERAL SURGERY,
ALBUQUERQUE, NM

## INTRODUCTION

Studying the distribution of disease and the factors that affect the health and illness of the population are increasingly important aspects in medicine. Careful compilation of medical data through local databases and national registries can help determine problematic trends. The pediatric population is a target of significant preventive medicine strategies, including bicycle helmets, car seats, and poison control. Epidemiology allows us to appropriately apply these preventative measures.

More attention has also been placed on preventing burn injuries. Burn injury is an important cause of morbidity in North America. The pediatric population and the elderly are at higher risks for burns. More so than in many other diseases or injuries, pediatric burn injury is a highly preventable injury. Initiatives and programs have been established to decrease the number of burn injuries through fire prevention, smoke alarm use, hot tap water temperature control, and increasing the general public awareness. By understanding the epidemiology of pediatric burn injury, we can better understand the risk factors for burn injury, identify specific and more cost-effective targets of prevention, reduce morbidity and mortality, and provide more effective methods for therapy, health care delivery, and resource utilization.

## EPIDEMIOLOGY

Burns are a significant cause of injury and one of the leading causes of death in the pediatric population. According to the Centers for Disease Control and Prevention, burn injury is the third most common cause of death in patients aged between 0 and 14 years. This number tapers off in the older pediatric population, and overall is the seventh most common cause of death between the ages of 0 and 18.[1] In 2004, data from the CDC reported 9339 total deaths from unintentional injuries in the pediatric population. Of these, burns and fires accounted for 5.7% of deaths, behind only motor vehicle accidents and drowning. In the pediatric population, burn injury accounts for 4.7%, 5.8%, 2.2%, and 0.5% mortality in the age groups of 0 to 4 years, 5 to 9 years, 10 to 14 years, and 15 to 18 years, respectively. The number of deaths from burns decreases with age in the pediatric population. In contrast, burn injury is only the sixth leading cause of unintentional death and is not within the top 20 causes of deaths in the overall population, accounting for only 0.1% of total deaths in 2004.[1]

In 2006, the CDC reported 9036931 nonfatal injuries in people between the ages of 0 and 18 years. Fire and burn injury accounted for 128182 incidents and represented 1.4% of total injuries. Between the ages of 1 to 4 years, fire and burn injury accounted for 2.6% of injuries, and between the ages of 5 to 9 years, 10 to 14 years, and 15 to 18 years, they accounted for 1.1%, 0.7%, and 1.1% of injuries, respectively. The incidence for fire and burn injury across all age groups is 1.4%.[1] Although the incidence between all age groups and in the 0- to 18-year-old group is almost equal, there is a higher mortality in the pediatric population.[1]

Overall, the number of deaths and incidents from fire and burn injury has been decreasing (Figures 1 and 2). In 1981, the CDC reported that of 15702 deaths in children younger than 19 years (Figure 3), fire and burn injury accounted for 1349, or 8.6% of these deaths. In 1990, of 11807 deaths, fire and burn injury accounted for 953, or 8.1% of deaths, and in 2000 there were 9778 deaths, of which 629, or 6.4%, were due to fire and burn injury. Over the 19-year period, burn-related mortality decreased by 53.4%, exceeding the decrease in overall mortality of 37.7%.[1]

The American Burn Association also maintains a database of patients hospitalized in burn centers, the National Burn Repository. Between 1997 and 2007, there were 181836 burn patients treated in US burn centers. Patients from the ages of 0 to 20 years accounted for 51211, or 32% of burn admissions.[2]

The most common causes of burn injury requiring admission were scalds and flames. Scalds accounted for nearly 28% of burn injury in 0- to 20-year-olds, while flames accounted for 18% of injuries. Flame injury is the more common etiology after the age of 5, and it is rare in children under the age of 2 (4.3%). In the 0- to 2-year age group, the second leading cause of injury after scalds is contact burns, accounting for 19% (of injuries in that age group.[2]

Reported incidence of burns from the CDC and National Burn Repository emphasize the importance of burn injury in the pediatric population. Although the number of burns

has decreased from decade to decade, burns remain an important target for preventative medicine.

Pediatric burn admissions vary according to availability of resources, cultural differences, and medical practice. There are a growing number of specialized burn care centers, but the majority of burn injuries are minor and can usually be managed on an outpatient basis.[3] Minor burn injuries are usually evaluated in emergency departments and urgent care clinics and followed with primary care physicians.

## BURN ETIOLOGIES

By understanding the causes and reasons for burn injury, we are able to more accurately prevent burn injury and identify better targets for prevention. The main causes of burns are scalds, contact/thermal burns, fire and fire-related injuries, fireworks-related injuries, and electrical injuries. Each cause has its own specific risk factors and age predominance. Understanding these risk factors is important for reducing the incidence of burn injuries and developing prevention strategies for specific target age groups. The American Burn Association recognized the importance of a age-specific stratification of the etiology of burns in children. Looking at the pediatric population as a whole does not give an accurate picture of the cause of childhood burns (figure 5 A)[2]. Prior to 2007, the National Burn Repository (NBR) reported burn etiology in ages 0–2, 2–5 and 5–20. This stratification was not sufficient to study the etiology of thermal injury in a developing pediatric population since it was recognized that the cause of the burn was age dependent. The current stratifications reported by the NBR in children are ages 0–1, 1–2, 2–5, 5–16 and 16–20.[2] This finer analysis will permit a better method of analyzing thermal injury in the dynamic development of children. As demonstrated, the incidence of scalds and contacts decrease with age and the incidence of fire and fire-related burns increasess (Figures 5B–5F).

## Scalds

Scald burns account for the majority of burn injuries in the pediatric age group, accounting for 30% to 50% of injuries.[4,5,6] Scald burns are of particular importance in patients aged from 0 to 5 years. An average of 8 children with scald burns die each year, with a majority of deaths occurring in children younger than 4 years.[7] The majority of scald burns occur when hot water is pulled from a pot off an elevated surface or when a container of hot water is overturned or spilled. The greatest risk comes to children younger than 2 years, with scalds accounting for nearly 65% of burn injuries in that age group. Two main injury patterns account for 52% of scalds. These injuries most commonly occur when a child reaches up and pulls down a pot from an elevated surface such as a stove or when a child grabs, overturns, or spills a pot onto himself or herself.[8] Another significant cause of scalds in patients younger than 15 months occurs when another person spills or splashes hot liquid on the child, accounting for 28% of scald injuries.[8] Males are more prone to scald injuries, accounting for 58% of scald incidents.[5,9,10]

The majority of scald injuries are treated and released without a hospital admission.[7] Injuries that require hospitalization involve higher percentage of total surface area burned or deeper burns. While scald burns are usually due to hot water pulled from an elevated surface, another significant cause of scald burns is hot tap water scalds. Hot tap water scalds account for nearly 25% of scald injuries and tend to be more severe and have a larger total body surface area burned compared to spills. Due to these factors, hot tap water scalds are associated with a higher hospitalization and mortality rate than other scald burns.[11,12] Up to 39% of tap water scalds involve a body surface area of at least 25%, and nearly one-third of these patients require hospitalizations. In addition, the occurrence of tap water scalds is more frequent in younger children, in which 88% of tap water scalds occurred by age 5.[12]

A survey of hot-water temperature in household bathtubs showed a mean of 142°F, with a range from 90°F to 168°F.[12] It has been shown that temperatures greater than 120°F can result in significant burns.[13] Temperatures at 140°F or higher can increase the risk of full-thickness burns if skin is exposed for more than 30 seconds.[13] In infants, this time is reduced to as little as 1 second (Table 1). Careful attention to the temperature of tap water should be taken to prevent tap water scalds. Surveys have demonstrated that very few people understand at what temperature a hot water heater should be set to prevent burn injury. This ignorance even extends to pediatric health care providers; 12 of 32 pediatric practitioners surveyed at one institution recommended that water heater temperatures be set above 130°F.[12] It is unclear whether their recommendations were related to insufficient knowledge of burn prevention tactics or whether they had some other reason to justify their decision (for example, risks of incubating *Legionella* at lower temperatures). Water at 130°F can cause significant burn injury.[13]

A possible explanation for a higher incidence of deeper scald injuries in children is that young children have thinner skin that sustains damage more quickly and at a lower temperature. Due to their age and development, children also have less awareness and coordination and lack the ability to react quickly to avoid a burn.[14,15] By nature, children are inquisitive and explore their environment through touch. They often learn to extend their hands to grab things, including pulling down pots filled with hot water. Because of their short stature, they are less aware of the contents in a pot or container that they pull down. In conjunction with the lack of a coordinated muscular system, they lack fine motor skills, making children at higher risk for scalds.

Some hot tap water scalds occur when an infant's caretaker fills a bathtub with hot water, not realizing that the water is too hot. In addition, he or she might leave the infant in a tub filled with hot water if there is a distraction in a different room or area, such as a telephone call or a cry for help from other persons. There are a high number of tap water scalds in toddlers/preschool ages when curiosity or abuse results in the child becoming trapped in hot water and unable to escape.[12]

## Contact Burns

Contact burns account for the second most common burn injury in young children. Among hospitalized burn victims, they accounted for 26% of injuries in children aged 0 to 1 years and 24% in children aged 1 to -2 years. This number decreases to 17% in ages 2 to 5, and 9% in ages 5 to 16.[2] The majority of contact burns occur from household appliances, including clothing irons, hair straighteners, hair curlers, stove tops, and room heaters. Contact burns are usually well defined, linear, and affect a small total body surface area. Nevertheless, due to the high temperature of some of these appliances, contact burns can often result in severe injury. Hot irons are a frequent offending agent. In the resting position, the hot surface is exposed, leaving it open to injury. One study revealed that the mean age of patients with thermal injury from a hot iron was 24 months, with children between 1 and 2 years most at risk for contact burn with a hot iron.[16] Males were again more likely to be burned than females.[16,17] Hair straighteners are an increasing cause of contact burn. Unlike an iron, hair straighteners have two hot surfaces that can heat up to 220°C, or 428°F. The resting and cooling positions leave the hot surfaces exposed and vulnerable to contact. Because of the two surfaces, they often cause thermal injury in two areas of the body.[18]

Injuries from hot appliances typically result in small burns. The total body surface area injury from contact burns averages 2.1%. Burn injury via this mechanism is usually partial thickness; however, children are vulnerable to full-thickness burns with prolonged contact.[17] Due to the severity of the injury, up to 36% of contact burns from hot appliances require surgical intervention.[19] The hands and fingers are the most frequent areas of injury.

Children aged between 1 and 2 years are at most risk for a contact injury from a hot item. Learning to ambulate, they need to steady themselves against stationary objects. One of these stationary objects may happen to be a hot appliance. Young children in their "exploratory years" are extremely curious. In addition, this age group is more ambulatory than the infant group but less aware of dangerous items than older children are. The combination of mobility and lack of awareness makes children aged 1 to 2 years more able to encounter and more vulnerable to injury from hot items such as irons, hair straighteners, and radiators. They also cannot react or withdraw as quickly to avoid serious burns. This is also demonstrated by the most injured area of the body from contact burns, the palm. Spending time in the kitchen with a parent who is preparing a meal places the child in an environment with hot objects that can cause injury.

## House Fires and Fire-Related Injuries

House fires account for approximately 3000 deaths and 17000 injuries a year in the United States.[20] Overall, house fires are the third leading cause of fatal home injuries.[21] Children under age 5 have double the risk of adults of death after injury in a house fire.[22] In 2003, residential fire-related injuries accounted for 261 deaths, representing 7.4% of all mortality between the ages of 0 and 4 years.[23] Although not as common as scalds and contact burns, fire and fire-related injury remain a leading cause of mortality in children. Of all mechanisms of burn injury, fire-related injury results in the highest mortality rates.[6] Fire and fire-related injury accounted for 40% of burn hospital admissions between 1997 and 2007 and 18% of pediatric burn admissions.[2] Unlike scalds and contact burns, burn injury from fires increases with age. Approximately 4% of admissions due to fire are for children younger than 2 years, and this increases to 18% in patients aged 2 to 5 years and 36% in patients aged 5 to 20 years. Males also tend to be at higher risk for fire-related injuries than females.[2]

Only 5% of house fires are due to fire-play by children. However, up to 42% of fire-related injuries are due to fire-play by children, including playing with matches or lighters. The majority of house fires are due to cigarette smoking, which accounts for over 50% of causes. Fires that start in the living room or bedroom are almost twice as likely to result in injury compared to fires started in the kitchen or other parts of the house.

Clothing ignition often occurs in the setting of fire and in flame injury. The number of pediatric burn injuries from clothing ignition is declining, but it remains a significant cause of mortality due to the thickness of the burn and the higher percentage of total body surface area burned as a result. The incidence for clothing ignition has decreased dramatically with the use of fire-resistant and flame-retardant fibers for clothing. Among these fire-resistant materials are polyester and other synthetic materials. Cotton and many natural fibers, on the other hand, have been shown to burn quite readily and quickly. The use of more snug and tighter-fitting clothing has decreased the incidence of clothing ignition.[24] Legislation related to fire prevention and children's clothing is discussed in more detail in the "Burn Prevention" section of this chapter.

Children are at higher risk for house fire injury for several reasons. First, they are more likely to play with fire. Second, they lack the comprehension for the potential dangers of playing with fire. Third, they are unable to react as well when circumstances are out of control and are unable to plan an escape. Lastly, although they may be aware of a fire, they often depend on others for escape.[25]

## Fireworks Burns

Burns from fireworks occur with less frequency than other types of burns. There were approximately 10800 people treated for fireworks-related injury in the United States in 2005, with only 4 mortalities.[26] This figure is slightly lower than an estimated 12600 people treated for fireworks-related injury in 1994. Children represent more than half of these patients.[27] Approximately 60% of fireworks-related injuries are burns, primarily from sparklers and firecrackers. Sparklers, popular among younger children, caused 20% of injuries. They were more prevalent in younger children, causing 46%, 25%, 15%, and 11% of burns in children aged 0 to 4, 5 to 9, 10 to 14, and 15 to 19 years, respectively. Firecrackers had a higher cause of injury in the older age groups, accounting for 24%, 34%, 32%, and 25% in those same age groups.[28] Also causing significant injury were aerial devices (ie, bottle rockets or Roman candles), often causing injuries other than burns, such as eye injuries.

The individual responsible for lighting the firework is most likely to sustain injury. However, bystanders are still at significant risk, with at least 22% of children sustaining injury from fireworks as bystanders. In addition, there is an overwhelmingly high rate of injury with fireworks in males, with males accounting for 77% of all fireworks-related injuries.[26]

The common sites of burns with fireworks are the hands, fingers, and eyes. The majority of fireworks-related burns are second degree, representing 37% of all injuries. First-degree burns occurred in 19% of injuries and third-degree in only 4% of incidents. The large part of fireworks injuries occur between June 18 and July 18, with 60% to 80% of injuries recorded around the Fourth of July. Over the last 15 years, there has been a steady decline in fireworks-related injuries in children.[26]

The majority of fireworks-related injuries do not require hospital admission. Greater than 90% are treated and discharged from the emergency department, and only 5% to 7% require hospitalization.[26]

## Electrical Burns

Electrical injuries are rare in children, accounting for only 1.1% of burn injuries between 1997 and 2007.[2] The incidence of electrical injury increases with age, accounting for 0.5%, 0.8%, 2%, 2.1%, and 2.6% of all electrical injuries occurring in the age groups of 0 to 1, 1 to 2, 2 to 5, 5 to 16 and 16 to 20 years, respectively. Electrical injuries can be divided in two categories, low voltage (<1000 volts, e.g., contact with electrical cords and appliances) and or high voltage (>1000 volts, e.g., or lighting strikes). The most common causes of electrical injuries are direct contact with electrical cords, up to 48%, or with faulty electrical appliances, 26%. Inserting a metal object into an electrical outlet accounts for approximately 18% of electrical burns.[29] Although the occurrence of electrical injuries is relatively low, up to 61% of electrical injuries require skin grafting. The most common areas affected by electrical injury are the hands, feet, and skull. These body parts represent areas of source and ground contact points. Younger children also have been linked to cord biting, causing burn injury around the oral orifice.[30] Cord biting has been shown to have a higher incidence in the Canadian population, up to 6%, but remains a concern regardless of geographic differences.[31] Males are more likely to have electrical injuries than females, with figures as high as 70%.[30] The greatest number of deaths from electrical injury occurred in older children, while, the majority of less severe injuries occurred in the younger population (0–4 years). Nonfatal electrical injuries tend to be caused by low-voltage current from household electrical outlets. In one study, most of the low-voltage injuries were minor, requiring minimal treatment.[31]

Injury from lightning strikes represents only a fraction, or approximately 1%, of all electrical injuries. However, lightning strikes are not required to be reported, and the number of injuries or deaths may be underestimated. Lightning strikes tend to be high voltage and account for a higher percentage of mortality. Nearly 25% of deaths secondary to electrical burns in children are due to lightning strikes. A report between 1980 and 1995 found mortality from lightning strikes to be greatest between patients aged 15 to 19 years. There is a high male prevalence of lightning strikes, with as much as 7 times the rate of that of females.[32,33] This mechanism of injury tends to occur in areas where thunderstorms are more prevalent: the South, the Rockies, and the Ohio and the Mississippi river valleys.[33]

## CHILD ABUSE

Abuse remains a significant cause of injury to children although it represents a completely preventable injury. The number of child abuse–related burns is underestimated but

may represent a significant fraction of burn injuries. Up to 20% to 30% of children with burn injury have evidence suggestive of abuse, neglect, or failure to thrive or have an old burn injury detectable on admission or in old records.[12,34] Burns caused by abuse are considered to be more indicative of premeditated attacks than other cases of abuse. Other violent acts are thought to be more spontaneous, as a result of and as a response to acts of anger, passion, or aggression.

Risk factors include single-parent families and parental drug abuse, and delay in seeking health care may be a sign of child abuse.[35] Ethnicity and social class have not been found to correlate with the incidence of child abuse. Abuse also has been found to be twice more common in males than in females. In cases of child abuse involving scalds, injuries usually include bilateral limbs or an isolated buttocks burn, have a clear tide mark, and exhibit symmetrical lesions.[36] Also indicative of abuse are scald injuries with stocking or glove patterns and a uniform thickness of burn. Splash marks are typically absent in abuse cases. One study revealed that burns inflicted by abuse had a higher mortality than accidental burns, required higher frequency of skin grafting, and had more intensive care admissions.[37]

## Risk Factors for Burns

Studies have shown a strong correlation between different socioeconomic classes, available health care resources, and mortality. The mortality from all injuries in children has been shown to be highest in the lowest socioeconomic class. Injuries from burns and fires also show a strong correlation among different socioeconomic classes.

A large-scale study evaluating burn injuries in the pediatric population in 2000 from the Healthcare Cost and Utilization Project Kids' Inpatient Database showed a significant difference in age, race, and income in the number of children requiring admission to hospitals following burn injuries.[6] Children younger than 2 years were more likely to require hospitalizations and were also more likely to be nonwhite. Risks of burn-related injuries were higher in Hispanics and blacks (Figure 6). Children living in areas of high poverty rates, single-parent families, and families with lower incomes also had a higher rate of burn injuries.[38,39,40]

The education level of the parents was also a significant factor in determining burns in children. Parents, whether one or both parents, with an education level higher than high school displayed a decreased risk for burns in children. Interestingly, the education of the father was less of a factor than that of the mother.[33]

Children living in crowded housing and areas where housing was more closely grouped together were also at higher risk for burn injury. This may be a reflection of the economic status of the family and the likelihood that burns occurred more frequently in urban areas than in rural areas.[40]

Protective factors for burns include families with a living room in the house, ownership of the house, and higher education of the parents. These are also indicators that higher socioeconomic status plays a role.[40] Many families with scald injuries in children were single-parent homes with little supervision. Families that did not have running water were at higher risks for scalds.[40]

As previously mentioned, contact burns are frequently due to irons, hair straighteners, and heaters. There is a higher incidence of contact burns in lower-income, single-parent, and single-child households.[41] In lower-income housing, it has been shown that many families do not use elevated ironing tables and often improvise by ironing on floors or tables, leaving hot irons exposed in easily accessible areas. In most cases, contact burns from irons and other appliances are often due to carelessness and neglect, with the parents unaware of the dangers from these hot appliances. This is especially true in single-child households, where many burns have been attributed to parental inexperience.[40]

House fire has been well studied due to the high morbidity and mortality of the related injury. House fires are commonly due to smoking, fire-play, arson, faulty electrical wiring, and heating equipment. One study revealed that at higher risk are houses built between the 1950s and 1960s, low-income families, and homes without smoke detectors. Families earning the lowest median income, less than $20000 a year, had an incidence of 9.9 injuries per 100000 compared to an incidence of only 2.3 injuries per 100000 people in families earning an income between $40000 and $60000. Families earning the lowest median income also had almost 150% higher incidence of house fires.[42]

Residents of central urban areas as well as rural areas were at higher risk for injury in a house fire. In addition, people living in the southern United States had a higher risk of house fire–related mortality.[43]

The risk of house fire injury is also greatly increased in nonwhite populations, especially in African American, Native American, and Hispanic populations. These groups tend to live in homes that are associated with a higher risk of fire-related injuries and fatalities, including mobile homes and apartment complexes. Mobile homes and apartment complexes fall in a category of homes that have been shown to be at higher risks for fire-related deaths. They have fewer exits, fewer windows, and oftentimes, out-of-date heating systems.

Smoke detectors have been highly linked to preventing fatal house fires. Smoke alarms have decreased the number of deaths by up to 60%. Nonwhite populations have been shown to have a lower rate of functional smoke detector use. This also has contributed to the higher risk of fire-related

injury in the nonwhite population. The protective effects of smoke alarms also depend on the cause of the house fire. In cases where fire-play was the cause of the house fire, smoke detectors did not show any difference in protection from injuries or fatalities. In all other causes, smoke detectors have been associated with a decrease in house-fire related injuries.[44]

Smoking and alcohol abuse are significant risk factors for house fires. Studies have found careless smoking to be responsible for a significant percentage of house fire–related deaths. Tobacco-related fires usually start with ignition of bedding or furniture when someone falls asleep while smoking. Alcohol intoxication is frequently associated with these fires.[45]

The greatest risk from fireworks-related injuries comes from lack of adult supervision. In more than 50% of cases, there was a lack of supervision possibly leading to inappropriate handling of fireworks. Recent studies, however, have also found that increased adult supervision may not prevent injury in children.[46]

## BURN PREVENTION

Burn injury is a highly preventable injury, especially in the pediatric population (Figure 7), as up to 64% of burns result from accidents. Improvements in survival from burns have been made over the last several decades due to advances in medical management, surgical intervention, nutrition, and resuscitation. The most effective way to improve survival, however, is likely through prevention of burn injuries.

A large amount of resources have been invested into prevention and education. The fire service, fire companies, American Burn Association, and individual burn centers have been primarily responsible for fire prevention. One of the most widely publicized, effective measures is the "stop, drop, and roll" fire safety technique. Some other methods involve active programs promoting the use of smoke detectors and carbon monoxide detectors. However, more educational programs and public awareness are being distributed through media outlets other than fire services. A joint effort by the media, health care services, educational services, and fire services would make a greater impact on public awareness and prevent unnecessary burn injury.

Currently, two major classes of burn prevention are utilized. Primary prevention involves preventing the event from occurring, whereas secondary prevention focuses on supportive therapy and reducing disability after the event.[47] Both active and passive prevention strategies exist as well. Passive prevention includes approaches that do not depend on individuals for prevention. Instead, standards and techniques that remove the human factor are implemented. Automobile airbags fall into the passive category. Active prevention requires behavioral adjustments and efforts by individuals to reduce the risks of danger. An example of active prevention is the use of seatbelts to reduce serious injury in car accidents. Active prevention measures are more difficult to implement due to the compliance and cooperation of the people involved. For pediatric burn prevention, compliance depends on both children and parents. In many cases, children are too young to comprehend the subject matter, and it is often difficult to persuade parents to approach matters differently. Successful prevention of burn injuries relies on well-structured implementation of both passive and active prevention measures.

One of the best examples of burn prevention includes the use of smoke detectors. The use of smoke detectors has decreased house fire–related injuries significantly and has arguably had the greatest impact on reducing fire-related mortality. One study estimated a decrease in mortality by 60%. Smoke detectors have been shown to reduce the risk of fire death by 13%.[48] Smoke detector giveaway programs have decreased the number of house fire-related injuries in high-risk populations. In addition, it has been found that giving away smoke detectors in high-risk communities is the most effective and cost-efficient measure to reach high-risk populations and reduce injury.[49]

Although the use of smoke detectors has decreased the number of house fire-related injuries, it has been found that many households do not have functional smoke detectors. One study found that about 71% of households polled reported having a functional smoke detector. However, when the households were physically surveyed, only 49% of houses had functional smoke detectors.[50] This finding points to the importance of campaigns to educate people about testing their smoke detectors and changing the batteries regularly, a program often led by fire services.

Although passive prevention with smoke detectors has been shown to be quite effective, education programs to reach children through schools, primary care physician office visits, and other community arenas are also important. These programs have been shown to be effective in increasing the knowledge about the dangers of fire and the importance of formulating escape plans.[51,52]

Efforts to reduce scald burns have included campaigns to educate the public about the dangers of scalds and ways to minimize exposure to hot water. Installation of water heater temperature regulators has also been evaluated. For tap water scalds, educational programs have not been shown to be effective.[53] Prevention programs utilizing both an educational component as well as installation of water heater temperature regulators that limit water temperatures to 120°F have been shown to be effective.[54,55] Legislative measures to require water heater temperatures to be preset at lower temperatures have decreased the number of injuries and the total body surface area burned when an injury does occur. Furthermore, these measures reduced mortality, length of hospital stay, and the number of surgical interventions required after thermal injury.[56]

Contact burns from hot irons are a preventable source of burns. The development of an "iron shoe" cooling device may help to dissipate heat and prevent contact burns. One such device uses a silicone polymer that shields the iron from the edges and surfaces of the iron and decreases the temperature of the iron from over 200°C to under 50°C. A prototype has been created and tested at our institution but has yet to be distributed to consumers. This device has potential to be an inexpensive method for preventing contact burns from irons.[57]

Measures to reduce firework injuries include educational campaigns as well as legislative interventions. States that have banned certain fireworks have seen a reduction in fireworks-related burns.[58] Programs to increase awareness of fireworks-related burns also need to be effective, abundant, and publicized during Fourth of July celebrations, when fireworks-related burns most commonly occur.[26] Other successful programs to reduce fire-related injuries include the implementation of child-safe lighters and legislative measures to use fire-resistant materials in clothing.

The use of fire-resistant and flame-retardant materials has led to a decline in the number of sleepwear-related burn injuries. Legislation in 1972 required that children's pajamas be made of flame-resistant materials, which resulted in an almost zero incidence of sleepwear-related burns. However, this was overturned in 1996 by the Consumer Product Safety Commission (CPSC). Since this policy reversal, recent surveys have shown that sleepwear-related burn injuries have increased by 157%.[59] Currently, the American Burn Association and several members of Congress are attempting to reenact legislation to require usage of fire-resistant and flame-retardant material in children's sleepwear. Currently the CPSC recommends that child sleepwear (for children greater than 9 months old) be either flame resistant or made of snug-fitting cotton.[60] Cotton is widely regarded as more comfortable than flame-retardant fabrics of the past, and snug-fitting clothes are less likely to hang and ignite. Time will tell whether this clothing strategy is effective.[60]

Future prevention programs should target the high-risk population. These include communities with a high number of low-income families, single-parent families, and a non-white population. Early and frequent educational programs for children are also important. In summary, burn prevention strategies involve primary, secondary, passive, and active techniques. When these preventative measures are backed by legislation, injuries are more effectively reduced.

## Burn Economics

Fire and burn injuries represent a significant burden to medical costs. Burns can have long-term impact on victims, including ongoing medical bills for follow-up care, rehabilitation, and scar revisions. Significant emotional stress and psychological trauma can also result from burn injury. The visible effects and scars from burns can be emotionally damaging, which may add up to extensive costs in clothing, make-up, and other cosmetic interventions. By evaluating the cost of burn injuries, decisions about health care resources and distribution can be better made. There is increasing pressure to reduce costs from insurance companies, third-party payers, and hospital administration.

Fire and burn injuries are estimated to cost over $2.1 billion annually in children younger than 19 years.[61] In the year 2000, the total charges for burn-associated hospitalizations totaled $211772700. The mean charge for each hospitalization was approximately $21800, with a median of $7700. Charges for individual hospitalizations ranged from $25 to $985951. However, approximately 10% of patients accrued more than $47300 of total charges.[6]

The extent of injury was associated with the length of stay and the expenses of hospitalization. First-degree injuries were associated with a shorter length of stay, 2.1 days, and a smaller total charge, $5430. As the injury became larger, the total charge increased dramatically. Second-degree burns had a length of stay of 4.1 days, totaling $11200, while third-degree burns had a mean length of stay of 11.7 days, with a mean charge of $43900.[6]

The same associations were also made with the percent total body surface area burned. The smaller the total body surface area burned, the shorter the length of stay and the lower the cost of the hospitalization. A burn less than 10% total body surface area had a mean hospitalization of 4.9 days with a charge of $13900.[6] Burns greater than 40% total body surface had a mean length of stay greater than 5 times that and charges more than 10 times that of a burn less than 10% total body surface area. The total charge for hospitalizations did not show any difference between gender, race, or hospital location.[6]

Patients that had minor burn injuries and were seen in the emergency department had an average hospital charge of $1185.[62] These patients had a mean total body surface area burned of 5.4%. Patients with minor burns seen in an outpatient burn clinic had an average total charge of $691 with a mean total surface area burned of 7.2%.[59] These statistics may represent a higher cost in the emergency department due to treatment time, laboratory tests, radiologic tests, and other diagnostic tests. Most of these tests may be unnecessary and superfluous expenses. Pharmacy represents one of the higher charges incurred to patients when visiting an outpatient burn clinic. There was a 76% greater charge for pharmacy services compared to that for patients seen in the emergency department.[59]

Specialized burn centers are larger and have higher staffing and a higher level of technology. These centers have better patient outcomes and survival despite treating sicker patients and more severe burns.[63] However, specialized burn centers typically have higher costs. The mean cost per patient in one study was $32033. The mean cost per hospital day was $477.[64] Factors that affected the total charge included timing of surgery and interventions. Early surgical interventions for severe burns reduced total charge.

The importance of analyzing burn economics is to provide better understanding for decisions for distribution of health care resources. Pressures to reduce health care costs are increasing. Specialized burn centers provide a higher level of care that has been shown to improve patient outcomes. Despite the high cost of hospitalization in specialized burn centers, they are a necessary resource to improve patient survival and allow patients to have a more productive life following their injury. Although many communities depend on emergency departments for burn care, minor burn injuries may be better treated through outpatient burn clinics. Such clinics have lower total charge while reducing unnecessary diagnostic tests and reserving health care resources. Data would suggest that more money and time should be placed into implementing outpatient burn clinics to reduce total expenses.

## Summary and Conclusion

Burn injury remains a significant burden in the pediatric population and is a large public health concern. It is one of the leading causes of injury and death in children, utilizing a significant amount of health care resources. Through the study of epidemiology, burn providers can identify and control health problems in the population. After problems are identified, steps can be taken to decrease the incidence and mortality of burns, improve the quality of life of burn victims, and allocate health care resources to more effectively to treat burns.

The current system creates enormous pressures for health care to be more efficient and less costly. Understanding the causes and risk factors for burns will determine better, targeted areas of prevention and treatment. Continued emphasis on tabulating patient factors and outcomes is needed to further the evolution of health care and burn treatment. This includes improving modes of health care delivery, improving resource allocation, and minimizing excessive and unnecessary health care dollars.

Prevention of burns remains a public health goal. The first step to decreasing the amount of burn injuries is prevention. Increasing public awareness and education has seen mixed results. In the future, better methods may utilize both passive and active preventative measures as well as legislation to reduce risks for burn injuries.

## KEY POINTS

- Epidemiology is a key component in medicine that helps to understand ways to prevent disease, reduce mortality, and improve patient outcomes. The etiology of thermal injury in pediatric patients is age dependent and prevention strategies need to target specific age groups in children.
- Burn and fire-related injuries are leading causes of injury and deaths in the pediatric population. They are the third leading cause of unintentional deaths in children younger than 14 years, only behind motor vehicle accidents and drownings.
- Scalds and fire-related burns comprise most of the burns in children.
- Scalds make up over 60% of burns in children younger than 2. The largest risk factors for scalds are children younger than 2, nonwhite families, and single-parent families.
- Scald burns are usually due to children pulling containers and pots filled with hot liquid from an elevated surface, splashes, and bathtubs filled with hot tap water.
- Contact thermal burns occur from exposure to irons, curling irons, hair straighteners, and stove tops. They often cause deeper burns due to the high temperatures that these appliances can reach.
- House fires do not occur as frequently as scalds or contact burns but are responsible for a higher mortality rate.
- Most house fires are due to cigarette use and children playing with fire.
- Fifty percent of fireworks-related burns are seen in children and occur mostly during the month surrounding the Fourth of July.

- Sparklers and firecrackers account for the majority of injuries. Sparklers cause more burn injuries in children younger than 5 years, while firecrackers are responsible for the majority of burns in the remaining pediatric age groups.
- Electrical injuries account for only a small portion of overall injuries and are due to contact with faulty electrical cords or to inserting metal objects into electrical outlets.
- Lightning injuries are rare but are responsible for nearly a quarter of deaths in electrical burns in children.
- Child abuse is a significant cause of burn injury in the pediatric population. Suspicious attributes include stocking and glove scald patterns with a uniform burn thickness, isolated buttocks burns, and symmetrical lesions.
- Risk factors for burns include low-income families, single-parent families, and nonwhite families. A poor maternal education also places children at higher risk for burns.
- Smoke detectors have reduced house fire injuries significantly. Families and communities without smoke detectors are at higher risks for house fire–related injuries.
- Prevention is a key component to limiting burn injury. A large number of resources have been placed towards burn prevention, including educational programs, smoke alarm giveaways, limiting firework sales, hot water heater temperature regulators, child-safe lighters, and fire-resistant fibers.
- The most effective prevention campaigns involve both active and passive prevention techniques. The combination of techniques should be applied towards future prevention programs where applicable.
- Burn injury consumes a large share of health expenses, and expenditures for health charges total $2.1 billion per year.
- Specialized burn centers, although more expensive, increase survival and patient quality of life. Outpatient clinics are less costly than emergency department visits and provide adequate and comparable care.

## FIGURES AND TABLES

### FIGURE 1
**Number of unintentional burns in children aged 0 to 19 years from 2000–2006.**

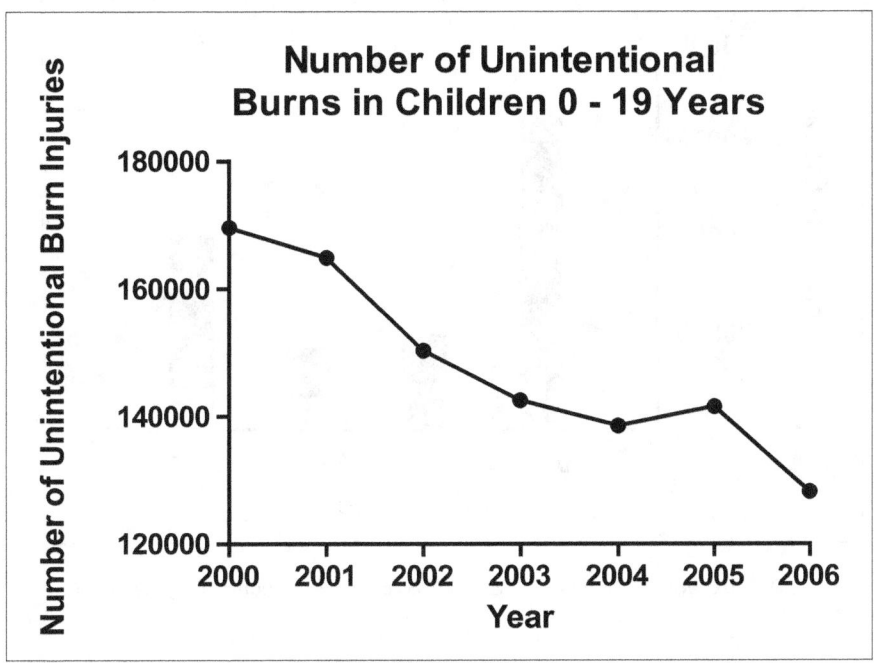

*Source.* Data extrapolated from CDC WISQARS database for nonfatal injuries 2006.

### FIGURE 2
**Deaths from burn injuries in children aged 0 to 19 years from 1981 to 2004.**

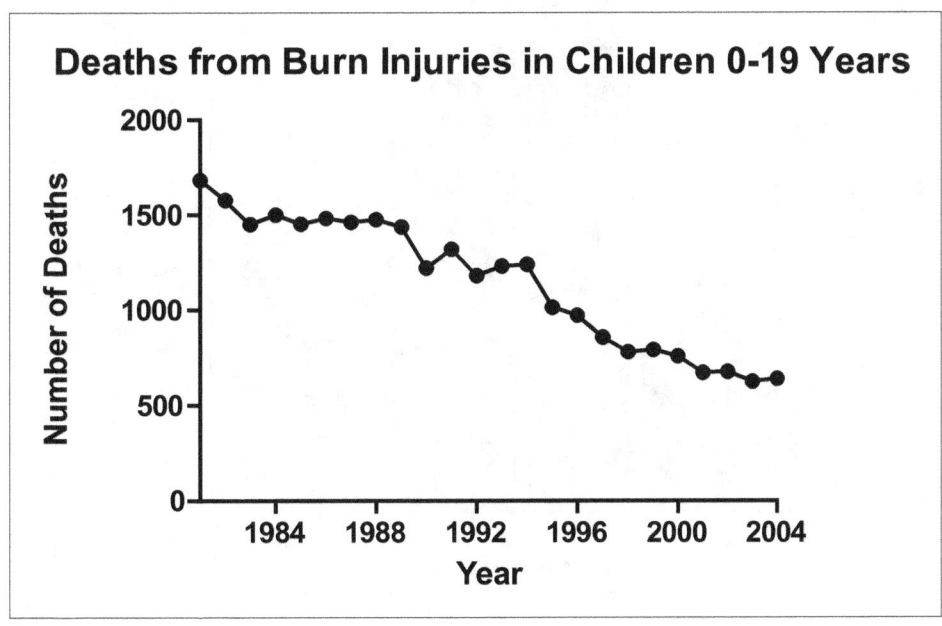

*Source.* Data extrapolated from CDC WISQARS database for fatal injuries.

**FIGURE 3**
**Number of burns in age groups 0 to 4, 5 to 9, 10 to 14, and 15 to 19 years in 2006.**

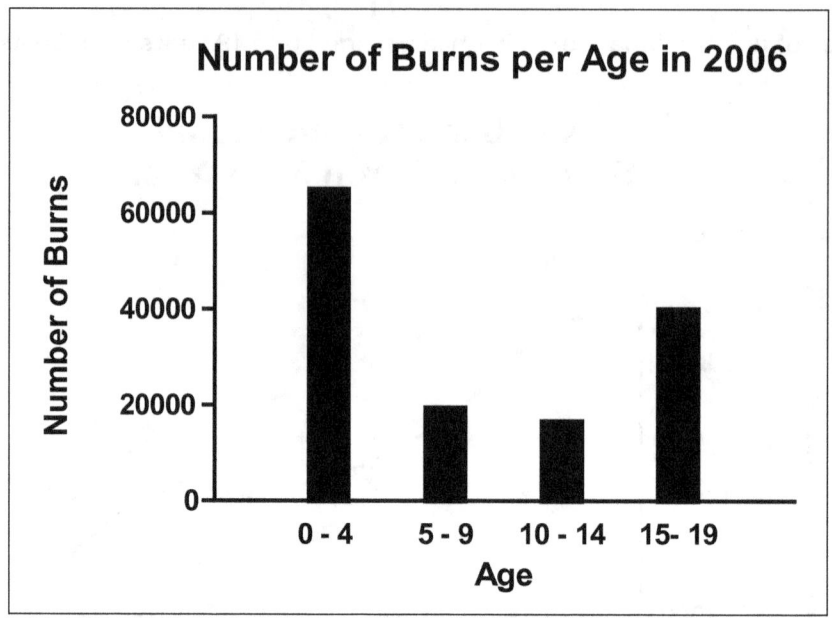

*Source.* Data extrapolated from CDC WISQARS database for nonfatal injuries 2006.

**FIGURE 4**
**Graph of incidence of burns by age and gender.**

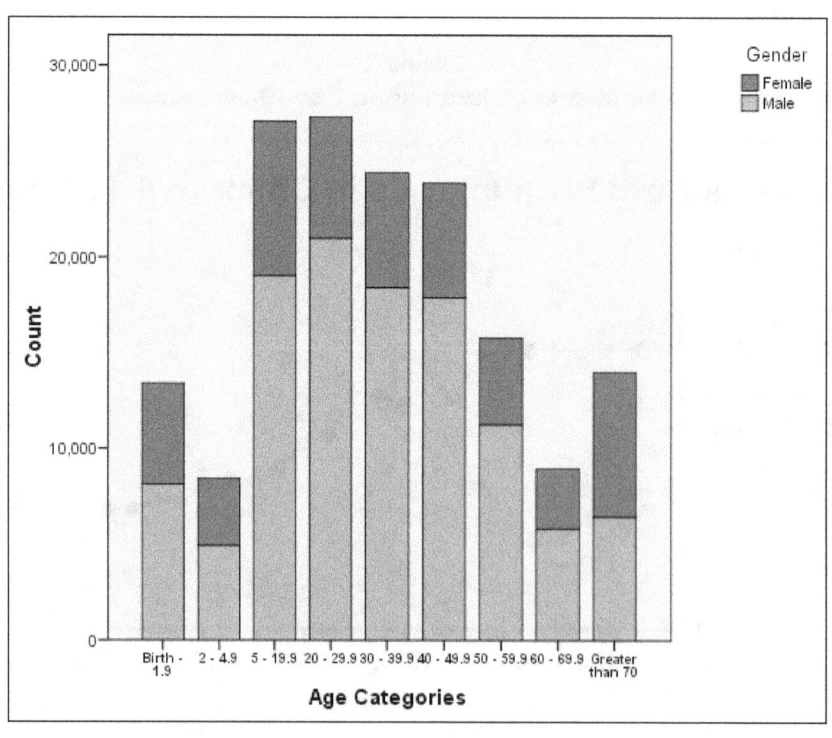

*Source.* Data from NBR 2007.

**FIGURE 5A**
**Burn etiologies in children from birth to 20 years, 1997–2007.**

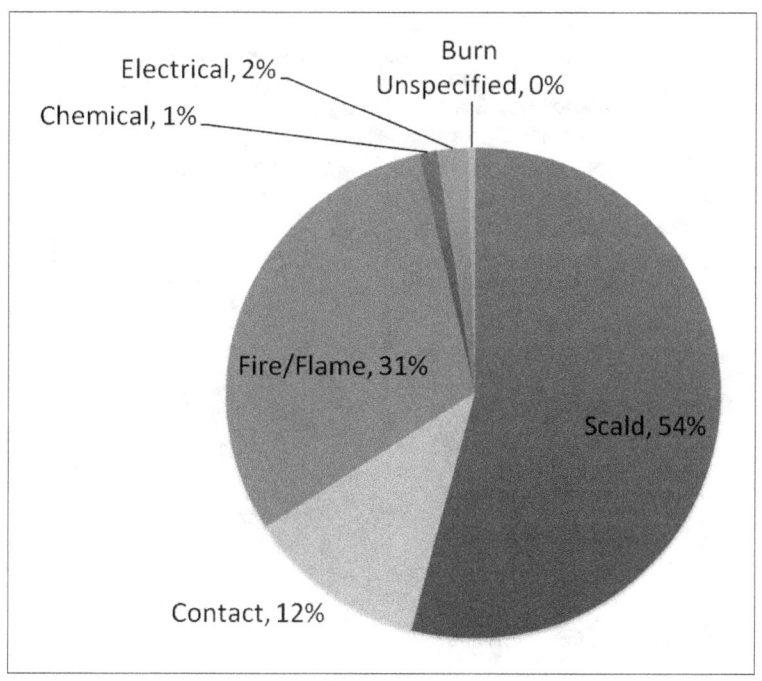

**FIGURE 5B**
**Burn etiologies in children from birth to 0.9 years, 1997–2007.**

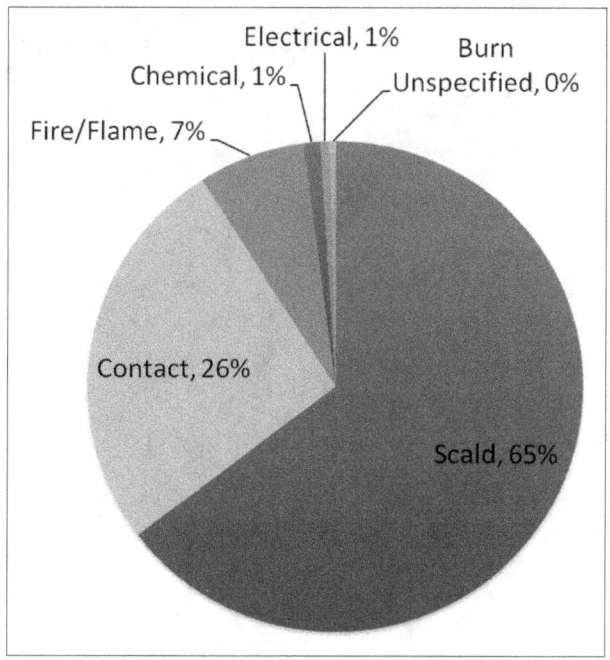

## FIGURE 6
## Ethnicity/race of burn patients.

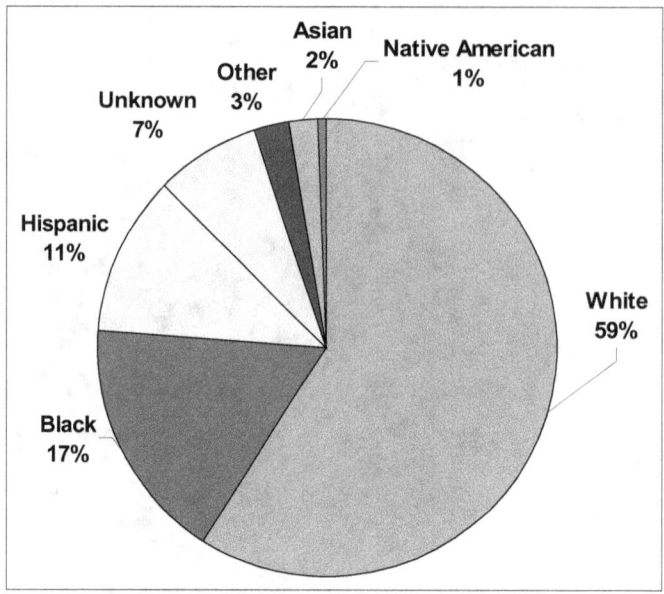

*Source.* Data from NBR 2007.

## FIGURE 7
## Categories of circumstances of burn injuries.

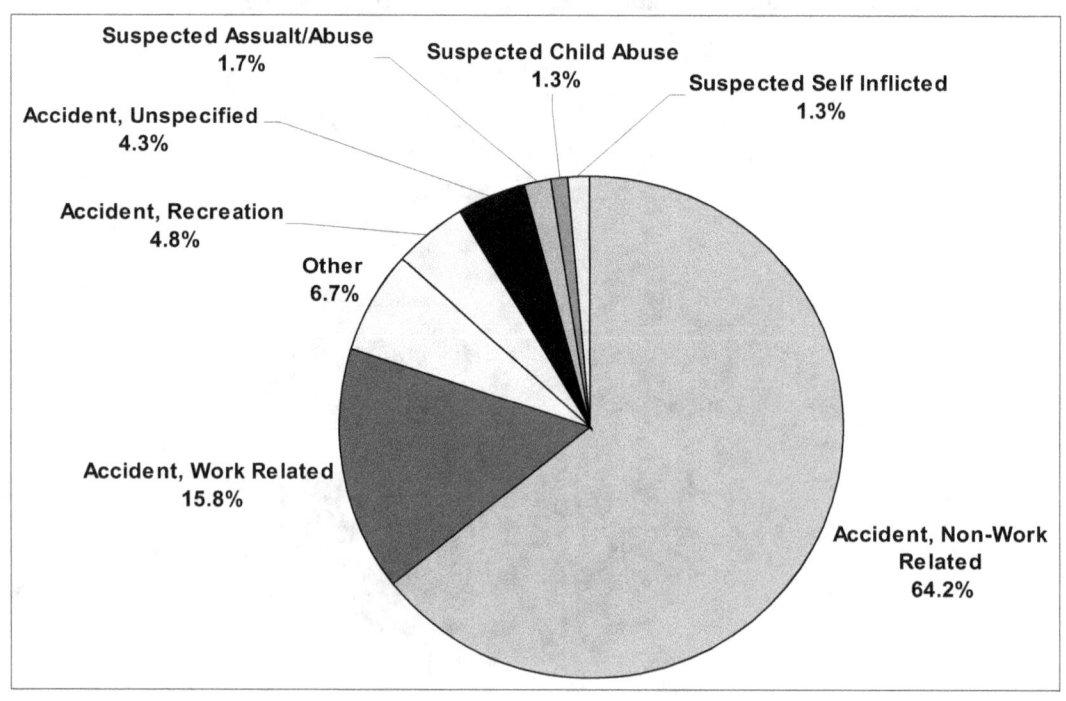

*Source.* Data from NBR 2007.

FIGURE 8
Categories of injury site.

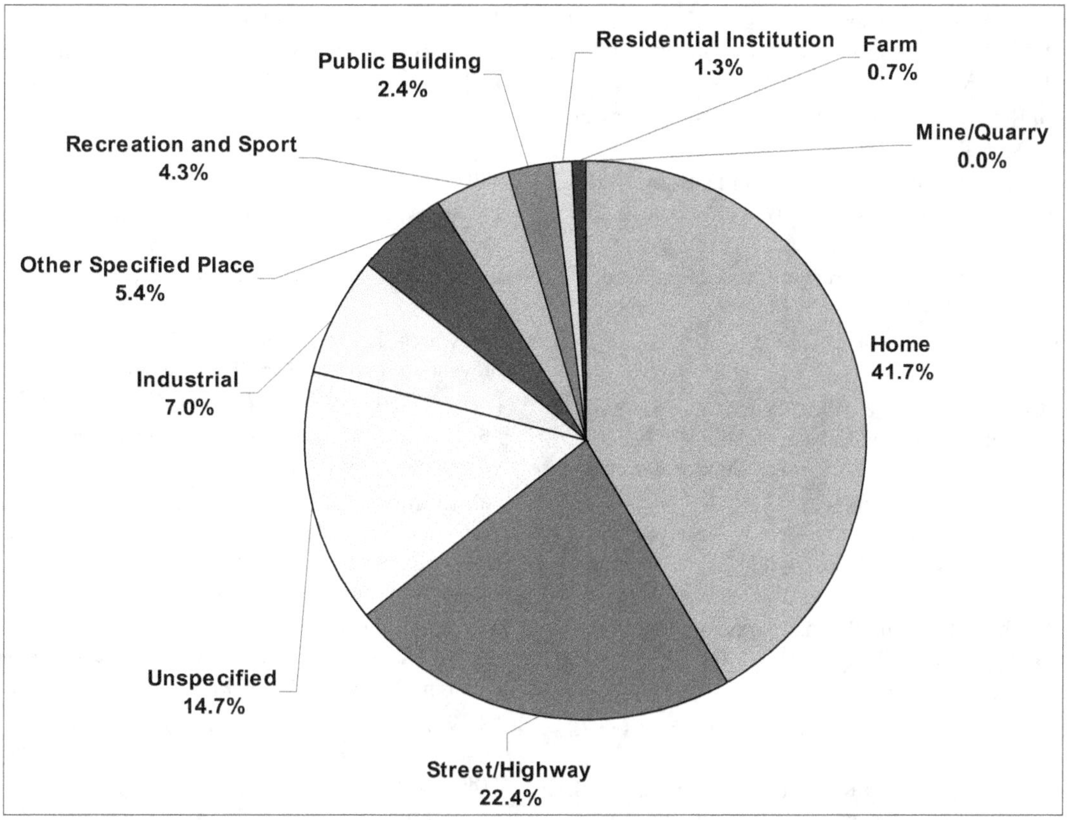

*Source.* Data from NBR 2007.

TABLE 1
Time exposure for second- and third-degree scald burns for various water temperatures.

| Temp °C | Temp °F | Time to Second-Degree Burns | Time to Third-Degree Burns |
|---|---|---|---|
| 40 | 104 | 100 min | 167 min |
| 45 | 113 | 2 min | 8 min |
| 50 | 122 | 11 sec | 20 sec |
| 55 | 131 | 2 sec | 5 sec |
| 60 | 140 | instant | 1 sec |
| 65 | 149 | instant | instant |
| 70 | 158 | instant | instant |

## REFERENCES

1. Data Collected from queries to WISQARS Injury Mortality Reports, 1999–2006 (http://webappa.cdc.gov/sasweb/ncipc/mortrate10_sy.html) National Center for Injury and Prevention and Control, Atlanta,GA.

2. National Burn Repository Report 2007, Dataset 4.0, American Burn Association, Chicago, IL, 2007.

3. Carlsson A, Uden G, Hakansson A, Karlsson ED. Burn injuries in small children, a population-based study in Sweden. *J Clin Nurs.* 2006; **15**(2): 129–134.

4. Smith EI. The epidemiology of burns: the cause and control of burns in children. *Pediatrics.* 1969; **44**: 821.

5. Safe Kids Worldwide. *Burn and Scalds Safety.* Washington, DC: SKW; 2007.

6. Shields BJ, Comstock RD, Fernandez SA, Xiang H, Smith GA. Healthcare resource utilization and epidemiology of pediatric burn-associated hospitalizations, United States, 2000. *J Burn Care Res.* 2007; **28**(6): 811–826.

7. Washington State Childhood Injury Report. *Fire and Burn.* Washington State Department of Health, Olympia, WA, November 2004.

8. Drago DA. Kitchen scalds and thermal burns in children five years and younger. *Pediatrics.* 2005; **115**(1): 10–16.

9. Banco L, Lapidus G, Zavoski R, Braddock M. Burn injuries among children in an urban emergency department. *Pediatr Emerg Care.* 1994; **10**(2): 98–101.

10. Quayle KS, Wick NA, Gnauck KA, Schootman M, Jaffe DM. Description of Missouri children who suffer burn injuries. *Inj Prev.* 2000; **6**(4): 255–258.

11. McLoughlin E, McGuire A. The causes, cost, and prevention of childhood burn injuries. *Am J Dis Child.* 1990; **144**(6): 677–683.

12. Feldman KW, Schaller RT, Feldman JA, McMillon M. Tap water scald burns in children. 1997. *Inj Prev.* 1998; **4**(3): 238–242.

13. Moritz AR, Henriques FC. Studies of thermal injury: the relative importance of time and surface temperature in the causation of cutaneous burns. *Am J Pathol.* 1947; **23**: 695.

14. Katcher ML. Scald burns from hot tap water. *JAMA.* 1981; **246**(11): 1219–1222.

15. American Burn Association. Scald injury prevention educator's guide. http://www.ameriburn.org/Preven/ScaldInjuryEducator's Guide.pdf., American Burn Association, Chicago, IL, 2010.

16. Gaffney P. The domestic iron. A danger to young children. *J Accid Emerg Med.* 2000; **17**(3): 199–200.

17. Qazi K, Gerson LW, Christopher NC, Kessler E, Ida N. Curling iron-related injuries presenting to US emergency departments. *Acad Emerg Med.* 2001; **8**(4): 395–397.

18. Duncan RA, Waterston S, Beattie TF, Stewart K. Contact burns from hair straighteners: a new hazard in the home. *Emerg Med J.* 2006; **23**(3): e21.

19. Alden NE, Rabbitts A, Yurt RW. Contact burns: is further prevention necessary? *J Burn Care Res.* 2006; **27**(4): 472–475.

20. Federal Emergency Management Agency. *Fire in the United States 1987–1996.* 11th ed. Emmitsburg, MD: National Fire Data Center, United States Fire Administrator and FEMA (produced by TriData Corporation, Arlington, VA); 1999.

21. Runyan CW, Bangdiwala SI, Linzer MA, Sacks JJ, Butts J. Risk factors for fatal residential fires. *N Engl J Med.* 1992; **327**(12): 859–863.

22. Safe Kids Worldwide. *Fire Safety.* Washington, DC: SKW; 2007.

23. Pressley JC, Barlow B, Kendig T, Paneth-Pollak R. Twenty-year trends in fatal injuries to very young children: the persistence of racial disparities. *Pediatrics.* 2007; **119**(4): e875–e884.

24. Warda L, Tenenbein M, Moffatt ME. House fire injury prevention update. Part II. A review of the effectiveness of preventive interventions. *Inj Prev.* 1999; **5**(3): 217–225.

25. Squires T, Busuttil A. Can child fatalities in house fires be prevented? *Inj Prev.* 1996; **2**(2): 109–113.

26. Greene MA, Joholske J. 2005 fireworks annual report; fireworks-related deaths, emergency department treated injuries, and enforcement activities during 2005. Washington, DC: US Consumer Product Safety Commission; 2006.

27. Smith GA, Knapp JF, Barnett TM, Shields BJ. The rockets' red glare, the bombs bursting in air: fireworks-related injuries to children. *Pediatrics.* 1996; **98**(1): 1–9.

28. Witsaman RJ, Comstock RD, Smith GA. Pediatric fireworks-related injuries in the United States: 1990–2003. *Pediatrics.* 2006; **118**(1): 296–303.

29. Lui P, Tildsley J, Fritsche M, Kimble RM. Electrical burns in children. *J Burns and Surg Wound Care.* 2003; **2**: 8.

30. Rabban JT, Blair JA, Rosen CL, Adler JN, Sheridan RL. Mechanisms of pediatric electrical injury. New implications for product safety and injury prevention. *Arch Pediatr Adolesc Med.* 1997; **151**(7): 696–700.

31. Nguyen BH, MacKay M, Bailey B, Klassen TP. Epidemiology of electrical and lightning related deaths and injuries among Canadian children and youth. *Inj Prev.* 2004; **10**(2): 122–124.

32. Lightning-associated deaths—United States 1980–1995. *MMWR.* 1998; **47**: 391–394.

33. Lopez RE, Holle RL. Demographics of lightning casualties. *Semin Neurol.* 1995; **15**(3): 286–295.

34. Rosenberg NM, Marino D. Frequency of suspected abuse/neglect in burn patients. *Pediatr Emerg Care.* 1989; **5**(4): 219–221.

35. Chester DL, Jose RM, Aldlyami E, King H, Moiemen NS. Non-accidental burns in children—are we neglecting neglect? *Burns.* 2006; **32**(2): 222–228.

36. Yeoh C, Nixon JW, Dickson W, Kemp A, Sibert JR. Patterns of scald injuries. *Arch Dis Child.* 1994; **71**(2): 156–158.

37. Andronicus M, Oates RK, Peat J, Spalding S, Martin H. Non-accidental burns in children. *Burns.* 1998; **24**(6): 552–558.

38. Simon PA, Baron RC. Age as a risk factor for burn injury requiring hospitalization during early childhood. *Arch Pediatr Adolesc Med.* 1994; **148**(4): 394–397.

39. Karr CJ, Rivara FP, Cummings P. Severe injury among Hispanic and non-Hispanic white children in Washington state. *Public Health Rep.* 2005; **120**(1): 19–24.

40. Delgado J, Ramirez-Cardich ME, Gilman RH, et al. Risk factors for burns in children: crowding, poverty, and poor maternal education. *Inj Prev.* 2002; **8**(1): 38–41.

41. Scholer SJ, Hickson GB, Mitchel EF Jr, Ray WA. Predictors of mortality from fires in young children. *Pediatrics.* 1998; **101**(5): E12.

42. Istre GR, McCoy MA, Osborn L, Barnard JJ, Bolton A. Deaths and injuries from house fires. *N Engl J Med.* 2001; **344**(25): 1911–1916.

43. Warda L, Tenenbein M, Moffatt ME. House fire injury prevention update. Part II. A review of the effectiveness of preventive interventions. *Inj Prev.* 1999; **5**(3): 217–225.

44. Istre GR, McCoy M, Carlin DK, McClain J. Residential fire related deaths and injuries among children: fireplay, smoke alarms, and prevention. *Inj Prev.* 2002; **8**(2): 128–132.

45. Barillo DJ, Goode R. Fire fatality study: demographics of fire victims. *Burns.* 1996; **22**(2): 85–88.

46. Baker SP. Childhood injuries: the community approach to prevention. *J Public Health Policy.* 1981; **2**(3): 235–246.

47. Hunt JL, Arnoldo BD, Purdue GF. Prevention of burn injuries. In: Herndon DN, ed. *Total Burn Care.* 3rd ed. Philadelphia: Saunders Elsevier; 2007: 33–42.

48. DiGuiseppi C, Roberts I, Li L. Smoke alarm ownership and house fire death rates in children. *J Epidemiol Community Health.* 1998; **52**(11): 760–761.

49. Douglas MR, Mallonee S, Istre GR. Comparison of community based smoke detector distribution methods in an urban community. *Inj Prev.* 1998; **4**(1): 28–32.

50. Douglas MR, Mallonee S, Istre GR. Estimating the proportion of homes with functioning smoke alarms: a comparison of telephone survey and household survey results. *Am J Public Health.* 1999; **89**(7): 1112–1114.

51. Varas R, Carbone R, Hammond JS. A one-hour burn prevention program for grade school children: its approach and success. *J Burn Care Rehabil.* 1988; **9**(1): 69–71.

52. Eckelt K, Fannon M, Blades B, Munster AM. A successful burn prevention program in elementary schools. *J Burn Care Rehabil.* 1985; **6**(6): 509–510.

53. Spallek M, Nixon J, Bain C, et al. Scald prevention campaigns: do they work? *J Burn Care Res.* 2007; **28**(2): 328–333.

54. Han RK, Ungar WJ, Macarthur C. Cost-effectiveness analysis of a proposed public health legislative/educational strategy to reduce tap water scald injuries in children. *Inj Prev.* 2007; **13**(4): 248–253.

55. Cagle KM, Davis JW, Dominic W, Gonzales W. Results of a focused scald-prevention program. *J Burn Care Res.* 2006; **27**(6): 859–863.

56. Erdmann TC, Feldman KW, Rivara FP, Heimbach DM, Wall HA. Tap water burn prevention: the effect of legislation. *Pediatrics.* 1991; **88**(3): 572–577.

57. Beers R, Anthamattan M, Reid D, Kahn S, Lentz C. Development of a safety device for preventing clothing iron contact burns. *J Burn Care Res.* 2009; **30**(1): 70–76.

58. Berger LR, Kalishman S, Rivara FP. Injuries from fireworks. *Pediatrics.* 1985; **75**(5): 877–882.

59. American Burn Association. Key legislative and policy issues. http://www.ameriburn.org/advocacy_safechildrenssleepwear.php. American Burn Association, Chicago IL, 2000.

60. US Consumer Product Safety Commission. NEWS from CPSC, New labels on children's sleepware alert parents to fire dangers, Washington, DC, 2000, http://www.cpsc.gov/cpscpub/prerel/prhtml00/00129.html.

61. Miller TR, Finkelstein AE, Zaloshnja E, Hendrie D. The cost of child and adolescent injuries and the savings from prevention. In: Liller KD, ed. *Injury Prevention for Children and Adolescents: Research, Practice, and Advocacy.* Washington, DC: American Public Health Association; 2006; 10–16.

62. Kagan RJ, Warden GD. Care of minor burn injuries: an analysis of burn clinic and emergency room charges. *J Burn Care Rehabil.* 2001; **22**(5): 337–340.

63. Pacella SJ, Butz DA, Comstock MC, Harkins DR, Kuzon WM Jr, Taheri PA. Hospital volume outcome and discharge disposition of burn patients. *Plast Reconstr Surg.* 2006; **117**(4): 1296–1305; discussion 306–307.

64. Sanchez JL, Pereperez SB, Bastida JL, Martinez MM. Cost-utility analysis applied to the treatment of burn patients in a specialized center. *Arch Surg.* 2007; **142**(1): 50–57; discussion 57.

# Skin: Structure, Development, and Healing

Naveed Saqib, MD, Department of Surgery Section of Burns
and Trauma, University of New Mexico HSC Albuquerque, NM

Thomas R. Howdieshell, MD, Professor of Surgery,
Department of Surgery Section of Burns and Trauma,
University of New Mexico HSC, Albuquerque, NM

## Introduction

Great improvements have been achieved over the past few decades to reduce morbidity and mortality related to burn injuries. Increasingly aggressive surgical approaches with early tangential excision and wound closure probably represent the most significant change in recent years, leading to improvement in mortality rates of burn victims at a substantially lower cost.[1,2,3] Early burn wound closure reduces the

infectious complications and shortens hospital stay. Faster healing decreases the severity of hypertrophic scarring, joint contractures, and joint stiffness and promotes quicker rehabilitation.[4] Therefore, a comprehensive and evolving knowledge of wound healing is of major importance to the survival and clinical outcome of burn patients.

Human skin is a complex structure with unusual functional diversity. Topologically, the skin is continuous with the lung and intestinal epithelia. Whereas the lung and gut are commonly viewed as exchange surfaces for gasses and nutrients, the skin is more commonly considered a barrier.[5,6] The concept of an integumental barrier emphasizes the role of the skin as a protective boundary between the organism and a potentially hostile environment. This protective role is evident at birth as the fetus abruptly transitions from the warm, wet, sterile, and protected milieu to a cold, dry, microbe-laden world filled with physical, chemical, and mechanical dangers. Focusing only on the barrier properties of the skin, however, de-emphasizes the important role of the skin in social communication, perception, and behavioral interactions. The skin, as the surface of the organism, is both a cellular and molecular structure as well as a perceptual and psychological interface.[7] This dual functionality befits a true boundary and must be kept in mind to fully appreciate the dynamic organization of the skin and its close kinship with the nervous system.

The skin also provides the physical scaffold that defines the form of the animal. Due to the action of the somatic musculature, a vertebrate's body continually changes shape, which is difficult in a dry, terrestrial environment. A wide variety of strategies have been devised by different animals to cope with the exigencies of different habitats.[8] Arthropods have a largely inflexible body surface, covered with an exoskeleton. Many vertebrates, such as amphibians, live on land but are confined to humid or wet microhabitats. Reptiles and fish have a skin surface covered predominantly with scales, birds have evolved feathers, and most mammals are covered with a protective mantle of fur. Among primates, humans are unique in possessing a nonfurred skin with a thick, stratified interfollicular epidermis and a well-developed stratum corneum.[9,10]

The question of the presumptive advantage of losing a protective and insulating coat of fur has long intrigued evolutionary biologists and physical anthropologists.[11] Three of the most distinctive physical features distinguished among human beings are a nonfurred skin surface; a large, versatile, highly organized brain; and opposable thumbs. The close embryologic connection between the epidermis and the brain (both are ectodermal derivatives) supports the contention that these peculiar structural aspects of human development have coevolved.

We have often overlooked the direct participation of the skin in higher-level functions such as perception and behavioral interactions.[12] Cutaneous attributes form the basis for many readily observed biologic distinctions, including age, race, and gender, as well as multiple overlapping sociocultural characteristics, including tattooing, cosmetics, and tanning.

Much of the complex structure of skin can be explained in terms of the function of its component cells, cellular organelles, and biochemical composition. This broad image has resulted from the application of immunology, biochemistry, physiology, transgenic models, biophysics, and molecular biology, often used in combination with various forms of microscopy.

## SKIN STRUCTURE

## Overview

The epidermis is a continually renewing, stratified squamous epithelium that keratinizes and gives rise to derivative structures (sebaceous glands, nails, hair follicles, and sweat glands) called appendages. The epidermis is approximately 0.4 mm to 1.5 mm in thickness, as compared to the 1.5 mm to 4 mm full-thickness skin. The majority of cells in the epidermis are keratinocytes that are organized into 4 layers named for either their position or a structural property of the cells. Viable cells move outwardly from the basal layer to form layers of progressively more differentiated cells; terminally differentiated keratinocytes are found in the stratum corneum. Intercalated among the keratinocytes at various levels in the epidermis are the immigrant cells—melanocytes, Langerhans cells, and Merkel cells. Melanocytes and Langerhans cells migrate into the epidermis during embryonic development, while Merkel cells probably differentiate in situ. Other cells, such as lymphocytes, are transient inhabitants of the epidermis and are extremely sparse in normal skin. The epidermis rests on and is attached to a basal lamina that separates epidermis and dermis and mediates their attachment. There are many regional variations in the structural properties of the epidermis and its appendages; some are apparent grossly, such as thickness, comparing palm with flexor forearm, while other regional differences are microscopic.[13]

## The Keratinocyte

The keratinocyte is an ectodermally derived cell that constitutes at least 80% of the epidermal cells. All keratinocytes contain cytoplasmic keratin intermediate filaments in their cytoplasm and form desmosomes or modified desmosomal junctions with adjacent cells. Other features of keratinocytes depend upon their location within the epidermis.[14]

Keratin filaments are a hallmark of the keratinocyte and other epithelial cells. Predominantly, they serve a structural (cytoskeletal) role in the cells. More than 30 different keratins, approximately 20 epithelial and 10 hair keratins, all within a range of 40 kDa to 70 kDa molecular mass, have been identified in epithelial cells, cataloged, and assigned a number. The keratins are separated into acidic (type I, cytokeratins K10 to K20) and basic to neutral (type II, cytokeratins K1 to K9) subfamilies based on their isoelectric points, immunoreactivity, and sequence homologies with type I and type II wool keratins.[15,16] Keratins assemble into filaments both within cells and when reconstituted in vitro as obligate heteropolymers, meaning that a member of each family (acidic and basic) must be coexpressed in order to form the filament structure. The coexpression of specific keratin pairs is dependent on cell type, tissue type, developmental stage, differentiation stage, and disease condition. Thus, understanding how keratin expression is regulated provides insight into epidermal differentiation.[17,18]

## Layers of the Epidermis

The basal layer, or stratum germinativum, contains mitotically active, columnar-shaped keratinocytes that attach to the basement membrane zone and give rise to cells of the more superficial epidermal layers. Basal cells contain a large nucleus with typical housekeeping organelles, including Golgi, rough endoplasmic reticulum, mitochondria, lysosomes, and ribosomes. In addition, there are membrane-bound vacuoles that contain pigmented melanosomes transferred from melanocytes by phagocytosis.[19]

The keratin filaments in basal cells are in fine bundles organized around the nucleus, and they insert into desmosomes and hemidesmosomes. The K5 and K14 pair of keratins are expressed in the basal layer of the epidermis and other stratifying epithelia. Other keratins are expressed in small subpopulations of basal keratinocytes, including K15 and K19, which are associated with putative stem cells.[20,21] Microfilaments (actin, myosin, and α-actinin) and microtubules are other cytoskeletal elements present in basal cells. Some of the microfilamentous components of the cytoskeleton are also important links with the external environment via their association with the integrin receptors present on basal keratinocytes. Integrins are a large family of cell surface molecules involved in cell-cell and cell-matrix interactions, including adhesion and initiation of terminal differentiation.[22]

Based on cell kinetic studies, 3 populations coexist within the basal layer: stem cells, transient amplifying cells, and postmitotic cells. Functional evidence for the existence of long-lived epidermal stem cells comes from both in vivo and in vitro studies.[23,24] Because epidermal cells isolated from small biopsy specimens can be expanded in tissue culture and can be used to reconstitute sufficient epidermis to cover the entire skin surface of burn patients, such a starting population must contain long-lived stem cells with extensive proliferative potential.

The tissue localization of putative epidermal stem cells has been based in part on stem cell characteristics defined in other self-renewing systems, such as bone marrow and fetal liver. Under stable conditions, stem cells cycle slowly; only under conditions requiring more extensive proliferative activity, such as during wound healing or after exposure to exogenous growth factors, do stem cells undergo multiple, rapid cell divisions. A large amount of data supports the existence of multipotent epidermal stem cells within the bulge region of the hair follicle based on these traits. Additional evidence suggests that a subpopulation of surface epidermal basal cells also possesses stem cell characteristics.[25,26,27]

The second type of basal cell, the transient amplifying cells of the stratum germinativum, arise as a subset of daughter cells produced by the infrequent division of stem cells. These transient amplifying cells provide the bulk of the cell divisions needed for stable self-renewal and are the most common cells in the basal compartment. After undergoing several cell divisions, these cells give rise to the third class of epidermal basal cells, the postmitotic cells. It is the postmitotic cells that undergo terminal differentiation, detaching from the basal lamina and migrating superficially, ultimately differentiating into a corneocyte. In humans, the normal transit time for a basal cell, from the time it detaches from the basal layer to the time it enters the stratum corneum, is at least 14 days. Transit through the stratum corneum and desquamation requires another 14 days.[28,29]

These 3 functional classes of epidermal basal cells (stem cells, transient amplifying cells, and postmitotic cells) are difficult to distinguish in situ based solely on morphology or protein expression. The term "epidermal proliferative unit" has been used to describe vertical columns of progressively differentiating cells in the epidermis.[30]

The shape, structure, and subcellular properties of spinous cells correlate with their position within the midepidermis. They are named for the spinelike appearance of the cell margins in histologic sections. Suprabasal spinous cells are polyhedral in shape and have a rounded nucleus. Cells of the upper spinous layers are larger, more flattened, and contain organelles called lamellar granules. The cells of all spinous layers contain large and conspicuous bundles of keratin filaments. As in basal cells, the filaments are organized concentrically around the nucleus and insert into desmosomes peripherally.[31]

The "spines" of spinous cells are the abundant desmosomes, calcium-dependent cell surface modifications that promote adhesion of epidermal cells and resistance to mechanical stresses. The molecular components of the desmosome have been well characterized.[32] Within each cell there is a desmosomal plaque associated with the internal surface of the plasma membrane. It is composed of 6 polypeptides: plakoglobin, desmoplakins I and II, keratocalmin, desmoyokin, and band 6 protein. Transmembrane glycoproteins of the cadherin family provide the adhesive properties on the external surface or core of the desmosome. These glycoproteins include desmogleins 1 and 3 and desmocollins I and II. The extracellular domains of these proteins form part of the core. The intracellular domains insert into the plaque, linking them to the intermediate filament (keratin) cytoskeleton.

E-cadherins, which are characteristic of adherens junctions, are associated with actin filaments via interaction with the catenins and may regulate the organization of adherens junctions and influence epidermal stratification. The differences in the proteins in the 2 types of cell attachment structures may be related to specific requirements for the adherens junction-actin relationship, as compared with the association of the desmosome proteins and keratin intermediate filaments.[33,34,35]

Lamellar granules deliver precursors of stratum corneum lipids into the intercellular space. The granules are first evident in the cytoplasm of the upper spinous cells, even though the primary site of their activity is at the granular-cornified layer interface.[36] They are 0.2 μm to 0.3 μm in diameter, membrane-bound, secretory organelles that contain a series of alternating thick and thin lamellae; these are folded sheets or disklike or liposomelike structures. Lamellar granules contain glycoproteins, glycolipids, phospholipids, free sterols, and a number of acid hydrolases, including lipases, proteases, acid phosphatase, and glycosidases. Glucosylceramides, the precursors to ceramides and the dominant component of the stratum corneum lipids, are found in lamellar granules. The enzymes indicate that lamellar granules are a type of lysosome with characteristics of both secretory granules and liposomes. Roles for the lamellar granule in providing the epidermal lipids responsible for the barrier properties of the stratum corneum, the synthesis and storage of cholesterol, and the adhesion/desquamation of cornified cells have been hypothesized.[37,38]

The granular layer is characterized by the buildup of components necessary to the process of programmed cell death and the formation of a superficial water-impermeable barrier.[39] The typical cytoplasmic organelles associated with an active synthetic metabolism are still evident within cells of the stratum granulosum, but the most apparent structures within these cells are the basophilic, keratohyalin granules. Keratohyalin granules are composed primarily of an electron-dense protein, profilaggrin, and keratin intermediate filaments. Loricrin, a protein of the cornified cell envelope, is also found within the keratohyalin granule.[40]

Other protein markers of keratinization are components of the cornified cell envelope (CE), a 7 nm- to 15 nm-thick dense protein layer deposited beneath the plasma membrane of cornified cells. Proteins of the CE constitute a significant fraction of the protein in the granular cell and are rendered insoluble by cross-linking via disulfide bonds and

(γ-glutamyl) lysine isopeptide bonds formed by transglutaminases. Involucrin, keratolinin, loricrin, small proline-rich proteins, the serine protease inhibitor elafin (SKALP), filaggrin linker-segment peptide, and envoplakin have all been found as components of the CE.[41]

The granular cell not only synthesizes, modifies, and/or cross-links new proteins involved in keratization, it also plays a role in its own programmed destruction. This occurs during the abrupt transition from a granular cell to a terminally differentiated cornified cell. The change involves the loss of the nucleus and virtually all of the cellular contents, with the exception of the keratin filaments and filaggrin matrix.[42]

Complete transition from a granular to a cornified cell is accompanied by a 45% to 85% loss in dry weight. The layers of resultant cornified, or horny, cells provide mechanical protection to the skin and a barrier to water loss and permeation of soluble substances from the environment. The stratum corneum barrier is formed by a 2-component system of lipid-depleted protein-enriched corneocytes surrounded by a continuous extracellular lipid matrix. The flattened, polyhedral-shaped cell is the largest cell of the epidermis. Its shape and surface features are adapted to maintain the integrity of the stratum corneum yet allow for desquamation. High molecular mass keratins stabilized by intermolecular disulfide bonds account for up to 80% of the cornified cell. The remainder of the cell content appears to be an electron-dense matrix material, probably filaggrin, surrounding the filaments. The nucleus is lost from normal stratum corneum cells, but it persists in incompletely keratinized cells, as seen in psoriasis. Remnants of organelles, especially profiles of membranes and melanin pigment, are occasionally present within the normal cell.[43,44] A rigid CE borders the outer stratum corneum cells. The stratum corneum cell retains some metabolic functions and thus is not the inert covering it has been previously considered.[45]

## Nonkeratinocytes of the Epidermis

The melanocyte is a dendritic, pigment-synthesizing cell derived from neural crest that is confined mainly to the basal layer.[46] In postnatal skin, the cell body of the melanocyte often extends toward the dermis below the level of the basal cell, but always superior to the lamina densa. Melanocyte processes contact keratinocytes in basal and more superficial layers but do not form junctions with them at any level. Melanocytes are recognized light microscopically by their pale-staining cytoplasm, ovoid nucleus, and the intrinsic color of the pigment-containing melanosomes. Differentiation of the melanocyte correlates with the acquisition of its primary functions: melanogenesis, arborization, and transfer of pigment to keratinocytes.[47,48] The melanosome is the distinctive organelle of the melanocyte. It is resolved at the ultrastructural level as an ovoid, membrane-bound structure within which a series of receptor-mediated, hormone-stimulated, enzyme-catalyzed reactions produce melanin.[49]

There are important organizational relationships and functional interactions between keratinocytes and melanocytes that the melanocyte depends on for differentiation and function.[50] Approximately 36 basal and suprabasal keratinocytes are thought to coexist functionally with each melanocyte in an epidermal-melanin unit, an organizational system that is mimicked in vitro when the 2 cell types are co-cultured. Within this aggregate, melanocytes transfer pigment to associated keratinocytes. As a result, pigment is distributed throughout the basal layer and, to a lesser extent, the more superficial layers, where it protects the skin by absorbing and scattering potentially harmful radiation.[51]

Merkel cells are slow-adapting, type I mechanoreceptors located in sites of high tactile sensitivity. They are present among basal keratinocytes in particular regions of the body.[52] Merkel cells receive stimuli as keratinocytes are deformed and respond by secretion of chemical transmitters. They are found both in hairy skin and in the glabrous skin of the digits, lips, regions of the oral cavity, and the outer root sheath of the hair follicle. In some of these sites, they are assembled in specialized structures called tactile discs or touch domes. Like other nonkeratinocytes, Merkel cells have a pale-staining cytoplasm. The nucleus is lobulated, and the margins of cells project cytoplasmic "spines" toward keratinocytes.[53] Merkel cells make synaptic contacts with nerve endings to form the Merkel cell-neurite complex. New evidence suggests that Merkel cells are the mechanoreceptors while the nerve terminals transduce the transient phase. The morphology of the contacting membranes of both the Merkel cell and neurite is similar to the presynaptic and postsynaptic modifications that are characteristic of a synapse. Moreover, the presence of neurotransmitter-like substances in the dense core granules suggests that the Merkel cell is the receptor that transmits a stimulus to the neurite via a chemical synapse.[54]

Langerhans cells are bone marrow–derived, antigen-processing, and antigen-presenting cells that are involved in a variety of T cell responses.[55] The Langerhans cell is not unique to the epidermis: it is found in other squamous epithelia, including the oral cavity, esophagus, and vagina; in lymphoid organs such as the spleen, thymus, and lymph node; and in the normal dermis.[56]

Langerhans cells migrate from the bone marrow to the circulation into the epidermis early in embryonic development and continue to repopulate the epidermis throughout life.[56] Langerhans cells are the primary cells in the epidermis responsible for the recognition, uptake, processing, and presentation of soluble antigen and haptens to sensitized T lymphocytes and are implicated in the pathologic mechanisms underlying allergic contact dermatitis, cutaneous leishmaniasis, and human immunodeficiency virus infection.[57]

## Dermal-Epidermal Junction

The dermal-epidermal junction (DEJ) is a basement membrane zone that forms an interface between the epidermis and dermis. The major function of the DEJ is to attach the epidermis and dermis to each other and to provide resistance against external sheering forces. It serves as a support for the epidermis, determines the polarity of growth, directs the organization of the cytoskeleton and basal cells, provides developmental signals, and serves as a semi-penetrable barrier. The structures of the DEJ are almost entirely products of basal keratinocytes, with minor contributions from dermal fibroblasts.[26,58]

The DEJ can be subdivided into 3 supramolecular networks: the hemidesmosome-anchoring filament complex, the basement membrane itself, and the anchoring fibrils. The localization of antigens, determination of composition, and the known affinities of matrix molecules present in the basement membrane zone for other matrix molecules (laminin and type IV collagen) are the basis for the structural models of this region of the skin and define its function and physical properties. The subdivisions coincide with areas of weakness that can result in dermal-epidermal separation under circumstances of physical stress, genetic disease, an autoimmune process, or trauma.[59]

The hemidesmosome-anchoring filament complex binds basal keratinocytes to the basement membrane. The importance of these structures and molecules in maintaining the integrity of the skin can be surmised from inherited and acquired disorders of the skin in which they are either destroyed, altered, or absent, thereby resulting in dermal-epidermal separation.[59] A similar, although more superficial blistering within the plane of the basal epidermal layer, occurs in patients with the various forms of epidermolysis bullosa simplex caused by mutations in genes that code for the K5 and/or K14 basal cell keratins or other structural proteins specific for this layer.[59]

## The Dermis

The dermis is an integrated system of fibrous, filamentous, and amorphous connective tissue that accommodates nerve and vascular networks, epidermally derived appendages, fibroblasts, macrophages, mast cells, and other blood-borne cells, including lymphocytes, plasma cells, and leukocytes, that enter the dermis in response to various stimuli. Dermis makes up the bulk of the skin and provides its pliability, elasticity, and tensile strength. It protects the body from mechanical injury, binds water, aids in thermal regulation, and includes receptors of sensory stimuli. The dermis interacts with the epidermis in maintaining the properties of both tissues, collaborates during development in the morphogenesis of the DEJ and epidermal appendages (teeth, nails, sebaceous structures, and sweat glands), and interacts in repairing and remodeling the skin as wounds are healed.[60]

Collagen and elastic connective tissue are the main types of fibrous connective tissue of the dermis. Collagen is the major dermal constituent. It accounts for approximately 75% of the dry weight of the skin and provides both tensile strength and elasticity. The periodically banded, interstitial collagens (types I, III, and V) account for the greatest proportion of the collagen in the adult dermis. Approximately 80% to 90% of the collagen is type I collagen, and 8% to 12% is type III collagen. Type V collagen, although less than 5%, co-distributes and assembles into fibrils with both types I and III collagen, in which it is believed to assist in regulating fibril diameter. Type V collagen is polymorphic in structure (granules, filaments) and has been immunolocalized primarily to the papillary dermis and the matrix surrounding basement membranes of vessels, nerves, epidermal appendages, and at the DEJ.[61] Type IV collagen of the skin is confined to the basal lamina of the DEJ vessels and epidermal appendages.[61]

The elastic connective tissue is a complex macromolecular mesh, assembled in a continuous network that extends from the lamina densa of the DEJ throughout the dermis and into the connective tissue of the hypodermis. Its organization and importance in the dermis is best appreciated when examining samples of skin that have been digested to remove the collagen and other structures of the dermis but retain the extraordinarily stable elastic fibers. Elastic fibers return the skin to its normal configuration after being stretched or deformed. Elastic fibers are also present in the walls of cutaneous blood vessels and lymphatics and in the sheaths of hair follicles. By dry weight, elastic connective tissue accounts for approximately 4% of the dermal matrix protein.[62,63]

Elastic fibers have microfibrillar and amorphous matrix components. Several glycoproteins have been identified as constituents of the microfibrils. Among the most characterized of these molecules is fibrillin, a 350 kDa molecule. Mutations in fibrillin have been identified in patients with Marfan's syndrome, an inherited connective tissue disease in which patients frequently die of aneurysm of the aorta.[63]

Several filamentous or amorphous matrix components are present in the dermis between the fibrous matrix elements, associated with the fibers themselves, organized on the surface of cells and in basement membranes. Proteoglycans (PG) and glycosaminoglycans (GAG) are the molecules of the "ground substance" that surrounds and embeds the fibrous components. They account for up to 0.2% dry weight of the dermis. PGs are unusually large molecules (100–2500 kDa) consisting of a core protein that is specific for the molecule and that determines which GAGs will be incorporated into the molecule. Hyaluronic acid usually binds to the core protein. The PGs/GAGs can bind up to 1000 times their own volume and thus regulate the water-binding capabilities of the dermis and influence dermal volume and compressibility; they also bind growth factors and link cells with the fibrillar and filamentous matrix, thereby influencing proliferation, differentiation, tissue repair, and morphogenesis. They are components of basement membranes and are present on surfaces of mesenchymal and epithelial cells.[64,65] The major PGs in the adult dermis are chondroitin sulfates/dermatan sulfates (biglycan, decorin, versican), heparan sulfate proteoglycans, and chondroitin-6 sulfate proteoglycans.[65]

Fibronectin (in the matrix), laminin (restricted to basement membranes), thrombospondin, vitronectin, and tenascin are glycoproteins found in the dermis, and like the PGs/GAGs, they interact with other matrix components and with cells through specific integrin receptors.[66,67] As a consequence of their binding to other glycoproteins, collagen and elastic fibers, PGs, and cells, glycoproteins are involved in cell attachment (adhesion), migration, spreading in vitro, morphogenesis (epithelial-mesenchymal interactions), and differentiation.[68]

Fibronectin is an insoluble, filamentous glycoprotein synthesized in the skin by both epithelial and mesenchymal cells; it ensheaths collagen fiber bundles and the elastic network, is associated with basal laminae, and appears on the surface of cells, where it is bound to the cell through 1 of multiple integrin receptors that mediate cell-matrix adhesion. Fibronectin also binds platelets to collagen, is found in fibrin-fibrinogen complexes, and plays a role in organizing the extracellular matrix.[69]

The dermis is organized into papillary and reticular regions; the distinction of the 2 zones is based largely on their differences in connective tissue organization, cell density, and nerve and vascular patterns.[70] Subdivisions of each of these regions are more or less apparent in mature skin, depending upon the individual. The papillary dermis is proximal to the epidermis, molds to its contours, and is usually no more than twice its thickness. The reticular dermis is the dominant region of the dermis and of the skin as a whole. A horizontal plane of vessels, the subpapillary plexus, marks the boundary between the papillary and reticular dermis. The deep boundary between the dermis and the hypodermis is defined by the transition from fibrous to adipose connective tissue.[71]

The papillary dermis is characterized by small bundles of small-diameter collagen fibrils and elastic fibers. Mature elastic fibers are usually not found in the normal papillary dermis. The papillary dermis also has a high density of fibroblasts that proliferate more rapidly, have a higher rate of metabolic activity, and synthesize different species of PGs as compared to those of the reticular dermis. Capillaries extending from the subpapillary plexus project toward the epidermis within the dermal papillae, fingerlike projections of papillary dermis that interdigitate with the rete pegs that project from the epidermis into the dermis.[72] The reticular dermis is composed primarily of large-diameter collagen fibrils organized into large, interwoven fiber bundles.

Fibroblasts, macrophages, and mast cells are regular residents of the dermis. They are found in greatest density in normal skin in the papillary region and surrounding vessels of the subpapillary plexus, but they also reside in the reticular dermis, where they are found in the interstices between collagen fiber bundles. Small numbers of lymphocytes collect around blood vessels in normal skin, and at a site of inflammation, lymphocytes and other leukocytes from the blood are prominent. Pericytes and veil cells ensheath the walls of blood vessels, and Schwann cells encompass nerve fibers.[73]

The fibroblast is a mesenchymally derived cell that migrates through the tissue and is responsible for the synthesis and degradation of fibrous and nonfibrous connective tissue matrix proteins and a number of soluble factors.[74] Most commonly, the function of fibroblasts is to provide a structural extracellular matrix framework as well as to promote interaction between epidermis and dermis by the synthesis of soluble factors.[60] The same fibroblast is capable of synthesizing more than 1 type of matrix protein simultaneously. The morphology of the fibroblast often suggests active synthetic activity; the cytoplasm includes multiple profiles of dilated rough endoplasmic reticulum and typically more than 1 Golgi complex.[75]

The monocytes, macrophages, and dermal dendrocytes are a heterogeneous collection of cells that constitute the mononuclear phagocytic system of cells in the skin. Macrophages have an expansive list of functions. They are phagocytic; they process and present antigen to immunocompetent lymphoid cells; they are microbicidal (through the production of lysozyme, peroxide, and superoxide), tumoricidal, secretory (growth factors, cytokines, and other immunomodulary molecules), and hematopoietic; and they are involved in coagulation, atherogenesis, wound healing, and tissue remodeling.[73,76]

Mast cells are specialized secretory cells distributed in connective tissue throughout the body, typically at sites adjacent to the interface of an organ and the environment. In the skin, mast cells are present in greatest density in the papillary dermis, near the DEJ, in sheaths of epidermal appendages, and around blood vessels and nerves of the subpapillary plexus.[77] The surface of dermal mast cells is modified by microvilli, and like fibroblasts, they are coated with fibronectin, which probably assists in securing the cells within the connective tissue matrix. Mast cells originate in the bone marrow from CD34 stem cells. Mast cell proliferation depends on the c-kit receptor and its ligand, SCF (stem cell factor).[78] Like basophils, mast cells also contain metachromatic granules and stores of histamines; both cells synthesize eosinophilic chemotactic factor and have IgE antibodies bound to their plasma membranes.

Mast cells synthesize an impressive repertoire of mediators. Some of them are preformed and stored in the granules. Histamine, heparin, tryptase, chymase, carboxypeptidase, neutrophil chemotatctic factor, and eosinophilic chemotactic factor of anaphylaxis are organized in the predominantly proteoglycan milieu of the granule in a manner that is suggested to retain enzymes in an inactive state prior to release.[77] The mast cell synthesizes and releases other molecules without storage, including a number of growth factors, cytokines (IL-1, IL-3, IL-4, IL-5, GM-CSF, and TNF-α), leukotrienes, and platelet-activating factors. Lysosomal granules in the cells contain acid hydrolases that degrade GAGs, PGs, and complex glycolipids intracellularly. Several additional enzymes are present in both the lysosomal and the secretory granules. These may be important in initiating the repair of damaged tissue and/or may help in degrading foreign material.[78]

The dendrocyte is a stellate, or sometimes spindle-shaped, highly phagocytic mixed connective tissue cell in the dermis of normal skin. Dermal dendrocytes are not specialized fibroblasts, but rather represent a subset of antigen-presenting macrophages or a distinct lineage that originates in the bone marrow. Similar to many other bone marrow–derived cells, dermal dendrocytes express factor XIIIa and the HLe-1 (CD45) antigen, and they lack typical markers of the fibroblastic cell (Te-7).[79] These cells are particularly abundant in the papillary dermis and upper reticular dermis, frequently in the proximity of vessels of the subpapillary dermis. Dermal dendrocytes are also present around vessels in the reticular dermis and in the subcutaneous fat. The number of dermal dendrocytes is elevated in fetal, infant, photoaged, and select pathologic adult skin and in association with sites of angiogenesis. Dermal dendrocytes are immunologically competent cells that function as effector cells in the afferent limb of an immune response.[80]

## Cutaneous Vasculature

The dermal microvascular unit represents an intricate assemblage of cells responsible not only for cutaneous nutrition but also for immune cell trafficking, regulation of vessel tone, and local hemostasis. The dermal microvasculature is divided into 2 important strata. First, the superficial vascular plexus defines the boundary between the papillary and reticular dermis and extends within an adventitial mantle to envelop adnexal structures. This subpapillary plexus forms a layer of anastomosing arterioles and venules in close approximation to the overlying epidermis and is normally surrounded by other cellular components of the dermal microvascular unit. Small capillary loops emanate from the superficial vascular plexus and extend into each dermal papilla. The capillaries that are present throughout the dermis, but especially in the papillary dermis, are composed of a layer of endothelial cells surrounded by an incomplete layer of pericytes. The second plexus, the deep vascular plexus, is connected to the first by vertically oriented reticular dermal vessels and separates the reticular dermis from the subcutaneous fat. Many of these vessels are of larger caliber and communicate with branches that extend within fibrous septa that separate lobules of underlying subcutaneous fat.[81,82]

A special vascular structure, the glomus, is located within the reticular dermis in certain areas. Glomus formations occur most abundantly in the pads and nail beds of the fingers and toes, but also on the volar aspect of the hands and feet, in the skin of the ears, and in the center of the face. The glomus is concerned with temperature regulation. It represents a special arteriovenous shunt that, without the interposition of capillaries, connects an arteriole and a venule. When open, these shunts cause a great increase in blood flow in the area.[83]

## Cutaneous Lymphatics

The lymph channels of the skin are important in regulating pressure of the interstitial fluid by resorption of fluid released from vessels and in clearing the tissue of cells, proteins, lipids, bacteria, and degraded substances. Lymph flow within the skin depends upon movements of the tissue caused by arterial pulsations and larger-scale muscle contractions and movement of the body. Bicuspid-like valves within the lymphatic vessels may help prevent backflow and stasis of fluid in the vessels.[84] The lymph capillaries drain into a horizontal plexus of larger lymph vessels located deep in the subpapillary venous plexus. Lymph vessels can be distinguished from blood vessels in the same position by a larger luminal diameter (often difficult to see in their normally collapsed state in the skin) and thinner wall that consists of an endothelium, discontinuous basal lamina, and elastic fibers.[84]

## Nerves and Receptors

The nerve networks of the skin contain somatic sensory and autonomic fibers. The sensory fibers alone (free nerve endings) or in conjunction with specialized structures (corpuscular receptors) function at every point of the body as receptors of touch, pain, temperature, itch, and mechanical stimuli. The density and types of receptors are regionally variable and specific, thus accounting for the variation in acuity at different sites of the body. Receptors are particularly dense in hairless areas such as the areola, labia, and glans penis. Sympathetic motor fibers are co-distributed with the sensory nerves in the dermis until they branch to innervate the sweat glands, vascular smooth muscle, arrector pili muscle of the hair follicles, and sebaceous glands.[85]

The skin is innervated by large, myelinated cutaneous branches of musculocutaneous nerves that arise segmentally from spinal nerves. Small branches that enter the deep dermis are surrounded by an epineurial sheath; perineurial and endoneurial sheaths and Schwann cells envelop fiber bundles and individual fibers, respectively. The pattern of nerve fibers in the skin is similar to the vascular patterns. Nerve fibers form a deep plexus, then ascend to a superficial, subpapillary plexus.[86]

The sensory nerves, in general, supply the skin segmentally (dermatomes), but the boundaries are imprecise and there is overlapping innervation to any given area. Autonomic innervation does not follow exactly the same pattern because the postganglionic fibers distributed in the skin originate in sympathetic chain ganglia where preganglionic fibers of several different spinal nerves synapse.[85] Free nerve endings are the most widespread and undoubtedly the most important sensory receptors of the body. In humans, they are always ensheathed by Schwann cells and a basal lamina. Free nerve endings are particularly common in the papillary dermis just beneath the epidermis, and the basal lamina of the fiber may merge with the lamina densa of the basement membrane zone.[86]

Corpuscular receptors have a capsule and an inner core and contain both neural and nonneural components. The capsule is a continuation of the perineurium, and the core includes preterminal and terminal portions of the fiber surrounded by laminated wrappings of Schwann cells. The Meissner's corpuscle is an elongated or ovoid mechanoreceptor located in the dermal papilla of digital skin and oriented vertically toward the epidermal surface. The Pacinian corpuscle lies in the deep dermis and subcutaneous tissue of skin that covers weight-bearing surfaces of the body. Pacinian corpuscles serve as rapidly adapting mechanoreceptors responding to vibrational stimuli.[87,88]

## Skin Appendages

The hair follicle, with its hair in longitudinal section, consists of 3 parts: the lower portion, extending from the base of the follicle to the insertion of the arrector pili muscle; the middle portion, or isthmus, a rather short section, extending from the insertion of the arrector pili to the entrance of the sebaceous duct; and the upper portion, or infundibulum, extending from the entrance of the sebaceous duct to the follicular orifice. The lower portion of the hair follicle is composed of 5 major portions: the dermal hair papilla; the hair matrix; the hair, consisting inward to outward of medulla, cortex, and hair cuticle; the inner root sheath, consisting inward to outward of inner root sheath cuticle, Huxley layer, and Henle layer; and the outer root sheath.[89]

It has been proposed that stem cells lie in a specialized region of the hair follicle outer root sheath (ORS) known as the bulge, and are ultimately responsible for replenishing the differentiated cells of the interfollicular epidermis in addition to generating all the hair lineages.[90] The bulge lies beneath the sebaceous gland at the point of insertion of the arrector pili muscle.

Communication with the underlying dermis plays an important role in regulating epidermal differentiation, with specialized mesenchymal cells of the dermal papilla at the base of the hair follicle providing the best-characterized microenvironment (often referred to as a niche) both in vivo and in vitro. Growth and differentiation of postnatal hair follicles are controlled by reciprocal interactions between the dermal papilla and the cells of the hair matrix.[91,92]

In human epidermis of non-hair-bearing skin, basal cells that are not actively cycling and that express several putative stem cell markers are found in clusters that have a specific topology with respect to the underlying connective tissue.[93] The stem cell clusters are surrounded by basal cells that are actively cycling and express markers of transient amplifying cells, and it is from within this latter compartment that cells committed to terminal differentiation move into the layers above.[94]

Sebaceous glands are an appendage of the hair follicle, located above the bulge and arrector pili muscle and just below the hair shaft orifice at the skin surface. Sebaceous gland progenitor cells emerge near the conclusion of embryogenesis, but the gland does not mature until just after birth. The main role of the gland is to generate terminally differentiated sebocytes, which produce lipids and sebum. When sebocytes disintegrate, they release these oils into the hair canal for lubrication and protection against bacterial infections. Sebaceous gland homeostasis necessitates a progenitor population of cells that gives rise to a continual flux of proliferating, differentiating, and, finally, dead cells that are lost through the hair canal.[95]

The apocrine glands differ from eccrine glands in origin, distribution, size, and mode of secretion. The eccrine glands primarily serve in the regulation of heat, and the apocrine glands represent scent glands. Eccrine glands are present everywhere in the human skin; however, they are absent in areas of modified skin that lack all cutaneous appendages,

that is, the vermillion border of the lips, the nail beds, the labia minora, the glans penis, and the inner aspect of the prepuce. They are found in greatest abundance on the palms and soles and in the axillae. The eccrine sweat gland is engineered for temperature regulation. With approximately 3 million glands in the human integument weighing 35 μg per gland, the average human boasts about 100 g of eccrine glands capable of producing a maximum of approximately 1.8 L of sweat per hour.[96]

Apocrine glands are encountered in only a few areas: in the axillae, in the anogenital region, as modified glands in the external ear canal (ceruminous glands), in the eyelid (Moll's glands), and in the breast (mammary glands). Occasionally, a few apocrine glands are found on the face, in the scalp, and on the abdomen; they usually are small and nonfunctional. Apocrine glands develop their secretory portion and become functional only at puberty. The reason for apocrine secretion in humans remains an enigma, although it may simply be an evolutionary vestige (musk glands of the deer and scent glands of the skunk are modified apocrine-type structures).[97]

The nail unit is a region of specialized keratinization of practical importance, since dermatoses, infections, and neoplasms may affect this site, prompting histologic sampling. The nail unit has 6 main components: (1) the nail matrix, which gives rise to the nail plate; (2) the nail plate; (3) the cuticular system, consisting of the dorsal component, or cuticle, and the distal component, or hyponichium; (4) the nail bed, which includes the dermis and underlying bone and soft tissue beneath the nail plate; (5) an anchoring system of ligaments between bone and matrix proximally and between grooves distally; and (6) the nail folds proximally, laterally, and distally.[98]

## DEVELOPMENT OF SKIN

## Overview

Significant advances in the understanding of the molecular processes responsible for the development of the skin have been made over the last several years. Such advances have significantly broadened our knowledge of wound healing and increased our understanding of the clinicopathologic correlation among inherited disorders of the skin, allowing for the early diagnosis and treatment of such diseases.[99]

Conceptually, fetal skin development can be divided into 3 distinct but temporally overlapping stages, those of specification, morphogenesis, and differentiation. These stages roughly correspond to the embryonic period (0–60 days), the early fetal period (2–5 months), and the late fetal period (5–9 months) of development. The earliest stage, specification, refers to the process by which the ectoderm lateral to the neural plate is committed to become epidermis and subsets of mesenchymal and neural crest cells are committed to form the dermis. It is at this time that patterning of the future layers and specialized structures of the skin occurs, often via a combination of gradients of proteins and cell-cell signals. The second stage, morphogenesis, is the process by which these committed tissues begin to form their specialized structures, including epidermal stratification, epidermal appendage formation, subdivision between the dermis and subcutis, and vascular formation. The last stage, differentiation, denotes the process by which these specialized tissues further develop and assume their mature forms.[100]

After gastrulation, the embryo surface emerges as a single layer of neuroectoderm, which will ultimately specify the nervous system and skin epithelium. At the crossroads of this decision is Wnt signaling, which blocks the ability of ectoderm to respond to fibroblast growth factors (FGFs). In the absence of FGF signaling, the cells express bone morphogenetic proteins (BMPs) and become fated to develop into epidermis. Conversely, the acquisition of neural fate arises when, in the absence of a Wnt signal, the ectoderm is able to receive and translate activating cues by FGFs, which then attenuate BMP signaling through inhibitory cues. The embryonic epidermis that results consists of a single layer of multipotent epithelial cells. It is covered by a transient protective layer of tightly connected squamous endodermislike cells, known as periderm, which is shed once the epidermis has stratified and differentiated.[101,102]

## Insights From Fetal Wound Healing

In mature skin, wound repair typically begins with hemostasis and inflammation. This is followed by a proliferative phase, with reepithelialization, angiogenesis, and collagen production, and ends with the generation of a permanent scar. However, animal studies and clinical observations have shown that a different type of healing occurs in fetal skin in the first 2 trimesters of development. In early fetal skin, wounds exhibit a unique pattern of wound healing leading to regeneration. Notably, repair in the fetus takes place with little or no inflammation, faster reepithelialization, and no scarring.[103] Insights into regenerative healing may provide information about how to accelerate postnatal wound healing as well as how to improve healing from a cosmetic standpoint. Future research directions include identification of the molecular controls responsible for scarless healing, with the intention that this new information will lead to improved therapeutic strategies for wound healing.[104]

As experimental studies have demonstrated, it is evident that fetal wounds heal differently depending upon the gestational age of the fetus. In the first and second trimesters of development, fetal skin undergoes rapid healing with

little or no inflammation and no scarring. Scarless healing in early fetal skin is a form of regeneration, with renewal of skin appendages such as hair follicles and sebaceous glands in addition to the restoration of a normal dermal matrix and no scar. Near the third trimester, a transition period occurs. At this point, the skin begins to lose its ability to regenerate and instead undergoes fibrotic healing similar to that in postnatal skin.[105] Pathology reports and basic research studies have shown that scarless healing occurs in fetal skin until around 22 weeks to 24 weeks of gestation in the human fetus.[106]

The uterine environment in which fetal wounds heal is unique, with amniotic fluid surrounding the healing wounds. Originally, this warm and sterile amniotic fluid, rich in growth factors and extracellular matrix components, was considered imperative for the scarless fetal healing process. Although it has been suggested that the sterile nature of amniotic fluid and anti-inflammatory factors that it contains may help facilitate noninflammatory, scarless healing, the amniotic fluid environment is not required for this process.[107] Studies utilizing the developing opossum indicate that amniotic fluid is not essential for scarless healing. In this marsupial model, offspring develop in a pouch instead of a uterine environment, but the developmental process in the pouch resembles the in utero development of a mammalian fetus with scarless healing.[108]

Transplantation studies have also been used to investigate the importance of amniotic fluid in scarless tissue repair. Studies in sheep have shown that wounds made in adult skin or late gestational fetal skin transplanted onto fetal lambs heal with a scar; therefore, skin beyond the transition to fibrotic healing continues to heal with a scar even if repair takes place in a fetal environment. In addition, early human fetal skin transplanted subcutaneously in nude mice heals without a scar after wounding, demonstrating that scarless healing in fetal skin is independent of amniotic fluid or perfusion by fetal serum.[103]

## Inflammation

One of the first distinguishing characteristics of scarless fetal healing identified was a lack of inflammation. A diminished inflammatory response in scarless fetal wounds has been demonstrated repeatedly in many different models of fetal wound healing.[109,110] The presence of inflammation during repair is believed to contribute to the transition from scarless to fibrotic healing in fetal skin because a significant inflammatory response to injury does not manifest until the third trimester, when the skin begins to heal with a scar.[104,108] Inducing inflammation with killed or live bacteria, chemical agents, or various mediators of inflammation, including cytokines, growth factors, and prostaglandins, in early fetal wounds results in the formation of a scar, when normally these wounds would have healed without a scar.[111,112]

Once the idea that minimal inflammation defined scarless fetal repair was accepted, studies focused on characterizing the specific inflammatory cell types that were missing and determining the mechanisms of reduced inflammation. Virtually all the cells involved in acute inflammation respond differently to injury in early fetal skin, including platelets, neutrophils, macrophages, and lymphocytes.[113]

## Reepithelialization

Martin et al, who conducted numerous studies on fetal wound reepithelialization, identified fundamental differences in the mechanics of reepithelialization in embryonic wounds. Although adult wounds have been shown to reepithelialize through extension of lamellipodia followed by epidermal cells at the wound edge crawling over the wound bed, embryonic wounds exhibit no signs of lamellipodia or filopodial extensions. Instead, epidermal cells at the edge of wounds in both chick and mouse embryos assemble an actin cable that contracts like a purse string to close the wound.[114,115]

## Angiogenesis

Angiogenesis, the process of new blood vessel growth, is a key element of the proliferative phase of healing in adult wounds. Until recently, no studies quantitatively comparing angiogenesis in early and late fetal wounds were available. Whitby and Ferguson reported a noticeable lack of neovascularization in fetal mouse wounds compared to adult wounds with immunostaining for collagen IV and laminin, both of which stain endothelial basement membranes.[116] In addition, in a rat model of fetal wound healing, investigators observed angiogenesis in day 19 fetal wounds but not in day 16 wounds.[117] Several proangiogenic factors have been found to be absent or present at lower levels in scarless wounds versus scar-forming wounds, including basic fibroblast growth factor (bFGF), transforming growth factor $\beta 1$ (TGF-$\beta 1$), platelet-derived growth factor (PDGF), and prostaglandin $E_2$ (PG $E_2$).[118,119] It has also been shown that the addition of substances capable of inducing angiogenesis in early fetal wounds (TGF-$\beta 1$, PDGF, PGE$_2$, and hyaluronidase) causes scar formation.[120,121]

## Extracellular Matrix

The most obvious difference between fetal and adult skin healing is the lack of dermal scar tissue formation. Instead of reducing a scar with a significantly altered extracellular matrix (ECM), fetal skin has the unique ability to lay down new ECM with a composition and arrangement similar to normal, unwounded skin, complete with the regeneration of hair follicles and other appendages.[122]

One of the first differences identified in the ECM of fetal wounds is the presence of high levels of glycosaminoglycans (GAGs). Glycosaminoglycans are polysaccharides comprised of repeating acidic and basic disaccharides found at high levels in connective tissues. Important GAGs in the skin include chondroitin sulfate, dermatan sulfate, heparan sulfate, heparin, and hyaluronic acid (HA).[123]

Many initial fetal wound healing studies focused on one particular GAG, hyaluronic acid, which appears to be present at the highest levels in fetal wounds. Hyaluronic acid can influence the structure, assembly, and hydration of the ECM and appears to support cell growth and migration, especially during development. Amniotic fluid has high levels of HA, especially earlier in gestation; high levels of hyaluronic acid stimulating activity (HASA), a factor that promotes HA deposition, also are present in amniotic fluid.[124,125] Fetal wounds also have less of the HA degrading enzyme hyaluronidase than adult wounds. Together, the high levels of HA and HASA, combined with low levels of hyaluronidase, are thought to be responsible for the persistent high levels of HA in fetal wounds.[126]

Collagen production obviously differs between scarless and scar-forming fetal wounds. In the first and second trimesters of development, fetal skin is capable of healing wounds with newly formed collagen in a fine reticular or basket-weave pattern identical to normal skin. This type of collagen network allows for regeneration rather than scar formation and is distinctly different from the thick, disorganized, parallel bundles of collagen that make up scar tissue.[127]

During normal adult wound repair, extensive ECM remodeling leads to collagen reorganization and formation of a mature scar. The remodeling process consists of both the production and the degradation of collagen and other ECM components; a relative imbalance in this process by either an abnormally high production of collagen or inadequate degradation could result in excessive scarring. According to a review of the subject, matrix metalloproteases (MMPs) and tissue inhibitors of the proteolytic activity of MMPs (TIMPs) are key to maintaining the appropriate balance between matrix production and degradation.[128] Bullard et al used immunochemistry to examine MMP levels in a model of subcutaneous transplantation of human fetal skin in immunodeficient mice and reported higher levels of MMP-1 (interstitial collagenase), MMP-2 (gelatinase A), and MMP-3 (stromelysin-1) in midgestation human fetal skin compared to adult skin. In addition, the authors showed that adding TGF-$\beta$ reduced MMP levels in fetal skin.[129] More recently, mRNA levels of a panel of MMPs and TIMPs were determined using scarless and fibrotic fetal wound healing in rat skin. Dang et al showed that scarless fetal wounds express MMP-1, MMP-9 (gelatinase B), and MMP-14 (membrane type 1 MMP) more quickly or at higher levels than fibrotic fetal wounds.[130]

## Growth Factors

Several growth factors with profibrotic properties have been studied in fetal wound healing. Many of the published fetal wound–healing experiments have focused on TGF-β family members because this family of proteins has been shown to have a defined role in fibrosis.[131] Differences in TGF-β expression, with lower levels and rapid clearance of TGF-β1 and TGF-β2 during scarless fetal repair compared to fibrotic healing, have been demonstrated repeatedly. In particular, reduced expression of TGF-β1 in early fetal wounds has been confirmed in incisional and excisional wounds in murine, rat, and human skin. The consistency of these findings in several diverse models suggests that minimal TGF-β1 expression in response to injury is a conserved response in early fetal skin.[132]

Numerous studies demonstrate that adding TGF-β causes a fibrotic healing response in early fetal skin that would normally heal scarlessly or without fibrosis, further solidifying a role for TGF-β and scar formation. The TGF-β3 isoform, which has antifibrotic effects in adult wounds, is reportedly higher in non-scarring fetal wounds. In addition, TGF-β receptors, TGF-βRI, and TGF-βRII are present at lower levels in scarless fetal wounds than in fibrotic wounds.[133,134]

## Fibroblasts and Myofibroblasts

The fibroblast is the primary cell type responsible for determining whether scarless or fibrotic healing will occur; therefore, regenerative fetal healing must ultimately depend on the ability of fetal fibroblasts to produce and arrange new collagen and other ECM components in similar quantities, ratios, and arrangements to unwounded skin. These characteristics appear to be unique to early gestation fetal fibroblasts because skin fibroblasts past the transition period lose the ability to make normal ECM in response to wounding. The critical role of the fetal fibroblast in scarless healing has been highlighted by Lorenz et al.[135] Human fetal skin retains the ability to heal scarlessly when transplanted subcutaneously in nude mice but heals with a scar when transplanted as a cutaneous graft. Utilizing antibodies specific for either mouse or human collagen types I and III, the authors demonstrated that the healed dermis in scarless, subcutaneous grafts was made up of human collagen. The collagen contained within the newly formed dermis of

the subcutaneous graft wounds was assessed histologically and found to be arranged in a reticular pattern similar to unwounded skin. The collagen in these scarless wounds was identified as human collagen and as such must have been produced by the human fetal fibroblasts. Conversely, the new matrix in cutaneous grafts that healed with a scar consisted of mouse collagen, suggesting that the murine adult fibroblasts, not the human fetal fibroblasts, were involved in the production of scar tissue. These studies underscore the unique ability of fetal fibroblasts to facilitate scarless healing in the fetus.[135]

Aside from normal fibroblasts, myofibroblasts, specialized contractile fibroblasts, also can contribute to wound repair. These cells express alpha smooth muscle actin (α-SMA) and are characterized using transmission electron microscopy by a well-developed rough endoplasmic reticulum, nuclei with irregular borders, secretory vesicles denoting active collagen synthesis, and organized microfilament bundles.[136] In fetal wounds, myofibroblast numbers appear to correlate with fibrotic healing. Studies in sheep have indicated that myofibroblasts are absent in early scarless fetal wounds but are present during healing at later stages, when permanent scarring occurs.[137] A lack of myofibroblasts has been reported in wounded mouse embryos. In addition, adding TGF-β1 to early fetal rabbit wounds induces fibrosis and increases the number of α-SMA-positive myofibroblasts in the wounds, further supporting the association of myofibroblasts with scar formation in fetal wounds.[138,139]

## Developmental Genes

A few studies have explored the potential involvement of developmental genes in scarless healing. The bone morphogenetic proteins (BMPs) belong to one family of developmental growth factors involved in skin and hair follicle development. Stelnicki et al demonstrated BMP-2 expression in the epidermis and developing hair follicles of human fetal skin. When exogenous BMP-2 was added to fetal lamb wounds, epidermal growth was augmented and the number of hair follicles and other skin appendages increased. However, fibroblast number and fibrosis also increased.[140] Stelnicki et al also found differential regulation of 2 homeobox genes, PRX-2 and HOXB-13, in a model of scarless fetal repair. Expression of PRX-2 was induced during scarless fetal wound healing, in contrast to adult wounds that displayed no increase in expression. In addition, expression of HOXB-13 was reduced during fetal wound healing compared to unwounded skin or adult wounds. Subsequent studies from the same group showed that deletion of the PRX-2 gene altered in vitro wound-healing parameters of fetal but not adult skin fibroblasts, which may have implications for the regulation of scarless healing.[141]

The Wnt signaling pathway also is known to be important for skin and hair follicle development. Recently, Colwell et al showed that Wnt-4 is expressed at higher levels in uninjured fetal skin than in postnatal skin. However, Wnt-4 expression increased during the healing of both fetal and postnatal wounds, suggesting that Wnt-4 is not likely to be an important mediator of scar tissue formation.[142]

## Cornified Envelope

During the latter part of gestation, epithelial surfaces at environmental interfaces undergo structural and functional changes, including synthesis of complex proteolipid materials. The stratum corneum is generally formed after 23 to 24 weeks of gestation. The formation of a barrier to water loss and infection is a sine qua non for survival in the extrauterine environment. Of note, synthesis and secretion of epidermal barrier lipids occurs in the form of lamellar bodies. This process is similar to that occurring over a parallel time frame in the developing lung.[143] The barrier lipids in the epidermis, unlike the lung, are generally devoid of phospholipids and consist primarily of free fatty acids, cholesterol, and ceramides.[5] Covalent cross-linking of structural proteins and ceramides results in formation of a highly insoluble cornified envelope, typical of the mature mammalian stratum corneum.[45] The cornified envelope, while only 10 nm to 15 nm thick and of uniform density, is highly insoluble, secondary to cross-linking by intracellular transglutaminases.[144]

## Biology of Vernix

The development of epidermal barrier function has many similarities to surfactant production and lung development. Both the epidermal keratinocyte and the type 2 alveolar cell are lipid-synthesizing cells that secrete barrier lipids in the form of lamellar bodies. Both interface with a gaseous environment under similar hormonal control at similar periods of development. There is a clear analogy between the mechanisms by which the lung develops a functionally mature epithelial surface ready for air adaptation and those by which the skin surface matures under total aqueous conditions for terrestrial adaptation to a dry environment. An unanswered question in epidermal biology, however, is by which mechanism the epidermal barrier forms under conditions of total aqueous emersion. Prolonged exposure of the skin surface to water in adults is harmful.[145]

Sebaceous glands are found in the skin of all mammals except whales and porpoises.[146] The primary function is the excretion of sebum, which is a complex mixture of relatively nonpolar lipids, most of which are synthesized de novo by the glands.[147] In newborn infants, sebaceous glands are well formed, hyperplastic, and macroscopically visible over certain body areas. The surge in sebaceous gland activity during the last trimester of pregnancy leads to production of a thick, lipid-rich, hydrophobic film (the vernix caseosa) overlying the developing stratum corneum.[148]

The amniotic fluid becomes turbid during the last trimester of pregnancy. In vitro, the addition of physiologically relevant amounts of pulmonary surfactant leads to emulsification and release of immobilized vernix. This finding is consistent with a mechanism by which vernix is progressively released from the skin surface after formation of an intact stratum corneum under the influence of lung-derived surfactant within the amniotic fluid. The fetus subsequently swallows the detached vernix. Measurements of the amino acids of vernix have demonstrated that it is rich in glutamine, a known trophic factor for the developing gut. Further work is required to establish the degree to which epithelial surfaces "cross-talk" in preparation for birth.[149,150]

## NORMAL WOUND HEALING

### Phases

Wound healing is a dynamic, interactive process involving soluble mediators, blood cells, extracellular matrix, and parenchymal and stem cells. Wound healing has 3 phases—inflammation, proliferation, and maturation—that overlap in time. During the first 4 to 5 days after closing an incision, little change in wound strength is noted. During this time, inflammatory cells invade the incision, so it is called the inflammatory or lag phase. After this period, there is a rapid increase in collagen content in the incision that is associated with a rapid increase in tensile strength. This phase is called the proliferative or collagen phase. Two key events occur during this phase, the deposition of the ECM and the ingrowth of new vessels. Finally, there is a prolonged phase where the incision continues to gain strength (up to approximately 80% of the original skin) but there is no increase in collagen content. Also during this maturation phase, the wound tends to become less cellular and vascular until a quiescent scar is formed.[151]

### Inflammation

Tissue injury causes the disruption of blood vessels and extravasation of blood constituents. The blood clot reestablishes hemostasis and provides a provisional extracellular matrix for cell migration. Platelets not only facilitate the formation of a hemostatic plug but also secrete several mediators of wound healing, such as PDGF, that attract and activate macrophages and fibroblasts.[152] However, in the absence of hemorrhage, platelets are not essential to wound healing. Numerous vasoactive mediators and chemotactic factors are generated by the coagulation and activated-complement pathways and by injured or activated parenchymal cells. These substances recruit inflammatory leucocytes to the site of injury.[153]

Infiltrating neutrophils cleanse the wound area of foreign particles and bacteria and are then extruded with the eschar or phagocytosed by macrophages. In response to specific chemoattractants, such as fragments of extracellular-matrix protein, TGF-β, and monocyte chemoattractant protein 1 (MCP-1), monocytes also infiltrate the wound site and become activated macrophages that release growth factors such as PDGF and vascular endothelial growth factor (VEGF), which initiate the formation of granulation tissue. Macrophages bind to specific proteins of the extracellular matrix by their integrin receptors, an action that stimulates phagocytosis of microorganisms and fragments of extracellular matrix by the macrophages.[154]

Adherence to the extracellular matrix also stimulates monocytes to undergo metamorphosis into inflammatory or reparative macrophages. Adherence induces monocytes and macrophages to express colony-stimulating factor 1 (CSF-1), a cytokine necessary for the survival of monocytes and macrophages; tumor necrosis factor α (TNF-α), a potent inflammatory cytokine; and PDGF, a potent chemoattractant and mitogen for fibroblasts. Other important cytokines expressed by monocytes and macrophages are transforming growth factor α (TGF-α), interleukin-1 (IL-1), TGF-β, and insulin-like growth factor 1 (IGF-1).[155] The monocyte-derived and macrophage-derived growth factors are almost certainly necessary for the initiation and propagation of new tissue formation in wounds, because macrophage-depleted animals have defective wound repair.[156] Thus, macrophages appear to have a pivotal role in the transition between inflammation and repair.[157]

## Epithelialization

When exposed to physical trauma and chemical assaults, the epidermis must protect itself, which it does by producing copious amounts of cytoplasmic heteropolymers, known as intermediate filaments, that are composed of keratin proteins. As cells exit from the basal layer and begin their journey to the skin surface, they switch from the expression of keratins K5 and K14 to K1 and K10. This switch was discovered more than 25 years ago and remains the most reliable indication that an epidermal cell has undergone a commitment to terminally differentiate.[158] The first suprabasal cells are known as spinous cells, reflecting their cytoskeleton of K1/K10 filament bundles connected to robust cell-cell junctions known as desmosomes. These connections provide a cohesive, integrative mechanical framework across and within stacks of epithelial sheets. K6, K16, and K17 are also expressed suprabasally, but only in hyperproliferative situations such as wound healing. This keratin network not only remodels the cytoskeleton for migration but also regulates cell growth through binding to adaptor protein 14–3–3σ and stimulating Akt/mTOR (mammalian target of rapamycin) signaling.[159]

As spinous cells progress to the granular layer, they produce electron-dense keratohyalin granules packed with the protein profilaggrin, which, when processed, bundles keratin intermediate filaments even more to generate large macrofibrillar cables. In addition, cornified envelope proteins, which are rich in glutamine and lysine residues, are synthesized and deposited under the plasma membrane of the granular cells. When the cells become permeabilized to calcium, they activate transglutaminase, generating γ-glutamyl ε-lysine cross-links to create an indestructible proteinaceous sac to hold the keratin macrofibrils. The final steps of terminal differentiation involve the destruction of cellular organelles, including the nucleus, and the extrusion of lipid bilayers, packaged in lamellar granules, onto the scaffold of the cornified envelope. The dead stratum corneum cells create an impenetrable seal that is continually replenished as inner layer cells move outwards and are sloughed from the skin surface.[160]

## Granulation Tissue Formation

New stroma, often called granulation tissue, begins to invade the wound space approximately 4 days after injury. Numerous new capillaries endow the new stroma with its granular appearance. Macrophages, fibroblasts, and blood vessels move into the wound space at the same time.[161] Macrophages provide a continuing source of growth factors necessary to stimulate fibroplasia and angiogenesis, the fibroblasts produce the new extracellular matrix necessary to support cell ingrowth, and blood vessels carry oxygen and nutrients necessary to sustain cell metabolism.

Growth factors, especially PDGF and TGF-β1, in concert with the extracellular matrix molecules, presumably stimulate fibroblasts of the tissue around the wound to proliferate, express appropriate integrin receptors, and migrate into the wound space.[162]

The structural molecules of newly formed extracellular matrix, termed the provisional matrix, contribute to the formation of granulation tissue by providing a scaffold or conduit for cell migration. These molecules include fibrin, fibronectin, and hyaluronic acid. In fact, the appearance of fibronectin and the appropriate integrin receptors that bind fibronectin, fibrin, or both on fibroblasts appears to be the rate-limiting step in the formation of granulation tissue.[163] The fibroblasts are responsible for the synthesis, deposition, and remodeling of the extracellular matrix.

Conversely, the extracellular matrix can have a positive or negative effect on the ability of fibroblasts to synthesize, deposit, remodel, and generally interact with the extracellular matrix.[162]

After migrating into wounds, fibroblasts commence the synthesis of extracellular matrix. The provisional extracellular matrix is gradually replaced with a collagenous matrix, perhaps as a result of the action of TGF-β1.[164] Once an abundant collagen matrix has been deposited in the wound, the fibroblasts stop producing collagen and the fibroblast-rich granulation tissue is replaced by a relatively acellular scar. Cells in the wound undergo apoptosis triggered by unknown signals. Dysregulation of these processes occurs in fibrotic disorders such as keloid formation and scleroderma.[165]

## Neovascularization

Adult neovascularization has traditionally been thought to be limited to angiogenesis, which can be defined as the sprouting of vessels from preexisting endothelial cells. Prior research has shown that this process is mediated by the release of angiogenic growth factors such as VEGF, PDGF, nitric oxide (NO), and FGF. These factors initiate local changes, including vasodilatation and increased vascular permeability, the activation of resident endothelial cells, and the degradation of the basement membrane. These cytokines/growth factors also stimulate endothelial cell migration and proliferation and the formation of capillary sprouts that ultimately lead to restored perfusion.[166]

Progenitor cells have been identified in adult bone marrow cells that possess the ability to replace resident cells throughout the human body.[167] Tissues in which bone marrow–derived stem cells have been identified include liver, brain, heart, and skeletal muscle.[168] While the contribution of progenitor cells is variable, it is becoming increasingly clear that wound healing in adults occurs by both differentiated resident cells and the recruitment of cells from the circulation.[169]

New blood vessel growth (neovascularization) is a process currently being reevaluated in light of recent advances in progenitor biology. With the identification of circulating endothelial progenitor cells (EPCs), neovascularization is now believed to occur via 2 possible mechanisms: the sprouting of preexisting resident endothelial cells (angiogenesis) or the recruitment of bone marrow–derived EPCs (vasculogenesis).[170] The participation of EPCs has been well documented in a number of conditions requiring neovascularization, including peripheral vascular disease, myocardial ischemia, stroke, retinopathy, tumor growth, and wound healing.[171,172] This has led to the examination of EPC transplantation in the treatment of ischemic conditions. Since human trials have already been initiated to investigate the

therapeutic and diagnostic utility of EPCs, it is important that their mechanism of action be more fully understood.[173]

It has been previously reported that EPCs are mobilized from bone marrow into circulation, home to sites of ischemia, undergo in situ differentiation, and ultimately participate in the formation of new blood vessels. This EPC mobilization cascade starts with peripheral hypoxia-induced tissue release of VEGF and subsequent activation of bone marrow stromal nitric oxide synthase (NOS), resulting in increased bone marrow NO levels. In this process, eNOS is essential in the bone marrow microenvironment, and increases in bone marrow NO levels result in mobilization of EPCs from bone marrow niches to circulation, ultimately allowing for their participation in tissue-level vasculogenesis in wound healing. At tissue level, EPC recruitment depends on ischemia-induced upregulation of stromal cell-derived factor-1α (SDF-1α). Impairments in eNOS function have been reported with hyperglycemia, insulin resistance, and in peripheral tissue from diabetic patients.[174,175,176]

## Wound Contraction and Extracellular Matrix Reorganization

Wound contraction involves a complex and superbly orchestrated interaction of cells, extracellular matrix, and cytokines. During the second week of healing, fibroblasts assume a myofibroblast phenotype characterized by large bundles of actin-containing microfilaments along the cytoplasmic face of the plasma membrane of the cells and by cell-cell and cell-matrix linkages.[177] The appearance of the myofibroblast corresponds with the commencement of connective tissue compaction and the contraction of the wound. The contraction probably requires stimulation by TGF β-1 or β-2 and PDGF, attachment of fibroblasts to the collagen matrix through integrin receptors, and cross-links between individual bundles of collagen.[178,179]

Collagen remodeling during the transition from granulation tissue to scar is dependent on continued synthesis and catabolism of collagen at a low rate. The degradation of collagen in the wound is controlled by several proteolytic enzymes, termed matrix metalloproteases, which are secreted by macrophages, epidermal cells, and endothelial cells as well as fibroblasts.[180] The various phases of wound repair rely on distinct combinations of matrix metalloproteases and tissue inhibitors of metalloproteases (TIMPs).[181]

Wounds gain only about 20% of their final strength in the first 3 weeks, during which time fibrillar collagen has accumulated relatively rapidly and has been remodeled by contraction of the wound. Thereafter, the rate at which wounds gain tensile strength is slow, reflecting a much slower rate of accumulation of collagen and, more importantly, collagen remodeling with the formation of larger collagen bundles and an increase in the number of intermolecular crosslinks.[182] Nevertheless, wounds never attain the same breaking strength (the tension at which skin breaks) as uninjured skin. At maximal strength, a scar is only 70% to 80% as strong as normal skin.[183]

## Epithelial-Mesenchymal Transition (EMT) and Endothelial-Mesenchymal Transition (EndMT) Concepts

Cell phenotype is the result of the dynamic equilibrium state reached between a cell's transcription and transduction machinery and the local environment. Cell phenotype transitions involving modulation of cell-cell adhesion occur during both physiological and pathological states. Epithelial cell subpopulations actively downregulate cell-cell adhesion systems during embryogenesis and wound healing and leave their "local neighborhood" to move into new microenvironments where they eventually differentiate into distinct cell types.[184]

Reepithelialization of cutaneous wounds involves extensive modulation of keratinocyte adhesion and motility. Intermediate filaments retract from keratinocyte surfaces, desmosomes and hemidesmosomes associated with these intermediate filaments are disrupted, partial or complete dissolution of the basement membrane occurs, and keratinocytes lose polarity.[185] These changes are accompanied by profound alterations in the actin-based cytoskeleton and occur concomitantly with an increase in migratory activity. In the final stages of reepithelialization, reversion to the differentiated epithelial phenotype occurs with formation of stable intercellular and cell-substrate contacts. The events taking place during wound reepithelialization are reminiscent of the developmental process of epithelial-mesenchymal transition (EMT). EMT is a dramatic phenotypic alteration characterized by transformation of anchored epithelial cells into migratory fibroblastlike individualized cells. EMT involves complete dissociation of intercellular adhesion structures (adherens junctions and desmosomes), cell elongation, and reorganization of the cytoskeleton.[184]

The Snail family of zinc finger transcription factors, including Snail and Slug, is involved in EMT during development. Slug was first described as a transcription factor expressed in cells undergoing EMT during gastrulation and neural crest emergence in chicken.[186] Both Snail and Slug induce EMT-like changes when overexpressed in epithelial cell lines, and both repress E-cadherin, a key molecule in cell adhesion, at the transcriptional level in vitro. Reepithelialization in the adult skin shares some features with EMT, such as modulation of the cytokeratin network, marked remodeling of cell-cell adhesion structures, and the emergence of cell motility.[187]

Traditionally, adult fibroblasts are considered to be derived directly from embryonic mesenchymal cells and to increase in number slowly as a result of the proliferation of resident fibroblasts.[188] However, recent studies in organs such as the kidney, lung, and liver and in metastatic tumors have shown that during fibrosis, in addition to the proliferation of resident fibroblasts, bone marrow–derived fibroblasts and epithelial cells contribute to fibroblast accumulation through EMT.[189]

Endothelial-mesenchymal transition (EndMT) is a form of EMT that occurs during the embryonic development of the heart. The mesenchymal cells that form the atrioventricular cushion, the primordia of the valves and septa of the adult heart, are derived from the endocardium by EndMT. Both EMT and EndMT appear to be important molecular mechanisms involved in wound healing.[190]

## ABNORMAL WOUND HEALING

### Introduction

For decades, hypertrophic scarring, contraction, and pigment abnormalities have altered the future for children and adults after thermal injury. The hard, raised, red and itchy scars, inelastic wounds, and hyperpigmented and hypopigmented scars are devastating to physical and psychosocial outcomes. The specific causes remain essentially unknown, and at present, prevention and treatment are symptomatic and marginal at best.[191]

Hypertrophic scarring after deep partial-thickness and full-thickness wounds is common. A review of the English literature on the prevalence of hypertrophic scarring reveals that children, young adults, and people with darker, more pigmented skin are particularly vulnerable, and in this subpopulation, the prevalence is as high as 75%.[192]

Hypertrophic scarring is devastating and can result in disfigurement and scarring that affects quality of life, which in turn can lead to a lowered self-esteem, social isolation, prejudicial societal reactions, and job discrimination. Scarring also has profound rehabilitation consequences, including loss of function, impairment, disability, and difficulties pursuing recreational and vocational pursuits.[193,194]

### Keloid Versus Hypertrophic Scar

Keloids and hypertrophic scars are separate clinical and histochemical entities. Clinically, hypertrophic scars remain within the confines of the original scar border, whereas keloids invade adjacent normal dermis. Hypertrophic scars generally arise within 4 weeks, grow intensely for several months, and then regress. In contrast, keloids may appear later, following the initial scar, and then gradually proliferate indefinitely. Although both keloids and hypertrophic scars have increased fibroblast density, only keloids have increased fibroblast proliferation rates. Collagen fibers in keloids are larger, thicker, and more wavy than those found in hypertrophic or normal scars and assume a random orientation, whereas those in hypertrophic scars orient parallel to the epidermal surface. Enzyme concentrations, such as alanine transaminase and metabolic activities marked by adenosine triphosphate, are elevated in keloids compared with normal scar tissue and hypertrophic scars. Fibroblasts isolated from keloid and hypertrophic scar tissue exhibit increased gene transcription of α-I procollagen. However, the increased mRNA concentration is compensated at the posttranscriptional level in hypertrophic scars, but not in keloids. The posttranscriptional difference results in an increased ratio of type I to type III collagen found in keloids, but not in hypertrophic scars.[195–200]

## Pathogenesis

Numerous hypotheses have been proposed for keloid formation and growth. The exuberant scar tissue found in keloids has been attributed to augmented growth factor activity (TGF-β and PDGF) and alterations in extracellular matrix (fibronectin, hyaluronic acid, and biglycan).[201]

TGF-β and PDGF are growth factors normally produced during the proliferative phase of wound healing and whose activities are most significantly abnormal in keloids. Keloid fibroblasts have heightened sensitivity to and dysfunctional regulation of TGF-β. Areas of enhanced proliferation and collagen deposition within keloid tissue have distinctly elevated levels of TGF-β. Similarly, keloid fibroblasts have 4-fold to 5-fold increased levels of PDGF receptor, and the growth-stimulatory effects are synergistic with TGF-β.[202]

The components of the extracellular matrix regulate growth factor activity. The extracellular matrix of keloids is abnormal, with elevated levels of fibronectin and certain proteoglycans and decreased levels of hyaluronic acid.[203] Fibronectin and hyaluronic acid are proteins expressed during normal wound healing, and their dysfunctional regulation in keloids contributes to the fibrotic phenotype. Biglycan and decorin are proteoglycans that bind collagen fibrils and influence collagen architecture. Keloids have aberrant production of these proteoglycans, resulting in disorganized extracellular matrix and collagen architecture.[204]

Epithelial-mesenchymal interactions likely play a fundamental role in keloid pathogenesis. Studies using keratinocyte-fibroblast in vitro co-culture systems have revealed that keloid keratinocytes can induce the keloid phenotype in normal fibroblasts. Furthermore, histologic changes in the epidermis of abnormal scars in vivo correlate with dermal fibroblast activity.[205] Proliferative pathways active in fetal cells and disabled in the adult possibly reemerge in the keloid. Unlike normal adult skin fibroblasts, fetal and keloid tissue can survive and proliferate in vitro in a reduced serum environment.[206] Hypoxia detected in keloid tissue has been reported to trigger the release of angiogenic growth factors, spurring endothelial proliferation, delayed wound maturation, and increased collagen production by fibroblasts. The hypoxia appears to be caused by endothelial overgrowth, partially to fully occluding the microvessel lumens in the keloids.[207,208]

Abnormal regulation of the collagen equilibrium leads to the characteristic physical appearance of a keloid, the large collagenous mass that distinguishes it from normal scar. Collagen content in keloids is elevated compared with normal tissue or scar tissue. Light and electron microscopic studies demonstrate that collagen in keloids is disorganized compared with normal skin. The collagen bundles are thicker and more wavy, and the keloids contain hallmark "collagen nodules" at the microstructural level. The ratio of type I to type III collagen is increased significantly in keloids compared with normal skin or scar, and this difference results from control at both the pretranscriptional and posttranscriptional levels.[209] Keloid fibroblasts have a greater capacity to proliferate because of a lower threshold to enter S phase and produce more collagen in an autonomous fashion.[210]

Matrix metalloproteases and their inhibitors (TIMPs) play a major role in keloid formation. Collagen is degraded by collagenase produced in fibroblasts and in inflammatory cells. Enzymes that inhibit or degrade collagenase exert an additional level of collagen regulation. Concentrations of collagenase inhibitors, alpha-globulins and plasminogen activator inhibitor-1, are consistently elevated in both in vitro and in vivo keloid samples, whereas levels of degradive enzymes are frequently decreased. Steroid-treated and irradiated keloids exhibit a decrease in collagenase inhibitors and an increase in apoptosis in fibroblasts, leading to normalization of net collagen levels.[211,212] Furthermore, matrix metalloprotease activity differs between keloid and normal fibroblasts, and these differences appear to directly affect phenotype. Because collagen predominates in the phenotypic appearance of keloids, collagen metabolism and particularly modulation of matrix metalloproteases serve as valuable targets of therapeutic intervention.[213]

An inherited abnormal immune response to dermal injury may cause keloid formation, as keloids are associated with particular human leukocyte antigen subtypes. Keloids tend to occur in darker-skinned individuals, and familial tendencies suggest a polygeneic inheritance pattern. However, darker complexion does not correlate directly with a higher rate of keloid formation, as seen in a study of 175 Malaysian keloid patients.[214] A genetic influence is probably directed through an immune phenotype. Studies suggest association of group A blood type and human leukocyte antigen B14, B21, BW35, DR5, and DQW3 in patients with a keloid diatheses.[215] Patients who develop keloids have a disproportionately high incidence of allergic diathesis and elevated levels of serum immunoglobin E. Multiple reports have found trends in patterns of serum complement, immunoglobin G, and immunoglobin M levels in patients with keloids, suggesting a systemic immune state genetically predisposed to keloid formation.[216]

Keloid formation has been considered an autoimmune connective tissue disease. Circulating non-complement-fixing antifibroblast antibodies bind to fibroblasts and stimulate proliferation and collagen production, similar to antithyroid antibodies in Hashimoto's thyroiditis. Keloids have been found associated with a number of other genetic connective tissue diseases, including Ehlers-Danlos syndrome, progeria, and scleroderma.[217]

Keloids can arise from an immune reaction to sebum. Dermal injury exposes the pilosebaceous unit to systemic circulation, and in individuals who retain T lymphocytes sensitive to sebum, a cell-mediated immune response is initiated.[218] Release of cytokines, in particular interleukins and TGF-β, stimulates mast cell chemotaxis and fibroblast production of collagen. As the keloid expands, further pilosebaceous units on the advancing border are disrupted and the process propagates. Keloids preferentially occur on anatomical sites with high concentrations of sebaceous glands, such as the chest wall, shoulder, and pubic area, and rarely occur on anatomical sites lacking sebaceous glands, such as the palm and the sole. The sebum reaction hypothesis explains why an individual with 2 otherwise identical incisions could develop 1 keloid and 1 normal scar.[219] The sebum reaction hypothesis also explains why only human beings, the only mammals with true sebaceous glands, are affected by keloid scarring. Patients with keloids demonstrate a positive skin reaction to intradermal sebum antigen and tend to have a greater resultant weal size than patients without a keloid diathesis. Furthermore, keloids can form following immunization with autologous skin, and a sebum vaccine can successfully desensitize select patients from keloid recurrence following excision.[220] The success of radiation therapy and steroids in the treatment of keloids, the former reducing sebum production and the latter inhibiting local lymphocyte activity, is consistent with a sebum reaction as the cause.[221] It has been speculated that ablation of the pilosebaceous unit before elective surgical excision may provide prophylaxis against the later formation of keloids.[219]

## BENCH TO BEDSIDE

Skin grafts have long been considered the standard for coverage of extensive soft-tissue defects such as burns and chronic wounds. However, autologous donor skin can be scarce, especially in large surface area burns. This has led to the development of alternative methods for wound coverage through tissue engineering of artificial skin.[222] Although much research has been performed, artificial skin equivalents have yet to demonstrate comparable clinical results to autologous skin grafts. One of the reasons for this is that the artificial skin lacks an intrinsic blood supply, whereas autologous skin has an extensive microvasculature consisting of, depending on thickness, a subpapillary dermal plexus and ascending capillary loops to the dermal papillae.[223,224] Attempts to enhance the process of angiogenesis using various growth factors such as VEGF have yielded an increase in survival and differentiation of endothelial cells in vitro and in vivo, but have not resulted in the production of a true vascularized construct.[225,226]

With the development of tissue-engineered skin replacements, the process of skin graft revascularization has become particularly relevant. The repeated failure of fabricated skin replacements to adequately revascularize has led to renewed efforts to definitively comprehend the process of autologous skin graft revascularization to tailor the creation of appropriate artificial skin equivalents.[227]

Early studies of skin graft revascularization suggested an early and direct connection between host and graft vessels (inosculation), before which graft survival was dependent on the process of inbibition (fluid absorption).[228] Recent research by Gurtner et al using transgenic rodent technology suggests that the potential mechanism of skin graft neovascularization occurs by means of an ordered process of recipient vascular ingrowth mirrored by donor vascular regression, eventually resulting in reconnection (inosculation) of the 2 separate vascular networks and restoration of circulatory continuity[229]. In addition, they demonstrated that postnatal vasculogenesis contributes to vascular growth and remodeling in a skin graft model, with up to 20% of new blood vessels formed from bone marrow–derived endothelial progenitor cells. This mechanism provides valuable insight into potential strategies for improving clinical success of larger composite grafts and tissue-engineered constructs.[229]

## CONCLUSION

Technologies for various molecular analyses (such as genomics, proteomics, transgenic mice), systems for sustained topical delivery (such as polymers and adenovirus vectors), major advances in tissue engineering (such as human skin engineering, cellular matrices, and bone marrow–derived cell therapy), novel discoveries of disease molecular pathogenesis from studies of patient biopsies and animal models, and developments in molecular targeting (in areas such as antisense oligonucleotides, siRNA, antibodies, and small molecules), coupled with breakthroughs in stem cell research, hold the promise of a bright future in wound-healing research. One of the major remaining steps is the integration of these resources into a coordinated effort to make the technology developed at the bench available to burn patients at the bedside.

## KEY POINTS

- Skin structures: epidermal-dermal junction, cutaneous vasculature, lymphatics, nerves, and appendages.
- Skin development including insights from fetal wound healing.
- Phases of normal wound healing.
- Abnormal wound healing to include keloid and hypertrophic scar pathogenesis.
- Current research and promise of the future.

## REFERENCES

1. Munster AM, Smith-Meek M, Sharkey P. The effect of early surgical intervention on mortality and cost-effectiveness in burn care (1978–1991). *Burns*. 1994; **20**: 61.

2. Lofts JA. Cost analysis of a major burn. *N Z Med J*. 1991; **16**: 488.

3. Ramzi PI, Barret JP, Herndon DN. Thermal injury. *Crit Care Clin*. 1999; **15**: 333.

4. Chia Chi K, Warren G. Acute burns. *Plast Reconstr Surg*. 2000; **105**: 2482.

5. Elias PM. The stratum corneum revisited. *J Dermatol*. 1996; **23**: 756.

6. Williams M, Feingold K. Barrier function of neonatal skin. *J Pediatr*. 1998; **133**: 467.

7. Hoath S, Visscher M, Heaton C, et al. Skin science and the future of dermatology. *J Cutan Med Surg*. 1998; **3**: 2.

8. Chuong GM, Nickoloff BJ, Elias PM, et al. What is the "true" function of skin? *Exp Dermatol*. 2002; **11**: 159.

9. Bereiter-Han J, Matoltsy A, Sylvia Richards K, eds. *Biology of the Integument: Vertebrates*. Berlin: Springer-Verlag; 1986.

10. Kligman A. The biology of the stratum corneum. In: Montagna W, Lobitz W, eds. *The Epidermis*. New York: Academic Press; 1964: 387–433.

11. Morris D. *The Naked Ape: A Zoologist's Study of the Human Animal*. New York: Random House; 1999.

12. Hoath S. The skin as a neurodevelopmental interface. *Neo-Reviews*. 2001; **2**: e292

13. Fuchs E, Byrne C. The epidermis: rising to the surface. *Curr Opin Genet Dev*. 1994; **4**: 725.

14. Steinhoff M, Brzoska T, Luger TA, et al. Keratinocytes in epidermal immune responses. *Curr Opin Allergy Clin Immunol*. 2001; **1**: 469.

15. Fuchs E. Keratins and the skin. *Annu Rev Cell Dev Biol*. 1995; **11**: 123.

16. Freedberg IM, Tomic-Canic M, Komine M, et al. Keratins and the keratinocyte activation cycle. *J Invest Dermatol*. 2001; **116**: 633.

17. Presland RB, Dale BA. Epithelial structural proteins of the skin and oral cavity: function in health and disease. *Crit Rev Oral Biol Med*. 2000; **11**: 383.

18. Elias PM, Feingold KR. Coordinate regulation of epidermal differentiation and barrier homeostasis. *Skin Pharmacol Appl Skin Physiol*. 2001; **14**(suppl 1): 28.

19. Nemes Z, Steinert PM. Bricks and mortar of the epidermal barrier. *Exp Mol Med*. 1999; **31**: 5.

20. Michel M, Torok N, Godbout MJ, et al. Keratin 19 as a biochemical marker of skin stem cells in vivo and in vitro: keratin 19 expressing cells are differentially localized in function of anatomic sites, and their number varies with donor age and culture stage. *J Cell Sci*. 1996; **109**: 1017.

21. Lyle S, Christofidou-Solomidou M, Liu Y, et al. The C8/144B monoclonal antibody recognizes cytokeratin 15 and defines the location of human hair follicle stem cells. *J Cell Sci*. 1998; **111**: 3179.

22. Tennenbaum T, Belanger AJ, Quaranta V, et al. Differential regulation of integrins and extracellular matrix binding in epidermal differentiation and squamous tumor progression. *J Investig Dermatol Symp Proc*. 1996; **1**: 157.

23. Watt FM. Stem cell fate and patterning in mammalian epidermis. *Curr Opin Genet Dev*. 2001; **11**: 410.

24. Nickoloff BJ, Denning M. Life and death signaling of epidermis: following a planned cell death pathway involving a trail that does not lead to skin cancer. *J Invest Dermatol*. 2001; **117**: 1.

25. Fuchs E, Merrill BJ, Jamora C, et al. At the roots of a never-ending cycle. *Dev Cell*. 2001; **1**: 13.

26. Ghohestani RF, Kehua L, Rousselle P, et al. Molecular organization of the cutaneous basement membrane zone. *Clin Dermatol*. 2001; **19**: 551.

27. Werner S, Somola H. Paracrine regulation of keratinocyte proliferation and differentiation. *Trends Cell Biol*. 2001; **11**: 143.

28. Spradling A, Drummond-Barbosa D, Kai T, et al. Stem cells find their niche. *Nature*. 2001; **414**: 98.

29. Jensen UB, Lowell S, Watt FM, et al. The spatial relationship between stem cells and their progeny in the basal layer of human epidermis. *Development*. 1999; **126**: 2409.

30. Cotsarelis G, Cheng SZ, Dong G, et al. Existence of slow-cycling limbal epithelial basal cells that can be preferentially stimulated to proliferate: implications on epithelial stem cells. *Cell*. 1989; **57**: 201.

31. Kowalczyk AP, Bornslaeger EA., Norvell SM, et al. Desmosomes: intercellular adhesive junctions specialized for attachment of intermediate filaments. *Int Rev Cytol*. 1999; **185**: 237.

32. Yap AS, Brieher WM, Gumbiner BM, et al. Molecular and functional analysis of cadherin-based adherens junctions. *Annu Rev Cell Dev Biol*. 1997; **13**: 119.

33. Lin MS, Wu T, Smith WC, et al. The desmosome and hemidesmosomes in cutaneous autoimmunity. *Clin Exp Immunol*. 1997; **107**(suppl 1): 9.

34. Hanakawa Y, Schechter NM, Lin C, et al. Molecular mechanisms of blister formation in bullous impetigo and staphylococcal scalded skin syndrome. *J Clin Invest*. 202; **110**: 53.

35. Richard G. Connexins: a connection with the skin. *Exp Dermatol*. 2000; **9**: 77.

36. Bos JD, Kapsenberg ML. The skin immune system: progress in cutaneous biology. *Immunol Today*. 1993; **14**: 75.

37. Elias PM, Goerke J, Friend DS. Mammalian epidermal barrier layer lipids: composition and influence on structure. *J Invest Dermatol*. 1977; **69**: 535.

38. Elias PM. Epidermal lipids, barrier function, and desquamation. *J Invest Dermatol*. 1983; **80**: 44.

39. Holbrook KA. Biologic structure and function: perspectives on morphologic approaches to the study of the granular layer keratinocyte. *J Invest Dermatol*. 1989; **92**: 84S.

40. Hynes RO. Cell adhesion: old and new questions. *Trends Cell Biol*. 1999; **9**: M33.

41. Kalinin AE, Kajava AV, Steinert PM, et al. Epithelial barrier function: assembly and structural features of the cornified cell envelope. *Bioessays*. 2002; **24**: 789.

42. Morasso MI, Markova NG, Sargent TD, et al. Regulation of epidermal differentiation by a distal-less homeodomain gene. *J Cell Biol*. 1996; **135**: 1879.

43. Tomic-Canic M, Komine M, Freedberg IM, et al. Epidermal signal transduction and transcription factor activation in activated keratinocytes. *J Dermatol Sci*. 1998; **17**: 167.

44. Hoath S, Leahy D. Formation and function of the stratum corneum. In: Marks E, Leveque JL, Voegeli R, eds. *The Essential Stratum Corneum*. London: Martin Dunitz Ltd; 2002: 31–40.

45. Kalinin A, Marekov LN, Steinert PM. Assembly of the epidermal cornified cell envelope. *J Cell Sci*. 2001; **114**(17): 3069.

46. Vancollie G, Lambert J, Nayaert JM. Melanocyte biology and its implications for the clinician. *Eur J Dermatol*. 1999; **9**: 241.

47. Seiberg M. Keratinocyte-melanocyte interactions during melanosome transfer. *Pigment Cell Res*. 2001; **14**: 236.

48. Mottaz JH, Zelickson AS. Melanin transfer: a possivle phagocytic process. *J Invest Dermatol*. 1967; **49**: 605.

49. Jimbow K, Quevedo WC Jr., Fitzpatrick TB, et al. Some aspects of melanin biology (review). *J Invest Dermatol*. 1976; **67**: 72.

50. Valyi-Nagy IT, Murphy GF, Mancianti ML, et al. Phenotypes and interactions of human melanocytes and keratinocytes in an epidermal reconstruction model. *Lab Invest*. 1990; **62**: 314.

51. Shibata T, Prota G, Mishima Y. Non-melanosomal regulatory factors in melanogenesis. *J Invest Dermatol*. 1993; **100s**: 274.

52. Ogawa H. The Merkel cell as a possible mechanoreceptor cell. *Prog Neurobiol*. 1996; **49**: 317.

53. Johnson KO. The roles and functions of cutaneous mechanoreceptors. *Curr Opin Neurobiol*. 2001; **11**: 455.

54. Smith KR Jr. The ultrastructure of the human Haarsheibe and Merkel cells. *J Invest Dermatol*. 1970; **54**: 150.

55. Jakob T, Udey MC. Epidermal Langerhans cells: from neurons to nature's adjuvants. *Adv Dermatol*. 1999; **14**: 209.

56. Foster A, Holbrook KA, Farr AG. Ontogeny of Langerhans cells in human embryonic and fetal skin. *J Invest Dermatol*. 1986; **86**: 240.

57. Murphy GF, Bhan AK, Sato S, et al. A new immunologic marker for human Langerhans cells. *N Engl J Med*. 1981; **304**: 791.

58. Burgeson RE, Christiano AM. The dermal-epidermal junction. *Curr Opin Cell Biol*. 1997; **9**: 651.

59. Uitto J, Pulkkinen L. Molecular genetics of heritable blistering disorders. *Arch Dermatol*. 2001; **137**: 1458.

60. Beer HD, Gassmann MG, Munz B, et al. Expression and function of keratinocyte growth factor and activin in skin morphogenesis and cutaneous wound repair. *J Investig Dermatol Symp Proc*. 2000; **5**: 34.

61. Burgeson RE, Nimni ME. Collagen types: Molecular structure and tissue distribution. *Clin Orthop*. 1992; **282**: 250.

62. Cristiano AM, Uitto J. Molecular pathology of the elastic fibers. *J Invest Dermatol*. 1994; **103**: 53S.

63. Kielty CM, Shuttleworth CA. Microfibrillar elements of the dermal matrix. *Microsc Res Tech*. 1997; **38**: 413.

64. Iozzo RV. Matrix proteoglycans: from molecular design to cellular function. *Annu Rev Biochem*. 1998; **67**: 609.

65. Scott JE. Supramolecular organization of extracellular matrix glycosaminoglycans in vitro and in the tissues. *FASEB J*. 1992; **6**: 2639.

66. Schwarzbauer JE, Sechler JL. Fibronectin fibrillogenesis: a paradigm for extracellular matrix assembly. *Curr Opin Cell Biol*. 1999; **11**: 622.

67. Aumailley M, Rousselle P. Laminins of the dermo-epidermal junction. *Matrix Biol*. 1999; **18**: 19.

68. Jones FS, Jones PL. The tenascin family of ECM glycoproteins: Structure, function, and regulation during embryonic development and tissue remodeling. *Dev Dyn*. 2000; **218**: 235.

69. Schvartz I, et al. Vitronectin. *Int J Biochem Cell Biol*. 1999; **31**: 539.

70. Holbrook KA, Byers PH. Diseases of the extracellular matrix: Structural alterations of collagen fibrils in skin. In: Uitto J, Perejda A, eds. *Connective Tissue Disease: Molecular Pathology of the Extracellular Matrix*. New York: Marcel Dekker; 1987: 10–25.

71. Uto J, Bernstein EF. Molecular mechanisms of cutaneous aging: connective tissue alterations in the dermis. *J Investig Dermatol Symp Proc*. 1998; **3**: 41.

72. Kobayasi T. Dermoepidermal junction of normal skin. *J Dermatol.* 1978; **5:** 157.

73. Cline MJ. Monocytes, macrophages, and their diseases in man. *J Invest Dermatol.* 1978; **71:** 56.

74. Falanga V, Zhou LH, Takagi H, et al. Human dermal fibroblast clones derived from single cells are heterogenous in the production of mRNAs for alpha 1(I) procollagen and transforming growth factor-beta 1. *J Invest Dermatol.* 1995; **105:** 27.

75. Wang R, Ghahary A, Shen Q, et al. Hypertrophic scar tissues and fibroblasts produce more transforming growth factor-beta 1 mRNA and protein than normal skin and cells. *Wound Repair Regen.* 2000; **8:** 128.

76. Weber-Matthiesen K, Sterry W. Organization of the monocyte/macrophage system of normal human skin. *J Invest Dermatol.* 1990; **95:** 83.

77. Church MK, Clough GF. Human skin mast cells: In vitro and in vivo studies. *Ann Allergy Asthma Immunol.* 1999; **83:** 471.

78. Nagata H, Okada T, Worobec AS, et al. c-Kit mutation in a population of patients with mastocytosis. *Int Arch Allergy Immunol.* 1997; **113:** 184.

79. Nemes Z, Thomázy V, Adány R, et al. Identification of histiocytic reticulum cells by the immuno-histochemical demonstration of factor XIII (F-XIIIa) in human lymph nodes. *J Pathol.* 1986; **149:** 121.

80. Cerio R, Griffiths CEM, Cooper KD, et al. Characterization of factor XIIIa positive dermal dendritic cells in normal and inflamed skin. *Br J Dermatol.* 1989; **121:** 421.

81. Yen A, Braverman IM. Ultrastructure of the human dermal microcirculation: The horizontal plexus of the papillary dermis. *J Invest Dermatol.* 1976; **66:** 131.

82. Braverman IM, Yen A. Ultrastructure of human dermal microcirculation II: The capillary loop of the dermal papillae. *J Invest Dermatol.* 1977; **68:** 44.

83. Pepper M, Laubenheimer R, Cripps DJ. Multiple glomus tumors. *J Cutan Pathol.* 1977; **4:** 244.

84. Ryan TJ. Structure and function of lymphatics. *J Invest Dermatol.* 1989; **93:** 18S.

85. Johansson O. The innervation of the human epidermis. *J Neurol Sci.* 1995; **130:** 228.

86. Arthur RP, Shelley WB. The innervation of human epidermis. *J Invest Dermatol.* 1959; **32:** 397.

87. Hashimoto K. Fine structure of the Meissner corpuscle of human palmar skin. *J Invest Dermatol.* 1973; **60:** 20.

88. Pease DC, Quilliam TA. Electron microscopy of the Pacinian corpuscle. *J Biophys Biochem Cytol.* 1957; **3:** 331.

89. Hardy MH. The secret life of the hair follicle. *Trends Genet.* 1992; **8:** 55.

90. Taylor G, Lehrer MS, Jensen PJ, et al. Involvement of follicular stem cells in forming not only the follicle but also the epidermis. *Cell.* 2000; **102:** 451.

91. Sengel P. Epidermal-dermal interactions. In: Bereiter-Hahn J, Matoltsy AG, Richards KS, eds. *Biology of the Integument: Vertebrates.* Vol 2. Berlin: Springer-Verlag; 1986: 374–408.

92. Watt FM, Hogan BLM. Out of Eden: stem cells and their niches. *Science.* 2000; **287:** 1427.

93. Potten CS. Cell replacement in epidermis via discrete units of proliferation. *Int Rev Cytol.* 1981; **69:** 271.

94. Fuchs E. Scratching the surface of skin development. *Nature.* 2007; **445:** 834.

95. Ito M, Suzuki M, Motoyoshi K, et al. New findings on the proteins of sebaceous glands. *J Invest Dermatol.* 1984; **82:** 381.

96. Sato K, Kane N, Soos G, et al. The eccrine sweat gland: basic science and disorders of eccrine sweating. *Prog Dermatol.* 1995; **29:** 1.

97. Schaumberg-Lever G, Lever WF. Secretion from human apocrine glands. *J Invest Dermatol.* 1975; **64:** 38.

98. Johnson M, Shuster S. Continuous formation of a nail along the bed. *Br J Dermatol.* 1993; **128:** 277.

99. Holbrook KA. Structure and function of the developing human skin. In: Goldsmith LA, ed. *Physiology, Biochemistry, and Molecular Biology of the Skin.* New York: Oxford Press; 1991: 63–75.

100. Loomis CA. Development and morphogenesis of the skin. *Adv Dermatol.* 2001; **17:** 183.

101. Stern CD. Neural induction: old problem, new findings, yet more questions. *Development.* 2005; **132:** 2007.

102. M'Boneko V, Merker HJ. Development and morphology of periderm of mouse embryos (days 9–12 of gestation). *Acta Anat (Basel).* 1988; **133:** 325.

103. Lorenz HP, Longaker MT, Perkocha LA, et al. Scarless wound repair: a human fetal skin model. *Development.* 1992; **114**(1): 253.

104. Steinicki EJ, Bullard KM, Harrison MR, et al. A new in vivo model for the study of fetal wound healing. *Ann Plast Surg.* 1997; **39**(4): 374.

105. Beanes SR, Hu FY, Soo C, et al. Confocal microscopic analysis of scarless repair in the fetal rat: defining the transition. *Plast Reconstr Surg.* 2002; **109**(1): 160.

106. Longaker MT, Whitby DJ, Adzick NS, et al. Studies in fetal wound healing, VI: second and early third trimester fetal wounds demonstrate rapid collagen deposition without scar formation. *J Pediatr Surg.* 1990; **25**(1): 63.

107. Morykwas MJ, Ledbetter MS, Ditesheim JA, et al. Cellular inflammation of fetal excisional wounds: effects of amniotic fluid exclusion. *Inflammation.* 1991; **15**(3): 173.

108. Armstrong JR, Ferguson MW. Ontogeny of the skin and the transition from scar-free to scarring phenotype during wound healing in the pouch of a young marsupial, Monodelphis domestica. *Dev Biol.* 1995; **169**(1): 242.

109. Wilgus TA, Bergdall VK, Tober KL, et al. The impact of cyclooxygenase-2 mediated inflammation on scarless fetal wound healing. *Am J Pathol.* 2004; **165**(3): 753.

110. Hopkinson-Woolley J, Hughes D, Gordon S, et al. Macrophage recruitment during limb development and wound healing in the embryonic and foetal mouse. *J Cell Sci.* 1994; **107**(5): 1159.

111. Kumta S, Ritz M, Hurley JV, et al. Acute inflammation in foetal and adult sheep: the response to subcutaneous injection of turpentine and carrageenan. *Br J Plast Surg.* 1994; **47**(5): 360.

112. Krummel TM, Michna BA, Thomas BL, et al. Transforming growth factor beta (TGF-beta) induces fibrosis in a fetal wound model. *J Pediatr Surg.* 1988; **23**(7): 647.

113. Adolph VR, DiSanto SK, Bleacher JC, et al. The potential role of the lymphocyte in fetal wound healing. *J Pediatr Surg.* 1993; **28**(10): 1316.

114. Martin P, Lewis J. Actin cables and epidermal movement in embryonic wound healing. *Nature.* 1992; **360**(6400): 179.

115. McCluskey J, Martin P. Analysis of the tissue movements of embryonic wound healing—DiI studies in the limb bud stage mouse embryo. *Dev Biol.* 1995; **170**(1): 102.

116. Whitby DJ, Ferguson MW. The extracellular matrix of lip wounds in fetal, neonatal and adult mice. *Development.* 1991; **112**(2): 651.

117. Ihara S, Motobayashi Y, Nagao E, et al. Ontogenic transition of wound healing pattern in rat skin occurring at the fetal stage. *Development.* 1990; **110**(3): 671.

118. Whitby DJ, Ferguson MW. Immunohistochemical localization of growth factors in fetal wound healing. *Dev Biol.* 1991; **147**(1): 207.

119. Sullivan KM, Lorenz HP, Meuli M, et al. A model of scarless human fetal wound repair is deficient in transforming growth factor beta. *J Pediatr Surg.* 1995; **30**(2): 198.

120. Lanning DA, Nwomeh BC, Montante SJ, et al. TGF-beta1 alters the healing of cutaneous fetal excisional wounds. *J Pediatr Surg.* 1999; **34**(5): 695.

121. Haynes JH, Johnson DE, Mast BA, et al. Platelet-derived growth factor induces fetal wound fibrosis. *J Pediatr Surg.* 1994; **29**(11): 1405.

122. DePalma RL, Krummel TM, Durham LA III, et al. Characterization and quantitation of wound matrix in the fetal rabbit. *Matrix.* 1989; **9**(3): 224.

123. Toole BP. Hyaluronan is not just a goo! *J Clin Invest.* 2000; **106**(3): 335.

124. Dahl L, Hopwood JJ, Laurent UB, et al. The concentration of hyaluronate in amniotic fluid. *Biochem Med.* 1983; **30**(3): 280.

125. Estes JM, Adzick NS, Harrison MR, et al. Hyaluronate metabolism undergoes an ontogenic transition during fetal development: implications for scar-free wound healing. *J Pediatr Surg.* 1993; **28**(10): 1227.

126. Longaker MT, Adzick NS, Hall JL, et al. Studies in fetal wound healing: Fetal wound healing may be modulated by hyaluronic acid stimulating activity in amniotic fluid. *J Pediatr Surg.* 1990; **25**(4): 430.

127. Longaker MT, Whitby DJ, Ferguson MW, et al. Adult skin wounds in fetal environment heal with scar formation. *Ann Surg.* 1994; **219**(1): 65.

128. Parks WC. Matrix metalloproteinases in repair. *Wound Repair Regen.* 1989; **7**(6): 423.

129. Bullard KM, Cass DL, Banda MJ, et al. Transforming growth factor beta-1 decreases interstitial collagenase in healing human fetal skin. *J Pediatr Surg.* 1997; **32**(7): 1023.

130. Dang CM, Beanes SR, Lee H, et al. Scarless fetal wounds are associated with an increased matrix metalloproteinase-to-tissue-derived inhibitor or metalloproteinase ratio. *Plast Reconstr Surg.* 2003: **111**(7): 2273.

131. Roberts AB, Sporn MB, Assoian RK, et al. Transforming growth factor beta: rapid induction of fibrosis and angiogenesis in vivo and stimulation of collagen formation in vitro. *Proc Natl Acad Sci U S A.* 1986; **83**(12): 4167.

132. Martin P, Dickson MC, Millan FA, et al. Rapid induction and clearance of TGF beta 1 is an early response to wounding in the mouse embryo. *Dev Genet.* 1993; **14**(3): 225.

133. Shah M, Foreman DM, Ferguson MW. Neutralisation of TGF-beta 1 and TGF-beta 2 or exogenous addition of TGF-beta 3 to cutaneous rat wounds reduces scarring. *J Cell Sci.* 1995; **108**(3): 985.

134. Soo C, Beanes SR, Hu FY, et al. Ontogenetic transition in fetal wound transforming growth factor-beta regulation correlates with collagen organization. *Am J Pathol.* 2003; **163**(6): 2459.

135. Lorenz HP, Lin RY, Longaker MT, et al. The fetal fibroblast: the effector cell of scarless fetal skin repair. *Plast Reconstr Surg.* 1995; **96**(6): 1251.

136. Longaker MT, Burd DA, Gown AM, et al. Midgestational excisional fetal lamb wounds contract in utero. *J Pediatr Surg.* 1991; **26**(8): 942.

137. Estes JM, Vande Berg JS, Adzick NS, et al. Phenotypic and functional features of myofibroblasts in sheep fetal wounds. *Differentiation.* 1994; **56**(3): 173.

138. Lanning DA, Diegelmann RF, Yager DR, et al. Myofibroblast induction with transforming growth factor-beta 1 and -beta 3 in cutaneous fetal excisional wounds. *J Pediatr Surg.* 2000; **35**(2): 183.

139. Cass DL, Sylvester KG, Yang EY, et al. Myofibroblast persistence in fetal sheep wounds is associated with scar formation. *J Pediatr Surg.* 1997; **32**(7): 1017.

140. Stelnicki EJ, Longaker MT, Holmes D, et al. Bone morphogenetic protein-2 induces scar formation and skin maturation in the second trimester fetus. *Plast Reconstr Surg.* 1998; **101**(1): 12.

141. Steinicki EJ, Arbeit J, Cass DL, et al. Modulation of the human homeobox genes PRX-2 and HOXB13 in scarless fetal wounds. *J Invest Dermatol.* 1998; **111**(1): 57.

142. Colwell AS, Krummel TM, Longaker MT, et al. Wnt-4 expression is increased in fibroblasts after TGF-beta 1 stimulation and during fetal and postnatal wound repair. *Plast Reconstr Surg.* 2006; **117**(7): 2297.

143. Williams M, Hanley K, Elias P, et al. Ontogeny of the epidermal permeability barrier. *J Investig Dermatol Symp Proc.* 1998; **3**: 75.

144. Kim SY, Jeitner TM, Steinert PM. Transglutaminases in disease. *Neurochem Int.* 2002; **40**: 85.

145. Warner RR, Boissy YL, Lilly NA, et al. Water disrupts stratum corneum lipid lamellae: damage is similar to surfactants. *J Invest Dermatol.* 1999; **113**: 960.

146. Montagna W. Comparative aspects of sebaceous glands. In: Montagna W, Ellis R, Silver A, eds. *Advances in the Biology of the Skin*. Vol 4. *The Sebaceous Glands*. Oxford: Pergamon Press; 1963: 32–45.

147. Zouboulis C, Fimmel S, Ortmann J, et al. Sebaceous glands. In: Hoath SB, Maibach H, eds. *Neonatal Skin: Structure and Function*. New York: Marcel Dekker; 2003: 59–88.

148. Hoath S, Pickens W. The biology of vernix. In: Hoath SB, Maibach H, eds. *Neonatal Skin: Structure and Function*. New York: Marcel Dekker; 2003: 193–210.

149. Narendran V, Pickens W, Wickett R, et al. Interaction between pulmonary surfactant and vernix: a potential mechanism for induction of amniotic fluid turbidity. *Pediatr Res*. 2000; **48**: 120.

150. Buchman AL. Glutamine: is it a conditionally required nutrient for the human gastrointestinal system? *J Am Col Nutr*. 1996; **15**: 199.

151. Woodley DT, O'Keefe EJ, Prunieras M. Cutaneous wound healing: a model for cell-matrix interactins. *J Am Acad Dermatol*. 1985; **12**: 420.

152. Heldin CH, Westermark B. Role of platelet-derived growth factor in vivo. In: Clark RAF, ed. *The Molecular and Cellular Biology of Wound Repair*. 2nd ed. New York: Plenum Press; 1996: 249–273.

153. Simpson DM, Ross R. The neutrophilic leukocyte in wound repair: a study with antineutrophil serum. *J Clin Invest*. 1972; **51**: 2009.

154. Brown EJ. Phagocytosis. *Bioessays*. 1995; **17**: 109.

155. Rappolee DA, Mark D, Banda MJ, et al. Wound macrophages express TGF-α and other growth factors in vivo: analysis by mRNA phenotyping. *Science*. 1988; **241**: 708.

156. Leibovich SJ, Ross R. The role of the macrophage in wound repair: a study with hydrocortisone and antimacrophage serum. *Am J Pathol*. 1975; **78**: 71.

157. Riches DWH. Macrophage involvement in wound repair, remodeling, and fibrosis. In: Clark RAF, ed. *The Molecular and Cellular Biology of Wound Repair*. 2nd ed. New York: Plenum Press; 1996: 95–141.

158. Fuchs E, Green H. Changes in keratin gene expression during terminal differentiation of the keratinocyte. *Cell*. 1980; **19**: 1033.

159. Kim S, Wong P, Coulombe PA. A keratin cytoskeletal protein regulates protein synthesis and epithelial cell growth. *Nature*. 2006; **441**: 362.

160. Coulombe PA, Wong P. Cytoplasmic intermediate filaments revealed as dynamic and multipurpose scaffolds. *Nat Cell Biol*. 2004; **6**: 699.

161. Clark RAF, Lanigan JM, DellaPelle P, et al. Fibronectin and fibrin provide a provisional matrix for epidermal cell migration during wound reepithelialization. *J Invest Dermatol*. 1982; **79**: 264.

162. Xu J, Clark RAF. Extracellular matrix alters PDGF regulation of fibroblast integrins. *J Cell Biol*. 1996; **132**: 239.

163. McClain SA, Simon M, Jones E, et al. Mesenchymal cell activation is the rate-limiting step of granulation tissue induction. *Am J Pathol*. 1996; **149**: 1257.

164. Clark RAF, Nielsen LD, Welch MP, et al. Collagen matrices attenuate the collagen-synthetic response of cultured fibroblasts to TGF-β. *J Cell Sci*. 1995; **108**: 1251.

165. Desmoulier A, Redard M, Darby T, et al. Apoptosis mediates the decrease in cellularity during the transition between granulation tissue and scar. *Am J Pathol*. 1995; **146**: 56.

166. Conway EM, Collen D, Carmeliet P. Molecular mechanisms of blood vessel growth. *Cardiovasc Res*. 2001; **49**: 507.

167. Fuchs E, Segre JA. Stem cells: a new lease on life. *Cell*. 2000; **100**: 143.

168. Krause DS, Theise ND, Collector MI, et al. Multi-organ, multi-lineage engraftment by a single bone marrow-derived stem cell. *Cell*. 2001; **105**: 369.

169. Ortic D, Kajstura J, Chimenti S, et al. Bone marrow cells regenerate infarcted myocardium. *Nature*. 2001; **410**: 701.

170. Isner JM, Asahara T. Angiogenesis and vasculogenesis as the therapeutic strategies for postnatal neovascularization. *J Clin Invest*. 1999; **103**: 1231.

171. Asahara T, Masuda H, Takahashi T, et al. Bone marrow origin of endothelial progenitor cells responsible for postnatal vasculogenesis in physiological and pathological neovascularization. *Circ Res*. 1999; **85**: 221.

172. Edelberg JM, Tang L, Hattori K, et al. Young adult bone marrow-derived endothelial precursor cells restore aging-impaired cardiac angiogenic function. *Circ Res*. 2002; **90**: E89.

173. Assmus B, Schachinger V, Teupe C, et al. Transplantation of progenitor cells and regeneration enhancement in acute myocardial infarction (TOPCARE-AMI). *Circulation*. 2002; **106**: 3009.

174. Takahashi T, Kalka C, Masuda H, et al. Ischemia- and cytokine-induced mobilization of bone marrow-derived endothelial progenitor cells for neovascularization. *Nat Med*. 1999; **5**: 434.

175. Ceradini DJ, Kulkarni AR, Callaghan MJ, et al. Progenitor cell trafficking is regulated by hypoxic gradients through H1F-1 induction of SDF-1. *Nat Med*. 2004; **10**: 858.

176. Du XL, Edelstein D, Dimmeler S, et al. Hyperglycemia inhibits endothelial nitric oxide synthase activity by post-translational modification at the Akt site. *J Clin Invest*. 2001; **108**: 1341.

177. Welch MP, Odland GF, Clark RAF. Temporal relationships of F-actin bundle formation, collagen and fibronectin matrix assembly, and fibronectin receptor expression to wound contraction. *J Cell Biol*. 1990; **110**: 133.

178. Montesano R, Orci L. Transforming growth factor-β stimulates collagen-matrix contraction by fibroblasts: implications for wound healing. *Proc Natl Acad Sci U S A*. 1988; **85**: 4894.

179. Chiro JA, Chan BMC, Roswit WT, et al. Integrin α2β1 (VLA-2) mediates reorganization and contraction of collagen matrices by human cells. *Cell*. 1991; **67**: 403.

180. Mignatti P, Rifkin DB, Welgus HG, et al. Proteinases and tissue remodeling. In: Clark RAF, ed. *The Molecular and Cellular Biology of Wound Repair*. 2nd ed. New York: Plenum Press; 1996: 171–194.

181. Madlener M, Parks WC, Werner S. Matrix metalloproteinases (MMPs) and their physiological inhibitors (TIMPs) are

differentially expressed during excisional skin wound repair. *Exp Cell Res.* 1998; **242:** 201.

182. Baily AJ, Bazin S, Sims TJ, et al. Characterization of the collagen of human hypertrophic and normal scars. *Biochim Biophys Acta.* 1975; **405:** 412.

183. Levenson SM, Geever EF, Crowley LV, et al. The healing of rat skin wounds. *Am Surg.* 1965; **161:** 293.

184. Savagner P. Leaving the neighborhood: molecular mechanisms involved during epithelial-mesenchymal transition. *BioEssays.* 2001; **23:** 912.

185. Martin P. Wound healing: aiming for perfect skin regeneration. *Science.* 1997; **276:** 75.

186. Nieto MA. The snail superfamily of zinc-finger transcription factors. *Nat Rev Mol Cell Biol.* 2002; **3:** 155.

187. Arnoux V, Côme C, Kusewitt DF, et al. Cutaneous wound healing: a partial and reversible EMT. In: Savagner P, ed. *Rise and Fall of the Epithelial Phenotype: Concepts of Epithelial-Mesenchymal Transition.* Austin, TX: Landes Bioscience; 2004: 110–120.

188. Weber, KT. Monitoring tissue repair and fibrosis from a distance. *Circulation.* 1997; **96:** 2488.

189. Iwano M, Plieth D, Danoff TM, et al. Evidence that fibroblasts derive from epithelium during tissue fibrosis. *J Clin Invest.* 2002; **110:** 341.

190. Eisenberg LM, Markwald RR. Molecular regulation of atrioventricular valvuloseptal morphogenesis. *Circ Res.* 1995; **77:** 1.

191. Engrav LH, Garner WL, Tredget EE. Hypertrophic scar, wound contraction and hyper-hypopigmentation. *J Burn Care Res.* 2007; **28:** 593.

192. Spurr ED, Shakespeare PG. Incidence of hypertrophic scarring in burn-injured children. *Burns.* 1990; **16:** 179.

193. Abdullah A, Blakeney P, Hunt R, et al. Visible scars and self-esteem in pediatric patients with burns. *J Burn Care Rehabil.* 1994; **15:** 164.

194. Van Loey NE, Van Son MJ. Psychopathology and psychological problems in patients with burn scars: epidemiology and management. *Am J Clin Dermatol.* 2003; **4:** 245.

195. Murray JC. Keloids and hypertrophic scars. *Clin Dermatol.* 1994; **12:** 27.

196. Muir IF. On the nature of keloid and hypertrophic scars. *Br J Plast Surg.* 1990; **43:** 61.

197. Ehrlich HP, Desmouliere A, Diegelmann R, et al. Morphological and immunochemical differences between keloid and hypertrophic scar. *Am J Pathol.* 1994; **145:** 105.

198. Hoopes JE, Su CT, Im MJ. Enzyme activities in hypertrophic scars and keloids. *Plast Reconstr Surg.* 1971; **47:** 132.

199. Ueda K, Furuya E, Yasuda Y, et al. Keloids have continuous high metabolic activity. *Plast Reconstr Surg.* 1999; **104:** 694.

200. Friedman DW, Boyd CD, Mackenzie JW, et al. Regulation of collagen gene expression in keloids and hypertrophic scars. *J Surg Res.* 1993; **55:** 214.

201. Pierce GF, Tarpley JE, Yanagihara D, et al. Platelet-derived growth factor (BB homodimer), transforming growth factor-beta 1, and basic fibroblast growth factor in dermal wound healing: neovessel and matrix formation and cessation of repair. *Am J Pathol.* 1992; **140:** 1375.

202. Younai S, Venters G, Vu S, et al. Role of growth factors in scar contraction: an in vitro analysis. *Ann Plast Surg.* 1996; **36:** 495.

203. Kischer CW, Wagner HN Jr., Pindur J, et al. Increased fibronectin production by cell lines from hypertrophic scar and keloid. *Connect Tissue Res.* 1989; **23:** 279.

204. Hunzelmann N, Anders S, Solberg S, et al. Co-ordinate induction of collagen type I and biglycan expression in keloids. *Br J Dermatol.* 1996; **135:** 394.

205. Andriessen MP, Niessen FB, Van de Kerkhof PC, et al. Hypertrophic scarring is associated with epidermal abnormalities: An immunohistochemical study. *J Pathol.* 1998; **186:** 192.

206. Russell SB, Trupin KM, Rodriguez-Eaton S, et al. Reduced growth-factor requirement of keloid-derived fibroblasts may account for tumor growth. *Proc Natl Acad Sci U S A.* 1988; **85:** 587.

207. Kischer CW. The microvessels in hypertrophic scars, keloids, and related lesions: a review. *J Submicrosc Cytol Pathol.* 1992; **24:** 281.

208. Kischer CW, Thies AC, Chvapil M. Perivascular myofibroblasts and microvascular occlusion in hypertrophic scars and keloids. *Hum Pathol.* 1982; **13:** 819.

209. Younai S, Nichter LS, Wellisz T, et al. Modulation of collagen synthesis by transforming growth factor-beta in keloid and hypertrophic scar fibroblasts. *Ann Plast Surg.* 1994; **33:** 148.

210. Nakaoka H, Miyauchi S, Miki Y. Proliferating activity of dermal fibroblasts in keloids and hypertrophic scars. *Acta Derm Venereol.* 1995; **75:** 102.

211. Luo S, Benathan M, Raffoul W, et al. Abnormal balance between proliferation and apoptotic cell death in fibroblasts derived from keloid lesions. *Plast Reconstr Surg.* 2001; **107:** 87.

212. Tuan TL, Zhu JY, Sun B, et al. Elevated levels of plasminogen activator inhibitor-1 may account for the altered fibrinolysis by keloid fibroblasts. *J Invest Dermatol.* 1996; **106:** 1007.

213. Uchida G, Yoshimura K, Kitano Y, et al. Tretinoin reverses upregulation of matrix metalloproteinase-13 in human keloid-derived fibroblasts. *Exp Dermatol.* 2003; **12:** 35.

214. Alhady SM, Sivanantharajah K. Keloids in various races: a review of 175 cases. *Plast Reconstr Surg.* 1969; **44:** 564.

215. Castagnoli C, Peruccio D, Stella M, et al. The HLA-DR beta 16 allogenotype constitutes a risk factor for hypertrophic scarring. *Hum Immunol.* 1990; **29:** 229.

216. Placik OJ, Lewis VL Jr. Immunologic associations of keloids. *Surg Gynecol Obstet.* 1992; **175:** 185.

217. Kazeem AA. The immunological aspects of keloid tumor formation. *J Surg Oncol.* 1988; **38:** 16.

218. Fong EP, Bay BH. Keloids: the sebum hypothesis revisited. *Med Hypotheses.* 2002; **58:** 264.

219. Fong EP, Chye LT, Tan WT. Keloids: time to dispel the myths? *Plast Reconstr Surg.* 1999; **104:** 1199.

**220.** Yagi KI, Dafalla AA, Osman AA. Does an immune reaction to sebum in wounds cause keloid scars? Beneficial effect of desensitization. *Br J Plast Surg.* 1979; **32:** 223.

**221.** Chytilova M, Kulhanek V, Horn V. Keloids as a form of auto-aggression in the scar. *Rozhl Chir.* 1960; **39:** 393.

**222.** Gallico GG III. Biologic skin substitutes. *Clin Plast Surg.* 1990; **17:** 519.

**223.** Braverman IM, Yen A. Ultrastructure of the human dermal microcirculation. II. The capillary loops of the dermal papillae. *J Invest Dermatol.* 1977; **68:** 44.

**224.** Braverman IM. The cutaneous microcirculation. *J Investig Dermatol Symp Proc.* 2000; **5:** 3.

**225.** Kaigler D, Krebsbach PH, Polferini PJ, et al. Role of vascular endothelial growth factor in bone marrow stromal cell modulation of endothelial cells. *Tissue Eng.* 2003; **9:** 95.

**226.** Taub PH, Marmur JD, Zhang WX, et al. Locally administered vascular endothelial growth factor cDNA increases survival of ischemic experimental skin flaps. *Plast Reconstr Surg.* 1998; **102:** 2033.

**227.** Supp DM, Supp AP, Bell SM, et al. Enhanced vascularization of cultured skin substitutes genetically modified to overexpress vascular endothelial growth factor. *J Invest Dermatol.* 2000; **114:** 5.

**228.** Haller J Jr., Billingham R. Studies of the origin of the vasculature in free skin grafts. *Ann Surg.* 1967; **166:** 896.

**229.** Capla JM, Ceradini DJ, Tepper OM, et al. Skin graft vascularization involves precisely regulated regression and replacement of endothelial cells through both angiogenesis and vasculogenesis. *Plast Reconstr Surg.* 2006; **117:** 836.

# CHAPTER FIVE

# ETIOLOGY OF IMMUNE DYSFUNCTION IN THERMAL INJURIES

DAIZHI PENG, MD, PhD, PROFESSOR OF SURGERY, DEPUTY DIRECTOR,
INSTITUTE OF BURN RESEARCH, SOUTHWEST HOSPITAL, STATE KEY LABORATORY OF TRAUMA,
BURNS AND COMBINED INJURY, THE THIRD MILITARY MEDICAL UNIVERSITY, CHONGQING, PR CHINA

WENHUA HUANG, MD, PROFESSOR OF CLINICAL IMMUNOLOGY, INSTITUTE OF BURN RESEARCH,
SOUTHWEST HOSPITAL, STATE KEY LABORATORY OF TRAUMA, BURNS AND COMBINED INJURY,
THE THIRD MILITARY MEDICAL UNIVERSITY, CHONGQING, PR CHINA

## INTRODUCTION

The skin is the largest organ of the body, consisting of epidermal and dermal layers. As the main target tissue of thermal injuries, it provides a formidable, and yet vulnerable, physical barrier. The epidermis consists of keratinocytes, Langerhans cells, intraepidermal lymphocytes, and melanocytes. The dermis contains capillaries and a variety of immune cells, including dendritic cells, macrophages, and dermal lymphocytes.[1-3] Comprising a mechanical barrier, the keratinocytes secrete or express a number of cytokines, chemokines, and other bioactive molecules, such as interleukin-1, macrophage inflammatory protein 3α (MIP-3α, CCL20), antimicrobial peptides, and receptor activator of NF-B ligand (RANKL).[3-6] RANKL overexpression in keratinocytes results in functional alterations of epidermal dendritic cells and systemic increases of regulatory CD4[+] and CD25[+] T cells.[5] Langerhans cells are attracted to the epidermis from the circulation by CCL20.[2] Langerhans and dermal dendritic cells act as antigen-presenting cells to initiate the adaptive immune response in the skin.[1,2]

Most of the skin-associated lymphocytes are CD8[+] cells with γδ T cell receptors (TCR).[7] Therefore, the skin, being the largest innate immune organ, plays an important role in local inherent and adaptive immunities of the host immune system.[1-7] Since burn injury directly destroys the skin, the balance between the body and environment is ultimately disturbed.

Despite significant advances in intensive care technology and antibiotic administration, infections and multiple organ failure are still the most common lethal complications of major burn patients.[8-11] Thermal injury causes not only local changes of the skin wound but also systemic pathophysiological disorders of various systems.[12-15] The immunological consequences following severe thermal injury are an important component of the systemic responses of the host. For nearly five decades it has been recognized that burn injury causes marked alterations of immune function, resulting in life-threatening systemic infections, tissue damage, and even death.[16-18] Extensive and deep burns have widespread and profound impact on the various cells and molecules of the innate and adaptive immune systems.[13-21]

The initial response to a severe burn injury is hyperinflammation, often referred to clinically as the systemic inflammatory response syndrome (SIRS). The function of innate immune cells, such as neutrophils, is suppressed during this period.[18–22] The adaptive immune response after burn injury begins with slightly increased lymphocyte activity and immunoglobulin responses, then converts to marked immunodepression of T and B lymphocytes.[23–26] Obviously, both innate and adaptive immunity have increased or depressed functions and variable amounts of different cells and molecules throughout the postburn period. The general characteristics of postburn immune dysfunction are a hyperinflammatory and hypoimmune response for the innate and adaptive immunities, respectively.[19,21] The main clinical outcomes of postburn immune dysfunction include tissue damage[18,22] and increased susceptibility to opportunistic pathogens caused by uncontrolled inflammation and suppressed adaptive immunity.[14,17,20] Furthermore, severely burned patients are predisposed to multiple organ damage and infection leading to increased mortality. In order to decrease the morbidity of these lethal complications, the mechanism of postburn immune dysfunction has been studied at both the cellular and molecular level.[27,28,29] However, restoration of immune dysfunction after burn injury has been a difficult task due to the complicated and sophisticated interactions among the immune cells and molecules within the immune system.

Stress, massive necrotic tissue, shock, infection, malnutrition, and other events sequentially appear in burn patients.[8,10,15,16,20,23] Subsequently, seriously burned patients undergo various therapeutic procedures, administration of medications, and surgical manipulations.[9,22] Based on etiologic considerations, all of these clinically relevant factors alter the microenvironment of the immune cells and molecules in which they reside, finally causing postburn immune dysfunction. In this chapter, we summarize recent advances of the above-mentioned factors in order to gain a greater understanding of the pathogenesis of this immune dysfunction. More attention should be paid to the immunologic effects of these factors in order to better improve immune function in the comprehensive treatment of seriously burned patients.

## STRESS REACTION

Complex interactions between the neuroendocrine and immune systems exist. The neuroendocrine system plays a predominant role in the regulation of immune responses, particularly during times of stress. It is well known that the hypothalamus controls the immune functions of the body via the hypothalamic-pituitary-adrenal (HPA) axis.[31] Recently, it has been shown that the afferent and efferent vagus nerve fibers have proinflammatory and anti-inflammatory effects, respectively. Neurotransmitters, neuropeptides, and stress hormones released by the activated autonomic nervous system and HPA axis act on the immune system.[32] Various stressors, including wound pain, necrotic tissue, shock, infection, and surgical procedures, can stimulate the neuroendocrine system and elicit stress reactions directed at neutralizing the initial insult to the body. Ample evidence exists regarding the influence of elevated levels of catecholamines, glucocorticoids, and ß-endorphins on spontaneous and mitogen-stimulated lymphocyte proliferation after injury or in vitro coculture.[23,33,34] Corticosteroids are also responsible for thymus atrophy and thymocyte apoptosis.[23,34,35] Thermal injury with sepsis is associated with both increased monocytopoiesis and increased release of LPS-stimulated macrophage cytokines. These actions are partly mediated by sympathetic activation and increased nerve-stimulated release of norepinephrine from the bone marrow.[36]

## INJURED TISSUES

Thermal injury involves the skin and underlying tissues, as well as the lungs when inhalation injury occurs. Immediately after thermal injury, viable tissue in the zone of stasis surrounds heat-coagulated tissue in the center of the burn wound.[12] The necrotic and apoptotic tissues caused by heat energy are the major pathogenic factors involved in postburn immune dysfunction. The injured tissues release large numbers of tissue thromboplastin, activated Factor XII, and denatured proteins. The extrinsic and intrinsic blood coagulation systems and complement system are directly activated,[18,37,38] followed thereafter by the fibrinolytic and kinin systems. Consequently, inflammatory mediators are generated as products of the activated components from these four systems.[37] The injured tissues robustly produce and/or release vasoactive amines and lipid mediators as well as proinflammatory and chemotaxtic cytokines such as histamine, platelet-activated factor (PAF), arachidonic acid products, tumor necrotic factor-α (TNF-α), and interleukin 8.37 The dead and dying cells in necrotic and apoptotic tissues release components of various cellular structures, particularly from the nucleus.[39,40] Recently, both host chromosomal high-mobility group box 1 protein (HMGB1) and genomic DNA are thought to trigger an inflammatory response.[39,40] From our experiments, we have observed that the elevated level of serum HMGB1 in scalded rats partially contributes to the direct release of dead or necrotic cells from the burn wound (D.P., W.H., unpublished data). These mediators not only initiate the local inflammatory response of thermally injured tissues but are also involved in the inflammation and tissue edema of remote organs when the burn injury is severe enough.[37] It has been experimentally proven that inhalation injury affecting one side of lung can induce edema of the other lung as well. Eschar toxin from a burn wound causes inhibition of mitochondrial respiratory function in hepatocytes, eliciting a stronger immunosuppressive effect on antibody formation and cell-mediated immunity than that of lipopolysaccharide (LPS).[41,42] The subeschar fluid from burned patients also inhibits lymphocyte proliferation.[43] In addition, the extent of burn injury profoundly impacts patient immune status by causing suppressed splenic T-cell proliferation.[44] Therefore, burn wounds are not only well recognized as a main source of inflammatory mediators which initiate the hyperinflammatory response, but are also an important arsenal of immunosuppressive substances that induce the hypoimmune response after burns.

## ISCHEMIA AND HYPOXIA

Burn trauma produces significant fluid shifts that in turn reduce cardiac output and tissue perfusion. Fluid resuscitation restores peripheral perfusion and increases oxygen delivery to previously hypoperfused tissue. While persistent tissue ischemia and hypoxia after burn injury can result in cell death, volume resuscitation may also exacerbate tissue injury by producing oxygen free radicals during reperfusion. Cell death and oxygen free radicals can subsequently initiate tissue inflammation. Hypoxia increases the TNF-α production of monocytes from healthy volunteers, whereas enhanced production of IL-1 and IL-6 only occurs after transient hypoxia and reoxygenation of monocytes.[45] Systemic hypoxia induces the microvascular inflammatory response mediated by mast cells.[46] Hypoxia also reduces the mitogen-stimulated proliferation and IL-2 and interferon-γ (IFN-γ) release of T cells, but not mitogen-stimulated B cell proliferation.[47] Burn trauma upregulates inflammatory cytokine synthesis of IL-1β, IL-6, and TNF-α by parenchymal cells of other tissues such as cardiomyocytes.[48] These results provide strong support to the idea that ischemia and hypoxia in lymphoid and other tissues during burn shock and volume resuscitation play a critical role in postburn immune dysfunction.

## BACTERIA AND THEIR COMPONENTS

Severe burn patients are particularly vulnerable to wound contamination, bacterial colonization, wound sepsis, and systemic infection.[8] There is extensive evidence from animal studies that translocation of bacteria and LPS from the intestine to intestinal lymph nodes, liver, and circulation occur in certain circumstances, such as severe burns, hemorrhagic shock, and malnutrition.[49] The ability

of pathogens to cause serious inflammation is due to the effects of their structural components acting upon the innate immune system of the host. These include bacterial DNA, proteins (exotoxin and hemolysin), flagella, pili, and LPS from gram-negative bacteria and teichoic acid, lipoteichoic acid, and peptidoglycan from gram-positive bacteria.[50–52] These components are released when bacterial cells are destroyed during their spontaneous growth and subsequently activate the immune cells, inducing vigorous production of inflammatory mediators by binding the relevant pattern recognition receptors on the surface of these cells.[53] The release of bacterial DNA molecules is obviously influenced by the different classes and dosages of antibiotics.[52] LPS stimulates the monocytes and macrophages to produce considerable inflammatory cytokines (TNF-α, IL-1, IL-6, IL-8, and HMGB1, a DNA-binding cytokine), anti-inflammatory mediators (IL-10, IL-13, IL-14, transforming growth factor ß [TGF-ß], and nitric oxide [NO]), and breakdown products of arachidonic acid (prostaglandin [PG] E2 and I2, thromboxane [TX] A2 and B2, and leukotriene [LT] C4, D4, and E4 ).[37,39,50] LPS also activates components of the complement system and allows them to split into fragments such as C5a, C3a, and C567. Furthermore, LPS enhances glucocorticoid release from the adrenal glands. These factors, including IL-10, TGF-β, NO, and PGE2, have immunosuppressive activities and contribute to the inhibitory effect of LPS on the adaptive immune response. The synergistic effect between bacterial DNA and LPS makes the diverse immunological consequences of LPS more powerful.[51] Burn victims with infection exhibit high levels of circulating cytokines such as TNF-α, IL-6, IL-8[55], and HMGB1. The bacterial quorum sensing system is particularly involved in the induction of cytokine expression during *Pseudomonas aeruginosa* infections of burn wounds.[55]

## NUTRITIONAL DEFICITS

The stress-induced metabolic alterations after burn injury lead to protein-calorie/protein malnutrition, which, along with micronutrient deficits, can induce immune function depression.[56] Furthermore, the hypermetabolism triggered from burn injury leads to specific nutrient deficits such as glutamine and arginine.[57–59] Glutamine and arginine are semidispensable amino acids with a number of beneficial effects on the immune response. The nutritional deficits which occur during burn injury contribute to the pathogenesis of alterations in both innate and adaptive immune defenses. It is generally accepted that high-protein diets improve immunologic functions and decrease infectious complications.

## THERAPEUTIC MEDICINES AND HOST FACTORS

Most burn patients require opiate analgesics for treatment of pain associated with the initial injury and postinjury procedures such as wound debridement and dressing changes. Severe burn patients often need blood transfusions due to extensive volume resuscitation and procedures such as escharectomy. Antibiotics are routinely used for the prophylaxis and treatment of infection in major burn patients. It is well documented that opiates, blood transfusions, antimicrobial agents, and the type of fluid used for resuscitation have profound immunomodulatory effects.[60–63] A number of host factors can also impact immune functional parameters following burn injury, including age, gender, and genetic background.[64–67] All of the above therapy-associated regimens and other factors can contribute to the development of immune dysfunction under a variety of circumstances following thermal injury.

## CONCLUSION

Severe burns directly cause extensive skin degeneration and necrosis and also induce a series of significant systemic responses, such as stress, ischemia and reperfusion, infection, and hypermetabolism. These factors, along with some of the relevant therapies used for the treatment of such patients, cause changes in the microenvironment surrounding the immune cells and immune molecules and also play critical roles in the pathogenesis of immune dysfunction after burns (Figure 1). Postburn immune dysfunction involves a number of cells and molecules not only in the immune system but in other systems as well. Attempting to modulate immune function by choosing appropriate target cells or molecules to decrease the degree of tissue damage and infection is a difficult task. According to the etiologic analysis of postburn immune dysfunction, efforts for improving immune dysfunction after burn injury have occurred at the global and integral level against pathogenic factors. These measures include amelioration of the stress reaction, prompt eschar excision for reducing release of biological factors or toxins from necrotic wound tissues, rapid fluid resuscitation for ameliorating ischemia and hypoxia, adequate antimicrobial chemotherapy with powerful bactericidal effects and less release of microbial components, and enteral nutritional supplementation combined with immunonutrients, prebiotics, and metabolically

relevant hormones such as growth hormone and insulin-like growth factor I.[68] The effect of these clinically relevant factors upon immune functions should be carefully considered during the treatment of major burn patients. The future comprehensive therapeutic protocol for massively burned patients should be updated with consideration of the advances in basic and clinical research in the field of immunology.

## KEY POINTS

- The skin is the largest innate immune organ of the body and also the main target tissue of thermal insults.
- Burn injury results in marked immune dysfunction, that predisposes patients to multiple organ damage and infection leading to increased mortality in seriously burned patients.
- Burn wounds are well recognized as a main storage of inflammatory mediators as well as an important arsenal of immunosuppressive substances.
- Ischemia and hypoxia in lymphoid and other tissues during burn shock and volume resuscitation play a critical role in the postburn immune dysfunction.
- Bacteria and their components from the gut and wounds following burns cause serious inflammation and have the inhibitory effects on the adaptive immune response.
- The nutritional deficits, various stressors, medications and patient-associated factors contribute to the development of immune dysfunction under a variety of circumstances following thermal injury.
- The effect of these clinically relevant factors upon the immune functions should be comprehensively considered during the treatment of massive burn patients for a higher survival rate.

## ACKNOWLEDGMENTS

This review article was supported by grants from the National Natural Science Foundation of China (Grand Program, No. 39290700-01), National Key Basic Research and Development Project of China (973 Project) (No. 2005CB522605), and National High Technology Research and Development Project of China (863 Project) ( No. 2006AA02A121).

**FIGURE**

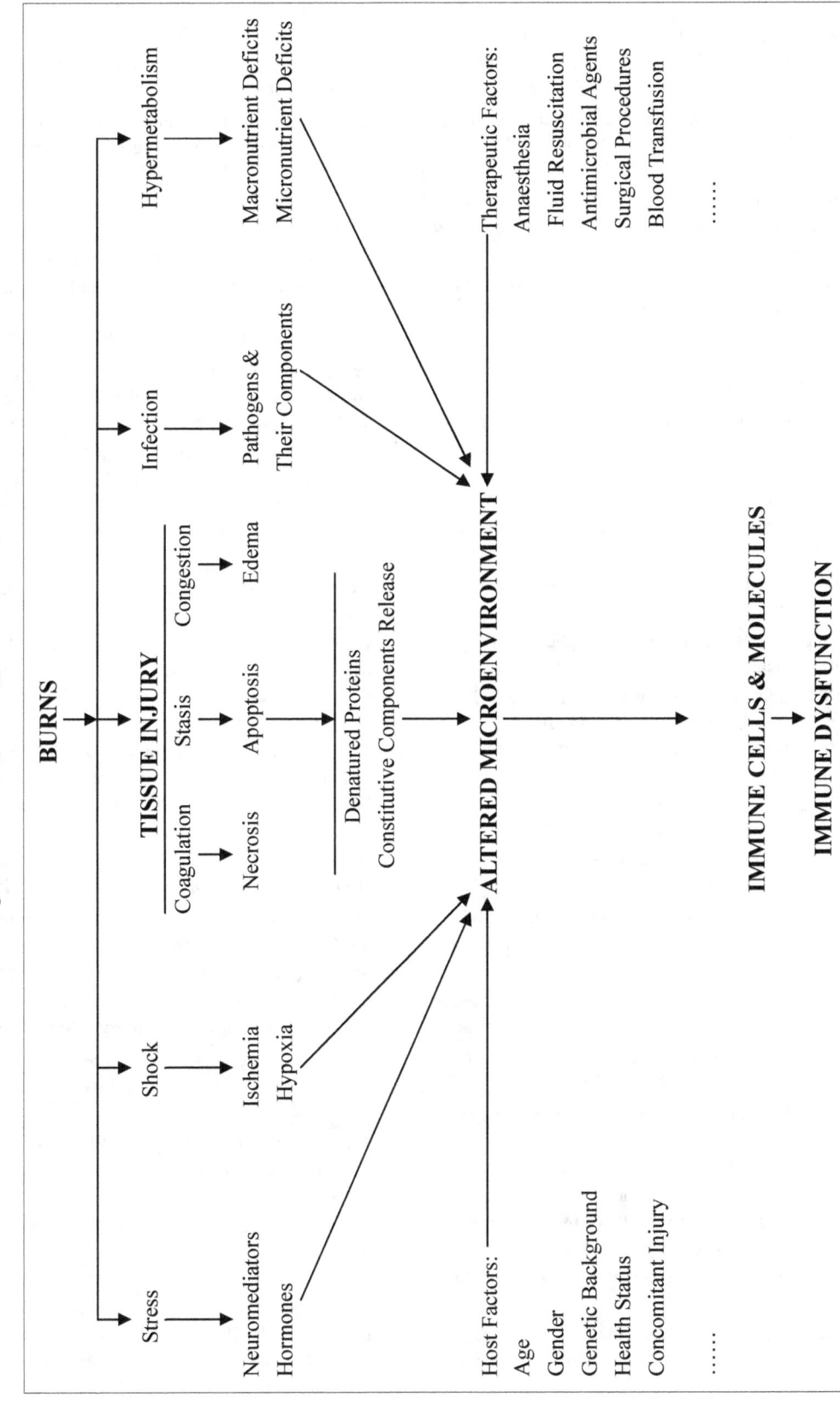

**FIGURE 1**
**Etiologic factors of postburn immune dysfunction.**

## REFERENCES

1. Yoshino M, Yamazaki H, Nakano H, et al. Distinct antigen trafficking from skin in the steady and active states. *Int Immunol.* 2003; **15**(6): 773–779.

2. Charbonnier AS, Kohrgruber N, Kriehuber E, et al. Macrophage inflammatory protein 3α is involved in the constitutive trafficking of epidermal Langerhans cells. *J Exp Med.* 1999; **190**(12): 1755–1767.

3. Loser K, Mehling A, Loeser S, et al. Regulatory CD4⁺CD25⁺ T cells are important in suppressing immune responses. *Nat Med.* 2006; **12**(12): 1372–1379.

4. Homey B, Alenius H, Muller A, et al. CCL27-CCR10 interactions regulate T cell-mediated skin inflammation. *Nat Med.* 2002; **8**(2): 157–165.

5. Yamaguchi T, Sakaguchi S. Skin controls immune regulators. *Nat Med.* 2006; **12**(12): 1358–1359.

6. Yue H, Peng D. Structure and function of CCL20. *Immunol J.* 2004; **20**(3)(suppl): S100–S102.

7. Lewis JM, Girardi M, Roberts SJ, Barbee SD, Hayday AC, Tigelaar RE. Selection of the cutaneous intraepithelial gammadelta+ T cell repertoire by a thymic stromal determinant. *Nat Immunol.* 2006; **7**(8): 843–850.

8. Pruitt BA, McManus AT, Kim SH, Goodwin CW. Burn wound infections: current status. *World J Surg.* 1998; **22**(2): 135–145.

9. Sharma BR, Singh VP, Bangar S, Gupta N. Septicemia: the principal killer of burns patients. *Am J Infect Dis.* 2005; **1**(3): 132–138.

10. Tatevossian RG, Shoemaker WC, Wo CCJ, Dang ABC, Velmahos GC, Demetriades D. Noninvasive hemodynamic monitoring for early warning of adult respiratory distress syndrome in trauma patients. *J Crit Care.* 2000; **15**(4): 151–159.

11. Hessen MT, Kaye D. Principals of selected and use of antibacterial agents. *Infect Dis Clin North Am.* 2000; **14**(2): 265–279.

12. Jackson DM. The diagnosis of the depth of burning. *Br J Surg.* 1953; **40**(164): 588–596.

13. Peng D, Huang W, Ai S, Wang S. Clinical significance of leukocyte infiltrative response in deep wound of patients with major burns. *Burns.* 2006; **32**(8): 946–950.

14. Munster AM. Immunologic response of trauma and burns: an overview. *Am J Med.* 1984; **76**: 142–145.

15. Abraham E. Host defense abnormalities after hemorrhage, trauma, and burns. *Crit Care Med.* 1989; **17**(9): 934–939.

16. Ninnemann JL. Trauma, sepsis, and the immune response. *J Burn Care Rehabil.* 1987; **8**(6): 462–468.

17. Alexander JW, Ogle CK, Stinnett JD, MacMillan BG. A sequential, prospective analysis of immunologic abnormalities and infection following severe thermal injury. *Ann Surg.* 1978; **188**(6): 809–816.

18. Hoesel LM, Niederbichler AD, Schaefer J, et al. C5a-blockade improves burn-induced cardiac dysfunction. *J Immunol.* 2007; **178**(12): 7902–7910.

19. Peng DZ, Huang WH, Li A. The roles of macrophage in immune dysfunction following severe thermal injury. *Chin J Surg.* 1994; **32**(5): 310–313.

20. Piccolo MTS, Sannomiya P. Inhibition of neutrophil chemotaxis by plasma of burned patients: effect of blood transfusion practice. *Burns.* 1995; **21**(8): 569–574.

21. Schwacha MG. Macrophages and post-burn immune dysfunction. *Burns.* 2003; **29**(1): 1–14.

22. Murphy TJ, Paterson HM, Kriynovich S, et al. Linking the "two-hit" response following injury to enhanced reactivity. *J Leukoc Biol.* 2005; **77**(1): 16–23.

23. Peng D, Huang W, Li A. Postburn kinetic changes of stress hormones and splenocyte immune function in rats. *Acta Acadiemiae Midicinae Militaris Teritae.* 1990; **12**(2): 100–103.

24. Yamamoto H, Hayes YO, deSerres S, Chang J, Tabata T, Meyer AA. Burn injury induces a biphasic immunoglobulin M response. *J Trauma.* 1995; **39**(2): 279–284.

25. De AK, Kodys KM, Pellegrini J, et al. Induction of global anergy rather than inhibitory Th2 lymphokines mediates posttrauma T cell immunodepression. *Clin Immunol.* 2000; **96**(1): 52–66.

26. Zheng J, Wu J, Peng D, et al. The postburn change in splenic T lymphocyte transmembrane signal transduction and its relationship with the secretion of IL-2 and IL-10 in severely scalded mice. *Chin J Burns.* 2000; **16**(6): 352–354.

27. Peng DZ, Wang XM, Luo GX, et al. Signal transduction of macrophages (MΦ) after burns. *Eur J Haematol.* 1996; **57**(59) (suppl): 5.

28. Fazal N, Choudhry MA, Sayeed MM. Inhibition of T cell MAPKs (Erk 1/2, p38) with thermal injury is related to down-regulation of $Ca^{2+}$ signaling. *Biochim Biophys Acta.* 2005; **1741**(1–2): 113–119.

29. Wang Y, Peng D, Huang W, Zhou X, Liu J, Fang Y. Mechanism of altered TNF-α expression by macrophage and the modulatory effect of Panax notoginseng saponins in scald mice. *Burns.* 2006; **32**(7): 846–852.

30. Besedovsky H, Sorkin E. Network of immune-neuroendocrine interaction. *Clin Exp Immunol.* 1977; **27**(10): 1–12.

31. Matthay MA, Ware LB. Can nicotine treat sepsis? *Nat Med.* 2004; **10**(11): 1161–1162.

32. Levy EM, McIntosh T, Black PH. Elevation of circulating ß-endorphin levels with concomitant depression of immune parameters after traumatic injury. 1986; **26**(3): 246–249.

33. Deitch EA, Bridges RM. Stress hormones modulate neutrophil and lymphocyte activity in vitro. *J Trauma.* 1987; **27**(10): 1146–1154.

34. Nakanishi T, Nishi Y, Sato EF, Ishii M, Hamada T, Inoue M. Thermal injury induces thymocyte apoptosis in the rat. *J Trauma.* 1998; **44**(1): 143–148.

35. Peng D, Huang W, Li A, Ye B. Kinetic changes of thymocyte responsiveness in vitro after thermal injury. *Chin J Surg.* 1993; **31**(8): 501–503.

36. Cohen MJ, Shankar R, Stevenson J, Fernandez R, Gamelli RL, Jones SB. Bone marrow norepinephrine mediates development of functionally different macrophages after thermal injury and sepsis. *Ann Surg.* 2004; **240**(1): 132–141.

37. Arturson G. Pathophysiology of the burn wound and pharmacological treatment. The Rudi Hermans Lecture 1995. *Burns.* 1996; **22**(4): 255–274.

38. Peng D, McManus AT, Hu Y, et al. Complement activation stimulate GTPase activity and secretory function of macrophages following burns. *J Burn Care Rehabil.* 2001; **22**(2)(suppl): 126.

39. Lotze MT, Tracy K. High-mobility group box 1 protein (HMGB1): nuclear weapon in the immune arsenal. *Nat Rev Immunol.* 2005; **5**(4): 331–342.

40. Jiang N, Pisetsky DS. The effect of inflammation on the generation of plasma DNA from dead and dying cells in peritoneum. *J Leukoc Biol.* 2005; **77**(3): 296–302.

41. Chen Z, Xiong Y, Lou S, Shu C, Liu X. Inhibition of mitochondrial respiratory function by an organic solvent extractable component from the extract of burn eschar. *Burns.* 1991; **17**(4): 282–287.

42. Monge G, Sparkes BG, Allgöwer M, Schoenenberger GA. Influence of burn-induced lipid-protein complex on IL1 secretion by PBMC in vitro. *Burns.* 1991; **17**(4): 269–275.

43. Ferrara JJ, Dyess DL, Luterman A, Peterson RD, Curreri PW. In vitro effect of complement inactivation upon burn-associated cell-mediated immunosuppression. *Ann Surg.* 1990; **56**(9): 571–574.

44. Alexander M, Chaudry IH, Schwacha MG. Relationships between burn size, immunosuppression, and macrophage hyperactivity in a murine model of thermal injury. *Cell Immunol.* 2002; **220**(1): 63–69.

45. Ertel W, Morrison AH, Ayala A, et al. Hypoxemia in the absence of blood loss or significant hypotension causes inflammatory cytokine release. *Am J Physiol.* 1995; **269**(1, pt 2): R160–R166.

46. Steiner DR, Gonzalez NC, Wood JG. Mast cells mediate the microvascular inflammatory response to systemic hypoxia. *J Appl Physiol.* 2003; **94**(1): 325–334.

47. Zuckerberg AL, Goldberg LI, Lederman HM. Effects of hypoxia on interleukin-2 mRNA expression by T lymphocytes. *Crit Care Med.* 1994; **22**(2): 197–203.

48. Niederbichler AD, Westfall MV, Su GL, et al. Cardiomyocyte function after burn injury and lipopolysaccharide exposure: single-cell contraction analysis and cytokine secretion profile. *Shock.* 2006; **25**(2): 176–183.

49. Kane TD, Alexander JW, Johannigman JA. The detection of microbial DNA in the blood: a sensitive method for diagnosing bacteremia and/or bacterial translocation in surgical patients. *Ann Surg.* 1998; **227**(1): 1–9.

50. de Haas CJ, van Leeuwen EM, van Bommel T, Verhoef J, van Kessel KP, van Strijp JA. Serum amyloid P component bound to gram-negative bacteria prevents lipopolysaccharide-mediated classical pathway complement activation. *Infect Immun.* 2000; **68**(4): 1753–1759.

51. Gao JJ, Xue Q, Papasian CJ, Morrison DC. Bacterial DNA and lipopolysaccharide induce synergistic production of TNF-alpha through a post-transcriptional mechanism. *J Immunol.* 2001; **166**(11): 6855–6860.

52. Peng D, Guymon CH, McManus AT, Xiao GX. Release of DNA from *Pseudomonas aerugisona* in vitro during spontaneous growth and treatment with ciprofloxacin. *Chin J Surg.* 2005; **43**(3): 178–181.

53. Takeda K, Kaisho T, Akira S. Toll-like receptors. *Annu Rev Immunol.* 2003; **21**: 335–376.

54. Yamada Y, Endo S, Inada K. Plasma cytokine levels in patients with severe burn injury—with reference to the relationship between infection and prognosis. *Burns.* 1996; **22**(8): 587–593.

55. Rumbaugh KP, Hamood AN, Griswold JA. Cytokine induction by the *P. aeruginosa* quorum sensing system during thermal injury. *J Surg Res.* 2004; **116**(1): 137–144.

56. Peng D. The effect of nutrition support on the modulation of immune disturbance after burns. *Chin J Burns.* 2006; **22**(6): 401–404.

57. Jeschke MG, Herndon DN, Ebener C, Barrow RE, Jauch KW. Nutritional intervention high in vitamins, protein, amino acids, and omega3 fatty acids improves protein metabolism during the hypermetabolic state after thermal injury. *Arch Surg.* 2001; **136**(11): 1301–1306.

58. Wang S, Li A. Gut-derived hypermetabolism after burns. *Chin J Burns.* 2001; **17**(4): 200–201.

59. Wischmeyer PE, Lynch J, Liedel J, et al. Glutamine administration reduces gram-negative bacteremia in severely burned patients: a prospective, randomized, double-blind trial versus isonitrogenous control. *Crit Care Med.* 2001; **29**(11): 2075–2080.

60. Alexander M, Daniel T, Chaudry IH, Schwacha MG. Opiate analgesics contribute to the development of post-injury immunosuppression. *J Surg Res.* 2005; **129**(1): 161–168.

61. Winslow GA, Shelby J, Nelson EW, Saffle JR. Influence of allogeneic blood transfusion on natural killer cell activity in burn-injured mice. *J Burn Care Rehabil.* 1996; **17**(2): 117–123.

62. Nau R, Eiffert H. Modulation of release of proinflammatory bacterial compounds by antibacterials: potential impact on course of inflammation and outcome in sepsis and meningitis. *Clin Microbiol Rev.* 2002; **15**(1): 95–110.

63. Horton JW, Maass DL, White DJ. Hypertonic saline dextran after burn injury decreases inflammatory cytokine responses to subsequent pneumonia-related sepsis. *Am J Physiol Heart Circ Physiol.* 2006; **290**(4): H1642–H1650.

64. Choudhry MA, Plackett TP, Schilling EM, Faunce DE, Gamelli RL, Kovacs EJ. Advanced age negatively influences mesenteric lymph node T cell responses after burn injury. *Immunol Lett.* 2003; **86**(2): 177–182.

65. Gregory MS, Duffner LA, Faunce DE, Kovacs EJ. Estrogen mediates the sex difference in post-burn immunosuppression. *J Endocrinol.* 2000; **164**(2): 129–138.

66. Schwacha MG, Holland LT, Chaudry IH, Messina JL. Genetic variability in the immune-inflammatory response after major burn injury. *Shock.* 2005; **23**(2): 123–128.

**67.** Barber RC, Aragaki CC, Rivera-Chavez FA, Purdue GF, Hunt JL, Horton JW. TLR4 and TNF-a polymorphisms are associated with an increased risk for severe sepsis following burn injury. *J Med Genet*. 2004; **41**(11): 808–813.

**68.** Jeschke MG, Barrow RE, Herndon DN. Recombinant human growth hormone treatment in pediatric burn patients and its role during the hepatic acute phase response. *Crit Care Med*. 2000; **28**(5): 1578–1584.

# CHAPTER SIX

# BURN PATHOPHYSIOLOGY

TODD F. HUZAR, MD, UNITED STATES ARMY INSTITUTE OF SURGICAL RESEARCH

EDWARD MALIN IV, MD, UNITED STATES ARMY INSTITUTE OF SURGICAL RESEARCH

STEVEN E. WOLF, MD, FACS, DEPARTMENT OF SURGERY,
UNIVERSITY OF TEXAS HEALTH SCIENCE CENTER—SAN ANTONIO

## INTRODUCTION

Injuries are common in the pediatric population and are associated with dramatic morbidity and mortality. In fact, unintentional injuries are a leading cause of injury and death among children. Historically, fires have been catastrophic to both health and home. In 2007, there were an estimated 1.6 million fires, causing over 17000 injuries and nearly 3500 deaths.[1] Death from fire and burn injuries was the second leading cause of nontransportation and unintentional fatalities in children 15 years of age and younger. Approximately 80% of all pediatric burns are unintentional, while the other 20% are associated with abuse or neglect.[2]

Death and injury from fire primarily affect children aged 4 years and younger.[3] These children face an increased risk in a fire because they are still somewhat dependent on others for their safety. Sadly enough, many of these children perish in their own homes because they are incapable of understanding the need to escape or how to do so quickly. In 2004, the National Fire Incident Reporting System (NFIRS) and the National Fire Protection Association (NFPA) found that 2007 children suffered thermal injuries, with 44% of burns and 50% of fire deaths occurring in the 4 years and younger age group.[3]

Small children should not be considered small adults. Young children are physiologically different compared to adults and even older children and often do not tolerate thermal injury well. Their thinner skin results in much deeper burns than in older children, and they are also more susceptible to the effects of smoke, which is associated with 48% of the fatalities found in children under the age of 15 years.[3] In addition, even small burns in children often require formal fluid resuscitation and more volume (cc/kg/TBSA) compared to adults with similar sized burns.

Scald burns are common in children and account for nearly 60% to 80% of burn injuries occurring worldwide.[4,5] In the United States, scalds are the leading cause of burns in children and account for approximately 65% of burns to children under the age of 5 years.[6] In fact, children aged 5 years and under have a risk of scald injury 3 to 4 times that of any other age group.[7] Hot tap water is associated with roughly 25% of all scald burns seen in children, which tend to be rather severe due to high temperatures causing deeper burns than other agents.[7] Feldman and others demonstrated that hot water scalds burn a larger body surface area, create more full-thickness injury, have a higher incidence of postburn scarring, and carry a higher mortality rate than other forms of scalds.[8]

Epidemiological studies have shown that children are vulnerable to the effects of thermal and nonthermal injury. However, most research involving the pathophysiology of burns has been reported in the adult literature. Interestingly, despite their differences, children exhibit many of the same physiologic, inflammatory, and immunological responses as adults.

## BURN DEPTH

The skin is the largest organ in the body and is composed of 2 layers: epidermis and dermis. The thickness of the epidermis varies depending on the region of the body (thin eyelids and thick soles). The dermis constitutes the majority of skin's thickness, which varies depending on age, gender, and location.[9] In addition to management of thermoregulation, the skin functions as a protective layer against fluid and electrolyte loss, infection, and exposure to radiant energy.

The epidermis is the superficial portion of skin, composed of 5 different layers. The innermost basal layer is composed of immature and undifferentiated keratinocytes (ectodermal origin). It takes approximately 2 to 4 weeks for keratinocytes to move from the basal layer to the stratum corneum, which is the most superficial and protective layer of the epidermis.[10,11] Other cell types present within the epidermis which serve to filter out ultraviolet light and phagocytize invading microorganisms are melanocytes and Langerhans cells, respectively. One of the more unique characteristics of the epidermis is its ability to regenerate from keratinocytes lining the dermal appendages and edges of the wound.

The dermis, on the other hand, is a thick (2–4 mm) layer of highly vascularized and innervated cells of mesodermal origin.[12] The dermis is composed of a papillary (superficial) and reticular (deeper) layer. The bulk of the dermis is made up of collagen fibers that are secreted by fibroblasts. Fiber orientation in the extracellular matrix allows for stretching and tensile strength.[13] The dermis contains adnexal structures (ie, sweat glands, hair follicles) that extend through the upper layers of the epidermis and supply reepithelializing keratinocytes after injury. Both the dermis and epidermis receive their blood supply from a dermal plexus of capillary vessels and the endothelial lining, which also secrete mediators of inflammation. These mediators regulate local and systemic inflammatory responses.[14] An abundance of sensory nerves are present in the dermal layer, and after injury they mediate pain and itching and influence local inflammation and wound healing.[15]

The major mechanisms of burns in children include thermal, chemical, and electrical injuries. Thermal injury is the most common form and occurs from excessive temperatures causing direct damage to skin and its underlying structures.[6,16] Injuries can result from direct contact with fire or an open flame, scalding from liquids, and contact with a superheated object causing coagulation necrosis of the skin and its elements. The depth of the burn varies according to the source of thermal injury and duration of exposure to the offending agent.

A chemical burn occurs from exposure to an alkali or acid and can be lethal due to the possibility of systemic absorption of the chemical as well as the depth/extent of the injury. The severity of the burn depends on the concentration and type of chemical in addition to the duration and degree of exposure.[17] Damage is created by direct injury to the cellular membranes and transfer of heat by chemical reactions within the skin. Chemical burns are initially difficult to assess because absorption can take hours to days before tissue damage is complete.[6] Although cutaneous chemical burns are uncommon in children, their risk for accidental ingestion of such compounds is greater.

Children are particularly vulnerable to electrical injuries in the household. Common injuries emanate from chewing on electrical cords and inserting metallic objects into electric sockets. Many of these injuries result from low-voltage electricity and cause small cutaneous burns; however, in the case of oral commissure burns, they have devastating complications, such as risk for late contractures.[18] Injury to the skin is mediated by direct injury to the cell membranes and generation of heat due to differences in resistance of the body's tissues.

The depth to which burns damage the skin and underlying tissues varies depending on the injurious agent. Some of the factors that can affect the depth of a burn should be mentioned. Medical personnel should consider the age of the patient in relation to the cause of an injury, because children under the age of 2 years have thinner skin than adults and thus suffer deeper burns in a relative sense.[6] The location of the burn itself may affect the depth due to variations in skin thickness by body region.[7] Additionally, the mechanism of the burn and duration of exposure to the injurious agent have significant impact on depth.[19]

Burn depth can be defined as the amount of tissue destroyed by heat, chemicals, or electricity.[20] Historically, burns have been classified as first, second, and third degree. Subsequently, a newer method was developed which is more accurate in classifying burn wound depth by describing the actual anatomic thickness of injured skin (Table 1).

Superficial burns (formerly first-degree) are confined only to the outer epidermal layers of skin. Since only the epidermis is injured, there is no disruption of skin integrity. These burns are characterized by pain and erythema without blistering or any open wounds. Pain from these burns is generated by injury to nerve endings found in the epidermis. A common cause of superficial burns is ultraviolet radiation (eg, sunburn). These injuries typically heal rapidly (< 1 week) without any scarring.

Second-degree or partial-thickness burns destroy the epidermis and also injure part of the dermis, including dermal appendages. They do not extend through the entire depth of the dermis. Partial-thickness burns can be further divided into 2 categories depending on the depth of dermal injury. Superficial partial-thickness burns destroy the entire epidermis as well as the upper portion of the dermis. Although the dermal skin appendages are damaged, many of them survive and participate in reepithelialization. Blisters are secondary to injury to the dermal capillaries and allow leakage of plasma that then separates the destroyed epidermis from the basement membrane. These blisters weep inflammatory fluid that contributes to further volume loss. Wounds tend to be bright red to mottled in appearance and wet to touch, with blisters as described. Pain can be quite severe in this particular type of burn due to exposure of dermal nerve endings to air.[15] Fortunately, these wounds tend to heal spontaneously in 1 to 2 weeks with minimal scarring.

Deep partial-thickness burns are of greater concern since they involve complete destruction of the epidermis and a majority of the dermis. Such severe dermal damage leaves few dermal appendages intact, which diminishes the ability to heal spontaneously. Wounds are described as dark red to yellowish-white in color and slightly moist, and they minimally blanch to pressure. There is decreased sensation to pinprick, although the perception to deep pressure may remain intact.[7] Blisters do not usually occur since close adherence between destroyed tissue and viable dermis prevents edema fluid from separating the epidermis from the dermis. Pain is minimal due to destruction of pain fibers in the dermis. Compromised blood flow to areas with deep partial-thickness burns allows for increased risk of infection and wound conversion to full-thickness injury. Excision and grafting is commonly warranted to expedite wound repair in these patients since healing can be delayed for months. Furthermore, the risk for development of hypertrophic scarring increases with nonoperative management.

Third-degree or full-thickness burns involve injury to the epidermis, dermis, and the underlying subcutaneous tissue. These wounds appear to be charred or white in color, dry, leathery, and insensate and contain thrombosed blood vessels that are visible through the burnt tissue. Necrotic skin (eschar) is a potent stimulator of the inflammatory response and is excellent pabulum for bacterial and fungal growth. Full-thickness burns do not heal spontaneously due to destruction of the dermis and are at high risk of hypertrophic scarring if allowed to heal by contraction. The inflammatory response is attenuated when early excision and grafting of full-thickness burns is performed. Subdermal burns, once called fourth-degree, occur with severe thermal injury and extend through subcutaneous tissue into connective tissue, muscle, and even bone. As expected, they present a significant challenge for even the most experienced burn surgeons.

## BURN SIZE

Proper sizing of burns assists with estimating the extent of injury. More importantly, it helps with determining the amount of fluid resuscitation required for patients with burn shock. Burn size is expressed as a percentage of total body surface area (%TBSA). When determining %TBSA, first-degree burns are not included in the tabulation. Adults can be initially mapped using the "rule of nines," which assigns certain percentages to different areas of the body.[21] However, this schema is inappropriate for use in children because the head and neck comprise a larger percentage of body surface area, with a smaller portion of body surface area encompassing the lower extremities. In 1944, Lund and Browder devised a new mapping system for children which took into account these differences in body proportions relative to age.[22] Most pediatric burn centers now employ a modified version of the Lund-Browder charting system (Table 2). This system can be difficult when mapping children with scald burns due to their noncontiguous nature.[23] Nagel et al described another method for measuring difficult burns by estimating the hand surface of a child (1–13 years of age) to approximate a 1% TBSA.[23]

## IMMUNE SYSTEM

Thermal and nonthermal burns to human tissue can have deleterious local and systemic effects on the immune system depending on the mechanism of injury, duration of contact, and associated secondary injuries. The immune system's response to burns has been extensively studied in the adult population. For various reasons, the pediatric literature is not as prolific. The unique qualities of the pediatric patient which will affect their response to burn injury include a discrepancy of body surface area (BSA) versus weight compared to adults, as well as the baseline hypermetabolic state seen in younger patients. Even though the pediatric literature has fewer entries on the subject, the overall response of the child's immune system to burns appears to be relatively similar to that of an adult.

## LOCAL CHANGES

Burns cause pathophysiologic changes in skin that can be characterized by the effects of the heat source in combination with acute inflammatory changes caused by the injury.[24] The mechanism by which burns cause injury is through coagulative necrosis of the epidermis and underlying deeper skin structures. The depth of injury is dependent on the substance's temperature, duration of exposure, and its specific heat (eg, grease burns cause more extensive damage compared to hot water burns at the same temperature and duration). The extent of exposure will dictate if the injury is limited locally or whether a systemic response is elicited. Burns greater than 10% total body surface area (TBSA) are more likely to produce a systemic response which is affected by immunoinflammatory factors, causing a dysfunction of the immune system. The disruption of immune function is proportional to the degree of burn injury.

The 2 layers of skin act as a "heat sink" to decrease the transfer of thermal energy to the underlying vital structures. Because of immediate changes in capacitance and temperature transmission, injury is mainly confined superficially. Sensory fibers in the skin sense changes in body surface temperature, leading to secretion of locally acting vasoactive mediators, which then cause vasodilation of dermal blood vessels in an attempt to dissipate thermal energy.[19] Injury to the skin and its structures from thermal energy releases acute inflammatory mediators from the injured cells and initiates the inflammatory response.[25]

After the thermal insult, inflammatory cells begin to demarginate from the bloodstream and migrate into the burned tissues. Large numbers of neutrophils are found within the dermis in the first few hours after superficial thermal injury, peak within 24 hours, and slowly retreat from the dermis in 72 hours.[26] However, deeper burns cause prolonged sequestration of neutrophils due to obliteration of vessels in the upper dermis and damage to deeper vessels.[27] Neutrophils are partly responsible for ischemic reperfusion injury due to release of free oxygen radicals. These then cause endothelial cell damage by increasing capillary permeability and provoking denaturation and fragmenting of collagen and extracellular matrix components.[28,29] Lymphocytes and macrophages begin to accumulate in the superficial burn at approximately 12 hours, but have not been found in deeper dermal burns.[30] Although the combination of inflammatory cells and mediators causes significant damage to the tissues in the thermally injured area, the inflammatory response can be seen throughout the entire human body.

The local tissue environment is overwhelmed with vasoactive mediators due to the combined effects of the local inflammatory response and release from injured cells. Substances such as cytokines, bradykinin, histamine, and arachidonic acid derivatives damage the capillaries and interstitium as a prelude to the formation of massive tissue edema.[25] Changes in the derivatives of Starling forces create favorable pressure gradients for capillary leakage of intravascular volume.[31,32] These forces result in loss of intravascular volume along capillary beds and produce an increased capacity of the interstitial space.[33] The formation of edema is relatively quick for smaller burns; however, the overall amount of edema fluid is less in larger burns, since large losses of intravascular volume lead to decreased blood flow to burned tissue and cause less edema formation.[34] Additionally, both formation and resorption of edema fluid occur faster in partial-thickness burns compared to full-thickness burns. This phenomenon is due to the greater vascular perfusion and larger number of intact lymphatics seen in partial-thickness burns.[25] Edema formation is decreased in deep thermal burns due to diminished vascular perfusion and limited resolution of formed edema secondary to damaged lymphatics.[35]

In 1953, Jackson described 3 concentric zones of thermal injury.[36] The innermost zone is that of coagulation, where cellular death occurs from direct tissue damage. In severe burns, it represents nonviable cells with no identifiable functioning vasculature. The middle area is the zone of stasis, containing a mixture of viable and nonviable cells with variable blood flow secondary to vasoconstriction, leading to ischemia. It is believed that thromboxane A2 is the cause of decreased blood flow in this zone.[25] Survival of cells in this zone is dependent upon adequate blood flow, prevention of infection, and prevention of desiccation, all of which could contribute to conversion of this zone to an area similar to the zone of coagulation.[37] The outermost area of injury is the zone of hyperemia, which is completely viable and shows signs of vasodilation due to inflammatory mediators. Discoloration of skin helps to delineate this area from noninjured tissue. This zone will usually recover and heal as long as hypotension and burn wound infection are avoided.[38] Changes of the microvasculature in the tissues surrounding the burn can cause extension of burn wound necrosis that can convert partial-thickness injuries to full-thickness burns.[39]

Additional factors involved in the body's response to local tissue trauma involve degranulation of mast cells that release multiple biologically active mediators, specifically histamine.[40] Vasodilation and vasoconstrictive factors both contribute to advancement of tissue damage due to an influx of inflammatory mediators and a decrease of perfusion, respectively. These vasoactive substances help mediate the flow of excess fluid into the interstitium. Consequently, histamine and its stimulation of xanthine oxidase produce an abundance of oxygen radicals, which results in more tissue damage and systemic consequences. If the burn is severe enough, the circulation of vasoactive substances, along with the decrease in intravascular volume, leads to the systemic process of "burn shock."

Animal research has broadened our understanding of histamine receptors and their role in regulating local edema after burn trauma. In one study comparing the function of histamine receptors on cellular permeability, H1, H2, and H3 receptors were not proven to be "important actors in the regulation of vascular patency permeability."[41] The clinical use of antihistamines in the treatment of edema has not provided much success either.

Several other vasoactive substances have been implicated in the systemic formation of hemodynamic alterations and have also contributed to the local effects of increased capillary permeability. These circulatory factors include serotonin, thromboxanes (TXA—from platelet activation), components of complement activation, products of arachidonic acid breakdown, bradykinin, and cortisol, as well as others.[26,42]

Regardless of the mechanism, insult and destruction of the skin's protective characteristics exposes the underlying tissue to a local inflammatory response. Furthermore, the extent of the injury determines the nature and degree of the systemic response.

## SYSTEMIC RESPONSE

The immune response elicited by burns involves a complex physiologic patchwork of proinflammatory reactions. Homeostasis of the existing immunoinflammatory and hematological systems are disrupted after a severe burn injury. The combination of cytokine release, activation of the complement system (C3a, C5a), platelet activation and the coagulation cascade, release of endothelial vasoactive substances (bradykinin, NO), influx of TXA and other by-products of arachidonic acid, response of the immune system to endotoxin, and the production of oxygen radicals all play a role in the clinical effects.[19] The baseline status of the patient dictates the effectiveness of his or her response; however, most children do not suffer from the same maladies of chronicity as the adult population.

The systemic response to severe burns can manifest in many ways. Clinically, the patient can exhibit signs of the systemic inflammatory response syndrome (SIRS). When there is a concomitant source of infection, sepsis can be diagnosed. Septic shock is described when factors contribute to the development of cardiovascular collapse. As the severity of the burn increases, so does the incidence of acute lung injury, renal failure, and multiple organ dysfunction syndrome (MODS), leading to increased morbidity and mortality.[43,44]

At the time of the injury, upregulation of macrophages initiates a cascade of cytokine release (eg, IL-1, IL-2, IL-6, IL-8, IL-10, TNF-α, TGF-β, and IFN-γ) and lymphocyte activation.[45] The corresponding cascade of immunoinflammatory mediators leads to immune dysfunction, with a resultant decreased resistance to infection, hemodynamic instability and shock, acute lung injury, and multiorgan failure.[46]

Over the last 2 decades, many studies have examined the role of cytokines with respect to trauma and burns. Stimulation of macrophages under these circumstances causes a release of proinflammatory cytokines not normally circulating in healthy patients. Significantly elevated levels of IL-1, IL-6, IL-8, and TNF-α have been measured in severely injured patients who also developed sepsis.[47,48,49] These cytokines were also associated with a higher incidence of mortality.

Deitch described a "two-hit" phenomenon which illustrates the effects of thermal injury on the immune system. The initial hit from a cutaneous burn primes the immune system to abnormally express proinflammatory factors and consequent anti-inflammatory mediators. Elevation of both leads to an inadequate response to a second insult, for example, wound infection. This is associated with a robust hypermetabolic state equipped with producing hemodynamic instability and further tissue injury.[50]

Research continues to explore the clinical applications in utilizing inflammatory and biological markers for the identification of sepsis. In a recent analysis of burn patients suffering from SIRS, sepsis, severe sepsis, or septic shock, the authors explored the utility of various laboratory values—C-reactive protein, WBC count, and procalcitonin—in diagnosing sepsis. The results revealed the presence of elevated procalcitonin levels in septic patients, which were superior to CRP or WBC in predicting sepsis.[51] An earlier retrospective study had also reported procalcitonin to have diagnostic value in evaluating for sepsis.[52] As prevention of sepsis and its early diagnosis are essential to the management of the severely burned patient, these conflicting studies reveal some of the challenges in establishing clear standards for monitoring the immunoinflammatory process.

Burn shock is the outcome of multiple factors characterized by the innate inflammatory response to severe injury. The roles of macrophages and the subsequent cascade of increasing cytokines contribute to instability of the body's homeostasis. As inadequate perfusion continues, additional local and systemic mediators further worsen the structure of microvascular permeability, causing a leak into the interstitial or "third" space. Oxygen radicals have been postulated to contribute to this process. Oxidative damage due to overproduction of oxygen radicals and its toxic effects have been implicated in "the local and distant pathophysiological events observed after burn."[53] The use of antioxidants such as vitamin C, vitamin E, and melatonin may have some clinical role in managing the toxic effects of free radicals—though no definitive consensus has been reached on their use in treating burns.[54,55] Some animal studies have even considered the use of induced hypothyroidism for managing the systemic response and resultant organ failure in severe burns.[56]

In severely burned patients with a significant systemic response, the mainstay of treatment is fluid resuscitation in order to maximize end-organ perfusion. An untoward consequence of high-volume crystalloid infusion can be intra-abdominal hypertension (IAH), with bladder pressures exceeding 25 mmHg.[57,58] Complications associated with abdominal compartment syndrome include elevated peak airway pressures, oliguria, and potential bowel ischemia. When decompressive laparotomy is required for severe cases of IAH, the patient's overall mortality is significantly increased. Some studies have demonstrated the use of colloids to be protective against the development of IAH.[59,60] Regardless of the type of fluid chosen, the effects of the initial resuscitation should be monitored closely.

## Hypermetabolism in Children

The human body is highly susceptible to injury that has effects both physically and metabolically. While there is a broad spectrum of injury we can endure, burns have one of the most severe impacts. Burns can scar physically and severely alter our metabolic capacity. Burn victims undergo intense hypermetabolic and catabolic states for weeks to months, and in extreme cases, these alterations can last for 1 to 2 years.[61]

Patients who are severely burned undergo a metabolic response initially characterized by a short, hypodynamic state after the initial injury. A hypermetabolic state ensues, with a hyperdynamic circulation delineated by increased body temperature, glycolysis, proteolysis, lipolysis, and futile substrate cycling.[62] These hypermetabolic patients undergo a significant reduction in lean body mass, muscle weakness, immunodepression, and poor wound healing.

Consequently, metabolism enters the "ebb" or shock phase, consisting of decreased blood pressure, cardiac output, body temperature, and oxygen consumption.[63] The ebb phase lasts for 12 to 24 hours and can be best described as depression of metabolic activity seen in early injury, including burns. Response to injury involves large increases in circulating levels of both catecholamines and vasopressin, with the level of response dependent on the severity of the injury.[64] Increased catecholamine activity in these patients leads to elevated levels of glucagon, which inhibits secretion of insulin, resulting in hyperglycemia. Due to relative insulin resistance, tissues which rely on glucose as a fuel must instead draw on whatever energy sources are available. The hypodynamic/hypovolemic state created by a severe burn causes increased vasopressin levels, leading to water retention. In addition, the renin-angiotensin system is activated in order to maintain intravascular volume, which tends to become rapidly diminished in severely burned patients.

After a period of time, metabolism enters the "flow" phase, characterized by hypermetabolism, increased cardiac output, increased urinary nitrogen losses, altered glucose metabolism, and accelerated tissue catabolism. Hypermetabolism can be defined as an increase in the basal metabolic rate above the predicted normal level. Thus, the overall increase in oxygen consumption, which can be related to the severity of the burn, occurs from elevations in both heart rate and myocardial contractility (cardiac output) in an attempt to deliver the optimal supply of energy and substrates to the burn wound at the expense of other tissues.[65]

The hypermetabolic or "flow" phase lasts from 9 to 12 months following a severe burn. The intensity of the catabolic state in these patients depends on the percentage of total body surface area burned. The resting metabolic rate in burn patients increases in a curvilinear fashion, dependent upon the %TBSA.[66] During this hypermetabolic phase, patients lose significant amounts of lean body mass, with even a 10% to 15% loss leading to increased infection rates and marked delays in wound healing.[57] The loss of lean mass directly results in muscle weakness, which can cause prolonged mechanical ventilation, diminished cough reflexes, and increased difficulty with ambulating protein-malnourished patients.[67]

A severe burn causes an imbalance between anabolism and catabolism by increasing the plasma levels of catecholamines. The surge in catecholamine levels directly increases levels of glucagon as compared to the already lower levels of insulin.[68] This difference in the glucagon to insulin ratio favors release of amino acids from skeletal muscle, which become a fuel in this hypermetabolic state.[57] Additionally, studies have shown that burn patients oxidize amino acids 50% faster than nonburn patients due to hypermetabolism. Another major metabolic disturbance caused by severe burns is the inability to utilize body fat stores for energy. During starvation, the body is normally able to utilize lipids as fuel and create a "protein sparing" effect. However, thermal injury inhibits fat utilization, and skeletal muscle subsequently undergoes proteolysis to meet the nitrogen needs of burn patients.[69] Negative net protein balance can be further enhanced by the development of sepsis, leaving open wounds, uncontrolled hyperglycemia, insulin resistance, and severe hypermetabolism.[70,71]

In studies by Gore et al and Flakoll et al, hyperglycemic patients tended to have increased rates of muscle protein breakdown.[72,73] Insulin use in hyperglycemic burn patients acts as a muscle protein anabolic agent.[74] Thomas et al showed that burned children started on low-dose insulin infusions (9–10 units/hr) experience substantial muscle anabolism.[75] Furthermore, the use of glucose coupled with insulin in burn patients can preserve body mass, reverse nitrogen balance, and retain energy stores, but unfortunately does not alter the hypermetabolic state.[76]

Patients with extensive burns can lose up to 25% of their premorbid body weight in the first 3 weeks due to flow phase hypermetabolism. Increased rates of catabolism seen in burn patients can be associated with larger percentage TBSA burns, heavier admission weights, and longer periods of time to primary wound excision and grafting. Early excision and grafting performed within the first 48 to 72 hours can decrease the metabolic rate by nearly 40%. In addition, patients started on enteral nutrition which delivers adequate amounts of kilocalories proportionate to their body weight and TBSA burned will have a diminished overall hypermetabolic status; however, early feeding and adequate calories do not abolish the hypermetabolic state. Enteral nutritional support is preferable to parenteral formulations due to the increased mortality, impaired liver function, and reduced immunocompetence seen with parenteral feeding.[53]

In many burn units, resting energy expenditure (REE) is estimated using the Harris-Benedict equation, which incorporates gender, age, weight, and height. The equations are

REE (males) = 10 × weight (kg) + 6.25 × height (cm) −
5 × age (y) + 5;
REE (females) = 10 × weight (kg) + 6.25 × height (cm) −
5 × age (y) − 161.[77]

Another method of determining REE is indirect calorimetry, which measures actual oxygen consumption and carbon dioxide production to derive energy utilization.

Burns can cause severe and prolonged metabolic disturbances that can last up to a year after the initial injury. The persistent and profound catabolism from this hypermetabolic state hampers rehabilitation efforts and delays the patient's return to a meaningful, functional life.[78] Although many anabolic strategies are employed to limit loss of lean body mass, the simplest and most effective is early burn excision and grafting of the wound. Other modalities used in an attempt to augment the tide of catabolism include beta blockers (propranolol), growth hormone, and synthetic testosterone analogues (ie, oxandrolone).

The use of beta blockers began from the belief that the most effective way of treating the catabolic state is by inhibiting catecholamines, catabolism of skeletal muscle, and the overall increase in basal energy expenditure. By blocking beta adrenergic receptors, there is a decrease in

thermogenesis, tachycardia, cardiac work, and resting energy expenditure. Barret et al found that long-term use of propranolol in burn patients (at doses reducing the heart rate by approximately 20%) was found to decrease overall cardiac work and decrease fatty infiltration of the liver.[79] Another study revealed that propranolol diminishes wasting of skeletal-muscle protein and raises lean body mass after major burns by causing enhanced intracellular recycling of free amino acids used in protein synthesis.[80]

Another drug used to augment the body's response to burn injury is growth hormone, which has been found to be useful in reducing wound healing at skin graft donor sites by nearly 25% and to improve the quality of wound healing with no increase in scar formation. The use of recombinant growth hormone has been shown to be extremely effective in children by increasing lean body mass, vertical bone growth, and bone mineral content even after being discontinued for years. Growth hormone also attenuates the initial acute response to thermal injuries and improves albumin production by the liver.[81] Growth hormone is not without its own side effects, specifically hyperglycemia, which can lead to increased morbidity and mortality.[82]

Oxandrolone, a steroid analogue which is 1/20 the strength of testosterone, has been used in burn patients. Studies of its use in young males with burn injury have shown a 2-fold improvement in protein synthetic insufficiency and a 2-fold decrease in protein breakdown.[83] At a dose of 0.1 mg/kg twice daily, oxandrolone was found to improve muscle protein metabolism in burn patients by enhancing the efficiency of protein synthesis. In 2003, Demling and De Santi showed that patients receiving oxandrolone and adequate nutrition regained weight and lean mass 2 to 3 times faster than with nutrition alone. At a 6-month follow up, these patients maintained their body weight and lean body mass.[84]

## EFFECTS ON THE RENAL SYSTEM

Severe burns have been implicated in causing a broad spectrum of local and widespread negative effects on the body. Acute renal failure secondary to burns is a well-known complication associated with portending a worse prognosis.[85] The incidence of this devastating complication has been noted in the literature to range from 1% to 30% of admitted patients, but its presence has an associated mortality of 70% to 100%.[86,87]

Acute renal failure has a multitude of definitions, but ours involves a sudden decrease in the glomerular filtration rate due to either intrinsic kidney disease or changes in intrarenal hemodynamics.[88] Diminished renal function leads to accumulation of cellular waste products (eg, urea, creatinine, and potassium) in the bloodstream, which can subsequently cause their own significant complications.

Burn patients are unique in their susceptibility to acute renal failure at 2 points during the postburn period: early and late.

Early renal failure can occur immediately after a severe burn secondary to decreases in renal perfusion due to hypovolemia or damage from intravascular pigments (eg, hemoglobin or myoglobin) that deposit in and occlude the renal tubules.[89] Hypovolemia from burn shock occurs as a consequence of excessive fluid loss from burn wounds, depletion of intravascular volume secondary to fluid shifts, and decreases in cardiac output from circulating vasogenic mediators.[83,84] Most importantly, delays in the initiation of aggressive fluid resuscitation may aggravate the profound hypovolemia due to the previously mentioned causes, and together lead to renal hypoperfusion and injury.[90] A study by Jeschke et al illustrated this point by showing that aggressive fluid resuscitation started within the first 2 hours after a burn injury in children resulted in significant improvement in the survival of patients with acute renal failure.[83]

Extensive depletion of intravascular volume and burn stress leads to a significant release in catecholamines and other stress hormones (eg, vasopressin and aldosterone). As a result, vasoconstriction and changes in regional blood flow to the kidneys occurs, which further exacerbates renal hypoperfusion.[85,91] The thermal cutaneous injury is thought to be the source of mediators that enhance the effects of stress-induced hormones. Many authors have proposed that cytokines (eg, interleukin-6, tumor necrosis factor) released from the burn wound itself interact with circulating stress-induced hormones and promote continuously unopposed vasoconstriction of the renal vasculature. Consequently, this event increases the chances of developing acute renal injury.[92,93]

The late form of acute renal failure is mainly attributed to systemic sepsis and manifests approximately 2 weeks after a burn. Severe sepsis and associated multiorgan failure associated with elevated levels of cytokines and other proinflammatory mediators can lead to increased vascular permeability and renal tissue damage.[83] Even the treatment of clinical sepsis can be a culprit in the initiation of late renal failure. For example, nephrotoxic antibiotics such as aminoglycosides can increase the risk of renal failure in septic burn patients.[94] The combination of sepsis and renal failure predicts a rather poor prognosis.[83,84]

As time progresses, it is hoped that advances in the management of acute renal failure will lead to decreases in morbidity and mortality. For now, early initiation of fluid resuscitation and aggressive management of sepsis can possibly spare burned children the added insult of renal failure and its dismal prognosis.

## EFFECTS ON THE GASTROINTESTINAL SYSTEM

A child exposed to a severe burn (> 20% TBSA) is at risk for developing secondary organ involvement, especially with the gastrointestinal tract, either directly or indirectly. In children, the accidental ingestion of caustic chemicals can have deleterious effects on the gastrointestinal system, ranging from minor oral cavity ulceration to full-thickness necrosis and perforation. Stress ulceration associated with burns was first described in the mid-eighteenth century by Curling, and its incidence has prompted the widespread use of prophylactic medications.[95] Another complex process which exists in the severely burned child is the extent of the external insult and its treatment influencing secondary injury to the intestine and further exacerbating the body's systemic response to the trauma.

The literature has sought to determine the etiology of gastrointestinal injury in burns and the clinical implications as related to sepsis. A phenomenon in which the mucosa of the gastrointestinal tract atrophies as result of a burn has been described. In animal studies, the intestinal weight of rats with burn trauma has been compared to those without such wounds. Injured animals were shown to have about 20% less intestinal weight than the control group secondary to a decrease in mucosa.[96] Additional studies examining the effects of burns on the gastrointestinal tract have further elucidated this process by proving disruption of the normal homeostatic balance of cell death and proliferation. Despite increased cell proliferation after scalding injury, the gut epithelium of mice revealed an overall decrease in cell number due to the overwhelming presence of diffuse apoptosis.[97] Follow-up studies showed this increase in cell death was less likely a result of hypoperfusion in mesenteric vessels and more likely secondary to the systemic inflammatory response after a severe burn.[98]

The clinical implications of gastrointestinal damage are quite significant when considering the development of burn sepsis. Some have demonstrated gut-derived sepsis may be directly related to an increase in gut permeability with paracellular translocation of gram-negative bacteria and release of endotoxin. Based on the fact that the extent of the burn directly correlates with the degree of permeability, a gut-lymph theory has evolved, describing a leaky gut that spills inflammatory factors into the lymphatic channels rather than the portal system.[99,100,101] In studies examining the effects of severe injury, it has been postulated that the process of lymphatic drainage of these inflammatory mediators via the thoracic duct may also contribute to shock-induced acute lung injury.[102]

Life-threatening sepsis can be attributed to many factors related to gastrointestinal injury: (1) microbial load and virulence, (2) status of the gut barrier, and (3) magnitude of the host's immunoinflammatory response.[103] Early enteral feeding has been speculated to be one of the ways to ameliorate the injurious systemic response to burns and also fortify the gastrointestinal tract's mucosal layer.[104]

Gastrointestinal problems, including gastrointestinal bleeding, Curling ulcers, pancreatitis, superior mesenteric artery syndrome, acalculous cholecystitis, intestinal necrosis, and paralytic ileus[105] are well-recognized complications associated with burns. Paralytic ileus and enteral feeding intolerance are often seen in burn patients as a prequel to the onset of sepsis; however, the exact etiology of these 2 conditions is unknown.[106] Tokyay et al and Reines et al showed that elevated thromboxane A2 levels in sepsis cause significant mesenteric vasoconstriction that limits mesenteric blood flow.[107,108] Decreased mesenteric perfusion possibly causes the intestinal neuroendocrine system to slow peristalsis, leading to ileus/feeding intolerance; malperfusion can directly alter mucosal fluid resorption, producing diarrhea.[106] Enteral feeding intolerance is an entity which should be monitored closely, as it may be the only early clinical sign of sepsis.

# INHALATION INJURY

Inhalation injury was first recognized in the first century AD in prisoners who were exposed to wood smoke as a method of execution. However, injury from smoke inhalation did not receive much public or scientific attention until the infamous Cocoanut Grove fire of 1942 occurred, killing 491 people.[109] Many of the victims of this fire suffered severe inhalation injury secondary to being trapped in an oxygen-deprived, confined space. Following this tragedy, there was a significant amount of research into the pathophysiology of inhalation injury.

Smoke inhalation has been found to be associated with 20% to 30% of major burns and increases the overall morbidity and mortality in severely burned patients.[110,111] Studies have shown that inhalation injury is an important contributor to mortality when also considering percentage of total body surface area involved and patient age.[112] The lethality of smoke inhalation is due to the combination of its components (eg, particulate matter and gases) affecting different levels of the respiratory tract. The composition of smoke depends on the type of combustible material and the room's oxygen content.[113] Some of the more dangerous gases found in smoke include sulfur dioxide, carbon monoxide, phosgene, acrolein, ammonia, hydrogen chloride, and hydrogen cyanide, all of which have different effects locally in the lungs and systemically.[103] Smoke inhalation has been found to have devastating effects on both the upper and lower airways.

The oropharynx and upper airways suffer the brunt of the heat from inhaled gases, with most of the large particulate matter trapped in the nasopharynx and oropharynx. Hot, inspired gases are rapidly cooled by the moist and well-vascularized mucosal surfaces of the mouth, tongue, and oropharynx. The exchange of thermal energy into these tissues causes rapid mucosal swelling as well as increased transvascular fluid migration due to higher flow of lymph fluid and blood into the injured mucosa.[114] As the injury progresses, cytokines released in response to tissue injury further compound airway swelling to the point that the airway begins to narrow. This then leads to a decreased ability to move air and secretions, which can ultimately result in asphyxiation.[115] Prophylactic intubation should be considered in patients with upper airway injury to prevent airway loss and the need for an emergency airway. Intubation, however, may itself cause further damage to the tracheal mucosa and even result in laryngeal injury.[116]

The action of the oropharynx and upper airways as a "heat sink" protects the lower airways from thermal injury; however, steam can bypass this cooling mechanism due to its greater heat-carrying capacity compared to "dry" smoke.[117] The inhaled steam remains "hot" and easily proceeds to the lower airways, where it causes blistering. Eventual sloughing of the bronchial mucosa leading to an intense inflammatory response with subsequent parenchymal damage is seen. This group of patients is at higher risk for the development of ARDS and pneumonia than those with smoke-related inhalation injuries.[118] Injuries from steam inhalation occur with less frequency in the pediatric population than in adults because this occurs more often in job-related incidents.

As smoke begins to percolate down the tracheobronchial tree, a mixture of particulate matter and toxins attack the ciliated, columnar epithelium, causing local vasodilation mediated by leukotrienes, histamine, neural neuropeptides, and nitric oxide (produced by nitric oxide synthase).[103,119] The effect of this rapid vasodilation is necrosis of the ciliated epithelium that precipitates separation from the tracheobronchial wall.[120] Simultaneously, smoke-borne toxins cause a massive release of inflammatory mediators that may lead to severe bronchoconstriction such that spontaneous breathing or mechanical ventilation may be extremely difficult.[121] The combination of damaged epithelium and increased flow of lymph and blood results in transudation of large amounts of protein-rich fluid from "leaky" capillaries into the airways. This transudative/exudative proteinaceous fluid mixes with inflammatory cells and sloughed-off tracheobronchial epithelium to form soft, bronchial casts.[122] In a few hours, these casts solidify and cause obstruction of small-caliber and medium-caliber airways, along with alveoli.[105,123] The formation of these obstructive casts is not uniform and can affect different segments of the lung. Bronchial casts cause distal airway atelectasis, precipitating ventilation/perfusion mismatch due to hypoventilation.[103] In normal lungs, hypoventilation causes hypoxic vasoconstriction of blood vessels in underventilated segments and shunts blood away from these areas, thus preventing ventilation/perfusion mismatching. However, circulating inflammatory mediators (eg, nitric oxide, a vasodilator) inhibit this mechanism and lead to continuous perfusion of these segments, which results in poor oxygenation of blood and eventual hypoxemia.[124] Mechanically ventilated patients may suffer a combination of barotrauma/volutrauma to nonoccluded pulmonary segments secondary to increased airway pressures from the ventilator attempting to overcome airway occlusion from these casts.[125]

The alveolus is the final stop in the pathway of destruction for smoke and its components. Gases and particulate matter directly damage the epithelial lining of the alveoli, while obstructive bronchial casts and sequelae of the inflammatory response cause indirect injury to these fragile structures. Particulate matter entering the alveolus activates pulmonary macrophages, which phagocytize debris and subsequently release oxygen free radicals (eg, superoxide) and lysozymes that injure both the macrophage and surrounding alveolar epithelium.[103] Pulmonary macrophages consequently lyse, releasing cytokines and proinflammatory mediators that enter the circulation and attract neutrophils into the alveoli, causing epithelial damage and further propagating the systemic inflammatory response.[126] Neutrophils secrete enzymes (eg, elastase, oxygen radicals) that cause disruption of the capillary endothelial junctions, allowing protein-rich plasma to enter the alveoli.[102] Plasma within the alveoli begins to clot as a result of the procoagulant nature of pulmonary epithelium; this causes dissolution of surfactant and eventual atelectasis of affected pulmonary segments.[127] As one would expect, pneumonia and ARDS are common complications of parenchymal injury and increase mortality in patients with severe inhalation injury.

A common and deadly component of smoke is carbon monoxide (CO). It is a product of incomplete combustion of many fuels commonly found in homes, including wood, paper, and cotton.[128] The toxic effect of carbon monoxide is mediated by its ability to bind to hemoglobin and make it unavailable for oxygen transport.[129] Since carbon monoxide's affinity for hemoglobin is 230 to 270 times greater than that of oxygen,[130] small concentrations of carbon monoxide give rise to high carboxyhemoglobin levels. This causes a left shift of the oxygen-hemoglobin curve and decreases the availability for oxygen to dissociate at the capillary level for a given partial pressure of oxygen.[131] The overall effect of carbon monoxide poisoning

is profound hypoxemia manifesting as cardiac and central nervous system symptoms, including coma, seizures, dysrhythmias, myocardial ischaemia, and hypotension.[132,133] Carbon monoxide also binds to intracellular cytochromes, which leads to electron transport chain dysfunction and finally, direct injury at the cellular level.[134] Also of great concern is carbon monoxide exposure to a fetus, which is more detrimental due to fetal hemoglobin's greater affinity for CO compared to adult hemoglobin. As a result, CO could cause more profound effects at lower concentrations.[135] Carbon monoxide poisoning can have long-term side effects such as psychiatric disorders and a fatal demyelination syndrome; however, longitudinal studies in the pediatric population are limited.[136,137,138]

## BACTEREMIA/SEPSIS

Skin provides a natural mechanical barrier to microbial invasion. In the event of a disruption in the skin's protective quality, as in a burn, the body is at risk for systemic infection. The consequences of bacteremia and subsequent sepsis can be minimized with aggressive resuscitation and timely treatment of burn wounds with early debridement. The pathogens responsible for bacteremia are vast and can often be identified based on the mode of exposure (ie, pulmonary, urinary, gastrointestinal, etc).[139]

Disruption of the skin's protective nature leads to penetration and exposure of normally sterile tissue space to bacteria, fungi, and viruses; the same process occurs to the mucosal lining of the respiratory tract in inhalation injury. The presence of necrotic tissue planes inhibits the effectiveness of innate antimicrobial responses. The issue of gut translocation has led to more speculation than confirmation regarding its contribution to bacteremia. The burn patient's physiologic status often masks the normal response to infection (eg, tachycardia, fever, leukocytosis, etc). These signs are also seen in most trauma patients; additionally, the pediatric burn patient's baseline hypermetabolic state provides an additional challenge in determining whether an infection is present. Important signs of systemic infection and sepsis such as hypotension, mental status changes, fluid sequestration, oliguria, and organ failure become more significant signals in light of the above discussion. Therefore, early detection and diagnosis with prompt treatment are essential in the management of bacteremia. In burn patients, sepsis usually precedes the development of multiple organ failure.[39] Even in the most severe cases of pediatric burn injury, early treatment with excision and grafting can minimize morbidity and mortality.[140,141] Other contributors to bacteremia include central line catheters, endotracheal tubes, disruption of the blood-brain barrier, urinary drainage tubes, and body cavity drains.

## ELECTRICAL BURNS

The US Consumer Product Safety Commission estimates that 4000 injuries associated with electric extension cords are treated in emergency departments each year. Half of these injuries involving young children resulted in burns to the mouth.[142] An additional 1000 children are injured secondary to electrocution after inserting an object into an electrical receptacle.[143] The pediatric population is particularly susceptible to injuries in the household, especially those which occur by exposure to electrical current.

The effects of these often preventable injuries can vary from minor trauma to even death. For the clinician, it is helpful to understand the effects of electrical exposure on the body in order to completely manage the sequelae of such injuries. The sources of electrical injury can vary widely: oral or hand contact, insertion of an object into an electrical outlet, direct contact with an industrial or household appliance, contact with high-voltage current secondary to an electrically charged rail, and contact with a high-powered wire while climbing a tree.[144] Young children are often exposed to electrical injury from biting electrical cords or placing objects into electrical outlets; however, older children are more frequently exposed to high-voltage injuries from power lines while climbing trees or utility poles.[145,146] Regardless of the mechanism, children experiencing electrical injuries can suffer devastating and disfiguring injuries.

Electrical injury can be divided into 2 categories: low-voltage and high-voltage. Low voltage is typically classified as energy less than 1000 volts (V) (eg, household current is 110V to 230V), and high voltage is considered greater than 1000V (eg, high-tension lines possess greater than 100000V and lightning strikes can exceed 10 million volts).[147] Block et al described 4 ways that electrical energy can cause injury: (1) direct injury to the electrical system of the heart, resulting in dysrhythmias; (2) blunt injury from high voltage strikes (eg, lightning), leading to falls; (3) transformation of electrical energy to thermal energy, causing cutaneous burns; and (4) electroporation in high-voltage injuries allowing formation of pores in the cell membrane, leading to cellular disruption and causing death without direct thermal insult.[148] One of the reasons why electrical injury is so devastating is because of the variety of ways in which tissue damage can occur.

Burns secondary to an electrical current often begin at the point of contact and travel through the path of least resistance along nerves, muscle, and blood vessels.[149] In electrical exposure, some claim that high-resistance tissues (eg, skin, bone, and fat) develop larger elevations in temperature and undergo coagulative necrosis, causing damage that is not visible by the naked eye.[150] However, because the duration of current is miniscule (in nanoseconds), it is difficult to justify this alone as the cause of injury. Skin has a wide range of electrical resistance, which can be altered by its external moisture content. For example, it has been demonstrated that dry skin has a higher resistance to electrical current compared to moist skin, and this results in a greater degree of superficial injury while more of the deeper structures are spared. On the other hand, less resistance is encountered with moist skin, which allows electrical current to easily reach deeper layers, causing injury to both those structures and internal organs.[147]

Injury from an electrical source has a wide variety of sequelae, and the amount of physiologic damage correlates with the current/voltage that flows through the body. Electricity can affect a majority of the body's organs, including the lungs, heart, central nervous system, and musculoskeletal system. The respiratory drive can become dysfunctional due to inhibition of the central nervous system, paralysis of the respiratory muscles, or cardiac arrest from an electrical shock; however, damage to the parenchyma is not commonplace.[150] The functions of the heart and brain can easily be disrupted since they rely on electrical impulses. As current makes its way through the heart it can cause arrhythmias, conduction abnormalities, and direct myocardial injury. Ventricular fibrillation is the most common arrhythmia seen in low alternating current (AC) voltage injuries. Higher rates of asystole are seen in patients receiving shocks from high AC voltage and direct current.[151,154] Sudden death is a direct complication of both these arrhythmias. Children rarely suffer from postelectrical injury arrhythmias; however, nonspecific ST segment/T wave abnormalities associated with premature ventricular and junctional complexes can be seen on an EKG.[145,152] Alternating current has been noted to cause sinus bradycardia and high-degree atrioventricular blockade by directly damaging the sinoatrial (SA) and atrioventricular (AV) nodes, respectively.[153] Direct injury to the myocardium has also been reported in the literature and is possibly due to conversion of electrical current to thermal energy or electroporation.[154]

As electrical current traverses the body, it travels through nerves and can damage both the peripheral and central nervous systems. Sensory deficits, memory loss, muscle paralysis, loss of consciousness, cerebral infarction, cerebral hemorrhage, and respiratory arrest can occur as a result of severe electrical shocks.[155] The musculoskeletal system can also be adversely affected. There have been reports of fractured bones and joint dislocations secondary to tetanic muscle contractions.[156] Muscle is also damaged from the conversion of electrical energy to thermal energy causing rhabdomyolysis and pigmenturia that can lead to subsequent renal failure.

Electrothermal injury has been well documented in the literature. In one of the earliest studies on the effects of electricity in animals, the pathophysiology of this type of burn was tested. The study examined the effects of alternating current at different voltage levels on the tissues of mongrel dogs and rats. Low-voltage exposure resulted in a superficial burn, while higher voltages translated into more extensive deep tissue and muscle injury. The relationship between temperature and amperage helped explain the extent of tissue damage. Small areas of electrical exposure translated into high electrical current and therefore a greater concentration of damage. Additional factors contributing to the degree of injury were linked to derivatives of Ohm's law, which relates the ratio of voltage to amperage as it is equal to resistance. The study found that as amperage increased, resistance of the tissue decreased to a point where "a rapid climb in amperage coincided with the complete breakdown of skin resistance."[157] Overall, the "general effects vary from a minimal tingling to that of death, depending on the type of current, frequency, duration, the pathway of the current and the amount of current."[158] The clinical implications of these findings help describe the injuries sustained by children.

A child who bites an electrical cord or inserts a pen into an electrical socket will most likely suffer from severe localized tissue injury. On the other hand, exposure of electrical energy to a broader surface, such as the back, will have greater dispersion of the current with less tissue injury; however, the effects on other organ systems may result in more severe damage and even death. It should be noted that either mechanism of electrical exposure can result in cardiac complications.

In the United States, households are powered with alternating current, which is considered more dangerous than direct current. Exposure to alternating current can cause repetitive muscle contractions, which can lead to sudden cardiac death secondary to ventricular fibrillation (more commonly in adults than children).[148,159] On the other hand, direct current affects muscle by creating a synchronous, forceful contraction which is able to throw the victim away from the electrical source, thus causing additional non-thermal trauma.[150] In addition, disruption of the electrical impulses that travel through the nervous system by electrical injury can lead to possible paralysis and subsequent respiratory arrest. All these factors contribute to the exceptionally dangerous nature of this form of injury.

## CHEMICAL BURNS

Chemical burns result from exposure to acid, alkali, or organic (hydrocarbon) compounds. The means of exposure can occur by direct contact through skin, ingestion, or inhalation. Factors involved in determining the extent of injury include the amount and concentration of a substance, its toxicity, the mechanism of injury, and the duration of exposure. Tissue destruction from these nonthermal burns will persist until the offending chemical has been removed or neutralized.

Acids produce coagulation of the surrounding tissue. By the process of hydrolysis, proteins precipitate into the extracellular space. Alkali burns are often more extensive, causing liquefactive necrosis and disruption of tissue planes. Most chemical burns of this nature result in full-thickness tissue damage. The lipid-soluble characteristics of organic solutions complicate the management of these exposures, as chemical absorption can lead to systemic toxicity.[160] In the example of hydrocarbons (eg, gasoline), the consequences of exposure can vary from a simple cutaneous burn to multiorgan failure from a more devastating systemic toxicity.[161] Also, it is possible that activation of some chemicals when exposed to tissue may cause an exothermic reaction resulting in thermal injury as well.

Most chemical burns can be managed with local wound care; however, a severe and extensive exposure can lead to a systemic response, as described previously in this chapter. In the event of an inhalation injury, early identification of the toxin and mechanism of exposure will be essential in the management of these patients. For example, the inhalation of ammonia within a confined space can have both short-term effects on the patient's respiratory status as well as producing long-standing parenchymal injury to the lung tissue. If a child ingests a toxin, the effects on the upper gastrointestinal (GI) system can range from mild erythema to perforation with contamination of the mediastinum. The management of this injury should be tailored to identifying the degree of injury and its location along the GI tract. The toxicity of the chemical is the key to understanding the extent of tissue damage. If a systemic response is clinically evident, the liver and kidney will be particularly affected as the body attempts to cleanse itself of the toxin.

Despite the presence of millions of different chemicals in the world in general, the pediatric patients' exposure to these substances occurs more often in their own homes. The presence of household cleaners and solutions supplies ample opportunity for unintended exposures to young children. In a retrospective analysis of children ingesting caustic substances, the majority of chemicals were alkali in nature, resulting in 87% of the identified esophageal burns.[162]

Despite the type of toxin, the initial treatment to topical exposure remains the same: immediate removal of the substance, either by brushing away excess powder and/or by thoroughly lavaging the area with several liters of fluid.[163] The goal is to neutralize the chemical by returning physiologic pH to the affected tissue in order to minimize denaturation of the cell's protein matrix. In the event of inhalation of chemicals, continuous monitoring in an ICU setting and possible early intubation are the mainstays to managing the latent progression of pulmonary injury and systemic complications.

## COLD INJURIES

Exposure to cold temperatures has similar effects on tissue as compared to thermal injury. The principles remain the same in that the degree and extent of tissue injury is related to the temperature (ie, the lower the temperature the more tissue damage) and the duration of exposure. In the case of frostbite, the extremities, especially the fingers and toes, are particularly susceptible to injury.

The mechanism of frostbite injury is a 2-hit phenomenon. The first hit causes direct cellular damage due to decreased tissue temperatures. As tissues reach freezing temperatures, ice crystals form within the extracellular spaces and cause structural damage to the cell membranes.[164] The resultant membrane damage results in intracellular dehydration due to changes in the electrochemical/osmotic gradient allowing free water to flow out of cells. Severe alterations in the concentrations of intracellular electrolytes can lead to cell death. Declining tissue temperature produces a precipitation of intracellular ice crystals that will eventually expand, destroying the cell.[165] In addition, alterations in blood flow to the skin due to tissue cooling result in cycles of alternating vasoconstriction and vasodilation, causing partial freezing and thawing that further enhances cellular damage.[166,167] The second hit is due to progressive dermal ischemia that is related to the repeated "freeze/thaw" cycles releasing a variety of inflammatory mediators (eg, prostaglandins, thromboxanes, bradykinin, and histamine). Consequently, significant endothelial injury, tissue edema, cessation of dermal blood flow, and eventual skin necrosis occurs.[164]

The damaged tissue can be graded according to its appearance by the following classification: first-degree— white, hard plaque; second-degree—clear fluid, superficial blisters; third-degree—purple fluid, deep blisters, and discolored skin; and fourth-degree—necrotic tissue.[145] The management and treatment of these injuries focuses on rapidly rewarming the tissue, maintaining aggressive wound care with debridement of nonviable tissue (if needed), and minimizing systemic effects.

## CONCLUSION

The pathophysiology of thermal and nonthermal burn injuries in the pediatric population is still not completely understood. In burn trauma, the complex balance of immunologic, hematological, and inflammatory systems is disrupted as the normally protective tissue planes in the body are destroyed. The mechanism of the injury and the duration of the exposure help dictate the extent of the burn. The key components to evaluating a burn are the following: establishing an accurate extent of the injury, understanding the local and systemic effects of burns, and recognizing the presence of secondary organ injury. The immunoinflammatory response to burn trauma will affect the patient's treatment and recovery. Much of the research on the immunoinflammatory system over the last 2 decades has helped to shed some light into this response. Inflammatory substances have been shown to play a major role in the local and systemic effects; however, more research is needed in these areas in order to transform the science into clinical application.

## KEY POINTS

- It is important for clinicians to understand the pathophysiology of burn injury when evaluating and treating pediatric burn patients.
- The severity of the injury can be measured by calculating the burn size, identifying the mechanism of injury and duration of exposure, and accounting for associated comorbidities.
- Mortality and morbidity are directly related to the severity of the injury.
- The immunoinflammatory system can produce both a local and a systemic response, which in turn can have deleterious effects on the body's organ systems—severe burns can lead to multiple organ dysfunction syndrome and death.
- More research on pediatric burns is required to further improve care in this population.

# TABLES

## TABLE 1
### Descriptions of burn depth.

| Burn Type | Definition | Physical Signs |
|---|---|---|
| **Superficial (First-Degree)** | Injury only to the epidermis | Skin is pink or slightly reddish, dry with no blister formation, mildly painful to touch. |
| **Partial-Thickness (Second-Degree)** | | |
| **1. Superficial**<br>**2. Deep** | 1. Injury to the epidermis and upper 1/3 of dermis<br>2. Injury to the epidermis, majority of dermis, and skin appendages | 1. Skin is bright red or mottled in color; presence of bullae/blisters, wet and weeping; blanches when touched; extremely painful to touch or with air movement.<br>2. Skin is dark red to whitish/yellowish; ruptured bullae and minimal moisture; less painful to touch compared to superficial partial-thickness burn; decreased sensation to pinprick, but intact to deep pressure. |
| **Full-Thickness (Third-Degree)** | Injury to epidermis, dermis, and subcutaneous tissue | Skin is charred or white in color with dry texture and leathery feel; thrombosed vessels visible through eschar; nonblanching and nonpainful; insensate to touch. |

## TABLE 2
### Body area versus appropriate body surface area percentage in pediatric patients.

| Area | Birth to 1 Year | 1–4 Years | 5–9 Years | 10–14 Years | 15 Years |
|---|---|---|---|---|---|
| **Head** | 19% | 17% | 13% | 11% | 9% |
| **Neck** | 2% | 2% | 2% | 2% | 2% |
| **Anterior Trunk** | 13% | 13% | 13% | 13% | 13% |
| **Posterior Trunk** | 13% | 13% | 13% | 13% | 13% |
| **Buttock (Left or Right)** | 2.5% each buttock | 2.5% each buttock | 2.5% each buttock | 2.5% each buttock | 2.5% each buttock |
| **Genitalia** | 1% | 1% | 1% | 1% | 1% |
| **Upper Arm (Left or Right)** | 4% each upper arm | 4% each upper arm | 4% each upper arm | 4% each upper arm | 4% each upper arm |
| **Lower Arm (Left or Right)** | 3% each lower arm | 3% each lower arm | 3% each lower arm | 3% each lower arm | 3% each lower arm |
| **Hand (Left or Right)** | 2.5% each hand | 2.5% each hand | 2.5% each hand | 2.5% each hand | 2.5% each hand |
| **Thigh (Left or Right)** | 5.5% each thigh | 6.5% each thigh | 8% each thigh | 8.5% each thigh | 9% each thigh |
| **Leg (Left or Right)** | 5% each leg | 5% each leg | 5.5% each leg | 6% each leg | 6.5% each leg |
| **Foot (Left or Right)** | 3.5% each foot | 3.5% each foot | 3.5% each foot | 3.5% each foot | 3.5% each foot |

# REFERENCES

1. National Center for Injury Preventions and Control. http://www.cdc.gov/homeandrecreationalsafety/fire-prevention/fires-factsheet.html. Sept 28, 2008.

2. US Fire Administration/National Fire Data Center. Residential fires and child casualties. *Topical Fire Research Series*. 2005; 5(2): 1–5.

3. US Fire Administration/National Fire Data Center. Risk to children in 2004. *Topical Fire Report Series*. 2008; 7(6): 1–6.

4. Drago DA. Kitchen scalds and thermal burns in children five years and younger. *Pediatrics*. 2005; 115: 10–16.

5. Tse T, Poon CH, Tse KH. Paediatric burn prevention: an epidemiological approach. *Burns*. 2006; 32: 229–234.

6. American Burn Association. National Burn Repository 2005 Report. www.ameriburn.org. Chicago: ABA website. 2006; Version 2.0.

7. Rimmer RB, Weigand S, Foster KN, et al. Scald burn in young children—a review of Arizona burn center pediatric patients and a proposal for prevention in the Hispanic community. *J Burn Care Res*. 2008; 29: 595–605.

8. Feldman KW, Schaller RT, Feldman JA, McMillon M. Tap water scald burns in children. *Pediatrics*. 1978; 62: 1–7.

9. Southwood WF. The thickness of the skin. *Plast Reconstr Surg*. 1955; 15(5): 423–429.

10. Rudolph R, Ballantyne DL Jr. Skin grafts. In: McCarthy J, ed. *Plastic Surgery*. Philadelphia: WB Saunders; 1990: 221–274.

11. Supple KG. Physiologic response to burn injury. *Crit Care Nurs Clin North Am*. 2004; 16: 119–126.

12. Bishop JF. Burn wound assessment and surgical management. *Crit Care Nurs Clin North Am*. 2004; 16: 145–177.

13. Yannas IV, Burke JF. Design of artificial skin I. Basic design principles. *J Biomed Mater Res*. 1980; 14(1): 65–81.

14. Gibran NS, Hemibach DM. Current status of burn wound pathophysiology. *Clin Plast Surg*. 2000; 27(1): 11–22.

15. Crowe R, Parkhouse N, McGrouther D, et al. Neuropeptide-containing nerves in painful hypertrophic scar tissue. *Br J Dermatol*. 1994; 130(4): 444–452.

16. Spinks A, Wasiak J, Cleland H, et al. Ten year epidemiological study of pediatric burns in Canada. *J Burn Care Res*. 2008; 29(3): 482–488.

17. *Advanced Burn Life Support Manual*. Chicago: American Burn Association; 2001.

18. Orgel MG, Brown HC, Woolhouse FM. Electrical burns of the mouth in children; a method for assessing results. *J Trauma*. 1975; 15(4): 285–289.

19. Sheridan RL. Evaluating and managing burn wounds. *Derm Nurs*. 2000; 12(1): 8–22.

20. DeSanti L. Pathophysiology and current management of burn injury. *Adv Skin Wound Care*. 2005; 18(6): 323–332.

21. Knaysi GA, Crikelair GF, Crosman B. The rule of nines: its history and accuracy. *Plast Reconstr Surg*. 1968; 41: 560–563.

22. Lund CC, Browder NC. The estimation of areas of burn. *Surg Gynecol Obstet*. 1944; 79: 352–358.

23. Nagel TR, Schunk JE. Using the hand to estimate the surface area of a burn in children. *Pediatr Emerg Care*. 1997; 13(4): 254–255.

24. Arturson G. Pathophysiology of the burn wound and pharmacological treatment. The Rudi Hermans lecture, 1995. *Burns*. 1996; 22(4): 255–274.

25. Artuson G. Pathophysiological aspects of the burn syndrome with special reference to liver injury and alterations of capillary permeability. *Acta Chir Scand*. 1961; 274(suppl): 55.

26. Mulligan MS, Till GO, Smith CW, et al. Role of leukocyte adhesion molecules in lung and dermal vascular injury after thermal trauma to skin. *Am J Pathol*. 1994; 144: 1008–1015.

27. Tyler M, Watts A, Perry M. Dermal cellular inflammation in burns: an insight into the function of dermal microvascular anatomy. *Burns*. 2001; 27: 433–438.

28. Balogh GT, Illes J, Szekely Z, Forrai E, Gere A. Effect of different metal ions on the oxidative damage and antioxidant capacity of hyaluronic acid. *Arch Biochem Biophys*. 2003; 410: 76–82.

29. Rees MD, Hawins CL, Davies MJ. Hypochlorite-mediated fragmentation of hyaluronan, chondroitin sulfates, at related N-acetyl glycosamines: evidence for chloramide intermediates, free radical transfer reactions, and site specific fragmentation. *J Am Chem Soc*. 2003; 125: 13719–13733.

30. Demling RH. The burn edema process: current concepts. *J Burn Care Rehabil*. 2005; 26: 207–227.

31. Ferrara JJ, Westervelt CL, Kukuy EL, et al. Burn edema reduction by methysergide is not due to control of regional vasodilation. *J Surg Res*. 1996; 61(1): 11–16.

32. Lund T, Onarheim H, Reed R. Pathogenesis of edema formation in burn injuries. *World J Surg*. 1992; 16(1): 2–9.

33. Ward PA, Till GO. Pathophysiologic events related to thermal injury of skin. *J Trauma*. 1990; 30(12)(suppl): S75–S79.

34. Saffle JR, Zeluff GR, Warden GD. Intramuscular pressure in the burned arm: measurement and response to escharotomy. *Am J Surg*. 1980; 140: 825–831.

35. Szabo G, Posch E, Magyar Z. Interstitial fluid, lymph, and edema formation. *Acta Physiol Acad Sci Hung*. 1980; 56: 367–378.

36. Jackson DM. The diagnosis of the depth of burning. *Br J Surg*. 1953; 40(164): 588–596.

37. Pham TN, Gibran NS, Heimbach DM. Evaluation of the burn wound: management decisions. In: Herndon DN, ed. *Total Burn Care*. London: WB Saunders; 2007: 119–126.

38. Khabl JS, Bauer W, Andel H, et al. Progression of burn wound depth by systemic application of a vasoconstrictor: an experimental study with a new rabbit model. *Burns*. 1999; 25(8): 715–721.

39. Boykin JV, Eriksson E, Pittman RN. In-vivo microcirculation of a scald burn and the progression of post-burn dermal ischemia. *Plast Reconstr Surg*. 1980; 66: 191–198.

40. Santos FX, Arroyo C, Garcia I, et al. Role of mast cells in the pathogenesis of post burn inflammatory response: reactive oxygen species as mast cell stimulators. *Burns*. 2000; **26**: 145–147.

41. Grantors J, Cassata J. Role of histamine receptors in the regulation of edema and circulation postburn. *Burns*. 2003; **29**: 769–777.

42. Holliman CJ, Meuleman TR, Larsen KR, et al. The effect of ketanserin, a specific serotonin antagonist, on burn shock hemodynamic parameters in a porcine burn model. *J Trauma*. 1983; **23**(10): 867–871.

43. Greenhalgh DG, Saffle JR, Holmes JH 4th, et al. American Burn Association consensus conference to define sepsis and infection in burns. *J Burn Care Res*. 2007; **28**(6): 776–790.

44. Fitzwater J, Purdue GF, Hunt JL, O'Keefe GE. The risk factors and time course of sepsis and organ dysfunction after burn trauma. *J Trauma*. 2003; **54**(5): 959–966.

45. Youn Y, LaLonde C, Demling R. The role of mediators in the response to thermal injury. *World J Surg*. 1992; **16**(1): 30–36.

46. Schwacha MG. Macrophages and post-burn immune dysfunction. *Burns*. 2003; **29**: 1–14.

47. Yeh FL, Lin WL, Shen HD, Fang RH. Changes in circulating levels of interlukin-6 in burned patients. *Burns*. 1999; **25**: 131–136.

48. Yeh FL, Lin WL, Shen HD, Fang RH. Changes in levels of serum IL-8 in burned patients. *Burns*. 1997; **23**(7/8): 555–559.

49. Vindenes H, Ulvestad E, Bjerknes R. Increased levels of circulating interlukin-8 in patients with large burns: relation to burn size and sepsis. *J Trauma*. 1995; **39**(4): 635–640.

50. Deitch EA. Multiple organ failure: pathophysiology and potential future therapy. *Ann Surg*. 1992; **216**: 117–134.

51. Bargues L, Chancerelle Y, Catineau J, Jault P, Carsin H. Evaluation of serum procalcitonin concentration in the ICU following severe burn. *Burns*. 2007; **33**(7): 860–864.

52. Sachse C, Machens HG, Felmerer G, et al. Procalcitonin as a marker for the early diagnosis of severe infection after thermal injury. *J Burn Care Rehabil*. 1999; **20**(5): 354–360.

53. Parihar A, Parihar MS, Milner S, Bhat S. Oxidative stress and anti-oxidative mobilization in burn injury. *Burns*. 2008; **34**: 6–17.

54. Maldonado M, Murillo-Cabezas F, Calvo J, et al. Melatonin as pharmacologic support in burn patients: a proposed solution to thermal injury–related lymphocytopenia and oxidative damage. *Crit Care Med*. 2007; **35**(4): 1177–1185.

55. Sener G, Sehirli A, Satiroglu H, Keyer-Uysal M, Yegen B. Melatonin improves oxidative organ damage in a rat model of thermal injury. *Burns*. 2002; **28**: 419–425.

56. Sener G, Sehirli A, Velioglu-Ogunc A, et al. Propylthiouracil (PTU)-induced hypothyroidism alleviates burn-induced multiple organ injury. *Burns*. 2006; **32**: 728–736.

57. Ivy ME, Possenti PP, Kepros J, et al. Abdominal compartment syndrome in patients with burns. *J Burn Care Rehabil*. 1999; **20**(5): 351–353.

58. Ivy ME, Atweh NA, Palmer J, Possenti PP, Pineau M, D'Aiuto M. Intra-abdominal hypertension and abdominal compartment syndrome in burn patients. *J Trauma*. 2000; **49**(3): 387–391.

59. Oda J, Ueyama M, Yamashita K, et al. Hypertonic lactated saline resuscitation reduces the risk of abdominal compartment syndrome in severely burned patients. *J Trauma*. 2006; **60**(1): 64–71.

60. O'Mara M, Slater H, Goldfarb IW, Caushaj P. A prospective, randomized evaluation of intra-abdominal pressures with crystalloid and colloid resuscitation in burn patients. *J Trauma*. 2005; **58**(5): 1011–1018.

61. Przkora R, Jeschke MG, Barrow RE, et al. Metabolic and hormonal changes of severely burned children receiving long-term oxandrolone treatment. *Ann Surg*. 2005; **242**: 384–389.

62. Pereira CT, Murphy K, Jeschke MG, Herndon DN. Post burn muscle wasting and the effects of treatments. *Int J Biochem Cell Biol*. 2005; **37**: 1948–1961.

63. Frankenfield DC, Smith JS, Cooney RN, et al. Relative association of fever and injury with hypermetabolism in critically ill patients. *Injury*. 1997; **28**: 617.

64. Stoner HB. Interpretation of the metabolic effects of trauma and sepsis. *J Clin Pathol*. 1987; **40**: 1108–1117.

65. Yu YM, Tompkins RG, Ryan CM, Young VR. The metabolic basis of the increase in energy expenditure in severely burned patients. *J Parenter Enteral Nutr*. 1999; **23**: 160–168.

66. Hart DW, Wolf SE, Chinkes DL, et al. Determinants of skeletal muscle catabolism after severe burn. *Ann Surg*. 2000; **232**: 455–465.

67. Arora NS, Rochester DF. Respiratory muscle strength and maximal voluntary ventilation in undernourished patients. *Am Rev Respir Dis*. 1982; **126**: 5–8.

68. Herndon DN. Mediators of metabolism. *J Trauma*. 1981; **21**: 701–705.

69. Bessey P, Jiang Z, Johnson D, Smith R, Wilmore D. Posttraumatic skeletal muscle proteolysis: the role of the hormonal environment. *World J Surg*. 1989; **13**: 465–470.

70. Hart DW, Wolf SE, Ramzy PI, et al. Anabolic effects of oxandrolone after severe burn. *Ann Surg*. 2000; **233**(4): 556–564.

71. Hart DW, Wolf SE, Mclak RP, et al. Persistence of muscle catabolism after severe burn. *Surgery*. 2000; **128**: 312–319.

72. Gore DC, Chinkes DL, Hart DW, Wolf SE, Herndon DN, Sanford AP. Hyperglycemia exacerbates muscle protein catabolism in burn-injured patients. *Crit Care Med*. 2002; **30**: 2438–2442.

73. Flakoll PJ, Kill JO, Abumrad NN. Acute hyperglycemia enhances proteolysis in normal man. *Am J Physiol*. 1993; **265**: E715–E721.

74. Jahoor F, Shangraw RE, Miyoshi H, Wallfish H, Herndon DN, Wolfe RR. Role of insulin and glucose oxidation in mediating the protein catabolism of burns and sepsis. *Am J Physiol*. 1989; **257**: E323–E331.

75. Thomas SJ, Morimoto K, Herndon DN, et al. The effect of prolonged euglcemic hyperinsulinemia on lean body mass after severe burn. *Surgery*. 2002; **132**: 341–347.

76. Wilmore DW, Curreri PW, Spitzer KW. Supranormal diet in thermally injured patients. *Surg Gynecol Obstet*. 1971; **132**: 881.

77. Mifflin MD, St Jeor ST, Hill LA, et al. A new predictive equation for resting energy expenditure in healthy individuals. *Am J Clin Nutr*. 1990; **51**(2): 241–247.

78. Herndon DN, Tompkins RG. Support of the metabolic response to burn injury. *Lancet*. 2004; **363**: 1895–1902.

79. Barret JP, Jeschke MG, Herndon DN. Fatty infiltration of the liver in severely burned pediatric patients: autopsy findings and clinical implications. *J Trauma*. 2001; **51**: 736–739.

80. Herndon DN, Hart DW, Wolf SE, Chinkes DL, Wolfe RR. Reversal of catabolism by beta-blockade after severe burns. *N Eng J Med*. 2001; **345**: 1223–1229.

81. Jeschke MG, Barrow RE, Herndon DN. Recombinant human growth hormone treatment in pediatric burn patients and its role during the hepatic acute phase response. *Crit Care Med*. 2000; **28**: 1578–1584.

82. Ramirez RJ, Wolf SE, Barrow RE, Herndon DN. Growth hormone treatment in pediatric burns: a safe therapeutic response. *Ann Surg*. 1998; **228**: 439–448.

83. Ferrando AA, Sheffield-Moore M, Wolf SE, Herndon DN, Wolfe DD. Testosterone administration in severe burns ameliorates muscle catabolism. *Crit Care Med*. 2001; **29**: 1936–1942.

84. Demling RH, DeSanti L. Oxandrolone induced lean mass gain during recovery from severe burns is maintained after discontinuation of the anabolic steroid. *Burns*. 2003; **29**: 793–797.

85. Holm C, Hörbrand F, von Donnersmarck GH, Mühlbauer W. Acute renal failure in severely burned patients. *Burns*. 1999; **25**(2): 171–178.

86. Schiavon M, DiLandro D, Baldo M, et al. A study of renal damage in seriously burned patients. *Burns*. 1994; **20**: 71–73.

87. Sawada Y, Momma S, Takamizawa A, et al. Survival from acute renal failure after severe burns. *Burns*. 1984; **11**: 143–147.

88. Jeschke MG, Barrow RE, Wolf SE, Herndon DN. Mortality in burned children with acute renal failure. *Arch Surg*. 1998; **133**(7): 752–756.

89. Chrysopoulo MT, Jeschke MG, Dziewulski P, Barrow RE, Herndon DN. Acute renal dysfunction in severely burned adults. *J Trauma*. 1999; **46**(1): 141–144.

90. Aikawa N, Wakabayashi G, Ueda M, et al. Regulation of renal function in thermal injury. *J Trauma*. 1990; **30**(suppl 12): 5174–5178.

91. Holm C, Hörbrand F, von Donnersmarck GH, et al. Acute renal failure in the severely burned. *Burns*. 1999; **25**: 171–178.

92. Herndon DN, Barrow RE, Rutan RL, et al. A comparison of conservative versus early excision. *Ann Surg*. 1989; **209**: 547–553.

93. Rodriguez JL, Miller CO, Garner WL, et al. Correlation of the local and systemic cytokine response with clinical outcome following thermal injury. *J Trauma*. 1993; **34**: 684–694.

94. Mustonen KM, Vuola J. Acute renal failure in intensive care burn patients. *J Burn Care Res*. 2008; **29**(1): 227–237.

95. Haubrich WS. Curling of Curling's ulcer. *Gastroenterology*. 1998; **114**(5): 901.

96. Carter EA, Udall JN, Kirkham SE, Walker WA. Thermal injury and gastrointestinal function. *J Burn Care Rehabil*. 1986; 7(6): 469–474.

97. Ramzy PI, Wolf SE, Irtun O, Hart DW, Thompson JC, Herndon DN. Gut epithelial apoptosis after severe burn: effects of gut hypoperfusion. *J Am Coll Surg*. 2000; **190**(3): 281–283.

98. Wolf SE, Ikeda H, Matin S, Debroy MA, Rajaraman S, Herndon DN. Cutaneous burn increases apoptosis in the gut epithelium of mice. *J Am Coll Surg*. 1999; **188**(1): 10–16.

99. Othman M, Aguero R, Lin H. Alterations in intestinal microbial flora and human disease. *Gastroenterology*. 2008; **24**(1): 11–16.

100. LeVoyer T, Cioffi WJ, Pratt L, et al. Alterations in intestinal permeability after thermal injury. *Arch Surg*. 1992; **127**: 26–29, discussion 29–30.

101. Ryan C, Yarmush M, Burke J, Tompkins R. Increased gut permeability early after burns correlates with the extent of burn injury. *Crit Care Med*. 1992; **20**: 1508–1512.

102. Magnotti L, Upperman J, Xu D, et al. Gut-derived mesenteric lymph but not portal blood increases endothelial cell permeability and promotes lung injury after hemorrhagic shock. *Ann Surg*. 1998; **228**: 518–527.

103. Epstein MD, Banducci DR, Manders EK. The role of the gastrointestinal tract in the development of burn sepsis. *Plast Reconstr Surg*. 1992; **90**(3): 524–531.

104. Wasiak J, Cleland H, Jeffery R. Early versus delayed enteral nutrition support for burn injuries. Cochrane Database of Systematic Reviews. Issue 3, Art. No.: CD005489. The Cochrane Library. http://www.cochrane.org/reviews. Jul 19, 2006.

105. Pruitt BA Jr. Complications of thermal injury. *Clin Plast Surg*. 1974; **1**: 667–691.

106. Wolf SE, Jeschke MG, Rose JK, Desai MH, Herndon DN. Enteral feeding intolerance: an indicator of sepsis-associated mortality in burned children. *Arch Surg*. 1997; **132**(12): 1310–1314.

107. Tokyay R, Loick HM, Traber DL, Heggers JP, Herndon DN. Effects of thromboxane synthetase inhibition on postburn mesenteric vascular resistance and the rate of bacterial translocation in a chronic porcine model. *Surg Gynecol Obstet*. 1992; **174**: 125–132.

108. Reines HD, Halushka PV, Cook JA. Plasma thromboxane concentrations are raised in patients dying with septic shock. *Lancet*. 1982; **2**: 174–175.

109. Zawacki BE, Jung RC, Joyce J, Rincon E. Smoke, burns, and the natural history of inhalation injury in fire victims: a correlation of experimental and clinical data. *Ann Surg*. 1977; **185**(1): 100–110.

110. Thompson PB, Herndon DN, Traber DL, et al. Effect on mortality of inhalation injury. *J Trauma*. 1986; **26**: 163–165.

111. Finnerty CC, Herndon DN, Jeschke MG. Inhalation injury in severely burned children does not augment the systemic inflammatory response. *Critical Care*. 2007; **11**(1): R22.

112. Fraser JF, Mullany D, Traber D. Inhalational lung injury in patients with severe thermal burns. *Contemp Crit Care*. 2007; **4**(9): 1–12.

113. Birky MM, Clarke FB. Inhalation of toxic products from fires. *Bull N Y Acad Med*. 1981; **57**: 997–1013.

114. Herndon DN, Traber LD, Linares H, et al. Etiology of the pulmonary pathophysiology associated with inhalation injury. *Resuscitation*. 1986; **14**: 43–59.

115. Herndon DN, Traber DL, Traber LD. The effect of resuscitation on inhalation injury. *Surgery*. 1986; **100**: 248–251.

116. Calhoun KH, Deskin RW, Garza C, et al. Long-term airway sequelae in a pediatric burn population. *Laryngoscope*. 1988; **98**: 721–725.

117. Merrel P, Mayo D. Inhalation injury in the burn patient. *Critical Care Nurs Clin North Am*. 2004; **16**: 27–38.

118. Still J, Friedman B, Law E, et al. Burns due to exposure to steam. *Burns*. 2001; **27**(4): 379–381.

119. Soejima K, McGuire R, Snyder NT, et al. The effect of inducible nitric oxide synthase (iNOS) inhibition on smoke inhalation injury in sheep. *Shock*. 2000; **13**: 261–266.

120. Linares HA, Herndon DN, Traber DL. Sequence of morphologic events in experimental smoke inhalation. *J Burn Care Rehabil*. 1989; **10**: 27–37.

121. Traber DL, Herndon DN, Stein MD, et al. The pulmonary lesion of smoke inhalation in the ovine model. *Circ Shock*. 1986; **18**: 311–323.

122. Herndon DN, Traber DL, Niehaus GD, et al. The pathophysiology of smoke inhalation in a sheep model. *J Trauma*. 1984; **24**: 1044–1051.

123. Cox RA, Burke AS, Soejima K, et al. Airway obstruction in sheep with burn and smoke inhalation injuries. *Am J Respir Cell Mol Biol*. 2003; **29**(3, pt 1): 295–302.

124. Enkhbaatar P, Traber DL. Pathophysiology of acute lung injury in combined burn and smoke inhalation injury. *Clin Sci*. 2004; **107**: 137–143.

125. Traber DL, Herndon DN, Enkhbaatar P, Maybauer MO, Maybauer DM. The pathophysiology of inhalation injury. In: Herndon DN, ed. *Total Burn Care*. London: WB Saunders; 2007: 248–261.

126. Youn YK, Lalonde C, Demling R. Oxidants and the pathophysiology of burn and smoke inhalation injury. *Free Radic Biol Med*. 1992; **12**: 409–415.

127. Seeger W, Stohr G, Wolf HR, Neuhof H. Alteration of surfactant function due to protein leakage: special interaction with fibrin monomer. *J Appl Physiol*. 1985; **58**: 326–338.

128. Terrill JB, Montgomery RR, Reinhardt CF. Toxic gases from fires. *Science*. 1978; **200**: 1343–1347.

129. Coburn RF, Forman HJ. Carbon monoxide toxicity. In: Fishman AP, ed. *Handbook of Physiology*. Vol. 4, *Gas Exchange*. Bethesda, MD: American Physiological Society; 1987: 439–456.

130. Myers RAM, Snyder SK, Lindberg S, et al. Value of hyperbaric oxygen in suspected carbon monoxide poisoning. *JAMA*. 1981; **264**: 2478–2481.

131. Roughton FJ, Darling RC. The effect of carbon monoxide on the oxyhemoglobin dissociation curve. *Am J Physiol*. 1944; **141**: 17–31.

132. Colburn RF, Mayers LB. Myglobin O2 tension determined from measurement of carboxymyoglobin in skeletal muscle. *Am J Physiol*. 1973; **220**: 66–74.

133. Cancio LC. Current concepts in the pathophysiology and treatment of inhalation injury. *Trauma*. 2005; **7**: 19–35.

134. Zhang J, Piantadosi CA. Mitochondrial oxidative stress after carbon monoxide hypoxia in the rat brain. *J Clin Invest*. 1992; **90**: 1193–1199.

135. Longo LD, Hill EP. Carbon monoxide uptake and elimination in fetal and maternal sheep. *Am J Physiol*. 1977; **232**: H324–H330.

136. Parrish RA. Smoke inhalation and carbon monoxide poisoning in children. *Pediatr Emerg Care*. 1986; **2**(1): 36–39.

137. Shillito F. The problem of nervous and mental sequelae in carbon monoxide poisoning. *JAMA*. 1936; **106**: 669–672.

138. Smith JS, Brandon S. Morbidity from acute carbon monoxide poisoning at a three year follow–up. *Br Med J*. 1973; **1**: 319–321.

139. Linares HA. A report of 115 consecutive autopsies in burned children: 1966–1980. *Burns*. 1982; **8**: 263–270.

140. Sheridan R, Remensnyder J, Prelack K, Petras L, Lydon M. Treatment of the seriously burned infant. *J Burn Care Rehabil*. 1998; **19**(2): 115–118.

141. Herndon, DN, Rutan, R, Rutan TC. Management of the pediatric patient with burns. *J Burn Care Rehabil*. 1993; **14**(1): 3–8.

142. Consumer Product Safety Commission. http://www.cpsc.gov/cpscpub/pubs/16.html. Sept 15, 2008.

143. Consumer Product Safety Commission. http://www.cpsc.gov/cpscpub/pubs/524.html. Sept 15, 2008

144. Rabban JT, Blair JA, Rosen CL, Adler JN, Sheridan RL. Mechanisms of pediatric electrical injury: new implications for product safety and injury prevention. *Arch Pediatr Adolesc Med*. 1997; **151**(7): 696–700.

145. Celik A, Ergün O, Ozok G. Pediatric electrical injuries: a review of 38 consecutive patients. *J Pediatr Surg*. 2004; **39**: 1233–1237.

146. Bingham H. Electrical burns. *Clin Plast Surg*. 1986; **13**: 75–85.

147. Jain S, Bandi V. Electrical and lightning injuries. *Crit Care Clin*. 199; **15**: 319–331.

148. Block TA, Aarsvold JN, Matthews KL II, et al. The 1995 Lindberg Award. Nonthermally mediated muscle injury and necrosis in electric trauma. *J Burn Care Rehabil*. 1995; **16**: 581–588.

149. Rouse RG, Dimick AR. The treatment of electrical injury compared to burn injury: a review of pathophysiology and

comparison of patient management protocols. *J Trauma.* 1978; **18**(1): 43–47.

**150.** Spies C, Trohman R. Narrative review: electrocution and life-threatening electrical injuries. *Ann Intern Med.* 2006; **145**(7): 531–537.

**151.** Solem L, Fischer RP, Strate RG. The natural history of electrical injury. *J Trauma.* 1977; **17**: 487–492.

**152.** Garcia CT, Smith GA, Cohen DM, Fernandez K. Electrical injuries in a pediatric emergency department. *Ann Emerg Med.* 1995; **26**: 604–608.

**153.** James TN, Riddick L, Embry JH. Cardiac abnormalities demonstrated post-mortem in four cases of accidental electrocution and their potential significance relative to nonfatal electrical injuries to the heart. *Am Heart J.* 1990; **120**: 143–157.

**154.** Ku CS, Lin SL, Hsu TL, Wang SP, Chang MS. Myocardial damage associated with electrical injury. *Am Heart J.* 1989; **118**: 621–624.

**155.** Cherington M. Neurologic manifestations of lightning strikes. *Neurology.* 2003; **60**: 182–185.

**156.** Butler ED, Gant TD. Electrical injuries with special reference to the upper extremities. A review of 182 cases. *Am J Surg.* 1977; **134**: 95–101

**157.** Hunt JL, Mason AR, Masterson TS, Pruitt BA. The pathophysiology of acute electric injuries. *J Trauma.* 1976; **16**(5): 335–340.

**158.** Thomson HG, Juckes AW, Farmer AW. Electric burns to the mouth in children. *Plast Reconstr Surg.* 1965; **35**(5): 466–477.

**159.** Lown B, Neuman J, Amarasigham R, et al. Comparison of alternating current with direct electroshock across the closed chest. *Am J Cardiol.* 1962; **10**(2): 223–233.

**160.** Winfree J, Barillo D. Nonthermal injuries. *Nurs Clin North Am.* 1997; **32**(2): 275–296.

**161.** Simpson LA, Cruse CW. Gasoline immersion injury. *Plast Reconstr Surg.* 1981; **67**(1): 54–57.

**162.** Bautista Casasnovas A, Estevez Martinez R, Varela Cives R, Villanueva Jeremias A, Tojo Sierra R, Cadranel S. A retrospective analysis of ingestion of caustic substances by children, ten-year statistics in Galicia. *Eur J Pediatr.* 1997; **156**: 410–414.

**163.** Mozingo DW, Smith AA, McManus WF, Pruitt BA, Mason AD. Chemical burns. *J Trauma.* 1988; **28**(5): 642–647.

**164.** Murphy JV, Banwell PE, Roberts HN, McGrouther DA. Frostbite: pathogenesis and treatment. *J Trauma.* 2000; **48**(1): 171–178.

**165.** Heggers JP, Robson MC, Manavalen K, et al. Experimental and clinical observations on frostbite. *Ann Emerg Med.* 1987; **16**: 1056–1062.

**166.** Washburn B. Frostbite. *N Engl J Med.* 1962; **266**: 974–989.

**167.** Britt LD, Dascombe WH, Rodriguez A. New horizons in management of hypothermia and frostbite injury. *Surg Clin North Am.* 1991; **71**: 345–370.

# CHAPTER SEVEN

# PEDIATRIC BURN RESUSCITATION

BRADLEY J. PHILLIPS, MD

## INTRODUCTION

### General Incidence and Mortality Figures

In the year 2000, an estimated 10000 children younger than the age of 18 years were hospitalized with burn-associated injuries in the United States.[1] Although the majority of pediatric burn patients survive and go on to lead healthy, productive lives, deaths from fire and burn-related injuries are still the second leading cause of unintentional death for 1- to 9-year-olds and the third leading cause for African American 10- to 19-year-olds.[2] Male pediatric burn patients considerably outnumber female patients,[1] and African Americans are disproportionately affected in the 1-to-9-year-old age group.[2] Most importantly, children under the age of 4 years continue to have a 2 to 2.7 higher risk of mortality (dependent upon age) as a result of burn-related injuries compared to older children.[3] However, data from the National Burn Repository for the years 1995 to 2005[4]

show a mortality rate of about 1.5%, which is about less than half the typical rate for the years 1982 to 1985.[5] This significant achievement is in part due to improvements in burn shock resuscitation and an aggressive approach to overall care, including intensivist-directed protocols.

### Early Studies in Brief

The first 48 hours of treating a pediatric burn patient are by far the most critical due to burn-induced hypovolemic shock and vascular compartmental imbalance. The extensive fluid loss that starts within minutes of the injury was first recognized by Underhill,[6] who in 1921 studied the victims of the Rialto Theater fire in New Haven, Connecticut. This concept was also understood by Cope, the senior surgeon at Massachusetts General Hospital, who, with assistance from Moore, his resident, treated many of the burn victims from the 1942 Cocoanut Grove nightclub fire in Boston. Their subsequent research led to an approach in which fluid was given to combat the consequences of the fast-developing edema and loss of intravascular volume.[7] A team led by Evans et al[8] from the Medical College of Richmond, however, was the first to report a simple surface area/weight-based formula that utilized a 1:1 ratio of intravenous electrolytes (crystalloid) and colloids (high-molecular-weight materials, such as proteins or dextrans) to guide resuscitation; this combination was then titrated to individual needs based upon urine output and hemoglobin concentration. The Evans formula, as it became known, was quickly revised by researchers at the Brooke Army Medical Center in San Antonio to include Ringer's lactate solution (the Brooke formula).[9] In part this was due to a recognition that metabolic acidosis played a role in burn shock and that adding sodium bicarbonate helped correct the base deficit.

## Development of Resuscitation Formulas

Based upon differing schools of thought, a number of resuscitation formulas and various methods for calculating their infusion rate were published from the 1950s to the 1970s. One of the most highly debated points was (and is) the use of colloid. A key study conducted by Baxter and Shires in 1968,[10] which employed radioisotope dilution techniques, demonstrated that the composition of edema fluid in early postburn wounds was isotonic with respect to plasma and that the protein concentrations in the two compartments were essentially similar. This led to the authors' conclusion that adding protein during resuscitation was futile because it simply escaped into the interstitial space, which was the primary reason why the formula that Baxter[11] later developed was colloid-free. This approach became known as the Parkland formula, named after the Parkland Hospital in Dallas, Texas, where Baxter practiced; at present, it is the most commonly used formula in the United States.

The Baxter-Parkland formula uses lactated Ringer's solution and is infused at a rate of 4 mL/kg/percent of burn area for the first 24 hours of resuscitation, with one half administered in the first 8 hours. A review conducted by Baxter[12] of 516 children under the age of 12 years admitted during the years 1973 to 1977 indicated that only 2% exceeded the guideline of 4 ± 0.3 mL, although the deviation rate for adults was 30%. In this review, resuscitation endpoints were urine output (>40 mL/hour) and cardiac output. Interestingly, only 4 deaths occurred in this pediatric group: all had burns exceeding 50% of TBSA (total body surface area), all were younger than 3 years, and all experienced a delay of 3 to 6 hours in resuscitation.

In their review of 177 children under the age of 13 years, conducted at the Intermountain Burn Center in Salt Lake City, Utah (1978-1985), Merrell et al[13] also employed the Parkland formula, modified to include basal fluid requirements.

Interestingly, their intravenous infusion rates were titrated to a urinary endpoint of 1 mL/kg/h. Clinical assessment included serum electrolyte levels and hematocrit, supported by data from urinary catheters, arterial lines, and at times CVP (central venous pressure) catheters. Children who required twice the predicted amount of crystalloid were switched to hypertonic lactated Ringer's solution (180-230 mEq/sodium/L), and exchange transfusion at 1.5 times the patient's calculated blood volume was initiated in unresponsive patients. In this study, resuscitation volumes for children versus adults were reversed compared to the study of Baxter,[12] with an average of 5.80 mL/kg/% BSA (burn surface area). Early mortality rate was 7% versus 15% for the final mortality rate.

Two points emerge from a comparison of these studies: (1) considerably higher resuscitation volumes were reported by Merrell et al, and (2) the mortality rates were much higher in the study of Merrell et al[13] compared to that of Baxter,[12] although not out of line with previously reported studies.[14,15] In addition, based upon regression analysis, Merrell et al[13] were among the first to question the long-held idea that the higher surface area to body weight ratio in children was responsible for the increased resuscitation volumes.

The higher resuscitation volumes reported by Merrell et al[13] also caused the investigators at the US Army Institute of Surgical Research to initiate a retrospective study of their patients.[16] This group utilized the modified Brooke formula, which is composed of lactated Ringer's solution at 3 mL/kg/percent of burn area—less than the Parkland formula—titrated to 1 ml/kg/h urine output. The formula was administered in the same manner as Parkland, although the calculation of maintenance fluid requirements was different. Even though the mean age of patients was much younger (2.2 years vs. 4 years), the injuries were more severe in terms of % BSA (41.7% vs. 27.3%), mean full-thickness percentage was greater (23.7% vs. 12.6%), and the associated inhalation injury rate was much higher (21% vs. 12%), the results demonstrated that the mean resuscitation volume was 3.91 mL/kg/percent of burn area, only a 30% excess compared to a 45% excess for Merrell et al.[13]

Do these results mean that groups of patients at different facilities were overresuscitated or underresuscitated with regard to volume compared to other groups? This is not an easy question to answer, but it is a key point, because the problem of overresuscitation has become increasingly frequent since the 1980s. Some investigators believe that more aggressive endpoints and inotropic treatment are the major causes, as exemplified by a recent study that randomized patients to 1 of 2 possible treatments.[17] In this trial, the control group was resuscitated with the Baxter-Parkland formula (4 mL/kg/percent of burn area; 5.6 mL/kg/percent of burn area in cases of verified inhalation injury) using conventional endpoints (minimum urine output 0.5 mL

/kg/h, mean arterial pressure >70 mmHg, and central venous pressure >2 cm $H_2O$ above PEEP [positive end-expiratory pressure]). In the experimental group, the endpoint goals were an intrathoracic blood volume index (ITBV) >800 mL/m$^2$ and a cardiac index >3.5 L/min/m$^2$. Although the mean age of the patients was 41.3 years, clearly marking this study as an adult investigation, the mean resuscitation volume during the first 24 hours of the control group almost matched the predicted volume based upon the Baxter formula (16.2 L vs. 16.0 L). However, the experimental group received 27.1 L. Mortality rates were slightly higher in the control group compared to the experimental group (40% vs. 32%). The message from this study seems to be that more aggressive endpoints may account for excessive crystalloid resuscitation, but even more importantly, may not confer a significant benefit when the risks of overresuscitation are taken into account. This point will be further discussed in the context of burn pathophysiology.

## Colloid

Not all burn specialists agree with just using the Parkland or modified Brooke formula to resuscitate pediatric burn patients during the first 24 hours. For example, the group at the Shriner's Burns Institute in Galveston by the late 1970s added both glucose and colloid to the basic lactated Ringer's solution (47.5 g/L glucose, 12.5 g/L albumin); significant amounts of antacids (Maalox, 30 mL/m$^2$ body surface area) were also given orally or through a nasogastric tube.[18] In this small study of 30 children, no mortality occurred as result of the treatment, although 17% later died of infectious complications. In addition, there was no reported overresuscitation, although this is hard to judge due to the presentation of the data and the fact that relatively vague endpoints were used.

The effect of adding colloid to the resuscitation formula was investigated on dogs by the same group to test the hypothesis that colloid added early after a burn could decrease the amount of plasma lost to interstitial spaces.[19] The results demonstrated that fluid loss 6 hours postburn was much higher when only lactated Ringer's solution was used compared to adding 5% albumin. The fluid loss was also inversely proportional to the amount of albumin administered. Furthermore, the severely depressed cardiac output that occurs after a burn was modestly increased relative to the output 2 hours postburn in proportion to the amount of albumin given. Hematocrit values were also much more normal in the group of dogs given albumin (likely a reflection of dilution in the LR group). The conclusion of these experiments—in agreement with previous observations and experiments—seemed to confirm the concept that adding colloid to the resuscitation approach decreased the amount of fluid escaping to the extravascular space.

Demling's group,[20] based in Boston, agreed with the general principle of adding colloid, but their experiments suggested that adding colloid was not helpful until recovery of membrane semipermeability began. Moreover, they favored the use of dextrans because of higher colloid osmotic pressure and lower expense compared to albumin. In fact, in a sheep model, using CVP and pulmonary wedge pressure (PWP) as endpoints, one group was resuscitated with lactated Ringer's solution commencing 2 hours postburn, while the experimental group received a 10% solution of low-molecular-weight dextran in saline. The findings were unequivocal: the control group required a resuscitation volume of 75 mL/kg while the experimental group required only 35 mL/kg, with mean urine outputs of 65 mL/kg and 40 mL/kg, respectively. The net fluid requirements translated to 3.5 mL/kg/% TBSA and 1.5 mL/kg/% TBSA, respectively.

By the mid-1980s, therefore, it should have been clear that adding colloids to the resuscitation approach—for example, 12 hours postburn—was a more effective method than just using isotonic crystalloid. Why did this not happen? Principally for 2 reasons: first, there was no evidence that adding colloid improved outcomes in terms of *mortality*—indeed, to the contrary, a meta-analysis conducted by Schierhout and Roberts[21] later showed that colloid administration was associated with an *increase* in mortality in critically ill patients (however, the majority of these were not burn patients); and second, a movement to use hypertonic saline had gained support.

## Hypertonic Saline

Based on earlier work, Monafo et al[22] published a key paper in 1973 which appeared to demonstrate that the use of hypertonic saline (240-300 mEq of sodium) could substantially reduce the amount of fluid necessary to resuscitate a patient while providing the same overall sodium load. The concept was a simple one: reduce the shift of intravascular water into extracellular spaces by increasing the osmolality of the plasma. One of the additional benefits was thought to be an increase in urine output because the kidneys are required to deal with a higher osmotic work load.

Although Monafo et al[22] were unable to observe a benefit with pediatric patients, Caldwell and Bowser[23] undertook a prospective study to determine if this was truly the case. Although a small study (N = 37) comparing the use of hypertonic saline (experimental) against lactated Ringer's solution (control), the authors reported that despite a 38% greater water load received by the control group, the cumulative urine volume was not significantly greater until 48 hours postburn (2.1 vs. 1.2 mL/kg/percent burn). Monafo et al[24] then published a subsequent study in

1984 that involved 74 patients with a greater burn injury (mean 63% TBSA) and a high percentage of inhalation injury (47%). Again, patients treated with hypertonic saline required significantly less fluid (44% less than a control group treated with lactated Ringer's solution). Water and sodium load requirements generally increased in concert with larger burns, although the correlation was poor. Patients older than 60 years required significantly higher water and sodium loads, although the authors reported no excess requirements regarding inhalation injury. Factors that accounted for the high mortality rate (42%) included advanced age and inhalation injury. While there was a significant difference between water and sodium loads required by survivors and nonsurvivors, there was no significant correlation between the amount of sodium administered in the resuscitation fluid and outcome, which used urine output as the endpoint and mortality rate as outcome.

Gunn et al[25] also studied adult burn patients using hypertonic lactated saline (HLS) and lactated Ringer's solutions (LR), although the study was smaller (N = 51) and the mean burned area was much smaller (23%). However, the investigators did not observe any significant difference in any of the parameters measured, except for differences in pulmonary artery wedge pressure (PAWP) and stroke volume index. What is also noteworthy in this trial is that patients received colloid (fresh frozen plasma) to maintain a serum albumin over 2 g/dL. In addition, many patients were given enteral feeding support during the first 24 hours. Since no mortality data were reported, it is difficult to correlate the resuscitation procedures with outcomes and compare this approach to other studies. Resuscitation volumes were 5.4 mL/kg/percent burn for both groups, which is much higher compared to other literature values of the time for HTS treatment, and ought to have been lower if the plasma given actually had a substantial impact. In conclusion, this was one of the first papers to report "disappointing" results with HTS.

In 1995, Huang et al[26] published an alarming report showing that resuscitation with HTS was associated with a 2-fold increase in mortality rate compared to patients resuscitated with LR. This was attributed in part to a 4-fold increase in renal failure. Moreover, while total resuscitation volumes were lower during the first 24 hours in the HTS group compared to the 2 LR groups, after 48 hours cumulative fluid loads were similar and total sodium load was higher in the hypertonic saline group.

The results of this study were unexpected given the outcomes of previous investigations, but in reality, no one had attempted such a rigorous examination of outcomes before. It had been known for some time that the consequences of hypernatremia could be devastating, even when guidelines restricting plasma sodium levels to less than 160 mEq/L

were followed.[24,25] In particular, subarachnoid and subdural hemorrhages were known risks associated with hypernatremia.[27] Moreover, correcting hypernatremia too quickly carries attendant penalties.[28,29] Despite minor deviations compared to previous hypertonic saline resuscitation protocols, the ensuing debate did not find any major flaws with the study, and the paper today remains a cautionary tale for all who still use HTS in resuscitating burn patients. Perhaps the most illuminating item to come from this investigation is that in hypovolemic patients, HTS infusions per se do not cause the kidney to increase its output, as will be discussed in a later section of this chapter.

## Endpoints

Prior to the late 1980s, clinicians principally used urinary and cardiac output parameters as their primary endpoints for resuscitation of burn patients during the first 48 hours, augmented by vital signs and mental status. However, a few practitioners had gained experience with invasive cardiac monitoring in difficult cases, and a key series was published by Dries and Waxman in 1991.[30] This review of 14 patients documented fluid challenges during resuscitation (boluses of fluid given within 30 minutes, varying from 0.5 L to 2 L) by observing urine output as well as hemodynamic and oxygen transport variables obtained from flow-directed, balloon-tip pulmonary artery catheters (PACs) and cardiac output parameters acquired by using the thermodilution technique. All the patients were critically ill, and 9 patients died of sepsis after the first 48 hours. After fluid challenge, both cardiac index (CI) and oxygen delivery ($DO_2$) increased, and in half of the patients, $VO_2$ (oxygen consumption) increased concurrently with fluid challenge, although changes in this parameter were not detected by vital signs or urine output. These findings suggested that in some patients, an apparently acceptable set of vital signs and urine output masked an inadequate plasma volume to meet increased oxygen and metabolic demands. In other words, a tissue oxygen deficit occurred in 50% of the patients—this was recognized only by invasive monitoring and would have gone unnoticed using traditional endpoints. Thus in theory, these authors suggested that invasive monitoring allows titration of resuscitation volumes, infusing additional volume in cases of tissue oxygen deficit, but minimizing volume in those cases in which it is not needed, thus potentially decreasing the edema. Against these new endpoints, however, must be weighed the attendant risks that invasive monitoring brings, especially in the young neonate or infant.

Similar invasive monitoring trials had been going on in the field of severe trauma, based on earlier work by Shoemaker and others.[31,32] For example, Fleming et al[33] conducted a randomized controlled trial (RCT) enrolling patients into either a control group (resuscitation guided by vital signs, hemoglobin levels, CVP, wedge pressure, and urine output) or an experimental group in which resuscitation was guided by achieving a $DO_2$ target of 670 mL/min/m², a $VO_2$ target of 166 mL/min/m², and a CI of 4.52 L/min within 24 hours of admission and maintaining these goals through the first 48 hours of resuscitation. The mortality rates were 23% for the experimental group and 44% for the control group, which was not statistically significant. However, for the 47 study patients that had more severe blood loss (3-10 L), the difference was more pronounced: 18% vs. 44%. Furthermore, in the 27 patients that reached supranormal values within 24 hours, the mortality rate (15%) was significantly lower compared to those patients who took longer to reach the targeted values (54%). Interestingly, mean cardiac and oxygen transport parameters for the control and experimental groups started diverging 8 hours postadmission.

These results encouraged similar studies to be undertaken in the field of burn resuscitation. For example, Schiller et al[34] undertook a retrospective review of patient records from 1990 to 1994 and divided them into 3 groups: (1) 53 patients for whom hyperdynamic circulatory endpoints were utilized by employing a PAC during 1992-1993 (index group); (2) a match-paired group of 33 patients in which traditional endpoints were utilized during 1990-1991 (control group); and (3) a third group of 30 patients designated as a protocol group, in which a written resuscitation protocol was utilized that incorporated lessons learned from previous experiences prior to 1994 following an aggressive series of oxygen transport and hemodynamic endpoints. Mortality steadily decreased over the time period studied, and the incidence of resuscitation failure and associated death significantly decreased during the same time period. Mortality rates were 48% for the control group, 32% for the index group, and 10% for the protocol group, despite comparable BSAs, age, and inhalation injuries. Resuscitation volumes for the control group were close to that predicted by the Parkland formula, whereas volumes for the other groups were much higher. The authors concluded that "resuscitation of burn victims to a higher circulatory standard improves microcirculatory flow, tissue perfusion, and tissue organization, thereby protecting organ function."[34(p14)]

Despite these and other encouraging studies, many clinicians were far from being persuaded that invasive monitoring, particularly that which required PACs, was the wave of the future, especially when the study of Connors et al[35] was published in *JAMA* in 1996.[36,37] Using case-matching analysis, Connors et al[35] found that patients with a PAC had an increased 30-day mortality (OR 1.24, 95% CI: 1.03-1.49; OR = odds ratio, CI = confidence interval). Moreover, the mean cost per hospital stay was $49300 with a PAC and

$35700 without it. This was a large (N = 5735), well-conducted study whose results were surprising, in part because no other study had so vividly demonstrated such a lack of cost-benefit, and there were no ready explanations for the increased mortality.

However, while this study raised the alarm concerning PACs, it did not impede advances in the search for less invasive and more elegant approaches to setting aggressive goals for burn resuscitation endpoints. One such approach is ITBV: intrathoracic blood volumes.

ITBV has most recently been measured by the transpulmonary double-indicator dilution (TPID) technique, which employs a CV catheter and an arterial fiberoptic thermistor catheter inserted into the femoral artery.[38] TPID utilizes both temperature and dye dilution principles to obtain a variety of cardiac parameters,[39] and includes the possibility to calculate extravascular lung water (EVLW), which can offer an accurate estimate of interstitial water in the lung.

A fair correlation between ITBV and CI was obtained ($R^2 = 0.445$) in an observational study of 24 burn patients, although the correlation between ITBV and $DO_2$ was poor ($R^2 = 0.247$), and there was no correlation between CVP and CI or $DO_2$. However, the correlation between ITBV and $DO_2$ did permit optimization of oxygen delivery, although the end result was a substantially larger resuscitation volume compared to the predicted volumes using the Parkland formula. Importantly, ITBV-guided resuscitation allowed preload restoration and peripheral oxygen delivery within 24 hours. EVLW did not increase in parallel with ITBV, suggesting, as other studies had found,[40,41] that pulmonary complications are less associated with crystalloid resuscitation per se than with sepsis or pulmonary capillary permeability. A more recent investigation has also studied the relationship between CVP and total circulating blood volume index (TBVI) during burn resuscitation,[42] its authors concluding that CVP is more influenced by external pressures, such as intra-abdominal pressure, rather than TBVI, and is not a good endpoint for resuscitation. On the other hand, TBVI correlated well with cardiac output and stroke volume ($R^2 = 0.550$, $R^2 = 0.606$, respectively).

## Overresuscitation and Complications

In recent years, a trend to much higher resuscitation volumes than was originally intended by Baxter has become apparent.[43,44] This phenomenon has been termed *fluid creep* by Pruitt.[45] Its origin is likely to be multifactorial and is probably caused by more aggressive endpoints and a higher use of opiates and other analgesics (which blunt systemic responses).[46] One consequence of these aggregate phenomena is a rise in the incidence of abdominal compartment syndromes. In 1995, Greenhalgh and Warden[47] highlighted this problem for the first time in burn patients by measuring the intra-abdominal pressure (IAP) in 30 children with large burns. They found that patients who had 1 or more measurements exceeding 30 mmHg during the monitoring period had (1) significantly larger burns, (2) an increase in septic episodes, and (3) a higher mortality rate. However, they also noted that relatively simple interventions, or even laparotomy (in order to relieve intra-abdominal pressure), could be instituted with good outcomes.

In 2005, O'Mara et al[48] reported the results of a randomized controlled trial (RCT) that was conducted to determine if the use of colloid (fresh frozen plasma, 75 mL/kg, titrated against urine output 0.5-1 mL/kg/h) and lactated Ringer's solutions (2 L over 24 hours) (experimental group) could lower intra-abdominal pressure in comparison to utilization of the Parkland formula in adult burn resuscitation. The results were startling: the mean IAP for the control group was 10.6 mm Hg vs. 26.5 mm Hg for the experimental group, and while 2 patients in the experimental group developed IAPs > 25 mm Hg, only 1 patient in the control group maintained an IAP of < 25 mm Hg. In addition, the control group required 24% more fluid than the experimental group. Mortality was 27% in the control group and 19% in the experimental group. Although this was a small trial in terms of numbers (N = 15 for the control group, N = 16 in the experimental group), and thus little emphasis should be placed on the difference between mortality rates, the study unequivocally showed a relationship between IAP and resuscitation volume. Although many other studies have confirmed this relationship, we do not know if excessive fluid is the only cause of ACS (abdominal compartmental syndrome). However, it is clear that should IAP rise above a certain critical level (most authors agree > 25 mm Hg), swift intervention should take place to ensure that ACS does not develop.

## GENERAL GOALS AND OBJECTIVES

Children are more sensitive than adults in regard to resuscitation, and since their physiological reserve is less, resuscitation must be more precise. The general goals for resuscitation during the first 48 hours are to attain correct vascular volume, maintain tissue perfusion, and improve acid-base balance—all goals to be achieved without exacerbating postburn edema, evidenced at the extreme by development of ACS. Addressing the oxygen deficit and restoring cardiac parameters to preburn levels are also important goals, although often these cannot be achieved within the first 48 hours due to physiological limitations.

As discussed earlier, how these goals are achieved is still a matter for debate since many options are viable. The classic endpoint for children weighing < 30 kg is still a urine

output of 1 mL/kg/hour, as was reiterated at the State of the Science meeting in 2006,[49] although in practice, a range of 1.0 to 1.5 mL/kg/hour is acceptable for the first 24 hours, provided that there are no concurrent signs of underresuscitation or overresuscitation.[16] Children approaching 50 kg in weight, however, are better served using adult endpoints. For the first several hours, urine output should be checked every 15 minutes.

Should other endpoints besides urinary output be utilized in resuscitation of children with severe burns? Given that invasive monitoring has not been validated in adults with regard to improved mortality either in burns or trauma,[50,51] this approach should be reserved for more serious cases. Pham et al[52] recently conducted a review of invasive monitoring in adults using the grading scheme of Sackett.[53] The level of evidence was mostly Class V. Their recommendation (grade level A) was to not use a preload-driven strategy, nor to use invasive monitoring in general unless special circumstances warrant.

In children, most providers use femoral or internal jugular triple lumen catheters to monitor CVP and oxygen parameters rather than pulmonary artery catheters. In addition, since children have significant cardiopulmonary reserve and reflex tachycardia is frequently present, mental clarity, pulse pressures, arterial blood gases, distal extremity color, capillary refill, and body temperature, as well as the modified Glasgow coma scale when appropriate, should all be assessed to further guide resuscitation.[56] In parallel to trauma studies, burn studies[57-60] have also shown that monitoring serum base deficit and lactate can provide additional information regarding the generalized state of burn shock. Although there is some dispute whether plasma lactate is a better predictor of outcome compared to base deficit, serial measurements of either of these variables seem to be superior to gastric tonometry[61] as a means of assessing burn-induced metabolic acidosis.

Several factors must also be considered when resuscitating children, since they will impact the methods by which goals are achieved: BSA percentage, presence of inhalation injury, electrolyte infusion rates, glycogen reserves, and time since the burn was inflicted. In terms of burned surface area, children are more at risk compared to adults. For example, in this age group, intravenous resuscitation is commonly required for burns with a surface area of 10% to 20%.[12,13,62] Children also require greater resuscitation volumes compared to adults because of larger maintenance volumes resulting from a higher surface to weight ratio.[13,16,63-65] Intravenous boluses should be avoided (if possible) during the resuscitation phase, since this method likely aggravates the escape of fluid into the extravascular space. If venous access is initially compromised, bone marrow compartments in the anterior tibial plateau, medial malleolus, anterior iliac crest, and distal femur can be safely infused for children up to 8 years of age using a gravity drip, provided the bone is sufficiently soft for needle penetration (ie, intraosseus infusion).[56,66]

After decompression of the stomach,[67] enteral nutrition should be established as soon as possible. This is particularly important for children with high TBSAs given the associated metabolic demands. Such feeding can prevent upper gastrointestinal bleeding, obviate the need for antacids, and may assist in preventing subsequent infection.[68] Although vomiting is always a risk factor in children, administration of antiemetics can be used to help facilitate overall management.[69] Various formulas are available for determination of caloric needs for different age groups and TBSA percentages.[70-72]

One overriding important message that has remained constant, despite the various formulas or fluids utilized, is this: fluid resuscitation and the restoration of intravascular volume should not be delayed. This might seem obvious, but one study demonstrated that the incidence of sepsis, renal failure, and mortality was significantly higher in burned children receiving fluid resuscitation 2 or more hours after the burn injury ($P < .0001$).[73]

## BURN SHOCK RESUSCITATION

### Pathophysiology in Brief

Although the pathophysiology of burn shock is covered in a later chapter, a short summary will help provide the basic understanding for fluid resuscitation and why some of its aspects are still contentious.

Burn injury comprises hypovolemic shock as well as direct injury at the cellular level. Although heat is responsible for most of the damage in burned tissue, the effects in cells distal to the burn are mediated by a host of entities, including histamine, bradykinin, vasoactive amines, hormones, prostaglandins, leukotrienes, and neutrophils.

Oxidative damage, including the release of lipid peroxidation products, results in endothelial cell damage, the most critical aspect of which is increased capillary permeability.[74] Matrix elements, such as collagen and hyaluronic acid,[75,76] are also degraded by pro-oxidants, which could be one cause of the negative interstitial pressure encountered.[74] Thus, treatment with antioxidants ought to reduce the edema associated with the burn, and many studies have reported such results, the most intriguing of which has been the use of high doses of vitamin C.[77] The vasoconstriction induced by thromboxane $TXA_2$, which is partly responsible for the ischemic flow in affected tissues, coupled with

the local vasodilation initiated by $PGI_2$, also potentiate the resultant edema.[74]

The vascular changes brought about by these mediators can be best understood through the Starling equation, which governs fluid movement in the capillary bed:[74]

$$Q = K_f (Pcap - Pi) + \sigma (\pi p - \pi i)$$

in which Q represents the fluid filtration rate that peaks 1 to 2 hours after the burn; $K_f$ is the capillary filtration coefficient, which increases 2 to 3 times because of the burn injury; Pcap is the capillary hydrostatic pressure, which typically increases from 24 mmHg to 48 mmHg postburn; Pi is the interstitial hydrostatic pressure, which changes from a slightly negative pressure to a much stronger one, chiefly as a result of collagen/hyaluronic acid degradation producing many osmotically active fragments; $\sigma$ is the reflection coefficient, a measure of semipermeability of the capillary membrane, which is reduced postburn; and $(\pi p - \pi i)$ represents the plasma colloid gradient (oncotic gradient), which opposes the hydrostatic gradient (Pcap - Pi) and approaches zero postburn.

Overall, the changes in the Starling equation are thus:

| | | |
|---|---|---|
| ↑ | $K_f$ | [increases] |
| ↑↑ | (Pcap - Pi) | [dramatically increases] |
| → 0 | $\sigma (\pi p - \pi i)$ | [becomes negligible] |

These changes cause the net fluid filtration rate (Q) to vastly increase. However, another factor, the interstitial compliance—a measure of how much pressure is required to change the volume of the interstitial space—dramatically increases as a result of damage to the mechanical (helical coiling) properties of the interstitial protein matrices. In other words, the initial edema makes it far easier for more edema to occur in the interstitial space. Finally, the lymphatic system has to drain the excess fluid from the interstitium, but is typically overwhelmed by the huge increases in flow rate. In addition, if dermal and subdermal lymphatics are damaged, this further decreases the ability of the lymphatic system to cope effectively.

The time course of edema formation following a partial-thickness burn is shown in Figure 3. As a rule, full-thickness burns cause less local edema (and slower-developing edema) than partial-thickness burns due to less vascular perfusion.[78,79] However, burns that destroy dermal lymphatics are likely to prolong the edema. Thus, the dynamics of the edema change in parallel with the type of burn and the amount of burn area as a result of differing changes in the elements of the Starling equation. Appreciating the changes that govern capillary and interstitial dynamics is helpful in comprehending the limitations of colloid addition during resuscitation.

Other important cellular changes that result from a severe burn include cell membrane depolarization, which is associated with an influx of sodium and water. This event seems to be mediated by at least one type of shock factor[80] and is likely related to burn-related inhibition of Na-K-ATPase[81,82] as well as calcium transport changes,[783] both of which seem to decrease cardiac function. There is also evidence that caspases, which are intracellular cysteine proteases involved in programmed cell death (apoptosis), provide a pivotal role in the disruption of homeostasis.[84] This body of evidence should give some pause to those that believe cardiac function can be completely restored through aggressive fluid resuscitation and inotropic support alone.

The acidosis that develops as a consequence of a severe burn has always been deemed an indicator of oxygen deficit, but this might not be entirely true; rather, it might be a consequence of increased glucose flux.[85] We do know that energy expenditure increases postburn and that there is a limitation to oxidative phosphorylation. However, there is preliminary evidence to suggest that the rate of glucose oxidation is not the limiting step, which indicates that another unidentified mechanism is at work.[86] These results imply that the increase in serum lactate is not entirely a result of oxygen deficit, and thus lactate levels should not *primarily* drive oxygen demand goals, although they should help in following overall perfusion status.

## Resuscitating the Burned Child

### Isotonic Crystalloid

As was noted earlier, lactated Ringer's solution has become the base crystalloid for resuscitation fluids. It is composed of 130 mmol/L of sodium, 109 mmol/L of chloride, 28 mmol/L lactate, 4 mmol/L of potassium, and 1.5 mmol/L of calcium (sodium chloride 0.6%, sodium lactate 0.31%, potassium chloride 0.03%, calcium chloride 0.015%), which is slightly different to the Hartman's solution that is commonly used in the United Kingdom (sodium chloride 0.6%, sodium lactate 0.25%, potassium chloride 0.04%, calcium chloride 0.027%). LR is isotonic with respect to plasma but also contains lactate, which is ultimately metabolized in the liver, effectively producing bicarbonate, and thus partially counteracts the metabolic acidosis induced by the burn. This bicarbonate formation is temporary, though, and through the enzymatic action of carbonic anhydrase, an equilibrium will tend to be maintained, thus forming more $CO_2$ and worsening the acidosis over time. If liver impairment is known prior to fluid resuscitation or discovered during resuscitation, LR should be immediately discontinued

in favor of normal saline; bicarbonate should then be used in place of the lactate, or Plasmalyte B can be started, taking care to ensure that metabolic alkalosis does not occur.

More effective replacements for lactate have been tested in hemorrhagic shock resuscitation, such as betahydroxybutyrate[87] and the L isomer of lactate (commercial lactated Ringer's solutions are racemic),[88] but this is still of question in the burn community. The rationale for testing such replacements is that racemic LR solutions can provoke inflammatory responses (ie, increase neutrophilic oxidative bursts), especially when large volumes are infused.

Plasmalyte B is another commonly used resuscitation fluid that more closely approximates plasma (sodium 140 mmol/L, chloride 98 mmol/L, potassium 5 mmol/L, bicarbonate 50 mmol/L), but since published trials of this fluid versus LR in burn resuscitations have taken place, its cost-effectiveness and overall utility are in doubt.

During fluid resuscitation with LR, it is also vital to monitor electrolytes to ensure that sodium and potassium plasma concentrations do not reach dangerously low or high concentrations. Typically, hypernatremia develops if fluid underresuscitation or sepsis occurs, although other causes are possible.[89] Hyponatremia is less common during the first 48 hours, but may be observed between the third and fifth day postburn, and is commonly due to overresuscitation;[12] however, its cause must be established before correcting it.

### Hypertonic Saline

Research regarding the use of hypertonic saline since the publication of the safety study of Huang et al[26] has been divided into animal experiments and human investigations. Several small experiments have been conducted on sheep, rats, and mice to compare various aspects of fluid resuscitation. Kinsky et al[90] compared the use of 7.5% saline and 6% dextran (HSD) versus LR in sheep and found that fluid requirements in the HSD group were 22% of the LR group, the water content of various organs was less in the HSD group, and plasma colloid osmotic pressure was 3 mm Hg to 5 mm Hg higher in the HSD group. Chen et al,[91] using mice, compared hypertonic to various hypotonic saline solutions and concluded that hypertonic saline (HTS) stimulated the toll-like receptors of inflammatory cells, which is an important measure of the host's response in bacterial challenge. Using rats, Kien et al[92] compared HTS to LR and confirmed the resuscitation volume ratios observed by Kinsky et al[90] and discovered that the HTS group had better cardiac and organ tissue perfusion compared to the LR group. Finally, Milner et al[93] compared HTS to LR in sheep and reported similar results to Kinsky et al[90] and Kien et al.[92] Although positive in outlook regarding the case for HTS, one criticism of these and other animal experiments is that the time course has been too short to determine whether the differential in observed fluid requirements is maintained over the long term.

A small study comparing fluid resuscitation in burned adults (N = 18, percentage TBSA > 35%) using an HTS bolus in conjunction with LR versus LR alone found little differences between most parameters with the exception of troponin I levels, which were significantly lower in the HTS bolus group, suggesting that cardiac dysfunction was not as severe in this group.[94] This was an interesting finding not previously seen in human studies, and could have a potential application, although we have no information in regard to mortality in burns patients using this method of HTS infusion.

A Japanese study that compared HTS versus LR in the resuscitation of burned adults (N = 36, percentage BSA > 40%) showed a significant resuscitation volume difference (3.1 mL/24 h/kg/% TBSA vs. 5.2 mL/24 h/kg/% TBSA) over the first 24 hours, but primarily investigated IAP, demonstrating a consistently lower bladder pressure in the HTS group but a consistently higher abdominal perfusion pressure.[95] The interpretation of these results suggested that the HTS group had a lower risk of developing ACS, which is consistent with the premise that higher resuscitation volumes do increase the chance that ACS might develop.

Pham et al[52] analyzed several prospective clinical studies of hypertonic saline resuscitation and determined that the level of evidence was mostly Class I and Class II. Their recommendation (grade level B) was that this technique should only be used by experienced burn physicians and that close monitoring of plasma sodium is required.

In 2004, the Cochrane group updated their latest findings with regard to burn resuscitation, comparing near isotonic crystalloid to hypertonic crystalloid.[100] Their meta-analysis reported that the pooled relative risk of mortality for resuscitation using HTS was 1.49 (95% CI: 0.56-3.95), which is lower than that reported by Huang et al,[26] but still elevated. Although the authors were conservative in their conclusion, the results suggest that resuscitation based upon HTS does carry a substantial increased risk of mortality compared to standard LR treatment. If this is so, by what mechanism could HTS cause mortality to rise?

For many years, it was thought that the increased levels of ADH (antidiuretic hormone) observed after major burns constituted a syndrome of inappropriate ADH secretion. However, in 1991, Cioffi et al[101] demonstrated that this concept was incorrect because the increased renal perfusion did not relate to total blood volume, which is the neuronal set point (a factor not measured prior to this study, and which was found to be relatively low). As Huang et al[26] have pointed out, hypovolemia and increased serum osmolality

further stimulate ADH release, but likely depress ANP (antinatriuretic peptide). In addition, following a severe burn, aldosterone levels are mildly elevated, aggravating sodium retention in the plasma. Consequently, serum sodium and osmolality can remain persistently elevated while urine output is significantly decreased, sometimes to the point of renal failure. This might be the "danger point" in some patients.

Summarizing, it is clear that while resuscitation using hypertonic saline may have some advantages on the battlefield and in mass casualty events,[87] the LR approach is preferable in burn units unless there are some specific concerns that might justify the increased risks, such as very high TBSA burns or failure to resuscitate with isotonic saline.

## Colloid

The rationale for using any kind of colloid has always centered on the concept that its addition to the plasma of burn patients will exert an oncotic force and perhaps ameliorate the oncotic gradient ($\pi p - \pi i$), which in burn patients tends to drastically decrease as the reflection coefficient, a measure of the semipermeability of the capillary membranes, worsens. Biochemically speaking, adding colloids will only help if a significant fraction of the oncotically active biomolecules are retained on the plasma side of the capillary membrane. Further, this concept only applies to partial-thickness burns and uninjured surrounding tissue, not full-thickness burns where the capillaries are quickly occluded.[74] While the burn itself was originally thought to be responsible for the change in the reflection coefficient, we now know that inflammatory mediators also contribute toward the alteration, thus opening the door to the possibility that if we can control the mediators, we may be able restore the permeability characteristics of the membrane more quickly.

The evidence to date suggests that until approximately 8 to 12 hours postburn, it is not worthwhile to add plasma or albumin to the fluid resuscitation regimen because the molecular size of albumin is too small in relation to the enlarged pore sizes of the semipermeable membrane.[74,102,103] In addition, early addition of albumin may increase the risk of bacterial translocation in the GI tract, thus inviting sepsis complications.[104] However, dextrans may be employed at a slightly earlier time because of their higher molecular size.

The meta-analysis of Schierhout and Roberts published in 1998,[21] which examined mortality rates in crystalloid versus colloid resuscitation in critically ill patients, had a chilling effect on the use of colloids in burn resuscitation, especially in the United Kingdom.[105] Based upon 4 studies, the analysis showed a pooled RR of 1.21 (95% CI: 0.88-1.66) in regard to mortality.[21] Ten years later, with more data, a different picture emerged for resuscitated critically ill patients[106]: (1) for colloid versus crystalloid resuscitation using albumin or plasma, the pooled RR was 1.01 (95% CI: 0.92-1.10); (2) for dextran versus crystalloid, the pooled RR was 1.24 (95% CI: 0.94-1.65); (3) for hydroxyethyl starch versus crystalloid, the pooled RR was 1.05 (95% CI: 0.63-1.75); (4) for modified gelatin versus crystalloid, the pooled RR was 0.91 (95% CI: 0.49-1.72); and (5) for colloid (dextran) plus hypertonic crystalloid versus isotonic crystalloid, the pooled RR was 0.88 (95% CI: 0.74-1.05). Although the burn care community has yet to comment on this recent meta-analysis, some tentative conclusions can be drawn. First, the use of plasma or albumin does not appear to pose a substantial risk of excess mortality. Second, the use of dextran appears to affect the mortality rate substantially, depending on how it is combined with other fluids. Finally, the majority of patients utilized in this meta-analysis were not burn patients, so these results should be applied with caution.

Based upon these findings, if a decision to use colloid is made, the options with the least question marks are plasma, albumin, or modified gelatin. The practice of using plasma in burn resuscitation dates back to the original Evans and Brooke formulas, which incorporate plasma at the specified colloid addition rate of 1 mL/kg/% TBSA. However, the use of plasma has not been systematically studied in humans via large clinical trials, although there is a wealth of animal and human case series data. For example, Du et al[107] conducted a small RCT to test the outcome of crystalloid plasma versus fresh frozen plasma (FFP), but extrapolation of the promising results to a general statement of the efficacy of plasma addition is difficult because of the small numbers involved. Reconstituted dried plasma and plasma protein fractions were in common use in the United Kingdom in the 1980s and 1990s (Mount Vernon, Muir, and Barclay formulas),[108-110] and FFP is still employed in some burn centers as an adjunct to resuscitation with crystalloid due to the expense of and shortages of albumin.

Albumin has been used as an adjunct to crystalloid fluid resuscitation since it became commercially available in the early 1950s. Following the early studies we have already described,[18,19] Goodwin et al conducted a burn resuscitation RCT in which young adults either received LR (N = 39; TBSA = 48%) or LR + 2.5% albumin (N = 40; TBSA = 53%) for the first 24 hours.[111] In the second 24 hours, plasma volume was replaced by colloid equivalent to plasma at a rate of 0.3 to 0.5 ml/kg body weight/% BSA. This was a well-designed study that evaluated cardiac functions and EVLW. The authors concluded that there were no differences in the cardiac parameters studied but a significant difference in the accumulation of EVLW over several days, with more water accumulating in the albumin-treated group. In comparison, an experiment conducted in sheep a few years later

using several protocols, including LR and LR plus albumin, showed a clear advantage for the albumin-treated group.[112] In any case, modern studies continue to demonstrate a lack of superior long-term outcome (eg, multiple organ dysfunction scores[113]) when comparing crystalloid plus albumin versus crystalloid-alone resuscitation. Further, long-term administration of albumin, even to reverse clinical hypoalbuminemia, does not appear to confer any advantages in previously healthy children receiving adequate nutrition.[114]

If albumin is selected, the amount of 5% albumin infusion required can be based upon the simple formula of 0.5 mL/kg/% TBSA or a more graduated approach in which more albumin is used (0.3 to 0.5 mL/kg/% TBSA) to match the amount of burned surface area (30 % to ≥ 70%).[115]

As early as 1995, a university hospital consortium using Delphi techniques produced a series of guidelines on the use of albumin,[116] which for burn resuscitation was phrased thus:

> Fluid resuscitation should be initiated with crystalloid solutions. If crystalloid resuscitation exceeds 4L in adults 18 to 26 hours postburn, and burns cover more than 30% of the patient's body surface area, non-protein colloids may be added. If non-protein colloids are contraindicated, albumin may be used.

This trend toward less usage of albumin was accentuated in the United Kingdom following a series of meta-analyses published by the Cochrane group which led to an interesting discussion in the *Journal of Critical Care* concerning the use of albumin in critically ill patients.[117,118]

Predictably, the issue continues to simmer. A recent case-controlled study published in 2007, for example, showed that albumin administered to burn patients with a TSBA ≥ 20% who were more ill compared to the control group (higher inhalation injury rate, higher initial serum lactate, and longer time to achieve resuscitation endpoint) was protective in a multivariate mode of mortality (OR: 0.27; 95% CI: 0.07-0.97).[119] This was a surprising result compared to the meta-analysis of Perel and Roberts.[106] Another factor is that the true incidence of excess mortality related to the product itself likely has steadily decreased over the last 20 years because manufacturing impurities have been progressively eliminated.[120]

In their evidence-based review of colloid resuscitation, Pham et al[52] listed 6 trials with Class I or Class II evidence, summing up the trials by suggesting that use of colloid can decrease total volume requirements, but that if it is employed, it should be given late in the first 24 hours (recommendation grade A). Again, it should be pointed out that none of these trials have demonstrated superior long-term outcome.

## Alternatives to Albumin or Plasma

Other colloids have been tested in burn resuscitation, primarily dextrans, which are polymerized high-molecular-weight glucose chains. However, the vast majority of experiments have been animal-based. As described previously, Murphy et al[94] conducted a small RCT testing hypertonic saline plus Dextran 70 (HSD) versus crystalloid, but since no data regarding long-term outcome were reported, conclusions regarding mortality cannot be drawn. Interestingly, one experiment conducted in sheep suggested that the volume-sparing effect produced by HSD is dependent on the dose, dosing interval, and infusion rate—that is, a continuously infused dose does not provide a prolonged reduction in volume resuscitation.[123] A single-dose approach was also utilized by Murphy et al.[94]

Hydroxyethyl starch (HES) has also been tested in both animals and humans. Early studies demonstrated that this material seemed equivalent to plasma or albumin, but the nature of the experimental design precluded exact conclusions.[124] A more recent and larger Chinese study also concluded that HES could partially substitute for plasma (patients were randomized to HES or plasma), and no adverse effects were reported.[125] However, it should be stressed that we still do not have any long-term outcome data using this material. Gelatin has not yet been used in burn resuscitation, although the mortality data associated with its use in trauma is favorable.[106]

Based upon his research and that of others, Demling[74] believes that colloids can only affect the edema situation in nonburned tissue, and that clinicians might further investigate antioxidants in lieu of using colloid. As with much other clinical science, the question of benefit using colloids during the critical phase of burn resuscitation will have to await answers from RCTs that employ reasonably large numbers.

## The Very Young Patient

The very young burn patient, typically aged 4 years or younger, deserves special consideration because, as mentioned previously, this age group is considered to be high risk in regard to mortality.[3] In a recent review of children admitted to a burn unit in Boston, 26 out of 1537 (1.7%) had all 3 risk factors that the authors identified as problematic: young age, inhalation injury, and large burns.[126] The authors reported not starting colloid administration until 18 to 24 hours postburn and using 5% albumin in LR at a dose of 0.5 to 0.7 mL/kg/percent burn for 24 hours "after the leak seals." In addition, supplemental albumin was given at a rate of 1 to 2 g/kg/day if serum albumin fell below 1 g/dL or below 1.5 g/dL in the presence of pulmonary dysfunction or enteral feeding intolerance. Enteral nutritional support

via gastric feeding tubes was also provided within 24 hours postburn. Anabolic agents, such as growth hormone or steroids, were not given, although the judicious use of these entities to improve healing rates is a longer-term question worthy of more research.[127]

Fluid losses in very young children are proportionately higher compared to older children, and most formulas will often miscalculate how much fluid should be given.[56] Based on the "rule of nines" for this age group (head: 19; body: 32; arms: 9.5 each; legs: 15 each), or preferably a nomogram, resuscitation should be accomplished by first calculating surface area. The Galveston approach uses a formula of 5000 mL/m² of BSA plus 2000 mL/m² BSA during the first 24 hours postburn, with half of the volume given during the first 8 hours.[18,56] The next 24 hours should employ 3750 mL/m² of BSA plus 1500 mL/m² of BSA for maintenance requirements. Another vital requirement is to start fluid resuscitation as soon as possible, since delays of an hour or more can mean the difference between survival and death.

Caloric needs are also an important consideration because very young children do not have sufficient glycogen stores to meet the metabolic demands imposed by burns during the first 24 hours. Enteral feeding should be started as soon as possible. Milk is well tolerated by young children, although its low sodium content may need to be compensated for with sodium supplementation[56] since urinary sodium losses can be substantial.

Although resuscitation goals for very young children are generally the same as for older children, any decision to use invasive hemodynamic monitoring must be carefully thought out, weighing the risks against benefits. While such monitoring is helpful at times, other, more indirect techniques, such as echo-Doppler devices,[128] may be useful in more severe cases.

## Inhalation Injury in Children

Inhalation injury is always a significant risk for mortality regardless of age or burn size, and if not recognized can lead to pulmonary failure. Therefore, children involved in any kind of flame injury should be promptly assessed. A large study (N = 12010) of children aged 1 to 14 years discharged from hospitals in 4 populous states after treatment for burns showed an incidence of 5.1% for inhalation injury.[129] Incidence of inhalation injury in children tends to increase in respect to age due to the nature of the burn injury (scalds are more common in younger children); a longitudinal study reported by Ryan et al found more than a doubling of the incidence of inhalation injury in an age group of 11 to 20 years compared to 1 to 10 years (19.0% vs. 8.1%).[130] Adding inhalation injury to a burn increases mortality by a factor of 5 to 9.[131,132]

The pathophysiology of inhalation injury has been described and will be a focus of another chapter. However, a recent study found that there were no increased levels of proinflammatory cytokines, indicating that inhalation injury in addition to a burn injury does not seem to augment the systemic inflammatory response.[133] An alternate hypothesis advanced by the same authors suggested that immunocompromise and immunodysfunction might be involved.

Intubation is required in many cases. A retrospective study of patients with smoke inhalation injury found that intubation was positively and significantly correlated with findings of soot in the oral cavity, facial burns, body burns, and fiberoptic laryngoscopic findings of edema in the true and false vocal cords.[134] However, the authors also discovered that classic symptoms of smoke inhalation—stridor, hoarseness, drooling, and dysphagia—had no correlation with intubation. Other signs that inhalation injury has occurred include carbonaceous sputum, abnormal mental status (agitation or stupor), respiratory distress, or elevated carboxyhemoglobin (> 10%).[135]

Controversies continue over airway management. When required, the ideal intubation uses an endotracheal tube, aided by bronchoscopy if needed. If this fails, tracheostomy should be performed between the second and third cervical ring,[56] since cricothyroidotomy for children under 12 years of age is not recommended.[136] A study of 38 children with an average BSA of 54%, of whom 63% had an inhalation injury and a tracheostomy performed, showed that tracheostomy was a safe procedure that resulted in improved ventilator management.[137]

In terms of pharmacological management, one study has shown that administration of heparin (5000 units) and 3 mL of a 20% solution of N-acetylcystine aerosolized every 4 hours the first 7 days after the injury can ameliorate casts produced from destroyed ciliated epithelial cells and reduce pulmonary failure secondary to smoke inhalation.[138] Experiments in sheep utilizing nebulized albuterol to mitigate the results of inhalation injury by improving airway clearance and decreased fluid flux (lower pause and peak inspiratory pressures, decreased pulmonary transvascular fluid flux, significantly higher $PaO_2/FiO_2$ ratio, and decreased shunt fraction at 48 hours postburn) have also been sufficiently promising.[139] However, in most centers this approach is still of question.

In terms of fluid requirements, it was always observed that inhalation injury increased fluid requirements.[140-142] However, a recent study conducted by Klein et al[143] that employed a more sophisticated regression analysis showed that this was not necessarily true. Rather, increased fluid requirements seem to be linked with intubation and ventilation need. As the vast majority of pediatric patients with inhalation injury are likely to be intubated and placed on a ventilator, it is not surprising that inhalation injury has become thought of as predictive of increased fluid requirements. In practical terms, despite conventional approaches and higher infusion formulas (eg, 6 ml/kg/% TBSA), there does not seem to be evidence to support an a priori adjustment of fluid rates in the setting of inhalation injury.

## Abdominal Compartment Syndrome

In the general burn population, about 1% of all patients develop ACS,[144] although Ivy et al report that it is a common problem in patients with TBSAs of 70% or more[145]; other studies suggest that its incidence rapidly increases with percentage of burned surface area, although this is not the only factor. The issue of abdominal compartment syndrome has not been thoroughly discussed in the literature with regard to children. Case studies demonstrate that compartmental syndromes can appear within several hours of a burn injury, but also may be delayed several days.[47] Aggressive intervention is vital because intra-abdominal hypertension (IAH) can swiftly prove fatal, with mortality rates of 50% to 60%.[47,144]

Early signs that can alert the clinician to the possibility of ACS include an unexplained drop in urine output associated with lack of response to volume loading, unexplained increases in peak inspiratory pressures, or decreases in cardiac performance. One simple way to estimate the intra-abdominal pressure is by attaching a pressure monitor to the Foley catheter.[47] If the bladder pressure is ≥ 30 mm Hg, a laparotomy should be immediately considered. Other specific indications reported by Ivy et al[145] (in adults) to start checking bladder pressures include (1) attainment of a fluid volume of 250 ml/kg body weight, and (2) peak inspiratory pressure exceeding 40 cm of water. Oda et al[146] noted similar results to the study of Ivy et al[145] and suggested that 300 ml/kg body weight (in the first 24 hours) and 70% BSA were the thresholds for developing ACS in adults.

Ivy et al[145] also define intra-abdominal hypertension as a bladder pressure > 25 mm Hg and point out that IAH is far more manageable than ACS. Thus the range in bladder pressure of 25 mm Hg to 30 mm Hg seems to be critical. Zak[147] has commented that abdominal ultrasounds and plain film abdominal and chest radiographs can be also useful in detecting the presence of ACS and reminds emergency room personnel that even "minor household accidents" in very young children, particularly with erythrematous but as yet nonblistered skin, can later develop ACS if not properly managed.

Although Oda et al[95] reported that during burn resuscitation of adults the development of ACS was far less when using hypertonic lactated Ringer's solution, there is a paucity of data in children on which to base such a fluid resuscitation strategy. It also remains unknown whether it would benefit a child to switch to such a fluid if the child started developing IAH.

## Choice of Fluids and Formulas

To date, there is no level I or level II evidence to support a single crystalloid-based resuscitation strategy[52]; as such, it seems that if resuscitation is conducted in a timely and efficient manner, the exact choice of fluids or the specific formula used may be less important than the overall clinical picture of organ perfusion. All formulas and protocols should be viewed as general "starting points" and placed in context with endpoint goals. Children with more severe burns and/or inhalation injuries will likely require more fluid compared to children with less severe burns or no inhalation injuries; this should be remembered at the bedside in order to avoid either underresuscitation or overresuscitation.

Some of the more common formulas used in the United States are shown in Table 4, and 3 specific formulas will be reviewed in more detail.

### Baxter-Parkland

In the United States, Ireland, and the United Kingdom, Parkland is the most commonly used formula.[148,149] However, surveys in the United States have found that practices at many burn units vary according to the experience of the director and experience gathered at the unit for many years.[148] Although many institutions consistently hold to the Parkland formula for the first 24 hours, there is considerable variation in regard to the second 24 hours, which reflects different ideas and practice methods.

As noted previously, in the last 2 decades, actual resuscitation volumes have often exceeded calculated requirements by a large margin,[150] and many clinicians have been rightly concerned about this trend, particularly with regard to complications such as ACS. However, provided that endpoints have been properly defined and followed, this large gap between observed and calculated fluid requirement should not dominate assessment in the first 24 hours. There is also some evidence to show that burn patients transferred to burn units from other outside hospitals in rural areas tended to be overresuscitated for small burns and underresuscitated for larger burns because of inaccurate estimation of burned area.[151] The former problem may not have major consequences, but the latter is far more serious. Maintenance fluids to replace insensible losses of water and salts in children can be calculated based on a straightforward approach—that is, the "4:2:1" (4 mL/kg for the first 10 kg of body weight; 2 mL/kg for the next 11-20 kg; and 1 mL/kg for weight above 20 kg).

Maintenance requirements can be met by intravenous infusion and/or enteral feedings.

In many centers, the second 24-hour period features the addition of colloid, although the permissible range is large and is adjusted according to the preferences of the burn unit. Within 48 hours, most children should be well resuscitated, and the process then shifts to the maintenance phase and protein replacement phase.

### Cincinnati

The major difference between the Parkland formula and the Cincinnati approach is that maintenance fluid volumes are calculated using actual body surface area. Originally in Cincinnati, maintenance levels in the first 24 hours were calculated using a formula of 1500 mL/m$^2$, but a newer formula has been added to account for evaporative water losses.[62] A further difference from Parkland is that colloid is added at the rate of 20% of calculated plasma volume during the second 24-hour period.

In very young children and in children with massive burns and/or severe inhalation injury, Warden have recommended the use of modified hypertonic saline (LR + 50 mEq sodium bicarbonate) for the first 8 hours as a means of reducing the fluid load and correcting for the more severe metabolic acidosis. After 8 hours, such patients are then given LR for 8 hours, and finally 5% albumin in LR for the final 8 hours of the first 24-hour period.[62]

### Galveston

The Galveston approach to calculating fluid requirements for burn resuscitation is also different than others. It employs a formula based upon the area of burned skin (5000 mL/m$^2$ of burn) and maintenance based on body surface area (2000 mL/m$^2$). In addition, albumin is added to maintain a serum albumin greater than 2.5 g/dL by using a solution consisting of 50 mL of 25% human serum albumin (12.5 g) added to 950 mL LR.[152] This seems to be a fundamental difference in opinion between the shrines in the application of colloid in the first 24 hours. For example, the Cincinnati approach does not espouse colloid addition during the first 24 hours because their researchers determined that addition of albumin to maintain a serum albumin level of 1.5 to 2.5 g/dL or 2.5 to 3.5 g/dL made no difference in outcome.[113]

## Vasopressors, Hemodynamics, and Adjunctive Measures

The use of inotropic or hemodynamic support has not been systematically studied in the burn literature, and the scattered results that do exist have been contradictory. For example, one study in sheep (60% BSA, full-thickness burn) demonstrated no advantage in outcome by using dobutamine,[153] whereas a small study of adults (N = 9) indicated that dobutamine infusions (5 µg/kg/min) given after the PAWP reached 15 mm Hg improved cardiac output parameters.[54] Other human studies of burn patients have also been supportive of dobutamine use: inotropic support with dobutamine and careful titration of volume infusion according to end-diastolic volumes improved hemodynamics, as demonstrated by significant increases in right ventricular ejection fractions in all patients without any changes in mean arterial pressures, urine output, or oxygenation.[154] In younger children, large-scale fluid resuscitation may cause a relative state of right-sided heart failure which can be improved with dobutamine.

Given that the study of inotropic/hemodynamic support has been far more extensive in the general sepsis/shock literature, and the supposition that it is reasonable to assume that conclusions from this body of literature are somewhat relevant to burn resuscitation, several guidelines have recently been proposed as part of evidence-based reviews.

First, vasopressor preference is norepinephrine or dopamine to maintain an initial target of mean arterial pressure ≥ 65 mm Hg. Second, dobutamine inotropic therapy is useful when cardiac output remains low despite fluid resuscitation and combined inotropic/vasopressor therapy. Both these recommendations are strong, but the quality of evidence for them is low (grade C).[155,156]

Other ideas for adjunctive therapy have also been advanced and some tested, including vitamin C therapy. It is likely that as we better understand the mediation of burn injury through signaling and inflammatory mediators, more precise adjunct therapy, including inotropic support, will be forthcoming.

## Failure of Resuscitation: Now What?

Assessing resuscitation is a continual process throughout the first 48 hours, given that approximately 13% of all patients die because of resuscitation failure.[157] Whereas a successful resuscitation will likely become apparent during this period (and can be predicted with good accuracy), it is extremely difficult to predict those patients that have a high risk of mortality based on standard variables.[158] If resuscitation is not successful, there are 3 general causes: (1) overresuscitation with respect to fluid volume, (2) underresuscitation, and (3) other etiologies.

Overresuscitation means that too much fluid has been infused, and several problems may be encountered. Klein et al[143] examined outcome and amount of fluid administration using both odds ratio and the equation [(fluids received – fluids predicted)/fluids predicted x 100] to define

3 categories: ≤ predicted; 0 to 25% of predicted; and > 25 % predicted. The authors found that using odd ratios, there was a significant increased risk of developing ARDS, pneumonia, bloodstream infections, multiple organ failure, and death with increasing fluid requirements. Use of the equation and adjusting for patient and injury characteristics, a logistical regression analysis also showed that when the measured infused volume was > 25 % of predicted volume, there was a trend (nonsignificant difference) toward increased risk of adverse outcome, including death. However, dichotomizing patients based on a 250 mL/kg of fluid received parameter[145] resulted in predictions that were more similar to odd ratios. Although there have been several investigations examining outcomes in relation to fluid amount given during resuscitation, the study of Klein et al[143] is probably one of the most illuminative and suggests that the benchmark figure of 250 mL/kg of fluid received devised by Ivy et al[145] is a useful indicator that overresuscitation has occurred.

If overresuscitation is suspected, the development of compartmental syndromes should be first confirmed or denied by measuring bladder pressure and treating excessive pressure accordingly, as has been previously described. In addition, intraocular pressure should be measured, as excessive pressure in the eye can be devastating. Sullivan et al[158] recommend lateral canthotomy in cases in which IOP exceeds 30 mm Hg.

If overresuscitation is suspected as the cause of resuscitation failure, in experienced centers, consideration should be given to switching to HTS treatment to minimize further fluid addition. In extreme cases, the use of plasma exchange as a means to combat resuscitation failure in burn patients could be initiated. Warden et al[159] reported that in resuscitation failure, defined as reaching twice the fluid requirements predicted by the Parkland formula as well as persistent metabolic acidosis and arterial hypotension and no improvement after switching to HTS, plasma exchange was successful in 16 out of 17 patients. This process involved a continuous blood cell separator and rejection of platelet-poor plasma fractions and addition of 1.5 times the calculated blood volume with type-specific fresh frozen plasma. Similar results were documented by Stratta et al,[160] who studied children, and Schnarrs et al,[161] who studied both adolescent children and adults. A small RCT was conducted by Kravitz et al[162] to test the outcome of crystalloid versus plasma exchange in burned adults, but the numbers were too small to draw any substantive conclusions despite promising results. A few centers are having anecdotal success employing continuous renal replacement therapy (CRRT) in this setting, although formal investigation is lacking.

Failure due to underresuscitation is rarer but can happen in patients in which the burned surface area is high (eg, > 70%), especially when inhalation injury is present and/or the burned child is very young. When one compares fluid requirements according to a particular formula and compares this figure against fluids administered, it is possible to have met the formula requirements and yet still have underresuscitated the child because burn surface area and/or severity of injury may have been underestimated or mistakes were made in calculations.[163] Therefore, how does one recognize underresuscitation? There is no single parameter that will provide an answer. Rather, several clinical markers may provide clues: insufficient urine output (eg, < 1.0–1.5 ml/kg/hour), very low cardiovascular indices, or a generalized delay in initiating resuscitation.[164] If underresuscitation is suspected, the immediate response should be to increase the rate of fluid infusion, using additional small boluses if required. A switch to another formula may also be beneficial, especially one that bases fluid requirements on burn area, is more generous with fluid maintenance requirements, or uses colloid.

If overresuscitation or underresuscitation has been ruled out and resuscitation failure is apparent (eg, respiratory distress [$PaO_2/FiO_2 \leq 200$ mm Hg], CVP > 10 mm Hg, or urine output < 1 mL/kg/h[164]), other etiologies are likely. One recent study has determined that failure to maintain a patent airway was the third most common cause of death in pediatric burn patients[165]; since this cause is preventable, a reassessment of the child's oxygenation status should quickly reveal whether this is the case. Another study has indicated that depressed ventricular function (left ventricular stroke work index of 19.9 g/m/m²; normal 44–68 19.9 g/m/m²) is common in children unresponsive to resuscitation but can be compensated for with the initiation of inotropes and vasopressors.[164] In younger children, clinically important right-sided heart failure can be seen on a transient basis, which further impedes efforts toward restoring global perfusion; in this setting, low-dose dobutamine may play a role by improving inotropy, as well as the microcirculatory flow via peripheral vasodilation. In an emergency, plasma exchange may be successful when resuscitation failure is due to excessive levels of inflammatory mediators or severe metabolic acidosis. But severe lung injury, which Gore et al[165] have identified as the most common cause of death, is still the greatest single challenge, and various modes of progressive mechanical support can be employed, including and up to extracorporeal membrane oxygenation (ECMO).

# Fluid Replacement Following the Resuscitation Phase

Successful resuscitations are usually complete within the first 48 hours following the burn injury. Once resuscitated,

patients will only need maintenance fluid and enteral support until their burns have been treated, either with excision and grafting or conventional wound care. A switchover from intravenous infusion to complete enteral feeding is possible 1 to 4 days after the burn depending on the percent TBSA and other injuries. However, a few other considerations are needed. First, if colloid has not been given, protein replacement may be required and the level of serum albumin can be used as a guide, with supplementation advised if the level is below 2 to 2.5 g/dL. Second, if a hypertonic saline approach was employed, more free water may be needed to reduce any hyperosmolar state induced. Potassium and magnesium supplementation are commonly required, and close monitoring (and control) of blood glucose should be undertaken.

# Conclusion

Burn injuries in children—even severe burns—can successfully be treated provided resuscitation is properly accomplished. Successful resuscitation also leads to fewer complications, such as organ dysfunction and sepsis. Although many different formulas can be employed during the resuscitation phase, in the last 2 decades there has been a tendency to use much higher volumes than calculated. This "fluid creep" can have serious consequences, especially in regard to the development of abdominal compartment syndrome. Mistakes in calculating fluid requirements from formulas or incorrectly estimating burn areas can also lead to underresuscitation or overresuscitation. Regardless of the fluid or formula chosen, starting fluid resuscitation as soon as possible is the key to successful resuscitation and outcome.

There is no consensus regarding the type of fluid (or formula) to be used in pediatric burn resuscitation. Most approaches use isotonic crystalloid, although some cases may benefit from hypertonic saline solutions if appropriate precautions are taken. The use of colloid is still controversial, with no demonstrated benefit in long-term outcome, although recent work indicates that judicious use may not adversely affect mortality rates. If colloid is chosen, plasma, albumin, or gelatin are the safest approaches to take.

Proper attention to endpoint titration rather than adhering to rigid parameters tends to lead to better resuscitation. Although classical endpoints such as urine output and cardiac indices are still important, other invasive means of assessing pulmonary or cardiovascular parameters should be used when there is uncertainty in assessment or in more severe cases. However, the decision to use invasive devices must always be balanced against risk engendered by their usage.

The use of adjunctive measures to support hemo-dynamics is encouraged, but should be conservative in approach. On the other hand, employing antioxidants, such as vitamin C, seems to be a safe and promising adjunct; it is likely that many more novel adjunctive treatments will be developed as research continues into better comprehension of the burn injury at the cellular level.

Perhaps the most important message of all is that there should be no grounds to refuse treatment to a badly burned child simply because of the nature of the injuries; even children with 98% TBSA injuries and inhalation injury have survived to lead productive lives.

## KEY POINTS

- There is no evidence that one particular formula is better than another; starting fluid resuscitation without delay is more critical than the formula chosen.
- Isotonic crystalloid formulas are most commonly used during the first 24 hours of burn resuscitation.
- In children, adequate maintenance volumes must be added to the resuscitation formulas.
- Hypertonic saline-based approaches should be reserved for those cases that may benefit (signs of overresuscitation, more severe injuries).
- The use of colloids is optional, but if chosen, should not be started until 8 to 12 hours postburn.
- The colloids with the least risk are plasma, albu-min, and gelatin.
- If colloids are not given during resuscitation, plasma protein replacement will be necessary in some children.
- Start enteral feeding as soon as the child can tolerate it—often within hours of the injury.
- Be mindful of caloric requirements, especially in high BSA cases.
- Ensure that burned areas are estimated and for-mulas calculated correctly; mistakes in calcula-tions can be very harmful.
- Resuscitate by means of endpoint titration.
- Classical endpoints such as urine output and car-diac output still remain the most useful; however, invasive monitoring can be employed in more severe cases where hemodynamic monitoring provides additional information.
- Watch out for overresuscitation.
- Overresuscitation can lead to the development of compartment syndromes or even intra-abdominal hypertension, which is often fatal if not aggres-sively treated.

- Underresuscitation may occur in patients with high (>70%) BSA and/or inhalation injury; hy-pertonic saline fluids may have a role to play in these patients.
- In cases of resuscitation failure when underre-suscitation or overresuscitation is not obvious, consider hypertonic saline use or even plasma exchange.
- Inhalation injuries require swift evaluation and frequently intubation or even tracheostomy.

## REFERENCES

1. Shields BJ, Comstock RD, Fernandez SA, et al. Healthcare resource utilization and epidemiology of pediatric burn-associat-ed hospitalizations, United States, 2000. *J Burn Care Res* 2007; **28**(6): 811–26.

2. Bernard SJ, Paulozzi LJ, Wallace LJD. Fatal injuries among children by race and ethnicity—United States, 1999–2002. *MMWR*. 2007; **56**: 1–16.

3. Thombs BD, Singh VA, Milner SM. Children under 4 years are at greater risk of mortality following acute burn injury: evidence from a national sample of 12,902 pediatric admissions. *Shock*. 2006; **26**: 348–352.

4. Miller SF, Kagan RJ, Jeng JC, et al; American Burn Associa-tion. National Burn Repository 2005 report, dataset version 2.0. http://www.ameriburn.org/NBR2005.pdf. Accessed December 14, 2007.

5. Herndon DN, Lemaster J, Beard S, et al. The quality of life after major thermal injury in children: an analysis of 12 survivors with ≥ 80% total body, 70% third-degree burns. *J Trauma*. 1986; **26**: 609–619.

6. Underhill FP. The significance of anhydremia in extensive sur-face burn. *JAMA*. 1930; **95**: 852–857.

7. Cope O, Moore FD. The redistribution of body water and fluid therapy of the burned patient. *Ann Surg*. 1947; **126**: 1010–1045.

8. Evans EI, Purnell OJ, Bobinett PW, Batchelor ADR, Martin M. Fluid and electrolyte requirements in severe burns. *Ann Surg*. 1952; **135**: 804–817.

9. Reiss E, Stirmann JA, Artz CP, Davis JH, Amspacher WH. Fluid and electrolyte balance in burns. *Ann Surg*. 1953; **137**: 456–464.

10. Baxter CR, Shires T. Physiological response to crystalloid resuscitation of severe burns. *Ann N Y Acad Sci*. 1968; **150**: 874–894.

11. Baxter CR. Fluid volume and electrolyte changes in the early post-burn period. *Clin Plast Surg*. 1974; **1**: 693–703.

12. Baxter CR. Problems and complications of burn shock resus-citation. *Surg Clin North Am*. 1978; **58**: 1313–1322.

13. Merrell SW, Saffle JR, Sullivan JJ, Navar PD, Kravtiz M, Warden GD. Fluid resuscitation in thermally injured children. *Am J Surg*. 1986; **152**: 664–669.

14. Curreri PW, Luterman A, Braun DW, Shires GT. Burn injury. Analysis of survival and hospitalization time for 937 patients. *Ann Surg*. 1980; **192**: 472–478.

15. Feller I, Flora JD Jr., Bawol R. Baseline results of therapy for burned patients. *JAMA*. 1976; **236**: 1943–1947.

16. Graves TA, Cioffi WG, McManus WF, Mason AD, Pruitt BA. Fluid resuscitation of infants and children with massive thermal injury. *J Trauma*. 1988; **28**: 1656–1659.

17. Holm C, Mayr M, Tegeler J, et al. A clinical randomized study on the effects of invasive monitoring on burn shock resuscitation. *Burns*. 2004; **30**: 798–807.

18. Carvajal HF. A physiologic approach to fluid therapy in severely burned children. *Surg Gynecol Obstet*. 1980; **150**: 379–384.

19. Hilton JG. Effects of fluid resuscitation on total fluid loss following thermal injury. *Surg Gynecol Obstet*. 1981; **152**: 441–447.

20. Demling RH, Kramer GC, Gunther R, Nerlich M. Effect of nonprotein colloid on postburn edema formation in soft tissues and lung. *Surgery*. 1984; **95**: 593–602.

21. Schierhout G, Roberts I. Fluid resuscitation with colloid or crystalloid solutions in critically ill patients: a systematic review of randomised trials. *BMJ*. 1998; **316**: 961–964.

22. Monafo WW, Chuntrasakul C, Ayvazian VH. Hypertonic sodium solutions in the treatment of burn shock. *Am J Surg*. 1973; **126**: 778–783.

23. Caldwell FT, Bowser BH. Critical evaluation of hypertonic and hypotonic solutions to resuscitate severely burned children: a prospective study. *Ann Surg*. 1979; **189**: 546–550.

24. Monafo WW, Halverson JD, Schechtman K. The role of concentrated sodium solutions in the resuscitation of patients with severe burns. *Surgery*. 1984; **95**: 129–135.

25. Gunn ML, Hansbrough JF, Davis JW, Furst SR, Field TO. Prospective, randomized trial of hypertonic sodium lactate versus lactated Ringer's solution for burn shock resuscitation. *J Trauma*. 1889; **29**: 1261–1267.

26. Huang PP, Stucky FS, Dimick AR, Treat RC, Bessey PQ, Rue LW. Hypertonic sodium resuscitation is associated with renal failure and death. *Ann Surg*. 1995; **221**: 543–557.

27. Finberg L, Luttrell CN, Redd H. Pathogenesis of lesions in the nervous system in hypernatremic states: experimental studies of gross anatomic changes and alterations of chemical composition of the tissues. *Pediatrics*. 1959; **23**: 46–53.

28. Morris-Jones PH, Houston IB, Evans RC. Prognosis of the neurological complications of acute hypernatraemia. *Lancet*. 1967; **2**: 1385–1389.

29. Shimizaki S, Yoshioka T, Tanaka N, et al. Body fluid changes during hypertonic lactated saline solution therapy for burn shock. *J Trauma*. 1977; **17**: 38–43.

30. Dries DJ, Waxman K. Adequate resuscitation of burn patients may not be measured by urine output and vital signs. *Crit Care Med*. 1991; **19**: 327–329.

31. Shoemaker WC, Montgomery ES, Kaplan E, Elwyn DH. Physiologic patterns in surviving and nonsurviving shock patients. Use of sequential cardiorespiratory variables in defining criteria for therapeutic goals and early warning of death. *Arch Surg*. 1973; **106**: 630–636.

32. Bland R, Shoemaker WC, Shabot MM. Physiologic monitoring goals for the critically ill patient. *Surg Gynecol Obstet*. 1978; **147**: 833–841.

33. Fleming A, Bishop M, Shoemaker W, et al. Prospective trial of supranormal values as goals of resuscitation in severe trauma. *Arch Surg*. 1992; **127**: 1175–1181.

34. Schiller WR, Bay RC, Garren RL, Parker I, Sagraves SG. Hyperdynamic resuscitation improves survival in patients with life-threatening burns. *J Burn Care Rehabil*. 1997; **18**: 10–16.

35. Connors AF, Speroff T, Dawson NV, et al. The effectiveness of right heart catheterization in the initial care of critically ill patients. *JAMA*. 1996; **276**: 889–897.

36. Soni N. Swan song for the Swan-Ganz catheter? *BMJ*. 1996; **313**: 763–764.

37. Dalen JE, Bone RC. Is it time to pull the pulmonary artery catheter? *JAMA*. 1996; **276**: 916–918.

38. Holm C, Melcer B, Hörbrand F, Wörl HH, von Donnersmarck GH, Mühlbauer W. Intrathoracic blood volume as an early end point in resuscitation of the severely burned: an observational study of 24 patients. *J Trauma*. 2000; **48**: 728–734.

39. Sakka SG, Reinhart K, Wegscheider K, Meier-Hellmann A. Comparison of cardiac output and circulatory blood volumes by transpulmonary thermo-dye dilution and transcutaneous indocyanine green measurement in critically ill patients. *Chest*. 2002; **121**: 559–565.

40. Pfeiffer UJ, Wisner-Euteneier AJ, Lichtwarck-Aschoff M, Zimmerman G, Blümel G. Less invasive monitoring of cardiac performance using arterial thermodilution. *Clin Intensive Care*. 1994; **5**: 28.

41. Godje O, Peyerl M, Seebauer T, Dewald O, Reichart B. Reproducibility of double indicator dilution measurements of intrathoracic blood volume compartments, extravascular lung water and liver function. *Chest*. 1998; **113**: 1070–1077.

42. Küntscher MV, Germann G, Hartmann B. Correlations between cardiac output, stroke volume, central venous pressure, intra-abdominal pressure and total circulating blood volume in resuscitation of major burns. *Resuscitation*. 2006; **70**: 37–43.

43. Engrav LH, Colscott PL, Kemalyan N, et al. A biopsy of the use of the Baxter formula to resuscitate burns or do we do it like Charlie did it? *J Burn Care Rehabil*. 2000; **21**: 91–95.

44. Friedrich JB, Sullivan SR, Engrav LH, et al. Is supra-Baxter resuscitation in burn patients a new phenomenon? *Burns*. 2004; **30**: 464–466.

45. Pruitt BA Jr. Protection from excessive resuscitation: "pushing the pendulum back." *J Trauma*. 2000; **49:** 567–568.

46. Sullivan SR, Friedrich JB, Engrav LH, et al. "Opioid creep" is real and may be the cause of "fluid creep." *Burns*. 2004; **30:** 583–590.

47. Greenhalgh DG, Warden GD. The importance of intra-abdominal pressure measurements in burned children. *J Trauma*. 1995; **36:** 685–690.

48. O'Mara MS, Slater H, Goldfarb IW, Caushaj PF. A prospective, randomized evaluation of intra-abdominal pressures with crystalloid and colloid resuscitation in burn patients. *J Trauma*. 2005; **58:** 1011–1018.

49. Greenhalgh DG. Burn resuscitation. *J Burn Care Res*. 2007; **28:** 555–565.

50. Gattinoni L, Brazzi L, Pelosi P, et al. A trial of goal-oriented hemodynamic therapy in critically ill patients. *N Engl J Med*. 1995; **333:** 1025–1032.

51. Ahrns KS. Trends in burn resuscitation: shifting the focus from fluids to adequate endpoint monitoring, edema control, and adjuvant therapies. *Crit Care Nurs Clin North Am*. 2004; **16:** 75–98.

52. Pham TN, Ciancio LC, Gibran NS. American Burn Association practice guidelines for burn shock resuscitation. *J Burn Care Res*. 2008; **29:** 257–266.

53. Sackett DL. Rules of evidence and clinical recommendations on the use of antithrombotic agents. *Chest*. 1989; **95:** 2S–4S.

54. Barton RG, Saffle JR, Morris SF, Mone M, Davis B, Shelby J. Resuscitation of thermally injured patients with oxygen transport criteria as goals of therapy. *J Burn Care Rehabil*. 1997; **181** (pt 1): 1–9.

55. Holm C, Melcer B, Horbrand F, et al. The relationship between oxygen delivery and oxygen consumption during fluid resuscitation of burn-related shock. *J Burn Care Rehabil*. 2000; **21:** 147–154.

56. Benjamin D, Herndon DN. Special considerations of age: the pediatric burned patients. In: Herndon DN, ed. *Total Burn Care*. 2nd ed. London: WB Saunders; 2001: 427–438.

57. Jeng JC, Lee K, Jablonski K, Jordan MH. Serum lactate and base deficit suggest inadequate resuscitation of patients with burn injuries: application of a point-of-care laboratory instrument. *J Burn Care Rehabil*. 1997; **18:** 402–405.

58. Choi J, Cooper A, Gomez M, Fish J, Cartotto R. The 2000 Moyer award. The relevance of base deficits after burn injuries. *J Burn Care Rehabil*. 2000; **21:** 499–505.

59. Jeng JC, Jablonski K, Bridgeman A, Jordan MH. Serum lactate, not base deficit, rapidly predicts survival after major burns. *Burns*. 2002; **28:** 161–166.

60. Andel D, Kamholz LP, Roka J, et al. Base deficit and lactate: early predictors of morbidity and mortality in patients with burns. *Burns*. 2007; **33:** 973–978.

61. Holm C, Hörbrand F, Mayr M, Henckel von Donnersmarck G, Mühlbauer W. Assessment of splanchnic perfusion by gastric tonometry in patients with acute hypovolemic burn shock. *Burns*. 2006; **32:** 689–694.

62. Warden GD. Burn shock resuscitation. *World J Surg*. 1992; **16:** 16–23.

63. Ahrns KS, Harkins DR. Initial resuscitation after burn injury: therapies, strategies, and controversies. *AACN Clin Issues*. 1999; **10:** 46–60.

64. Diller KR. Adapting adult scald safety standards to children. *J Burn Care Res*. 2006; **27:** 314–324.

65. Drago DA. Kitchen scalds and thermal burns in children five years and younger. *Pediatrics*. 2005; **115:** 10–16.

66. Fiser HD. Intraosseous infusion. *N Engl J Med*. 1990; **322:** 1579–1581.

67. Mlcak R, Cortiella J, Desai MH, Herndon DN. Emergency management of pediatric burn victims. *Pediatr Emerg Care*. 1998; **14:** 51–54.

68. McDonald WS, Sharp CW, Deitch EA. Immediate enteral feeding in burn patients is safe and effective. *Ann Surg*. 1991; **213:** 177–183.

69. Brown TL, Hernon C, Owens B. Incidence of vomiting in burns and implications for mass burn casualty management. *Burns*. 2003; **29:** 159–162.

70. Hildreth MA, Herndon DN, Desai MH, Broemeling LD. Current treatment reduces calories required to maintain weight in pediatric patients with burns. *J Burn Care Rehabil*. 1990; **11:** 405–409.

71. Hildreth MA, Herndon DN, Desai MH, Duke MA. Caloric needs of adolescent patients with burns. *J Burn Care Rehabil*. 1989; **10:** 523–526.

72. Gore DC, Rutan RL, Hildreth M, Desai MH, Herndon DN. Comparison of resting energy expenditures and caloric intake in children with severe burns. *J Burn Care Rehabil*. 1990; **11:** 400–404.

73. Barrow RE, Jeschke MG, Herndon DN. Early fluid resuscitation improves outcomes in severely burned children. *Resuscitation*. 2000; **45:** 91–96.

74. Demling RH. The burn edema process: current concepts. *J Burn Care Rehabil*. 2005; **26:** 207–227.

75. Mendoza G, Alvarez AI, Pulido MM, et al. Inhibitory effects of different antioxidants on hyaluronan depolymerization. *Carbohydr Res*. 2007; **342:** 96–102.

76. Sener G, Sehirli O, Erkanli G, Cetinel S, Gedik N, Yeğen B. 2-Mercaptoethane sulfonate (MESNA) protects against burn-induced renal injury in rats. *Burns*. 2004; **30:** 557–564.

77. Tanaka H, Matsuda T, Miyagantani Y, Yukioka T, Matsuda H, Shimazaki S. Reduction of resuscitation fluid volumes in severely burned patients using ascorbic acid administration: a randomized, prospective study. *Arch Surg*. 2000; **135:** 326–331.

78. Carvajal HF, Linares HA, Brouhard BH. Relationship of burn size to vascular permeability changes in rats. *Surg Gynecol Obstet*. 1979; **149:** 193–202.

79. Demling R, Mazzess R, Witt R, Wolberg W. The study of burn edema using dichromatic absorptiometry. *J Trauma*. 1978; **18**: 124–128.

80. Button B, Baker RD, Vertrees RA, et al. Quantitative assessment of a circulating depolarizing factor. *Shock*. 2001; **15**: 239–244.

81. Horton JW, Tan J, White DJ, Maass DL. Burn injury decreases myocardial Na-K-ATPase activity: the role of PKC inhibition. *Am J Physiol Regul Integr Comp Physiol*. 2007; **293**: R1684–R1692.

82. Yu YM, Tompkins RG, Ryan CM, Young VR. *JPEN J Parenter Enteral Nutr*. 1999; **23**: 160–168.

83. Ballard-Croft C, Maass DL, Sikes PJ, Horton JW. Sepsis and burn complicated by sepsis after cardiac transporter expression. *Burns*. 2007; **33**: 72–80.

84. Carlson DL, Maass DL, White J, Sikes P, Horton JW. Caspase inhibition reduces cardiac myocyte dyshomeostasis and improves cardiac contractile function after major burn injury. *J Appl Physiol*. 2007; **103**: 323–330.

85. Gore DC, Ferrando A, Barnett J, et al. Influence of glucose kinetics on plasma lactate concentration and energy expenditure in severely burned patients. *J Trauma*. 2000; **49**: 677–678.

86. Gore DC, Rinehart A, Asimakis G. Temporal changes in cellular energy following burn injury. *Burns*. 2005; **31**: 998–1002.

87. Rhee P, Koustova E, Alam HB. Searching for the optimal resuscitation method: recommendations for the initial fluid resuscitation of combat casualties. *J Trauma*. 2003; **54**: S52–S62.

88. Watters JM, Brundage SI, Todd SR, et al. Resuscitation with lactated Ringer's does not increase inflammatory response in a swine model of uncontrolled hemorrhagic shock. *Shock*. 2004; **22**: 283–287.

89. Pruitt BA. Fluid and electrolyte replacement in the burned patient. *Surg Clin North Am*. 1978; **58**: 1291–1312.

90. Kinsky MP, Milner SM, Button B, Dubick MA, Kramer GC. Resuscitation of severe thermal injury with hypertonic saline dextran: effects on peripheral and visceral edema in sheep. *J Trauma*. 2000; **49**: 844–853.

91. Chen LW, Huang HL, Lee IT, Hsu CM, Lu PJ. Hypertonic saline enhances host defense to bacterial challenge by augmenting toll-like receptors. *Crit Care Med*. 2006; **34**: 1758–1768.

92. Kien ND, Antognini JF, Reilly DA, Moore PG. Small-volume resuscitation using hypertonic saline improves organ perfusion in burned rats. *Anesth Analg*. 1996; **83**: 782–788.

93. Milner SM, Kinsky MP, Guha SC, Herndon DN, Phillips LG, Kramer GC. A comparison of two different 2400 mOsm solutions for resuscitation of major burns. *J Burn Care Rehabil*. 1997; **18**: 109–115.

94. Murphy JT, Horton JW, Purdue GF, Hunt JL. Cardiovascular effect of 7.5% sodium chloride-dextran infusion after thermal injury. *Arch Surg*. 1999; **134**: 1091–1097.

95. Oda J, Ueyama M, Yamashita K, et al. Hypertonic lactated saline resuscitation reduces the risk of abdominal compartment syndrome in severely burned patients. *J Trauma*. 2006; **60**: 64–71.

96. Jelenko C III, Williams JB, Wheeler ML, et al. Studies in shock and resuscitation, I: use of a hypertonic, albumin-containing, fluid demand regimen (HALFD) in resuscitation. *Crit Care Med*. 1979; **7**: 157–167.

97. Bowser-Wallace BH, Caldwell FT Jr. A prospective analysis of hypertonic lactated saline v. Ringer's lactate-colloid for the resuscitation of severely burned children. *Burns Incl Therm Inj*. 1986; **12**: 402–409.

98. Shimazaki S, Yukioka T, Matuda H. Fluid distribution and pulmonary dysfunction following burn shock. *J Trauma*. 1991; **31**: 623–626.

99. Bortolani A, Governa M, Barisoni D. Fluid replacement in burned patients. *Acta Chir Plast*. 1996; **38**: 132–136.

100. Bunn F, Roberts I, Tasker R, Akpa E. Hypertonic versus near isotonic crystalloid for fluid resuscitation in critically ill patients. *Cochrane Database Syst Rev*. 2004; CD002045.

101. Cioffi G Jr., Vaughan GM, Heironimus JD, Jordan BS, Mason AD, Pruitt BA Jr. Dissociation of blood volume and flow in regulation of salt and water balance in burn patients. *Ann Surg*. 1991; **214**: 213–220.

102. Harms BA, Bodai BI, Kramer GC, Demling RH. Microvascular fluid and protein flux in pulmonary and systemic circulation after thermal injury. *Microvasc Res*. 1982; **23**: 77–86.

103. Reed RK, Bowen BD, Bert JL. Microvascular exchange and interstitial volume regulation in the rat: implications of the model. *Am J Physiol*. 1989; **2157**: H2081–H2089.

104. Chen LW, Wang JS, Hwang B, Chen JS, Hsu CM. Reversal of the effect of albumin on gut barrier function in burn by the inhibition of inducible isoform of nitric oxide synthase. *Arch Surg*. 2003; **138**: 1219–1225.

105. Fogarty BJ, Khan K. Multicentre randomised controlled trial is needed before changing resuscitation formulas for major burns [letter]. *BMJ*. 1999; **318**: 1215.

106. Perel P, Roberts I. Colloids versus crystalloids for fluid resuscitation in critically ill patients. *Cochrane Database Syst Rev*. 2007; CD000567.

107. Du GB, Slater H, Goldfarb IW. Influences of different resuscitation regimens on acute early weight gain in extensively burned patients. *Burns*. 1991; **17**: 147–150.

108. Muir I. The use of the Mount Vernon formula in the treatment of burn shock. *Intensive Care Med*. 1981; **7**: 49–53.

109. Hughes KR, Armstrong RF, Brough MD, Parkhouse N. Fluid requirements of patients with burns and inhalation injuries in an intensive care unit. *Intensive Care Med*. 1989; **15**: 464–466.

110. Murison MS, Laitung JK, Pigott RW. Effectiveness of burns resuscitation using two different formulas. *Burns*. 1991; **17**: 484–489.

111. Goodwin CW, Dorethy J, Lam V, Pruitt BA Jr. Randomized trial of efficacy of crystalloid and colloid resuscitation on hemodynamic response and lung water following thermal injury. *Ann Surg*. 1983; **197**: 520–531.

112. Carvajal HF, Parks DH. Optimal composition of burn resuscitation fluids. *Crit Care Med.* 1988; **16**: 695–700.

113. Greenhalgh DG, Housinger TA, Kagan RJ, et al. Maintenance of serum albumin levels in pediatric burn patients: a prospective randomized trial. *J Trauma.* 1995; **39**: 67–74.

114. Sheridan RL, Pelack K, Cunningham JJ. Physiologic hypoalbuminemia is well tolerated by severely burned children. *J Trauma.* 1997; **43**: 448–452.

115. Oliver RI Jr., Spain D, Stadelmann RW. Burns, resuscitation and early management. *eMedicine 2006.* http://www.emedicine.com/plastic/topic159.htm. Accessed December 18, 2007.

116. Vermeulen LC Jr., Ratko TA, Erstad BL, Brecher ME, Matuszewski KA. A paradigm for consensus. The University Hospital Consortium guidelines for the use of albumin, nonprotein colloid, and crystalloid. *Arch Intern Med.* 1995; **155**: 373–379.

117. Pulimood TB, Park GR. Debate: albumin administration should be avoided in the critically ill. *Crit Care.* 2000; **4**: 151–155.

118. Webb AR. The appropriate role of colloids in managing fluid imbalance: a critical review of recent meta-analytic findings. *Crit Care.* 2000; **4**(2): S26–S32.

119. Cochran A, Morris SE, Edelman LS, Saffle JR. Burn patient characteristics and outcomes following resuscitation with albumin. *Burns.* 2007; **33**: 25–30.

120. Matejtschuk P, Dash CH, Gascoigne EW. Production of human albumin solution: a continually developing colloid. *Br J Anaesth.* 2000; **85**: 887–895.

121. Bocanegra M, Hinostroza F, Kefalides NA, et al. A long-term study of early fluid therapy in severely burned adults. III. Simultaneous comparison of saline solutions alone, or combined with plasma. *JAMA.* 1966; **195**: 268–274.

122. Waxman K, Holness R, Tominaga G, Chela P, Grimes J. Hemodynamic and oxygen transport effects in burn resuscitation. *Ann Surg.* 1989; **209**: 341–345.

123. Elgjo GI, Traber DL, Hawkins HK, Kramer GC. Burn resuscitation with two doses of 4 mL/kg hypertonic saline dextran provides sustained fluid sparing: a 48-hour prospective study in conscious sheep. *J Trauma.* 2000; **49**: 251–265.

124. Waters LM, Christensen MA, Sato RM. Hetastarch: an alternative colloid to burn shock management. *J Burn Care Rehabil.* 1989; **10**: 11–16.

125. Chen J, Han CM, Xia SC, Tang ZJ, Su SJ. Evaluation of effectiveness and safety of a new hydroxyethyl starch used in resuscitation of burn shock [in Chinese]. *Zhonghua Shao Shang Za Zhi.* 2006; **22**: 333–336.

126. Sheridan RL, Schnitzer JJ. Management of the high-risk pediatric burn patient. *J Pediatr Surg.* 2001; **36**: 1308–1312.

127. Herndon DN, Hawkins HK, Nguyen TT, et al. Characterization of growth hormone enhanced donor site healing in patients with large cutaneous burns. *Ann Surg.* 1995; **221**: 849–856.

128. Gueugniaud PY, David JS, Petit P. Early hemodynamic variations assessed by an echo-Doppler aortic blood flow device in a severely burned infant: correlation with the circulating cytokines. *Pediatr Emerg Care.* 1998; **14**: 282–284.

129. Bessey PQ, Arons RR, DiMaggio CJ, Yurt RW. The vulnerabilities of age: burns in children and older adults. *Surgery.* 2006; **140**: 705–717.

130. Ryan CM, Schoenfeld DA, Thorpe WP, Sheridan RL, Cassem EH, Tompkins RG. Objective estimates of the probability of death from burn injuries. *N Engl J Med.* 1998; **338**: 362–366.

131. Barrow RE, Spies M, Barrow LN, Herndon DN. Influence of demographics and inhalation injury on burn mortality in children. *Burns.* 2004; **30**: 72–77.

132. Meshulam-Derazon S, Nachumovsky S, Ad-El D, Sulkes J, Hauben DJ. Prediction of morbidity and mortality on admission to a burn unit. *Plast Reconstr Surg.* 2006; **118**: 116–120.

133. Finnerty CC, Herndon DN, Jeschke MG. Inhalation injury in severely burned children does not augment the systemic inflammatory response. *Crit Care.* 2007; **11**: R22.

134. Madnani DD, Steele NP, de Vries E. Factors that predict the need for intubation in patients with smoke inhalation injury. *Ear Nose Throat J.* 2006; **85**: 278–280.

135. Bennett JDC, Milner SM, Gheranrdini G, Phillips LG, Herndon DN. Burn inhalation injury. *Emerg Med.* 1997; **12**: 22–24,31,32.

136. Magnason DK, Maier RV. Pathophysiology of injury. In: Eichelberger MR, ed. *Pediatric Trauma: Prevention, Acute Care, and Rehabilitation.* St. Louis, MO: Mosby Year Book, 1993: 61.

137. Palmieri TL, Jackson W, Greenhalgh DG. Benefits of early tracheostomy in severely burned children. *Crit Care Med.* 2002; **30**: 922–924.

138. Desai MH, Mlcak R, Richardson J, Nichols R, Herndon DN. Reduction in mortality in pediatric patients with inhalation injury with aerosolized heparin/N-acetylcystine therapy. *J Burn Care Rehabil.* 1998; **19**: 210–212.

139. Palmieri TL, Enkhbaatar P, Bayliss R, et al. Continuous nebulized albuterol attenuates acute lung injury in an ovine model of combined burn and smoke inhalation. *Crit Care Med.* 2006; **34**: 1719–1724.

140. Herndon DN, Barrow RE, Linares HA, et al. Inhalation injury in burned patients: effects and treatment. *Burns Incl Therm Inj.* 1988; **14**: 349–356.

141. Navar PD, Saffle JR, Warden GD. Effect of inhalation injury on fluid resuscitation requirements after thermal injury. *Am J Surg.* 1985; **150**: 716–720.

142. Dai NT, Chen TM, Cheng TY, et al. The comparison of early fluid therapy in extensive flame burns between inhalation and non-inhalation injuries. *Burns.* 1998; **24**: 671–675.

143. Klein MB, Hayden D, Elson C, et al. The association between fluid administration and outcome following major burn: a multicenter study. *Ann Surg.* 2007; **245**: 622–628.

144. Hobson KG, Young KM, Ciraulo A, Palmieri TL, Greenhalgh DG. Release of abdominal compartment syndrome improves survival in patients with burn injury. *J Trauma.* 2002; **53**: 1129–1134.

**145.** Ivy ME, Atweh NA, Palmer J, Possenti PP, Pineau M, D'Aiuto M. Intra-abdominal hypertension and abdominal compartment syndrome in burn patients. *J Trauma*. 2000; **49:** 387–391.

**146.** Oda J, Yamashita K, Inoue T, et al. Resuscitation fluid volume and abdominal compartment syndrome in patients with major burns. *Burns*. 2006; **32:** 151–154.

**147.** Zak AL. Acute respiratory failure that complicates the resuscitation of pediatric patients with scald injuries [letter]. *J Burn Care Rehabil*. 2000; **21:** 290.

**148.** Fakhry SM, Alexander J, Smith D, Meyer AA, Peterson HD. Regional and institutional variation in burn care. *J Burn Care Rehabil*. 1995; **16:** 85–90.

**149.** Baker RH, Akhavani MA, Jallali N. Resuscitation of thermal injuries in the United Kingdom and Ireland. *J Plast Reconstr Aesthet Surg*. 2007; **60:** 682–685.

**150.** Blumetti J, Hunt JL, Arnoldo BD, Parkas JK, Purdue GF. The Parkland formula under fire: is the criticism justified? *J Burn Care Res*. 2008; **29:** 1801–1886.

**151.** Freiburg C, Igneri P, Sartorelli K, Rogers F. Effects of differences in percent total body surface area estimation on fluid resuscitation of transferred burn patients. *J Burn Care Res*. 2007; **28:** 42–48.

**152.** Warden GD. Fluid resuscitation and early management. In: Herndon DN, ed. *Total Burn Care*. 2nd ed. London: WB Saunders; 2001: 88–97.

**153.** Shah A, Connolly CM, Kirschner RA, Herndon DN, Kramer GC. Evaluation of hyperdynamic resuscitation in 60% TBSA burn-injured sheep. *Shock*. 2004; **21:** 86–92.

**154.** Schultz AM, Werba A, Wolrab C. Early cardiorespiratory patterns in severely burned patients with concomitant inhalation injury. *Burns*. 1997; **23:** 421–425.

**155.** Beale RJ, Hollenberg SM, Vincent JL, Parrillo JE. Vasopressor and inotropic support in septic shock: an evidence-based review. *Crit Care Med*. 2004; 32(11).

**156.** Dellinger RP, Levy MM, Carlet JM, et al. Surviving sepsis campaign: international guidelines for management of severe sepsis and septic shock: 2008. *Crit Care Med*. 2008; **36:** 296–327.

**157.** Cancio LC, Reifenberg L, Barillo DJ, et al. Standard variables fail to identify who will not respond to fluid resuscitation following thermal injury: brief report. *Burns*. 2005; **31:** 358–365.

**158.** Sullivan SR, Ahmadi AJ, Singh CN, et al. Elevated orbital pressure: another untoward effect of massive resuscitation after burn injury. *J Trauma*. 2006; **60:** 72–76.

**159.** Warden GD, Stratta RJ, Saffle JR, Kravitz M, Ninneman JL. Plasma exchange therapy in patients failing to resuscitate from burn shock. *J Trauma*. 1983; **23:** 945–951.

**160.** Stratta RJ, Saffle JR, Kravitz M, Ninneman JL, Warden GD. Exchange transfusion therapy in pediatric burn shock. *Circ Shock*. 1984; **12:** 203–212.

**161.** Schnarrs RH, Cline CW, Goldfarb IW, et al. Plasma exchange for failure of early resuscitation in thermal injuries. *J Burn Care Rehabil*. 1986; **7:** 230–233.

**162.** Kravitz M, Warden GD, Sullivan JJ, Saffle JR. A randomized trial of plasma exchange in the treatment of burn shock. *J Burn Care Rehabil*. 1989; **10:** 17–26.

**163.** Bhat S, Humphries YM, Gulati S. The problems of burn resuscitation formulae: a need for a simplified guideline. *J Burns Wounds*. 2004; 3: 7. http://www.journalofburnsandwounds.com/volume03/volume03_article06.pdf. Accessed January 22, 2008.

**164.** Reynolds EM, Ryan DP, Sheridan RL, Doody DP. Left ventricular failure complicating severe pediatric burn injuries. *J Pediatr Surg*. 1995; **30:** 264–270.

**165.** Gore DC, Hawkins HK, Chinkes DL, et al. Assessment of adverse events in the demise of pediatric burn patients. *J Trauma*. 2007; **63:** 814–818.

# CHAPTER EIGHT

# BURN CRITICAL CARE

ROB SHERIDAN, MD, BURN SURGERY SERVICE, SHRINERS HOSPITAL FOR CHILDREN, BOSTON, MA

## INTRODUCTION

The probability of survival and the quality of life for burned children has substantially improved over the years. This is largely the result of surgical maneuvers that change the natural history of burns by identification and excision of deep wounds and biologic closure of generated wounds before uncontrolled sepsis and systemic inflammation occur. However, in order to be successful, these physiologically stressful operations, and the burn resuscitation that usually precedes them, require sophisticated critical care management. Although many components of critical care in general apply to burn patients, this chapter will attempt to concisely summarize those critical care issues which are unique to the burn population.

## MANAGEMENT STRATEGY

Organizing the overall care of patients with large burns can be difficult, and is therefore best divided into phases.[1] One such organizational plan is outlined in Table 1. During the initial evaluation and resuscitation phase, which typically occurs from days 0 through 3, the patient and injury are thoroughly evaluated, associated injuries and comorbid conditions are identified, and an accurate individualized fluid resuscitation is carried out. During the second phase, the natural history of burns is changed by identification, excision, and biologic closure of deep wounds. In patients with larger wounds, this may require a series of staged operations during the first 3 to 7 days after injury. During the third phase of definitive wound closure, temporary coverages are replaced with autograft, and acute reconstruction of the hands, face, genitals, and feet are completed. The final stage of care is rehabilitation and reconstruction, which involves ranging, splinting, and antideformity positioning. In actual practice, this phase begins during resuscitation, but becomes increasingly involved and time-consuming towards the end of the acute hospital stay. In patients with serious injuries, this phase of care may continue for years after discharge and include scar management, reconstructive surgery, and emotional recovery.

## Burn Physiology as It Applies to Critical Care

A unique and important aspect of caring for seriously burned children in the intensive care unit involves recognition of a predictable sequence of major physiologic changes (Table 2), which should be anticipated and accurately supported to optimize outcome. These changes were described by Cuthbertson as the "ebb" and "flow" phases of injury.[2] The ebb phase describes the period in the first 24 hours following injury, characterized by a hypodynamic state which is addressed with fluid resuscitation. The physiology of the postresuscitation period, or flow phase, describes the subsequent development of high cardiac output, reduced peripheral resistance, fever, and muscle catabolism. This hypermetabolic phase is profound in patients with large burns and will persist until well after wound closure. The increased need for nutritional support in this latter phase has major implications for burned patients.[3] This period can be significantly exaggerated by delayed wound closure and sepsis.

### Physiology of the Resuscitation Period

After sustaining serious burns, patients develop a diffuse capillary leak that is relatively unique to this population. This is thought to be secondary to a poorly described group of wound-released mediators which results in extravasation of fluids, electrolytes, and even moderate-sized colloid molecules into the interstitial tissues for a number of hours after injury. The clinical consequence of this physiology is the need for fluid resuscitation. A variety of body-size-and-burn-size-based resuscitation formulas have been developed over the past several decades to address this problem. However,

all are inherently inaccurate, as multiple other variables can affect the degree and duration of this leak, including delays in resuscitation, inhalation injury, and the depth and vapor transmission characteristics of the wound. No formula accurately predicts volume requirements in all patients, and unfortunately, inaccurate resuscitation is associated with substantial morbidity. Therefore, burn resuscitation is ideally guided by hourly reevaluation of resuscitation endpoints, with formulas serving only to help determine initial volume infusion rates and roughly predict overall volume requirements.

## Postresuscitation Physiology

After a successful resuscitation, the diffuse capillary leak predictably abates and fluid needs abruptly decline 18 to 24 hours after injury. Over the next 2 or 3 days, a systemic inflammatory state evolves which is manifested clinically by a hyperdynamic circulation, fever, and increased protein catabolism. The etiology of this physiology is also poorly characterized but is felt to be driven by a combination of cortisol, catecholamines, glucagon, and bacteria and their by-products from the wound as well as a compromised gastrointestinal barrier, pain, and evaporative temperature loss.

The clinical consequences during this phase involve cachexia and compromised wound healing if adequate nutritional support is not provided. Other important considerations are control of environmental temperature, prompt removal of nonviable tissue with physiologic wound closure, and management of pain and anxiety. Although these maneuvers will reduce the degree of systemic inflammation and hypermetabolism, there is no known method by which this physiology can be eliminated.

## Intensive Care Unit Admission and Resuscitation

Burn patients should be approached as having sustained potential multiple traumas. Their evaluation should follow guidelines established by the advanced trauma life support (ATLS) course of the American College of Surgeons Committee on Trauma.[4] In many if not most cases, burn patients will not be completely evaluated for trauma prior to their arrival in the intensive care unit. This need for a thorough evaluation and tertiary survey is an important consideration during initial care in the ICU.

### Admission Evaluation

A special point of emphasis regarding the primary survey of burn patients includes airway evaluation and control. Progressive mucosal edema can compromise airway patency over the first few postinjury hours, especially in young children. The safety and control of the airway should be evaluated as soon as burn patients arrive in the ICU. Swelling of the face, tongue, or neck or the presence of soot in the airway should prompt concern. A large surface burn in conjunction with these findings can portend rapid airway compromise. Facial and airway edema can make the burned child challenging to intubate. If the child's airway is edematous and appears likely to be difficult, requesting extra help is advisable prior to initiating intubation efforts. Proper tube security is critical since inadvertent extubation in the patient with a burned, swollen face and airway is potentially lethal. A harness system using umbilical ties is one method of proven efficacy. Secure, reliable vascular access is also an essential component of the initial evaluation. In children with significant burns, this usually requires central venous access. In an emergent situation, intraosseous access is a useful bridge, although it is important to confirm proper placement of these lines in order to avoid infusion into soft tissues. A number of burn-specific issues which commonly arise during the secondary survey of burn patients should be considered during the admission of seriously burned children to the ICU (Table 3).

## Initial Resuscitation

Shortly after the burn injury, wound-released mediators are absorbed into the systemic circulation, leading to stress-triggered and pain-triggered hormonal release. These changes drive a diffuse loss of capillary integrity and secondary extravasation of fluids, electrolytes, and moderate-sized colloid molecules. Increased permeability is seen in children whose resuscitation has been delayed or who have suffered inhalation injury. A number of burn resuscitation formulas based on body size and burn extent have evolved over the past 40 years to assist in estimating the fluid needs of these patients. However, since other variables that impact fluid needs are not considered, all the formulas are inherently inaccurate. The modified Brooke is a common consensus resuscitation formula (Table 4). Although somewhat controversial, many centers practice early colloid administration to reduce overall volume needs and reduce edema.

Burn resuscitation should be guided by hourly reevaluation of resuscitation endpoints (Table 5). At any point during resuscitation, the total 24-hour volume can be predicted based on the known volume infused and the current rate of infusion. If this number exceeds 6 ml/kg/% burn/24 h, it is likely that the resuscitation is not proceeding optimally. At this point one can consider the use of low-dose dopamine, colloid administration, echocardiography, or placement of a pulmonary artery catheter to gather additional information regarding the adequacy of ventricular filling and myocardial contractility.

## BURN INTENSIVE CARE ISSUES BY SYSTEM

As care in the intensive care unit proceeds, multiple burn-specific issues can be expected. ICU length of stay for burn patients is typically longer compared to those associated with most other disease processes, as children undergo the trial of staged wound closure.

## Neurologic Issues in the Burn ICU

Neurologic issues that should be addressed on a regular basis include management of pain and anxiety, the exposed globe, and peripheral neuropathies. Significant pain and anxiety accompany virtually all burn injuries and can have adverse short-term and long-term physiologic and psychological consequences. Post-traumatic stress syndrome is described in approximately a third of patients surviving serious burns.[5] In the past, suboptimal control of predictable injury-related pain and treatment-related pain and anxiety was very common. This is a legacy that the current generation of burn intensivists endeavors to correct. Given the rapid development of opiate and benzodiazepine tolerance in patients with serious burns, as well as the fear of respiratory depression, addiction, and litigation, significant undermedication in this unique population of patients with severe pain has resulted, along with an often protracted need for intensive care.[6] However, addiction is rare, and medication requirements typically rapidly decrease after wound closure, particularly in children. Successful management is facilitated by organized pharmacological guidelines.[7] Selected nonpharmacological measures can be useful adjuncts to pain control, but opiate and benzodiazepine synergy remains the cornerstone at this time.

In children with deep facial burns and large surface burns, intraocular hypertension can occur because of retrobulbar (with generalized) edema in the setting of a noncompliant deeply burned face. When detected, this should be addressed with lateral canthotomy to reduce intraocular pressure and decrease the chance of visual loss. Progressive contraction of the burned eyelids and periocular skin can cause exposure of the globe. This predictably results in desiccation, which is followed by keratitis, ulceration, and globe-threatening infection. To address these issues, frequent lubrication with hourly application of ocular lubricants suffices in most situations. If this is inadequate and keratitis develops, acute lid release is indicated. Tarsorrhaphy is rarely adequate treatment and can damage the lids, as the power of contraction will often cause tarsorrhaphy sutures to pull through.

Peripheral neuropathies occur in critically ill children in the burn intensive care unit because of direct thermal damage to peripheral nerves, metabolic derangements associated with critical illness, or secondary to pressure from positioning or splinting. With careful attention to prompt decompression of tight compartments and proper positioning and splint fitting, many peripheral neuropathies can be avoided. Diligent monitoring of extremity perfusion with prompt escharotomy and/or fasciotomy will avoid the morbidity of constricting eschar and missed compartment syndromes. Properly applied and fitting splints will avoid pressure-induced neuropathies. Careful positioning of deeply sedated or anesthetized patients will prevent traction and pressure injuries.

## Pulmonary Issues in the Burn ICU

Pulmonary issues often dominate the critical care needs of children with burns. These include airway control, inhalation injury, pulmonary infection, respiratory failure, and in some, carbon monoxide intoxication. The highest priority, the "most important vital sign," is security of the airway. Security of the endotracheal tube or tracheostomy should be regularly evaluated and verified. The unit staff should be equipped to deal with sudden airway emergencies. Indications for intubation include impending or established airway edema, respiratory failure, and in some patients, the need for frequent trips to the operating room. Inhalation injury alone, in the absence of complications such as airway obstruction, pneumonia, or respiratory failure, is not an indication for intubation.

### Inhalation Injury

Inhalation injury is a clinical diagnosis based on a history of closed space exposure presence of burned nasal hairs, and carbonaceous sputum. Fiberoptic bronchoscopy facilitates diagnosis in equivocal cases, may help document laryngeal edema, and can also be useful when making decisions regarding preemptive intubation for evolving upper airway edema. Inhalation injury is commonly associated with five issues in the intensive care unit: initial large airway obstruction and bronchospasm, followed later by small airway obstruction, infection, and respiratory failure.

Initially, facial and oropharyngeal edema leads to acute upper airway obstruction, which is more common in smaller children. When anticipated, intubation in this setting is often not emergent, allowing for carefully performed procedures with proper staff and equipment. Bronchospasm caused by aerosolized irritants is a common occurrence in the first 24 to 48 hours, especially in young children. Although it usually responds well to inhaled beta-2

adrenergic agonists, children will occasionally require intravenous bronchodilators such as terbutaline or low-dose epinephrine infusions. Steroids can be useful in rare instances of recalcitrant bronchospasm. If mechanical ventilatory support is necessary, it is important to use ventilation techniques that minimize auto-PEEP in order to avoid an otherwise common and difficult complication.

In the later phases of care, small airway obstruction may develop as necrotic endobronchial debris sloughs, and the ciliary clearance mechanism is usually simultaneously impaired. Small airway obstruction is followed by pulmonary infection (pneumonia or tracheobronchitis) in approximately 30% to 50% of children with inhalation injury.[8] Differentiating between pneumonia and tracheobronchitis (purulent infection of the denuded tracheobronchial tree) is difficult, but the difference is generally not important. Any patient with inhalation injury who develops newly purulent sputum, fever, and impaired gas exchange is likely to have pulmonary infection and should probably be treated with pulmonary toilet and antibiotics adjusted to sputum gram stain and culture.[9] Pulmonary toilet is particularly important because inhalation injury to bronchial mucosa greatly impairs mucocilliary clearance. In most cases, shorter antibiotic courses combined with pulmonary toilet are effective therapy. Since small endotracheal tubes can become suddenly occluded, it is important to be prepared to evaluate acute deterioration of intubated children with inhalation injury (Table 6). In older children with larger endotracheal tubes, therapeutic bronchoscopy can help maintain clearance of more distal airways.

Respiratory failure in burn patients is managed as for other etiologies. Patients generally do well with a pressure-limited ventilation strategy based on permissive hypercapnia.[10] Even if fluid balance is accurate and pulmonary toilet vigorous, some children will fail with this approach and may need to be considered for innovative methods of support, such as extracorporeal support or inhaled nitric oxide.[9] Some patients, especially those with extensive burns and generalized systemic inflammation, will develop ARDS in the absence of infection. These children should be managed with ventilatory strategies that limit inflating pressures. When instituting a strategy of permissive hypercapnia, it is useful to remember that topical sulfamylon is a carbonic anhydrase inhibitor which can limit the ability of the kidneys to generate bicarbonate.

### Carbon Monoxide Poisoning

Carbon monoxide (CO) exposures are not uncommon in structural fires. By binding heme-containing enzymes, notably hemoglobin and the cytochromes, carbon monoxide causes a deficiency of both oxygen delivery and utilization, resulting in cellular hypoxia. There may also be other associated cellular damage due to lipid peroxidation, although this is less well described. It has been reported that a small percentage of patients with serious CO exposures may develop delayed neurologic sequelae. Although cyanide has been detected in some patients with inhalation injury, it is rapidly metabolized and very rarely a cause for concern. Therefore, routine treatment with amyl nitrate and sodium thiosulfate is not justified unless uncorrectable acidosis raises unusual suspicion of severe exposure.

Differentiating serious CO exposures from obtundation due to hypoxia, alcohol, drugs, head injury, or hypotension can be difficult. The issue of whether hyperbaric oxygen may improve the prognosis of those suffering serious isolated CO exposures remains controversial. Rather, the practical question is, when the resource is available, which CO-exposed patients should be treated with hyperbaric oxygen versus 100% normobaric oxygen for 6 hours.[8] Hyperbaric oxygen (HBO) treatments vary, but an exposure to 3 atmospheres for 90 minutes, with 3 10-minute "air breaks," is typical. Especially in monoplace chambers, patient access and monitoring are compromised, so unstable patients are often not good candidates. Relative contraindications include wheezing or air trapping, which increases the risk of pneumothorax, and high fever, due to the increased risk of seizures. Before HBO treatment is begun, endotracheal tube balloons should be filled with saline to avoid balloon compression and associated air leaks, and the possibility of occult pneumothorax from central line placement should be reasonably excluded. Myringotomies are required in unconscious patients. Since there is data both supporting and refuting the utility of HBO in treating CO exposures, each patient should be considered individually with documentation of thoughtful judgment.

## Gastrointestinal Issues in the Burn ICU

Gut failure has a number of presentations common in patients with serious burns. Varieties of gut failure include both solid and hollow organ dysfunctions.

Perhaps the most commonly affected solid organ is the liver, which is manifested in 3 basic forms: early transaminase elevations, cholestasis, and hepatic synthetic failure. It is very common for patients with large burns to develop transaminase elevations in the first days after injury. This is thought to be secondary to early splanchnic ischemia and hepatocellular injury. It usually resolves in the days following successful resuscitation and is rarely associated with synthetic dysfunction. Cholestasis commonly accompanies septic episodes later in the course of burn care and can be differentiated from obstructive phenomena by ultrasound.

Successful treatment requires identification and eradication of the often distant septic focus. Hepatic synthetic failure can occur if septic foci are not identified and controlled. Both cholestasis and hepatic synthetic dysfunction are occasionally caused by overfeeding via the parenteral route, with secondary fatty infiltration. However, cholestasis leading to synthetic failure can also be characteristic of end-stage organ dysfunction. Rising hepatocellular chemistries and associated synthetic dysfunction are a cause of great concern.

Pancreatitis is occasionally seen, usually as a complication of splanchnic ischemia during resuscitation. It presents with enteral feeding intolerance, ileus, and upper abdominal pain. Laboratory findings include amylase and lipase elevations. Rarely, progression to hemorrhagic pancreatitis occurs.[12] Most patients will tolerate enteral postpyloric feedings if carefully monitored, although some may require temporary parenteral support.

Burn patients demonstrate a propensity for a remarkable ulcer diathesis (Curling's ulcers) that historically was a common cause of death due to perforation, peritonitis, or bleeding. It seems likely that this is secondary to reduced splanchnic flow. Prophylactic treatment is advisable in most children with serious burns until physiologic wound closure is accomplished and patients are tolerating tube feedings. Cholecystitis is rarely seen in children, although it should be sought (generally by ultrasound) in the setting of obstructive chemistries and upper abdominal pain. Bedside drainage is possible in critically ill patients.[13]

Enteral dysfunction in the form of ileus commonly accompanies septic episodes and generally resolves with identification and treatment of the septic focus. Rare children will develop significant enteral ischemia associated with resuscitation failure or severe unremitting sepsis. Initially this will present as ileus but can progress to abdominal distension and recalcitrant septic shock. It is a common autopsy finding in burn patients.[14] Varieties of infectious colitis, most commonly *Clostridium difficile*, are occasionally seen in the burn unit. This usually presents as diarrhea but can progress to colonic dilatation and necrosis. Diagnosis is by stool titer, and effective treatment includes enteral administration of metronidazole or vancomycin. Finally, diarrhea is common in the burn unit and is commonly an artifact of hyperosmolar enteral feedings, but infectious etiologies must be excluded.

## Nutritional Support in the Burn ICU

Hypermetabolic burn patients become rapidly catabolic without nutritional support.[14] The optimal route of feeding is enteral. Most children will tolerate intragastric continuous tube feedings beginning at a low rate during resuscitation and advanced as tolerated. Initially, a sump nasogastric tube can be used to monitor gastric residuals and help determine feeding tolerance. Subsequently, soft-weighted tubes can be placed. Postpyloric feedings are better tolerated by some patients, particularly if gastric motility is compromised. It is important to ensure that an ileus is not present when administering postpyloric feedings. Monitoring abdominal distention and bowel sounds is important. Parenteral nutrition can be initiated if tube feedings are not tolerated.

Whether feeding parenterally or enterally, it is prudent to monitor and control serum glucose. The hormonal milieu after burns predisposes even healthy children to hyperglycemia. It has been shown that persistent hyperglycemia can contribute to negative outcomes.[15] Insulin infusions can be helpful in this regard, but they must be used cautiously and in conjunction with close monitoring as well as specific unit policies and procedures in order to avoid the dangerous consequences of hypoglycemia.

Both underfeeding and overfeeding have adverse sequelae. Underfeeding results in muscle catabolism and immune compromise. Overfeeding results in fatty liver infiltration and excessive $CO_2$ production. Nutritional support should be designed to meet individual needs. A large number of formulas have been developed to predict individual requirements, but they vary widely in their predictions. The current consensus suggests that in most children, protein needs are about 2.5 gm/kg/day and caloric needs are between 1.5 and 1.7 times the calculated basal metabolic rate (BMR), or 1.3 to 1.5 times measured resting energy expenditure (REE). BMR is generally calculated from equations such as the Harris-Benedict equation, whereas REE is generally measured by indirect calorimetry. Physical examination, quality of wound healing, and nitrogen balance can be used to clinically monitor the adequacy of nutritional support over the long course of a burn hospitalization.

## Infectious Disease Issues in the Burn ICU

The most effective way of minimizing sepsis in burn patients is through prompt excision and closure of their wounds, but topical agents are helpful in slowing the inevitable development of infection in deep wounds. Common topical wound agents relatively unique to the burn ICU environment have critical care implications. Mafenide acetate as an 11% cream or a 5% aqueous solution may be painful upon application but has excellent eschar penetration and a broad antibacterial spectrum. It is absorbed systemically and is a moderately strong carbonic anhydrase inhibitor, compromising renal bicarbonate production. Aqueous silver nitrate as a 0.5% solution is painless on application, with a broad antibacterial and antifungal spectrum. It does not penetrate thick eschar

well and tends to leach electrolytes, contributing to hyponatremia and hypokalemia. If silver sulfadiazine is used as the topical agent, trans-eschar free water losses can be very high, and serum sodium should be closely monitored.

It is tempting to overuse antibiotics in critically ill burn patients. However, antibiotics are two-edged swords. Hypermetabolic burn patients are routinely moderately febrile, so this sign is insensitive in its association with infection. When unexpected high fever develops, a complete physical exam should be performed, lines inspected for infection, wounds evaluated for sepsis, supportive labs and radiographs taken, and cultures of blood, urine, and sputum sent. If no clear focus of infection is seen and the child appears unstable, hypotensive, or with very high fever or leukocytosis, empiric broad-spectrum antibiotic administration is a reasonable precaution pending return of culture data. If no focus of infection is documented, antibiotics can be stopped after a 48-hour to 72-hour course. Reflexive prolonged antibiotic administration for moderate fever in this setting may lead to development of resistant organisms.

Burn patients referred after receiving care in outside facilities may bring with them not only their wounds but also resistant organisms unique to the referring institution. Relatively rigid infection control practices should be a routine part of care in all burn units to minimize the occurrence of cross-infection. Although it is probably not possible to completely eliminate this problem in real life, universal precautions and compulsive hand washing will go a long way toward minimizing it.

## Combined Burns and Trauma in the Burn ICU

Children with combined burns and trauma present unique challenges to the burn ICU team. Typically, these patients present as management conflicts when the priorities of the burn struggle with those of the nonburn traumatic injuries. Thoughtful judgment is required in every case and is facilitated by clear identification of the conflict. A common scenario involves children with burns and head injury or anoxic injury who must have cerebral edema controlled during resuscitation. However, placing intracranial pressure monitors through burns increases the risk of infection. While every case is unique, a reasonable compromise often includes very tightly controlled resuscitation with short-term placement of indicated pressure monitors under proper precautions and antibiotic coverage. Children with blunt chest injuries and overlying burns may require chest tubes which traverse burned areas and increase the risk of empyema. Moreover, tubes may be difficult to secure and the tracts may not close well at the time of removal. One approach might involve use of a long subcutaneous tunnel to reduce trouble closing the tract and timely tube removal to reduce the chance of empyema. Children with blunt or penetrating abdominal injury and burns may have their visceral injuries masked and thereby detected late. Furthermore, there is a higher incidence of wound dehiscence when operating through a burned abdominal wall. While every case is different, liberal use of imaging will detect otherwise occult injuries when the mechanism of injury is consistent with abdominal trauma. In those requiring operative intervention, one can consider placing retention sutures after laparotomy. Children with simultaneous fractures may have fracture management compromised by an overlying burn. Although internal fixation through burned skin is not an optimal option, many burned and fractured extremities can be managed with external fixation followed by prompt wound excision and closure.

## Rehabilitation in the Burn ICU

Rehabilitation efforts should ideally begin during resuscitation and continue, as much as is practical, during critical illness. Both physical and occupational therapists should be involved, initially with twice-daily passive ranging of joints and static antideformity positioning to prevent the otherwise inevitable development of contractures. Therapists should be informed of the sequence of planned operations in order to modify therapy to support these procedures. Therapists should be encouraged to range patients under anesthesia and to use this valuable time to fabricate custom splints. These efforts during the acute period will pay great dividends later in the hospitalization.

## COMMON COMPLICATIONS IN THE BURN ICU

Successful management of complications in the burn ICU is facilitated by a high index of suspicion. Management of patients with serious injuries often requires that a series of complications are successfully addressed as the wound is progressively closed. Compulsive attention to changes in the patient's clinical status will facilitate early detection and successful intervention.

## Neurologic Complications in the Burn ICU

Transient delirium occurs in as many as 30% of children at some point during their hospitalization.[16] Immediate care involves elimination and/or management of hypoxia, metabolic disturbances, or structural injuries. In some children this will require neuroimaging. Seizures are occasionally seen as

the result of hyponatremia or as a consequence of too-rapid weaning of benzodiazepines. They are generally prevented or managed with correction of these issues. Peripheral nerve injuries can be discovered late in the course of therapy. They are usually a consequence of direct thermal injury, compression from compartment syndrome or overlying inelastic eschar, metabolic disturbances, or improper splinting techniques. In most children, these resolve or improve with supportive therapy, although liberal decompression, careful positioning, and splinting will minimize their occurrence.

## Cardiovascular Complications in the Burn ICU

Serious cardiovascular complications are rare. Intravascular infections, including endocarditis and suppurative thrombophlebitis, present with fever and recurrent bacteremia without signs of local infection. Examination of peripheral and central intravenous sites and use of ultrasound facilitate diagnosis. While infected peripheral veins can be excised, the treatment of infected central venous clots or endocarditis usually requires protracted antibiotic therapy with judicious use of long-term anticoagulation. Hypertension occurs in up to 20% of recovering seriously burned children and is generally well managed with beta-adrenergic blockers. As venous thromboembolic complications are surprisingly infrequent in children with serious burns, routine prophylaxis is not currently standard-of-care. However, this practice is controversial in older children and adults, and many facilities have guidelines for formal prophylaxis. We recommend this be individualized to both the patient and program. Iatrogenic catheter insertion complications, such as vascular lacerations, are minimized by careful technique and should occur infrequently.[17]

## Pulmonary Complications in the Burn ICU

Pulmonary complications are common, particularly in children with inhalation injury. Up to 50% of children with serious inhalation injuries will develop pneumonia, which is frequently successfully managed with pulmonary toilet and focused antibiotics.[18] Respiratory failure may occur early in the absence of infection secondary to inhalation of noxious chemicals or later in the course secondary to sepsis or pneumonia. Lung protective ventilation strategies can facilitate recovery and minimize further complications. Some children will require innovative methods of support.[19] Finally, children will occasionally present with carbon monoxide intoxication, which is usually well managed with 6 hours of 100% oxygen. Some children may benefit from hyperbaric oxygen treatment, but this therapy is not without risk and should be considered on a case-by-case basis.

## Hematologic Complications in the Burn ICU

Neutropenia can be seen in two settings. In the first days after resuscitation, some children will develop worrisome neutropenia in the absence of infection. If the absolute neutrophil count is concerning, this is usually managed with prophylactic antibiotics. Later, neutropenia can occur with sepsis and is especially worrisome. Often the harbinger of sepsis, thrombobcytopenia is a particularly concerning development. Disseminated intravascular coagulation also frequently accompanies uncontrolled sepsis and should prompt preemptive antibiotic therapy and focused investigation for a septic focus. Global immunologic deficits are associated with serious burns and can contribute to a high rate of infectious complications.

## Otologic Complications in the Burn ICU

Denuded cartilage is susceptible to auricular chondritis secondary to bacterial invasion. This can result in rapid loss of viable cartilage and severe aesthetic deformity. It can often be prevented by routine use of topical mafenide acetate on all burned ears, as this agent will penetrate the underlying relatively avascular cartilage. Sinusitis and otitis media can complicate transnasal instrumentation with endotracheal and enteral tubes. When this occurs, drainage of these spaces can be restored by relocation of tubes. Infections are treated with antibiotics and topical decongestants. Rarely, surgical drainage is needed. Many children who require prolonged airway access may experience such complications as nasal alar and septal necrosis, vocal cord erosions and ulcerations, tracheal stenosis, and tracheoesophageal and tracheo-innominate artery fistulae. All these complications are minimized by frequent attention to tube position and cuff pressures, avoidance of oversized tubes, and regular inspection of tube-securing straps and devices.

## Enteric Complications in the Burn ICU

Early hepatic dysfunction is usually secondary to splanchnic ischemia and results in transient transaminase elevations. It is extremely common during resuscitation from large burns and resolves after resuscitation. Hepatic failure which develops later in a patient's course is usually a late-stage manifestation of sepsis and multiorgan failure. It begins with elevation of cholestatic chemistries and progresses to coagulopathy and synthetic failure. Pancreatitis which begins with elevations of amylase and lipase can lead to ileus and hemorrhagic pancreatitis. It reflects another manifestation of splanchnic flow deficits early and sepsis-induced organ failures later in the hospital course. Sepsis without localizing signs but with rising cholestatic chemistries can be suggestive of acalculous cholecystitis. It can be diagnosed by examination and ultrasound and managed with antibiotics, percutaneous cholecystostomy, or surgery. Gastroduodenal ulceration, also related to splanchnic flow deficits that impair mucosal defenses, is common, but is prevented in most patients with routine use of proton pump inhibitors, histamine receptor blockers, or antacids. Intestinal ischemia and infarction is secondary to inadequate resuscitation, sepsis, or as a late-stage manifestation of multiorgan failure.

## Ophthalmic Complications in the Burn ICU

Acute intraocular hypertension can occur during resuscitation if the face has been deeply burned and there is a large overall surface burn causing diffuse, retrobulbar edema.[20] In worrisome circumstances, it can be quickly diagnosed by tonometry and treated by lateral canthotomy, a bedside procedure. Ectropia results from contraction of burned tissues around the eye. This can occur surprisingly rapidly during the first weeks after injury if the face has been burned and will result in exposure of the globe. This will predictably lead to keratitis and desiccation of the globe, which can cause ulceration and perforation. In order to prevent this very serious complication, modest exposure can be managed with topical ophthalmic lubricants. More severe exposure, however, should prompt acute lid release. Tarsorrhaphy is rarely helpful as the force of contraction will pull out tarsorrhaphy sutures. Children with Toxic Epidermal Necrolysis (TENS) can develop symblepharon, or scarring of the lid to the denuded conjunctiva. This can be minimized through daily examinations and mechanical adhesion disruption.

## Renal/Adrenal and Genitourinary Complications in the Burn ICU

Renal complications include both early and delayed renal insufficiency.[21] Early acute renal failure follows inadequate perfusion during resuscitation or is a consequence of myoglobinuria. Late renal failure can be seen as a complication of sepsis, multiorgan failure, or the use of nephrotoxic agents. In most children, management with careful fluid and electrolyte support suffices. Occasional patients will require transient continuous or intermittent renal replacement therapy. Survivors rarely need long-term dialysis.

Acute adrenal insufficiency rarely occurs in children secondary to hemorrhage into the gland.[22] It presents with cryptic hypotension, fevers, hyponatremia, and hyperkalemia. The electrolyte abnormalities may be obscured by electrolyte replacement therapy. Screening is performed by obtaining a random cortisol level, and diagnosis is confirmed by ACTH stimulation testing. Therapy involves glucocorticoid replacement, which can usually be tapered in most patients during the recovery period.

Urinary tract infections are minimized by using bladder catheters only when absolutely necessary. Such infections are treated with focused antibiotics. Children with even severe perineal and genital burns do not generally require colonic diversion or catheterization. *Candida* cystitis is usually seen in those with bladder catheters who have undergone treatment with broad-spectrum antibiotics. Changing the catheter and Amphotericin irrigation are generally successful. If infections are recurrent, the upper urinary tracts should be screened with ultrasound.

## Musculoskeletal Complications in the Burn ICU

Exposed bone is common in severe burn injuries. In many children, small areas can be debrided with a powered bit until viable cortical bone is reached and subsequently allowed to granulate. Vacuum-assisted dressings can speed granulation of many of these wounds until autografts can be done. Some children will need local or distant flaps. Simultaneously fractured and burned extremities are best immobilized with external fixators while overlying burns are grafted. Heterotopic ossification develops weeks after injury, especially in deeply burned elbows. Most patients respond to physical therapy, but some require excision of heterotopic bone to achieve full function. Unusual pain with passive motion during ranging in the burn ICU should prompt radiographic investigation.

## CONCLUSION

Seriously burned children require a high level of skill and attention from the multidisciplinary critical care team in order to achieve favorable outcomes. However, survival is not the only consideration. Thoughtful, coordinated efforts in the ICU enhance both survival and the quality of ultimate recovery of children suffering serious burns.

## KEY POINTS

- Intensive Care is an essential element of acute burn management.
- An organized, systematic approach to these complex patients facilitates good outcomes.

# TABLES

## TABLE 1
### Phases of burn care.

| Phase | Objectives | Time Period |
|---|---|---|
| Initial Evaluation and Resuscitation | Accurate fluid resuscitation and thorough evaluation | 0–72 hours |
| Initial Wound Excision and Biologic Closure | Exactly identify and remove all full-thickness wounds and achieve biologic closure | Days 1–7 |
| Definitive Wound Closure | Replace temporary with definitive covers and close small complex wounds | Day 7–Week 6 |
| Rehabilitation, Reconstruction, and Reintegration | Initially to maintain range and reduce edema, subsequently to strengthen and facilitate return to home, work, school | Day 1 through discharge |

## TABLE 2
### Predictable physiologic changes in burn patients.

| Period | Physiologic Changes | Clinical Implications |
|---|---|---|
| Resuscitation Period (days 0 to 3) | Massive capillary leak | Closely monitor fluid resuscitation |
| Postresuscitation Period (day 3 until 95% definitive wound closure) | Hyperdynamic and catabolic state with high risk of infection | Remove and close wounds to avoid sepsis; nutritional support is essential |
| Recovery Period (95% wound closure until one year after injury) | Continued catabolic state and risk of nonwound septic events | Accurate nutritional support essential; anticipate and treat complications |

TABLE 3
Burn-specific issues in the secondary survey.

| | |
|---|---|
| **HISTORY** | 1. Important points include the mechanism of injury, closed space exposure, extrication time, delay in seeking attention, fluid given during transport, and prior illnesses and injuries. |
| **HEENT** | 1. The globes should be examined and the corneal epithelium stained with fluorescein before adnexal swelling makes examination difficult. Adnexal swelling provides excellent coverage and protection of the globe during the first days after injury. Tarsorrhaphy is virtually never indicated acutely. |
| | 2. Corneal epithelial loss can be overt, giving a clouded appearance to the cornea, but is more often subtle, requiring fluorescein staining for documentation. Topical ophthalmic antibiotics constitute optimal initial treatment. |
| | 3. Very deep burns of the face in association with diffuse and retrobulbar edema can cause intraocular hypertension. This should be checked in this setting, and if pressures are elevated, lateral canthotomy should be performed. |
| | 4. Signs of airway involvement include perioral and intraoral burns or carbonaceous material and progressive hoarseness. |
| | 5. Hot liquid can be aspirated in conjunction with a facial scald injury and can result in acute airway compromise requiring urgent intubation. |
| | 6. Endotracheal tube security is crucial and is best maintained with an umbilical tape harness, rather than adhesive tape, on the burned face. |
| **NECK** | 1. The radiographic evaluation is driven by the mechanism of injury. |
| | 2. Rarely, in patients with very deep burns, neck escharotomies are needed to facilitate venous drainage of the head. |
| **CARDIAC** | 1. The cardiac rhythm should be monitored for 24 to 72 hours in those with electrical injury. |
| | 2. Although elderly patients may develop transient atrial fibrillation if modestly overresuscitated, significant dysrhythmias are unusual if intravascular volume and oxygenation are adequately supported. |
| | 3. Those with a prior history of myocardial infarction may reinfarct with the hemodynamic stress associated with the injury and should be appropriately monitored. |
| **PULMONARY** | 1. Ensure inflating pressures are less than 40 cm $H_2O$ by performing chest escharotomies when needed. |
| | 2. Severe inhalation injury may lead to slough of endobronchial mucosa and thick bronchial secretions that can occlude the endotracheal tube; one should be prepared for sudden endotracheal tube occlusions. |
| **VASCULAR** | 1. The perfusion of burned extremities should be vigilantly monitored by serial examinations. Indications for escharotomy include decreasing temperature, increasing consistency, slowed capillary refill, and diminished Doppler flow in the digital vessels. One should not wait until flow in named vessels is compromised to decompress the extremity. |
| | 2. Fasciotomy is indicated after electrical injury or deep thermal injury when distal flow is compromised on clinical examination. Compartment pressures can be helpful, but clinically worrisome extremities should be decompressed regardless of compartment pressure readings. |
| **ABDOMEN** | 1. Nasogastric tubes should be in place and their function verified, particularly prior to air transport in unpressurized helicopters. |
| | 2. An inappropriate resuscitative volume requirement may be a sign of an occult intra-abdominal injury. |
| | 3. Torso escharotomies may be required to facilitate ventilation in the presence of deep circumferential abdominal wall burns. |
| | 4. Immediate ulcer prophylaxis with histamine receptor blockers and antacids is indicated in all patients with serious burns. |

*(continued on next page)*

## TABLE 3 (continued)

| | |
|---|---|
| **GENITOURI-NARY** | 1. Bladder catheterization facilitates using urinary output as a resuscitation endpoint and is appropriate in all who require a fluid resuscitation. |
| | 2. It is important to ensure that the foreskin is reduced over the bladder catheter after insertion, as progressive swelling may otherwise result in paraphimosis. |
| **NEUROLOGIC** | 1. An early neurologic evaluation is important, as the patient's sensorium is often progressively compromised by medication or hemodynamic instability during the hours after injury. This may require CT scanning in those with a mechanism of injury consistent with head trauma. |
| | 2. Patients who require neuromuscular blockade for transport should also receive adequate sedation and analgesia. |
| **EXTREMITIES** | 1. Extremities that are at risk for ischemia, particularly those with circumferential thermal burns or those with electrical injury, should be promptly decompressed by escharotomy and/or fasciotomy when clinical examination reveals increasing consistency, decreasing temperature, and diminished Doppler flow in digital vessels. Limbs at risk should be dressed so they can be frequently examined. |
| | 2. The need for escharotomy usually becomes evident during the early hours of resuscitation. Many escharotomies can be delayed until transport has been effected if transport times will not extend beyond 6 hours postinjury. |
| | 3. Burned extremities should be elevated and splinted in a position of function. |
| **WOUND** | 1. Wounds, although often underestimated in depth and overestimated in size on initial examination, should be evaluated for size, depth, and the presence of circumferential components. |
| **LABORATORY** | 1. Arterial blood gas analysis is important when airway compromise or inhalation injury is present. |
| | 2. A normal admission carboxyhemoglobin concentration does not eliminate the possibility of a significant exposure, as the half-life of carboxyhemoglobin is 30 to 40 minutes in those effectively ventilated with 100% oxygen. |
| | 3. Baseline hemoglobin and electrolytes can be helpful later during resuscitation. |
| | 4. Urinalysis for occult blood should be sent in those with deep thermal injuries or electrical injuries. |
| **RADIOGRAPH** | 1. The radiographic evaluation is driven by the mechanism of injury and the need to document placement of supportive cannulae. |
| **ELECTRIC** | 1. Monitor cardiac rhythm in high-voltage (greater than 1000 volt) or intermediate-voltage (greater that 220 volt) exposures for 24 to 72 hours. |
| | 2. Low-voltage and intermediate-voltage exposures can cause locally destructive injuries, but uncommonly result in systemic sequelae. |
| | 3. After high-voltage exposures, delayed neurologic and ocular sequelae can occur, so a carefully documented neurologic and ocular examination is an important part of the initial assessment. |
| | 4. Injured extremities should be serially evaluated for intracompartmental edema and promptly decompressed when it develops. |
| | 5. Bladder catheters should be placed in all patients suffering high-voltage exposure to document the presence or absence of pigmenturia. This is treated adequately with volume loading in most patients. |
| **CHEMICAL** | 1. Irrigate wounds with tap water for at least 30 minutes. Irrigate the globe with isotonic crystalloid solution. Blepharospasm may require ocular anesthetic administration. |
| | 2. Exposures to hydrofluoric acid may be complicated by life-threatening hypocalcemia, particularly exposures to concentrated or anhydrous solutions. Such patients should have serum calcium closely monitored and supplemented. Subeschar injection of 10% calcium gluconate solution is appropriate after exposure to highly concentrated or anhydrous solutions. |
| **TAR** | 1. Tar should be initially cooled with tap water irrigation and later removed with a lipophilic solvent. |

TABLE 4
**A consensus resuscitation formula.**

| | |
|---|---|
| **FIRST 24 HOURS** | Adults and Children > 20 kg: |
| | **Ringer's Lactate**: 2-4 cc/kg/%burn/24 h (first half in first 8 hours) |
| | **Colloid\***: none, but many practitioners would advise 5% albumin at 1 x maintenance rate if burn is over 30% TBSA |
| | Children < 20 kg: |
| | **Ringer's Lactate**: 2-3 cc/kg/%burn/24 h (first half in first 8 hours) |
| | **Ringer's Lactate with 5% Dextrose**: maintenance rate (approximately 4 cc/kg/h for the first 10 kg, 2 cc/kg/h for the next 10 kg, and 1 cc/kg/h for weight over 20 kg) |
| | **Colloid\***: none, but many practitioners would advise 5% albumin at 1 x maintenance rate if burn is over 30% TBSA |
| **SECOND 24 HOURS** | All patients: |
| | **Crystalloid**: To maintain urine output, commonly requiring approximately 1.5 x maintenance rate. If silver nitrate is used, sodium leeching will mandate continued isotonic crystalloid. If other topical is used, free water requirement is significant. Serum sodium should be monitored closely. Nutritional support should begin, ideally by the enteral route. |
| | **Colloid\* (5% albumin in Ringer's lactate to maintain serum albumin at or above 2.0 gm/dl):** |
| | 0%–30% burn:   none |
| | 30%–50% burn:   0.3 cc/kg/%burn/24 h |
| | 50%–70% burn:   0.4 cc/kg/%burn/24 h |
| | 70%–100% burn:   0.5 cc/kg/%burn/24 h |

\* The role of colloid is an area of controversy. Check with the program to which the patient will be referred for its recommendations. This author routinely administers 5% albumin at a maintenance rate to patients with burns over 40% of the body surface.

TABLE 5
**Age-specific resuscitation endpoints.**

Sensorium: arousable and comfortable
Temperature: warm centrally and peripherally
Systolic Blood Pressure: for infants, 60 mmHg systolic; for older children, 70 to 90 plus 2 x age in years mmHg; for adults, mean arterial pressure over 60 mmHg
Pulse: 80-180 per minute (age dependent)
Urine Output: 0.5-1 cc/kg/h (glucose negative)
Base Deficit: less than 2

# REFERENCES

1. Sheridan RL. Burn care: results of technical and organizational progress. *JAMA Contemp Update*. 2003: **290**(6): 719–722.

2. Cuthbertson D. The physiology of convalescence after injury. *Br Med Bull*. 1945; **3**: 96–102.

3. Jeschke MG, Mlcak RP, Finnerty CC, et al. Burn size determines the inflammatory and hypermetabolic response. *Crit Care*. 2007; **11**(4): R90.

4. Kennedy D, Gentleman D. The ATLS course, a survey of 228 ATLS providers. *Emerg Med J*. 2001; **18**(1): 55–58.

5. Stoddard FJ, Ronfeldt H, Kagan J, et al. Young burned children: the course of acute stress and physiological and behavioral responses. *Am J Psychiatry*. 2006; **163**(6): 1084–1090.

6. Saxe G, Stoddard F, Courtney D, et al. Relationship between acute morphine and the course of PTSD in children with burns. *J Am Acad Child Adolesc Psychiatry*. 2001; **40**(8): 915–921.

7. Sheridan RL, Hinson M, Blanquierre M, et al. Development of a pediatric burn pain and anxiety management program. *J Burn Care Rehabil*. 1997; **18**: 455–459.

8. Mlcak RP, Suman OE, Herndon DN. Respiratory management of inhalation injury. *Burns*. 2007; **33**(1): 2–13.

9. Pham TN, Neff MJ, Simmons JM, Gibran NS, Heimbach DM, Klein MB. The clinical pulmonary infection score poorly predicts pneumonia in patients with burns. *J Burn Care Res*. 2007; **28**(1): 76–79.

10. Hollingsed TC, Saffle JR, Barton RG, Craft WB, Morris SE. Etiology and consequences of respiratory failure in thermally injured patients. *Am J Surg*. 1993; **166**(6): 592–596, discussion 596–597.

11. Sheridan RL, Shank ES. Hyperbaric oxygen treatment: a brief overview of a controversial topic. *J Trauma*. 1999; **47**(2): 426–435.

12. Ryan CM, Sheridan RL, Schoenfeld DA, Warshaw AL, Tompkins RG. Postburn pancreatitis. *Ann Surg*. 1995; **222**(2): 163–170.

13. Sheridan RL, Ryan CM, Lee MJ, Mueller PR, Tompkins RG. Percutaneous cholecystostomy in the critically ill burn patient. *J Trauma*. 1995; **38**: 248–251.

14. Prelack K, Dwyer J, Dallal GE, et al. Growth deceleration and restoration after serious burn injury. *J Burn Care Res*. 2007; **28**(2): 262–268.

15. Hemmila MR, Taddonio MA, Arbabi S, Maggio PM, Wahl WL. Intensive insulin therapy is associated with reduced infectious complications in burn patients. *Surgery*. 2008; **144**(4): 629–635.

16. Ilechukwu ST. Psychiatry of the medically ill in the burn unit. *Psychiatr Clin North Am*. 2002; **25**(1): 129–147.

17. Sheridan RL, Weber JM. Mechanical and infectious complications of pediatric central venous cannulation: lessons learned from a 10-year experience placing over 1000 central venous catheters in children. *J Burn Care Res*. 2006; **27**(5): 713–718.

18. Edelman DA, Khan N, Kempf K, White MT. Pneumonia after inhalation injury. *J Burn Care Res*. 2007; **28**(2): 241–246.

19. Sheridan RL, Hess D. Inhaled nitric oxide in inhalation injury. *J Burn Care Res*. 2009; **30**(1): 162–164.

20. Sullivan SR, Ahmadi AJ, Singh CN, et al. Elevated orbital pressure: another untoward effect of massive resuscitation after burn injury. *J Trauma*. 2006; **60**(1): 72–76.

21. Steinvall I, Bak Z, Sjoberg F. Acute kidney injury is common, parallels organ dysfunction or failure, and carries appreciable mortality in patients with major burns: a prospective exploratory cohort study. *Crit Care*. 2008; **12**(5): R124.

22. Reiff DA, Harkins CL, McGwin G Jr, Cross JM, Rue LW III. Risk factors associated with adrenal insufficiency in severely injured burn patients. *J Burn Care Res*. 2007; **28**(6): 854–858.

23. Rosenkrantz K, Sheridan RL. Management of the burned trauma patient: balancing conflicting priorities. *Burns*. 2002; **28**(7): 665–669.

24. Neugebauer CT, Serghiou M, Herndon DN, Suman OE. Effects of a 12-week rehabilitation program with music & exercise groups on range of motion in young children with severe burns. *J Burn Care Res*. 2008; **29**(6): 939–948.

25. Sheridan RL, Hinson, MM, Liang MM, Mulligan JL, Ryan CM, Tompkins RG. Long-term outcome of children surviving massive burns. *JAMA*. 2000; **283**(1): 69–73.

CHAPTER NINE

# COMMON PITFALLS OF PEDIATRIC BURN CARE

J. KEVIN BAILEY, MD, FACS, ASSISTANT PROFESSOR OF SURGERY,
UNIVERSITY OF CINCINNATI COLLEGE OF MEDICINE;
STAFF SURGEON, SHRINERS HOSPITALS FOR CHILDREN;
ASSOCIATE DIRECTOR, UNIVERSITY HOSPITAL BURN CENTER; CINCINNATI, OH

RICHARD J. KAGAN, MD, FACS, PROFESSOR OF SURGERY,
UNIVERSITY OF CINCINNATI COLLEGE OF MEDICINE;
CHIEF OF STAFF, SHRINERS HOSPITALS FOR CHILDREN;
DIRECTOR, UNIVERSITY HOSPITAL BURN CENTER; CINCINNATI, OH

PETRA WARNER, MD, FACS, ASSOCIATE PROFESSOR OF SURGERY,
UNIVERSITY OF CINCINNATI COLLEGE OF MEDICINE;
ASSISTANT CHIEF OF STAFF, SHRINERS HOSPITALS FOR CHILDREN; CINCINNATI, OH

## INTRODUCTION

In the majority of cases, treatment of acute thermal injury is relatively straightforward, particularly with pediatric injuries. However, the relative resilience of children may lead to a false sense of security. This patient population can tolerate a degree of less-than-optimal management up until the point of disaster. Therefore, avoiding these pitfalls is clearly preferable in order to minimize morbidity and mortality.

## PITFALLS OF INITIAL CARE AND RESUSCITATION (THE EMERGENT SETTING)

The initial step in evaluation and management of any emergent patient care dilemma is security of the airway.

The foremost question is "Does the patient have a patent airway?" followed by "If so, will the patient be able to maintain the airway, and for how long?" A stepwise approach should allow for timely treatment and avoidance of airway emergencies.

Patency of the airway in the emergent setting is assessed similar to nonburn scenarios. If the child's level of consciousness is markedly depressed or if there are concerns regarding the ability of the patient to protect his or her airway, then intubation is indicated.[1] Simultaneously, the patient should be assessed for audible breathing, such as stridor or wheezing. The presence of stridor is relatively infrequent, but in cases of inhalation injury, it is a specific sign.[2, 3] In cases of stridor which indicate impending airway loss, plans should turn towards immediate intubation. When maintainability of the airway is in question or there is evidence of impending respiratory failure, consultation with the definitive burn care team should be sought if possible. Otherwise, it is prudent to proceed with definitive airway management rather than risk the possibility of dealing with an emergent situation. The unique anatomic differences of the pediatric airway are critical to keep in mind when assessing and managing airway, breathing, and ventilation issues in children. The shorter tracheal length, larger tongue size, and the more anterior/superior location of the glottic opening are key points to remember when attempting intubation in children. Because the pediatric epiglottis is less cartilaginous, use of a straight laryngoscope blade may facilitate intubation. The quality of the voice and some gauge of the ability to move air into and out of the lungs can be assessed with interrogation of the patient. Clearly, this may be slightly less fruitful in nonverbal patients. The assessment can then quickly proceed to evaluation of the general effort involved in air exchange. Important elements of the examination include evidence of tachypnea, retractions, or use of accessory muscles. Without preexisting respiratory disease, such as asthma, these findings suggest inhalation injury until proven otherwise.[2] The sense of urgency should be tempered by the fact that progression of respiratory failure is usually observable over a period of hours. The pitfall can occur from failure to recognize the potential for disaster and not maintaining a vigilant posture.

During assessment of the patient's breathing, the physician should also obtain a sense of the size of the burn and the circumstances surrounding the injury. With burns greater than 30% total body surface area (TBSA) in children, significant swelling will be expected. The edema may eventually lead to a disproportionately larger decrease in the cross-sectional area of the child's trachea compared to adults. At this point, the astute physician must balance the competing needs of the patient—assessment of the relative size of the burn, the possible need for intubation, and the pressing urgency to avoid hypothermia. Historic factors may weigh in the decision as well, such as mechanism of injury (entrapment in a burning building), preexisting medical disease, or polytrauma.

It is noteworthy to discuss the problems encountered in securing the airway of a child who has suffered facial burns. Tape will not adhere to the moist wound bed incurred from partial-thickness burns, to eschar, or to areas treated with topical antibiotic ointment. However, a number of commercial devices are available which function well. Alternate strategies include the use of twill tape secured around the head, although care must be taken to guard against pressure on the oral commisures or ears (particularly as swelling occurs). A second method is to apply adhesive tape to the endotracheal tube and then simply staple the tape to the

face.[4] Although this strategy has little drawback in cases of full-thickness burns, one must use caution in cases of partial-thickness burns in order to avoid scarring from the staples themselves (Figure 1). If facial burns are not clearly full thickness, then staples should be replaced in 3 to 5 days.

Following confirmation of a secure airway, attention is then directed towards assessment of breathing. Supplemental oxygen should be administered in all cases, since the addition of oxygen not only addresses hypoxia, but is also the first-line treatment for carbon monoxide (CO) toxicity. If the possibility of CO poisoning is raised, then hyperbaric oxygen therapy (HBO) may be suggested by a member of the initial care team. In critically burned patients, however, hyperbaric oxygen treatment is not indicated for 2 reasons. First, any potential efficacy of treatment must be weighed against the increased risk created by isolating the patient from the full support of the burn care team.[5] Moreover, if transfer is indicated, then definitive care may be delayed. Secondly, despite several studies regarding use of HBO for carbon monoxide poisoning, its efficacy remains uncertain.[6] Suffice it to say, the decision regarding HBO therapy should be deferred to the burn surgeon.

The next issue involved in the initial care of a burned child will be obtaining intravenous access. Any burn greater than 10% TBSA in a child should suggest the possible need for ongoing fluid administration/resuscitation.[7] In addition, IV access is often necessary for administration of analgesics. In children, initial access can be peripheral, central, or intraosseous (IO). During the acute burn injury, collapsed vessels due to hypovolemia can make intravenous access difficult. In this scenario, intraosseous access should be considered. Recent amendment of the PALS (Pediatric Advanced Life Support) guidelines now has no age restrictions for intraosseous line placement. The only clinical contraindications are suspected tibial fracture or traumatic disruption of the venous return proximal to the site of IO insertion. If IO access is not an option, rehydration can be initiated with a feeding tube until intravenous access is obtained. In general, guidelines for the choice of access follow those elaborated by the American College of Surgeons (ACS), the Advanced Trauma Life Support® (ATLS®).[1] In the emergent setting, peripheral access would be the first choice, followed by central access via the femoral vein, although the internal jugular and subclavian vessels are also options. Additional areas of access include the scalp vein or a saphenous vein cutdown. A temporary alternative route for IV access in the neonate involves catheterization of the umbilical artery or vein. Central line placement in a child under the age of 5 years can be daunting due to the small vessel sizes; however, the technique is essentially identical to that used in adults.

With the availability of ultrasound technology, it is probably worth noting the growing emphasis of this technique; not only has its use been recently encouraged by the American College of Surgeons,[8] but it has been shown to decrease complications rates.[9] It also offers the opportunity to more effectively monitor the procedure during training, as the instructor can hold the ultrasound probe for the trainee and track the course of the needle's point as it moves through the soft tissue. Given the greater benefits of utilizing ultrasound compared to the risks of performing a blind procedure, along with support from the ACS, Leapfrog Group for Patient Safety, and insurance companies, it is likely that this technique will become the standard of care for placement of central lines in the near future.

Invariably, once intravenous access is gained, the next potential pitfall will present itself. The question will be raised as some variant of "What fluids do you want and how fast do you want to run them?" Essentially, the options fall into the broad choices of "too fast," "too slow," and "just right." "Just right" is the most tempting. Every practitioner has at least a vague recollection of the Parkland formula. However, in order to calculate the appropriate volume of fluid to administer, the size of the burn must be estimated. The pitfall occurs by exposing the patient for assessment of the burn wound and the distraction of the burn team by the injury. This is then followed by a period in which the calculations for an estimation of the fluid rate occur, which will then be taken as gospel until the patient reaches definitive care. Meanwhile, the team is still working on the "ABC's" of trauma care.[1] So, "just right" comes at the risk of rushing assessment of the injury, exposing the patient to hypothermia an additional time (as there will be a thorough head-to-toe evaluation with the secondary exam), and the potential for erroneous estimation that will remain in place until a fresh set of eyes reassesses the situation. Key in management is to remember that the patient is first a trauma patient, then a burn patient. Once the trauma workup has been completed, assessment of the burn can be performed. While trying to determine the exact extent of burn injury and its associated depth, significant time can pass, thus increasing the time of exposure and subsequent risk of hypothermia.

Multiple authors have remarked on the disparity between the initial estimation and the final determination of burn size in the burn unit.[10, 11] Much of this difference probably arises from the approach of estimating burn size too early in the course of care. Given the immediate sense of urgency, alternate solutions for fluid management include arbitrary boluses of crystalloid. And, in fact, ATLS and PALS both support this method in their algorithms; however, PALS categorizes burn shock as "hypovolemic," and this oversimplification of the pathophysiology can lead to the somewhat common approach of recommending successive boluses of 10 ml/kg to 20 ml/kg.[12] Rather, the challenge of burn shock management is probably more akin to that of septic shock. As such, fluid administration must be somewhat judicious, and treatment may sometimes necessitate the careful use of vasopressors, as in sepsis.[13, 14] One must remember that there may be a price to be paid for overaggressive fluid administration, which is often not evident in the emergency room.[15, 16]

An alternative strategy to consider is the following: for infants, order isotonic intravenous fluids (e.g., lactated Ringer's) at a rate of 125 ml/hr; for children, begin IVF at a rate of 250 ml/hr; and for teens, begin at 500 ml/hr.[17] This strategy will accomplish several objectives. First, once IV access is obtained, it will quickly answer the question of fluids, and the resuscitation team can maintain their focus on the orderly evaluation and care of the trauma patient. Examination of the child should remain deliberate and organized, hopefully decreasing the time of exposure and risk of hypothermia. Secondly, if there are significant differences between this arbitrary rate and that derived from the Parkland formula, then the relative excess or deficiency of fluid will have been given for a short time (perhaps 15 minutes to an hour). Thus, this strategy avoids bolus therapy and potential overresuscitation. Finally, because the fluid administration rate is temporary, the rate will need to be confirmed and adjusted by monitoring urine output. This method emphasizes the need to continuously reassess the volume status of the patient and avoids the pitfall of trying to use algebra (the Parkland formula) to solve a calculus problem (the rate of flow out of the intravascular space due to the injury, or third spacing). Ultimately, even in the burn center, the key is to frequently adjust the rate of fluid administration to achieve adequate resuscitation as judged by adequate urine output and other indices of tissue perfusion.

## PITFALLS DURING THE SECONDARY EXAM

As resuscitation begins and evaluation of the patient progresses, a more detailed examination of the patient is conducted by the team. At this point, the goal is 2-fold. First, all injuries need to be appreciated and the severity of each injury assessed.[14] This may require the team to deliberately ignore the burn injury for a brief period of time in order to focus specifically on the possibility of missed injuries. Secondly, the circumstances regarding the history of the injury can be sought at this point. These details are of particular importance when there is any possibility of abuse. It is worth noting and documenting details of the events so that any changes in the reported history can be clearly tracked. Although it would seem relatively simple, a word of caution is warranted. When seeking and documenting a clear history, one must avoid inferring information and introducing bias—particularly in cases of possible abuse.

Fortunately, missed injuries concomitant with thermal injuries are rare. This is probably due to a number of reasons. First, in order to sustain blunt or penetrating injuries with burns, the patient is usually a victim of an explosion, fall, or motor vehicle collision. In such cases, first responders alert emergency care teams fairly predictably. Consequently, there is a search for injury patterns common to the mechanism. For example, patients burned in motor vehicle collisions are more prone to blunt trauma, and the emergency room team has experience with motor vehicle collision injury patterns. The challenge occurs when the medical team or patient becomes distracted by the injury; when the patient is the victim of an unwitnessed accident (e.g., the patient is presumed to have walked out of an open front door instead of falling through the broken second-story window) or assault (where fire was started in an attempt to cover up evidence or cause harm in addition to penetrating trauma); or when initial circumstances are not clearly communicated (the presence of an explosion with significant concussive force) (Figure 2).

In general, the larger the burn injury, the more distracting it is for both the patient and the care team. ATLS® lists burns as distracting injuries, so that the physical exam alone is insufficient to detect intra-abdominal injuries. Just as any other type of grotesque traumatic injury (amputated limb, severe facial trauma, or gross soft tissue loss) may divert the care team, so, too, can a burn. Therefore, attention may be prematurely focused on the more obvious injury (the burn) and transfer arranged without obtaining a full history or fully examining a patient. A penetrating injury may be completely overlooked by this omission. Part of the reluctance to complete the exam may stem from a concern of causing more pain by moving the patient or manipulating burned skin. However, this is a necessary discomfort in any case where the existence of additional injury is uncertain.

At this point, a more concerted effort to quantify the burn can occur. Numerous methods have been devised to estimate the size of a burn. The 3 most useful tools are the "rule of nines," the Lund-Browder chart, and the "rule of palms." Each requires some knowledge of the tool and its correct use. The rule of nines divides the body into regions which have a percentage of the total body surface somewhere close to a multiple of 9.[18] The Lund-Browder chart and its derivations divide the body into smaller regions with

the intent of arriving at a more precise percentage of the burned area (Figure 3).[19] The rule of palms essentially states that the patient's palm (exclusive of the fingers and thumb) is equal to about one-half of a percent of the total body surface area, or that the entire palmar surface of the hand and fingers approximates 1% of the patient's total body surface area.[20]

There are numerous reports regarding the discrepancy in estimation of burn size between the emergency department and burn centers. The differences result from unappreciated burns, areas erroneously thought burned (perhaps covered by soot), and misapplication of the tools. Burns are somewhat dynamic in that blisters develop over time and wounds change as the patient progresses through the medical system. It is also probably unwise to expect burn patients to be cleaned (potentiating hypothermia) in the emergency department. However, there is merit to emphasizing that with both the rule of nines and the Lund-Browder chart, the areas circumscribed on the chart can be divided further. For example, if only one-third of the anterior torso is burned, then the area involved would approximate one-third of 18% (or 6%) rather than rounding up to 18% as the estimated area of involvement. In addition, if the estimation is conducted during the secondary exam, there may be less urgency to force more gross approximations. Finally, it should be emphasized again that if adjustments are made to the intravenous fluid administration rate based on the patient's response, then any gross errors in estimation of burn size or estimated fluid needs will be mitigated.

There are additional elements of the secondary exam that are important. First, the patient's immunization history should be obtained, and if doubt exists, confirmed later. Burns are tetanus-prone wounds, which warrant appropriate prophylaxis. Second, the condition of the eyes should be documented with facial burns since the incidence of corneal abrasion may be as high as 13% in such patients.[21] Specific evidence of corneal abrasion or conjunctival irritation should be sought, such as foreign body sensation or photophobia. If the patient cannot supply appropriate responses, or if any uncertainty exists, then fluorescein examination of the cornea is indicated. This is particularly important in victims with extensive or severe facial burns, as the rapid development of periorbital edema may preclude an adequate exam for days. If there is evidence of ocular trauma, then consultation from an ophthalmologist should be sought early in order to afford the consultant the ability to examine the patient.

Finally, neuromuscular function of the extremities should be specifically examined and thoroughly documented. This information is vital in assessing for clinical evidence of compartment syndrome, which can develop insidiously and generally is not present during the time a patient is in the emergency department (during the first few hours after injury). Therefore, it can be a pitfall of resuscitation during the first 24 to 36 hours.

## PITFALLS DURING THE INITIAL RESUSCITATION AND EARLY DEFINITIVE CARE

As care of the burned child progresses through the first 24 to 48 hours, a concerted effort to minimize the amount of fluid given should be maintained. Details regarding the experimental and clinical evidence supporting a judicious and systematic approach to resuscitation are explored elsewhere in this textbook. It is worthwhile to echo the concerns, as there is evidence of morbidity induced by "overresuscitation." The complications associated with greater volumes of resuscitative fluid include the development of pulmonary edema, abdominal compartment syndrome, and compartment syndromes of the extremities.

The development of a compartment syndrome has the potential to greatly increase the morbidity of a thermal injury. The pressure threshold at which ischemia develops has been debated for a number of years. Experimental work in animals has demonstrated that normal muscle metabolism requires a perfusion pressure (the difference between the mean arterial pressure and compartment pressure) of 30 mmHg in normal muscle and 40 mmHg in moderately injured muscle.[22] Deep-tissue ischemia results from tissue pressures exceeding capillary perfusion pressure (conservatively estimated as 30 mmHg).[23] As tissue edema develops beneath the eschar (or deep dermal burns) and fascia of the extremities, one or the other layer may become restrictive enough to prevent any further change in the volume of the muscular compartments. At this point, further development of edema is hypothesized to result in increased compartment pressures. Regardless of the exact mechanism, management is relatively straightforward.

The most important component in the management of compartment syndrome is diagnosis. If a patient can accurately report pain with passive stretch of the muscle group, pain at rest (deep muscular pain), or paresthesias, then this is sufficient cause for objective confirmation. If a patient cannot reliably report neurological symptoms, then a screening examination looking for evidence of pain with passive motion at the joints and increased firmness of the compartment can be done. However, it is a pitfall to rely solely on these maneuvers. Furthermore, the mere presence of pulses (either by palpation or Doppler) should not be

accepted as evidence that a compartment syndrome is not present. The muscle of entire compartments may die even if a palpable pulse is present more distally on the extremity (Figure 4). Finally, it is possible to miss the window of increased pain, which may only last for approximately 1 hour.[24] Measurement of compartment pressures is the most reliable, objective measure to predict the development of a compartment syndrome. Available methods for measurement include the use of a Stryker® device or simply using an 18-gauge needle attached to a pressure monitor, as found at the bedside of most modern critical care rooms. Pressures of 30mm Hg or greater are considered elevated.

Once there is evidence of elevated pressures, intervention is guided by the clinical situation. If there is overlying eschar or deeply burned skin, then an escharotomy should be performed expeditiously. Once completed, the physician must document that the pressure has been adequately released by repeated measurement of the compartment. If compartment hypertension has been inadequately treated, then an appropriate fasciotomy should be considered. Admittedly, there is some debate as to whether an absolute pressure should be used as the sole indication for fasciotomy or if the difference between the diastolic blood pressure (or mean arterial pressure) and the compartment pressure should be used. In our experience, children who have elevated compartment pressures after escharotomy are victims of large burns, have large fluid requirements, and usually have circumferential third-degree burns of the extremities. The need to avoid the pitfall of a missed compartment syndrome in this group more than outweighs any small potential benefit of trying to avoid a fasciotomy. Few outcomes are more disheartening than saving a child from the mortality of a large burn, only to realize the most morbid injury is a missed compartment syndrome—possibly requiring amputation of the extremity. A fasciotomy performed for questionable indications is preferable to the consequences that might occur by delaying treatment while awaiting absolute diagnostic certainty.

With respect to avoidable morbidity, the burn surgeon treating the child and coordinating care should also avoid the pitfall of allowing consultants to make conservative care decisions without being challenged. For example, an orthopedic surgeon may advise against operative fixation of a fracture. The rationale may involve unfamiliarity with improved outcomes from burn injury in recent years, so that a child with a large burn and associated injuries may erroneously be judged to have a low chance of survival. Furthermore, the decision may be based on a desire to avoid infection of hardware, in which case the burn surgeon may be able to redouble efforts to excise all full-thickness burns in a timely manner and thus allow for propitious fixation. This is greatly preferable to delaying specialty treatment that might have better results with earlier intervention.

## CONCLUSION

As in other forms of trauma, the key to expert burn care is adherence to a systematic approach that seeks to minimize the chances of avoidable or missed injuries. The fundamental elements include strong consideration of early respiratory support (especially in cases of suspected inhalation injury), deliberate avoidance of tunnel vision focused only on the cutaneous injury, and cautious administration of resuscitative fluid, with sensitivity to the consequences of overly vigorous resuscitation. Finally, it is worth noting

the benefits of early consultation with staff at a burn center verified by the American Burn Association.

## KEY POINTS

- Initial care of the trauma/burn patient should follow guidelines established by the American College of Surgeons' program, ATLS®.
- Care should be exercised to avoid overresuscitation, particularly avoiding fluid boluses unless the patient is hypotensive.
- A focused search for associated injuries may require deliberately ignoring the burn wound for a short time, while avoiding hypothermia.
- Missed compartment syndrome is the most debilitating preventable complication of burn injury, and avoidance requires vigilance on the part of the entire team.

## FIGURES

### FIGURE 1
In cases where facial burns are involved, it can be particularly challenging to effectively secure endotracheal tubes. One alternative is to use adhesive tape, and then secure the tape to the patient with staples. In areas of the face not involved with full-thickness burn, the staples can be replaced every few days to avoid scarring.

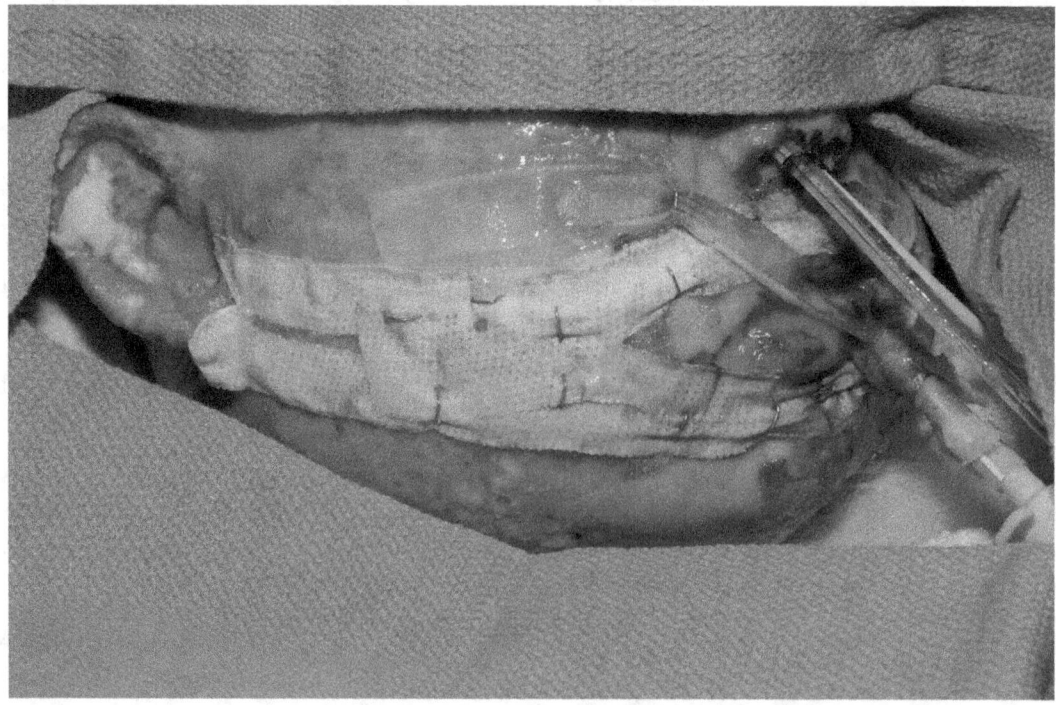

FIGURE 2
A graphic reminder that burn patients are trauma patients and subject to the same pitfall of missed injury. A young man ignited acetylene when he tried to start his car. The condition of the vehicle and injury circumstances were incompletely communicated, such that associated injuries—pulmonary contusion, three fractured ribs, and vague abdominal pain—were not initially addressed in the emergency department.

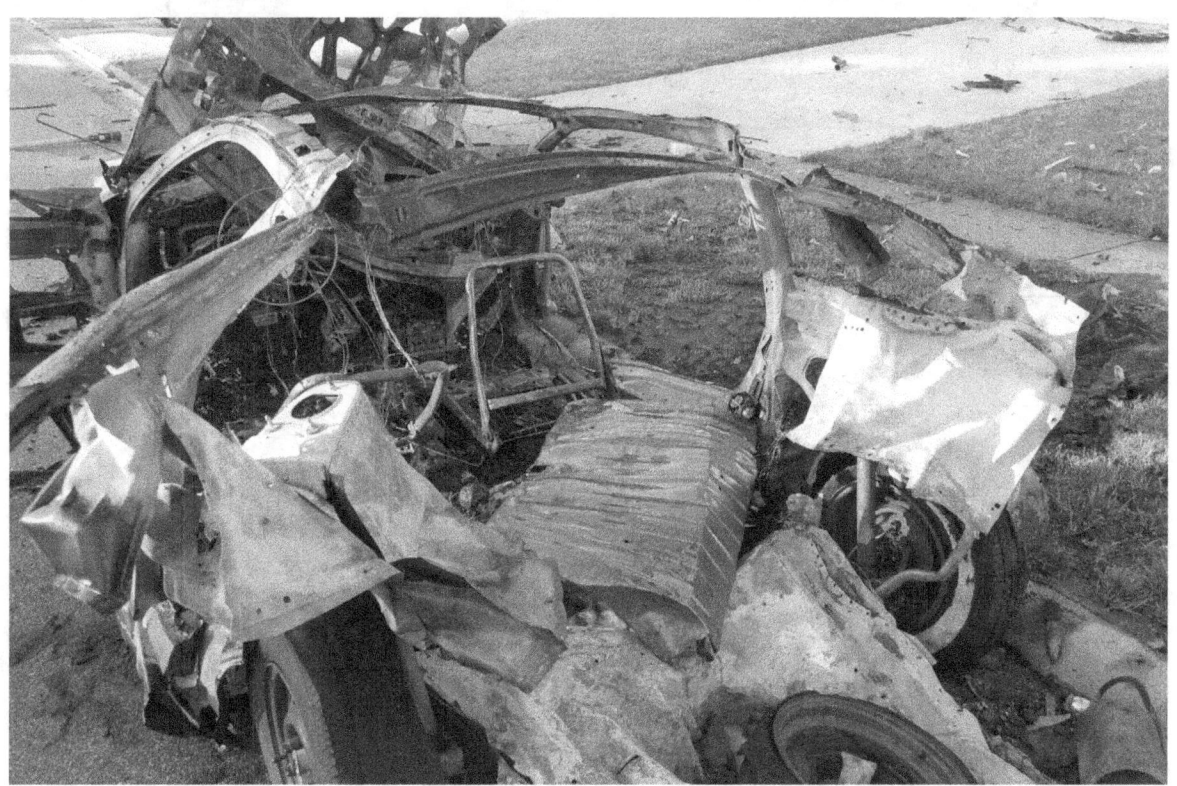

**FIGURE 3**
Example of Lund-Browder chart. Advantage of this type of diagram is more precise documentation of extent of injury and geometric pattern.

## Burn Estimate and Diagram
### Age vs Area
### Initial Evaluation

Cause of burn_____

Date of Burn_____

Time of Burn_____

Age_____

Sex_____

Weight_____

Date of Admission_____

Signature_____

Date_____

## Burn Diagram

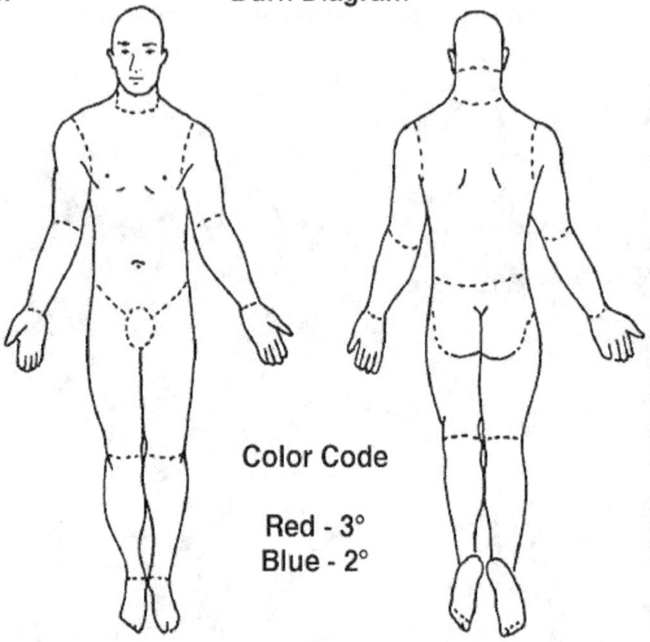

### Color Code

Red - 3°
Blue - 2°

| Area | Birth 1 yr. | 1-4 yrs. | 5-9 yrs. | 10-14 yrs. | 15 yrs. | Adult | 2° | 3° | Total | Donor Areas |
|------|------|------|------|------|------|------|------|------|------|------|
| Head | 19 | 17 | 13 | 11 | 9 | 7 | | | | |
| Neck | 2 | 2 | 2 | 2 | 2 | 2 | | | | |
| Ant. Trunk | 13 | 13 | 13 | 13 | 13 | 13 | | | | |
| Post. Trunk | 13 | 13 | 13 | 13 | 13 | 13 | | | | |
| R. Buttock | 2 1/2 | 2 1/2 | 2 1/2 | 2 1/2 | 2 1/2 | 2 1/2 | | | | |
| L. Buttock | 2 1/2 | 2 1/2 | 2 1/2 | 2 1/2 | 2 1/2 | 2 1/2 | | | | |
| Genitalia | 1 | 1 | 1 | 1 | 1 | 1 | | | | |
| R.U. Arm | 4 | 4 | 4 | 4 | 4 | 4 | | | | |
| L.U. Arm | 4 | 4 | 4 | 4 | 4 | 4 | | | | |
| R.L. Arm | 3 | 3 | 3 | 3 | 3 | 3 | | | | |
| L.L. Arm | 3 | 3 | 3 | 3 | 3 | 3 | | | | |
| R. Hand | 2 1/2 | 2 1/2 | 2 1/2 | 2 1/2 | 2 1/2 | 2 1/2 | | | | |
| L. Hand | 2 1/2 | 2 1/2 | 2 1/2 | 2 1/2 | 2 1/2 | 2 1/2 | | | | |
| R. Thigh | 5 1/2 | 6 1/2 | 8 | 8 1/2 | 9 | 9 1/2 | | | | |
| L. Thigh | 5 1/2 | 6 1/2 | 8 | 8 1/2 | 9 | 9 1/2 | | | | |
| R. Leg | 5 | 5 | 5 1/2 | 6 | 6 1/2 | 7 | | | | |
| L. Leg | 5 | 5 | 5 1/2 | 6 | 6 1/2 | 7 | | | | |
| R. Foot | 3 1/2 | 3 1/2 | 3 1/2 | 3 1/2 | 3 1/2 | 3 1/2 | | | | |
| L. Foot | 3 1/2 | 3 1/2 | 3 1/2 | 3 1/2 | 3 1/2 | 3 1/2 | | | | |
| | | | | | **Total** | | | | | |

### FIGURE 4
### Unfortunate example of missed compartment syndrome of anterior compartment (note remarkable difference between necrotic muscle in the most superior portion of the photograph and viable muscle running parallel in the more inferior portion of the field). This photograph is of an unburned extremity, with the most likely contributor being an aggressive fluid resuscitation.

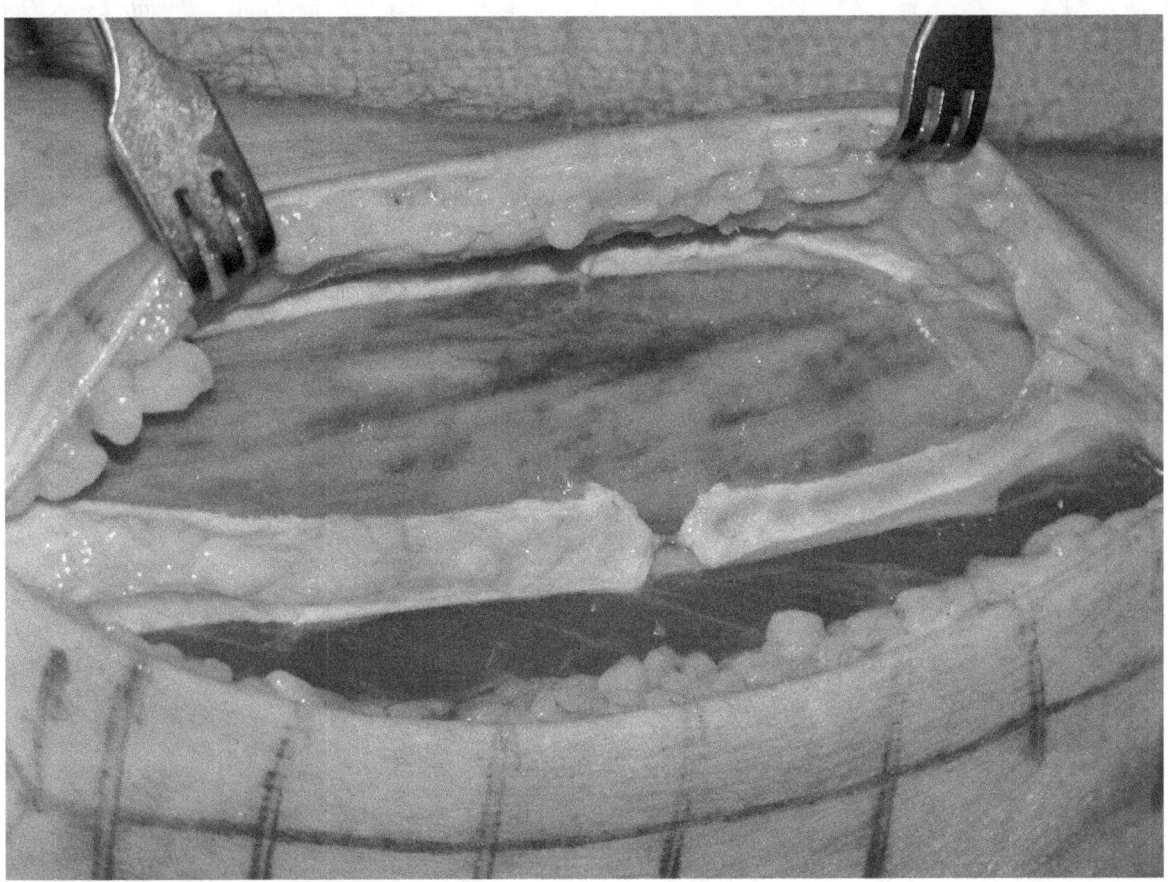

## REFERENCES

1. Trauma ACoSCo. *Advanced Trauma Life Support® for Doctors*. 7th ed. Chicago: American College of Surgeons; 2004.

2. Clark WR, Bonaventura M, Myers W. Smoke inhalation and airway management at a regional burn unit: 1974–1983. Part I: diagnosis and consequences of smoke inhalation. *J Burn Care Rehabil*. 1989; **10:** 52–62.

3. Madnani DD, Steele NP, de Vries E. Factors that predict the need for intubation in patients with smoke inhalation injury. *Ear Nose Throat J*. 2006; **85:** 278–280.

4. McCall JE, Cahill TJ. Respiratory care of the burn patient. *J Burn Care Rehabil*. 2005; **26:** 200–206.

5. Grube BJ, Marvin JA, Heimbach DM. Therapeutic hyperbaric oxygen: help or hindrance in burn patients with carbon monoxide poisoning? *J Burn Care Rehabil*. 1988; **9:** 249–252.

6. Juurlink DN, Buckley N, Stanbrook MB, Isbister GK, Bennett M, McGuigan MA. Hyperbaric oxygen for carbon monoxide poisoning. *Cochrane Database Syst Rev*. 2005; (1): CD002041. DOI: 10.1002/14651858.cd002041.pub2.

7. Merrell SW, Saffle JR, Sullivan JJ, Navar PD, Kravitz M, Warden GD. Fluid resuscitation in thermally injured children. *Am J Surg*. 1986; **152:** 664–669.

8. Statement on recommendations for uniform use of real-time ultrasound guidance for placement of central venous catheters. *Bull Am Coll Surg*. 2008; **93:** 35–36.

9. Leyvi G, Taylor DG, Reith E, Wasnick JD. Utility of ultrasound-guided central venous cannulation in pediatric surgical patients: a clinical series. *Paediatr Anaesth*. 2005; **15:** 953–958.

10. Collis N, Smith G, Fenton OM. Accuracy of burn size estimation and subsequent fluid resuscitation prior to arrival at the Yorkshire Regional Burns Unit. A three year retrospective study. *Burns*. 1999; **25:** 345–351.

11. Freiburg C, Igneri P, Sartorelli K, Rogers F. Effects of differences in percent total body surface area estimation on fluid resuscitation of transferred burn patients. *J Burn Care Res.* 2007; **28:** 42–48.

12. Ralston M, Gonzales L, Fuchs S, Simon W, et al. *Pediatric Advanced Life Support.* Dallas, TX: American Heart Association; 2006.

13. Dellinger RP, Levy MM, Carlet JM, et al. Surviving Sepsis Campaign: international guidelines for management of severe sepsis and septic shock: 2008. *Crit Care Med.* 2008; **36:** 296–327.

14. White CE, Renz EM. Advances in surgical care: management of severe burn injury. *Crit Care Med.* 2008; **36:** S318–S324.

15. Pruitt BA Jr. Protection from excessive resuscitation: "pushing the pendulum back." *J Trauma.* 2000; **49:** 567–568.

16. Klein MB, Hayden D, Elson C, et al. The association between fluid administration and outcome following major burn: a multicenter study. *Ann Surg.* 2007; **245:** 622–628.

17. Cancio LC, Mozingo DW, Pruitt BA Jr. Administering effective emergency care for severe thermal injuries. *J Crit Illn.* 1977; **12:** 85–95.

18. Knaysi GA, Crikelair GF, Cosman B. The rule of nines: its history and accuracy. *Plast Reconstr Surg.* 1968; **41:** 560–563.

19. Lund C, Browder NC. The estimation of areas of burns. *Surg Gynecol Obstet.* 1944; **79:** 352–358.

20. Nagel TR, Schunk JE. Using the hand to estimate the surface area of a burn in children. *Pediatr Emerg Care.* 1997; **13:** 254–255.

21. Lipshy KA, Wheeler WE, Denning DE. Ophthalmic thermal injuries. *Am Surg.* 1996; **62:** 481–483.

22. Heppenstall RB, Sapega AA, Scott R, et al. The compartment syndrome. An experimental and clinical study of muscular energy metabolism using phosphorus nuclear magnetic resonance spectroscopy. *Clin Orthop Relat Res.* 1988; **226:** 138–55.

23. Musgrave DS, Mendelson SA. Pediatric orthopedic trauma: principles in management. *Crit Care Med.* 2002; **30:** S431–S443.

24. Whitesides TE, Heckman MM. Acute compartment syndrome: update on diagnosis and treatment. *J Am Acad Orthop Surg.* 1996; **4:** 209–218.

# CHAPTER TEN

# ANESTHESIA FOR PEDIATRIC BURN PATIENTS

CHRISTINA FIDKOWSKI, MD, MASSACHUSETTS GENERAL HOSPITAL,
AND GENNADIY FUZAYLOV, MD, HARVARD MEDICAL SCHOOL

## INTRODUCTION

Major burn injuries are a significant cause of morbidity and mortality in many pediatric patients. Serious morbidity is more common than mortality. In the United States, pediatric burn injuries generate medical costs exceeding 2 billion dollars per year.[1] The majority of burns are due to thermal injuries, either from contact with hot liquids or vapors, from fires, or from direct contact with hot surfaces.[1] Electrical burns usually cause tissue destruction by direct thermal damage and associated injuries. For chemical burns, the degree of injury depends on the chemical, its concentration, and the duration of exposure.

Burn injury is characterized by depth of the burn, total body surface area (TBSA) involved, and the presence or absence of inhalational injury. The characterization of burn

depth is shown in Table 1. First-degree and superficial second-degree burns heal spontaneously, while deep second-degree, third-degree, and fourth-degree burns require excision and grafting surgery. The TBSA is approximated by the rule of nines in adults, as shown in Figure 1. This rule, however, does not accurately approximate TBSA in children because a child's head size is disproportionately larger than the body as compared to an adult. An approximation of TBSA in children of various ages is shown in Figure 1. The definition of a major burn injury as classified by depth, TBSA, and the location of burn injury is shown in Table 2.[2] It is important to note that severe burns in infants and neonates occur with a smaller TBSA burn injury due to immaturity of the organ systems and the subsequent difficulty maintaining homeostasis.[3] The prognosis following burn injury is determined by age, size and depth of the burn, associated injuries, and preexisting disease.

Pediatric burn patients present many anesthetic challenges, such as difficult airways, difficult vascular access, fluid and electrolyte imbalances, altered temperature regulation, sepsis, cardiovascular instability, and increased requirements of muscle relaxants and opioids. The anesthesia provider participates in the care of these critically ill pediatric patients with the initial resuscitation, intraoperative management, intensive care management, and pain control. The relevant pathophysiologic and pharmacologic changes from burn injury as well as guidelines for intraoperative management and pain control are discussed in this chapter.

## RELEVANT PATHOPHYSIOLOGY

The skin serves as a barrier to protect the host from infection as well as from heat and fluid losses. The destruction of this protective barrier by burn injury leads to infection and altered heat and fluid regulation. Children are particularly prone to these alterations because of their high surface area to volume ratio as compared to adults.

A major burn injury not only destroys the protective skin layer but also leads to the release of local and systemic mediators that produce systemic hypermetabolism and immunosuppression. These mediators also cause localized and systemic capillary leak with resultant edema. Local mediators include prostaglandins, leukotrienes, bradykinin, nitric oxide, histamine, and oxygen free radicals.[4] Systemic mediators include interleukin (IL) 1, IL-6, IL-8, IL-10, and tumor necrosis factor α (TNF-α).[4] The resultant hypermetabolism from systemic mediators begins within the first 3 to 5 days after thermal injury and continues for an extended period of time, up to many months postinjury.[5] The degree of hypermetabolism increases with an increase in burn size.[6] Females over the age of 3 years appear to have a decreased hypermetabolic response compared to their male counterparts.[7]

Along with the hypermetabolism associated with major thermal injury, pathophysiologic changes occur in all organ systems. Generally, these alterations only occur in the setting of a severe burn injury. The changes which are relevant to the anesthetic management of burn-injured patients are discussed below and summarized in Table 3.

## Cardiovascular

The acute phase of a burn injury starts immediately after the injury and resolves within 24 to 48 hours postinjury. During this time, patients have a transiently decreased cardiac output due to depressed myocardial function, increased

blood viscosity, and increased systemic vascular resistance from the release of vasoactive substances. Initially, patients develop burn shock primarily due to hypovolemia from the loss of intravascular volume to extravascular edema. Persistent hypovolemia and burn shock subsequently result in decreased tissue perfusion. This state of shock is treated with adequate fluid resuscitation to maintain urine output greater than 1 mL/kg/h.[8] Patients with severe burns may develop overt ventricular failure[6] and may benefit from inotropic support with dobutamine or dopamine. Placement of a pulmonary artery catheter may also be helpful to tailor therapy.[9]

A systemic inflammatory response is seen around 3 to 5 days postinjury (the second phase of burn injury) as patients become hypermetabolic. As a result, their cardiac output increases and systemic vascular resistance decreases, which allows for increased blood flow to organs and tissues. Clinically, patients may develop persistent tachycardia and systemic hypertension.

## Pulmonary

Altered pulmonary physiology results from both direct and indirect injury. Direct pulmonary injury occurs from the inhalation of flames, smoke, or toxic gases. Inhalational injury causes tissue edema with potential airway obstruction that may lead to respiratory distress. Carbon monoxide poisoning and cyanide toxicity can also contribute to respiratory compromise. Indirect causes of pulmonary compromise include systemic mediator–induced pulmonary hypertension, pulmonary edema, and decreased chest wall compliance from circumferential burns.

### Direct Pulmonary Injury

Direct pulmonary injury results from both thermal and chemical irritation.[10,11,12] Because the respiratory tract is an efficient heat exchanger, only the upper respiratory tract is affected by direct thermal injury. Direct injury to the upper respiratory tract results in edema and mucosal sloughing, which can eventually lead to airway obstruction. Damage to both the upper and lower respiratory tracts occurs by chemical irritation from products of combustion, such as oxides of nitrogen and sulfur, aldehydes, and hydrochloric acid. Injury to the lower respiratory tract results in inactivation of surfactant and the formation of interstitial edema. Clinically, the patient may develop bronchospasm, pulmonary edema, decreased pulmonary compliance, and ventilation-perfusion mismatch.

Inhalational burn injury is suggested by singed nasal hairs, carbonaceous secretions, sooty sputum, respiratory distress, wheezing, and facial burns. The diagnosis of upper airway injury is made by direct visualization using fiberoptic bronchoscopy. Xenon scanning and transthoracic thermal dilution techniques to calculate extravascular lung water may be used to determine the extent of parenchymal injury.[12]

The treatment for inhalational injury is ventilatory support. Treatment should be aggressive with early intervention since children can deteriorate more quickly than adults. If inhalational injury is suspected, the airway should be immediately secured by endotracheal intubation since edema formation during the first 24 to 72 hours postinjury could compromise the airway. This statement is especially pertinent in children because of their smaller airway diameters. Since resistance is indirectly proportional to the diameter to the fourth power, even a small amount of mucosal edema will cause a significant increase in airway resistance.

Pharmacologic treatment options include bronchodilators, racemic epinephrine, aerosolized n-acetylcysteine, and/or aerosolized heparin.[12] There appears to be no long-term benefit of treatment with corticosteroids.[13]

## Carbon Monoxide Poisoning

Carbon monoxide poisoning should be suspected in any patient with inhalational injury or with burns from open fires. Carbon monoxide binds to heme-containing proteins such as hemoglobin, cytochromes, and myoglobin.[14] The affinity of carbon monoxide for hemoglobin is 200 times stronger than that of oxygen. Carbon monoxide not only displaces oxygen from hemoglobin but also shifts the oxygen dissociation curve to the left. As a result, tissue oxygen delivery is decreased. The binding of carbon monoxide to cytochromes decreases cellular metabolism and tissue oxygenation. The binding of carbon monoxide to myoglobin decreases oxygen tension in cardiac and skeletal muscles, which can lead to cardiac dysfunction and rhabdomyolysis.

The diagnosis of carbon monoxide poisoning is confirmed by carboxy-hemoglobin levels and cooximetry.[14] The presence of carboxy-hemoglobin adversely affects the accuracy of conventional 2-wavelength pulse oximetry, which results in falsely high readings. The carboxy-hemoglobin level is dependent on both the concentration and duration of exposure. Normal carboxy-hemoglobin levels are in the range of 1% to 3%. Typically, patients with a level less than 20% present with mild symptoms such as nausea and headache.[14] Levels greater than 60% to 70% are often fatal due to coma, seizure, or cardiopulmonary arrest.[14] Treatment should not be delayed if there is a high suspicion of carbon monoxide poisoning. The mainstay of treatment is exposure to high concentrations

of inspired oxygen. The half-life of carboxy-hemoglobin is 240 to 320 minutes when breathing room air but decreases to 40 to 80 minutes when breathing 100% oxygen.[14] While treatment with hyperbaric oxygen is controversial, it can be considered for patients with a history of loss of consciousness, neurologic sequela, metabolic acidosis, or cardiopulmonary compromise or for patients at the extremes of age. The half-life of carboxy-hemoglobin decreases to 20 minutes when breathing 100% oxygen at 2.5 to 3 atmospheres.

## Cyanide Toxicity

Clinicians should be suspicious of cyanide toxicity when patients present with inhalational injury. Patients are exposed to cyanide during open fires involving nitrogen-containing plastics. Cyanide binds to cytochrome oxidase and impairs tissue oxygenation by converting intracellular aerobic metabolism to anaerobic metabolism.[15,16]

Since cyanide levels cannot be obtained in a timely manner, it is not practical to await test results prior to commencing treatment. Therefore, other signs, such as an elevated venous oxygen level and lactic acidosis that does not improve with oxygen administration, are suggestive of cyanide toxicity.[15] Initial treatment consists of 100% oxygen and supportive measures. Cyanide is metabolized slowly by the liver to the nontoxic thiocyanate. The administration of sodium thiosulfate, which serves as a sulfate donor, increases this conversion. The administration of nitrites such as amyl nitrite and sodium nitrite increases the amount of methemoglobin, which competes for cyanide binding from cytochrome oxidase. The induction of methemoglobin may be dangerous with inhalational injuries because of coexisting carboxy-hemoglobin. Young children are particularly sensitive to nitrite administration since fetal hemoglobin more easily converts to methemoglobin and since children have lower levels of methemoglobin reductase in comparison to adults. A recently approved antidote for cyanide toxicity in the United States is hydroxocobalamin, a precursor to vitamin B12.[16] The cobalt moiety of hydroxocobalamin readily binds intracellular cyanide to form the nontoxic cyanocobalamin (vitamin B12). This treatment may be more advantageous in children with smoke inhalation since it does not induce methemoglobinemia and has a rapid onset of action.

## Indirect Pulmonary Injury

Pulmonary injury can occur with severe burns in the absence of inhalational injury.[17] During the initial 24 to 72 hours postinjury, hypoproteinemia and decreased plasma oncotic pressure contribute to pulmonary edema formation. Additionally, inflammatory mediators such as TNF-α contribute to increased pulmonary capillary permeability. Clinically, the patient may develop tachypnea, dyspnea, and pneumonia as a result of increased pulmonary vascular resistance, interstitial edema, and decreased pulmonary compliance. Aggressive management of this pulmonary dysfunction with early endotracheal intubation or tracheostomy and mechanical ventilation is appropriate.

## Renal

In the acute phase of burn injury, the glomerular filtration rate is decreased due to a combination of decreased cardiac output and increased vascular tone from circulating catecholamines, vasopressin, and renin-angiotensin-aldosterone.[18] During the hypermetabolic phase, glomerular filtration increases due to increased cardiac output, but tubular dysfunction may occur. As a result, the exact effect on renal function and creatinine clearance is variable among patients.

Burn-injured patients, particularly those with electrical or crush injuries, are at risk for myoglobin release from damaged muscle cells. The subsequent myoglobinuria can lead to tubular damage and renal dysfunction.

## Endocrine and Metabolic

After the acute phase of burn injury, there is a massive release of stress hormones, which include catecholamines, antidiuretic hormone, renin, angiotensin, aldosterone, glucagon, and cortisol.[19,20,21] The amount of stress hormones released increases with the TBSA of burn injury.[22] This milieu of circulating stress hormones drives the hypermetabolic state that manifests clinically with increases in resting energy expenditure, core body temperature, muscle catabolism, lipolysis, glucolysis, futile substrate cycling, and insulin resistance.[19,20,21] While it was initially thought that this hypermetabolic state subsided with wound closure, there is evidence that it persists for at least 9 to 12 months postinjury. For children with greater than 40% TBSA burns, resting energy expenditure is 179% that of normal controls 1 week postinjury. This rate decreases to 153% at the time of wound closure and gradually declines to 115% at 12 months postinjury.[23]

Current efforts are focused on attenuating this hypermetabolic response.[19,20,21] Nonpharmacologic methods of decreasing hypermetabolism include early excision and wound closure, aggressive treatment of sepsis, high protein and carbohydrate enteral feeds, environmental temperature elevation, and a resistive exercise program. Pharmacologic agents that may attenuate hypermetabolism include anabolic proteins (growth hormone, insulinlike growth factor, and insulin), anabolic steroids (oxandrolone), and catecholamine antagonists (propranolol). Insulin,[24] oxandrolone,[25,26,27,28] and propranolol[29] are the most cost-effective pharmacologic treatments. Although the beneficial effects of these agents are not definitively established, they appear to be useful in certain circumstances.

In addition to hypermetabolism from stress hormone release, other endocrine derangements include decreased levels of thyroid hormones (T3 and T4) and vitamin D.[30,31] Hypovitaminosis D is secondary to acquired hypoparathyroidism in burn-injured children.[32] The resultant hypocalcemia and hypomagnesemia should be aggressively treated to prevent adverse cardiovascular effects such as hypotension and dysrhythmias.

## Hepatic

During the acute phase of burn injury, the liver is subjected to hypoperfusion from hypovolemia and depressed cardiac output. Hypoperfusion, along with ischemia-reperfusion injury and circulating inflammatory cytokines, leads to hepatic cell apoptosis.[33] Elevated levels of liver enzymes such as ALT, AST, and bilirubin are suggestive of this hepatic injury. These enzymes are elevated immediately postburn and typically return to normal within 2 to 6 weeks postinjury. Persistent or severe hepatic dysfunction is associated with worse outcomes.

Hepatic enlargement occurs due to intrahepatic fat and edema. There is also a decrease in the intrinsic hepatic proteins albumin and transferrin, as well as an increase in acute phase reactants, haptoglobin, C-reactive protein, and complement. These changes can persist for up to 6 to 12 months postinjury.

## Hematologic

During the acute phase of injury, systemic edema causes hemoconcentration with a resultant increased hematocrit and increased blood viscosity. After the initial resuscitation, patients develop anemia from a combination of dilution from resuscitation, blood loss at wound sites, and hemolysis from heat-damaged erythrocytes.[34] In the absence of other illness, patients can tolerate a low hematocrit (20%–25% range); however, in severely burn-injured children, a higher hematocrit may be desirable due to persistent blood loss.

After burn injury, thrombocytopenia occurs due to platelet aggregation at wound sites and damaged microvasculature. The body responds by increasing production of clotting factors, which leads to the development of a hypercoagulable state and may give rise to disseminated intravascular coagulation (DIC). Generally, patients do not require platelet transfusion.

## Gastrointestinal

The gastrointestinal tract is also susceptible to damage from hypoperfusion, ischemia-reperfusion injury, and circulating inflammatory mediators. Specifically, the intestinal mucosal barrier is easily damaged and becomes permeable to bacteria and endotoxins.[35] There is evidence that early enteral nutrition minimizes mucosal damage, decreases endotoxinemia, and reduces TNF-α levels.[35,36]

Burn-injured patients are at risk for developing gastric and duodenal stress ulcers, referred to as Curling's ulcers, which may lead to gastrointestinal bleeding.[2] Prophylactic treatment with H2-antagonists or proton pump inhibitors may be beneficial. These patients can also develop acute enterocolitis with resultant abdominal distention, hypotension, and bloody diarrhea. Additionally, severely burned patients can develop adynamic ileus and may benefit from gastric decompression. Acalculous cholecystitis can develop during the second and third week postinjury.

## Neurologic

Burn encephalopathy is described in the literature as a syndrome that includes hallucination, personality change, delirium, seizure, and coma. One study of 140 burn-injured children reports 20 cases of burn encephalopathy.[37] The most common causes of encephalopathy in that study are hypoxia followed by sepsis, hyponatremia, hypovolemia, and cortical vein thrombosis. Hypoxic neurologic insult results in a 33% chance of permanent cognitive deficits.[38] Another source of neurologic derangement is cerebral edema and elevated intracranial pressure, which are shown to occur during days 1 through 3 postinjury.[39] Hypertensive encephalopathy with resultant seizures is shown to occur in 7% of hypertensive pediatric burn patients.[40] The incidence of seizures in burn patients is roughly 1.5%, and risk factors include hyponatremia, a history of epilepsy, hypoxia, sepsis, and drug effects.[41]

Patients with electrical burns are at risk for developing direct neurologic injury. Depending on the entry and exit sites of the electrical current, paraplegia and quadriplegia from spinal cord damage are described in the literature.[42,43] Direct brain injury can also occur.[44]

## RELEVANT PHARMACOLOGY

Burn injury results in altered pharmacokinetics of many anesthetic drugs due to changes in the volume of distribution, protein binding, and metabolism.[45] The volume of distribution increases with the increased extracellular volume due to capillary leak. The free fraction of drug is altered with increased $\alpha_1$-acid glycoprotein and decreased albu-

min concentrations. Drug clearance is also altered by the metabolic derangements of burn injury. Specifically, during the acute phase (24-48 hours), decreased cardiac output and hypoperfusion to the liver and kidneys can result in decreased drug clearance. During the hypermetabolic phase (> 48 hours), renal and hepatic clearance increases. In addition to altered pharmacokinetics, burn physiology causes alterations in drug receptors that affect the pharmacodynamics of some anesthetic agents, such as the neuromuscular blockers.[46] The pharmacology of anesthetic agents relevant to the management of burn-injured patients is discussed below.

## Inhalational Anesthetic Agents

Potent inhalational anesthetic agents, which include halothane, isoflurane, sevoflurane, and desflurane, can be used for the induction and/or maintenance of general anesthesia. Children have an increased requirement of inhalational agents as compared to adults. The requirement of inhalational agents peaks in infants aged between 1 and 6 months and decreases through adulthood.[47] All potent inhalational agents have cardio-depressant properties that may not be tolerated by burn patients with hemodynamic compromise. Halothane is a safe and effective agent that is classically used in pediatric anesthesia because it enables a rapid inhalational induction without airway irritation.[47] However, the use of halothane in patients who require hemodynamic support, have metabolic or respiratory acidosis, or receive epinephrine-containing tumescent solutions may lead to further cardiac depression and arrhythmias. Although halothane hepatitis is reported in adult populations, pediatric burn patients do not appear to be at risk for this disease.[48] Isoflurane has fewer cardio-depressant properties compared to halothane; however, it does not allow for a rapid inhalational induction. Sevoflurane also has decreased cardio-depressant properties compared to halothane and is suitable for inhalational inductions due to its rapid onset, pleasant smell, and low airway irritability. Desflurane provides a rapid induction and emergence; however, it is a potent airway irritant and should not be used for inhalational inductions.

Nitrous oxide is a weak inhalational anesthetic agent and potent analgesic with minimal respiratory and cardiac depressant effects; therefore, it is a suitable adjunct to other anesthetic agents.

## Intravenous Anesthetic Agents

Thiopental, propofol, and ketamine are intravenous agents that can be used in pediatric burn patients for the induction and maintenance of anesthesia. Thiopental is a barbiturate with cardio-depressant properties that may lead to hypotension in hemodynamically unstable patients. The pharmacology of thiopental is altered in burn patients such that higher doses even up to 1 year postinjury may be required.[49] Propofol is a sedative-hypnotic agent that also possesses cardio-depressant properties. These 2 agents can be safely used in burn patients when the dose is titrated to effect. Ketamine, an N-methyl-D-aspartate (NMDA) antagonist, does not have respiratory depressant properties. Its cardio-depressant properties are typically balanced by its sympathomimetic effect; therefore, it may be more suitable for induction and maintenance of anesthesia in unstable patients. However, caution is warranted when using this agent for patients with a high sympathetic tone, as its cardio-depressant properties will become more prominent.

## Neuromuscular Blockers

Burn injury causes an upregulation of extrajunctional nicotinic acetylcholine receptors (AChRs) in the muscle membrane.[46] These extrajunctional receptors are mainly immature, with an altered response to ligand binding. This proliferation of immature receptors, which occurs within 48 to 72 hours after a burn injury, places the patient at risk for hyperkalemia from succinylcholine. Resistance to nondepolarizing muscle relaxants also occurs due to these receptor changes.[46,50]

Because of its rapid onset and short duration of effect, the depolarizing relaxant succinylcholine is often used for rapid sequence intubations or airway emergencies. While use of succinylcholine during the first 24 to 48 hours after burn injury is acceptable, it should be avoided after that time.[50] The upregulation of extrajunctional AChRs allows for a larger efflux of potassium from the intracellular to the extracellular space. Additionally, the immature receptors remain open longer, which also allows a larger efflux of potassium from the cell. It is hypothesized that once wounds are healed and functional mobility is regained, the patient is no longer at risk for lethal hyperkalemia.[50] Since conversion back to normal pharmacodynamics can take 1 to 2 years, succinylcholine should be avoided during that time.

Burn patients develop resistance to nondepolarizing muscle relaxants approximately 48 to 72 hours after injury due to AChR changes.[50] As a result, these drugs have a prolonged time to onset of effect and a shorter duration of action. This phenomenon is shown clinically with the steroidal nondepolarizing relaxants vecuronium and rocuronium.[51,52] Dose escalation of rocuronium to 0.9 mg/kg or 1.2 mg/kg prolongs its duration of action and decreases the time to onset, which may make it a suitable alternative

to succinylcholine for urgent intubations.[52] With the exception of atracurium and cisatracurium, which are metabolized by Hoffman elimination in the plasma, the nondepolarizing relaxants undergo renal and hepatic clearance, which can be significantly altered in burn patients based on their renal and hepatic function.[46]

## Antibiotics

The pharmacokinetics of many classes of antibiotics are altered in burn patients.[53] Aminoglycosides are shown to have a larger volume of distribution and an increased clearance, which may require elevated dosages at more frequent intervals.[54] β-lactams also have an increased volume of distribution and an increased clearance.[55,56] Vancomycin and the carbapenem imipenem are shown to have altered clearance that correlates with creatinine clearance.[53,57] The pharmacokinetics of the quinolone levofloxacin in burn patients is shown not to differ significantly from that of normal controls.[58] These studies also demonstrate large intrapatient and interpatient variability. Because of the unpredictable nature of antibiotic pharmacokinetics, certain antibiotic levels should be monitored. More specifically, intraoperative antibiotic dosing regimens may need to be altered to ensure adequate prophylaxis.[56]

## Opioids

Patients with burn injury typically require large amounts of opioids for pain control. A morphine infusion is commonly used to control baseline pain. Initial pharmacokinetic studies of morphine in burn patients showed a decreased clearance, a decreased half-life, and a decreased volume of distribution.[59] More recent studies reveal morphine clearance in burned patients is the same, if not slightly increased, compared to that of nonburned patients.[60,61] Therefore, large morphine requirements are likely due to severe pain or pharmacodynamic changes. Doses of morphine should be adjusted based on clinical needs. A recent study of bolus dose fentanyl in burn patients demonstrates an increased clearance and increased volume of distribution.[62] This finding is consistent with the larger fentanyl doses that are needed to achieve the same clinical effect.

## Opioid Adjuncts

### Ketamine

Since burn patients require high doses of opioid analgesics, which are associated with undesirable side effects such as gastrointestinal dysmotility and respiratory depression, opioid adjuncts are sometimes necessary for pain control. Ketamine, an NMDA antagonist, produces dissociative amnesia, analgesia, and sedation without hemodynamic or respiratory depression.[63] Oral and intramuscular ketamine are both shown to be effective for painful bedside procedures in pediatric burn patients.[64,65] In a case report, long-term intravenous ketamine is shown to be an effective opioid adjunct in a pediatric burn patient without tolerance or psychomimetic side effects.[66]

## Alpha-2 Agonists

Alpha-2 (α2) agonists are also used as opioid adjuncts in pediatric burn patients.[67] The α2-agonists act at the locus caeruleus to modulate pain perception. Potential side effects of these agents include hypotension and bradycardia. Clonidine is used orally and epidurally as an analgesic adjunct. Case reports show that clonidine reduces opioid requirements in both adult and pediatric burn patients.[68,69] In comparison to clonidine, dexmedetomidine (Precedex) is a newer α2-agonist that is 8 times more selective for α2 receptors than for α1 receptors. A recent retrospective study of pediatric burn patients shows that dexmedetomidine infusions in conjunction with opioids provide adequate analgesia when opioid infusions alone were inadequate.[70] Since dexmedetomidine has a relatively short half-life (2 hours), it is easily titrated during continuous infusions.

## Benzodiazepines

Benzodiazepines are sedative-hypnotic agents that act by potentiating the inhibitory action of gamma-aminobutyric acid (GABA) receptors. Parenteral benzodiazepines, such as diazepam, lorazepam, and midazolam, are used as anxiolytics. The clearance of diazepam is decreased in burn-injured children,[71] whereas that of lorazepam is increased.[72] While the clearance of midazolam is decreased in critically ill pediatric patients, its elimination half-life during continuous infusions is significantly shorter than that of other benzodiazepines. As a result, midazolam infusions are readily titratable and useful in the management of ventilated pediatric burn patients.[73]

## ANESTHETIC MANAGEMENT FOR ACUTE BURN PROCEDURES

The management of pediatric burn patients provides challenges for the anesthesiologist. In the acute phase of injury, attention must be paid to the patients' physiologic and pharmacologic changes described above. These patients are often critically ill with hemodynamic and respiratory

compromise; however, operative management cannot be delayed since procedures such as excision and grafting are the only treatment for their illness. General principles for the anesthetic management of these patients are described in the literature and summarized below.[2,74,75,76,77]

## Preoperative Assessment and Management

The preoperative assessment of a burn patient begins with an evaluation of the type of burn and the extent and depth of the burn, as well as any associated injuries. Patients with minor burns and a TBSA less than 10% typically do not require formal resuscitation, whereas those with major burns, with a TBSA greater than 30%, develop the systemic physiologic changes described above and require resuscitation. Patients with burn injury between these extremes require resuscitation but do not develop the systemic physiologic changes. The patient's medical history should be reviewed, as significant medical illness may merit more aggressive treatment and resuscitation even with minor burns. A review of previous anesthetic records is useful since these patients undergo frequent trips to the operating room. The patient's current physiologic state is determined by assessing the patient's present hemodynamics and/or pressor requirements, pulmonary compliance and ventilator settings, and volume status and urine output.

The physical exam should include a thorough airway evaluation, as many of these patients have distorted anatomy and are potential difficult intubations. Even if the patient is already intubated, the airway should be evaluated, as there may be a requirement for reintubation due to a ventilation leak around the endotracheal tube or an accidental extubation. The size and location of intravenous access and invasive monitoring is also noted on physical exam.

Because these patients have high metabolic demands, enteral nutrition should be continued as long as possible preoperatively.[78] Parenteral nutrition can be continued intraoperatively. Burn patients do not have evidence of delayed gastric emptying; therefore, stopping clear liquids 2 hours preoperatively or discontinuing enteral feeds 1 to 2 hours preoperatively is adequate.[79] See Table 4 for traditional preoperative NPO guidelines. Traditional preoperative fasting is waived for burn patients receiving continuous enteral tube feeds since this practice is not associated with increased morbidity or increased risk of aspiration in these patients.[80] For enteral feeds, the nasogastric tube is suctioned preoperatively and left open to gravity intraoperatively to minimize the risk of aspiration.

Laboratory studies, including complete blood count, electrolytes, coagulation studies, and BUN/creatinine, should be noted. Special emphasis should be placed on correcting any acid-base disturbances during the acute phase. If a blood bank sample is not current, one should be sent prior to the operation. A chest radiograph should be obtained in patients suspected of smoke inhalation. The positioning of central access is also evaluated with the chest radiograph. In the presence of carbon monoxide poisoning, the pulse oximeter may overestimate the saturation of hemoglobin; therefore, a carboxyhemoglobin level or co-oximetry should be used to assess the degree of carbon monoxide poisoning and guide treatment. Upon completion of the initial assessment, the anesthetic plan is reviewed with the parent and informed consent is obtained. At that point, the patient is ready for transport to the operating room.

Transport to the operating room requires the presence of at least 1 if not 2 skilled anesthesia providers. A transport monitor is utilized to monitor the electrocardiogram (EKG), blood pressure, and oxygen saturation. If the patient is intubated, an oxygen supply as well as an ambu bag or transport ventilator must be available. A PEEP valve should be used if the patient requires PEEP to maintain oxygenation. During transport, resuscitation medications and emergency airway equipment should be available.

## Monitoring and Access

Monitors for burn surgery include the ASA standard monitors for general anesthesia (Table 5). Many patients have large areas of burn injury, which may make standard monitor placement difficult. Large thorax burns may necessitate creative, nonstandard-surface electrode placement for EKG monitoring. Esophageal EKG monitoring is another option.[81] Peripheral pulse oximetry monitoring may be unreliable with extensive burn injury, hypoperfusion, or hypothermia. Alternative sites of probe placement include the ear lobe, buccal mucosa, tongue, and esophagus.[82,83,84] Blood pressure is monitored either invasively or noninvasively. Invasive blood pressure monitoring is advantageous if the extremities are injured or if large fluid shifts or blood loss are expected. End-tidal carbon dioxide monitoring allows for assessment of adequate ventilation given the increased carbon dioxide production from hypermetabolism. If the patient has pulmonary injury, an arteriolar-alveolar gradient may be present; therefore, arterial carbon dioxide measurements may be more appropriate than end-tidal carbon dioxide measurements for assessment of the adequacy of ventilation. Temperature should be monitored given the propensity for heat loss. Invasive central venous pressure monitoring along with urine output measurements provide insight into the patient's volume status.

Obtaining intravascular access can be challenging in burn patients. Large-bore peripheral intravenous lines are ideal for fluid replacement, especially with the large blood loss from excision and grafting surgery. Multilumen central catheters are satisfactory for drug infusions but may not be adequate for rapid fluid replacement given their high resistance. The femoral vein is our preferred site for central access. The subclavian vein and internal jugular vein are our second and third choices, respectively. Ideally, intravenous and intra-arterial access should be placed through noninjured tissue. If intravenous access cannot be obtained and the child needs access emergently for fluid resuscitation or medications, intraosseous access can be obtained rapidly in the anterior medial tibia, distal femur, or sternum as a temporary measure.[85] Complications from intraosseous access, such as osteomyelitis, are rare (~0.6%).[86]

## Airway Management

Pediatric airway anatomy differs from that of an adult, as shown in Table 6.[87] Laryngoscopy may be more difficult in a child due to a relatively large tongue which is difficult to manipulate, a relatively high glottic opening that is difficult to visualize, and an angled epiglottis that is difficult to lift during laryngoscopy. Passing the endotracheal tube through the glottic opening may be difficult since the opening is not perpendicular to the trachea. As the narrowest part of the pediatric airway is at the level of the cricoid cartilage, an endotracheal tube may be too large even if it passes easily through the vocal cords. These anatomical airway differences are most notable during infancy and gradually disappear as the child ages. Because of these airway differences, straight laryngoscope blades are more effective in pediatric patients. A summary of suggested laryngoscope blades and endotracheal tube sizes for children of various ages is shown in Table 7.

Securing the airway in a pediatric burn patient is challenging. Within the first 24 hours, succinylcholine is safe to use. Previously, the standard practice in pediatric patients was to place uncuffed endotracheal tubes to prevent mucosal damage. However, recent evidence suggests that low-pressure, high-volume cuffed endotracheal tubes should be used.[88] Patients who have suffered inhalational injury may develop decreased compliance, which requires higher ventilatory pressures that can cause leaks around uncuffed tubes.

Most patients presenting to the operating room during the acute phase will already have a secured airway, either an endotracheal tube or a tracheostomy. In those instances, the airway should be adequately secured prior to positioning the patient on the operating room table to prevent unintentional dislodgement.

In the acute phase, patients may have facial and airway edema that distorts the normal airway anatomy. In addition, patients may have limited neck mobility and mouth opening. All pediatric burn patients with face, neck, or upper chest injuries should be approached as potentially difficult airways. A thorough preoperative assessment should be performed, with a plan for securing the airway. Adequate instruments, such as laryngeal mask airways (LMAs), lighted stylets, fiberoptic bronchoscopes, and a surgeon capable of performing an emergent surgical airway, should be readily available.

An organized approach to evaluate the airway is to consider securing the airway through the nose, mouth, or trachea while the patient is awake, sedated, or anesthetized. If the patient has severe craniofacial abnormalities which suggest difficult mask ventilation, securing the airway while the patient is awake may be prudent. However, this option is only practical for older and cooperative patients. Awake nasal or oral intubations are performed with adequate local anesthetic to suppress airway reflexes. To secure the airway under sedation, agents such as ketamine (0.5-2 mg/kg) or dexmedetomidine (0.5-1 mcg/kg over 10 minutes followed by 0.2-0.7 mcg/kg/h) are used to ensure that respiratory depression does not occur. To secure the airway under general anesthesia, either an inhalational or an intravenous induction can be used as long as the patient is spontaneously ventilating until a definitive airway can be established.

The approach to the airway through the nose includes blind nasal intubation, which is reserved for extreme emergencies, and fiberoptic guided nasal intubation. The approach to the airway through the mouth includes direct laryngoscopy with endotracheal intubation, lighted stylet blind oral-tracheal intubation, bougie-guided endotracheal intubation under direct vision, fiberoptic intubation, and LMA insertion. The approach to securing the airway through the trachea includes emergent and elective surgical airways.

If both oral and nasal intubation techniques are viable options, we prefer oral intubation since the nasal route carries a risk of sinus infection. Additionally, we prefer oral intubation over early tracheostomy. Although early tracheostomy is shown to be safe and efficacious in pediatric burn patients,[89] we choose a more conservative approach to minimize tracheostomy site infections and pulmonary infections.

## Induction and Maintenance

The choice of anesthetic agents for a burn patient depends on the patient's current condition and the anesthesia provider's preference. Prior to induction, the patient should be adequately fluid resuscitated to prevent hemodynamic compromise with the anesthetic agents. If the patient is not already intubated, either an inhalational induction with halothane or sevoflurane or an intravenous induction with ketamine, thiopental, or propofol are good options. The dose ranges of intravenous anesthetic agents suitable for inducing general anesthesia are shown in Table 8. It is possible to induce the child prior to transfer to the operating room table to minimize pain and discomfort if his or her airway does not appear difficult.

Maintenance of anesthesia is accomplished with potent inhalational agents, a nitrous-narcotic technique, or a total intravenous anesthetic (TIVA). Patients in the acute phase of their injury may be too hemodynamically unstable to tolerate potent inhalational agents; therefore, the nitrous-narcotic technique with or without ketamine supplementation might be preferred. With the latter technique, muscle relaxants might be required to prevent movement due to spinal cord reflexes.

Regardless of which induction or maintenance agents are chosen, all medications should be titrated to effect since these patients demonstrate altered physiology. The anesthesia provider should also be aware of the pharmacologic changes discussed above, such as resistance to nondepolarizing muscle relaxants and requirements of higher narcotic doses.

## Fluid Management

Large intraoperative fluid losses are predictable during major burn surgeries. Not only are there insensible evaporative losses from the burn wounds, but there is also the potential for massive blood loss from excised wounds and donor sites.

There is limited data to approximate the amount of blood loss during excision and grafting procedures. Expected blood loss increases each day postinjury as the wound becomes more hyperemic. An estimation of blood loss during excision and grafting surgery based on the number of days postinjury is shown in Table 9.[90] The amount of blood loss is greater for tangential excisions as compared to fascial excisions and is approximated as 4 ml/cm$^2$ and 1.5 ml/cm$^2$, respectively.[77] Blood loss is also greater in infected wounds. Since these numbers are only approximations of blood loss, frequent hematocrit and hemoglobin measurements are necessary to determine blood loss for each individual patient.

While burn surgery has the reputation for massive blood loss, current surgical practice is aimed at reducing blood loss.[91] Such measures include infiltration with vasoconstrictors, limb tourniquets, compressive dressings, electrocautery, and maintaining euthermia. While large-volume infiltration with tumescent solutions containing vasoconstrictors is beneficial for minimizing blood loss, there is potential for systemic absorption with resultant fluid overload.[92] We limit the amount of tumescent solution, which contains 2 mcg/mL to 3 mcg/mL epinephrine, to 10 mL/kg to 40 mL/kg. While there is no current data to predict the amount of systemic absorption from tumescent solution, there is evidence that burn patients have altered body fluid water composition. In the acute setting, extracellular water is increased while intracellular water is decreased.[93] With these alterations in fluid balance, the patient's volume status should be monitored closely perioperatively.

In addition to blood loss, patients also have insensible fluid losses. During the initial resuscitation phase, fluid replacement is approximated by the Parkland formula, which is 4 mL/(kg x % BSA burned), in addition to standard maintenance fluids. When the patient has been adequately resuscitated prior to coming to the operating room, fluid replacement is best guided by indicators of organ perfusion, such as urine output, acid-base status, central venous pressure, blood pressure, and arterial pressure waveforms.

Intraoperative fluid losses are initially replaced with crystalloid and colloid solutions. We prefer colloid, in the form of 5% albumin, instead of crystalloid for fluid replacement. Packed red cell transfusions may be appropriate based on the patient's starting hemoglobin, estimated blood loss, and lowest tolerable hemoglobin. If the patient has received multiple units of red cells, the additional transfusion of coagulation factors may be warranted.

## Temperature Regulation

Burn patients are at great risk for intraoperative heat loss due to lack of an intact skin layer. In comparison to adults, pediatric patients are at a higher risk for intraoperative heat loss due to their larger surface area to volume ratio. When these patients become hypothermic, their metabolism increases heat production.[94] As a result, metabolic energy is diverted from other areas, such as wound healing. Therefore, one must take care to prevent intraoperative heat loss in these patients, even if these measures result in the operating room becoming uncomfortably warm.

Heat loss occurs by 4 mechanisms: radiation, convection, conduction, and evaporation. Radiation heat loss is the transfer of electromagnetic radiation from a warm patient to the cooler surrounding objects. Convective heat loss is the transfer of heat to cool air as it flows over the body surface. Conductive heat loss is the direct transfer of heat to objects in contact with the body surface. Evaporative heat loss is the transfer of heat to vaporize liquid water on the body surface. For a nude adult in a room at ambient temperature, heat losses from radiation, convection, conduction, and evaporation are approximately 60%, 12%, 3%, and 25%, respectively.[95] With loss of the dry protective skin barrier, evaporative losses become more significant in burn patients.

Heat loss can be minimized intraoperatively by many different interventions. Radiation heat loss is diminished by warming the operating room to decrease the temperature gradient between the patient and surroundings, by using heat lamps, and by placing reflective barriers such as mylar over the patient. Convective heat loss is minimized by warming the operating room, while conductive heat loss is reduced by placing the patient on warming blankets or other insulated materials. Evaporative heat loss is limited by covering the patient with impermeable materials such as plastic sheets or by humidifying anesthetic gases. Other methods to minimize heat loss include intravenous fluid and blood warmers and forced-air warming blankets to maintain euthermia.

## ANESTHETIC MANAGEMENT FOR RECONSTRUCTIVE PROCEDURES

Burn patients often return to the operating room multiple times for reconstructive procedures, such as scar revisions, reexcisions, and grafting. At the time of these reconstructive procedures, the primary wound is healed. Therefore, the patient may no longer exhibit the extreme physiologic and pharmacologic changes. Controversy remains as to when these patients are no longer susceptible to hyperkalemia from succinylcholine. A reasonable guideline is that once the wounds are healed and the patient is mobile, the patient is no longer susceptible to hyperkalemia.[46]

The anesthetic management for these procedures is similar to that for other plastic surgical operations. Since these patients typically undergo multiple reconstructive procedures, the preoperative assessment should focus on major changes in health since the last anesthetic and a careful airway evaluation. The previous anesthetic records should be reviewed to gain information on previous airway management and opioid requirements. Since these procedures are elective, the patient should be appropriately fasted, as shown in Table 4.

Since these patients undergo multiple anesthetics for reconstructive procedures, anxiolysis may be required prior to entering the operating room. Examples of premedication for younger children who do not have intravenous access include oral midazolam, oral or intramuscular ketamine, and oral clonidine. Older children who have intravenous access can benefit from intravenous benzodiazepines or opioids. Appropriate dose ranges for these agents are shown in Table 10.

Reconstructive procedures typically do not result in large amounts of blood loss or extensive fluid shifts. Therefore, a single peripheral intravenous line and standard ASA monitors for general anesthesia are adequate. Since the patient's primary wounds are healed, excessive fluid or heat loss is less of a concern. Fluid replacement should be based on maintenance fluid requirements. Temperature can be monitored, with warming blankets used as needed.

The choice of anesthetic is based on the surgical procedure. Minor surgical procedures such as suture removal can be performed with sedation. Ketamine may provide adequate analgesia and sedation for such procedures. A general anesthetic may be required for more invasive procedures. The choice of induction, either inhalational or intravenous, is made partially based on the patient's age and preference. The aim of this practice is to make the experience as pleasant as possible so that the child will not shy away when it is time for a repeat procedure.

After induction, the airway is secured. Based on the surgical location and procedure duration, an LMA is often adequate for securing the airway. If the patient has face or neck contractures, scar tissue may distort the airway, resulting in fixed flexion abnormalities and limited mouth opening. Severe neck contractures can limit placement of an LMA, in which case, the upside-down intubating LMA technique is an effective alternative.[96,97] If an LMA is not adequate, use of adjunctive airway equipment such as a fiberoptic bronchoscope or lighted stylet may be necessary. In extreme cases, a surgical neck release may be required prior to induction of anesthesia. Surgical neck release prior to intubation is performed with either local or general anesthesia with spontaneous mask ventilation.[98] In an extreme case of craniofacial deformity, extracorporeal membrane oxygenation (ECMO) is described in a case report as a bridge to securing the airway until neck release could be performed.[99]

Maintenance of anesthesia is performed with either potent inhalational agents, a nitrous-narcotic technique, or a total intravenous anesthetic per the anesthesia provider's preference. Emergence from anesthesia should be focused on patient comfort and adequate analgesia. These patients have a tendency to develop opioid tolerance, so these agents should be titrated to clinical effect.

Throughout the entire perioperative period, attention should be paid to the patient's comfort and anxiolysis. One example of providing pain-free care is using local anesthetics prior to intravenous placement. While there is concern for adverse psychological outcome from multiple general anesthetics, there appears to be no evidence of adverse psychological impact provided that adequate precautions are taken, such as premedication as needed.[100]

## PAIN MANAGEMENT

The ability to assess and treat pain in pediatric patients can be challenging, especially since younger children are not able to directly communicate their pain levels. Burn pain is a combination of background pain, procedure-related pain, and postoperative pain. Guidelines for the management of pain in pediatric burn patients are described in the literature.[101,102]

Background pain is the constant and variable pain from the burn injury itself. From our experience, this pain is proportional to the size of the thermal injury. While background pain from smaller TBSA burns may be controlled with intermittent boluses of opioids, pain control for larger TBSA burns may require opioid infusions. For a bolus dose, we typically start with 0.1 mg/kg/dose morphine every 2 hours as needed for pain control. Morphine infusions are started at 0.05 mg/kg/h for nonintubated patients and at 1 mg/kg/h for intubated patients. These patients do develop tolerance to opioids; therefore, doses should be reassessed frequently and titrated to patient comfort.

In order to minimize the escalation of opioid doses, other agents can be used as analgesic adjuncts. Acetaminophen, either oral or rectal, is one such opioid adjunct for pain control.[103] A ketamine infusion is also shown to be an effective analgesic adjunct.[66] For intubated patients, we use ketamine infusions at a rate of 0.5 to 3 mg/kg/h. We also use dexmedetomidine infusions starting at 0.5 mcg/kg/h, with titration up to a maximum of 2.5 mcg/kg/h.

Other factors, such as anxiety and pruritis, contribute to pain perception; therefore, treatment of these factors can better control the patient's pain. Benzodiazepines, such as oral or intravenous lorazepam (0.05 mg/kg/dose up to 1-2 mg/dose) or intravenous midazolam (0.02-0.04 mg/kg/dose) are effective in treating anxiety. Based on the patient's needs, a midazolam infusion can be started at 0.01 to 0.02 mg/kg/h for nonintubated patients and at 0.05 to 1 mg/kg/h for intubated patients. Pruritis is effectively treated with oral or intravenous diphenhydramine (1.25 mg/kg/dose up to 25-50 mg/dose) or with oral hydroxyzine (0.5 mg/kg/dose up to 25 mg/dose).

Burn patients also experience pain with procedures such as dressing changes. Background pain should be adequately controlled in order to have effective control of procedural pain. Procedure-related pain is controlled with additional boluses of opioids, benzodiazepines, and/or ketamine (0.5-2 mg/kg/dose).

As an adjunct to opioids, postoperative pain can be managed with regional anesthetic techniques. Choices of regional anesthesia for postoperative pain control in pediatric patients include epidural anesthesia via the caudal, lumbar, or thoracic approach and peripheral nerve blocks.[104]

While a case report of epidural anesthesia for a burned child is reported in the literature, there is limited data on the efficacy of this technique in pediatric burn patients.[105] Similarly, there is limited data on the use of peripheral nerve blocks for postoperative pain control in this population. A case report demonstrates the use of 2 continuous nerve blocks, axillary and sciatic, for postoperative pain control in a 3-year-old burned child.[106] Both continuous and single-shot fascia iliaca compartment blocks are efficacious in the treatment of donor site pain in the adult burn population.[107,108] A fascia iliaca compartment block is also shown to decrease pain from femur fractures in pediatric patients.[109] Therefore, this block may be beneficial in the pediatric burn population. While regional anesthesia techniques offer benefits for pain control, we typically do not use these techniques. For severe burns in the acute setting, it may be difficult to find sites for regional anesthesia that are free from burn injury. Additionally, regional techniques may not reliably provide analgesia during the many weeks in which excision and grafting procedures are performed. In the reconstructive phase, most operations are superficial plastic surgical procedures that do not require aggressive pain control postoperatively. Therefore, the benefits of regional anesthesia techniques may not outweigh the risks.

Another form of regional anesthesia is the intraoperative use of a dilute local anesthetic tumescent solution with epinephrine. In a prospective study of 30 children with less than 20% TBSA burn who received intraoperative dilute lidocaine tumescent solution, 80% did not require supplemental analgesics and 20% required only supplemental acetaminophen in the first 24 hours postoperatively.[110] It is essential to use dilute local anesthetics in the tumescent solution so that the total dose remains under the toxic dose limit of 7 to 10 mg/kg. Interestingly, systemic toxicity is less likely to occur in the burn population since the free fraction of local anesthetics is decreased due to increased levels of α1-glycoprotein.

Regardless of the agents and/or techniques used for pain control in pediatric burn patients, attention must be paid to the alterations in pharmacokinetics and pharmacodynamics. Specific examples of these alterations include tolerance to opioids and the decreased plasma free fraction of local anesthetics. Therefore, pain medications should be titrated to clinical effect.

## CONCLUSION

Pediatric burn patients provide significant challenges to the anesthesia provider. In order to provide safe and effective care for these patients, attention must be paid to the physiologic and pharmacologic changes that occur with burn injury. While attention to the technical details of airway management, fluid resuscitation, and temperature regulation are important, one must not overlook the importance of analgesia and patient comfort for these critically ill children. Following these principles will lead to a successful anesthetic.

## Acknowledgments

The authors wish to thank Nishan Goudsouzian, MD, Hemanth Baboolal, MD, and David Moss, MD, of the Department of Anesthesia and Critical Care, Massachusetts General Hospital, Boston, MA, USA, for their review of this chapter.

## TABLES

### TABLE 1
### Depth of burn injury.

| | |
|---|---|
| First Degree | Epidermis |
| Second Degree | |
| Superficial | Epidermis and superficial dermis |
| Deep | Epidermis and deep dermis |
| Third Degree | Epidermis and full-thickness dermis |
| Fourth Degree | Fascia, muscle, and bone |

TABLE 2
Definition of major burn injury.

Greater than 10% TBSA of third-degree burns
Greater than 25% TBSA of second-degree burns
Greater than 20% TBSA of second-degree burns in infants and neonates
Burn injuries involving the face, hands, feet, or perineum
Inhalational burn injuries
Chemical or electrical burns

TABLE 3
Pathophysiologic changes from burn injury.

|  | Early | Late |
|---|---|---|
| Cardiovascular | ↓ Cardiac output<br>↑ Systemic vascular resistance<br>Hypovolemia | ↑ Cardiac output<br>Tachycardia<br>Systemic hypertension |
| Pulmonary | Airway obstruction and edema<br>Carbon monoxide poisoning<br>Cyanide toxicity<br>Pulmonary edema | Chest wall restriction<br>Tracheal stenosis<br>Infection |
| Renal | ↓ Glomerular filtration rate<br>Myoglobinuria | ↑ Glomerular filtration rate<br>↑ Tubular dysfunction |
| Endocrine and Metabolic |  | ↑ Metabolic rate<br>↑ Core body temperature<br>↑ Muscle catabolism<br>↑ Lipolysis<br>↑ Glucolysis<br>↑ Futile substrate cycling<br>↑ Insulin resistance<br>↓ Thyroid hormones<br>↓ Vitamin D<br>↓ Parathyroid hormone |
| Hepatic | ↓ Perfusion<br>Hepatic apoptosis with ↑ AST, ALT, bilirubin<br>↑ Intrahepatic fat and edema | ↑ Perfusion<br>↑ Metabolism |
| Hematologic | Hemoconcentration<br>Hemolysis<br>Thrombocytopenia | Anemia |
| Gastrointestinal | ↓ Perfusion with mucosal damage<br>Endotoxinemia | Stress ulcers<br>Adynamic ileus<br>Acalculous cholecystitis |
| Neurologic | ↑ Cerebral edema<br>↑ Intracranial pressure | Hallucination<br>Personality change<br>Delirium<br>Seizure<br>Coma |

TABLE 4
**Preoperative NPO guidelines for pediatric patients accepted at MGH.**

| | |
|---|---|
| Clear liquids | 2 hours |
| Breast milk | 4 hours |
| Infant formula | 6 hours |
| Nonhuman milk | 6 hours |
| Light meal (crackers or dry toast) | 6 hours |
| Solids | 8 hours |

TABLE 5
**ASA standards for basic anesthetic monitoring for general anesthesia.**

| | |
|---|---|
| Oxygenation | Measurement of oxygen concentration in inspired gas<br>Quantitative measurement of blood oxygenation<br>Ability to assess patient color |
| Ventilation | Qualitative assessment by chest wall excursion or breath sounds<br>Quantitative assessment by expired carbon dioxide and volume of expired gas<br>Continual end-tidal carbon dioxide measurement by capnography, capnometry, or spectroscopy<br>System alarm to signal disconnection from mechanical ventilator |
| Circulation | Continuous electrocardiogram<br>Arterial blood pressure and heart rate determinations every 5 minutes<br>At least one of the following: palpation of pulse, auscultation of heart sounds, intra-arterial pulse tracing, ultrasound peripheral pulse monitoring, or pulse plethysmography or oximetry |
| Temperature | Monitoring of temperature for anticipated changes in body temperature |

TABLE 6
**Anatomical differences of the pediatric airway as compared to the adult airway.**

Relatively large head in comparison to body size

Relatively large tongue in comparison to other airway structures

Prominent tonsils and adenoids

Presence of deciduous teeth that can be loose

Narrow nasal passages

Larynx that lies higher in the neck—at the level of C3-C4 in infancy

Long, narrow, and angulated epiglottis in infancy

Vocal cords have a lower attachment anteriorly than posteriorly in infancy

Cricoid cartilage is the narrowest portion of airway in infancy

Short, narrow, and posteriorly angulated trachea in infancy

Narrow airway diameters

Relatively floppy pharyngeal muscles that are more sensitive to laryngospasm

TABLE 7
Suggested laryngoscope blades and endotracheal tube sizes for pediatric patients.

|  | Laryngoscope Blades | Endotracheal Tube Sizes |
|---|---|---|
| Premature and term neonate | Miller 0 | 2.5–3.0 |
| Neonate to 9 months | Miller 0–1 | 3.5 |
| 9 to 24 months | Miller 1, Wis-Hipple 1.5 | 4.0–4.5 |
| 2 to 5 years | Miller 1–1.5, Macintosh 1 | 4 + [Age(years) / 4] |
| 5 to 12 years | Miller 2, Macintosh 2 | 4 + [Age(years) / 4] |
| Adolescent to adult | Miller 2, Macintosh 3 | 7.0–7.5 |

TABLE 8
Induction doses for commonly used intravenous anesthetic agents.

| Ketamine | 1–2 mg/kg |
|---|---|
| Thiopental | 5–8 mg/kg |
| Propofol | 2.5–3.5 mg/kg |

TABLE 9
Prediction of blood loss during excision and grafting.

| TBSA > 30% | |
|---|---|
| 0–1 days postinjury | 0.41 mL blood loss/cm$^2$ excised |
| 2–16 days postinjury | 0.72 mL blood loss/cm$^2$ excised |
| > 16 days postinjury | 0.49 mL blood loss/cm$^2$ excised |
| TBSA < 30% | |
| Anytime postinjury | 1.2 mL blood loss/cm$^2$ excised |

TABLE 10
Doses for commonly used premedication agents.

| Midazolam | IV: 0.02-0.1 mg/kg<br>PO: 0.25-0.75 mg/kg |
|---|---|
| Fentanyl | IV: 1-4 mcg/kg |
| Ketamine | PO: 3-6 mg/kg<br>IM: 2-10 mg/kg |
| Clonidine | PO: 2-4 mcg/kg |

155

# REFERENCES

1. Shields BJ, Comstock D, Fernandez SA, Xiang H, Smith GA. Healthcare resource utilization and epidemiology of pediatric burn-associated hospitalizations, United States, 2000. *J Burn Care Res*. 2007; **28**(6): 811–826.

2. Stoelting RK, Diedorf SF. Diseases presenting in pediatric patients (burn injuries). In: Stoelting RK, Diedorf SF, eds. *Anesthesia and Co-Existing Disease*. 4th ed. New York: Churchill Livingston; 2002: 725–734.

3. Sun B-W, Zhou X-Q, Xia C-L, Chen Y-L. Management of severe burn injuries in neonates. *J Burn Care Rehabil*. 2004; **25**: 219–223.

4. Arturson G. Pathophysiology of the burn wound and pharmacological treatment. The Rudi Hermans Lecture, 1995. *Burns*. 1996; **22**(4): 255–274.

5. Jeschke MG, Barrow RE, Herndon DN. Extended hypermetabolic response of the liver in severely burned pediatric patients. *Arch Surg*. 2004; **139**: 641–647.

6. Jeschke MG, Mlcak RP, Finnerty CC, et al. Burn size determines the inflammatory and hypermetabolic response. *Crit Care*. 2007; **11**(4). DOI: 10.1186/cc6102.

7. Mlcak RP, Jeschke MG, Barrow RE, Herndon DN. The influence of age and gender on resting energy expenditure in severely burned children. *Ann Surg*. 2006; **244**(1): 121–130.

8. Monafo WW. Initial management of burns. *N Engl J Med*. 1996; **335**(21): 1581–1586.

9. Reynolds EM, Ryan DP, Sheridan RL, Doody DP. Left ventricular failure complicating severe pediatric burn injuries. *J Pediatr Surg*. 1995; **30**(2): 264–270.

10. Mlcak R, Cortiella J, Desai M, Herdon D. Lung compliance, airway resistance and work of breathing in children after inhalation injury. *J Burn Care Rehabil*. 1997; **18**(6): 531–534.

11. Irrazabal CL, Capdevila AA, Revich L, et al. Early and late complications among 15 victims exposed to indoor fire and smoke inhalation. *Burns*. 2008; **34**(4): 533–538.

12. Mlcak RP, Suman OE, Herdon DN. Respiratory management of inhalation injury. *Burns*. 2007; **33**: 2–13.

13. Cha SI, Kim CH, Lee JH, et al. Isolated smoke inhalation injuries: acute respiratory dysfunction, clinical outcomes, and short-term evolution of pulmonary functions with the effects of steroids. *Burns*. 2007; **33**: 200–208.

14. Kao LW, Nanagas KA. Carbon monoxide poisoning. *Med Clin North Am*. 2005; **89**: 1161–1194.

15. Geller RJ, Barthhold C, Saiers JA, Hall AH. Pediatric cyanide poisoning: causes, manifestations, management, and unmet needs. *Pediatrics*. 2006; **118**: 2146–2158.

16. Shepherd G, Velez LI. Role of hydoxocobalamin in acute cyanide poisoning. *Ann Pharmacother*. 2008; **42**: 661–669. DOI: 10.1345/aph.1K559.

17. Turnage RH, Nwariaku F, Murphy J, Schulman C, Wright K, Yin H. Mechanisms of pulmonary microvascular dysfunction during severe burn injury. *World J Surg*. 2002; **26**: 848–853.

18. Aikawa N, Wakabayashi G, Ueda M, Shinozawa Y. Regulation of renal function in thermal injury. *J Trauma*. 1990; **30**(12): S174–S178.

19. Herdon DN, Tompkins RG. Support of the metabolic response to burn injury. *Lancet*. 2004; **363**: 1895–1902.

20. Pereira CT, Murphy KD, Herdon DN. Altering metabolism. *J Burn Care Rehabil*. 2005; **26**(3): 194–199.

21. Pereira C, Murphy K, Jeschke M, Herndon DN. Post burn muscle wasting and the effects of treatments. *Int J Biochem Cell Biol*. 2005; **37**: 1948–1961.

22. Smith A, Barclay C, Quaba A, et al. The bigger the burn, the greater the stress. *Burns*. 1997; **23**(4): 291–294.

23. Hart DW, Wolf SE, Mlcak R, et al. Persistence of muscle catabolism after severe burn. *Surgery*. 2000; **128**: 312–319.

24. Pidcoke HF, Wade CE, Wolf SE. Insulin and the burned patient. *Crit Care Med*. 2007; **35**(9): S524–S530.

25. Thomas S, Wolf SE, Murphy KD, Chinker DL, Herndon DN. The long-term effect of oxandrolone on hepatic acute phase proteins in severely burned children. *J Trauma Inj Infect Crit Care*. 2004; **56**: 37–44.

26. Przkora R, Jeschke MG, Barrow RE, et al. Metabolic and hormonal changes of severely burned children receiving long-term oxandrolone treatment. *Ann Surg*. 2005; **242**(3): 384–391.

27. Jeschke MG, Finnerty CC, Suman OE, Kulp G, Mlcak RP, Herndon DN. The effect of oxandrolone on the endocrinologic, inflammatory, and hypermetabolic responses during the acute phase postburn. *Ann Surg*. 2007; **246**(3): 351–362.

28. Przkora R, Herndon DN, Suman OE. The effects of oxandrolone and exercise on muscle mass and function in children with severe burns. *Pediatrics*. 2007; **119**: e109–e116.

29. Jeschke M, Norbury WB, Finnerty CC, Branski LK, Herndon DN. Propranolol does not increase inflammation, sepsis, or infectious episodes in severely burned children. *J Trauma Inj Infect Crit Care*. 2007; **62**(3): 676–681.

30. Klein GL, Langman CB, Herndon DN. Vitamin D depletion following burning injury in children: a possible factor in post-burn osteopenia. *J Trauma Inj Infect Crit Care*. 2002; **52**: 346–350.

31. Gottschlich MM, Mayes T, Khoury J, Warden GD. Hypovitaminosis D in acutely injured pediatric burn patients. *J Am Diet Assoc*. 2004; **104**: 931–941.

32. Klein G, Langman CB, Herndon DN. Persistent hypoparathyroidism following magnesium repletion in burn-injured children. *Pediatr Nephrol*. 2000; **14**: 301–304.

33. Jeschke MG, Micak RP, Finnerty CC, Herndon DN. Changes in liver function and size after a severe thermal injury. *Shock*. 2007; **28**(2): 172–177.

34. Lawrence C, Atac B. Hematologic changes in massive burn injury. *Crit Care Med*. 1992; **20**(9): 1284–1288.

35. Venter M, Rode H, Sive A, Visser M. Enteral resuscitation and early enteral feeding in children with major burns—effect on McFarlane response to stress. *Burns*. 2007; **33**: 464–471.

**36.** Chen A, Wang S, Yu B, Li A. A comparison study between early enteral nutrition and parenteral nutrition in severe burn patients. *Burns.* 2007; **33:** 708–712.

**37.** Antoon AY, Volpe JJ, Crawford JD. Burn encephalopathy in children. *Pediatrics.* 1972; **50**(4): 609–616.

**38.** Rosenberg M, Robertson C, Murphy KD, et al. Neuropsychological outcomes of pediatric burn patients who sustained hypoxic episodes. *Burns.* 2005; **31:** 883–889.

**39.** Gueugniaud PY, Jauffray M, Bertin-Maghit M, et al. Cerebral oedema after extensive thermal injury: prognostic significance of early intracranial and cerebral perfusion pressures. *Ann Burns Fire Disasters.* 1997; **10**(2): 72.

**40.** Popp MB, Friedberg DL, MacMillan BG. Clinical characteristics of hypertension in burned children. *Ann Surg.* 1980; **191**(4): 473–478.

**41.** Mukhdomi GJ, Desai MH, Herndon DN. Seizure disorders in burned children: a retrospective review. *Burns.* 1996; **22**(4): 316–319.

**42.** Ko SH, Chun W, Kim HC. Delayed spinal cord injury following electrical burns: a 7-year experience. *Burns.* 2004; **30:** 691–695.

**43.** Arevalo JM, Lorente JA, Balseiro-Gomez J. Spinal cord injury after electrical trauma treated in a burn unit. *Burns.* 1999; **25:** 449–552.

**44.** Scholz T, Rippmann V, Wojtecki L, Perbix W, Rothschild MA, Spilker G. Severe brain damage by current flow after electrical burn injury. *J Burn Care Res.* 2006; **27:** 917–922.

**45.** Jaehde U, Sorqel F. Clinical pharmacokinetics in patients with burns. *Clin Pharmacokinet.* 1995; **29**(1): 15–28.

**46.** Martyn JA, Fukushima Y, Chon J-Y, Yang HS. Muscle relaxants in burns, trauma, and critical illness. *Int Anesthesiol Clin.* 2006; **44**(2): 123–143.

**47.** Cote CJ, Lugo RA, Ward RM. Pharmacokinetics and pharmacology of drugs in children. In: Cote CJ, Todres DI, Goudsouzian NG, Ryan JF, eds. *A Practice of Anesthesia in Infants and Children.* Philadelphia, PA: Saunders; 2001 :121–171.

**48.** Martyn JA. Clinical pharmacology and drug therapy in the burned patient. *Anesthesiology.* 1986; **65:** 67–75.

**49.** Cote CJ, Petkau AJ. Thiopental requirements may be increased in children reanesthetized at least one year after recovery from extensive thermal injury. *Anesth Analogues.* 1985; **64**(12): 1156–1160.

**50.** Martyn JA, Richtsfeld M. Succinylcholine-induced hyperkalemia in acquired and pathologic states. *Anesthesiology.* 2006; **104:** 158–169.

**51.** Uyar M, Epaguslar E, Ugur G, Balcioglu T. Resistance to vecuronium in burned children. *Pediatr Anesth.* 1999; **9:** 115–118.

**52.** Han TH, Kim HS, Bae JY, Kim KM, Martyn JA. Neuromuscular pharmacodynamics of rocuronium in patients with major burns. *Anesth Analogues.* 2004; **99:** 386–392.

**53.** Weinbren MJ. Pharmacokinetics of antibiotics in burn patients. *J Antimicrob Chemother.* 1999; **44:** 319–327.

**54.** Hoey LL, Tschida SJ, Rotschafer JC, Guay DRP, Vance-Bryan K. Wide variation in single, daily dose aminoglycoside pharmacokinetics in patients with burn injuries. *J Burn Care Rehabil.* 1997; **18**(2): 116–124.

**55.** Dailly E, Pannier M, Jolliet P, Bourin M. Population pharmacokinetics of ceftazidime in burn patients. *Br J Clin Pharmacol.* 2003; **56:** 629–634.

**56.** Dalley AJ, Lipman J, Venkatesh B, Rudd M, Roberts MS, Cross SE. Inadequate antimicrobial prophylaxis during surgery: a study of β-lactams levels during burn debridement. *J Antimicrob Chemother.* 2007; **60:** 166–169.

**57.** Dailly E, Kergueris MF, Pannier M, Jolliet P, Bourin M. Population pharmacokinetics of imipenem in burn patients. *Fundam Clin Pharmacol.* 2003; **17:** 645–650.

**58.** Kiser TH, Hoody DW, Obritsch MD, Wegzyn CO, Bauling PC, Fish DN. Levofloxacin pharmacokinetics and pharmacodynamics in patients with severe burn injury. *Amtimicrob Agents Chemother.* 2006; **50**(6): 1937–1945.

**59.** Furman WR, Munster AM, Cone EJ. Morphine pharmacokinetics during anesthesia and surgery in patients with burns. *J Burn Care Rehabil.* 1990; **11**(5): 391–394.

**60.** Herman RA, Veng-Pedersen P, Miotto J, Komorowski J, Kealey GP. Pharmacokinetics of morphine sulfate in patients with burns. *J Burn Care Rehabil.* 1994; **15**(2): 95–103.

**61.** Perreault S, Choiniere M, duSouich PB, Bellavance F, Beauregard G. Pharmacokinetics of morphine and its glucuronidated metabolites in burn injuries. *Ann Pharmacother.* 2001; **35:** 1588–1592.

**62.** Han T, Harmatz JS, Greenblatt DJ, Martyn JA. Fentanyl clearance and volume of distribution are increased in patients with major burns. *J Clin Pharmacol.* 2007; **47:** 674–680.

**63.** Martyn JA. Ketamine pharmacology and therapeutics. *J Burn Care Rehabil.* 1987; **8**(2): 146–148.

**64.** Humphries Y, Melson M, Gore D. Superiority of oral ketamine as an analgesic and sedative for wound care procedures in the pediatric patient with burns. *J Burn Care Rehabil.* 1997; **18**(1): 34–36.

**65.** Owens VF, Palmieri TL, Comroe CM, Conroy JM, Scavone JA, Greenhalgh DG. Ketamine: a safe and effective agent for painful procedures in the pediatric burn patient. *J Burn Res.* 2006; **27:** 211–216.

**66.** White MC, Karsli C. Long-term use of an intravenous ketamine infusion in a child with significant burns. *Pediatr Anesth.* 2007; **17:** 1102–1104.

**67.** Pal SK, Cortiella J, Herndon D. Adjunctive methods of pain control in burns. *Burns.* 1997; **23**(5): 404–412.

**68.** Kariya N, Shindoh M, Nishi S, Yukioka H, Asada A. Oral clonidine for sedation and analgesia in a burn patient. *J Clin Anesth.* 1998; **10:** 514–517.

**69.** Lyons B, Casey W, Doherty P, McHugh M, Moore KP. Pain relief with low-dose intravenous clonidine in a child with severe burns. *Intensive Care Med.* 1996; **22**(3): 249–251.

70. Walker J, MacCallum M, Fischer C, Kopcha R, Saylors R, McCall J. Sedation using dexmedetomidine in pediatric burn patients. *J Burn Care Res.* 2006; **27**(2): 206–210.

71. Martyn JA, Greenblatt DJ, Quinby WC. Diazepam kinetics in patients with severe burns. *Anesth Analg.* 1983; **62**: 293–297.

72. Martyn JA, Greenblatt DJ. Lorazepam conjugation is unimpaired in burn trauma. *Clin Pharmacol Ther.* 1988; **43**(3) :250–255.

73. Sheridan RL, McEttrick M, Bacha G, Stoddard F, Tompkin RG. Midazolam infusion in pediatric patients with burns who are undergoing mechanical ventilation. *J Burn Care Rehabil.* 1994; **15**: 515–518.

74. Beushausen T, Mucke K. Anesthesia management in pediatric burn patients. *Pediatr Surg Int.* 1997; **12**: 327–333.

75. MacLennan N, Heimback DM, Cullen BF. Anesthesia for major thermal injury. *Anesthesiology.* 1998; **89**(3): 749–770.

76. Pearson KS, Furman WR. Anesthesia for patients with major burns. In: Longnecker DE, Tinker JH, Morgan GE, eds. *Principles and Practice of Anesthesiology.* St. Louis, MO: Mosby Year-Book; 1998: 2165–2180.

77. Szyfelbein SK, Martyn JA, Sheridan RL, Cote CJ. Anesthesia for children with burn injuries. In: Cote CJ, Todres DI, Goudsouzian NG, Ryan JF, eds. *A Practice of Anesthesia in Infants and Children.* Philadelphia, PA: Saunders; 2001: 522–543.

78. Hu OY-P, Ho S-T, Wang J-J, Ho W, Wang H-J, Lin C-Y. Evaluation of gastric emptying in severe, burn-injured patients. *Crit Care Med.* 1993; **21**(4): 527–531.

79. Hildreth MA, Herndon DN, Desai MH, Broemeling LD. Caloric requirements of patients with burns under one year of age. *J Burn Care Rehabil.* 1993; **14**(1): 108–112.

80. Fisher C, Jenkins M, Gottschlich M. Perioperative enteral nutrition in the pediatric burn patient. *Anesthesiology.* 1995;83:A1164.

81. Reid M, Shaw P, Taylor RH. Oesophageal ECG in a child for burns surgery. *Paediatr Anaesth.* 1997; **7**(1): 73–76.

82. Pal SK, Kyriacou PA, Kumaran S, et al. Evaluation of oesophageal reflectance pulse oximetry in major burns patients. *Burns.* 2005; **31**: 337–341.

83. Kyriacou PA. Pulse oximetry in the oesophagus. *Physiol Meas.* 2006; **27**: R1–R35.

84. Cote CJ, Daniels AL, Connolly M, Szyfelbein SK, Wickens CD. Tongue oximetry in children with extensive thermal injury: comparison with peripheral oximetry. *Can J Anaesth.* 1992; **39**(5, pt 1): 454–457.

85. Evans RJ, Jewkes F, Owen G, McCabe M, Palmer D. Intraosseous infusion—a technique available for intravascular administration of drugs and fluids in the child with burns. *Burns.* 1995; **21**(7): 552–553.

86. Hurren JS, Dunn KW. Intraosseous infusions for burns resuscitation. *Burns.* 1995; **21**(4): 285–287.

87. Wheeler M, Cote CJ, Todres D. Pediatric airway. In: Cote CJ, Todres DI, Goudsouzian NG, Ryan JF, eds. *A Practice of Anesthesia in Infants and Children.* Philadelphia, PA: Saunders; 2001: 79–120.

88. Sheridon RL. Uncuffed endotracheal tubes should not be used in seriously burned children. *Pediatric Crit Care Med.* 2006; **7**(3): 258–259.

89. Palmieri TL, Jackson W, Greenhalgh DG. Benefits of early tracheostomy in severely burned children. *Crit Care Med.* 2002; **30**: 922–924.

90. Desai MH, Herndon DN, Broemeling L, Barrow RE, Nichols RJ, Rutan RL. Early burn wound excision significantly reduces blood loss. *Ann Surg.* 1990; **211**(6): 753–759.

91. Losee JE, Fox I, Hua LB, Cladis FP, Serletti JM. Transfusion-free pediatric burn surgery. *Ann Plast Surg.* 2005; **54**(2): 165–171.

92. Gilliland MD, Coates N. Tumescent liposuction complicated by pulmonary edema. *Plast Reconstr Surg.* 1997; **99**: 215–219.

93. Prelack K, Dwyer J, Sheridan R, et al. Body water in children during recovery from severe burn injury using a combined tracer dilution method. *J Burn Care Rehabil.* 2005; **26**: 67–74.

94. Crabtree JH, Bowser BH, Campbell JW, Gulnee WS, Caldwell FT. Energy metabolism in anesthetized children with burns. *Am J Surg.* 1980; **140**: 832–835.

95. Chinyanga HM. Temperature regulation and anesthesia. *Pharmacol Ther.* 1984; **26**(2): 147–161.

96. Khan RM, Verma V, Bhradwaj A, et al. Difficult laryngeal mask airway placement in a pediatric-burned patient: a new solution to an old problem. *Pediatr Anesth.* 2006; **16**: 360–361.

97. Kumar R, Prashast, Wadhwa A, Akhtar S. The upside-down intubating laryngeal mask airway: a technique for cases of fixed flexed neck deformity. *Anesth Analogues.* 2002; **95**: 1454–1458.

98. Kreulen M, Mackie DP, Kreis RW, Groenevelt F. Surgical release for intubation purposes in postburn contractures of the neck. *Burns.* 1996; **22**(4): 310–312.

99. Sheridan RL, Ryan DP, Fuzaylov G, Nimkin K, Martyn JA. An 18-month-old girl with an advanced neck contracture after a burn. *N Engl J Med.* 2008; **358**: 729–735.

100. Kayaalp L, Bozkurt P, Odabasi G, et al. Psychological effects of repeated general anesthesia in children. *Pediatr Anesth.* 2006; **16**: 822–827.

101. Ratcliff SL, Brown A, Rosenberg L, et al. The effectiveness of a pain and anxiety protocol to treat the acute pediatric burn patient. *Burns.* 2006; **32**: 554–562.

102. Sheridan R, Stoddard F, Querzoli E. Management of background pain and anxiety in critically burned children requiring protracted mechanical ventilation. *J Burn Care Rehabil.* 2001; **22**(2): 150–153.

103. Meyer WJ, Nichols RJ, Cortiella J, et al. Acetaminophen in the management of background pain in children post-burn. *J Pain Symptom Manage.* 1997; **13**(1): 50–55.

104. Polaner DM, Suresh S, Cote CJ. Pediatric regional anesthesia. In: Cote CJ, Todres DI, Goudsouzian NG, Ryan JF, eds.

*A Practice of Anesthesia in Infants and Children.* Philadelphia, PA: Saunders; 2001: 636–674.

**105.** Teixidor AP, Mabrok MM, Valls MJ, Garcia MV. Anesthesia and lumbar epidural anesthesia in an infant with third-degree burns. *Rev Esp Anestesiol Reanim.* 1989; **36**(5): 288–290.

**106.** Dadure C, Acosta C, Capdevila X. Perioperative pain management of a complex orthopedic surgical procedure with double continuous nerve blocks in a burned child. *Anesth Analogues.* 2004; **98**: 1653–1655.

**107.** Cuignet O, Pirson J, Boughrough J, Duville D. The efficacy of continuous fascia iliaca compartment blocks for pain management in burn patients undergoing skin grafting procedures. *Anesth Analogues.* 2004; **98**: 1077–1081.

**108.** Cuignet O, Mbuyamba J, Pirson J. The long-term analgesic efficacy of a single-shot iliaca compartment block in burn patients undergoing skin-grafting procedures. *J Burn Care Rehabil.* 2005; **26**: 409–415.

**109.** Wathen JE, Gao D, Merritt G, Georgopoulos G, Battan FK. A randomized controlled trial comparing a fascia iliaca compartment nerve block to a traditional systemic analgesic for femur fractures in a pediatric emergency department. *Ann Emerg Med.* 2007; **50**: 162–171.

**110.** Bussolin L, Busoni P, Giorgi L, Crescioli M, Messeri A. Tumescent local anesthesia for the surgical treatments of burns and postburn sequelae in pediatric patients. *Anesthesiology.* 2003; **99**: 1371–1375.

# CHAPTER ELEVEN

# ACUTE BURN EXCISION

ROB SHERIDAN, MD,
BURN SURGERY SERVICE, SHRINERS HOSPITAL FOR CHILDREN, BOSTON, MA

## ACUTE BURN EXCISION

At the heart of the past few decades' revolution in burn care is early excision and biologic closure of deep burn wounds.[1] Historically, deep burns were allowed to liquefy and separate over a period of weeks, leaving granulating wounds that might be autografted in those who survived the accompanying systemic infection and inflammation. In the 1970s and 1980s, the concept of early excision of deep burns prior to the development of local and systemic infection evolved due to the hard work of a number of important clinician-investigators caring for burn patients. The techniques have subsequently matured, but we owe these earlier pioneers a great debt of gratitude, as do our current patients.

## THE OPERATING ROOM ENVIRONMENT

Excision and biologic closure of burn wounds is conceptually simple but can be quite hazardous to patients if not prudently practiced. The operating room environment is a critical consideration.[2] This begins with transport to and from the operating room, which must be carefully planned and attended by experienced personnel.[3] Particular attention is required to avoid dislodgement of airway and vascular access devices. In order to maintain the child's body temperature, a careful but brisk transport is optimal to minimize the

complications associated with disruption of access devices and hypothermia.

The operating room environment must be carefully controlled, particularly with regards to heating capability if operations of any magnitude are to be successfully performed in critically injured children with large burns. Intraoperative hypothermia leads to acidosis, poor peripheral perfusion, and coagulopathy.[4] If the operating room can be adequately heated, this complication should essentially never occur. In addition, all intravenous and topical fluids should be warmed. Operating room personnel should become accustomed to any discomfort associated with extreme operating room temperatures.

Constant, respectful communication between surgical, nursing, and anesthesia personnel is essential[5] in order to ensure the child's critical care proceeds smoothly throughout the operation. Anesthesia should be familiar with the operative plan so fluid and blood needs can be planned accordingly. The level of stimulation changes substantially during burn cases, increasing rapidly during donor skin procurement. This, as well as the possibility of substantial blood loss, should be anticipated by the anesthesia team. The surgeon should frequently inform those assisting with the operation of current and future events as well.

Burn operations often require relative extremes of positioning, as no surface is immune to thermal injury. In addition to added heating circuits, burn operating rooms are ideally equipped with positioning aids such as overhead suspension systems. A number of devices, such as an overheat track system, are available and can substantially reduce operative time.

## WOUND EVALUATION

Appropriate intraoperative decisions regarding burn excision assume an ability to accurately determine burn depth, or more importantly, to determine the likelihood that a burn will heal.[6] In general, only burns of deep second-degree or deeper are excised and grafted. As superficial second-degree burns will heal in most patients within 3 weeks, they are for the most part left alone (sometimes assisted with topical agents or membrane dressings). Superficial second-degree burns tend to be moist and painful. Deep second-degree and third-degree burns tend to be leathery, dry, insensate, depressed, and waxy or leathery. Fourth-degree burns involve subcutaneous tissue, tendon, or bone and can have a charred appearance. It can sometimes be difficult, even for an experienced examiner, to accurately determine burn depth on initial examination. As a general rule, burns are often underestimated in depth initially.[7]

In the operating room, a very light pass with a hand-held dermatome over a representative area can give useful guidance, with viable superficial dermis identified by fine capillary bleeding. Many investigators have attempted to develop tools to assist the surgeon in determining which areas will not heal and will require excision. Unfortunately, none have met with wide success. Therefore, the eye of an experienced examiner remains the standard of burn-depth evaluation and provides the most reliable basis for operative decision making. In situations of mixed-depth injury, time spent in thoughtful planning before the initial excision will speed overall operative time and reduce intraoperative physiologic stress to the patient.

## DETERMINATION OF NEED AND TIMING OF OPERATION

Injuries vary in the physiologic threat they present to an injured child, and this is the principal consideration when deciding upon the need for and timing of operative intervention. In otherwise healthy children, the physiologic threat presented by the injury is primarily a function of injury size more than depth.[8] Children with deep dermal or full-thickness burns involving more than perhaps 20% of the body surface are at risk for the rapid development of wound infection and subsequently systemic infection, which is best avoided by early excision.

When children have large burns of indeterminate depth, it is often prudent to excise those areas that appear deep, acknowledging that subsequent excision may be required. In such cases, when it is unclear whether a substantial amount of wound will need excision and grafting, the operating room provides an optimal environment in which to assess wound depth.

Quite often, children will present with small indeterminate-depth wounds, most often from scalding injuries. Initially, many are best managed nonoperatively while wounds evolve and depth becomes more clear.[9] Generally, wounds are ideally left alone if capable of healing in less than 3 weeks since they are unlikely to become hypertrophic. A common approach to these small mixed-depth wounds is to treat them with topical therapy for approximately 3 to 5 days. During this period, wound depth becomes apparent, and it is usually quite clear which, if any, components of the wound need to be excised and grafted. Often, this can be accomplished in the outpatient setting. In this way, all grafts, donor sites, and second-degree burns can be healed within 3 weeks. Children with small but obviously full-thickness burns, commonly from contact injuries, are best served by early operative intervention.

Children with large mixed-depth burns greater than 20% of the body surface often benefit from a more aggressive surgical approach, as the injury size alone presents a physiological threat. Ideally, full-thickness components are excised and closed before wound colonization and systemic inflammation occur. The operative goal is to identify, excise, and close all full-thickness components. In those with very large burns, perhaps greater than 40%, this may require serial operations. In these children, temporary biologic closure can be achieved with human allograft, Integra®, or other temporary membranes. These wounds can subsequently be definitively closed with autograft when donor sites have healed or patients are more stable.

The definition of "early" in "early excision" is often debated. Most would probably agree that "early" is prior to the occurrence of local infection and systemic inflammation. Many practitioners define "early" as within 1 to 7 days after injury. The primary advantage of waiting toward the end of this window is that burn wounds have evolved to the point that intraoperative decision making is easier since burn depth is clearer and the level of viable excision is more reliably appreciated. However, in the hands of experienced practitioners, where children are well monitored and supported, excision and closure within hours of injury can be safely and effectively performed.[10]

A final, relatively common issue is the child who presents with a smaller injury complicated by localized wound sepsis. The important decision in this situation is whether excision is needed to facilitate control of infection. This is generally advisable with full-thickness burns. If burns are partial thickness, most cases of simple cellulitis can be effectively treated with topical antimicrobials and systemic antibiotics.[11]

## TECHNIQUES OF BURN WOUND EXCISION

Superficial wounds deemed likely to heal should not be excised. They need only be cleansed and treated with topical medications or temporary biologic dressings to prevent desiccation and minimize superinfection. Scattered reports have advocated very superficial excisions of such wounds, but there are no data that convincingly support this potentially morbid and expensive practice. Although topical proteolytic enzymes may have a limited role in superficial injuries, it is unclear if this practice improves on the results obtained by supportive care only.

After initial decompression is assured via escharotomy and/or fasciotomy, acute burns are generally addressed operatively in 1 of 5 ways, which vary with the depth of the wounds and the clinical status of the patient. These include sharp debridement of loose devitalized tissue, layered deep dermal excision, layered excision to viable subcutaneous fat, fascial excision, or subfascial excision.

Layered excision to viable deep dermis is a proper approach to deep second-degree burns which are unlikely to heal in less than 3 weeks. Although they may eventually heal, such wounds frequently become very hypertrophic and pruritic, particularly where skin is thin and has few appendages, such as the upper inner thigh or arm. If too superficial a burn is managed by mid-dermal excision followed by sheet grafting, bothersome sub-graft cyst formation commonly occurs as viable skin appendages lose their natural drainage. Dermal excisions are best reserved for those situations where it is evident that the bulk of the dermis is not viable. Layered deep dermal excisions can be done with hand-held dermatomes or with dermatomes powered by electricity or compressed nitrogen. Deep dermal excisions can be associated with substantial capillary bleeding, so it is important to use techniques to minimize blood loss, including subeschar dilute epinephrine clysis and exsanguination with proximal tourniquet inflation on extremities.[12] Perhaps the most useful technique is careful planning, including delineation of surgical margins, followed by swift excision.

Layered excision to viable subcutaneous fat is a useful technique in full-thickness cutaneous burns. When successfully applied, this method normalizes subsequent contour, appearance, and function. There is less bleeding than in deep

dermal excision because of reduced capillary density. The conventional wisdom that fat accepts grafts less reliably is probably not true. Rather, it may be more difficult to appreciate the viability of fat, and the bed tolerates desiccation poorly because of the reduced capillary density. Careful evaluation of the wound bed while minimizing open interstices results in reliably good graft take in most situations. These excisions can also be done with hand-held or powered dermatomes. Coverage of a well-excised subcutaneous bed with sheet grafts or minimally expanded meshed grafts usually produces excellent results. It is essential that grafts conform to the many small irregularities in beds of subcutaneous fat and that fat is not left exposed to desiccate. Widely meshed grafts do poorly on beds of subcutaneous fat.

Fascial excisions are not often required, having been more commonly done in the early years of acute excisional burn surgery. However, they are indicated if burns involve subcutaneous fat. Some patients with massive full-thickness burns seem best served with fascial excisions to minimize the chance of autograft loss on beds of subcutaneous fat. Also, some fragile elderly patients may be candidates for fascial excision as this technique minimizes blood loss and provides a highly reliable bed for autograft coverage. The disadvantage of major contour deformity must be considered. Fascial excision seems best performed with traction and coagulating electrocautery, which provides excellent hemostasis and a well-defined wound bed. The electrocautery plume can be substantial but can be minimized with high-efficiency suction devices, many of which are incorporated into the electrocautery hand-piece.

Subfascial excision of devitalized deep tissue is required in high-voltage injury, soft-tissue trauma, or occasionally in very deep thermal burns. Muscle compartments can be explored through standard fasciotomy incisions, allowing simultaneous decompression and debridement. Vacuum-assisted closure devices can be useful in preparing such wounds for grafting. Local or distant flaps may be used in other wounds. Definitive closure of such complex wounds can be difficult, and closure should be addressed on a case-by-case basis.

Throughout the operative event, the patient's condition should be continuously monitored and evaluated. Constant communication between the surgical and anesthetic teams is required to maintain optimal physiologic stability in acute burn operations of the magnitude done today. In particular, hypothermia must be anticipated and prevented, as loss of temperature control risks coagulopathy and instability that will compromise the operative event. This is best achieved by heating the operating room, as the degree of patient exposure needed often renders other devices to maintain temperature ineffective.

## TECHNIQUES TO MINIMIZE BLOOD LOSS

Acute burn excisions have a reputation for creating substantial blood loss, largely secondary to use of bleeding as the primary indicator of wound bed viability during excision. Estimates in the range of 3.5% to 5% of the blood volume for every 1% of the body surface excised have been published.[13] Other ways to determine viability of the bed during wound excision include bright, moist, yellow fat patent small blood vessels, absence of thrombosis of small vessels, and lack of extravascular hemoglobin staining. Accurate identification of tissue viability without the presence of free bleeding is an acquired skill that is difficult to master or maintain if these operations are not performed on a regular basis.

Intraoperative bleeding can be substantially reduced by planning careful excision prior to incision, use of proximal pneumatic tourniquets for extremity excisions, use of subeschar dilute epinephrine clysis for torso and head excisions, use of coagulating electrocautery for fascial excision, and maintaining intraoperative normothermia.[14] Further, less blood loss occurs when layered excisions are briskly performed in the first days following injury, when wounds are less hyperemic. Moreover, clear planning of excision margins using a variety of hand-held, gas-powered, or electric dermatomes can also facilitate the procedure. Fascial excisions using traction and coagulating electrocautery result in less blood loss. Maintenance of patient normothermia during large-burn operations may require operating room temperatures of 90°F to 120°F.

## GRAFT STABILIZATION AND CARE

Although methods of graft stabilization vary, all need to eliminate shear between grafts and underlying wounds, prevent desiccation and colonization of interstices, and minimize blood and serous collections beneath grafts. Ideally, postoperative dressings minimize the degree to which patients must be immobilized after surgery, allowing physical therapy and rehabilitation to continue as much as possible. Even though some of these techniques are time-consuming, it is time well spent if graft take is improved and postoperative immobility is minimized.

On most extremities, simple but very carefully applied gauze wraps which avoid causing distal ischemia suffice. On the anterior torso, moderately tightly stretched mesh can be secured over grafts, resulting in excellent fixation and minimal bulk. On the posterior torso, grafts can be stabilized with multi-ply layered gauze secured to the underlying soft tissues. This technique is suitable for extensive meshed grafts and also allows application of topical

agents.[15] Furthermore, prone positioning is not required and therapy can continue immediately after surgery. Standard tie-over dressings are suitable for small grafts in a wide variety of locations. Ideally, nonabsorbable sutures and staples are used judiciously, as removal can be time-consuming and painful. Carefully constructed and applied operative dressings as well as judicious use of tissue glues are excellent substitutes which minimize the need for these devices.

## DONOR SITE MANAGEMENT

Donor sites can be dressed by open or closed techniques. Open techniques include any nonocclusive dressing, such as fine-mesh gauze or Vaseline-impregnated dressings. Open management is forgiving of donor site colonization and fluid collections. The major disadvantage is the significant and predictable discomfort that occurs for the first few days until the dressing dries and forms a scablike barrier over the wound. Closed techniques include a wide variety of occlusive membranes and hydrocolloid dressings. The major advantage of this style of donor site management is a significant reduction in pain when they perform as hoped. The primary disadvantage is a relative inability to tolerate fluid collections and wound colonization. When this occurs, commonly in larger and posterior donors, membranes often need to be unroofed or removed, which itself can be unpleasant and uncomfortable.

In posterior and/or large donor sites, open donor site management seems more practical, anticipating and pharmacologically treating the predictable pain with techniques such as injection of long-acting anesthetics prior to emergence from anesthesia. For small anterior donor sites, closed management can be quite successful. Scalp donor sites in young children should be harvested relatively thin to minimize donor alopecia and transplantation of scalp hair.

## CONCLUSION

Most of the progress in burn care over the past 30 years has been a direct result of advances in the operative approach to acute burn wounds. Important adjuncts have included advances in blood banking and anesthetic techniques, but the core change has been early identification and excision of deep wounds prior to the development of sepsis and systemic inflammation. These operations, however, can be physiologically stressful to the point where more harm than good can occur unless careful planning and meticulous technique are diligently practiced. When we approach acute burn excisions with such care and consideration, our patients accrue major benefits.

## REFERENCES

**1.** Sheridan RL. Burn care: results of technical and organizational progress. *JAMA Contemp Update*. 2003; **290**(6): 719–722.

**2.** Sheridan RL. Comprehensive management of burns. *Curr Probl Surg*. 2001; **38**(9): 641–756.

**3.** Beckmann U, Gillies DM, Berenholtz SM, Wu AW, Pronovost P. Incidents relating to the intra-hospital transfer of critically ill patients. An analysis of the reports submitted to the Australian Incident Monitoring Study in Intensive Care. *Intensive Care Med*. 2004; **30**(8): 1579–1585.

**4.** Inaba K, Teixeira PG, Rhee P, et al. Mortality impact of hypothermia after cavitary explorations in trauma. *World J Surg*. 2009; **33**(4): 864–869.

**5.** Elks KN, Riley RH. A survey of anaesthetists' perspectives of communication in the operating suite. *Anaesth Intensive Care*. 2009; **37**(1): 108–111.

**6.** Heimbach D, Engrav L, Grube B, Marvin J. Burn depth: a review. *World J Surg*. 1992; **16**: 10–15.

**7.** Sheridan RL. Evaluating and managing burn wounds. *Dermatol Nurs*. 2000; **12**(1): 17–31.

**8.** Klein GL, Herndon DN. Burns. *Pediatr Rev*. 2004; **25**(12): 411–417.

**9.** Desai MH, Rutan RL, Herndon DN. Conservative treatment of scald burns is superior to early excision. *J Burn Care Rehabil*. 1991; **12**(5): 482–484.

**10.** Barret JP, Herndon DN. Modulation of inflammatory and catabolic responses in severely burned children by early burn wound excision in the first 24 hours. *Arch Surg*. 2003; **138**(2): 127–132.

**11.** Sheridan RL. Sepsis in pediatric burn patients. *Pediatr Crit Care Med*. 2005; **6**(3): S112–S119.

**12.** Sheridan RL, Szyfelbein SK. Staged high-dose epinephrine clysis is safe and effective in extensive tangential burn excisions in children. *Burns*. 1999; **25**: 745–748.

**13.** Housinger TA, Lang D, Warden GD. A prospective study of blood loss with excisional therapy in pediatric burn patients. *J Trauma*. 1993; **34**: 262–263.

**14.** White CE, Renz EM. Advances in surgical care: management of severe burn injury. *Crit Care Med*. 2008; **36**(7)(suppl): S318–S324.

**15.** Sheridan RL, Behringer GE, Ryan CM, et al. Effective postoperative protection for grafted posterior surfaces: the quilted dressing. *J Burn Care Rehabil*. 1995; **16**: 607–609.

# CHAPTER TWELVE

# BLOOD TRANSFUSION IN CHILDREN WITH BURN INJURY

TINA L. PALMIERI, MD, FACS, FCCM, SHRINERS HOSPITAL FOR CHILDREN, NORTHERN CALIFORNIA, AND THE UNIVERSITY OF CALIFORNIA DAVIS, SACRAMENTO, CA

## INTRODUCTION

Anemia is a common occurrence in critically ill patients, with approximately 25% receiving a blood transfusion.[1] Anemia is also frequent after major burn injury, which results in prolonged critical illness and hospitalization. Postburn hemolysis, surgical blood loss, the hypermetabolic state, sepsis, and decreased red cell production all contribute to postburn anemia. Children with major burn injury are no exception; approximately 25% of these children receive a blood transfusion.[2] Because every transfusion is associated with both risks and benefits, it is important to understand the history, salutary effects, and risks of transfusion for both adults and children with burns. Knowledge of the physiologic and anatomic differences between children and adults with respect to response to injury will help guide the decision-making process regarding blood transfusion. The goal of this chapter is to provide the burn practitioner with a fundamental knowledge base for transfusion in burned children based on patient physiology and blood product characteristics.

## HISTORY OF BLOOD TRANSFUSION

Many of our current transfusion practices are rooted in the historical development of blood transfusion as a therapeutic modality. Appreciation of the implications of this procedure requires a thorough understanding of how current blood transfusion practices were developed. Although the technique is relatively simple, the use of blood transfusion in clinical practice has been widely employed for less than 100 years.[3] Blood-letting as a therapeutic modality can be traced back to Hippocrates in 430 BC; however, the infusion of blood was delayed for several reasons. First, both the Romans and Greeks held to the humoral theory, which maintained that all living beings consisted of the balance of 4 elements: black bile, blood, phlegm, and yellow bile.[4] Illness was due to an imbalance of these elements, which could be corrected with proper diet and environmental alterations. Second, the physiology of circulation, which is the crux of transfusion medicine, needed to be recognized. Blood circulation physiology was first reported by William Harvey in 1628. This laid the groundwork for further advances in transfusion therapy.

The first blood transfusion experiments were conducted in the 1650s by members of the Oxford Experimental Philosophy Club, which consisted of such preeminent scientists as Robert Boyle, Thomas Willis, Christopher Wren, and Robert Hook. Wren demonstrated that substances injected intravenously could yield systemic effects. In 1666, Richard Lower successfully transfused blood from one dog to another venisected dog. Jean Denis, professor of philosophy and mathematics at Montpellier in France, began the practice of transfusion of blood from calves and lambs into humans, usually for the treatment of mental disorders.[5] Although this became popularized in Europe, others were not successful with interspecies blood transfusion in humans. Subsequently, blood transfusion fell into disfavor by the end of the century due to its high mortality rate.

The pioneer of modern blood transfusion therapy is James Blundell (1790–1878), an obstetrician at Gary's and St Thomas' hospitals in London.[6] Dr Blundell is credited with identifying 2 key concepts: (1) blood transfusion needs to occur between 2 members within the same species, and (2) blood transfusion requires specialized and appropriate medical equipment. Before applying these principles in people, Dr Blundell demonstrated through multiple canine experiments that intraspecies (ie, dog to dog) transfusion could be successful. He also demonstrated that interspecies (human to dog) transfusion was not feasible, a great accomplishment given that the concept of antibodies had not yet been introduced. Dr Blundell reported 10 successful human-to-human blood transfusions, primarily in postpartum hemorrhage, between 1818 and 1829.[7] He published these findings in the *Lancet* and retired 5 years later.[8] However, the adoption of this concept was slow, and by 1849 only 44 individuals had received blood transfusions.

The consistent success of blood transfusion in humans required further elucidation of the A, B, O, and ABO blood groups. Karl Landsteiner (1868–1943), an assistant in the Pathological-Anatomical Institute in Vienna, described clumping of red cells when serum of one individual was added to others. He attributed this reaction to an immunologic response and consequently reported 3 different blood groups in 1901. Although his work went unrecognized until the 1920s, he was eventually awarded the Nobel Prize in 1930. Multiple investigators developed different blood group categories, and it was not until the 1937 Congress of the International Society of Blood Transfusion that the ABO terminology was universally adopted.[3]

Twenty-five years later, other blood group antigens were identified, including Rhesus antibodies. Interestingly, the systems used to designate blood antigens are derived from the first patient described with the syndrome, rather than the investigator. Examples include the Kell system (infant with hematologic disease), Duffy (named after patient Joseph Duffy), and Kidd (named after a child of Mrs. Kidd with hematologic disease of the newborn).[9]

Once the major blood antigens were identified, the next challenge facing the widespread application of blood transfusion in clinical practice was to prevent blood coagulation during transfusion. In March 1908, Alexis Carrel (1873–1948) was the first physician to partially solve this problem when he successfully anastomosed the left radial artery of a father with a vein in the leg of his infant. When the transfusion was judged to be complete, Dr Carrel tied off both the artery and vein.[10] Both father and infant survived. This practice had several limitations, not the least of which was the inability to judge the volume of blood transfused, as well as the loss of the donor's vessel for further blood donation. It became clear that an anticoagulant needed to be added to donated blood to prevent clot formation. Richard Lewinsohn of Mount Sinai Hospital in New York performed a series of experiments which demonstrated that a 0.2% solution of sodium citrate was effective in preventing blood from clotting without causing systemic toxicity.[11] Later studies of dextrose and phosphate led to the current practice of using a citrate-phosphate-dextrose (CPD) solution to store blood safely for up to 28 days.[12]

The advent of World War I brought further advances in blood transfusion medicine. As it was not practical to bring blood donors to the front lines, a blood bank needed to be formed. The first blood bank was established in 1937 by Bernard Fantus at Cook County Hospital in Chicago.[13] The Second World War reinforced the need for blood banks as well as for fractionated blood products. Edwin Cohn, a professor at Harvard, isolated fractions of plasma (including albumin, fibrinogen, and immunoglobulin) by using serial additions of ethyl alcohol.[14] Cryoprecipitate was developed by Judith Pool in 1964 from the insoluble fraction of fresh quick-frozen plasma.[15]

The use of blood and blood products has expanded markedly since the initial transfusion experiments. Each year in the United States approximately 50% of children hospitalized in an intensive care unit receive a blood transfusion.[16,17] The use of fresh frozen plasma (FFP) has also increased steadily in the United States in the past 20 years. In 1979, one unit of FFP was transfused for every 6.6 units of packed red blood cells (PRBC), while in 2001, one FFP was transfused for every 3.6 units PRBC.[18] The ratio of FFP to PRBC continues to increase, especially in military medicine.

## HEMATOLOGIC AND PHYSIOLOGIC DIFFERENCES BETWEEN CHILDREN AND ADULTS

Children and adults differ both in their physiology and in their response to injury and illness. These differences influence both the timing and volume of transfusion. Rational administration of blood and blood products in children relies on an understanding of basic pediatric cardiovascular physiology.

## Physical Characteristics of Children

Children differ from adults with respect to cardiac physiology and function. For example, children have a higher resting heart rate than adults. The normal resting heart rate for a newborn infant is 100 to 160 beats per minute. This decreases to 70 to 120 beats per minute for children aged 1 to 10 years. After 10 years, the normal heart rate of a child approaches the adult norm of 60 to 100 beats per minute. Cardiac function also differs with age. Unlike an adult, the newborn's myocardium operates at near-maximum function at baseline. Therefore, a newborn may have difficulty increasing cardiac output to compensate for decreased oxygen carrying capacity.[19] In other words, infants cannot increase cardiac contractility to augment cardiac output; instead, they tend to increase heart rate. It is far more difficult for a burned child who already has tachycardia due to burn hypermetabolism to increase cardiac output by further raising heart rate. Infants with a burn may subsequently develop heart failure due to the increased metabolic demands of their injury.[20] In addition, decreased oxygen delivery capacity could result in myocardial ischemia in the newborn or very young infant. This may partly account for the increased mortality of burned children younger than 2 years.[21]

Despite being physically smaller than adults, children have a greater blood volume per unit mass. The mean blood volume for a child is 70 mL/kg, while the entire intravascular volume of an adult is 7% of total body weight. The increased blood volume per unit mass in children results in higher oxygen consumption and an elevated cardiac output per unit blood volume than adults.[22,23] This higher oxygen consumption can result in the need for greater oxygen delivery during times of critical illness, which can be ameliorated only by a blood transfusion.

Normal hemoglobin levels are also age-dependent. A child's normal hemoglobin reaches its nadir of 11.2 g/dL at approximately 2 to 3 months of age[24] (Table 1). Fetal hemoglobin, which decreases red blood cell life span from 120 to 90 days and shifts the oxygen-hemoglobin dissociation curve to the left, also plays a role in oxygen delivery in infants. Although fetal hemoglobin comprises 70% of hemoglobin at birth, only a fraction remains at 6 months of age.[25,26] In addition, critically ill infants with sepsis or polytrauma have a decreased production of erythropoietin in response to hypoxia or anemia.[27] Finally, children have a higher metabolic rate than adults, a difference that is exacerbated after burn injury.

## METABOLIC CONSEQUENCES AND RISKS OF BLOOD TRANSFUSION IN CHILDREN

Because children have a higher blood transfusion unit per volume ratio, they are at higher risk for metabolic perturbations after blood transfusion due to both the properties of red blood cells and the substrates used to help preserve red blood cells. These risks include hypocalcemia, hyperkalemia, hypomagnesemia, hypothermia, acidosis, and oxygen-hemoglobin dissociation curve shifts.

Ionized calcium is an important cofactor in many aspects of the coagulation cascade, as well as for myocardial contractility in the infant.[28] Hypocalcemia poses a greater risk to the neonate since the reduced sarcoplasmic reticulum in neonate myocardium makes cardiac contractility and relaxation dependent on ionized calcium concentration. The mechanism of action of citrate, which is used in blood storage, is to chelate calcium to prevent clot formation. As a result, transfusion can result in hypocalcemia. The degree of hypocalcemia is dependent on several factors, including the type of blood product transfused, the rate of the transfusion, and hepatic function.[29,30] Transfusion of whole blood and FFP results in the highest risk for development of hypocalcemia due to the higher concentration of citrate per unit volume. Hypocalcemia has been demonstrated following FFP administration during massive resuscitation in burns.[31] Decreasing the rate of blood transfusion to less than 1 mL/kg/min may ameliorate this hypocalcemic effect. Hypocalcemia can be corrected with either calcium chloride (5–10 mg/kg) or calcium gluconate (15–30 mg/kg). Calcium should never be administered through the same line as blood, as it may result in clot formation.

Hypomagnesemia may also occur after massive transfusion due to citrate toxicity. Because magnesium stabilizes resting membrane potential, hypomagnesemia may result in a life-threatening arrhythmia. If ventricular fibrillation or ventricular tachycardia refractory to calcium administration occurs after transfusion, intravenous magnesium sulfate in a dose of 25 to 50 mg/kg may be helpful.

Hyperkalemia has been implicated as a cause of cardiac arrest in children and infants during intraoperative transfusion of large amounts of blood products and during exchange transfusions.[32,33] Children with small blood volumes are at particularly high risk for hyperkalemia. The blood components with the highest levels of potassium include whole blood, irradiated units, and units nearing expiration (ie, "old blood").[34,35] Methods to decrease the risk of hyperkalemic cardiac arrest include using PRBC < 7 days old, avoiding whole blood in small infants, and washing erythrocytes. Large blood volumes infused rapidly can result in life-threatening arrhythmias.[32,35] Administration of calcium can help to resolve these arrhythmias by opposing the electrophysiologic effects of hyperkalemia; however, additional measures to lower serum potassium, such as glucose, insulin, albuterol, and Kayexalate, need to be administered to definitively resolve hyperkalemia.

Acidosis may also occur after blood transfusion. Stored blood cells initially undergo aerobic metabolism, but eventually anaerobic metabolism develops and increases lactic acid. The greatest risk for developing life-threatening acidosis occurs during rapid transfusion for massive blood loss in a hypovolemic patient. In the setting of burn injury, this is most likely to occur during extensive excision of the burn wound. Frequent measurement of acid/base status during burn excision and grafting will allow treatment of metabolic acidosis. Several days after a massive transfusion, it is not unusual for patients to develop metabolic alkalosis from metabolism of citrate in the blood products previously administered.

Hypothermia after blood transfusion in children requires special note. Children, due to their large surface area to body ratio, are predisposed to heat loss. Children with burn injury, due to loss of skin integrity, open wounds, and exposed tissue, are at an even higher risk for hypothermia. This increases oxygen consumption, exacerbates coagulopathy, and increases mortality.[36,37] The use of blood warmers during transfusion may decrease the incidence of hypothermia, as will maintenance of a warm operating room environment.

## INFECTIOUS DISEASE TRANSMISSION

Although the incidence of infectious disease transmission via blood transfusion is now lower than that for metabolic or immunologic complications, it remains an important consideration for children requiring blood transfusion.[38] Parents in particular are extremely concerned about the transmission of hepatitis and human immunodeficiency virus (HIV). Current blood screening tests include hepatitis B surface and core antigen, hepatitis C virus (HCV) antibody, HIV-1

and HIV-2 antibody, human T-lymphotrophic virus (HTLV) types I and II antibody, and nucleic acid amplification testing for HIV-1, HCV, syphilis, and West Nile virus. In addition to these commonly tested viral infections, bacteria can also infect blood products. The incidence of bacterial contamination is highest for platelets.[39,40,41] The incidence of infection from blood transfusion includes hepatitis C (1/1,600,000), hepatitis A (1/1,000,000), hepatitis B (1/220,000), HIV (1/1,900,000), bacterial contamination of blood (1/500,000), and blood type mismatch (1/14,000).[42] Other potential infections that could be transmitted via transfusion but are not tested for include HTLV, West Nile virus, babesiosis, Chagas disease, Lyme disease, malaria, Creutzfeldt-Jakob disease, and severe acute respiratory syndrome (SARS).

## INCOMPATIBILITY/IMMUNOLOGIC FACTORS

Acute hemolytic reactions generally occur when ABO incompatibility results in immunologic destruction of red cells. Despite the careful application of compatibility testing, these reactions continue to occur. Clerical error remains the leading cause of blood mismatch transfusion reactions. It is particularly important for 2 medical professionals to check the unit with both the blood bank paperwork and the patient's arm band in order to verify that the correct unit is truly intended for that patient. Strict adherence to transfusion protocols is important to avoid this iatrogenic complication.

Acute hemolytic reactions can also occur due to serologic incompatibilities of minor antigens not detected by current screening techniques. Fortunately, anaphylactic reactions rarely occur. Transfusion-related graft versus host reaction, in which lymphocytes in the transfused blood cause host cell destruction, occurs primarily in immunocompromised patients.[43,44] This condition can also happen primarily in premature infants or children with rapid acute blood loss, cardiopulmonary bypass, cancer, or severe systemic illness.[45] Thus, children with burn injury are at risk for this complication since they are immunosuppressed and often receive large volumes of blood in the operating room. Transfusion-related graft-versus-host disease can be minimized by using irradiated units, which effectively decreases the lymphocyte count. However, potassium levels must be monitored closely since irradiated blood has a higher potassium concentration.

Acute transfusion reactions are not infrequent in children. A recent study in a pediatric intensive care unit reported a 1.6% rate of acute transfusion reactions in 2500 transfusions, with 15% being immediately life-threatening.[46] Transfusion-related acute lung injury (TRALI), the onset of pulmonary insufficiency within 6 hours of transfusion, is estimated to occur in approximately 1 in every 5000 units transfused.[47] Children need to be monitored closely for these complications.

## DETERMINING HOW AND WHEN TO TRANSFUSE A CHILD

The blood volume of a child varies with age and weight, which impacts how much blood a child should receive during acute blood loss. The highest blood volume per unit weight is for a premature infant, at 90 to 100 mL/kg, while the lowest is for a very obese child, at 65 mL/kg. A term infant has a blood volume of 80 to 90 mL/kg until the age of 3 months, after which the total blood volume drops to 70 mL/kg.[48] The lower total blood volume of an infant relative to an adult is an important consideration in determining the amount of blood to give a child. During massive blood loss (defined as blood loss greater than 1 blood volume) in a child without preexisting anemia, the blood loss at which transfusion should be started (maximal allowable blood loss, or MABL) can be calculated from the following formula:

$$MABL = [(Hct_{start} - Hct_{target})/Hct_{start}] \times EBV$$

where EBV is estimated blood volume, $Hct_{target}$ is hematocrit goal, and $Hct_{start}$ is starting hematocrit.

In theory, blood loss to the level of MABL can be replaced by either crystalloid or colloid, with blood transfusion reserved for larger losses. Since the hematocrit in packed RBCs averages 70%, approximately 0.5 ml of packed RBCs should be transfused for each milliliter of blood loss beyond the MABL. Although this formula is attractive, it is merely an estimate and must be applied with caution. This formula can be problematic in the burned child, who has elevated red cell destruction and decreased red cell production. In general, during burn excision, a child loses 5% of his or her blood volume per percent burn excised on the face and 2% of his or her blood volume per percent burn excised on other areas.[49] Thus, an infant undergoing burn excision of the entire head could potentially lose 18% (body surface area of head) x 5 ml/% (blood volume lost per percent excision of head), which is 90% of the child's total blood volume. Adequate amounts of blood products should be ordered and readily available prior to the onset of surgery.

## Coagulopathy of Transfusion

Massive blood transfusion may result in coagulopathy due to a variety of reasons. First, thrombocytopenia may be caused by dilution of platelets during transfusion. In general,

a patient will lose 40% of the starting platelet count in the first blood volume lost, with loss of an additional 20% of the initial count at the second blood volume.[50] A preoperative platelet count measurement can be particularly valuable in this regard, especially in major burn excision cases. A child with sepsis and thrombocytopenia is more likely to require platelets than a child with a high or normal platelet count.

The second cause of coagulopathy during massive blood transfusion is depletion of clotting factors. Currently, packed red blood cells (PRBC) are the predominant form of red cell transfusion in the United States. Since 80% of the coagulation factors have been separated from packed RBCs, clotting factor deficiency will occur at approximately 1 blood volume.[50] If whole blood is used, all clotting factors except labile factors V and VIII will be transfused at normal levels. Thus, coagulation abnormalities tend to occur later (>3 blood volumes) when using whole blood.[51]

## SPECIFIC COMPONENT THERAPY CONSIDERATIONS

### Red Cell Transfusions

PRBC transfusion is used to augment hemodynamic status in more than 3 million patients per year, and an estimated 11 million units of PRBCs are transfused every year in the United States.[52] Approximately one-quarter of patients in the intensive care unit receive blood transfusions to ameliorate the effects of anemia.[53] Although PRBC transfusion has many beneficial effects, it is not without complications. Commonly cited adverse effects include infection, pulmonary edema, immune suppression, and microcirculatory alterations.[54] Blood transfusion has been associated with increased risk of nosocomial infections in the critically ill, including patients with burn injury.[55,56] Increased complications, including death, after transfusion have been associated with older and nonleukoreduced blood.[57-59]

Several methods have been advocated to reduce the complication rate of PRBC transfusion. In particular, some have advocated the use of "young" packed red blood cells (ie, less than 2 weeks after donation). After 15 days, stored red blood cells undergo a variety of morphologic and functional changes, including decreased deformability, depletion of 2,3-diphosphoglycerate, decreased ability to offload oxygen, reduction in adenosine triphosphate, loss of endogenous red blood cell antioxidants, and red cell sludging.[60] In addition, leukoreduction of packed red blood cells has been proposed as a possible method of decreasing the adverse outcomes after PRBC transfusion. Since the white blood cells present in both PRBC and platelet preparations can result in immunologic and physiologic dysfunction in the recipient,[61,62] reduction of leukocytes may mitigate these alterations.

Traditionally, blood has been transfused in both adults and children to maintain a hemoglobin level of at least 10 g/dL or hematocrit of 30%, to assure "optimal" oxygen delivery. However, the Transfusion Requirements in Critical Care (TRICC) study, a multicenter, prospective, randomized study of ICU patients, challenges this standard.[63] A total of 838 patients were randomized to receive blood transfusion based on a liberal (maintain hemoglobin 10–12 g/dL) versus a restrictive (maintain hemoglobin 7–8 g/dL) strategy. The restrictive strategy was found to be at least as effective as the liberal strategy in critically ill patients. Parameters such as in-hospital mortality, cardiac complications, and organ dysfunction were lower in the restrictive group. A similar study performed in children by many of the same investigators found that a restrictive transfusion policy could also be applied in children without increasing the incidence of adverse outcomes.[64] These findings are especially relevant since numerous studies have documented increased mortality and infection rates in children and adults receiving blood transfusions.[65,66,67]

## Red Cell Transfusion and Burns

The previously performed randomized trials evaluating blood transfusion practices have limited applicability to the burn population, since patients were excluded if they had a drop in hemoglobin of 3 g/dL or had ongoing blood loss. In the acute resuscitative phase, burn patients often have a significant reduction in hemoglobin due to ongoing blood loss (other trauma, escharotomies), hemodilution, or hemolysis. Neither study indicated whether or not burn patients were included. Of the 838 patients enrolled in the adult study, only 165 comprised the trauma category, and in the pediatric study, only 93 patients were in the surgery group, of which burn injury would have been a minor component. Hence, an adequate sample size to determine the outcome of a restrictive strategy in children with burn injury did not exist. Finally, the effects of a restrictive strategy on wound healing or infection were not assessed. Both of these variables are major considerations in children with burns.

Data on the ideal blood transfusion threshold in burns remain limited. In one study by Sittig and Deitch, a total of 14 patients admitted to a burn center during a 6-month interval were transfused if their hemoglobin level was <6.0 g/dL.[68] The outcomes of patients with >20% total body surface area (TBSA) burns or patients requiring excision and grafting of >10% TBSA were retrospectively compared to a matched group of 38 patients treated the previous year using a nonrestrictive policy (hemoglobin maintained above

9.5–10 g/dL). No differences existed in hospital length of stay. The patients treated with the traditional strategy received 3.5 times more blood than their restrictive counterparts. A more recent study evaluating the blood transfusion practices of 21 burn centers throughout the United States reported that for patients with burn injury >20% TBSA, mortality was related to age, TBSA burn, inhalation injury, the number of units of blood transfused in the burn intensive care unit, and the total number of units transfused.[69] The infection rate was also influenced by the number of blood transfusions: each transfusion increased the risk of infection by 11%. Thus, there appears to be an association between the volume of blood transfused with both infection and mortality.

The data for blood transfusions in burned children are limited primarily to single-center retrospective observational studies. Several studies have demonstrated that children are more likely to develop sepsis and/or infection if they receive a larger number of blood products.[2,70] In addition, these studies demonstrate that more complications occur in children receiving a greater number of blood transfusions. Hence, packed red blood cell transfusions should be administered judiciously. To date, the "optimal" transfusion threshold has not been defined for children with burn injury.

The use of whole blood transfusion after injury increased due to several reports of improved outcomes in soldiers with severe hemorrhage and burn injury during military conflicts.[71,72] A single case series report on the use of reconstituted whole blood during early burn excision in 20 children reported no increased risk of infectious episodes or coagulopathy during near-total-body burn excision.[73] Although intriguing, neither of these studies is prospective nor adequately powered to draw meaningful conclusions regarding the use of whole blood in burned children.

## Platelet Transfusions

Platelets, which are produced in the bone marrow and destroyed by the spleen, have an average lifespan of 9 to 10 days. They are obtained in 1 of 2 ways: the first method involves centrifugation of whole blood into platelet-rich plasma, which is again centrifuged to obtain platelets. In the second method, dubbed apheresis or plasmapheresis, blood is taken from a single donor, run through an apheresis unit (which separates the blood via centrifugation), and all components except for platelets are returned to the donor. The resulting apheresis unit has 6 times the number of platelets as whole blood and can be stored at room temperature for up to 5 days.[74]

Platelets play an important role in coagulation. However, the administration of platelets also carries multiple risks.[75] One study cited a 30% incidence of a transfusion reaction from platelets compared to 6.8% for red blood cells.[76] The age of the blood product is a predominant factor increasing the incidence of transfusion reaction: the older the blood product, the greater the risk. Platelets also have the highest bacterial contamination rate of all blood products. In patients who have active bleeding or are in need of surgical intervention, such as children with burn injury, the platelet count should be greater than 50,000/μL at the beginning of the procedure.[77]

## Fresh Frozen Plasma

Fresh frozen plasma (FFP) is perhaps the most commonly used plasma product to correct clotting factor abnormalities.[78] In general, FFP administration is indicated in patients with factor XI deficiency, active bleeding with an INR of >2, and patients with disseminated intravascular coagulation (DIC). Children with major burn injury frequently develop clotting abnormalities as well. Shortly after burn injury, a consumptive coagulopathy, together with microangiopathic destruction of red blood cells, occurs.[78,79] This results in anemia, thrombocytopenia, and coagulopathy. In addition, sepsis can result in DIC and a decreased platelet count.[80] Although FFP transfusion has traditionally been advocated for documented clotting abnormalities, studies of massive transfusion from the military have suggested improved survival if FFP is administered in a 1:1 ratio with packed red blood cells during times of massive blood loss.[81] The use of this strategy in children with burns has not been fully assessed.

## Cryoprecipitate and Factor Concentrates

Cryoprecipitate, rich in factor VIII, factor XIII, fibrinogen, and von Willebrand factor, is created by freezing and then slowly thawing plasma. The components of cryoprecipitate are more highly concentrated than in fresh frozen plasma; hence, a smaller volume is needed. A 10 to 15 mL bag of cryoprecipitate contains approximately 200 mg of fibrinogen.[77] The smaller volume needed to replete factors may be important for children, who have smaller blood volumes than adults and are less likely to tolerate large fluid volumes.

Recombinant factor VIIa (rFVIIa), originally developed to treat bleeding in patients with hemophilia, has also been used in the setting of massive hemorrhage. In critically ill patients, rFVIIa has been used successfully in a variety of disorders, including massively transfused trauma patients, cardiopulmonary bypass, liver injury or transplantation, and uncontrolled gastrointestinal hemorrhage.[82,83,84] rFVIIa decreases prothrombin time and improves hemostasis in

adults. Several papers describing the use of rFVIIa in burn excision and grafting have suggested that it may decrease the blood loss associated with burn wound excision.[85,86] However, the routine use of rFVIIa in burn excision cannot be recommended at this time.

## Erythropoietin

One method of potentially decreasing the need for red blood cell transfusion is the use of recombinant human erythropoietin (rHuEPO). In patients with responsive progenitor cells and adequate iron stores, rHuEPO may stimulate increased erythropoiesis. Several studies have reported the use of rHuEPO in critically ill patients. One prospective randomized study demonstrated a 10% decrease in allogeneic blood transfusion in critically ill patients receiving rHuEPO.[87] Its use in burns may be problematic due to the decreased iron stores and red cell production as well as the increased red cell destruction after burn injury. One prospective study of rHuEPO in burns showed no difference in the development of postburn anemia or transfusion requirements.[88] However, this study was probably underpowered to detect significant differences between groups with respect to mortality.

## DECREASING INTRAOPERATIVE BLOOD LOSS IN BURN SURGERY

Several simple techniques can be employed to decrease major blood loss due to massive excision of burn wounds. First, early excision has been demonstrated to reduce the blood loss associated with burn surgery.[89] This may be due in part to the effects of vasoactive mediators and edema associated with the early phases of burn injury. In addition, the neovascularization that accompanies wound healing will be far less extensive in the first few days postinjury. Other methods reported to decrease blood loss during burn excision include the use of limb tourniquets, subcutaneous tumescence or topical placement of vasoconstrictors, topical application of thrombin or fibrin, dermabrasion, and a 2-stage operative technique (burn excision 1 day, skin harvest and grafting the next).[90,91,92] Children in particular are well suited to the 2-stage approach, as it limits operating room time and the development of hypothermia, thus enabling massive early excision to be performed safely.

## CONCLUSIONS

Children with burn injuries pose challenges in multiple areas, including the use of blood transfusions. Age-related differences between adults and children impact the decision for transfusion. The indications for transfusion, type of transfusion, volume of transfusion, and potential side effects need to be scrutinized for every child with a burn injury in order to maximize the efficacy and minimize the complications associated with blood transfusion. Furthermore, minimizing blood loss during burn care treatment may decrease transfusion requirements and improve patient outcomes.

## TABLE

### TABLE 1
### Normal infant hemoglobin levels.

| Age | Hemoglobin (g/dL) |
|---|---|
| Birth | 19.3 |
| 2 weeks | 16.6 |
| 1 month | 13.9 |
| 3 months | 11.2 |
| 4 months | 12.2 |
| 6 months | 12.5 |
| 1 year | 12.5 |
| 9 years | 13.5 |

## REFERENCES

1. Wallace EL, Churchill WH, Surgenor DM, Cho GS, McGurk S. Collection and transfusion of blood and blood components in the United States, 1994. *Transfusion*. 1998; **38**: 625–636.

2. Palmieri TL, Lee T, O'Mara MS, Greenhalgh DG. Effects of a restrictive blood transfusion policy on outcomes in children with burn injury. *J Burn Care Res*. 2007; **28**: 65–70.

3. Giangrande PL. The history of blood transfusion. *Br J Haematol*. 2000; **110**: 758–767.

4. Lloyd, GER, ed. *Hippocratic Writings*. London: Penguin; 1978.

5. Keynes G. Tercentenary of blood transfusion. *BMJ*. 1967; **4**: 410–411.

6. Dzik WH. The James Blundell award lecture 2006; transfusion and the treatment of haemorrhage: past, present, and future. *Transfus Med*. 2007; **17**: 367–374.

7. Learoyd P. *A Short History of Blood Transfusion*. Leeds, UK: National Blood Service, Leeds Blood Center; 2006.

8. Blundell J. Observations on transfusion of blood. *Lancet*. 1828b; **1**: 431.

9. Coombs, RRA, Mourant AE, Race RR. In-vivo isosensitization of red cells in babies with haemolytic disease. *Lancet*. 1946; **i**: 264–266.

10. Clark TW. The birth of transfusion. *J Hist Med*. 1949; **4**: 337–338.

11. Lewinsohn R. Blood transfusion by the citrate method. *Surg Gynecol Obstet*. 1915; **21**: 37–47.

12. Gibson JG, Gregory CB, Button LN. Citrate-phosphate-dextrose solution for preservation of human blood: a further report. *Transfusion*. 1961; **1**: 280–287.

13. Fantus B. The therapy of the Cook County Hospital. *JAMA*. 1937; **109**: 128–131.

14. Cohn EF, Strong LE, Hughes WL, et al. Preparation and properties of serum and plasma proteins. *J Am Chem Soc*. 1946; **68**: 459–475.

15. Pool JG, Shannon AE. Production of high-potency concentrates of antihemophilic globulin in a closed bag system. *N Engl J Med* 1965; **273**: 1443–1444.

16. Armano R, Gauvin F, Ducruet T, et al. Determinants of red blood cell transfusions in a pediatric critical care unit: a perspective descriptive epidemiological study. *Crit Care Med*. 2005: **33**: 2637–2644.

17. Morris KP, Naqvi N, Davies P, et al. A new formula for blood transfusion volume in the critically ill. *Arch Dis Child*. 2005; **90**: 724–728.

18. Wallis JP, Kzik WH. Is fresh frozen plasma overtransfused in the United States? *Transfusion*. 2004: **44**: 1674–1675.

19. Barcelona SL, Thompson AA, Cote CJ. Intraoperative pediatric blood transfusion therapy: a review of common issues. Part I. *Pediatr Anesth.* 2005; **15**: 716–726.

20. Reynolds EM, Ryan DP, Sheridan RL. Left ventricular failure complicating severe pediatric burn injuries. *J Pediatr Surg.* 1995; **30**: 264–270.

21. Wolf SE, Rose JK, Desai MH, et al. Mortality determinants in massive pediatric burns: an analysis of 103 children with >=80% TBSA burns. *Ann Surg.* 1997; **225**: 554–569.

22. Cross KW, Tizard JP, Trythall DA. The gaseous metabolism of the newborn infant breathing 15% oxygen. *Acta Paediatr.* 1958; **47**: 217–237.

23. Cross KW, Flynn DM, Hill JR. Oxygen consumption in normal newborn infants during moderate hypoxia in warm and cool environments. *Pediatrics.* 1966; **37**: 565–576.

24. Barcelona SL, Cote CJ. Pediatric resuscitation in the operating room. *Anesthesiol Clin North Am.* 2001; **19**: 339–365.

25. Brown MS. Physiologic anemia of infancy: normal red-cell values and physiology of neonatal erythropoiesis. In: Stockman JA III, Pochedly C, eds. *Developmental and Neonatal Hematology.* New York, NY: Raven Press: 1988: 249–274.

26. Nathan DG, Orkin SH. *Nathan and Oski's Hematology of Infancy and Childhood.* 5th ed. Philadelphia, PA: WB Saunders Company; 1998.

27. Hobisch-Hagan P, Wiedermann F, Mayr A, Fries D, et al. Blunted erythropoietic response to anemia in multiply traumatized patients. *Crit Care Med.* 2001; **29**: 743–747.

28. Butenas S, Mann KG. Blood coagulation. *Biochemistry.* 2002; **67**: 3–12.

29. Barcelona SL, Cote CJ. Pediatric resuscitation in the operating room. *Anesthesiol Clin North Am.* 2001; **19**: 339–365.

30. Borland LM, Roule M, Cook DR. Anesthesia for pediatric orthotopic liver transplantation. *Anesth Analg.* 1985; **64**: 117–124.

31. Cote CJ, Drop LJ, Hoaglin DC, et al. Ionized hypocalcemia after fresh frozen plasma administration to thermally injured children: effects of infusion rate, duration, and treatment with calcium chloride. *Anesth Analg.* 1988; **67**: 152–160.

32. Brown KA, Bissonnette B, McIntyre B. Hyperkalaemia during rapid blood transfusion and hypovolaemic cardiac arrest in children. *Can J Anaesth.* 1990; **37**: 747–754.

33. Scanlon JW, Krakaur R. Hyperkalemia following exchange transfusion. *J Pediatr.* 1980; **96**: 108–110.

34. Fukuoka Y, Ishiyama T, Oguchi T, et al. Hyperkamemia after irradiated blood transfusion. *Masue.* 1999; **48**: 192–194.

35. Thorp JA, Plapp FV, Cohen CG, et al. Hyperkalemia after irradiation of packed red blood cells: possible effects with intravascular fetal transfusion. *Am J Obstet Gynecol.* 1990; **163**: 607–609.

36. Johnston TD, Chen Y, Reed RL. Functional equivalence of hypothermia to specific clotting factor deficiencies. *J Trauma.* 1994; **37**: 413–417.

37. Jurkovich GJ, Greiser WB, Luterman A, et al. Hypothermia in trauma victims: an ominous predictor of survival. *J Trauma.* 1987; **27**: 1019–1024.

38. Barcelona SL, Thompson AA, Cote CJ. Intraoperative pediatric blood transfusion therapy: a review of common issues. Part I: hematologic and physiologic differences from adults; metabolic and infectious risks. *Pediatr Anesth.* 2005; **15**: 716–726.

39. Smith LA, Wright-Kanuth MS. Bacterial contamination of blood components. *Clin Lab Sci.* 2003; **16**: 230–238.

40. Bell CE, Botteman MF, Gao X, et al. Cost-effectiveness of transfusion of platelet components prepared with pathogen inactivation treatment in the United States. *Clin Ther.* 2003; **25**: 2464–2486.

41. Goodnough LT, Kuter D, McCullough J, et al. Apheresis platelets: emerging issues related to donor platelet count, apheresis platelet yield, and platelet transfusion dose. *J Clin Apheresis.* 1998; **13**: 114–119.

42. Goodnough LT, Brecher MD, Kanter MH, et al. Transfusion medicine: part I: blood transfusion. *N Engl J Med.* 1999; **340**: 438–447.

43. Cohen A, Manno C. Transfusion practices in infants receiving assisted ventilation. *Clin Perinatol.* 1998; **25**: 97–111.

44. Warren LJ, Simmer K, Roxby D, et al. DNA Polymorphism analysis in transfusion-associated graft-versus-host disease. *J Paediatr Child Health.* 1999; **35**: 98–101.

45. Warren A. DePalma L, Yu M, McIntosh CL, et al. Changes in lymphocyte subpopulations as a result of cardiopulmonary bypass. The effect of blood transfusion. *J Thorac Cardiovasc Surg.* 1991; **101**: 240–244.

46. Gauvin F, Lacroix J, Pierre Robillard, et al. Acute transfusion reactions in the pediatric intensive care unit. *Transfusion.* 2006; **46**: 1899–1908.

47. Popovsky MA, Moore SB. Diagnostic and patholgenetic considerations in transfusion-related acute lung injury. *Transfusion.* 1985; **25**: 573–577.

48. Barcelona SL, Thompson AA, Cote CJ. Intraoperative pediatric blood transfusion therapy: a review of common issues. Part II: transfusion therapy, special considerations, and reduction of allogenic blood transfusions. *Pediatr Anesth.* 2005; **15**: 814–830.

49. Housinger TA, Lang D, Warden GD. A prospective study of blood loss with excisional therapy in pediatric burn patients. *J Trauma.* 1993; **34**: 262–263.

50. Cote CJ, Liu LM, Szyfelbein SK, et al. Changes in serial platelet counts following massive blood transfusion in pediatric patients. *Anesthesiology.* 1985; **62**: 197–201.

51. Miller RD. Complications of massive blood transfusions. *Anesthesiology.* 1973; **39**: 82–93.

52. Wallace EL, Churchill WH, Surgenor DM, Cho GS, McGurk S. Collection and transfusion of blood and blood components in the United States, 1994. *Transfusion.* 1998; **38**: 625–636.

53. Hebert PC, Wells G, Martin C, et al. A Canadian survey of transfusion practices in critically ill patients. *Crit Care Med*. 1998; **26**: 482–487.

54. Alvarez G, Hebert PC, Szick S. Debate: transfusing to normal haemoglobin levels will not improve outcome. *Crit Care*. 2001; **5**(2): 56–63.

55. Graves TA, Cioffi WE, Mason AD Jr, et al. Relationship of transfusion and infection in a burn population. *J Trauma*. 1989; **29**: 948–952.

56. Nichols RL, Smith JW, Klein DB, et al. Risk of infection after penetrating abdominal trauma. *N Engl J Med*. 1984; **311**: 1065–1070.

57. Weinberg JA, McGwin G Jr, Griffin RL, et al. Age of transfused blood: an independent predictor of mortality despite universal leukoreduction. *J Trauma*. 2008; **65**: 279–284.

58. Offner PJ, Moore EE, Biffl WL, et al. Increased rate of infection associated with transfusion of old blood after severe injury. *Arch Surg*. 2002; **137**: 711–716.

59. Nathens AB, Nester TA, Rubenfeld GD, et al. The effects of leukoreduced blood transfusion on infection risk following injury: a randomized controlled trial. *Shock*. 2006; **26**: 342–347.

60. Raghavan M, Marik PE. Anemia, allogenic blood transfusion, and immunomodulation in the critically ill. *Chest*. 2005; **127**: 295–307.

61. Bordin JO, Heddle NM, Blajchman MA. Biologic effects of leukocytes present in transfused cellular blood products. *Blood*. 1994; **84**: 1703–1721.

62. Jensen LS, Kissmeyer-Nielsen P, Wolff B, et al. Randomised comparison of leucocyte-depleted versus buffy-coat-poor blood transfusion and complications after colorectal surgery. *Lancet*. 1996; **348**: 841–845.

63. Hebert PC, Wells G, Blajchman MA, et al. A multicenter, randomized controlled clinical trial of transfusion requirements in critical care. *N Engl J Med*. 1999; **340**: 409–417.

64. Lacroix J, Hebert PC, Hutchison JS, et al. Transfusion strategies for patients in pediatric intensive care units. *N Engl J Med*. 2007; **356**: 1609–1619.

65. Kneyber MC, Hersi MI, Twisk JW, Markhorst DG. Red blood cell transfusion in critically ill children is independently associated with increased mortality. *Intensive Care Med*. 2007; **33**: 1414–1422.

66. Moore FA, Moore EE, Sauaia A. Blood transfusion: an independent risk factor for postinjury multiple organ failure. *Arch Surg*. 1997; **132**: 620–625.

67. Shorr AF, Duh M, Kelly KM, et al. Red blood cell transfusion and ventilator-associated pneumonia: a potential link? *Crit Care Med*. 2004; **32**: 666–674.

68. Sittig KM, Deitch EA. Blood transfusions: for the thermally injured or for the doctor? *J Trauma*. 1994; **36**(3): 369–372.

69. Palmieri TL, Caruso DM, Foster KN, et al. Blood transfusion practices in major burn injury: a multicenter study. *Crit Care Med*. 2006; **34**: 1602–1607.

70. Jeschke MG, Chinkes DL, Finnerty CC, et al. Blood transfusions are associated with increased risk for development of sepsis in severely burned pediatric patients. *Crit Care Med*. 2007; **35**: 579–583.

71. Spinella PC. Warm fresh whole blood transfusion for severe hemorrhage: U.S. military and potential civilian applications. *Crit Care Med*. 2008; **36**: S340–S345.

72. Repine TB, Perkins JG, Kauvar DS, et al. The use of fresh whole blood in massive transfusion. *J Trauma*. 2006; **60**: S59–S69.

73. Barret JP, Desai MH, Herndon DN. Massive transfusion of reconstituted whole blood is well tolerated in pediatric burn surgery. *J Trauma*. 1999; **47**: 31–38.

74. www.aabb.org/Content/About_Blood /Facts_About_Blood_ and_Blood_Banking. Accessed September 10, 2008.

75. Kruskall MS. The perils of platelet transfusions. *N Engl J Med*. 1997; **337**: 1914–1915.

76. Heddle NM, Klama LN, Griffith L, et al. Prospective study to identify the risk factors associated with acute reactions to platelet and red cell transfusions. *Transfusion*. 2003; **33**: 794–797.

77. Drews RE. Critical issues in hematology: anemia, thrombocytopenia, coagulopathy, and blood product transfusions in critically ill patients. *Clin Chest Med*. 2003; **24**: 607–622.

78. Curreri PW, Hicks JE, Aronoff RJ, et al. Inhibition of active sodium transport in erythrocytes from burned patients. *Surg Gynecol Obstet*. 1974; **139**: 538–540.

79. Simon TL, Curreri PW, Harker LA. Kinetic characterization of hemostasis in thermal injury. *J Lab Clin Med*. 1977; **89**: 702–711.

80. Cullen JJ, Murray DJ, Kealey GP. Changes in coagulation factors in patients with burns during acute blood loss. *J Burn Care Rehabil*. 1989; **10**: 517–522.

81. Kashuk JL, Moore EE, Lohnson JL, et al. Postinjury life threatening coagulopathy: is 1: 1 fresh frozen plasma: Packed red blood cells the answer? *J Trauma*. 2008; **65**: 261–271.

82. Lynn M, Jeroukhimov I, Klein Y, et al. Updates in the management of severe coagulopathy in trauma patients. *Intensive Care Med*. 2002; **28**: S241–S247.

83. White B, McHale J, Ravi N, et al. Successful use of recombinant FVIIa (Novoseven) in the management of intractable post-surgical intra-abdominal haemorrhage. *Br J Haematol*. 1999; **107**: 677–678.

84. Markiewicz M, Kalicinski P, Kaminski A, et al. Acute coagulopathy after reperfusion of the liver graft in children correction with recombinant activated factor VII. *Transplant Proc*. 2003; **35**: 2318–2319.

85. Johansson PI, Eriksen K, Nielsen SL, et al. Recombinant FVIIa decreases perioperative blood transfusion requirement in burn patients undergoing excision and skin grafting—results of a single center pilot study. *Burns*. 2007; **33**: 435–440.

86. Johansson PI, Eriksen K, Alsbjorn B. Rescue treatment with recombinant factor VIIa is effective in patients with life-threatening bleedings secondary to major wound excision: a report of four cases. *J Trauma*. 2006; **61**: 1016–1018.

**87.** Corwin HL, Gettinger A, Pearl RG, et al. Efficacy of recombinant human erythropoietin in critically ill patients: a randomized controlled trial. *JAMA*. 2002; **288:** 2827–2835.

**88.** Still JM Jr, Belcher K, Law EJ, et al. A double-blinded prospective evaluation of recombinant human erythropoietin in acutely burned patients. *J Trauma*. 1995; **38:** 233–236.

**89.** Desai MH, Herndon DN, Broemeling L, et al. Early burn wound excision significantly reduces blood loss. *Ann Surg*. 1990; **211:** 753–762.

**90.** Losee JE, Fox I, Hua LB, et al. Transfusion-free pediatric burn surgery: techniques and strategies. *Ann Plast Surg*. 2005; **54:** 165–171.

**91.** Djurickovic S, Snelling CFT, Boyle JC. Tourniquet and subcutaneous epinephrine reduce blood loss during burn excision and immediate autografting. *J Burn Care Rehab*. 2001; **22:** 1–5.

**92.** Warden GD, Saffle JR, Kravitz M. A two-stage technique for excision and grafting of burn wounds. *J Trauma*. 1982; **22:** 98–103.

# CHAPTER THIRTEEN

# INFECTIONS IN PATIENTS WITH SEVERE BURNS: DIAGNOSTIC AND MANAGEMENT APPROACH

JONATHAN M. ZENILMAN, MD, PROFESSOR OF MEDICINE, DIVISION OF INFECTIOUS DISEASES,
JOHNS HOPKINS BAYVIEW MEDICAL CENTER, BALTIMORE, MD

## INTRODUCTION

In the United States and other developed countries, aggressive resuscitation of patients with severe burns and rapid transport to specialized regional burn centers have essentially eliminated early hospital mortality. The major cause of death after the acute admission phase is sepsis, typically caused by nosocomially acquired organisms that are frequently resistant to multiple antimicrobials. Even if patients with burn injuries have few or no concurrent illnesses, they are nonetheless susceptible to infection because of large wound exposure, prolonged hospital stays, and use of invasive monitoring devices.

The incidence of infection in burn patients is high.[1] Palmieri et al reviewed 199 patients with toxic epidermal necrolysis at 15 major burn centers between 1995 and 2000 and found an overall mortality of 32%.[2] Sepsis accounted for the majority of early deaths in 33% of patients. In an additional 33%, multisystem organ failure primarily attributable to sepsis was the immediate cause. Weber et al reported on a series of children (< 18 years old) seen between 1996 and 2000 and found that the incidence of serious invasive infection for patients with > 30% body surface area (BSA) burns was 55 out of 60 (92%).[3] De Macedo et al[4] reviewed 252 unselected burn patients in Brazil between 2001 and 2002 and described a sepsis rate of 19% during hospitalization.

## MICROBIOLOGY OF BURN SEPSIS

The microbiology of burn wound infections and burn sepsis has changed dramatically over the past 25 years. In the 1960s and 1970s, burn wound cellulitis and impetigo was common, caused largely by gram-positive organisms, especially streptococci and staphylococci. With the evolution of silver-containing and more effective antibacterial dressings,[5,6,7] *Pseudomonas* and other hospital-acquired gram-negatives became the predominant organism. *Pseudomonas* is particularly well suited to establish wound infection because it easily forms biofilms on wound surfaces and has a natural reservoir in water, which is widely used for burn wound irrigation. Between 1997 and 2002, the Chandigarh, India Burn Center found *Pseudomonas* to be the most common isolate, followed by *Staphylococcus* and *Acinetobacter*.[8] Our results at the Hopkins Center were essentially similar, except for staphylococci being more common due to line infections. Evolution of *Pseudomonas* strains resistant to multiple antibiotics, including the carbapenems, has also evolved as a major problem in many centers.[9–11]

In most cases, the burn surface is initially sterile because of the thermal injury. However, subsequent interventions may result in inoculation of unusual organisms. For example, if a patient was immediately immersed in nonenvironmental water sources (such as a pond or river), the array of possible microorganisms can be expansive. It is therefore important to obtain a detailed history of postinjury events from the patient, family, and first responders. Absent unusual environmental exposures, the microbial evolution is typically from normal skin flora, primarily gram-positive cocci. Gram-negative organisms become more prevalent as the individual becomes colonized. The surface microbiology in 51 patients with a mean BSA burn of 23% who were hospitalized for at least 3 weeks was evaluated by Erol et al.[17] Gram-positive cocci, predominantly *Staphylococcus* species, were most prevalent on admission, but the flora shifted to *Pseudomonas* and other gram-negatives within a week after admission.

Since 2000, *Acinetobacter* has become a major pathogen, which is highly problematic because of its propensity to acquire multiple resistance determinants and therefore develop resistance to nearly all antibiotic classes.[9,12-16,18] These organisms are found in the environment and water sources and are particularly well suited to the biofilm environment which develops in patients with large BSA burns. *Acinetobacter* is frequently isolated from burn patients and severely injured/trauma patients who have long exposures to broad-spectrum antimicrobials. Despite these concerns, clinical experience has shown that the organism is not as virulent as other pyogenic bacteria.[19,20] However, differentiation of colonization from invasive disease can be extremely difficult in such critically ill patients. Davis et al from the US Army reported on patients with multidrug-resistant *Acinetobacter* infections from Iraq during 2003 through 2005, including 18 with osteomyelitis, 2 with burn infections, and 3 with deep wound infections.[21] Because the organism can be found on numerous fomites in the ICU setting,[22] it has been difficult to eradicate even with aggressive infection-control measures.

Besides *Acinetobacter*, enteric bacteria with multiple resistance determinants are increasingly encountered. Three emerging groups of particular concern are

- *Pseudomonas* and *Serratia*. These classical nosocomial organisms share the ability to acquire or evolve resistant determinants under antibiotic pressure. *Pseudomonas* expresses a variety of toxins and is the most common cause of invasive local infections in burn centers.
- Organisms with extended spectrum beta-lactamases (ESBL).[9,23] These are organisms with plasmids which encode beta-lactamases that have the capability of hydrolyzing second-generation and third-generation cephalosporins. There are over 100 types of ESBL that have been identified in the literature. These organisms are especially concerning from an infection-control perspective because the plasmids can potentially be transferred to other bacteria via conjugation.
- *Klebsiella pneumoniae* carbapenemase (KPC). Because this newly emergent organism encodes enzymes which hydrolyze carbapenems[24,25] such as meropenem and imipenem, it affords relatively few treatment options. In contrast to *Acinetobacter*, these organisms have been associated with as much as a 3-fold increase in mortality compared to other patients with bacteremia. Whether this is due to intrinsic pathogenicity or whether infection is a surrogate for more severe illness remains to be elucidated.

Fungal infections are a feared complication in severely injured patients with prolonged hospital stays.[1,26] Cochran reported on 44 patients with an average 49% BSA burn and *Candida* infection (defined as either candidemia or positive cultures from > 2 body sites). Patients with *Candida* received an average of 72 days of systemic antibiotics, while controls only had 36 days. Moreover, patients with multiple sites of *Candida* were more likely to receive broad-spectrum antibiotics. In intensive care settings, aggressive antimicrobial parsimony and fluconazole prophylaxis[27] have reduced candidemia as a nosocomial infection.

Morbidity, and especially mortality, from fungal infections is increasingly due to filamentous fungi (molds), especially *Fusariaum*, *Aspergillus*, and *Zygomeces* species.[1,28,29] These organisms have a particular predilection for areas of necrotic tissue and almost exclusively occur in patients on prolonged courses of broad-spectrum antibiotics. Diagnosis is often difficult, and careful examination of the tissue during dressing changes is critical. Mortality from these infections can reach over 50%.

## DIFFERENTIATING SEPSIS FROM BURN-INDUCED SIRS

Sepsis and inflammation due to thermal injury can cause the systemic inflammatory response syndrome (SIRS). The American Burn Association (ABA) consensus statement on burns and SIRS succinctly summarized the problem:[30]

Burn patients lose their primary barrier to microorganism invasion so they are constantly and chronically exposed to the environment. In response to this exposure, inflammatory mediators that change the baseline metabolic profile of the burn patient are continuously released. The baseline temperature is reset to about 38.5°C, and tachycardia and tachypnea persist for months....

The current definition of SIRS was created by a consensus conference of critical care and trauma physicians more than a decade ago. SIRS is considered to be present when a patient demonstrates 2 or more of the following:

- Temperature above 38°C or below 36°C
- Heart rate > 90 beats per minute (bpm) or > 2 SD above age-specific norms (85% age-adjusted maximum heart rate)
- Respiratory rate > 20 breaths per minute or maintenance of $PaCO2 < 32$ mm Hg. (children > 2 SD above age-specific norms)
- WBC count > 12000/mm3 or < 4000/mm3, or left shift defined as > 10% bands

Clinically differentiating sepsis in burn patients from burn-associated SIRS is not possible, as both have similar presentations. However, sepsis should always be suspected whenever there is an acute change in a patient's status. Other factors suggesting sepsis include

- hyperglycemia and insulin resistance
- thrombocytopenia
- abdominal distension
- enteral feeding intolerance
- diarrhea
- acute renal failure

A substantial clinical issue surrounding sepsis is the lack of reliability of the classical clinical markers. A study conducted by the US Army Burn Center evaluating 591 blood cultures from 129 patients with severe burns demonstrated that fever and hypothermia are neither sensitive nor specific as a predictor of bacteremia.[31] Similarly, a study conducted by Keen et al[32] between 1993 and 1997 at the Salt Lake City Burn Center found no relationship between bacteremia and the clinical signs of either fever or leukocytosis. SIRS independently induces an inflammatory response which can result in fever, leukocytosis, or other signs of inflammation. Hypothermia is commonly encountered in patients with large BSA burns because of loss of skin thermoregulation.

## BURN WOUND INFECTION

Burn wound infection has been classified into 3 major categories representing stages in the evolution of the burn wound. These consensus definitions have recently been extensively reviewed by Church et al[1] and modified for children by Upperman et al.[33,34]

## Burn Impetigo

Primary impetigo can also be seen in patients with partial-thickness burns, particularly of the scalp, and is often associated with *Staphylococcus aureus* and *Streptococcus pyogenes*. In hospitalized patients, impetigo involves loss of epithelium from a previously reepithelialized surface, such as grafted burns, partial-thickness burns allowed to close by secondary intention, or healed donor sites. Burn wound impetigo is not related to inadequate excision of the burn, mechanical disruption of the graft, or hematoma formation. Aggressive management is required with appropriate antibiotics in order to avoid graft failure.

## Burn Wound Cellulitis

Burn wound cellulitis is a spreading dermal infection in uninjured skin around a burn wound or donor site, characterized by erythema, tenderness, and induration with an advancing border. It is commonly caused by *S pyogenes*, and the diagnosis is usually based on clinical examination, as cultures are difficult to obtain.[35] In children, toxic shock syndrome needs to be a concern, as this may be their initial presentation. In hospitalized patients, streptococcal infections are much less common, as gram-negative rods and staphylococci are more typical. Gram-negative rods that produce exotoxins, such as *Pseudomonas*, are particularly prone to cause burn wound cellulitis. *Candida* is also a pathogen in patients who have had prolonged courses of antimicrobials, and may be particularly problematic at venous access sites.

## Invasive Burn Wound Infection

Invasive burn wound infection involves invasion of subcutaneous fascia, muscle, or healthy tissue beneath a wound from colonization/infection of overlying eschar. Its incidence is proportional to burn wound size, BSA involvement, and length of time before full coverage. Such patients are usually systemically toxic, with bacteremia and hypotension. The controversy regarding establishing a diagnosis of invasive burn wound infection is discussed in the following section. Since current surgical practice involves early, aggressive excision of burns, invasive infection usually occurs after debridement and is almost always due to gram-negative nosocomial pathogens. Clinical signs of invasive infection in the setting of a toxic patient include a change in the wound's appearance, such as hemorrhage, change in color, drainage, and liquefactive necrosis. In patients who have had recent skin grafts, development of a dusky appearance and separation of the graft is usually the first indication of invasive wound infection. Similarly, underlying infection in patients with allograft should be suspected if discharge is present or if there is clear separation of the allograft from the underlying tissue. Definite invasive burn wound infection is heralded by a change in wound appearance with punctate hemorrhages or rapid liquefaction, systemic toxicity, and positive blood cultures.

## THE DIAGNOSTIC CHALLENGE OF DIFFERENTIATING WOUND COLONIZATION VERSUS INFECTION

As all patients with severe burns become colonized with gram-negative organisms and clinical signs of invasive infection are difficult to discern in these very critically ill patients, determining true infection versus colonization remains challenging. Furthermore, there are no accurate, sensitive, or specific clinical features which can assist clinicians with the decision to initiate antibiotic therapy.

### Quantitative Cultures

Starting in the late 1960s, obtaining tissue biopsy specimens for histological examination and quantitative wound cultures of burns became widely used.[7,36,37] Diagnostic criteria included histological evidence of bacterial invasion beyond the burn eschar and bacteriological criteria of $10^4$ to $10^5$ organisms per gram of tissue. These empirically derived criteria were established during the period before burn excision became the standard of care. Since then, these criteria have been challenged as being overly empiric. Danilla evaluated[38] concordance between 1443 pairs of superficial and quantitative cultures and found mixed results.[38] Steer and colleagues collected 69 paired biopsy samples from 47 patients and found that there was no relationship between

clinical outcome and bacterial counts obtained either by biopsy or by total white cell count.[39,40] From an operational standpoint, quantitative cultures are expensive and involve tissue excision biopsies and complex processing by the clinical microbiology lab. Moreover, results from quantitative cultures using standard bacteriological techniques are typically not available for 3 to 4 days. By this time, the patient's status may have dramatically changed. Because of these problems, some experts, such as Mayhall, have questioned the utility of the procedure.[5] The issue of quantitative culture needs to be revisited for the following reasons:

- The studies which developed the technique were all performed in the clinical era before aggressive surgical excision, where the tissue culture was often burn eschar.
- There are critical clinical questions in learning how to differentiate colonization versus invasive infection, which can be answered by the use of animal models and molecular techniques.
- Development of newer, rapid quantitative molecular techniques can substantially shorten the turnaround time from days to hours.

### Pulmonary Issues

In patients with inhalation injury, pneumonia or tracheobronchitis occurs in approximately 30% of patients.[1,41,42] In our center, we have discovered upper respiratory flora are rapidly replaced with staphylococcal species (including methicillin-resistant *S aureus*, or MRSA) and gram-negative rods. Therefore, vigorous pulmonary toilet is critical, even early in the clinical course. Clinical signs of pulmonary infection may be subtle due to aggressive resuscitation efforts, large fluid shifts, and potential underlying diseases. In addition, trauma and high transfusion requirements in some cases may predispose to acute respiratory distress syndrome (ARDS), which can be very difficult to differentiate from pneumonia.

### Toxic Shock Syndrome in Burns

Toxic shock syndrome (TSS) is a burn complication almost exclusively seen in children.[43,44] TSS should be suspected when there is a sudden unexplained clinical deterioration with findings of fever, poor perfusion, hyponatremia, lymphopenia, and coagulopathy. Mucositis and a macular erythematous rash may be seen on intact skin and mucosal areas. The burn wound itself does not have a characteristic appearance, and the actual burn injury may be minor. Multiple organisms have been implicated in expressing the

179

TSS-associated toxins, including Group A *Streptococcus*, *S aureus*, and some *Pseudomonas* and *Klebsiella* strains. Young and Thornton[43] have proposed that children are susceptible to burn TSS because

- loss of protective skin barrier allows entry of the organisms
- there is functional immunosuppression
- the burn wound provides an ideal environment for toxin production
- pyrexia favors toxin production
- interstitial edema and disruption of surface and vascular clearance mechanisms are present
- the prevalence of antibodies to TSS toxin are directly proportional to age, which explains why burn TSS is almost never seen in adults

## Infectious Complications in the Head and Neck

In burns to the head, neck, and scalp, careful evaluation of the mucous membranes, eyes, ears, and surrounding structures should be performed early,[41,42] as formation of edema can interfere with pertinent findings. The eyes should be promptly evaluated by an ophthalmologist, preferably with fluorescein staining. Careful attention is required throughout the hospital course for development of keratitis, which can be catastrophic if caused by organisms such as *Pseudomonas*. Similarly, burns of the external ear and nose, especially in younger patients, can be complicated by suppurative chondritis. Topical prophylaxis of the eyes with antimicrobial-containing drops which provide high local concentrations and application of topical silver or mafenide acetate to the cartilaginous surfaces largely prevents these complications.

## Nosocomial Infections in Burns

Patients with severe burns often require hospitalization for prolonged periods, with long-term indwelling vascular access devices, urinary catheters, and endotracheal tubes. They are thus susceptible to the complications related to these interventions.

Catheter-associated BSI rates for burn intensive care units (ICUs) enrolled in the CDC's National Nosocomial Infections Surveillance (NNIS) System from January 1995 to June 2002 were 8.8 per 1000 central venous catheter (CVC) days, compared with pooled mean rates of 7.4 for pediatric ICUs, 7.9 for trauma ICUs, and 5.2 for surgical ICUs. These estimates include both the adult and pediatric burn population.[45] The incidence of all complications is higher in patients with larger BSA burns, as demonstrated from a recent study in 2005, which reported blood stream infection at 4.9 episodes per 1000 days, ventilator-associated pneumonia at 11.4 episodes per 1000 days, and urinary tract infections at 13.2 cases per 1000 days.[46] Often overlooked complications of intubation include otitis and sinusitis, which should always be kept in mind when evaluating patients with suspected sepsis.

Bloodstream infections due to *S aureus*, particularly MRSA, have increased. In our current environment, these infections are typically nosocomially acquired and related to indwelling lines rather than to the burn wound itself. MRSA now accounts for up to 70% of all staphylococci isolated in the United States and has become highly virulent.[47,48,49] Endocarditis due to these organisms is a particular concern, as they have a predilection for endocardial tissue. A case series of burn patients with endocarditis has demonstrated that those with staphylococcal bacteremia are particularly susceptible, with an appreciable increase in mortality. Current recommendations for staphylococcal bacteremia include treatment for a minimum of 4 weeks unless endocarditis can be conclusively ruled out.

All patients who remain hospitalized for prolonged periods and are exposed to broad-spectrum antibiotics are at increased risk for *Clostridium difficile* colitis.[50,51] This is less of an issue in the pediatric population than in adults, but can still cause appreciable morbidity and mortality. Prevention of *C difficile* colitis involves aggressive antimicrobial management, minimizing antibiotic exposure, and strict infection control measures. Clinically, *C difficile* colitis should be suspected in any patient with diarrhea and leukocytosis. Diagnosis requires identification of the toxin by cytotoxic assay. Empiric therapy with orally administered metronidazole or vancomycin should be initiated and continued for 10 to 14 days if the diagnosis is confirmed.

## Noninfectious Masqueraders

Acute hypotension in critically ill patients can also be caused by underlying noninfectious medical conditions. Critically ill patients, and burn patients in particular, may not necessarily manifest any symptoms, and diseases with cutaneous manifestations may not be evident because of the burn injury. In particular, the clinician should be attuned to

- Hypovolemia. Insensate fluid losses can be enormous, and fluid management, even in the most closely monitored circumstances, may be inadequate. Burn patients with SIRS-induced fever and hypovolemia can be misdiagnosed with sepsis and even septic shock.

- Endocrinopathies. Hypothyroidism and hypoadrenalism may result in hypotension and cardiovascular lability, including low cardiac output. In particular, patients without prior disease who have minimal thyroid or adrenal function can be tipped into crisis by the extreme metabolic demands of a burn injury. Clinicians should have a low threshold for evaluating the thyroid and adrenal axis.
- Hyperthyroidism/Thyroid Storm. This will present with persistent tachycardia, fever, and leukocytosis. Thyroid storm can be precipitated in patients with underlying hyperthyroidism who suffer a major injury. Patients exhibiting persistent tachycardia even after euvolemia is achieved should be suspected of manifesting thyroid dysfunction.

## PRINCIPLES OF DIAGNOSIS AND TREATMENT

The approach to managing infections in burn patients is predicated on the following principles:

- In the majority of cases, pediatric burn patients have minimal underlying disease and can manifest a robust inflammatory response.
- Surveillance cultures are obtained to identify existing organisms in case the patient becomes clinically septic. Treatment decisions, however, are not based on surveillance cultures alone.
- Patients with major BSA injuries will have a prolonged hospitalization and are susceptible to infection because of interruption of the skin barrier and multiple invasive devices.
- Antimicrobials, and especially broad-spectrum drugs, are critical for treating documented or highly suspected infection. Prolonged courses of these drugs will subsequently result in selection of antimicrobial-resistant organisms, predilection to fungal infection, and complications such as *C difficile*. Therefore, the shortest course of therapy should be used.
- Since patients will be colonized with multiple organisms, the decision to treat an infection should not be based solely on a culture that shows organisms. Rather, clinical indicators of infection need to be present as well.
- Differentiating SIRS from infection can be difficult, especially early in the patient's course. Furthermore, fever and leukocytosis have poor predictive value for sepsis. The likelihood of infection is low in patients with fever and leukocytosis if the following are not present:

  - hypotension
  - infiltrate on chest X-ray (for intubated patients)
  - clinical diagnosis of invasive wound infection

- Empiric treatment for burn infection or sepsis often involves use of broad-spectrum antimicrobials. Therapy should be "trimmed and tailored" to be as narrow spectrum as possible once an etiological diagnosis is made.
- With the exception of staphylococcal bacteremia, there is no prescribed time course for treatment. Once a removable source is debrided or drained, then antimicrobials can be discontinued 24 to 48 hours afterwards. Gram-negative bacteremia should be treated with courses of therapy for 5 to 7 days after documented clearance, assuming that all removable sources have been addressed.

## CLINICAL STRATEGIES AND APPROACH TO SPECIFIC PROBLEMS

Patients admitted to any burn facility should receive tetanus prophylaxis. Burn management, including excision, debridement, and coverage, is the most important aspect of infection prevention and management. Patients admitted to the ICU who are intubated or expected to have prolonged stays for multiple excisions should be considered for fluconazole prophylaxis.[27]

### Surveillance Cultures

Cultures of skin and other suspicious sites should be performed on admission to the facility in order to ascertain what organisms are colonizing the host skin, such as MRSA. This is particularly important if there are postburn environmental exposures or if the burn itself was related to water exposure (scald) where waterborne organisms may be involved. Biweekly surveillance cultures should be obtained in intubated patients (tracheal aspirates) and from burn wound sites, preferably by swab after debridement. As noted above, the utility of quantitative cultures for clinical decision making is controversial.

### Management Strategies

**Days 1 to 3 of hospitalization.** During the early hospitalization, infectious complications of burns are rare. Nearly all episodes of fever and leukocytosis during this time are due to burn-induced SIRS. Antimicrobials should not be administered unless there is a clear indication of sepsis.

**Days 4 to 7 of hospitalization.** During this period, discriminating burn-induced SIRS from infectious complications is difficult. In our experience, most infections during this period are caused by community-acquired organisms, although there is substantial local variation. Infections due to complications from indwelling catheters begin to arise. Appropriate cultures should be obtained, and regimens with effectiveness against *Pseudomonas* and resistant staphylococci should be initiated. Initial regimens used in our center include

- vancomycin + piperacillin/tazobactam
- vancomycin + ceftazidime
- vancomycin + cefipime

Vancomycin can be discontinued if cultures do not reveal staphylococci within 48 hours.

After obtaining cultures, it is necessary to ensure they are monitored. In our experience, over half of such cultures indicate sensitive organisms such as gram-negative enterics. In these cases, we recommend changing antibiotic coverage to the narrowest coverage possible in order to reduce the pressure for selection of more resistant organisms. For example, if blood or fluid cultures grow *Escherichia coli*–sensitive to first-generation cephalosporins, we would reduce coverage to maximal dose cefazolin. Second- and third-generation cephalosporin drugs such as cefotetan, ceftriaxone, or ampicillin/clavulanate are appropriate if the organisms' susceptibility is demonstrated.

**After day 7 of hospitalization.** At this point in time, burn-induced SIRS becomes less relevant, although increases in temperature and leukocytosis following debridement are more common. Colonization of the burn wound by nosocomial gram-negative organisms is nearly universal. Treatment for infection should be initiated if there are systemic signs of persistent fever (> 39°C), episodes of hypotension, or evidence of burn wound infection, such as indications of burn wound cellulitis or invasive burn wound infection or skin graft failure.

Management strategies should include source control, particularly excision of wound surfaces that are clinically infected. After cultures are obtained from all sources, empiric antimicrobials should be initiated. Our practice is to initiate treatment with a carbapenem, such as imipenem, meropenem, or doripenem, in combination with vancomycin. Treatment should be guided by knowledge of the surveillance wound or other source cultures if results are < 24 hours old. As above, reducing coverage to the narrowest regimen as soon as is appropriate is highly encouraged.

## Special Circumstances

**Surgical prophylaxis.** As standard surgical prophylaxis regimens predebridement are relatively ineffective against most burn-associated pathogens, such practice is not generally advised.

**Intubated patients with inhalation injury.** Inhalation injury produces an inflammatory response, especially if caustic substances are involved. We do not routinely recommend antimicrobial prophylaxis, but prefer close observation. After initial stabilization, daily Gram stains and sputum cultures of tracheal aspirates are recommended. In > 80% of patients who remain intubated, tracheitis or tracheobronchitis will occur, typically due to *S aureus* at days 5 to 7. This should be treated with a short course of antimicrobials (5-7 days) guided by susceptibility reports.

**Bacteremia.** When bacteremia is documented, all indwelling intravascular catheters should be changed, if feasible. Since burn patients often have very poor vascular access, if changing access sites is not possible, then the catheters should be changed over guidewires. Some data suggests lower rates of infection with silver-impregnated catheters.

**Staphylococcal bacteremia.** *S aureus* is a highly invasive organism which is particularly prone to cause metastatic infection and involve the endocardium.[52] Echocardiography, preferably trans-esophageal echocardiography, should be performed in all cases of staphylococcal bacteremia. In patients who remain bacteremic after 24 hours of therapy, occult abscesses and additional sources of infection should be considered; this includes careful physical examination and tomographic scanning of the chest, abdomen, and pelvis.

**Pneumonia.** Pneumonia in critically ill hospitalized patients should be managed using protocols for ventilator-associated pneumonia. Empiric antimicrobials should be included in such protocols as well.

***Pseudomonas* wound infection.** Burn patients are particularly at risk for wound infection due to *Pseudomonas*. These should be aggressively treated with local debridement and systemic antimicrobial therapy. Dual therapy with aminoglycoside and beta-lactam combinations is not indicated in most cases.[53-55] However, deterioration of renal function should prompt reevaluation and potential discontinuation.

## Prevention of Burn Infections

The pathogenesis of burn infections is clearly related to disruption of the surface epithelium, which allows access of microorganisms. Early excision, aggressive debridement of necrotic tissue, and rapid progress towards grafting is critical. However, these steps take time, especially in patients with extensive injuries.

**Topical dressings.**[56,57] Topical dressings are used ubiquitously, and silver-containing dressings have been largely credited with reducing morbidity and mortality from burn sepsis since the 1960s.

Silver sulfadiazine is a widely used agent with excellent broad-spectrum activity which is used in the United States for second- and third-degree burns. Its silver ions bind to nucleic acids of individual microorganisms and release sulfadiazine, which poisons the microbe's metabolism. The major complication of silver-containing dressings is silver-induced leukopenia. Although this can occur at any time, it is typically seen within the first week of use and manifests as a progressive decrease in the leukocyte count. Thought to be due to bone marrow suppression, it is reversible with discontinuation of silver-containing dressings. In severe cases of leukopenia, use of Neupogen as a temporizing measure can be considered if leukocyte counts are < 1000.

Mafenide acetate (Sulfamylon) has predominantly bacteriostatic activity against gram-negative bacteria, including *Pseudomonas*, as well as anaerobes such as *Clostridium*. There is little activity against gram-positive organisms such as *S aureus* or fungi. Mafenide is indicated for bacterial invasion of second- and third-degree wounds. Because of its high soft tissue and cartilage penetration, it is particularly useful in settings where underlying tissue may be involved, such as deep burns, or in burns overlying cartilaginous areas, such as the ear or nose. Although resistance to mafenide is rare, it needs to be used with care because it is painful on application and has been associated with impaired wound healing. Patients with large burns are at risk for metabolic acidosis since the drug is an inhibitor of carbonic anhydrase.

Bacitracin/neomycin/polymyxin B is frequently used for superficial burn wounds, but can be employed as a second-line dressing in patients who have experienced adverse effects to silver or mafenide. It has antimicrobial activity against gram-positive bacteria; the addition of neomycin and polymyxin B bolsters gram-negative coverage.

## Isolation and Infection Control[58]

In an ideal setting, all patients would have 1:1 nursing and implementation of barrier contact precautions. Since this is not feasible, standard precautions, which include aggressive compliance monitoring for hand washing, checklist procedures for insertion and maintenance of catheters and other invasive devices, and scrupulous attention to respiratory hygiene and wound care, should be followed when caring for all patients with burn injury.

Pediatric burn patients should also have policies restricting the presence of nonwashable toys such as stuffed animals and cloth objects, which can harbor large numbers of bacteria and can be difficult to disinfect. Toys should be nonporous and washable, designated for individual patient use, and thoroughly disinfected after use and before being given to another child. Paper items, such as storybooks and coloring books, should always be designated for single-patient use and should be disposed of if they become grossly contaminated or when the child is discharged.

In summary, burn infections in pediatric patients cause substantial morbidity and mortality. The menu of organisms involved is diverse, and treatment can be complex.

# TABLE

## TABLE 1
**Microorganisms causing invasive burn wound infections.**

**Gram-positive Organisms**

*Streptococcus pyogenes*

*Staphylococcus aureus*

Methicillin-resistant *S aureus*

*Enterococcus* species

Vancomycin-resistant enterococci

**Gram-negative Organisms**

*Pseudomonas aeruginosa*

*Escherichia coli* and other entericsi

*Klebsiella pneumoniae*

*Serratia marcescens*

*Enterobacter* species

*Proteus* species

*Acinetobacter* species

*Bacteroides* species

**MDR-resistant Species**

MDR-*Acinetobacter*

MDR-*Serratia*

MDR-*Pseudomonas*

ESBL-*Enterobacter*

KPC-*Klebsiella*

**Fungi**

*Candida* species

*Aspergillus* species

*Fusarium* species

*Alternaria* species

*Rhizopus* species

*Mucor* species

**Dosing Recommendations (Maximal Dosing for Suspected Sepsis in Burns)**

Amikacin: 5 mg/kg first dose; subsequent 5 to 7.5 mg/kg every 8 hours; adjust dose to maintain trough 2 to 5 µg/ml

Cefipime: 50 mg/kg every 8 hours

Ceftazidime: 50 mg/kg every 8 hours

Imipenem: 25 mg/kg every 6 hours

Meropenem: 20 mg/kg every 8 hours

Piperacillin/Tazobactam: 100 mg (piperacillin) every 8 hours up to maximal adult dose

Vancomycin: 15 mg/kg every 6 hours—dose by level

# REFERENCES

1. Church D, Elsayed S, Reid O, Winston B, Lindsay R. Burn wound infections. *Clin Microbiol Rev.* 2006; **19**: 403–434.

2. Palmieri TL, Greenhalgh DG, Saffle JR, et al. A multicenter review of toxic epidermal necrolysis treated in U.S. burn centers at the end of the twentieth century. *J Burn Care Rehabil.* 2002; **23**: 87–96.

3. Weber JM, Sheridan RL, Schulz JT, Tompkins RG, Ryan CM. Effectiveness of bacteria-controlled nursing units in preventing cross-colonization with resistant bacteria in severely burned children. *Infect Control Hosp Epidemiol.* 2002; **23**: 549–551.

4. de Macedo JL, Rosa SC, Castro C. Sepsis in burned patients. *Rev Soc Bras Med Trop.* 2003; **36**: 647–652.

5. Mayhall CG. The epidemiology of burn wound infections: then and now. *Clin Infect Dis.* 2003; **37**: 543–550.

6. Atiyeh BS, Gunn SW, Hayek SN. State of the art in burn treatment. *World J Surg.* 2005; **29**: 131–148.

7. Pruitt BA Jr, McManus AT, Kim SH, Goodwin CW. Burn wound infections: current status. *World J Surg.* 1998; **22**: 135–145.

8. Agnihotri N, Gupta V, Joshi RM. Aerobic bacterial isolates from burn wound infections and their antibiograms—a five-year study. *Burns.* 2004; **30**: 241–243.

9. Bonomo RA, Szabo D. Mechanisms of multidrug resistance in *Acinetobacter* species and *Pseudomonas aeruginosa. Clin Infect Dis.* 2006; **43**(suppl 2): S49–S56.

10. Paterson DL. The epidemiological profile of infections with multidrug-resistant *Pseudomonas aeruginosa* and *Acinetobacter* species. *Clin Infect Dis.* 2006; **43**(suppl 2): S43–S48.

11. Ozkurt Z, Ertek M, Erol S, Altoparlak U, Akcay MN. The risk factors for acquisition of imipenem-resistant *Pseudomonas aeruginosa* in the burn unit. *Burns.* 2005; **31**: 870–873.

12. Wong TH, Tan BH, Ling ML, Song C. Multi-resistant *Acinetobacter baumannii* on a burns unit—clinical risk factors and prognosis. *Burns.* 2002; **28**: 349–357.

13. Bayat A, Shaaban H, Dodgson A, Dunn KW. Implications for burns unit design following outbreak of multi-resistant *Acinetobacter* infection in ICU and burns unit. *Burns.* 2003; **29**: 303–306.

14. Griffith ME, Gonzalez RS, Holcomb JB, Hospenthal DR, Wortmann GW, Murray CK. Factors associated with recovery of *Acinetobacter baumannii* in a combat support hospital. *Infect Control Hosp Epidemiol.* 2008; **29**: 664–666.

15. Maragakis LL, Perl TM. *Acinetobacter baumannii*: epidemiology, antimicrobial resistance, and treatment options. *Clin Infect Dis.* 2008; **46**: 1254–1263.

16. Munoz-Price LS, Weinstein RA. *Acinetobacter* infection. *N Engl J Med.* 2008; **358**: 1271–1281.

17. Erol S, Altoparlak U, Akcay MN, Celebi F, Parlak M. Changes of microbial flora and wound colonization in burned patients. *Burns.* 2004; **30**: 357–361.

18. Landman D, Butnariu M, Bratu S, Quale J. Genetic relatedness of multidrug-resistant *Acinetobacter baumannii* endemic to New York City. *Epidemiol Infect.* 2009; **137**: 174–180.

19. Murray CK, Hospenthal DR. *Acinetobacter* infection in the ICU. *Crit Care Clin.* 2008; **24**: 237–248.

20. Murray CK, Hospenthal DR. Treatment of multidrug resistant *Acinetobacter. Curr Opin Infect Dis.* 2005; **18**: 502–506.

21. Davis KA, Moran KA, McAllister CK, Gray PJ. Multidrug-resistant *Acinetobacter* extremity infections in soldiers. *Emerg Infect Dis.* 2005; **11**: 1218–1224.

22. Herruzo R, de la Cruz J, Fernandez-Acenero MJ, Garcia-Caballero J. Two consecutive outbreaks of *Acinetobacter baumanii* 1-a in a burn intensive care unit for adults. *Burns.* 2004; **30**: 419–423.

23. Paterson DL, Bonomo RA. Extended-spectrum beta-lactamases: a clinical update. *Clin Microbiol Rev.* 2005; **18**: 657–686.

24. Walsh TR. Clinically significant carbapenemases: an update. *Curr Opin Infect Dis.* 2008; **21**: 367–371.

25. Pournaras S, Markogiannakis A, Ikonomidis A, et al. Outbreak of multiple clones of imipenem-resistant *Acinetobacter baumannii* isolates expressing OXA-58 carbapenemase in an intensive care unit. *J Antimicrob Chemother.* 2006; **57**: 557–561.

26. Cochran A, Morris SE, Edelman LS, Saffle JR. Systemic *Candida* infection in burn patients: a case-control study of management patterns and outcomes. *Surg Infect (Larchmt).* 2002; **3**: 367–374.

27. Pelz RK, Hendrix CW, Swoboda SM, et al. Double-blind placebo-controlled trial of fluconazole to prevent candidal infections in critically ill surgical patients. *Ann Surg.* 2001; 233: 542–548.

28. Murray CK, Loo FL, Hospenthal DR, et al. Incidence of systemic fungal infection and related mortality following severe burns. *Burns.* 2008; **34**: 1108–1112.

29. Ribes JA, Vanover-Sams CL, Baker DJ. Zygomycetes in human disease. *Clin Microbiol Rev.* 2000; **13**: 236–301.

30. Greenhalgh DG, Saffle JR, Holmes JH IV, et al. American Burn Association consensus conference to define sepsis and infection in burns. *J Burn Care Res.* 2007; **28**: 776–790.

31. Murray CK, Hoffmaster RM, Schmit DR, Hospenthal DR, Ward JA, Cancio LC, Wolf SE. Evaluation of white blood cell count, neutrophil percentage, and elevated temperature as predictors of bloodstream infection in burn patients. Arch Surg. 2007 Jul; **142**(7): 639–642.

32. Keen A, Knoblock L, Edelman L, Saffle J. Effective limitation of blood culture use in the burn unit. *J Burn Care Rehabil.* 2002; **23**: 183–189.

33. Upperman JS, Sheridan RL. Pediatric trauma susceptibility to sepsis. *Pediatr Crit Care Med.* 2005; **6**: S108–S111.

34. Upperman JS, Sheridan RL, Marshall J. Pediatric surgical site and soft tissue infections. *Pediatr Crit Care Med.* 2005; **6**: S36–S41.

35. Edwards-Jones V, Greenwood JE; Manchester Burns Research Group. What's new in burn microbiology? James Laing Memorial Prize Essay 2000. *Burns.* 2003; **29**: 15–24.

36. Robson MC, Heggers JP. Bacterial quantification of open wounds. *Mil Med*. 1969; **134**: 19–24.

37. Robson MC, Heggers JP. Delayed wound closure based on bacterial counts. *J Surg Oncol*. 1970; **2**: 379–383.

38. Danilla S, Andrades P, Gomez ME, et al. Concordance between qualitative and quantitative cultures in burned patients. Analysis of 2886 cultures. *Burns*. 2005; **31**: 967–971.

39. Steer JA, Papini RP, Wilson AP, McGrouther DA, Parkhouse N. Quantitative microbiology in the management of burn patients. II. Relationship between bacterial counts obtained by burn wound biopsy culture and surface alginate swab culture, with clinical outcome following burn surgery and change of dressings. *Burns*. 1996; **22**: 177–181.

40. Steer JA, Papini RP, Wilson AP, McGrouther DA, Parkhouse N. Quantitative microbiology in the management of burn patients. I. Correlation between quantitative and qualitative burn wound biopsy culture and surface alginate swab culture. *Burns*. 1996; **22**: 173–176.

41. Sheridan RL. Burns. *Crit Care Med*. 2002; **30**: S500–S514.

42. Sheridan RL. Comprehensive treatment of burns. *Curr Probl Surg*. 2001; **38**: 657–756.

43. Young AE, Thornton KL. Toxic shock syndrome in burns: diagnosis and management. *Arch Dis Child Educ Pract Ed*. 2007; **92**: ep97–ep100.

44. White MC, Thornton K, Young AE. Early diagnosis and treatment of toxic shock syndrome in paediatric burns. *Burns*. 2005; **31**: 193–197.

45. Weber J, McManus A; Nursing Committee of the International Society for Burn Injuries. Infection control in burn patients. *Burns*. 2004; **30**: A16–A24.

46. Wisplinghoff H, Bischoff T, Tallent SM, Seifert H, Wenzel RP, Edmond MB. Nosocomial bloodstream infections in US hospitals: analysis of 24,179 cases from a prospective nationwide surveillance study. *Clin Infect Dis*. 2004; **39**: 309–317.

47. Daum RS. Clinical practice. Skin and soft-tissue infections caused by methicillin-resistant *Staphylococcus aureus*. *N Engl J Med*. 2007; **357**: 380–390.

48. Burton DC, Edwards JR, Horan TC, Jernigan JA, Fridkin SK. Methicillin-resistant *Staphylococcus aureus* central line-associated bloodstream infections in US intensive care units, 1997–2007. *JAMA*. 2009; **301**: 727–736.

49. Klevens RM, Morrison MA, Nadle J, et al. Invasive methicillin-resistant *Staphylococcus aureus* infections in the United States. *JAMA*. 2007; **298**: 1763–1771.

50. Rice LB. The Maxwell Finland lecture: for the duration-rational antibiotic administration in an era of antimicrobial resistance and *Clostridium difficile*. *Clin Infect Dis*. 2008; **46**: 491–496.

51. Owens RC Jr, Donskey CJ, Gaynes RP, Loo VG, Muto CA. Antimicrobial-associated risk factors for *Clostridium difficile* infection. *Clin Infect Dis*. 2008; **46**(suppl 1): S19–S31.

52. Baddour LM, Wilson WR, Bayer AS, et al. Infective endocarditis: diagnosis, antimicrobial therapy, and management of complications: a statement for healthcare professionals from the Committee on Rheumatic Fever, Endocarditis, and Kawasaki Disease, Council on Cardiovascular Disease in the Young, and the Councils on Clinical Cardiology, Stroke, and Cardiovascular Surgery and Anesthesia, American Heart Association: endorsed by the Infectious Diseases Society of America. *Circulation*. 2005; **111**: e394–e434.

53. Magnotti LJ, Schroeppel TJ, Clement LP, et al. Efficacy of monotherapy in the treatment of *Pseudomonas* ventilator-associated pneumonia in patients with trauma. *J Trauma*. 2009; **66**: 8,1052, discussion 1058–1059.

54. Paul M, Silbiger I, Grozinsky S, Soares-Weiser K, Leibovici L. Beta lactam antibiotic monotherapy versus beta lactam-aminoglycoside antibiotic combination therapy for sepsis. *Cochrane Database Syst Rev*. 2006; **1**: CD003344.

55. Goverman J, Weber JM, Keaney TJ, Sheridan RL. Intravenous colistin for the treatment of multi-drug resistant, gram-negative infection in the pediatric burn population. *J Burn Care Res*. 2007; **28**: 421–426.

56. Patel PP, Vasquez SA, Granick MS, Rhee ST. Topical antimicrobials in pediatric burn wound management. *J Craniofac Surg*. 2008; **19**: 913–922.

57. D'Avignon LC, Saffle JR, Chung KK, Cancio LC. Prevention and management of infections associated with burns in the combat casualty. *J Trauma*. 2008; **64**: S277–S286.

58. Weber J, McManus A; Nursing Committee of the International Society for Burn Injuries. Infection control in burn patients. *Burns*. 2004; **30**: A16–A24.

# CHAPTER FOURTEEN

# FUNGAL INFECTIONS

BRADLEY J. PHILLIPS, MD

MARISSA CARTER, PHD

## INTRODUCTION

Fungal infections are always a source of concern in burn patients due to their underlying dysfunctional immune system, particularly when the burned area is extensive (> 60% TBSA—total body surface area). Besides the issue of immunocompetence, other sources of infection, including central venous lines, urinary catheters, prolonged mechanical ventilation, and broad-spectrum antibiotics, make burn patients one of the highest at-risk groups for invasive infection.[1,2] While newer antifungal agents have added to the armory available for clinicians to combat infection, certain fungal species still present problems, and the possibility of drug resistance must be borne in mind. An appreciation of the problem is best attained by examining both the past and current incidence of fungal infection as well as ascertaining trends from the data over the last 40 years. However, since pediatric-specific evidence is sparse in terms of fungal burn infection, we will try to draw lessons from the adult literature whenever possible.

## Incidence of Fungal Infections in Burn Patients

When assessing fungal infections over the past few decades in order to draw meaningful conclusions, one has to appreciate the progress of scientific technique. In this case, this translates to understanding that the characterization methods used today were less sophisticated 30 years ago. Furthermore, management of bacterial and fungal infections was different in terms of available options, and this in turn affected both the incidence and type of infection reported.

### Reports Prior to 1986

MacMillan et al[3] were among the first to publish data on candidiasis in burn patients based on a data collection period from 1964 through 1971. Of their 427 patients, 63.5% had at least one positive *Candida* culture, and 54.6% had positive cultures on more than one occasion. *Candida albicans* was the most common species isolated (43%). Although the

*Candida* organism was cultured from wounds in 58.6% of patients, 12% of positive cultures were obtained from urine, 11% from stools, and 9% from intravenous catheters. Of the 22 patients who developed *Candida* septicemia, 14 died (64%). A follow-up study by the same group at the Shriners Burns Institute in Cincinnati revealed that of 12 patients diagnosed with candidemia who had burns >30% TBSA, 5 patients had infections from *C albicans* and 7 patients' infections were from *C tropicalis*.[4] In the United Kingdom, Kidson and Lowbury[5] reported a 12.9% incidence of positive *Candida* cultures from wound isolates in 922 burn patients over a period of 2 years during the mid- to late 1970s. Of these cultures, 69% were due to *C albicans*, 12% to *C parapsilosis*, 5% to *C stellatoidea*, 4% each to *C krusei* and *C pseudotropicalis*, and 2% to *C tropicalis*. The authors also noted a positive association between percentage of TBSA burned and the appearance of positive cultures. Their explanation for the lower rate of positive *Candida* cultures compared to MacMillan et al[3] was due to a lower proportion of severely burned patients.

In 1979, Stone et al[6] reported the first study on *Aspergillus* infection in burn patients for the period 1963 through 1977, calculating an incidence rate of 0.5%. The authors also noted a much higher average TBSA burned (54%) and percentage of full-thickness injury (42%) in these patients compared to the general burn patient population. From an epidemiological viewpoint, the *Aspergillus* infections were episodic in 13 of the 18 cases, with the first outbreak involving 6 patients due to colonized air-conditioning ducts and filters in the burn unit. Although a maintenance cleaning schedule was initiated, new filters were still not available several years later. Therefore, the old filters were cleaned *in situ*, which resulted in an immediate cluster of 4 separate wound colonizations with the organism. Although this study was not the first to investigate the source of fungal infections, it remains a vivid illustration of the importance of maintaining good hygiene in burn units.

The experience of Spebar and Pruitt[7] in regard to candidiasis in the burned patient at the US Army Institute of Surgical Research at Fort Sam Houston, Texas, which spanned a time period from 1973 through 1978, was similar to previous reports.[3,5] Of the 1513 patients admitted for treatment, 521 (34.4%) had positive fungal cultures, and 86.7% of these patients were positive for *Candida*. While only 36 patients developed burn wound infection, 75% of these patients had candidemia, with a mortality rate for the entire group (36 patients) of 92%. The higher mortality rate was initially ascribed to the prolonged time (1 week) required to identify *Candida* in blood cultures and the delay in initiating amphotericin B treatment. However, the authors also pointed out that the invasive phase was invariably caused by an episode of bacterial sepsis, hemorrhage, or

hypotension that permitted existing colonization to expand out of control.

## 1986 through 1995

In their review of patients with thermal burns during 1984 and 1985, Pensler et al[8] noted an increased incidence of fungal sepsis with a mortality rate of 32%. Furthermore, they found that capricious use of broad-spectrum antibiotics aggravated the establishment of sepsis after wound colonization by fungi. Similar to previous studies, Desai et al[9] reported that 31.8% of their burn patients had a positive *Candida* culture during hospitalization. However, they observed a trend toward earlier *Candida* septicemia, which was ascribed to early, repeated surgical interventions, large transfusions, and more widespread use of broad-spectrum antibiotics in massively burned, immunosuppressed patients. Prevention, early detection, and aggressive treatment of candidiasis were promoted by Prasad et al,[10] who reported lower overall culture rates (13.5%), but higher rates of mortality (54%). However, these authors also reported that death in the majority of cases was due to bacterial septicemia or multiple organ failure (MOF). Similar positive *Candida* rates were reported in a much smaller study, but with much lower sepsis and mortality rates.[11]

During the mid- to late 1980s, there was a surge in the use of nystatin. By 1983, Desai and Herndon[12] reported the incidence of *Candida* burn wound infection had been steadily increasing at the Shriners Burns Institute in Galveston, Texas. This resulted in a change of practice in late 1984 to oral nystatin use ("swish and swallow") as well as for wound treatment. According to the authors of this study, this resulted in an order of magnitude decrease in *Candida* cultures and also eliminated cases of *Candida*-related septicemia. An extension of this study, in which burn patients admitted from 1980 through 1984 served as case controls versus patients admitted from 1985 through 1990 who were treated with nystatin, seemed to confirm these findings. A reduction in *Candida* colonization from 26.6% to 15.6% and a reduction in *Candida* sepsis rate from 3.3% to 0% was observed, as well as a reduction in patients with infection from 5.7% to 1.6%.[13] Dubé et al[14] also reported a reduction in *Candida*-positive cultures in burn patients from 15.5% to 10.5% as a result of the institution of nystatin therapy. However, the introduction of nystatin into the burn environment also resulted in a shift of *Candida* species, with a predominance of nystatin-resistant *C rugosa*.

Characterization of *Candida* isolates during this period of time showed small to moderate differences from previously reported results[3-5]: *C albicans* 72.6%; *C tropicalis* 9.7%; *C parapsilosis* 5.3%; multiple *Candida* species 11.5% (pediatric patients)[15]; and *C albicans* 75%; *C parapsilosis* 13%;

*C tropicalis* 6%; *C glabrata* 6% (adults).[16] A serotype/biotype analysis also revealed significant differences between burn and nonburn populations regarding metabolism (ability to utilize citrate). It further suggested that the partial -57 *C albicans* biotype might be either more common or more virulent compared to other biotypes.[15]

A follow-up review from 1979 through 1989 at the US Army Institute of Surgical Research revealed a rate of fungal wound infection of 6.7%,[17] with a mortality rate of 75% for this group of patients. While the rate of bacterial infections decreased during this period, the fungal infection rate remained steady. Although the causative agent of the infections could not be identified in many cases, the majority were caused by *Aspergillus* and *Fusarium* (68%), followed by *Candida* species (18%), *Mucor* and *Rhizopus* (9.1%), and *Microspora* and *Alternaria* species (each causing < 5% of infections). This pattern of infection was quite different from those reported by other studies. The authors also commented that, in their opinion, a previous study[12] which claimed that nystatin was effective against candidal infections was flawed due to diagnostic and procedural issues. A preference for amphotericin B, in combination with other antifungal agents, was noted by Becker et al.[17]

Another study conducted over 3¼ years on the management of *Candida* septicemia in burn patients reported a combined rate of bacterial/fungal infection of 6.9%, with almost one-third of these patients having positive blood cultures for *Candida*.[18] The species breakdown was *C albicans* 48%; *C parapsilosis* 28%; and *C tropicalis* 14%, with multiple species causing 10% of *Candida* infections. The *Candida* colonization rates reported over 5 years in a pediatric investigation during a similar time frame were 14.4%, but only 12% of these children developed candidemia.[19] A mortality rate of 24% was recorded, despite administration of nystatin (enteral), amphotericin B, and other antifungal drugs. The proportions of *Candida* species were similar to the study of Still et al.[18] Furthermore, the researchers demonstrated that recovery of fungal organisms at multiple sites was associated with candidemia.

## *1996 Onward*

To a large extent, the fungal species that cause burn wound infections are a reflection of their presence in the immediate environment. An Iraqi study documented that of 132 patients, 21.2% developed a fungal infection, and all except 1 were coinfected with bacterial species. *Aspergillus* was the most common fungal organism (53%), followed by *Candida* (31%)—of which *C krusei* and *C tropicalis* were the most common species—then *Penicillium* spp and *Zygomycetes* spp (8% each).[21] Although *A Niger* was the most common isolate in patients and burn care units, *A terreus*,

*Penicillium*, *Fusarium*, and *Zygomycetes* spp were more commonly found in burn wards compared to control sites, and were also isolated from patients. This indicates that dissemination of fungi from wounds to surroundings and reintroduction into patients was probably occurring.

A Brazilian investigation of patients (N = 203) with a mean TBSA burn of 15% conducted from February 2004 to February 2005 sampled wounds and cultured fungal organisms 4 times over a period of 1 month.[21] Approximately 12% of patients had a positive culture from the first swab, with *C tropicalis* and *C parapsilosis* accounting for the majority of organisms; however, by the time of the second swab, *C tropicalis* was dominant. The relatively high incidence of *C tropicalis* was considered alarming, as the species was not considered commensal and was nearly always associated with deep fungal infections. Interestingly, a similarly sized Indian study (N = 220) demonstrated a much higher colonization rate (63%) and a different prevalence of *Candida* species: *C albicans* (45%), *C tropicalis* (33%), *C glabrata* (13.5%), *C parapsilosis* (4%), *C krusei* (2.8%), and *C kefyr* (1.8%).[22]

The most recent study of fungal infection, which comprised 15 institutions and 6918 burn patients over the period 2003-2004, indicated an overall infection rate of 6.3% for patients admitted for acute burns.[2] Of those with a positive fungal infection, *Candida* was documented in 85.3% of patients, *Aspergillus* in 13.1%, unspecified yeast infections in 21.5%, other types of molds in 9.0%, and unidentified fungal species in 1.4%. Interestingly, 26.7% of patients had more than one organism cultured, with wounds, respiratory, urine, and blood being the most common sites of infection. The overall mortality rate in culture-positive patients was 13.3%, but was higher (21.2%) for the subgroup in which systematic antifungal treatment was instituted. The mortality rate was 11.6% for candidal infection, 25% for *Aspergillus*, and 41% for molds. This disturbing result for molds translated into an odds ratio (OR) of 11.99 in regard to mortality.

## Trends in the Last 40 Years

Since the introduction of broad-spectrum antibiotics and better care, there is no doubt that the incidence of bacterial wound infections has substantially decreased. While fungal infections were considered more of a nuisance prior to 1970, the advent of effective topical antibiotics, such as mafenide acetate, had serious consequences. Subsequently, fungal colonization of burn wounds became a serious problem during the 1970s and 1980s, with as many as 85% of patients affected.[2,23] Moreover, the change in the prevalence of fungal species, part of which may have resulted from the widespread use of nystatin, has presented challenging problems. The explanation for these observations is complex and is best understood by the interaction of fungi with changing drug patterns and practices as well as environments. In addition, the appearance of high-risk populations with compromised immune systems has had an impact on the prevalence of fungal infection.[24]

Although candidemia rates in acute, nonburn clinical settings rose during the 1980s and appeared to peak with a downward trend in the last few years,[24-26] a similar trend in burn units does not appear to have happened. Rather, although infection rates in most burn units rose during the 1970s and 1980s but declined thereafter, such rates appear to be holding steady around 5% to 8% for the last 10 to 15 years (with some exceptions reported of lower or higher rates). Also of concern is the appearance of other *Candida* spp, such as *C tropicalis*, *C parapsilosis*, *C glabrata*, and *C krusei*, whose increase in prevalence has in some instances caused treatment problems due to drug resistance.

The most important statistic, however, is the mortality rate from fungal wound infections. This appears to have remained unchanged in recent years despite the introduction of newer antifungal agents, such as the echinocandins.[27] Again, this is not a universal experience in all burn units, which may represent different practices, such as more aggressive treatment or prophylaxis, that are more effective in their settings. In the future, the challenge for burn specialists will be learning and incorporating techniques that effectively reduce colonization, infection, and mortality from fungal species.

## PATHOPHYSIOLOGY

### Candida

Even though more than 200 species of *Candida* are known, 99% of cases seen in the burn unit will be confined to about half a dozen species. Although most fungi are dimorphic, existing in the yeast and mycelial or filamentous hyphae form and switching from the filamentous to yeast form in the body, *Candida* is an exception. Instead, it propagates in the yeast form in the environment, then reproduces as blastospores in the body, which elongate and stick together to produce hyphae and pseudohyphae (a combination of yeast and filamentous forms). Most *Candida* species are commensal inhabitants of skin as well as the mucosal membranes of the respiratory, gastrointestinal, and genitourinary tracts. Many *Candida* species have been isolated from the environment as well. Thus, in burn patients, who have compromised immune systems, colonization normally proceeds from an endogenous source. However, several studies have demonstrated that infection

from exogenous sources does occur in hospital settings, even in specialized units where scrupulous hygiene is practiced.[26] This further emphasizes the susceptibility of burn patients to fungal infections, especially those whose percentage of TBSA burned is high. For example, a French study that utilized random amplified polymorphic DNA as a typing method to track *C albicans* in a burn unit found that some profiles of isolates showed a particular geographic pattern within the unit, suggesting room-to-room transmission.[28] The possibility of *C albicans* transmission at the Shriners Burns Institute in Cincinnati, Ohio, was also raised from the finding that 20 out of 96 pediatric patients over a 3-year period possessed the same serotype and biotype.[29]

Although the detailed biochemical pathophysiology of *Candida* infection is beyond the scope of this chapter, there are some important findings worth detailing in the context of burn wounds. Early work in animal models subjected to thermal injury suggested the virulence of *C albicans* strains was related to their ability to generate proteases. For example, proteinase augmentation of burned mice challenged with the low-virulence MY 1044 strain increased the mortality rate, whereas proteinase inhibition treatment of burned mice challenged with the high-virulence strain MY 1044 decreased it.[30] Both in vivo and in vitro studies also demonstrated that growth of the organism was related to its ability to project proteases into the surrounding environment and thus provide a source of amino acids from nearby proteins.[31] Degradation of immunoglobulins or activation of the kininogen-kinin cascade system would further lower the immune response to fungal growth. More recent work has focused on the synthesis, characterization, and substrate definition of these proteases in terms of understanding the virulence of different *C albicans* strains as well as other *Candida* species.

In the chapter discussing the hypothalamic-pituitary-adrenal axis, it was noted that suppression of type 1 Th cells occurs following thermal injury while the Th2 response is enhanced, and this shift favors *C albicans* infection. For example, Kobayashi et al[32] demonstrated that when SCID mice were inoculated with peripheral blood lymphocytes (PBLs) from burned patients, there was no resistance to infection. However, when PBLs were depleted of CD30+ cells, the mice survived infection.

CD30 is a surface antigen and member of the tumor necrosis factor receptor superfamily whose high serum concentration is found in several type 2 Th–related disorders and immune-mediated diseases, including rheumatoid arthritis. It appears to have a counter-regulatory function during chronic inflammation. More recent work has also demonstrated that soluble, T-cell-derived antigen binding molecules (TABMs) are another group of immunoproteins associated with type 1 Th cell suppression, cell-mediated immunity. In a study that characterized *C albicans* mannan-specific production (mannan is a polysaccharide) in patients who had invasive candidiasis, fungal colonization, or no colonization and healthy patients,[33] it was determined that the TABM specific to *C albicans* mannan was highest in patients with invasive candidiasis. Thus, it has been conjectured that the yeast form is recognized by dendritic cells (DCs) via toll-like receptor 4 (TLR4), which leads to candidal growth restriction and a type 1 Th response. However, in burn patients with cell-mediated immune response depression, the transition to the hyphal form is encouraged, with TLR2-mediated DC activation leading to T regulatory cell upregulation and invasive infection.

Of interest is that growth of *Candida* spp in burn wounds is often inhibited by the presence of other bacteria. Gupta et al[34] demonstrated that *Pseudomonas* spp inhibit the growth of *Candida* spp in burn patients 8 to 10 days postburn with TBSA burns varying from 15% to 90%. Previous in vitro studies[35] had suggested that *Pseudomonas* can form biofilms on *Candida* cells, thus killing them. This apparent toxicity, which is probably related to sterol metabolism, only affects the filamentous and not the yeast form due to differences in cell wall composition.

Depending on geographic location, the most common candidal species *after C albicans likely to be present in burn wounds are C parapsilosis, C tropicalis, and C glabrata. Candida parapsilosis* is common in infections associated with central lines and patients receiving TPN.[36] Although infections associated with this species are generally less virulent, invasive infection and death are possible with involvement of the respiratory system.[37] Resistance to amphotericin B[37] and 5-fluorocytosine[38] has been reported, and a recent examination of the susceptibility of the organism to 9371 isolates showed that resistance to fluconazole also occurred. However, concern regarding resistance to voriconazole or the echinocandins appeared unwarranted.[39] *While C tropicalis* has been considered an important cause of candidemia in patients with leukemia and other hematopoetic malignancies, as well as those who have undergone bone marrow transplantation, its mortality rate is comparable to *C albicans*.[40] Thus, it is not considered a major threat to burn units, even though its prevalence has been increasing. The prevalence of *C glabrata*, formerly known as *Torulopsis glabrata*, has also been increasing, with some concern regarding its resistance to fluconazole. Generally, it is not considered any more virulent than *C albicans*; it is commonly found in immunocompromised patients and patients with uncontrolled diabetes, and is often associated with diabetic renal infection. On the other hand, *C kruzei*, which is commonly associated with hematology-oncology services, has an intrinsic resistance to ketoconazole and fluconazole. It is also less susceptible to other antifungals, although response to the echinocandins so far has been excellent.[41]

## Aspergillus

As with *Candida*, more than 200 species of *Aspergillus* are known, but in general burn units typically see infection due to 3 or 4 species, with *A fumigatus*, *A niger*, *A terreus*, and *A flavus* most commonly identified. In comparison to *Candida*, *Aspergillus* spp produce thin, septate hyphae of approximately the same diameter, with acute branching angles of approximately 45°. The incidence of invasive aspergillosis has been increasing and carries a high mortality rate. Therefore, *Aspergillus* filamentous fungal infections in wounds should be considered life threatening. For example, Stone et al[6] reported a mortality rate of 78% in 18 burn patients with documented *Aspergillus* infection and recommended amputation of a single extremity in which infection was localized in order to improve the patient's prognosis. Recently, Murray et al[42] attempted to determine the relationship between fungal elements discovered at autopsy and mortality. While they noted that *Aspergillus* and *Candida* were the most frequently recovered fungi, *Aspergillus* was recovered in 13 of the 14 cases in which fungal infection was identified as an attributed cause of death. The implication is that *Aspergillus* has a greater propensity for directly causing mortality. Ballard et al[2] also reported a 12-fold increase in mortality when finding *Aspergillus* or other mold at any infection site. In addition, the authors considered the fact that slightly less than half of the mold and *Aspergillus* cultures reported in their review were from patients who were not receiving systemic treatment. Both these studies imply that prompt aggressive treatment is not being undertaken in some burn units.

Delineating the pathobiology of *Aspergillus* infections has been challenging. One recent study suggests that in *A fumigatus*, gliotoxin, a cytotoxic secondary metabolite produced by the organism, appears to induce apoptotic cell death by activating the proapoptotic Bcl-2 gene family member Bak. This elicits generation of reactive oxygen species, mitochondrial release of apoptogenic factors, and caspase-3 activation.[43] In essence, the toxin causes otherwise healthy cells to prematurely die. Another line of research suggests that the virulence of *Aspergillus* spp depends on its ability to acquire iron, either by using reductive iron assimilation (RIA) or by employing siderophore-assisted iron uptake[44] (siderophores are low-molecular-mass, ferric-iron-specific chelators). Because effectively combating aspergillosis with the current antifungal agents is difficult, prevention of extracellular siderophore biosynthesis via novel inhibitors, which leads to reduced virulence, looks to be a promising avenue.

## Fusarium

*Fusarium* is another organism that has been reported periodically in both case series[45,46] and review studies[17,21] of fungal infections in burn patients. Although the incidence of colonization and infection is less than *Aspergillus*, progression to invasive or disseminated infections is often fatal. Infection is possible in healthy, immunocompetent patients but is usually localized, often to limbs, and rarely fatal; however, when significant comorbid factors are present, such as chronic renal failure, ischemic heart disease, or diabetes, the risk of mortality increases.[47] Four *Fusarium* species are commonly pathogenic in humans: *F solani*, *F oxysporum*, *F verticilliodes*, and *F proliferatum*; *F solani* has been determined to be the most virulent in a murine model,[48] but due to the paucity of data, it is undetermined whether this is the case in humans.

Several mycotoxins are produced by *Fusarium* spp, including fumonisin B1, produced by *F verticillioides* in corn, which targets the liver and kidneys. A recent study also demonstrated that it induces expression of TNFα, IFNγ, and IL-12 in mouse liver, and that macrophages and liver epithelial cells interact in response to fumonisin B1 to augment cytokine expression.[49] The trichothenes inhibit eukaryotic protein synthesis, depress cell-mediated immunity and the humoral response to T-dependent antigens, and increase the susceptibility to candidiasis and cryptococcosis; these actions are mediated primarily via lymphocytes.[50] Given the impaired immune response and problems with protein biosynthesis observed in burn patients, it can be readily appreciated why these toxins are so deadly.

## Other Fungal Infections

It has been noted that previously rare fungal infections started to appear in the 1980s and continue to appear more frequently in burn units. For example, Becker et al reported the presence of both *Mucor* and *Rhizopus* spp in patients with disseminated fungal disease during the period 1979 through 1989.[17] While there are likely several factors contributing to this situation, the largest has been, and continues to be, the increase in the immunocompromised population, including HIV patients or organ transplant recipients.[26,51] It can then be conjectured that these "rare" fungi become more established in the environment of acute and long-term care facilities caring for these patients, and thus chances for opportunistic infection are enhanced. Again, it should be stressed that these types of fungal infections are normally absent in immunocompetent individuals, but patients with severe burns are more vulnerable to developing significant infections from these organisms.

Zygomycosis is an acute inflammation of the soft tissues, often associated with fungal invasion of the vasculature.

The zygomycete organisms commonly responsible, *Rhizopus*, *Mucor*, and *Absidia* spp, are ubiquitous in the environment. They produce a cottonlike growth on decaying vegetable matter or bread, which is composed of wide, ribbonlike, aseptate (hyphae or spore cells that lack cross-walls) hyaline hyphae with wide or right-angle branching.[52] With proper sectioning and staining, this morphology enables a relative easy distinction under the microscope between these species and other filamentous fungi which have pseudohyphae, such as *Aspergillus* and *Candida* species.

Transmission of these zygomycetes has been linked to spore-contaminated adhesive bandages,[53] catheter sites, electrodes, and contaminated surgical equipment or air-conditioner filters, but can also occur via the respiratory tract.[52] Typically, the infection site is cutaneous in burn patients, but cases of rhinocerebral mucormycosis, in which infection is initiated in the sinal or palate mucosa and progresses to the retro-orbital area and brain via the facial nerves, blood vessels, or cartilage, have occurred. For example, Stern and Kagan[54] reported the case of a 62-year-old diabetic male who had 29% TBSA burn injury after being involved in an airplane crash. Although successfully resuscitated, he later died of a massive cerebral vascular accident (CVA) with necrosis of the right temporal, right frontal, and parietal lobes. An autopsy and histopathological examination of the affected tissues revealed the presence of zygomycetal organisms. Another case involving ischemic necrosis of the upper extremities in a patient caused by invasive mucormycosis following soil contamination of severe burn wounds also highlights the aggressive measures that must be taken following diagnosis if the patient is to survive.[55]

The most recent review of the literature involving cutaneous mucormycosis indicated a mortality rate of 31%.[56] Ballard et al[2] recorded a mortality rate of 28% due to molds. Horvath et al[27] also noted that 30% of fungal wound infections had *Mucor*-like morphology—a high percentage—and using regression analysis determined that patients older than 40 years were the most vulnerable in terms of mortality. However, these authors also showed that mortality increased with decreasing age below 20 years, with infants predicted to have a mortality rate of nearly 10%. *Absidia corymbifera*, which can invade intact skin by using proteolytic enzymes, has also been reported in burn patients. This organism also exemplifies the difficulty in treating such cases, as it possesses a propensity for growth via the vasculature.[57]

## DIAGNOSIS

## Clinical Signs

The diagnosis of fungal infections is always difficult due to the variety of presenting clinical signs as well as the common finding that symptoms may not occur until the infection is well advanced. Moreover, uniform criteria for diagnosis are lacking.[2] Although colonization by *Candida* spp has been found to precede invasive sepsis, in 80% of patients this had no effect on their clinical course.[7] Thus, in some cases, an overtaxed immune system will tip the balance towards a critical event and cause an infection to propagate from a colonization site.

Generally, manifestations of candidemia include pyelonephritis, peritonitis, arthritis, hepatosplenic abscesses, pneumonitis, myositis, macronodular skin lesions, osteomyelitis, endophthalmitis, meningitis, and/or multiorgan involvement.[26] However, the progression from infection to invasive fungemia affects different organs according to the route of infection. For example, translocation from the gut will likely involve the liver and splenic tissues, whereas infection from a central line will often lead to endocarditis and renal problems. Patients with candidemia or disseminated infection will also develop fever and leukocytosis (leukocyte count typically above $15 \times 10^9$/L) unless they are taking immunosuppressive medications. Candidemia is most likely to occur 2 to 7 weeks postburn.[58] Fever also tends to be constant (101°F to 105°F, 24.1°C to 26.3°C) rather than variable, as is often observed with many bacterial infections. Fungemia-induced fever should not be confused with the metabolically related increase in temperature often seen for the first several days postburn in children. Another clue to the presence of candidiasis may be irresolution of a chronic episode of gram-negative sepsis.[58] When *Candida* is suspected, clinicians should also consult the risk factors associated with candidemia, which are described in a later section, as such factors can be informative.

Depending upon the age of a child and severity of infection, *Malassezia* yeast spp may induce temperature instability, bradycardia, thrombocytopenia, respiratory distress, or merely fever with mild illness.[26]

Although candidiasis is a very serious condition in a severely burned child, early recognition of *Aspergillus* or zygomycetes infections is more critical, as they carry a poorer prognosis once dissemination occurs. The classical route for aspergillosis is the respiratory tract through inhalation of fungal conida,[26] but in burned children this is unlikely unless an inhalation injury is present.[2] Early symptoms of invasive pulmonary aspergillosis include cough, fever, hemoptysis, and hypoxia, with variable chest radiographic changes.[24] Of note, one-third of patients may be asymptomatic.

Aspergillosis in the majority of pediatric burn patients is initially cutaneous. The first clinical presentation begins with erythrematous fluctuant nodules or plaques that progress to necrosis and/or eschar formation in a burn wound.[59] When changes in the character of a wound surface suddenly change—notably, swelling, induration, and tenderness accompanied by fever—cutaneous aspergillosis should

be added to the list of "usual suspects."[60] Generally, erythema and induration appear when the site of infection is an intravenous catheter, followed by progressive necrosis that develops radially.[60]

In a case study of 5 adults and 1 child with primary cutaneous aspergillosis, the diagnosis was made at approximately 6 weeks postburn.[59] Absolute neutrophil (polymorphonuclear cells) count in these patients was depressed (mean: 1058 per μL), but not classified as neutropenia. Although half of these patients were successfully treated, the remainder developed invasive aspergillosis and died. Typically, cutaneous aspergillosis develops 10 to 35 days postburn in patients with burns of 50% to 60% TBSA, but it can still occur even when burn wounds are nearly healed. For example, Williams et al[61] reported that a 4-year-old female with an 80% TBSA scald burn was treated successfully, even though she had multiple positive blood cultures for gram-positive and gram-negative organisms. Prior to discharge, however, she suddenly developed fulminant gram-negative sepsis thought to be unrelated to the healed scald. While this episode was also well managed, small, dark, necrotic ulcers started to extensively appear over the scalded area. Despite intensive antifungal treatment, fascial excision of involved tissue, and coverage with Integra, she developed MOF and died. This case study is an extremely unusual illustration of Koebner's phenomenon—the development of lesions in previously normal skin that has been internally or externally traumatized. Another case study documented the very rare development of aspergillosis in the GI tract.[62]

*Fusarium* infections can initiate in the skin, respiratory tract, extremities, eyes, GI tract, or the peritoneum.[47] Skin infections usually present as ulceration. In one case of *Fusarium* infection involving an adult male with a 73% TBSA hot grease scald injury, the process started with colonization of the wound 30 days postburn and progressed to fulminant, disseminated infection within 1 week to the thighs, legs, and thence to the feet, groin, and abdomen.[46] Disseminated, reddish, elevated boils infiltrated with *Fusarium* also appeared on his arms in the terminal phase. Despite attempts to halt the infection with below-the-knee amputations and aggressive antifungal treatment, he subsequently died.

While some *Mucor* infections are likely to manifest symptoms similar to cutaneous aspergillosis (central, black necrotic eschars surrounded by a margin of red to purple edematous cellulitis[54]), pulmonary, rhinocerebral, rhino-orbital, and gastrointestinal cases are possible.[52] Gastrointestinal manifestations include abdominal pain with hepatic abscesses, necrotic stomach wall ulcerations, diarrhea, paralytic ileus, and appendiceal masses. The diagnosis of rhinocerebral mucormycosis is difficult, although CT scans may assist in defining soft tissue abnormalities. Magnetic resonance imaging, however, is superior in demonstrating intracranial complications caused by fungal invasion.[54]

*Trichosporon* spp normally cause superficial infections of the hair shaft known as white piedra. It can also cause bloodstream infections in burn patients, resulting in endocarditis or peritonitis if dialysis is being performed.[26] In addition, wounds may be infected with results similar to aspergillosis.

## Laboratory and Culture Tests

Culturing fungal species is still an art which can be difficult in many instances, particularly when infections are due to more than one species. Moreover, as resources at some burn units may be limited, there are 3 important questions which a burn clinician should address: (1) Under what circumstances is it appropriate to culture fluids or tissues from a patient? (2) From what fluids or tissues should biopsies or swabs be taken? (3) How should the results be utilized?

Although some burn units have policies regarding routine fungal cultures, at a minimum, cultures should be obtained when (1) the patient is judged to be at high risk for a fungal infection, or (2) when suspicion is high that a fungal infection may be present. In the first instance, sampling should commence at least 1 week after burn injury, since this is the beginning of the fungal infection "envelope," unless there is already suspicion of an infection. Risks of infection may also change during the course of burn treatment and should therefore be frequently reevaluated. As we have previously seen, an individual who is progressing well can develop a defining event, or series of events, that may predispose him or her to infection. Such events include, but may not be limited to, bacterial sepsis; prolonged, extensive, and multiple surgeries involving debridement or excision; development of compartment syndromes or respiratory distress; or hypotensive episodes.

What constitutes "high suspicion"? Any prolonged fever accompanied by leukocytosis which is not explainable by bacterial infection is one possibility; another is a suspected or confirmed bacterial infection that fails to resolve after appropriate antibiotic treatment. In addition, appearance of any of the clinical signs or symptoms that have already been described, and which cannot be explained by other factors, should alert the clinician to the possibility of fungal infection.

There is a considerable difference between colonization and infection of a wound. Fungal colonization is not uncommon and usually goes unrecognized; generally, it is defined as observation of fungal elements in the burn eschar without penetration to the level of viable tissue. Fungal infection, on the other hand, has been defined as fungal invasion into viable tissue below the eschar.[64] Moreover, in terms of quantitative colony-forming culture analysis (defined as

$\log_{10}$ colony-forming units per gram of disrupted tissue), Horvath et al[27] highlighted the finding that infection, but not colonization, is independently associated with higher mortality. However, colonization may be an important finding in a high-risk patient who warrants early presumptive treatment to prevent infection. In addition, if resources permit, obtaining wound swabs on a periodic basis (for example, every 1 to 3 years) can help identify shifts in fungal colonization patterns that may be reflective of changes in the burn unit environment.

Swabs of the wound or other affected tissues are the most important sites to sample; blood, urine, and sputum cultures may also be helpful in confirmation of infection. However, results of cultures from such specimens by themselves can be misleading either because of contamination, especially from *Candida*, or because of failure to grow cultures, such as zygomycetes, even though fungi may be present.[52] In general, attempting to culture fungi from cerebrospinal fluid (CSF) specimens is not recommended[64]; in the case of meningitis, the combined use of the cryptococcal antigen test and bacterial cultures of CSF can replace routine fungal cultures of CSF, unless experience in the burn unit suggests that fungal pathogens other than *Cryptococcus* and *Candida* remain important causes of meningitis. When equipment or devices, such as catheters, are suspected as the source of a fungal infection (eg, intravenous site infection), a swab of the surface should also be taken.

Newer techniques, such as real-time PCR (polymerase chain reaction), are beginning to make inroads as an adjunct to the classical fungal culture methods.[66] In particular, *Aspergillus* spp have been targeted because of their high morbidity and mortality. Compared to current ELISA tests for galactomannan and tests for $(1 \rightarrow 3)$-$\beta$-D-glucan, the results of one PCR test were available 2.8 and 6.5 days earlier than the other tests, with a sensitivity of 79% vs 58% and 67%, and a specificity of 92% vs 97% and 84%, respectively, for the other tests.[67] However, such PCR tests are limited because most are only targeted toward one particular species. PCR tests targeted toward *Candida* identification are focused on the 6 or 7 most common species.[66] The initial results have been promising, but it will most likely be at least another decade before such tests are commonly available. Ultimately, the approach could be combined with array ("chip") technology to allow simultaneous detection of many fungal species.

Currently, many of the laboratories used by burn units only identify genera, rather than individual species of fungi. This approach is still helpful since it can differentiate between *Candida*, *Aspergillus*, or zygomycetes infection. More sophisticated analysis allows for species identification, which can aid in tailoring empirical treatment based on clinical suspicion alone. In interpreting results, it is important to keep in mind the definitions of infection and consider laboratory findings in the context of clinical findings. For example, an isolated urine sample positive for *Candida* does not necessarily mean that an infection is present. On the other hand, positive findings of a given fungal genus or species from multiple samples can assure the clinician that an infection is present and must be addressed.

## Making the Diagnosis

Making a diagnosis of fungal infection or fungal involvement requiring action is challenging because (1) if there is an infection, treatment should be initiated without waiting for culture or laboratory tests, (2) giving a patient antifungal treatment is not without risk, and (3) equivocal culture results are not helpful. For high-risk patients who have been already started on prophylactic antifungal agents, suspicion regarding a possible infection suggests the situation is likely to be serious. However, for lower-risk patients, there is no consensus on how to proceed. Ballard et al[2] expressed concern, based on their review of 2114 burn patients, that almost half of the cultures positive for molds or *Aspergillus* were from patients in whom systemic antifungal treatment had *not* been initiated. Should this result be interpreted as laxness by the attending clinicians or as their inability to judge whether an infection was really present given the clinical signs and symptoms (if any) that were present? In terms of interpreting equivocal culture results, Ballard et al[2] also encapsulate the dilemma faced in burn units with such questions as "Do positive blood cultures, or cultures of mold or *Aspergillus*, mandate treatment? When can cultures of *Candida* from urine or sputum be ignored?"

At this time, the best advice is to allow the patient's status to guide therapeutic decisions. Where strong suspicion has been elicited regarding infection, it is wiser to begin empirical therapy given that the risks involved in instituting antifungal treatment far outweigh those posed by infection. Moreover, while antifungal treatment can always be discontinued if unwarranted, one cannot gain the time lost from delayed treatment if a serious infection is present.

## TREATMENT

### Considerations

Although many case reports and studies have been published over the years regarding antifungal treatments for burn patients, all the efficacy studies of antifungal agents (eg, randomized controlled trials—RCTs) have been conducted in patients with other diseases or conditions. That is not to say the results of such trials are inapplicable, but rather that they should be interpreted with caution since the course of a *Candida* infection in a severely burned patient is not identical to that in a patient with HIV or cancer.

In general, the treatment of fungal infections relies upon a combination of debridement or more extensive excision of infected tissue where necessary (including amputation of extremities in life-threatening situations), surgical drainage, and systemic antifungal therapy. Removal of catheters and/or prosthetics may also be necessary if these are implicated in the infection.

There are 4 indications for administration of antifungal agents: (1) prophylaxis in the case of high-risk patients, (2) early presumptive treatment in the case of documented fungal colonization in which the risk and consequences of developing an invasive or disseminating infection are judged serious, (3) topical therapy for localized infection, and (4) systematic therapy for invasive infection or situations to prevent invasive fungemia.[67]

Empirical treatment (ie, treatment without obtaining a culture) should be initiated whenever patients have 3 or more of the following risk factors:

(1) 1 or more weeks of antibiotic therapy
(2) immunosuppression (prior condition or laboratory tests indicating it is present)
(3) long-term intravenous catheters
(4) violation of the GI tract
(5) intra-abdominal abscesses
(6) prolonged hospitalization (ie, several weeks)
(7) SIRS or multisystem organ failure

Empirical treatment should generally utilize the most effective agents until such time as culture results can provide more definitive information that might allow a more tailored response. For example, intravenous fluconazole (800 mg/day as a loading dose) can be started, followed by 400 mg/day for 7 days (IV). Renal failure patients should be treated according to their creatinine clearance: (1) > 50 mL/min—400 mg/day; (2) 20 to 50 mL/min—200 mg/day; and (3) 10 to 20 mL/min—100 mg/day. For patients undergoing dialysis, administering 400 mg after dialysis is recommended.

In the following sections, some of the major trials of different antifungal agents are described, along with a consensus of use against different fungal infections when available.

## Amphotericin B

Amphotericin B (amp B) is a polyene that has been used for several decades to treat fungal infections and is regarded as the "gold standard" drug against which newer agents are compared. It has a broad spectrum of activity, although its efficacy against *C lusitaniae*, *C guillermondi*, *A terreus*, and *Scedosporium* spp is limited.[24] Currently, it is considered a "second-line" drug due to its potential toxicity and side effects and is often used as a back-up when newer first-line drugs fail to resolve an infection. For example, in a recent expert panel consensus,[25] 17 out of 20 experts would choose a regimen of amp B in *Candida* infections if fluconazole treatment had already been tried, even if the patient was stable.

Side effects observed in 50% to 90% of cases include fever, chills, nausea, vomiting, and hypotension. More serious adverse effects include nephrotoxicity or are infusion-related. Amp B's nephrotoxic effects are potentiated by a high dosage and/or long duration, as well as other nephrotoxic drugs and diuretics. Alternate-day dosing, combinations with 5-fluorocytosine (at lower doses), and continuous infusion have all been attempted to moderate toxicity,[24] but the newer lipid-formulated versions (liposome) appear to be the most promising.

Although case reports from the early 1970s indicated that amp B was generally successful at clearing *Candida* infections from the blood, most patients subsequently died[3,4]; our opinion is that treatment was given too late to be effective. More recent RCTs comparing conventional amp B against its liposomal formulation suggest that timely treatment is effective. For example, a 1999 neutropenic sepsis RCT (empirical antifungal therapy for patients with persistent fever following antibacterial treatment) showed a 90% survival rate for the conventional amp B group vs 93% for the liposomal amp B group after 1 week. Moreover, fewer proven breakthrough fungal infections occurred in the liposomal amp B group.[69] Most importantly, significantly fewer adverse events and side effects occurred in the liposomal amp B group compared to the conventional amp B group. However, a more recent RCT tested a high-loading dose regimen (10 mg/day) of liposomal amp B against a standard dose (3 mg/day), followed by 3 mg/day for 2 weeks in patients with definite or presumed invasive/mold aspergillosis. No benefit was demonstrated in regard to higher dosing, with respective survival rates of 59% and 72% after 12 weeks.[70]

Three liposomal amp B formulations are currently available: ABLC-Abelcet, ABCD-Amphocil, and L-AmB-AmBisome. While a meta-analysis indicated that such formulations can reduce all-cause mortality for invasive fungal infections by 30% compared to conventional amp B, there appears to be no difference regarding efficacy between the 3 formulations.[71] The overall NNT (number needed to treat) figure calculated when using liposomal formulations of amp B (versus conventional amp B) to prevent 1 death was 31, which indicates little difference in effects. However, further RCTs[72,73] have revealed differences in tolerability of the formulations; combined adverse events were lowest with L-AmB (12%), intermediate with ABLC (32%), and highest with ABCD (41%).[24]

## Nystatin

Nystatin is a polyene that was brought into use during the mid-1950s for topical treatment of fungal infections and was found to be effective in treating *Histoplasma* and *Cryptococcus* infections as well. In the 1960s, burn units began employing it against *Candida* strains. Because of its limited solubility in water as well as serious side effects of nephrotoxicity and hemolytic toxicity when used parenterally, it is used in topical ointment form or taken as an oral suspension. Like other polyene macrolides, it acts by binding ergosterol, the primary fungal steroid, in the cell walls of fungi, causing formation of pores and apoptosis.

During the 1970s and 1980s, nystatin use was common in many burn units, either as a topical agent in conjunction with amphotericin B in cases of aspergillosis or *Candida*, or as prophylaxis in high-risk patients to prevent candidiasis by using the so-called "swish and swallow" technique.[6,11,12] However, besides issues of patient compliance, there were doubts of its efficacy. The case series of Heggers et al[74] suggested some efficacy when nystatin was used as a topical agent in combination with antimicrobial drugs. The case control design of Desai et al, which tested use of "swish and swallow" prophylactic nystatin, was more convincing, with a reduction of *Candida* colonization from 26.7% to 15.6%, *Candida* infection from 21.3% to 10.0%, and sepsis from 12.2% to 0%.[13] While the experience of Dubé et al[14] was similar to that of Heggers et al,[74] the authors raised the suggestion of topical nystatin use increasing fungemias and colonization caused by nystatin-resistant, amphotericin B–susceptible *C rugosa*. In 1999, Barret et al[75] reported the cases of 4 severely burned children in which excision of fungi-affected tissue, as well as use of amphotericin B and other agents, proved ineffective against *Fusarium* and *Aspergillus* angioinvasive infections. In order to save lives, they treated wounds with topical nystatin powder at $6 \times 10^6$ units/g, which was found to eradicate invasive clusters of fungi in deep wound tissues.

A recent RCT tested prophylactic fluconazole (200 μg/day) against nystatin suspension (6,000,000 IU/day) to prevent fungal infections in patients with leukemia undergoing remission induction chemotherapy.[76] The results showed that fluconazole was more successful in preventing fungal infections (68% of the fluconazole-treated patients vs 47% of the nystatin-treated patients, $P = .03$). The result of this clinical trial (and others) is one reason why nystatin is not routinely used as prophylaxis in current burn unit practice. However, some burn units choose to add the drug to other agents to prevent wound infection. Moreover, as Barret et al[75] have shown, its use may have some utility in *Fusarium*, *Aspergillus*, or infections due to rarer fungi in cases in which newer antifungal agents have limited activity.

# 5-fluorocytosine

5-fluorocytosine (flucytosine) is a fluorinated analog of cytosine that is deamidated intrafungally to 5-fluorouracil, which is subsequently phosphorylated and incorporated into fungal RNA, inhibiting protein synthesis. In addition, it is converted to 5-fluorodeoxyuridine-monophosphate, which inhibits fungal DNA synthesis. In the treatment of fungal infections in burn patients, flucytosine has not been used extensively due to its relatively weak antifungal activity.[14] Moreover, some fungi can become rapidly resistant to the drug when used alone.[24] As a result, it must always be used in combination with other antifungal agents. In combination with amphotericin B, it may be particularly useful in meningitis and endocarditis caused by *Candida* species.[77]

# The Azoles

The azoles include the imidazoles, ketoconazole and miconazole, and the triazoles, itraconazole, fluconazole, and voriconazole. The latter 2 azoles have constituted the mainstay of systemic antifungal treatment, largely because of their efficacy and lower toxicity compared to amphotericin B, and will thus be examined in terms of their efficacy.

Many trials involving fluconazole have been conducted, particularly in regard to cancer. Many of these studies have been ignored, however, in part because the "treatment model" is less applicable to burn patients and because several trials had major design flaws.[78] Instead, we shall focus on broader-applicability trials. Several early RCTs[79-81] of fluconazole versus amphotericin B for treatment of candidemia were designed as noninferiority trials, meaning they were designed to show equivalency. In strict terms, while at least 2 trials[79,80] might have been underpowered in our opinion, overall, they did show that fluconazole was an excellent substitute for amphotericin B, given that much data was missing regarding evaluability of the trials. Another trial revealed that the addition of amphotericin B to fluconazole appeared to improve outcomes, even though it was too underpowered to demonstrate this conclusion statistically.[82] However, the use of fluconazole in preventing fungal infections in critically ill patients was less unambiguous, with one trial[83] suggesting a positive benefit in regard to *Candida* infection and the other suggesting no benefit.[84] A 2-cohort study of 99 and 38 patients, respectively, also buttressed the findings of the Schuster et al RCT.[84] Furthermore, they suggested that, in concert with previous findings, broad use of prophylactic fluconazole in ICUs was increasing both the incidence of fluconazole-resistant *Candida* organisms as well as bacterial resistance of other microorganisms toward broad-spectrum antibiotics.[85] In addition, before the second trial[84] was conducted,

a consensus conference on candidal infection had already unanimously recommended that antifungal prophylaxis *not* be given on a routine basis.[25] We would agree and suggest that prophylaxis be undertaken only in high-risk, severely burned patients.

Voriconazole is a second-generation azole, and several trials were conducted to determine its efficacy compared to amphotericin B, or to a sequence of amphotericin B followed by fluconazole. Both the RCTs conducted by Walsh et al[86] and Herbrecht et al[87] suffered major problems. In the first instance, the outcome of the trial clearly showed that voriconazole was inferior to liposomal amphotericin B by composite endpoint. However, the claimed significant reduction in breakthrough infections disappeared when infections arbitrarily excluded from analysis were included.[78] The second trial,[87] which followed treatment for invasive aspergillosis, suffered from protocol design flaws that did not include premedication (steroids) to prevent infusion-related adverse events or the addition of fluid and electrolytes to minimize nephrotoxicity in the amphotericin B arm. Most importantly, the duration of treatments was vastly different, with a median duration of 77 days for the voriconazole group and 10 days for the amphotericin B group. This factor alone renders comparison between the groups meaningless. The third RCT, which compared voriconazole against a short course of amphotericin B (average duration 4 days) followed by fluconazole to treat candidemia,[88] also failed to show unequivocal equivalency, because although the outcomes were equivalent at 12 weeks according to the analysis protocol, they were not at the last available follow-up.

The incidence of adverse events related to administration of voriconazole appears to be less than for amphotericin B. They include visual disturbances (6%-45%), rashes, Stevens Johnson syndrome, toxic epidermal necrolysis, pancreatitis, hepatitis, and jaundice.[87,89,90] In addition, because voriconazole is metabolized via the cytochrome P450 isoenzymes CYP2C19, CYP2C9, and CYP3A4, the potential for drug interactions is high. Therefore, monitoring liver function and serum levels of the drug where possible, as well as adjusting dosages with coadministration of other medications, is required.[24,89]

Posaconazole has a broad spectrum of activity akin to voriconazole, but the latter is available only in oral form. In an RCT comparing posaconazole against fluconazole and itraconazole as prophylactic treatment to prevent fungal infection in patients undergoing chemotherapy, posaconazole demonstrated superior results in regard to proven or probable invasive fungal infections (2% vs 8% in the fluconazole/itraconazole groups).[91] Survival rates were significantly better in the posaconazole group, but serious adverse events possibly or probably related to treatment were also significantly higher in this group. Thus far, this drug has not been widely studied in burn patients. Although it appears to be a promising candidate for treating invasive infections, it should probably be reserved for salvage therapy in refractory or resistant infections or used as an alternative agent in zygomycosis, fusariosis, cryptococcal meningitis, coccidioidomycosis, or histoplasmosis until more data are available.[92] Several other azoles, including isavuconazole, ravuconazole, and albaconazole, are in various phases of clinical testing, and data on these drugs should be available in the near future. Albaconazole in particular has shown very potent activity against species of *Candida*, *Cryptococcus*, and *Aspergillus*.[93]

## The Echinocandins

Caspofungin, micafungin, and anidulafungin are lipopeptides that block the synthesis of glucan in the cell wall and are the result of several decades of research to find low-toxicity compounds in the echinocandin group. Due to low oral bioavailability, they must be given intravenously.

Several RCTs have tested the efficacy of the echinocandins. Mora-Duarte et al[94] conducted a double-blind trial of intravenous caspofungin against amphotericin B for the treatment of invasive candidiasis (N = 239). Successful outcomes were demonstrated in 73% of the caspofungin patients vs 62% in the amphotericin B group (ITT analysis, after therapy). Moreover, a significant difference in outcomes was noted in the per protocol analysis both after the end of therapy and 6 to 8 weeks after treatment. The results showed that caspofungin was at least as effective as amphotericin B, while causing significantly fewer adverse events. A similar but much larger trial (N = 1095) using caspofungin and liposomal amphotericin B to empirically treat patients with persistent fever and neutropenia confirmed the noninferiority of caspofungin (33.9% success rate vs 33.7% for amphotericin B) as well as a lower incidence of adverse events.[95]

Concerns arose regarding the fact that the first trial did not employ fluconazole (the preferred drug of choice at the time) rather than amphotericin B as the drug that should have been compared against caspofungin.[96] Subsequently, a RCT comparing anidulafungin against fluconazole in the treatment of patients with invasive candidiasis (N = 245) was undertaken.[97] In the modified ITT analysis, successful outcomes after the end of therapy and at a 2-week follow-up showed a significant difference in favor of anidulafungin (74% vs 57%, and 65% vs 49%, respectively), but were not significantly different after 6 weeks. Adverse events were generally similar, and the Kaplan-Meier estimates of survival showed a nonsignificant trend in favor of anidulafungin. Micafungin (low and high dosages of 100 mg and 150 mg daily) was also tested against caspofungin (70 mg, then 50 mg daily) for treatment of candidemia and other forms of invasive candidiasis in a large trial (N = 595).[98] Successful outcomes were recorded in 76.4% of the low-dose micafungin group, 71.4% in the high-dose micafungin group, and 72.3% in the caspofungin group. Again, adverse events were similar across all groups. The results of these trials suggest that the echinocandins are at least as efficacious in treating candidiasis as fluconazole; they may be superior under certain circumstances, but this will need to be confirmed with more data.

## Drug Interactions

The interactions between amphotericin B and other drugs have not been studied as extensively as for the azoles, but in general, other nephrotoxic drugs, such as aminoglycosides, cidofovir, or foscarnet, should be avoided. In addition, amphotericin B has the potential to induce potassium depletion, which may increase digitalis toxicity or enhance the curariform effect of skeletal muscle relaxants. Many of these effects, including the nephrotoxicity of amphotericin B, can be avoided through careful monitoring and the addition of fluids and electrolytes.

If flucytosine is used, caution must be employed with concomitant administration of myelosuppressive drugs, since cytarabine can reduce levels of flucytosine.[24]

Because triazoles inhibit a number of CYP isoenzymes, major drug-drug interactions will occur if a patient receives any other drugs metabolized by these enzymes in the liver.[99] Both itraconazole and voriconazole have the greatest potential in this regard, while fluconazole and posaconazole have less potential.[99,100]

Animal data and small case reports indicate that concentrations of caspofungin in the blood can be reduced by rifampicin after prompting an initial rise, whereas cyclosporin can cause a sustained elevation in caspofungin levels.[24] Increases in caspofungin clearance have also been noted when given concurrently with carbamazepine, dexamethasone, efavirenz, nelfinavir, nevirapine, or phenytoin. In these instances, increasing the dosage of caspofungin may be required.[101] Furthermore, caspofungin can cause reduced blood concentrations of tacrolimus, and thus monitoring of tacrolimus levels is advised.

## Specific Recommendations

As iterated at the beginning of this section, empirical treatment with fluconazole can be instituted while awaiting results of cultures. However, once identification of the genus or species has been accomplished, more refined treatment can begin. This does not preclude interim changes if the patient is not responding to fluconazole.

It is useful to begin by understanding the spectrum of activity of the antifungal agent classes and the specific species in which resistance has been observed. If a *Candida* species is confirmed as being responsible for the infection, treatment changes are appropriate for certain species. For example, if *C glabrata* is confirmed, asking the laboratory to conduct an MIC study is warranted: a continuing dosage of 400 mg/day of fluconazole is appropriate for an MIC of < 16, but values of 16 to 32 may indicate doubling the dosage to 800 mg/day; values > 32 suggests switching to an alternative treatment, such as amphotericin B at 0.5 to 1.0 mg/kg per day, would be beneficial. If *C krusei* is confirmed, treatment should be changed to 1 of the echinocandins, voriconazole, or amphotericin B. Finally, if endocarditis, meningitis, or endophthalmitis is present with a definite *Candida* infection, adding flucytosine may be of benefit.[77] If infection with *Cryptococcus neoformans* is confirmed, fluconazole therapy should be maintained since it demonstrates good activity against this organism.[99]

Proven *Aspergillus* infections are best treated with caspofungin or amphotericin B, respectively, although amphotericin B should not be used in cases of infection due to *A terreus*.[24,63] Infections due to *Fusarium* or *Scedosporium* spp are best treated with voriconazole or posaconazole.[24] Zygomycete infections are usually treated with liposomal variants of amphotericin B, although posaconazole may be a good alternative, despite the fact that it is only currently available in oral form.[100] It should also be remembered that amphotericin B has inconsistent activity against *Trichosporon* species and *Pseudallescheria boydi*[63]; in the latter case, voriconazole is appropriate, whereas in the former case, a combination of high-dosage fluconazole and amphotericin B may be the best strategy at this time.[102]

Since consensus guidelines regarding treatment of fungal infections in burn patients are lacking, management of such infections is largely influenced by local practice. As has been demonstrated, fungal infection patterns can differ considerably between burn units. Therefore, a comprehensive history of such infections in each unit can provide valuable information in terms of predicting the probability of infections due to certain species, the appearance of resistance to certain antifungal agents, and successful management options in difficult cases.

## SPECIAL TOPICS

### Risk Factors

Candidemia is the most studied model in terms of determining risk factors for fungal infection. Unfortunately, no published studies have specifically examined the burn patient population. In a case control study of 30 cancer patients and 58 controls, Karabinis et al determined that positive peripheral cultures for *Candida* spp, central catheterization, and neutropenia were the principal risk factors from

a multivariate logistic model.[103] A similarly designed study of 48 patients with leukemia (and 48 controls) revealed the following major risk factors from the logistic regression model: presence of a central line, bladder catheter, administration of 2 or more antibiotics, uremia, transfer from another hospital, diarrhea, and candiduria.[104] Conversely, prior surgical procedures reduced the odds of acquiring a candidal infection by a factor of 10, which implies that surgical patients receiving such treatments were protected to some extent. A larger case-control study (N = 88 for each arm) of hospital-acquired candidemia found that, from a multivariate analysis, the number of antibiotics administered prior to infection, isolation of *Candida* species from areas other than blood, prior hemodialysis, and prior use of a Hickman catheter were the major risk factors.[105] A large prospective cohort study that tracked the development of candidal bloodstream infections in a SICU for > 48 hours over a 2-year period, however, found that prior surgery, acute renal failure, parenteral nutrition, and the presence of a triple lumen catheter were major risk factors in patients who underwent surgery.[106] Ballard et al,[2] specifically studying burn patients, reported the incidence of many of the risk factors identified from these studies, indicating that the presence of catheters and central lines, systemic use of antibiotics, and need for ventilatory support were the most common occurrences. Reviewing all these studies together, the 3 likely factors predisposing toward *Candida* infections are high utilization of antibiotics, the presence of catheters, and total parenteral nutrition. In addition, hyperglycemia (> 180 mg/dL) and possibly APACHE scores should be considered as additional factors in the development of any type of fungal infection.[107]

Perhaps the best approach to encompassing use of risk factors in defining a high-risk population who will require prophylactic antifungal agents after completing resuscitation is to compile a short in-house list and define vulnerable patients as those who have 3 or more risk factors, such as were outlined at the beginning of the treatment section.

### Prophylaxis

The decision whether to empirically administer antifungal agents to patients at high risk of developing a fungal infection, and what drugs should be used, is not an easy one, even when addressing candidemia.[25] In addition to defining the high-risk patient, such factors as the presence of diabetes, the percentage of burned total body surface area, degree of immunosuppression, and age must be considered. Part of the problem is lack of an inherently safe antifungal agent which can cover all possibilities. Fluconazole is reasonably effective against some *Candida* species, but not all, and overuse may lead to increasing resistance in the burn unit. Moreover, fluconazole is ineffective against most molds.

Low prophylactic doses of amphotericin B have been utilized in neutropenic bone marrow transplant recipients to prevent aspergillosis in units where *Aspergillus* infections are common, but this strategy remains controversial.[107] Likewise, investigators have published findings on the prophylactic use of itraconazole and ketoconazole, but there is no agreement whether this is effective.

What would be useful are case control studies investigating prophylaxis in high-risk burn patients in regard to incidence of infection, outcomes, and mortality. However, until these studies are performed, the decision to institute prophylaxis will remain in the hands of burn unit policies, guided by local patterns and prior experience.

## Eliminating Sources of Fungal Infection

As has been discussed earlier, many episodes of fungal infection can be traced to the presence of specific fungal organisms in the environment or to patient-caregiver interactions. Although one cannot eliminate all sources of fungal infections—for example, many candidal sources originate from within the body—there are several practices that can minimize infection and certainly prevent nosocomial outbreaks.

First and foremost is hygiene. Poor hygiene and cross-contamination from within units or personnel adjacent to burn units are frequently cited as sources of infection that can be eliminated or certainly minimized. Both the biotyping analysis conducted by Neely et al[15] and the study of Mousa et al[20] offer insight into the mechanism of in-house transmission between patients and suggest that regular decontamination of units may pay dividends, particularly if clusters of infections are observed. Routine, careful cleaning of air-conditioning filters can also hinder dissemination of fungi.

Since structural changes to burn units or adjacent facilities can also cause airborne transportation of fungi, provision for monitoring the environment should be undertaken during these renovations. Instruments, catheters, and other surgical supplies can also be occasionally contaminated, either in an "as received" condition from the manufacturer or during use. Monitoring the frequency and site of fungal infections, as well as noting the species responsible for infections from month to month, can also provide valuable clues in regard to sources of infection. Clusters of cases should be promptly investigated, as such occurrences may signify an ongoing transmission that is beyond the "normal" background.

## Conclusion

Since the introduction of broad-spectrum antibiotics in burn units, the incidence of fungal infections has increased, although the overall rate seems to have stabilized in recent years. However, the incidence of candidal infections due to other species besides *C Albicans* has increased, as has resistance to the most popular antifungal agent, fluconazole. Moreover, the incidence of aspergillosis and infections due to other fungi, such as zygomycetes, is becoming more common. This has increased difficulty in both diagnosis and treatment. Diagnosis still relies heavily on clinical suspicion since laboratory cultures take several days to process. Such results can subsequently be used to refine empirical treatment with fluconazole. Due to the high morbidity and mortality of fungal infections, suspected or probable infections should be treated immediately, especially in high-risk patients, as delays in instituting treatment can prove fatal. Although the introduction of fluconazole, voriconazole, posaconazole, and caspofungin has shifted the role of amphotericin B to second-line and salvage use, it will still continue to be used for the treatment of zygomycetes infections until more data on posaconazole are available. As relevant data and consensus on prophylaxis, diagnosis, and treatment in the burn patient population are lacking, management of fungal infections will depend on local experience for the foreseeable future. Data suggest that paying particular attention to hygiene, changes in the environment, catheters, and central lines, as well as classifying the risk of patients upon admission to burn units, will all assist in the challenging process of reducing fungal infections and their significant consequences.

## Key Points

- Although the current incidence of fungal infections is approximately 6% to 7%, the proportion of noncandidal infections is probably around 40%, with high (proportional) rates of mold and *Aspergillus* infections reported in some burn units.
- For candidal infection, the mortality rate is approximately 10% to 15%, but mortality rates are much higher for *Aspergillus* and molds (25%–40%).
- A substantial proportion of *Candida* infections today are due to species other than *C albicans*. Both *C glabrata* and *C krusei* are increasingly resistant to fluconazole and require a switch to amphotericin B or one of the echinocandins.
- Once rare, infections due to zygomycetes, *Trichosporon*, and other molds and yeasts are becoming more common, in part due to the rise in immunocompromised populations.
- Diagnosis should be made on clinical suspicion; culture of patient isolates can confirm infection

and help refine subsequent treatment, but treatment should not await culture results.

- Any prolonged fever that is not due to bacterial infection, confirmed bacterial infection unresolved by antibiotics, or appearance of other clinical signs/symptoms that cannot be explained by other causes should cause the clinician to consider fungal infection as a possibility.

- *Candida* infections are often preceded by a major event that temporarily destabilizes the patient's condition—for example, surgery, sepsis from bacterial infection, or extensive antibiotic therapy.

- Drug-drug interactions are very important when azoles are used and require careful management and monitoring; such interactions are less important for the polyenes and echinocandins.

- *Aspergillus* infections are best treated with caspofungin; amphotericin B does not have activity against *A terreus*.

- Infections due to *Fusarium* or *Scedosporium* are best treated with voriconazole or posaconazole.

- Zygomycete infections are usually treated with liposomal variants of amphotericin B, although posaconazole may be a satisfactory alternative.

- Voriconazole is appropriate for *P boydi* infections, while a combination of high-dosage fluconazole and amphotericin B is recommended for *Trichosporon* infections.

- Burn patients should be classified as high risk or low risk upon admission to the burn unit. There is no consensus or strong evidence that prophylaxis with fluconazole or amphotericin B reduces the incidence of fungal infections in high-risk patients, but in severely burned patients there may be circumstances in which possible benefits outweigh the risks.

# REFERENCES

1. Cochran A, Morris SE, Edelman LS, Saffle JR. Systematic *Candida* infection in burn patients: a case-control study of management patterns and outcomes. *Surg Infect (Larchmt)*. 2002; 3: 367–374.

2. Ballard J, Edelman L, Saffle J, et al. Positive fungal cultures in burn patients: a multicenter review. *J Burn Care Res*. 2008; 29: 213–221.

3. MacMillan BG, Law EJ, Holder IA. Experience with *Candida* infections in the burn patient. *Arch Surg*. 1972; 104: 509–514.

4. Stieritz DD, Law EJ, Holder IA. Speciation and amphotericin B sensitivity studies on blood isolates of *Candida* from burned patients. *J Clin Path*. 1973; 26: 405–408.

5. Kidson A, Lowbury EJ. *Candida* infection in burns. *Burns*. 1979; 6: 228–230.

6. Stone HH, Cuzzell JZ, Kolb LD, Moskowitz MS, McGowan JE Jr. *Aspergillus* infection of the burn wound. *J Trauma*. 1979; 19: 765–767.

7. Spebar MJ, Pruitt BA Jr. Candidiasis in the burned patient. *J Trauma*. 1981; 21: 237–239.

8. Pensler JM, Herndon DN, Ptak H, et al. Fungal sepsis: an increasing problem in major thermal injuries. *J Burn Care Res*. 1986; 7: 488–491.

9. Desai MH, Herndon DN, Abston S. *Candida* infection in massively burned patients. *J Trauma*. 1987; 27: 1186–1188.

10. Prasad JK, Feller I, Thomson PD. A ten-year review of *Candida* sepsis and mortality in burn patients. *Surgery*. 1987; 101: 213–216.

11. Grube BJ, Marvin JA, Heimbach DM. *Candida*. A decreasing problem for the burned patient? *Arch Surg*. 1988; 123: 194–196.

12. Desai MH, Herndon DN. Eradication of *Candida* burn wound septicemia in massively burned patients. *J Trauma*. 1988; 28: 140–145.

13. Desai MH, Rutan RL, Heggers JP, Herndon DN. *Candida* infection with and without nystatin prophylaxis. An 11-year experience with patients with burn injury. *Arch Surg*. 1992; 127: 159–162.

14. Dubé MP, Heseltine PNR, Rinaldi RG, Evans S, Zawacki B. Fungemia and colonization with nystatin-resistant *Candida rugosa* in a burn unit. *Clin Infect Dis*. 1994; 18: 77–82.

15. Neely AN, Odds FC, Basatia BK, Holder IA. Characterization of *Candida* isolates from pediatric burn patients. *J Clin Microbiol*. 1988; 26: 1645–1649.

16. Ekenna O, Sherertz RJ, Bingham H. Natural history of bloodstream infections in a burn patient population: the importance of candidemia. *Am J Infect Control*. 1993; 21: 189–195.

17. Becker WK, Cioffi WG Jr, McManus AT, et al. Fungal burn wound infection. A 10-year experience. *Arch Surg*. 1991; 126: 44–48.

18. Still JM Jr, Belcher K, Law EJ. Management of *Candida* septicemia in a regional burn unit. *Burns*. 1995; 21: 594–596.

19. Sheridan RL, Weber JM, Budkevich LG, Tompkins RG. Candidemia in the pediatric patient with burns. *J Burn Care Rehabil*. 1995; 16: 440–443.

20. Mousa HAL, Al-Bader SM, Hassan DA. Correlation between fungi isolated from burn wounds and burn care units. *Burns*. 1999; 25: 145–147.

21. de Macedo JLS, Santos JB. Bacterial and fungal colonization of burn wounds. *Mem Inst Oswaldo Cruz*. 2005; 100: 535–539.

22. Gupta N, Haque A, Latiff AA, Narayan RP, Mukhopadhyay G, Prsad R. Epidemiology and molecular typing of *Candida* isolates from burn patients. *Mycopathologia*. 2004; 158: 397–405.

23. Law EJ, Kim OJ, Stieritz DD, MacMillan BG. Experience with systemic candidiasis in the burned patient. *J Trauma*. 1972; 12: 543–542.

24. Enoch DA, Ludlam HA, Brown NM. Invasive fungal infections: a review of epidemiology and management options. *J Med Microbiol.* 2006; **55**: 809–818.

25. Edwards JE Jr, Bodey GP, Bowden RA, et al. International Conference for the Development of a Consensus on the Management and Prevention of Severe Candidal Infections. *Clin Infect Dis.* 1997; **25**: 43–59.

26. Fridkin SK, Jarvis WR. Epidemiology of nosocomial fungal infections. *Clin Microbiol Rev.* 1996; **9**: 499–511.

27. Horvath EE, Murray CK, Vaughan GM, et al. Fungal wound infection (not colonization) is independently associated with mortality in burn patients. *Ann Surg.* 2007; **245**: 978–985.

28. Robert F, Lebreton F, Bougnoux ME, et al. Use of a random amplified polymorphic DNA as a typing method for *Candida albicans* in epidemiological surveillance of a burn unit. *J Clin Microbiol.* 1995; **33**: 2366–2371.

29. Neely AN, Odds FC, Basatia BK, Holder IA. Characterization of *Candida* isolates from pediatric burn patients. *J Clin Microbiol.* 1988; **26**: 1645–1649.

30. Neely AN, Holder IA. Effect of proteolytic activity on the virulence of *Candida albicans* in burned mice. *Infect Immun.* 1991; **59**: 1576–1578.

31. Neely AN, Orloff MM, Holder IA. *Candida albicans* growth studies: a hypothesis for the pathogenesis of *Candida* infections in burns. *J Burn Care Rehabil.* 1992; **13**: 323–329.

32. Kobayashi M, Kobayashi H, Herndon DN, Pollard RB, Suzuki F. Burn-associated *Candida albicans* infection caused by CD30⁺ type 2 T cells. *J Leukocyte Biol.* 1998; **83**: 723–731.

33. Kosonen J, Rantala A, Little CH, et al. Increased levels of *Candida albicans* mannan-specific T-cell-derived antigen binding molecules in patients with invasive candidiasis. *Clin Vaccine Immunol.* 2006; **13**: 467–474.

34. Gupta N, Haque A, Mukhopadhyay G, Narayan RP, Prasad R. Interactions between bacteria and *Candida* in the burn wound. *Burns.* 2005; **31**: 375–378.

35. Hogan DA, Kolter R. *Pseudomonas-Candida* interactions: an ecological role for virulence factors. *Science.* 2002; **296**: 2229–2231.

36. Plouffe JF, Brown DG, Silva J, et al. Nosocomial outbreak of *Candida parapsilosis* fungemia related to intravenous infusions. *Arch Intern Med.* 1977; **137**: 1686–1689.

37. Green D, Still JM Jr, Law EJ. *Candida parapsilosis* sepsis in patients with burns: report of six cases. *J Burn Care Rehabil.* 1994; **15**: 240–243.

38. Hoeprich PD, Ingraham JL, Kjcker B, Winship M. Development of resistance to five fluorocytosine in *Candida parapsilosis*. *J Infect Dis.* 1974; **130**: 112–118.

39. Pfaller MA, Diekema DJ, Gibbs DL, et al. Geographic and temporal trends in isolation and antifungal susceptibility of *Candida parapsilosis*: a global assessment from the ARTEMIS DISK Antifungal Surveillance Program, 2001 to 2005. *J Clin Microbiol.* 2008; **46**: 842–849.

40. Krcmery V, Barnes AJ. Non-*albicans Candida* spp causing fungaemia: pathogenicity and antifungal resistance. *J Hosp Infect.* 2002; **50**: 243–260.

41. Pfaller MA, Diekema DJ, Gibbs DL, et al. *Candida krusei*, a multidrug-resistant opportunistic fungal pathogen: geographic and temporal trends from the ARTEMIS DISK Antifungal Surveillance Program, 2001 to 2005. *J Clin Microbiol.* 2008; **46**: 515–521.

42. Murray CK, Loo FL, Hospenthal DR, et al. Incidence of systemic fungal infection and related mortality following severe burns [published online ahead of print August 6, 2008]. *Burns.* 2008; **34**(8): 1108–1112. DOI: 10.1016/j.burns.2008.04.007.

43. Pardo J, Urban C, Galvez EM, et al. The mitochondrial protein Bak is pivotal for gliotoxin-induced apoptosis and a critical host factor of *Aspergillus* fumigatus virulence in mice. *J Cell Biol.* 2006; **174**: 509–519.

44. Schrettl M, Bignell E, Kragl C, et al. Distinct roles for intra- and extracellular siderophores during *Aspergillus fumigatus* infection. *PLoS Pathog.* 2007; **3**: 1195–1207.

45. Wheeler MS, McGinnis MR, Schell WA, Walker DH. *Fusarium* infection in burned patients. *Am J Clin Pathol.* 1981; **75**: 304–311.

46. Latenser BA. *Fusarium* infections in burn patients: a case report and review of the literature. *J Burn Care Rehabil.* 2003; **24**: 285–288.

47. Nir-Paz R, Strahilevitz J, Shapiro M, et al. Clinical and epidemiological aspects of infections caused by *Fusarium* species: a collaborative study from Israel. *J Clin Microbiol.* 2004; **42**: 3456–3461.

48. Mayayo E, Pujol I, Guarro J. Experimental pathogenicity of four opportunist *Fusarium* species in a murine model. *J Med Microbiol.* 1999; **48**: 363–366.

49. Sharma N, He Q, Sharma RP. Augmented fumonisin B1 toxicity in co-cultures: evidence for crosstalk between macrophages and non-parenchymatous liver epithelial cells involving proinflammatory cytokines. *Toxicology.* 2004; **203**: 239–251.

50. Nelson PE, Dignani MC, Anaissie EJ. Taxonomy, biology, and clinical aspects of *Fusarium* species. *Clin Microbiol Rev.* 1994; **7**: 479–504.

51. Crameri R, Blaser K. Allergy and immunity to fungal infections and colonization. *Eur Respir J.* 2002; **19**: 151–157.

52. Ribes JA, Vanover-Sams CL, Baker DJ. Zygomycetes in human disease. *Clin Microbiol Rev.* 2000; **13**: 236–301.

53. Christiaens G, Hayette MP, Jacquemin D, Melin P, Mutsers J, De Mol P. An outbreak of *Absidia corymbifera* infection associated with bandage contamination in a burns unit. *J Hosp Infect.* 2005; **61**: 88.

54. Stern LE, Kagan RJ. Rhinocerebral mucormycosis in patients with burns: case report and reviews of the literature. *J Burn Care Rehabil.* 1999; **20**: 303–306.

55. Kraut EJ, Jordan MH, Steiner CR III. Arterial occlusion and progressive gangrene caused by mucormycosis in a patient with burns. *J Burn Care Rehabil.* 1993; **14**: 552–556.

56. Ledgard JP, van Hal S, Greenwood JE. Primary cutaneous zygomycosis in a burns patient: a review. *J Burn Care Res*. 2008; **29**: 286–290.

57. Constantinides J, Misra A, Nassab R, Wilson Y. *J Burn Care Res*. 2008; **29**: 416–419.

58. Stone HH, Kolb LD, Currie CA, Geheber CE, Cuzzell JZ. *Candida* sepsis: pathogenesis and principles of treatment. *Ann Surg*. 1974; **179**: 697–710.

59. Chakrabarti A, Gupta V, Biswas G, Kumar B, Sakhuja VK. Primary cutaneous aspergillosis: our experience in 10 years. *J Infect*. 1998; **37**: 24–27.

60. van Burik JH, Colven R, Spach DH. Cutaneous aspergillosis. *J Clin Microbiol*. 1998; **36**: 3115–3121.

61. Williams G, Moiemen N, Frame JD. Aspergillosis presenting as Koebner's phenomenon in a healed scald. *Burns*. 2000; **26**: 92–96.

62. Andres LA, Ford RD, Wilcox RM. Necrotizing colitis caused by systemic aspergillosis in a burn patient. *J Burn Care Res*. 2007; **28**: 918–921.

63. Schofield CM, Murray CK, Horvath EE, et al. Correlation of culture with histopathology in fungal burn wound colonization and infection. *Burns*. 2007; **33**: 341–346.

64. Barenfanger J, Lawhorn J, Drake C. Nonvalue of culturing cerebrospinal fluid for fungi. *J Clin Microbiol*. 2004; **42**: 236–238.

65. Espy MJ, Uhl JR, Sloan LM, et al. Real-time PCR in clinical microbiology: applications for routine laboratory testing. *Clin Microbiol Rev*. 2006; **19**: 165–256.

66. Kami M, Fukui T, Ogawa S, et al. Use of real-time PCR on blood samples for diagnosis of invasive aspergillosis. *Clin Infect Dis*. 2001; **33**: 1504–1512.

67. Dean DA, Burchard KW. Fungal infection in surgical patients. *Am J Surg*. 1996; **171**: 374–382.

68. Walsh TJ, Finberg RW, Arndt C, et al. Liposomal amphotericin B for empirical therapy in patients with persistent fever and neutropenia. *N Engl J Med*. 1999; **340**: 764–771.

69. Cornely OA, Maertens J, Bresnik M, et al. Liposomal amphotericin B as initial therapy for invasive mold infection: a randomized trial comparing a high-loading dose regimen with standard dosing (A,BiLpad trial). *Clin Infect Dis*. 2007; **44**: 1289–1297.

70. Barrett JP, Vardulaki KA, Conlon C, et al. A systematic review of the antifungal effectiveness and tolerability of amphotericin B formulations. *Clin Ther*. 2003; **25**: 1295–1320.

71. White MH, Bowden RA, Sandler ES, et al. Randomized, double-blind clinical trial of amphotericin B colloidal dispersion vs. amphotericin B in the empirical treatment of fever and neutropenia. *Clin Infect Dis*. 1998; **27**: 296–302.

72. Wingard JR, White MH, Anaissie E, et al. A randomized, double-blind comparative trial evaluating the safety of liposomal amphotericin B versus amphotericin B lipid complex in the empirical treatment of febrile neutropenia. *Clin Infect Dis*. 2000; **31**: 1155–1163.

73. Heggers JP, Robson MC, Herndon DN, Desai MH. The efficacy of nystatin combined with topical microbial agents in the treatment of burn wound sepsis. *J Burn Care Rehabil*. 1989; **10**: 508–511.

74. Barret JP, Ramzy PI, Heggers JP, Villareal C, Herndon DN, Desai MH. Topical nystatin powder in severe burns: a new treatment for angioinvasive fungal infections refractory to other topical and systemic agents. *Burns*. 1999; **25**: 505–508.

75. Young GA, Bosly A, Gibbs DL, Durrant S. A double-blind comparison of fluconazole and nystatin in the prevention of candidiasis in patients with leukaemia. *Eur J Cancer*. 1999; **35**: 1208–1213.

76. Pappas PG, Rex JH, Sobel JD, et al. Guidelines for treatment of candidiasis. *Clin Infect Dis*. 2004; **38**: 161–189.

77. Johansen HK, Gotzsche PC. Problems in the design and reporting of trials of antifungal agents encountered during meta-analysis. *JAMA*. 1999; **282**: 1752–1759.

78. Rex JH, Bennett JE, Sugar AM, et al. A randomized trial comparing fluconazole with amphotericin B for the treatment of candidemia in patients without neutropenia. *New Engl J Med*. 1994; **331**: 1325–1330.

79. Anaissie EJ, Darouiche RO, Abi-Said D, et al. Management of invasive candidal infections: results of a prospective, randomized, multicenter study of fluconazole versus amphotericin B and review of the literature. *Clin Infect Dis*. 1996; **23**: 964–972.

80. Phillips P, Shafran S, Garber G, et al. Multicenter randomized trial of fluconazole versus amphotericin B for treatment of candidemia in non-neutropenic patients. *Eur J Clin Microbiol Infect Dis*. 1997; **16**: 337–345.

81. Rex JH, Pappas PG, Karchmer AW, et al. A randomized and blinded multicenter trial of high-dose fluconazole plus placebo versus fluconazole plus amphotericin B as therapy for candidemia and its consequences in nonneutropenic subjects. *Clin Infect Dis*. 2003; **36**: 1221–1228.

82. Pelz RK, Hendrix CW, Swoboda SM, et al. Double-blind placebo-controlled trial of fluconazole to prevent candidal infections in critically ill patients. *Ann Surg*. 2001; **233**: 542–548.

83. Schuster MG, Edwards JE Jr, Sobel JD, et al. Empirical fluconazole versus placebo for intensive care unit patients: a randomized trial. *Ann Intern Med*. 2008; **149**: 83–90.

84. Rocco TR, Reinert SE, Simms HH. Effects of fluconazole administration in critically ill patients: Analysis of bacterial and fungal resistance. *Arch Surg*. 2000; **135**: 160–165.

85. Walsh TJ, Pappas P, Winston DJ, et al. Voriconazole compared with liposomal amphotericin B for empirical antifungal therapy in patients with neutropenia and persistent fever. *New Engl J Med*. 2002; **346**: 225–234.

86. Herbrecht R, Denning DW, Patterson TF, et al. Voriconazole versus amphotericin B for primary therapy of invasive aspergillosis. *New Eng J Med*. 2002; **347**: 408–415.

87. Kullberg BJ, Sobel JD, Ruhnke M, et al. Voriconazole versus a regimen of amphotericin B followed by fluconazole for candidaemia in non-neutropenic patients: a randomised non-inferiority trial. *Lancet*. 2005; **366**: 1435–1442.

**88.** Johnson LB, Kauffman CA. Voriconazole: a new triazole antifungal agent. *Clin Infect Dis.* 2003; **36:** 630–637.

**89.** Vehreschild JJ, Böhme A, Reichert D, et al. Treatment of invasive fungal infections in clinical practice: a multi-centre survey on customary dosing, treatment indications, efficacy and safety of voriconazole. *Int J Hematol.* 2008; **87:** 126–131.

**90.** Cornely OA, Maertens J, Winston DJ, et al. Posaconazole vs. fluconazole or itraconazole prophylaxis in patients with neutropenia. *New Engl J Med.* 2007; **356:** 348–359.

**91.** Rachwalski EJ, Wieczorkiewicz JT, Scheetz MH. Posaconazole: an oral triazole with an extended spectrum of activity (October) (CE) [published online ahead of print August 19, 2008]. *Ann Pharmacother.* 2008; **42**(10): 1429–1438. DOI: 10.1345/aph.1L005.

**92.** Pasqualotto AC, Denning DW. New and emerging treatments for fungal infections. *J Antimicrob Chemother.* 2008; **61**(suppl 1): i19–i30.

**93.** Mora-Duarte J, Bette R, Rotstein C, et al. Comparison of caspofungin and amphotericin B for invasive candidiasis. *New Engl J Med.* 2002; **347:** 2020–2029.

**94.** Walsh TJ, Teppler H, Donowitz GR, et al. Caspofungin versus liposomal amphotericin B for empirical antifungal therapy in patients with persistent fever and neutropenia. *New Engl J Med.* 2004; **351:** 1391–1402.

**95.** Brown AL, Greig JR. Caspofungin versus amphotericin B for invasive candidiasis. *New Engl J Med.* 2003; **348:** 1287.

**96.** Reboli AC, Rotstein C, Pappas PG, et al. Anidulafungin versus fluconazole for invasive candidiasis. *New Engl J Med.* 2007; **356;** 2472–2482.

**97.** Pappas PG, Rotstein CM, Betts RF, et al. Micafungin versus caspofungin for treatment of candidemia and other forms of invasive candidiasis. *Clin Infect Dis.* 2007; **45:** 883–893.

**98.** Chen SCA, Sorrell TC. Antifungal agents. *Med J.* 2007; **187:** 404–409.

**99.** Torres HA, Hachem RY, Chemaly RF, et al. Posaconazole: a broad-spectrum triazole antifungal. *Lancet Infect Dis.* 2005; **5:** 775–785.

**100.** Denning DW. Echinocandin antifungal drugs. *Lancet.* 2003; **362:** 1142–1151.

**101.** Cawley MJ, Braxton GR, Haith LR, Reilly KJ, Guilday RE, Patton ML. *Trichosporon beigelii* infection: experience in a regional burn center. *Burns.* 2000; **26:** 483–486.

**102.** Karabinis A, Hill C, Leclercq B, Tancrède C, Baume D, Andremont A. Risk factors for candidemia in cancer patients: a case-control study. *J Clin Microbiol.* 1988; **26:** 429–432.

**103.** Wey SB, Mori M, Pfaller MA, Woolson RF, Wenzel RP. Risk factors for hospital-acquired candidemia. A matched case-control study. *Arch Intern Med.* 1989; **149:** 2349–2353.

**104.** Blumberg HM, Jarvis WR, Soucie JM, et al. Risk factors for candidal bloodstream infections in surgical intensive care unit patients: the NEMIS prospective multicenter study. *Clin Infect Dis.* 2001; **33:** 177–186.

**105.** Tufano F. Focus on risk factors for fungal infections in ICU patients. *Minerva Anestesiol.* 2002; **68:** 269–272.

**106.** Perfect JR, Klotman ME, Gilbert CC, et al. Prophylactic intravenous amphotericin B in neutropenic autologous bone marrow transplant recipients. *J Infect Dis.* 1992; **165:** 891–897.

# CHAPTER FIFTEEN

# INHALATION INJURY

TISHA K FUJII, DO

STEVEN J. SCHWARTZ, MD, ASSISTANT PROFESSOR OF ANESTHESIOLOGY,
ADULT CRITICAL CARE AND SURGERY JOHNS HOPKINS HOSPITAL

BRADLEY J. PHILLIPS, MD

## INTRODUCTION

Although children are less likely than adults to suffer from inhalation injury, smoke inhalation nonetheless remains a serious and life-threatening problem. Young children are particularly vulnerable to smoke and other toxins because they are less likely to escape a confined space and because they have a higher minute ventilation and lower physiological reserve compared to teens and adults. In addition, relatively smaller airways may be more severely affected by airway edema and obstructing material. Inhaled toxins cause one of the most critical injuries following a thermal insult—the syndrome of "inhalation injury." The supraglottic region can be injured by both thermal and chemical components, whereas tracheobronchial and parenchymal injuries more commonly occur as a result of direct chemical damage. Inhalation injury is implicated in approximately 50% of all deaths from burn injury and has therefore become one of the most frequent causes of death. Early hypoxemia contributes to over 50% of smoke inhalation deaths, with carbon monoxide intoxication accounting for as many as 80% of fatalities.[1]

While progress has been made in improving the care and outcomes for burn patients, inhalation injury continues to challenge clinicians. Some reasons for the lack of formal data and studies in this area include the difficulty for a single center to perform a randomized, controlled, prospective trial as well as a lack of specific definitions and diagnostic criteria of the syndrome. A panel of experts at the Inhalation Consensus Conference evaluated the major unresolved issues regarding inhalation injury.[1] Research priorities were ranked for both adults and children. Many topics were similar for both populations, with the need for diagnostic and grading criteria and Beta-2 agonist nebulizer therapy serving as the 2 top priorities. However, research into heparinized nebulizer therapy was considered the third most important topic in the pediatric population.[1]

Over time, the development of advanced pediatric burn care has led to the formation of specialized units and teams who recognize the unique physiology of and needs in caring for critically ill children. Approaching the pediatric population as comprising children and not merely small adults can prove critical to preventing therapeutic errors that can result in disastrous iatrogenic complications.

Since studies regarding many aspects of inhalation injury in children are lacking, Palmieri et al conducted a retrospective review of children (0-18 years) admitted to 1 of 4 burn centers with a diagnosis of inhalation injury between 1997 and 2007.[2] Data were gathered for 3 categories: demographics, injury characteristics, and hospital course. Inhalation injury was primarily diagnosed by bronchoscopy (71%), followed by clinical exam/history (25%) and elevated carboxyhemoglobin levels (4%). A total of 850 patients were admitted during the study period; the mean age was 7 to 9 years +/- 0.2, with a preponderance of males. The mean TBSA burned was 48.6% +/- 0.9. Although the time from injury to admission was shorter in nonsurvivors (2.8 hrs +/- 0.6 vs 4.4 hrs +/- 0.4), they suffered more full-thickness burns (61.9%TBSA +/- 2.3%TBSA vs 35.4 +/- 1.0), had larger TBSA burns (68.5% +/- 1.9 vs 44.6% +/- 0.9), and spent more time on the ventilator. Significant differences in the group of nonsurvivors were seen with regard to burn size ($P < .001$), full-thickness burns ($P < .001$), and shorter hospital length of stay (LOS) ($P < .001$). The majority of nonsurvivors succumbed to respiratory dysfunction (36%), followed by sepsis (22%), multisystem organ failure (11%), and anoxic injury (11%). In conclusion, the major factors associated with increased mortality in pediatric patients suffering an inhalation injury were TBSA burned and full-thickness burns. In this review, mortality was 16%, and death occurred approximately 3 weeks following the initial injury. Although this was a retrospective study, it provides insight into the features that may assist clinicians with the difficult task of recognizing factors in inhalation injury which contribute to increased mortality.[2]

## PATHOPHYSIOLOGY

Injury to the tracheobronchial system is principally chemical in nature, as heat is primarily dispersed in the upper airways; direct thermal damage to the distal bronchi is seen only on occasion. Inhalants are classified as irritants, asphyxiates, or systemic toxins. Irritants such as ammonia, chlorine, sulfur dioxide, and carbon monoxide cause extensive cell injury within the respiratory tract. Every fire is unique with regards to the damage sustained to the respiratory system by the involvement of different chemicals and materials. For instance, combustion of cellulose, nylon, wool, silk, asphalt, and polyurethane increase the risk of hydrogen cyanide poisoning. Hydrogen cyanide, sulfide, and hydrocarbons are examples of asphyxiates which interrupt the delivery of oxygen to the tissues. Systemic toxins, meanwhile, can be absorbed through the respiratory endothelium. Damage correlates with the particular inhalants' chemical activity, size, solubility, temperature, and the duration and concentration of exposure. Upper airway injuries tend to be caused by more irritating, water-soluble, larger particles, whereas substances of smaller size and lower water solubility cause alveolar and parenchymal injury. Although gasoline self-extinguishes

when the oxygen concentration falls below 15%, other substances may continue to undergo thermal decomposition and further decrease ambient oxygen tension. Hypoxemia can result from a decrease in inspired oxygen concentration at the scene of injury, a mechanical inability of gas exchange because of airway obstruction or parenchymal pulmonary disease, or the inhibition of oxygen delivery and tissue use by toxins. Although early hypoxemia contributes to mortality from smoke inhalation, it is the presence of multiorgan dysfunction, a common sequela of hypoxia, which leads to a substantial increase in morbidity and mortality.

The immediate physiological response to smoke inhalation is a significant increase in bronchial blood flow and pulmonary lymph flow.[3,4,5,6] Heat from a thermal insult initially denatures protein and leads to complement activation.[3,7,8] This subsequently sets off a cascade of events involving histamine release, conversion of xanthine oxidase, and production of oxygen-derived free radicals.[3,7,9,10,11,12] As a result, increased permeability to protein and elevated microvascular pressure cause the characteristic formation of edema seen in this type of injury. The lymph content in this situation is similar to serum, thus indicating that permeability at the capillary level is markedly increased. The resulting edema is associated with an increase in neutrophils, postulated to be the primary mediators of pulmonary damage through release of proteases and free radicals, which can produce conjugated dienes via lipid peroxidation.[3,13,14,15] High concentrations of conjugated dienes present in pulmonary lymph fluid after inhalation injury support this theory.[3,16,17,18]

Besides edema formation, another hallmark of inhalation injury is the separation of ciliated epithelial cells from the basement membrane, followed by the formation of exudate within the bronchi.[19,20] This protein-rich exudate eventually coalesces to form fibrin casts which can be difficult to clear with standard airway suction techniques. Oftentimes, bronchoscopic removal is necessary. These casts also contribute to barotrauma within localized areas of the lung by producing a "ball-valve" effect. During inspiration, airway diameter increases and air flows past the cast into the distal airways; when the diameter decreases during expiration, the cast effectively occludes the airway, thereby preventing inhaled air from escaping. The subsequent increase in volume leads to localized elevations in pressure that are associated with numerous complications, including pneumothorax and decreased lung compliance.

The full extent of airway compromise may not be evident until 12 to 24 hours after the initial injury. For patients with extensive surface burns, chest wall restriction may occur because of eschar formation. Reflexive bronchoconstriction can further exacerbate this obstructive process. Both inspiratory and expiratory resistance can be increased with premature closure of tertiary bronchi leading to hyperinflation and air trapping. Surfactant production and activity are both impaired, which worsens alveolar collapse and segmental atelectasis. Low-pressure pulmonary edema seems to also play an important role in the development of lung injury from smoke inhalation. Damage to the alveolar-capillary membrane increases permeability, with ensuing intravascular leakage into the pulmonary interstitium. Eventually, increased lymphatic flow exacerbates alveolar edema. Loss of compliance, further atelectasis, and increasing edema can result in severe ventilation-perfusion mismatch and hypoxemia.

Pulmonary insufficiency related to inhalation injury can be broadly categorized as the result of thermal or chemical damage to the epithelial surfaces of the intrathoracic and extrathoracic airways. Pneumonia can then cause a secondary insult, sometimes days after the initial injury, leading to further cytotoxic damage. Accumulation of airway debris occurs due to impaired function of the cilia and the inflammatory cascade, which initiates neutrophil activation and leads to the destruction of alveolar-based macrophages and subsequent proliferation of bacteria. Overt respiratory failure with acute respiratory distress syndrome (ARDS) can develop at any time during this process. Ascertaining whether respiratory insufficiency is due to direct pulmonary injury or is the result of extensive metabolic, hemodynamic, and subsequent infectious complications related to the loss of integument surface can be challenging.

## CLINICAL PRESENTATION

The clinical presentation of inhalation victims can range from mild to severe. In most cases, the presentation of a person injured in a fire is obvious. When the patient is unable to provide a history, further details of the event and additional information can often be obtained from witnesses and first providers.

Patients with inhalation injury may present with various airway and pulmonary symptoms. A strong suspicion of smoke inhalation should be raised with signs of singed facial hair or eyebrows, eye irritations, facial burns, and soot marks. Patients presenting with shortness of breath, hoarseness, cough, hemoptysis, or facial burns should be admitted for observation. If tachypnea, rhonchi, wheezes, rales, or production of carbonaceous sputum are also present, then admission to a monitored unit is more appropriate. It is imperative to recognize that it may take several hours for upper airway swelling to develop. In general, facial burns, hoarseness, stridor, carbonaceous sputum, or upper airway injury with mucosal lesions identified upon oral examination are indications to promptly perform intubation. Symptoms

indicative of lower respiratory tract injury include tachypnea, dyspnea, cough, decreased breath sounds, wheezing, rales, rhonchi, and chest wall retractions. Cyanosis is an unreliable marker of underlying hypoxemia because of the bright-red ("cherry-pink") color imparted to the skin with elevated carboxyhemoglobin levels. Red retinal veins resulting from elevated venous oxyhemoglobin saturation may be noted on fundoscopic examination.

Neurologic injury, which may not be immediately evident, can occur from hypoxemia either at the time of injury or from pulmonary dysfunction. In the burned child, fear, pain, and obtundation from inadequate perfusion may cloud the clinical picture. Performing serial examinations with repeated assessments may improve one's ability to follow sensory changes and help guide initial resuscitation and stabilization. Victims who have not lost consciousness and with a normal neurologic examination on admission almost always recover without need for treatment beyond the administration of supplemental oxygen. Cyanide toxicity should be suspected in a child whose sensorium remains clouded despite oxygen therapy. The presence of coma following exposure to fire is nearly always indicative of carbon monoxide (CO) poisoning and should be promptly treated with 100% oxygen for at least 4 hours.

Although cardiovascular injury itself is usually not a focus in inhalation injury, complex cardiovascular changes with surface burns may coexist with smoke inhalation. Heart rate, capillary refill, warmth of unburned extremities, and blood pressure should be promptly evaluated at presentation and closely followed during the initial stabilization. Carbon monoxide poisoning should be suspected in young people with healthy hearts who demonstrate ischemic changes on an EKG. Narrowed pulse pressure may indicate inadequate volume resuscitation and should necessitate reevaluation of a patient's perfusion and fluid requirements. A low blood pressure is invariably a late finding of volume loss.

## INITIAL EVALUATION AND MANAGEMENT

The first priority when assessing a patient with a potential inhalation injury is to assess the airway and determine the need for intubation. Signs of partial obstruction, such as hoarseness, stridor, and expiratory wheezes, suggest a significant risk of progression to complete obstruction.[21] A study by Rue et al in 1995 revealed that up to 80% of patients with inhalation injury required endotracheal intubation for inhalation injury, even if only for short-term airway management.[22] In general, the indications for intubation in patients with inhalation injury are no different from general guidelines. The benefits of securing the airway with endotracheal intubation include provision of a secure airway, facilitating pulmonary toilet (suctioning, bronchodilator administration, etc), and addressing oxygenation and ventilation issues in a more direct fashion. As with all medical interventions, endotracheal intubation is not without risks, which include barotrauma, anatomical damage, increased risk of ventilator-associated pneumonia, tracheobronchitis, tracheomalacia, subglottic stenosis, and innominate or esophageal fistula formation. Until further studies are designed to answer the question of which patients might benefit from intubation, each patient must continue to be assessed individually.

Once patients have been intubated, the clinician must decide which mode of mechanical ventilatory support to institute. This becomes particularly relevant when dealing with patients who are significantly hypoxemic or who meet criteria for acute lung injury (ALI) or ARDS. While the ARDSnet study in 2000 has changed the way such patients are now managed (lung protective strategy utilizing low tidal volumes and maintaining low plateau pressures), it remains unclear how the results of these studies can or should be applied to children with inhalation injury. High-frequency oscillatory ventilation (HFOV), commonly used in neonates with ARDS, has been attempted in critically ill patients with ARDS as well, usually as a rescue therapy. Even though HFOV has been shown to consistently improve oxygenation, studies thus far have not revealed a consistency with improved outcomes. Specifically in burn patients, HFOV studies thus far include one animal experiment, a pediatric case report, and unpublished data from 19 adult burn patients with inhalation injury. HFOV is essentially a form of lung protective mechanical ventilation, which utilizes small tidal volumes at high frequencies (3-15 Hz), along with sustained high mean arterial pressures (30-40 cm $H_2O$). Concerns of HFOV include

(1) small airway obstruction due to edema/spasm and sloughing of mucosal carbonaceous debris;
(2) trouble managing gas trapping and hypercapnea;
(3) difficulty instituting adequate pulmonary toilet and other modalities (bronchodilators); and
(4) consideration that ARDS due to inhalation injury may produce different pathophysiologic changes as compared to other diseases.[23]

Understandably, questions remain as to the utility of HFOV in burns, whether instituted as a rescue therapy or as an earlier approach. Of note, high-frequency percussive ventilation has shown proven benefit when instituted immediately following smoke inhalation.[24-26] However, further studies are required to determine the exact role of this unique ventilatory modality.

As with all patients, obtaining a complete medical history is important. The presence of underlying lung disease, including simple asthma, can make a child more susceptible to airway irritation. It is valuable to remember that a child and an adult simultaneously exposed to smoke inhalation can present with notably different disease severity. Pediatric patients have an increased minute ventilation and a smaller body size compared to adults, which may increase toxin exposure. Children may also become disoriented more easily than adults, thus delaying escape from a poisonous environment and prolonging exposure. When documenting the history, it is important to explore the duration of exposure and, if possible, the actual toxins of exposure to help determine toxicity. A description of the mechanism of injury should include the location (ie, closed space) as well. With a smoky fire, any victim trapped in an enclosed space or exhibiting neurologic symptoms should receive 100% oxygen with a tight-fitting mask for at least 4 hours. Carbon monoxide, a colorless, odorless gas, is a major component of the smoke produced by incomplete combustion of carbon-containing compounds, such as wood, coal, and gasoline. A significant carbon monoxide exposure can occur even in the absence of flames, as with malfunctioning domestic equipment (eg, poorly ventilated space heaters, cooking gas) and exposure to automobile exhaust fumes, either from a suicide attempt (not uncommon amongst teenagers) or accidentally, from poor ventilation.

A complete physical examination should be performed as soon as possible, with careful inspection of the mouth and pharynx. Although copious mucus production and carbonaceous sputum are signs of inhalation injury, their absence does not rule out the diagnosis. In addition to carboxyhemoglobin (CO-Hb) levels, arterial blood gases should be drawn on anyone with suspected smoke poisoning in order to more accurately assess oxygenation. One of the earliest indicators of pulmonary compromise is an abnormal $PaO_2$ to $FIO_2$ ratio (the P/F ratio). A normal ratio is 400 to 500, whereas patients with respiratory insufficiency may demonstrate a ratio of less than 300 (eg, a $PaO_2$ of less than 120 with a $FIO_2$ of 0.40). A ratio of less than 250 is an indication for vigorous respiratory support rather than merely increasing the inspired oxygen concentration.

Once a patient is admitted to the burn unit, a standard approach to monitoring and further management should be followed. All patients should have continuous pulse oximetry. Cutaneous pulse oximetry uses a dual-wavelength technique of light refractance to measure hemoglobin saturation. Because it is falsely elevated by CO-Hb, all patients should have direct measurements of carboxyhemoglobin and oxyhemoglobin. Once the CO-Hb level has reached the reference range, pulse oximetry can be relied upon. All patients should have arterial blood gases drawn upon admission and as necessary thereafter, because CO-oximetry (arterial blood) uses a 4-wavelength technique of light refractance which allows accurate measurements of carboxyhemoglobin, oxyhemoglobin, deoxyhemoglobin, and methemoglobin. However, arterial oxygen tension does not accurately reflect the degree of carbon monoxide poisoning or cellular hypoxia. The $PaO_2$ level reflects the oxygen dissolved in blood that is not altered by the hemoglobin-bound carbon monoxide. Since dissolved oxygen makes up only a small fraction of arterial oxygen content, a $PaO_2$ level within the reference range may lead to a serious underestimation of oxygen delivery and the associated degree of hypoxia at the cellular level. Most blood gas machines calculate the oxygen saturation based on the $PaO_2$ level. Nonetheless, ABG measurements are useful to assess the adequacy of pulmonary gas exchange. Although the presence of a $PaO_2$ level within the reference range may not exclude significant tissue hypoxia due to the effects of carbon monoxide, the presence of a low $PaO_2$ (< 60 mm Hg) or hypercarbia ($PaCO_2$ level of 50 mm Hg or greater) is indicative of significant respiratory insufficiency. The workup should also include basic chemistry and complete blood counts in order to correct and follow underlying electrolyte imbalances and aid in fluid management.

## DIAGNOSTIC TOOLS

Inhalation injury is often suspected with a clinical history of exposure to smoke in a closed space, facial burns, singed nasal hair, hoarseness, wheezing, and carbonaceous sputum. As useful as these signs and symptoms or a suggestive history may be for identifying inhalation injury, they all possess poor sensitivity and specificity. A routine chest radiograph is also insensitive in diagnosing inhalation injury but may be useful as a baseline measure in the event of clinical deterioration. In addition, computed tomography has a limited role in diagnosis, though it may help delineate such pathology as atelectasis, effusions, consolidation, or the presence of a pneumothorax.

Therefore, more definitive methods, such as bronchoscopy and xenon 133 ($^{133}Xe$) scanning, which are more than 90% accurate in determining the presence of inhalation injury, should be employed. The fiberoptic bronchoscope, perhaps the most useful and successful modality, allows direct visualization of the supraglottic airway and tracheobronchial tree.[21] Bronchoscopic examination of the airway at the bedside (avoiding the need to transport critically ill patients) is usually sufficient to identify airway edema and inflammatory changes of the tracheal mucosa, such as hyperemia, mucosal ulceration, and sloughing. These findings, together with the clinical manifestations, can usually verify the presence of inhalation injury. Bronchoscopy can also be helpful in assisting with intubation during situations where

a difficult airway may be encountered. Complications of bronchoscopy are rare but include pneumothorax, infection, hypoxemia, arrhythmias, and death. Nonetheless, studies have determined that such complications are quite infrequent and the benefits usually outweigh the risks.[3,27,28,29] At this time, bronchoscopy remains the gold standard for diagnosing inhalation injury, even though it has limitations in identifying the full extent of pulmonary parenchymal damage. Bronchoscopic findings, however, do not correlate with clinical severity but are an objective measurement of initial exposure. Ventilation scanning with $^{133}Xe$ reveals areas of the lung that retain isotope 90 seconds after IV injection, thus indicating segmental airway obstruction. Although infrequently utilized for diagnosing inhalation injury, it may be valuable as an adjunctive modality in those cases where high clinical suspicion remains in the setting of an unremarkable bronchoscopic examination. It has been shown that utilizing both techniques produces 93% accuracy in the diagnosis of smoke inhalation.[3]

## CARBON MONOXIDE

Carbon monoxide intoxication is a particularly serious consequence of smoke inhalation and may account for up to 80% of fatalities. As such, carboxyhemoglobin level should be measured in all patients. Elevated levels or any clinical symptoms of CO poisoning are presumptive evidence of poisoning. In very smoky fires, CO-Hb levels of 40% to 50% may be reached after only 2 to 3 minutes of exposure. Neurologic dysfunction of carbon monoxide poisoning is classified into 2 syndromes: (1) persistent neurologic sequelae, which may improve over time, and (2) delayed neurologic sequelae, which occur after an initial period of improvement.[30] Up to one-third of patients with significant carbon monoxide exposure will develop long-term neurologic deficits.

Carbon monoxide binds to iron-containing compounds such as hemoglobin and cytochromes. Compared to molecular oxygen, CO possesses a much higher affinity (210 times as much) for the binding site on the hemoglobin moiety.[30] By causing a leftward shift of the oxyhemoglobin dissociation curve, a diminished amount of oxygen is off-loaded at the cellular level. Administering 100% oxygen decreases the elimination half-life of carbon monoxide, which is dependent on oxygen tension.

It should be kept in mind that smokers may have baseline CO levels up to 5% to 10% and therefore may experience worsening symptoms for the same level of exposure as nonsmokers. Also, blood carboxyhemoglobin levels may underestimate the degree of CO intoxication because of oxygen administration before arrival to the hospital. Unfortunately, low or normal levels do not rule out inhalation injuries, nor do they indicate the severity of poisoning or assist with determining treatment or prognosis.[31] Victims who remain comatose once CO-Hb levels have returned to normal carry a poor prognosis. The use of nomograms to extrapolate levels to the time of rescue has been shown to provide greater prognostic value. Factors that contribute to the extent of injury include the duration of exposure, concentration of CO, and premorbid condition of the victim.[32] The symptoms in relation to carboxyhemoglobin concentration are as follows:[3,33,34]

- Carboxyhemoglobin level of 0%–10%
  -Usually asymptomatic
- Carboxyhemoglobin level of 10%–20%
  -Mild headache, atypical dyspnea
- Carboxyhemoglobin level of 20%–30%
  -Throbbing headache, impaired concentration
- Carboxyhemoglobin level of 30%–40%
  -Severe headache, impaired thinking
- Carboxyhemoglobin level of 40%–50%
  -Confusion, lethargy, syncope
- Carboxyhemoglobin level of 50%–60%
  -Respiratory failure, seizures
- Carboxyhemoglobin level > 70%
  -Coma, death

Initial management of suspected CO toxicity includes supportive care and 100% oxygen. The basis for supplemental oxygen administration is the decreased half-life from 90 minutes (room air) to 20 to 30 minutes (high-flow $O_2$).[35] Although enthusiasts for hyperbaric oxygen treatment (HBOT) consider it a standard of care for CO poisoning, many physicians are skeptical. Several trials have been performed exploring the effects of hyperbaric therapy on CO poisoning; of the 7 randomized controlled trials, 4 did not find HBO beneficial in terms of improving neurologic sequelae, 2 reported a benefit, and 1 did not state outcomes.[32] Furthermore, when associated with a major burn injury, transport to a hyperbaric chamber may delay definitive burn care. One must also weigh the benefit with such possible complications as emesis, seizures, eustachian tube occlusion, aspiration, agitation requiring restraints or sedation, hypotension, tension pneumothorax, and cardiac arrhythmia or arrest. A recent retrospective study by Hampson et al [36] has revisited the question of HBOT in carbon monoxide poisoning. The records of 1505 patients with acute CO poisoning from 1978 through 2005 who received HBOT were reviewed. This study revealed a mortality rate similar to that previously reported, at 2.6%. Factors associated with increased mortality included decreased level of consciousness, fire as the source of CO, carboxyhemoglobin level, presence of endotracheal intubation during

HBOT, and severe metabolic acidosis. In a follow-up paper for the same group of patients, Hampson et al determined an increased risk of long-term mortality in adult survivors of acute carbon monoxide poisoning who were treated with HBOT.[37] While these results do not definitively answer questions, they do provide a basis for further investigation. The issue of whether, and at what time in the progression of CO poisoning, HBOT is of value will undoubtedly continue to be studied and debated.

## CYANIDE

Approximately one-third of patients with smoke inhalation from domestic fires will be exposed to cyanide (CN). Although laboratory confirmation may be delayed, CN levels should be sent at time of admission, even though the clinical significance of such levels is unknown. Persistent neurologic dysfunction unresponsive to supplemental oxygen, cardiac dysfunction, hypoxemia, unexplained metabolic acidosis, and severe lactic acidosis, particularly in the presence of high mixed venous oxygen saturation, are indicative of CN intoxication. Moreover, the unique odor of bitter almonds has been described with CN toxicity as well.[3,38,39]

CN causes tissue asphyxiation through inhibition of intracellular cytochrome oxidase. CN blocks the final step in oxidative phosphorylation and prevents mitochondrial oxygen use. Affected cells convert to anaerobic metabolism, and lactic acidosis ensues. The central nervous system (CNS) and the myocardium are most sensitive to cellular hypoxia. The CNS reacts to low concentrations of CN by inducing tachypnea and clinically apparent hyperventilation, which increases further exposure. Death is subsequently due to respiratory center paralysis.

In a setting consistent with potential CN exposure, one should consider instituting specific empiric therapy while awaiting laboratory confirmation of the diagnosis. Therapy with CN antidotes versus aggressive supportive care remains controversial. The basis for treatment is to oxidize hemoglobin to methemoglobin, which preferentially binds CN to form cyanmethemoglobin. This then dissociates and is metabolized by hepatic mitochondria to thiocyanate, which is excreted in the urine.[40] Since amyl nitrate or sodium nitrate can both cause cardiac irritability and hypotension, their use should be carefully considered in an often hypovolemic burn patient.

## EXPERIMENTAL THERAPIES

Antithrombin (AT) III is a serine protease inhibitor produced in the liver which complexes with and inhibits thrombin activity. Besides being a major physiologic anti-coagulant, it also possesses anti-inflammatory properties. Studies thus far have primarily focused on AT for congenital AT III deficiency, sepsis, and DIC. Thermal injury is a type of acquired AT deficiency due to multiple factors. The deficiency is usually seen postburn days 1 through 5 and is an independent predictor of length of stay and mortality.[41] Studies in burn patients have been performed, and there is promise in the potential of AT for improving outcomes in thermal injury (perhaps inhalation injury as well); however, further research is required in order to determine whether this will provide clinicians with another option in the challenging treatment of such patients.

Tocopherols are scavengers of reactive oxygen and nitrogen species. Large burns are associated with significant tissue oxidation and alpha tocopherol depletion. In addition, studies in animals have shown depletion of liver stores of vitamin E with skin and lung injury.[42] Morita et al subsequently studied nebulized and oral tocopherol in an animal model and discovered they were both effective in reducing the associated pathophysiologic responses of burns and smoke inhalation.[43,44] These studies provide interesting thoughts into the use of tocopherol for patients suffering burn and inhalation injury; however, once again, further studies are necessary before any recommendations can be made.

Since smoke inhalation injury is characterized by inflammation with oxidative damage, interest in the possible beneficial effects of vitamin C is increasing. In 2000 Tanaka et al performed a clinical trial of severely burned patients who were given high-dose vitamin C during resuscitation.[45] Thirty-seven patients with an average > 30% TBSA burn received either placebo or 66 mg/kg/h vitamin C for 24 hours. No differences in heart rate, blood pressure, base deficit, central venous pressure, or urine output were noted. Although the resuscitation volume after 24 hours was 40% lower in the vitamin C group, there was no difference in mortality. Of note is that 73% of these patients were diagnosed with inhalation injury by bronchoscopy at admission, with an equal distribution in both groups. There was no difference in PEEP or $FIO_2$ requirements in the first 96 hours, although a significant difference in $PaO_2/FIO_2$ was noted from 18 through 96 hours, as well in as the number of ventilator days.[45] A study by Dubick et al from San Antonio revealed similar findings in a 40% TBSA burn sheep model comparing placebo versus high-dose vitamin C (10 gm/first 500 cc resuscitation volume, followed by a 15 mg/kg infusion x 48 hours), with a 40% decrease in total fluid requirements noted.[46] Another study exploring the effects of vitamin C on smoke inhalation injury in 42 dogs by Jiang showed a reduction in extravascular lung water volume, PVR, carboxemia, hypoxia, and acidosis.[47] More impressive was the reduction in mortality

from 47.6% in the control group to 19.1% for the treatment group. Unfortunately, this study was only available in abstract form and utilized a treatment cocktail that included other substances. Therefore, conclusions are difficult to ascertain, and the role of vitamin C in inhalation injury remains elusive at this time.[47,48]

Steroids have been studied for years in the treatment of ARDS due to their anti-inflammatory effects. Concerns regarding the risks, such as infections, hypothalamic axis dysfunction, neuromuscular dysfunction, and osteoporosis, however, have tempered enthusiasm for their use. Despite multiple studies, steroids have not consistently proven beneficial in patients with ARDS. However, hope springs eternal, and proponents of steroid therapy continue to advocate their use. A recent systemic review and meta-analysis reexplored the controversy of whether corticosteroids are beneficial in acute lung injury and ARDS.[49] Five cohort studies and 4 randomized, controlled trials revealed a trend toward improvement in ventilator-free days, ICU stay, $PaO_2/FIO_2$, multiple organ dysfunction syndrome and lung injury scores, and mortality, without an increase in any significant complications. The authors concluded that these findings suggest a benefit of steroids in such patients, although confirmation is required by further studies.[49] Research involving steroids for inhalation injury has thus far been disappointing, and further research is necessary before any conclusions can be drawn.

The characteristic finding of alveolar fibrin deposition in ALI/ARDS is also seen in burn patients. Fibrin contributes to ventilation perfusion mismatch, atelectasis (through inhibition of surfactant), and attraction of inflammatory cells to the injury site. As such, anticoagulants have been theorized to possibly play a role in the pathophysiology of smoke inhalation. A study by Enkhbaatar et al revealed that an aerosolized fibrinolytic agent (tPA) improved pulmonary function in an ovine model of ALI following inhalation injury.[50] In 1988, Brown et al first reported on aerosolized heparin with and without dimethyl sulfoxide (DMSO) for smoke-inhalation-induced ALI in an ovine model. Decreased mortality was seen with heparin, and the effects were potentiated with the addition of DMSO.[51] A study by Murakami et al in 2003 of smoke inhalation in an ovine model revealed heparin nebulization to be beneficial;[52] however, another similar study of ARDS from smoke inhalation did not show any benefit with regards to improvement in pulmonary function. These findings were explained by the presence of decreased antithrombin levels in the broncho-alveolar lavage (BAL) of animals with ARDS.[53] In children with massive burns and inhalation injury, Desai et al in 1998 found that nebulized heparin along with aerosolized N-acetylcysteine significantly reduced the rates of reintubation, atelectasis, and mortality.[54] Thus far, the potential benefits of heparin for inhalation injury have been limited to animal and single-center studies. As with most other promising treatments, further studies need to be performed to better understand the effects before any recommendations can be postulated.

Inhaled nitric oxide (INO) is utilized as a treatment modality for pulmonary hypertension, particularly in neonates. It is also indicated for hypoxemic respiratory failure in newborns. INO is a potent, short-acting pulmonary vasodilator which increases cyclic guanosine monophosphate in smooth muscle. Risks associated with its use include methemoglobinemia and rebound hypoxemia after discontinuation. Use of INO in animal models with smoke inhalation revealed decreased pulmonary hypertension associated with inhalation injury, with variable effects regarding improvement of pulmonary shunting. Human studies include 2 adult and 1 children single-institution series that included patients with large burns and inhalation injury with respiratory failure. These studies demonstrated increased $PaO_2/FIO_2$ in two-thirds of patients, with a marginal improvement in the oxygenation ratio in the remainder of patients. Responses were usually seen within 60 minutes at doses of 20 ppm. No complications were reported, and survival was more common in those who demonstrated increases in the $PaO_2/FIO_2$ ratio.[55,56,57] A 2007 *BMJ* meta-analysis showed no survival benefit of INO in critically ill patients with oxygenation failure, despite an improvement in oxygenation.[58] With respect to burn patients with inhalation injury, INO improved oxygenation in some patients at doses of 5 to 20 ppm. This has prompted consideration for use in those patients who have otherwise failed conventional measures. Until further studies can explore the effects of INO for this population, no conclusions can be drawn.

Currently, the management and treatment for inhalation injuries is primarily supportive. The effort to develop new strategies and techniques continues to expand and includes areas of research into systemic as well as local response to thermal injuries. The core to such research is a better understanding of the basic but complex pathophysiology of the body's response to this type of presentation as well as the way in which the respiratory system responds. Much of the emphasis is placed on trying different methods of ventilatory support, focusing on improving ways to oxygenate and ventilate the child. The challenge involves optimizing these parameters while maintaining low airway pressures to minimize barotrauma.

Methods such as HFPV and airway pressure release ventilation (APRV) appear to recruit alveoli and allow efficient gas exchange while simultaneously using lower peak airway pressures when compared to conventional mechanical ventilation.[59] For severe respiratory failure, extracorporeal membrane oxygenation (ECMO) has been used in both the pediatric and adult population.[60] Another new and experimental technique called arteriovenous carbon dioxide removal ($AVCO_2R$) utilizes an extracorporeal membrane gas exchanger to remove $CO_2$ while oxygen diffuses across the native alveoli by low-frequency positive-pressure ventilation.[61] This method has been shown to significantly reduce ventilatory requirements and improve arterial blood pH levels.[62]

As overall patient survival continues to improve, pulmonary function as the child grows and develops is another challenge. In one study, hyperreactive airways along with inflammatory changes in the bronchial mucosa and elevated inflammatory cytokines have been shown to last up to 6 months, even with normal pulmonary function tests.[63] Other studies have shown development of restrictive and obstructive patterns on pulmonary function testing, with no appreciable return to normal lung function.[64] Still, further studies have revealed that children are quite resilient and exhibit a relatively good functional status, albeit with higher respiratory rates; moreover, some adults have shown no evidence of exercise compromise or any alteration in function post–inhalation injury.[65] Determining survival from inhalation injuries and returning to premorbid functioning is dependent on further investigation involving trials of newer agents and novel ventilatory strategies.

## CONCLUSION

The presence of smoke inhalation substantially increases morbidity and mortality of burn patients. Despite significant advances in overall care, the specific management of inhalation injury remains supportive. Furthermore, direct treatments remain elusive, partly due to the complexities involved in balancing a lung protective strategy with the risks of causing damage to at-risk pulmonary tissue. To further complicate matters, there are the multiple confounding factors commonly encountered in burn patients, such as infection, sepsis, and the hypermetabolic response.

The long-term outcome of children with inhalation injury is unknown with regards to general health measures, quality of life, physiological effects, and social adaptation. Small case studies comprise the majority of data on long-term pulmonary function after exposure. The available literature reveals that airway obstruction may occur for a prolonged period of time following smoke inhalation and that the extent of obstruction is proportional to the amount inhaled.[66] In particular, the effects on children are concerning since lung development continues until midchildhood. Until further studies are designed to determine the long-term physical and psychosocial effects of inhalation injury, caregivers must continue to strive for the best possible outcomes to allow these children to live happy and productive lives.

# REFERENCES

1. Pamieri T. Inhalation injury consensus conference: conclusions. *J Burn Care Res*. 2009; **30**(1): 209–210.

2. Palmieri T, Warner P, Mlcak R, et al. Inhalation injury in children: a 10 year experience at Shriners Hospitals for Children. *J Burn Care Res*. 2009; **30**(1): 1–3.

3. Herndon D, ed. *Total Burn Care*. 2nd ed. London: WB Saunders; 2002; 223–225.

4. Abdi S, Herndon D, Mcguire J, Traber L, Traber DL. Time course of alterations in lung lymph and bronchial blood flows after inhalation injury. *J Burn Care Rehabil*. 1990; **11**: 510–515.

5. Stothert JC Jr, Ashley KD, Kramer GC, et al. Intrapulmonary distribution of bronchial blood flow after moderate smoke inhalation. *J Appl Physiol*. 1990; **69**: 1734–1739.

6. Hales CA, Barkin P, Jung W, et al. Bronchial artery ligation modifies pulmonary edema after exposure to smoke with acrolein. *J Appl Physiol*. 1989; **67**: 1001–1006.

7. Friedl HP, Till GO, Trentz O, et al. Roles of histamine, complement and xanthine oxidase in thermal injury of skin. *Am J Pathol*. 1989; **135**: 203–217.

8. Oldham KT, Guice KS, Till GO, et al. Activation of complement by hydroxyl radical in thermal injury. *Surgery*. 1988; **104**: 272–279.

9. Ward PA, Till GO. Pathophysiologic events related to thermal injury of skin. *J Trauma*. 1990; **30**: S75–S79.

10. Schlayer HJ, Laaff H, Peters T, et al. Involvement of TNF in endotoxin triggered neutrophil adherence to sinusoidal endothelial cells of mouse liver and its modulation in acute phase. *J Hepatol*. 1988; **7**: 239–249.

11. Granger D, Rutili G, McCord J. Superoxide radicals in feline intestinal ischemia. *Gastroenterology*. 1981; **81**: 22–29.

12. Granger DN, McCord JM, Parks DA, et al. Xanthine oxidase inhibitors attenuate ischemia induced vascular permeability changes in the cat intestine. *Gastroenterology*. 1986; **90**: 80–84.

13. Traber DL, Schlag G, Redl H, et al. Pulmonary edema and compliance changes following smoke inhalation. *J Burn Care Rehabil*. 1985; **6**: 490–494.

14. Linares HA, Herndon DN, Traber DL, et al. Experimental inhalation injury: histopathological evaluation. *Annu Meet Am Burn Assoc*. 1983; **15**: 90–91.

15. Loick HM, Herndon DN, Traber LD, et al. Thromboxane receptor blockade with BM 13,177 following toxic airway damage by smoke inhalation in sheep. *Eur J Pharmacol*. 1993; **248**: 75–83.

16. Basadre JO, Sugi K, Traber DL, et al. The effect of leukocyte depletion on smoke inhalation injury in sheep. *Surgery*. 1988; **104**: 208–215.

17. Isago T, Fujioka K, Traber LD, et al. Pulmonary capillary pressure changes following smoke inhalation in sheep. *Anesthesiology*. 1990; **73**: A1234.

18. Loick HM, Traber LD, Tokyay R, et al. Mechanical alteration of blood flow in smoked and unsmoked lung areas after inhalation injury. *J Appl Physiol*. 1992; **72**: 1692–1700.

19. Abdi S, Evans MJ, Cox RA, et al. Inhalation injury to tracheal epithelium in an ovine model of cotton smoke exposure. Early phase (30 minutes). *Am Rev Respir Dis*. 1990; **142**: 1436–1439.

20. Barrow RE, Wang CZ, Cox RA, et al. Cellular sequence of tracheal repair in sheep after smoke inhalation injury. *Lung*. 1992: **170**: 331–338.

21. Sheridan RL. Airway management and respiratory care of the burn patient. *Int Anesthesiol Clin*. 2000; **38**(3): 129–145.

22. Rue LW, Dioffi WG, Mason A, McManus W, Pruitt BA. The risk of pneumonia in thermally injured patients requiring ventilatory support. *J Burn Care Res*. 1995; **16**: 262–268.

23. Cartotto R. Use of high frequency oscillatory ventilation in inhalation injury. *J Burn Care Res*. 2009; **30**(1): 1–4.

24. Cioffi WG, Loring WR, Graves TA, McManus WF, Mason AD, Pruitt BA. Prophylactic use of high frequency percussive ventilation in patients with inhalation injury. *Ann Surg*. 1991; **213**: 575–582.

25. Reper P, Wibauz O, VanLaeka P, Vandeenan D, Duinslager L, Vanderkelen A. High frequency percussive ventilation and conventional ventilation after smoke inhalation: a randomized study. *Burns*. 2002; **28**: 503–508.

26. Hall JJ, Hunt JL, Arnoldo BD, Purdue GF. Use of high frequency percussive ventilation in inhalation injuries. *J Burn Care Res*. 2007; **28**: 396–400.

27. Suratt PM, Smiddy JF, Gruber B. Deaths and complications associated with fiberoptic bronchoscopy. *Chest*. 1976; **69**: 747–751.

28. Credle WF Jr, Smiddy JF, Elliott RC. Complications of fiberoptic bronchoscopy. *Am Rev Respir Dis*. 1974; **109**: 67–72.

29. Pereira W Jr, Kovnat DM, Snider GL. A prospective cooperative study of complications following flexible fiberoptic bronchoscopy. *Chest*. 1978; **73**: 813–816.

30. Weaver LK. Carbon monoxide poisoning. *Crit Care Clin*. 1999; **15**: 297–317.

31. Hardy DR, Thom SR. Pathophysiology and treatment of carbon monoxide poisoning. *J Toxicol Clin Toxicol*. 1994; **32**: 613–629.

32. Kealey GP. Carbon monoxide toxicity. *J Burn Care Res*. 2009; **30**(1): 146–147.

33. Pitkanen J, Lund T, Aanderud L, Reed RK. Transcapillary colloid osmotic pressures in injured and non-injured skin of seriously burned patients. *Burns Incl Therm Inj*. 1987; **13**: 198–203.

34. Demling RH, Smith M, Gunther R, et al. Use of chronic prefemoral lymphatic fistula for monitoring systemic capillary integrity in unanesthetized sheep. *J Surg Res*. 1981; **31**(2): 136–144.

35. Crapo RO. Smoke inhalation injuries. *JAMA*. 1981; **246**: 1694–1696.

36. Hampson NB, Hauff NM. Risk factors for short-term mortality from carbon monoxide poisoning treated with hyperbaric oxygen. *Crit Care Med.* 2008; **36**(9): 2523–2527.

37. Hampson NB, Rudd RA, Hauff NM. Increased long term mortality among survivors of acute carbon monoxide poisoning. *Crit Care Med.* 2009; **37**(6): 1941–1947.

38. Clark CJ, Cambell D, Reid WH. Blood carboxyhemoglobin and cyanide levels in fire survivors. *Lancet.* 1981; **1**: 1332–1335.

39. Baud FJ, Barriot P, Toffis V, et al. Elevated blood cyanide concentrations in victims of smoke inhalation. *N Engl J Med.* 1991; **325**: 1761–1766.

40. Prein T, Traber DL. Toxic smoke compounds and inhalation injury—a review. *Burns Incl Therm Inj.* 1988; **14**: 451–460.

41. Latenser B. Use of antithrombin III in inhalation injury. *J Burn Care Res.* 2009; **30**(1): 186–188.

42. Traber MG, Shimoda K, Murakami K, et al. Burn and smoke inhalation injury in sheep depletes vitamin E: kinetic studies using deuterated tocopherols. *Free Radic Biol Med.* 2007; **42**(9): 1421–1429.

43. Morita N, Traber MG, Enkhbaatar P, et al. Aerosolized alpha tocopherol ameliorates acute lung injury following combined burn and smoke inhalation in sheep. *Shock.* 2006; **25**: 277–282.

44. Morita N, Shimoda K, Traber MG, et al. Vitamin E attenuates acute lung injury in sheep with burn and smoke inhalation injury. *Redox Rep.* 2006; **11**: 61–70.

45. Tanaka H, Matsuda T, Miyagantani Y, Yukioka T, Matsuda H, Shimazaki S. Reduction of resuscitation fluid volumes in severely burned patients using ascorbic acid administration. *Arch Surg.* 2000; **135**: 326–331.

46. Dubick MA, Williams C, Elgjo GI, Kramer GC. High dose vitamin C infusion reduces fluid requirements in the resuscitation of burn injured sheep. *Shock.* 2005; **24**: 139–144.

47. Jiang KY. Experimental study on combined treatment in smoke inhalation injury. *Zhonghua Zheng Xing Shao Shang Wai Ke Az Zhi.* 1991; **7**: 278–281.

48. Wolf S. Vitamin C and smoke inhalation injury. *J Burn Care Res.* 2009; **30**(1): 1–3.

49. Tang BMP, Craig JC, Eslick GD, et al. Use of corticosteroids in acute lung injury and acute respiratory distress syndrome: a systemic review and meta-analysis. *Crit Care Med.* 2009; **37**(5): 1594–1603.

50. Enkhbaatar P, Murakami K, Cox R, et al. Aerosolized tissue plasminogen activator improves pulmonary function in sheep with burn and smoke inhalation. *Shock.* 2004; **22**: 70–75.

51. Brown M, Desai M, Traber LD, Herndon DN, Traber DL. Dimethylsulfoxide with heparin in the treatment of smoke inhalation injury. *J Burn Care Rehabil.* 1988; **9**: 22–25.

52. Murakami K, Enkhbaatar P, Shimoda K, et al. High dose heparin fails to improve acute lung injury following smoke inhalation in sheep. *Clin Sci (London).* 2003; **104**: 349–356.

53. Murakami K, Enkhbaatar P, Morita N, et al. The elevation of airway antithrombin level in smoke inhalation with pneumonia in sheep. *Crit Care Med.* 2003; **31**: A28.

54. Desai MH, Mlcak R, Richardson J, Nichols R, Herndon DN. Reduction of mortality in pediatric patients with inhalation injury with aerosolized heparin/N-acetylcysteine therapy. *J Burn Care Rehabil.* 1998; **19**: 210–212.

55. Musgrave MA, Fingland R, Gomez M, Fish J, Cartotto R. The use of inhaled NO as adjuvant therapy in patients with burn injuries and respiratory failure. *J Burn Care Rehabil.* 2000; **21**: 551–557.

56. Sheridan RL, Zapol WM, Ritz RH, Tompkins RG. Low dose inhaled nitric oxide in acutely burned children with profound respiratory failure. *Surgery.* 1999; **126**: 856–862.

57. Sheridan RL, Hurford WE, Kacmarek RM, et al. Inhaled nitric oxide in burn patients with respiratory failure. *J Trauma.* 1997; **42**: 629–634.

58. Adhikari NK, Burns KE, Friedrich JO, Granton JT, Cook DJ, Meade MO. Effect of nitric oxide on oxygenation and mortality in acute lung injury: systemic review and meta-analysis. *BMJ.* 2007; **334**: 779.

59. Reper P, Van Bos R, Van Loey K, et al. High frequency percussive ventilation in burn patients: hemodynamics and gas exchange. *Burns.* 2003; **29**: 603–608.

60. Thompson JT, Molner JA, Hines MH, et al. Successful management of adult smoke inhalation with extracorporeal membrane oxygenation. *J Burn Care Rehabil.* 2005; **26**: 62–66.

61. Casper JK, Clark WR, Kelley RT, et al. Laryngeal and phonatory status after burn/inhalation injury: a long term follow-up study. *J Burn Care Rehabil.* 2002; **23**: 235–243.

62. Conrad SA, Zwischenberger JB, Grier LR, et al. Total extracorporeal arteriovenous carbon dioxide removal in acute respiratory failure: a phase 1 clinical study. *Intensive Care Med.* 2001; **27**: 1340–1351.

63. Park GY, Prk JW, Jeong DH, et al. Prolonged airway and systemic reactions after smoke inhalation. *Chest.* 2003; **123**: 475–480.

64. Desai MH, Micak RP, Robinson E, et al. Does inhalation injury limit exercise tolerance in children convalescing from thermal injury? *J Burn Care Rehabil.* 1993; **14**: 16–20.

65. Bourbeau J, Lacasse Y, Rouleau MY, et al. Combined smoke inhalation and body surface burns injury does not necessarily imply long-term respiratory health consequences. *Eur Respir J.* 1996; **9**: 1470–1474.

66. Palmieri T. Long term outcomes after inhalation injury. *J Burn Care Res.* 2009; **30**(1): 201–203.

# CHAPTER SIXTEEN

# METABOLIC RESPONSE TO BURNS

DAVID G. GREENHALGH, MD, FACS, SHRINERS HOSPITALS FOR CHILDREN NORTHERN CALIFORNIA
AND DEPARTMENT OF SURGERY, UNIVERSITY OF CALIFORNIA, DAVIS

## INTRODUCTION

The most profound response to any insult occurs after a major burn. The metabolic response leads to most of the hurdles and complications that a person must overcome in order to survive a major burn. In order to treat a burn patient, a caregiver must understand how the body responds to severe stress and then develop strategies to deal with the metabolic changes. The goal of this chapter will be to review the metabolic changes, ranging from the global changes to the molecular responses, which occur in response to a major insult. The second goal will be to discuss new theories that are being developed to explain why an older person is less capable of surviving a burn than a child is. The most important aspect of metabolic support, nutritional support, will be mentioned. The final section will examine the means of supporting or even reducing the hypermetabolic response so that patients will have a better chance of surviving. The goal will be to present new techniques that might further improve our ability to reverse the hypermetabolic response to burn injury.

## RESPONSE TO INJURY

All injury induces a local response that was described centuries ago by the Greeks. The classic "rubor, calor, dolor, tumor" (redness, warmth, pain, and swelling) responses are known by all health providers. It is interesting that the Greeks were also correct about the causes of these responses. Their "evil humors" are now called *cytokines* and other such mediators. Most of the time the inflammatory response remains a local response, but at times the response becomes systemic (meaning that all organs of the body become affected). When does a systemic response occur? It appears that there is a threshold magnitude of injury that is required for a systemic response. Since burns can be quantified based on the total body surface area (TBSA) involved, burn researchers have found that the hypermetabolic response occurs after a burn of around 15% to 20% TBSA. For children, the systemic response may occur after a smaller injury (as little as 10% TBSA). Other factors that contribute to the severity of injury, such as the depth of injury, associated injuries, smoke inhalation injury, and delay in resuscitation, may increase the odds of developing a systemic response to injury.

The systemic responses to a sizeable burn injury are frequently the same signs used as indicators of infection in other medical or surgical patients. These signs are the typical indicators that incite a caregiver to seek a source of infection in surgical or medical patients. In the burn patient, however, these perturbations are routine and expected findings. These "normal" changes in response to a major burn include a reset in the baseline temperature of the patient to approximately 38.5°C. As a matter of fact, most caregivers do not consider a burn patient to have a fever until he or she reaches around 39°C. Other signs of the hypermetabolic response include persistent tachycardia, tachypnea, increased calorie requirements, increased glucose flux, and protein catabolism. Since burn patients have these baseline hypermetabolic responses, they are usually excluded from studies related to the treatment of sepsis. If burn patients are to be involved in clinical trials, better criteria for sepsis need to be developed. Since standard hypermetabolic signs do not incite a seeking of a source of infection, members of the American Burn Association recently held a consensus conference to define sepsis and infection in burns.[1] These definitions now allow for standard definitions that may be used for clinical trials (see Table). Indicators that initiate a search for causes of infection or sepsis include a temperature > 39.0°C, increased fluid requirement, worsening pulmonary function, confusion, dropping platelet count, hyperglycemia, and feeding intolerance.

## HISTORY OF THE HYPERMETABOLIC RESPONSE TO BURNS

Researchers became aware of the signs and symptoms of the systemic response to injury decades ago. Cuthbertson gave a classic description of sepsis back in the 1970s when he described the "ebb" and "flow" phases of the response to significant injury.[2] The ebb phase describes the initial response to a profound injury when the body has not had time to compensate to the loss of intravascular volume. This phase is marked by vasoconstriction and a low-flow state associated with a marked hypometabolism as the body tries to compensate for the injury. In patients with profound burns who are not resuscitated, the body eventually shuts down as they quietly expire. If the patient is resuscitated, then the flow phase is initiated, with increased temperature, tachycardia, tachypnea, and massive fluxes in glucose and protein metabolism. This phase persists until months after the patient heals or until he or she expires.

Another description of the response to injury was reported by Selye, who described the response to extensive injury as "alarm, resistance, and exhaustion phases."[3] The alarm reaction can be equated with the ebb phase, while the resistance phase describes the patient's attempt to fight the insult and is similar to the flow phase. The exhaustion phase describes a patient dying of multiple organ dysfunction syndrome (MODS). These historic descriptions provide fairly accurate accounts of the common events observed in the response to injury. Interestingly, Leo Tolstoy in *War and Peace* gave a fairly accurate account of one of his protagonists dying of MODS after being injured in battle.

## INITIATORS OF THE RESPONSE TO INJURY

There are many signals that are released after an injury that initiate a local response. When the size of injury reaches a threshold magnitude, then a systemic or total body response is induced. Pain is one of the obvious immediate responses to injury. Damage to tissues initiates sensory neurons to release local mediators such as S-100 and other local mediators.[4] But an intact sensory system is not required for local inflammation, since paraplegics still respond despite loss of sensation. Local mediators such as epinephrine and norepinephrine are released to initiate vasoconstriction to stop bleeding. Soon after vasoconstriction, other local mediators induce vasodilation and increased permeability. These mediators, which induce local edema, include histamine, bradykinin, serotonin, prostaglandins, leukotrienes, nitric oxide, and many others. When the insult is large enough, such as after a burn > 20% TBSA or during sepsis, a systemic capillary leak develops that requires a formal resuscitation. All burn doctors know that the extent of capillary leak is proportional to the extent and depth of burn injury.

At the same time, damage to the endothelial cell surface of the vasculature exposes platelets to factors (such as collagen type I, activated adhesion molecules) that initiate platelet binding and release of their α-granules. α-Granules contain many mediators, such as platelet activating factor, growth factors (platelet-derived growth factor, transforming growth factor-β), platelet factor 4, and many other factors, that attract inflammatory cells into the wound. Tissue factor (factor VII) is released from damaged tissues to initiate the clotting cascade. By-products of thrombosis, including thrombin and fibrin, also are chemotactic for inflammatory cells. The complement cascade is initiated, and the release of C3a and C5a attracts more inflammatory cells into the wound. The first inflammatory cells to arrive are the neutrophils, which in turn release oxygen free radicals and proteases to "fight" invading organisms. Soon, macrophages arrive to begin, along with resident dendritic cells, phagocytosis of foreign antigens. Both cell types are involved in the release of other cytokines and growth factors that attract more inflammatory cells and fibroblasts and induce angiogenesis. In addition, both cells are involved with antigen processing to initiate the adaptive immune response with lymphocytes. The T lymphocytes are then involved in cell-mediated immune responses in addition to initiating the B cell production of antibodies. The details of the adaptive immune response are too detailed to describe here.

All organisms have developed a cellular recognition system, called the *innate immune system*.[5] Inflammatory cells, such as macrophages, have developed receptors that recognize components of foreign molecules, called *pathogen-associated molecular patterns* (PAMPs). These receptors, called *pathogen-recognition receptors* (PRRs), recognize products of bacteria (cell wall, flagella) or viruses (RNA, DNA) to initiate a cellular response. The best described receptor is the toll-like receptor-4 (TLR4) of advanced vertebrates (Figure 1). This receptor is the main responder to the by-product of the gram-negative cell wall—lipopolysaccharide (LPS). LPS is bound in the serum by LPS-binding protein (LBP), which in turn binds to membrane-bound CD14. CD14 has no signaling component, but instead it binds to TLR4, which is involved in intracellular signaling. The entire complex forms a dimer which has associated membrane proteins (MD2 and adapter proteins such as MyD88). An intracellular cascade is initiated, which passes through the key signaling complex, NF-κB. NF-κB is inhibited from traveling into the nucleus by binding to IκB, which is degraded after signaling through the TLR4 pathway. Free NF-κB travels into the nucleus to bind to its response element on DNA to induce the production of various cytokines, of which tumor necrosis factor α (TNF-α), interleukin 1 (IL-1), and interleukin 6 (IL-6) are the best described. To add to the complexity of the response system, if different adapter proteins are bound to the TLR4 complex, then different intracellular signaling pathways are induced to produce different cytokines (such as interferon β).[6] While TLR4 is the key responder to LPS of gram-negative bacteria, the key receptor for gram-positive organisms is TLR2. Humans have 10 toll-like receptors which respond to different bacteria or viral components. In addition, there are other foreign molecule receptors (RIG-1, MDA5, NOD-1, NOD-2) that are not included in the TLR family.

In response to binding to the innate immune receptor system, multiple proteins (cytokines, chemokines, and growth factors) are released. For small injuries, these dozens of cytokines lead to the classical local inflammatory responses of pain, erythema, warmth, and swelling (dolor, rubor, calor, and tumor). When the insult is greater than a threshold amount, the cytokines spill into the systemic circulation and are detected in the central nervous system. In essence, danger signals are transmitted to the brain. It is not clear which cytokines are danger signals, but it is clear that the message is picked up in parts of the brain, including the hypothalamus. Recent evidence suggests that one mode of responding to stress is through the vagus, to warn the body of impending stress.[7] The other well-described response is called the hypothalamic-pituitary-adrenal (HPA) axis.[8] The stress message is transmitted as corticotrophin-releasing hormone (CRH) to the pituitary, which in turn releases adrenocorticotrophic hormonecorticotrophin (ACTH) to induce signaling to the adrenal gland. In response to ACTH, cortisol is released in the adrenal cortex. The adrenal medulla is also induced to release epinephrine, norepinephrine, and vasopressin. Sympathetic activation leads to the tachycardia, tachypnea, and other signs of increased metabolic rate seen in burn patients. The increased metabolic rate increases the set temperature of the patient so he or she typically has a low-grade fever of around 38.5°C.

The catecholamine response to stress has been well studied.[9-11] There is stimulation of the $\alpha_1$ and $\beta_1$ adrenergic receptors (AR). The $\beta_1$ adrenergic receptor is activated with higher levels of epinephrine and norepinephrine. This receptor is classically involved in vasoconstriction, especially during the initial shock phase of burn injury. The $\beta_1$ adrenergic receptor is activated with lower levels of catecholamines and is involved in the longer-lasting effects of stress. The $\beta_1$ adrenergic receptor is involved in inducing increased heart rate, respiratory rate, and cardiac output, along with the decrease in systemic vascular resistance seen in burn patients during the "flow" phase of shock. The $\beta_1$ adrenergic receptor is also responsible for increased heat production and thus for the increase in the set temperature of patients with large burns. The increase in metabolic rate also leads to increased oxygen consumption and calorie requirements. These increased metabolic needs stress the importance of aggressive nutritional support when treating the patient with massive burns. The $\beta_1$ adrenergic receptor also has a profound influence on glucose metabolism. There is increased glucose production that is needed to "feed" the cells attempting to heal the wounds. Stimulation of the $\beta_1$ adrenergic receptor leads to increased gluconeogenesis, glycogenolysis, lipolysis, and lactate production. In addition, there is decreased insulin-mediated glycogenesis.

The stimulation of the adrenal cortex leads to cortisol release, which has profound effects on the metabolic rate of the burn patient.[12-15] The glucocorticoid response also contributes to the increase in oxygen consumption and resting energy expenditure. Like catecholamines, glucocorticoids affect many pathways to increase glucose levels. They increase glucagon levels while increasing insulin resistance. Glycogenolysis, gluconeogenesis, and lipolysis are all increased. Glucocorticoids also affect protein metabolism. Proteins are broken down from one of the largest sources in the body—skeletal muscle. Proteins are broken down to release alanine and glutamine, which can be turned into glucose. Proteolysis leads to increased nitrogen excretion.[16] Substrate cycling is increased to a great extent. In essence, the body is sacrificing muscle to feed the cells involved in fighting infection and healing the wound. While fat is also utilized, it is not used as much as the skeletal muscle. In addition to hormone induction of muscle breakdown, inactivity also contributes to the loss of muscle mass during a burn injury. Studies are now suggesting that exercise programs may prevent some of the muscle loss of extensive injury.[17,18] Even the bone is affected: bone mass is reduced as a response to the stimulation of glucocorticoids.[19]

The release of cortisol also leads to a switch in the type of proteins that are synthesized by the liver. Instead of producing structural proteins, the liver switches production to the synthesis of acute phase proteins.[20] Acute phase proteins assist the body with dealing with invading organisms and healing the wound. Some key acute phase proteins include C-reactive protein, serum amyloid A, complement (C3), haptoglobin, and fibrinogen.[21] Many of these proteins, such as C-reactive protein and complement, are needed to deal with infections.[21]

Not all of the actions of glucocorticoids are adverse (Figure 2). Clearly, cortisol is essential to handling any form of stress.[22] Cortisol is needed for optimal response to catecholamines and thus allows for a better response to stress. Cortisol stabilizes cell membranes and may decrease the amount of edema after an injury. The release of cytokines leads to the systemic inflammatory response syndrome (SIRS). This continuous inflammatory response is a key moderator of the prolonged hypermetabolic response. Glucocorticoids are produced to counteract inflammation.[23] The anti-inflammatory effects occur by many mechanisms. First of all, glucocorticoids inhibit the synthesis of proinflammatory proteins. In addition, corticosteroids binding to the glucocorticoid receptor then enter the nucleus to bind to the glucocorticoid response element to increase the synthesis of anti-inflammatory mediators. In essence, glucocorticoid production must be closely regulated since too much or too little leads to adverse outcomes.

Insulin is a key hormone in the response to injury.[24,25] While insulin levels are increased after a burn injury, the relative increase is less than that of the hormones (such as glucagon) that counter the effects of insulin. The other factor is that burn patients or other stressed patients develop a relative resistance to insulin. Cortisol is involved in this insulin resistance. Cortisol tends to interfere with the effects of insulinlike growth factor 1 (IGF-1). IGF-1, or somatotropin-C, is an important anabolic hormone.[26-28] IGF-1 and insulin will bind both the insulin receptor and the IGF-1 receptor. To understand how insulin affects glucose regulation, it is helpful to understand how glucose enters the cell. Glucose enters cells through carrier proteins called glucose transporters 1-4 (GLUT1-GLUT4).[25,29] GLUT1 through GLUT3 are not influenced by insulin, while GLUT4, which is primarily in the liver, skeletal muscle, and adipocytes, requires insulin for activity. When insulin binds the insulin receptor, a tyrosine on the intracellular portion of the receptor is phosphorylated. This phosphorylation leads to intracellular signaling through the IRS complex to turn on phosphoinositol 3 kinase (PI3K), and ultimately GLUT4 is activated to transport glucose into the cell. It turns out that tyrosine autophosphorylation leads to stimulation glucose transportation. If, however, a serine is autophosphorylated, then resistance to insulin is developed. How a burn or cortisol affects this process is just beginning to be established.

As stated before, protein breakdown is a key problem in the response to injury. Protein synthesis is actually increased to produce acute phase and wound healing proteins, but synthesis is considerably below the extent of breakdown. We know that if a person loses more than 25% of his or her protein stores, he or she rarely survives.[30,31] If a patient with a large burn is not fed, he or she could lose 25% of his or her protein stores in 3 to 4 weeks.[31] Before aggressive feeding was a standard practice in burn units, patients with large burns would waste away, develop diarrhea and pneumonia, and ultimately die. These are the same symptoms of starving to death. Aggressive nutritional support is obviously very important.

More is currently known about the mechanisms of protein breakdown.[16,31,32] The preferred source for protein after injury is skeletal muscle. Protein is broken down to various components, with alanine being sent to the liver to be broken down into pyruvate. Glutamine is sent to the gut for conversion to glucose. The only amino acid that is not degraded is phenylalanine, which can be measured in the serum as an indicator of the degree of protein breakdown.

Once the proteolysis begins, any protein fragment is bound by ubiquitin through an adenosine triphosphate–dependent process. The process is initiated by activation of the ubiquitin-activating enzyme (E1), which transfers ubiquitin to a ubiquitin-conjugating enzyme (E2). The protein is presented by ubiquitin ligase E3, with the interaction between E2 and E3 leading to "tagging" of the protein with ubiquitins. Multiple ubiquitins bind the protein fragment, and the complex is passed through the 26S proteosome complex to be broken into peptide pieces in an energy-dependent process. Peptides are then sent to an extralysosomal proteolytic complex, tripeptidyl peptidase II (TPP II), which is, like the 26S proteosome, a giant peptidase composed of multiple subunits that form a central channel. This TPP II complex, which appears to be dependent on glucocorticoids, breaks peptide pieces into tripeptides. After this, the tripeptides are converted into single amino acids by aminopeptidase and other exopeptidases. There are also separate pathways of muscle breakdown that may occur before, concurrently with, or after proteosomal breakdown. The calcium-calpain system appears to be one of these alternative pathways.

Sepsis increases available calcium, which increases calpain activity. The calpains are involved in the release of myofilaments from myofibrils of muscle. For a review of the complex mechanisms of muscle breakdown, excellent reviews are available.[16,33]

## METABOLISM AND END ORGAN DYSFUNCTION

There are 2 main theories that explain why burns or major injuries lead to multiple organ dysfunction: the microvascular hypothesis and the cytopathic hypoxia hypothesis.[34,35] In reality, both concepts contribute to an understanding of organ dysfunction. The microvascular hypothesis suggests that localized, unregulated thrombosis leads to altered perfusion to various capillary beds, leading to poor perfusion of multiple capillary beds. The microscopic areas of poor perfusion are significant causes of pockets of hypoxia, which in turn lead to vasodilation in an attempt to perfuse those areas.[36,37] This vasodilation leads to the well-known decrease of systemic vascular resistance during the flow phase of septic shock.

The other pathophysiologic explanation for MODS is related to a phenomenon known as *metabolic failure*. The cytopathic hypoxia hypothesis suggests that organs develop dysfunction because cells "run out of gas."[35,38,39] Fink has termed this type of metabolic collapse "mitochondrial cytopathy."[38] In essence, there is inefficient use of the metabolic substrate. We know that burns increase the demands for calories to up to twice normal resting levels. The cytopathic hypoxia hypothesis suggests that the cell's ability to meet this energy demand fails, leading to gradual cellular and tissue damage. This metabolic failure leads to gradual organ failure and the situation that kills most burn patients, MODS. Current thinking suggests that an important part of the defect is due to failure at the mitochondrial level.

To better understand this form of metabolic failure, one must review some of the basics of mitochondrial function[40,41]. Interestingly, mitochondria originally evolved from bacteria invading cells. Mitochondria still contain the DNA of these ancestral bacteria. These bacteria set up a beneficial symbiotic relationship that ultimately allowed cells to utilize energy in a much more efficient manner. Now, we cannot live without these former microbes. Mitochondria have multiple essential functions, including producing > 95% of the adenosine triphosphate (ATP) in organisms. In addition, mitochondria control apoptosis and necrosis death pathways. They also regulate intracellular calcium flux, oxygen sensing, steroidogenesis, and signaling through reactive oxygen species. The dominant function of mitochondria is respiration through the respiratory chain complexes.

During normal respiration, glucose is converted to pyruvate, which is transferred into the mitochondria to produce cyclic adenosine monophosphate (cAMP), which enters the Krebs (citric acid) cycle to produce NADH and $FADH_2$. Fatty acids also enter the nucleus to undergo beta-oxidation to produce cAMP to produce the same factors. There are 5 respiratory chain complexes that function to oxidize NADH and $FADH_2$ to produce ATP. They also reduce cellular oxygen levels and maintain a proton-motive force that moves protons out and then back into the nucleus. These complexes also produce reactive oxygen species, especially superoxide. While the details of this process are beyond the scope of this chapter, excellent reviews are available.[40-42]

During sepsis there are changes that are noted in the structure of mitochondria.[39,42-44] Mitochondria lose their structural integrity and become enlarged. There is fragmentation of their inner membrane and distortion of their cristae. There is a decrease in oxygen utilization, ATP synthesis, and calcium-transport functions. Some have stated that the mitochondria are induced into a hibernation state.[45,46] The mitochondrial function worsens with deconditioning, which suggests that conditioning can improve the outcome of dealing with stress. These mitochondrial changes are being examined in patients with cardiac conditions, such as after myocardial infarction or cardiomyopathy. Neubauer has described the condition of an "engine out of fuel" as a major cause of cardiomyopathy.[47] Defects in the mitochondria include respiratory chain proton pump "slipping," mitochondrial membrane proton leakage (uncoupling oxygen consumption from ATP synthesis), and alterations in the supply of electrons to the respiratory chain complexes. The details are quite complex, but in simple terms, there are uncoupling proteins that are involved in shifting the utilization of oxygen from respiration to the production of heat.[48,49] These proteins may contribute to the changes observed in fevers and sepsis. Some suggest that specific respiratory chain complexes (complexes 1 and 4) may have a greater role in altering the response to sepsis.[35,38,50,51]

One can break up energy utilization into 3 components.[47] The first is substrate utilization, which is creating energy out of the fuel that we consume. This involves glycolysis and ATP synthesis from the Krebs cycle. Beta-oxidation of fatty acids is another form of substrate utilization. The second form is oxidative phosphorylation, which involves the creation of energy (ATP) by the mitochondrial respiratory chain complex. Finally, energy must be transferred to the recipient tissues (especially muscle) in order for the energy to be utilized. For muscle, transfer of energy occurs via the creatine energy transfer shuttle. Phosphate from ATP is transferred to creatine (to form phosphocreatine), and creatine kinase transfers phosphate back to ATP in the myocyte to allow for muscle contraction. Creatine is produced in the liver and transferred to the cells via a plasma membrane creatine transporter. To further complicate matters, there are molecular regulators of energy metabolism. There are nuclear-receptor transcription factors that are activated by lipid metabolites to tie gene expression and metabolism to substrate availability. There are nuclear receptors of the peroxisome proliferator-activated receptor (PPAR) family (PPARα, PPARβ, PPARγ), which tightly regulate substrate utilization and energy production. PPARα is a key regulator of enzymes of fatty acid oxidation. The nuclear-receptor coactivator PPARγ has been called the "master regulator of metabolic function in mitochondria."[47] All of these mechanisms tightly regulate metabolic rate in normal and pathologic conditions.

When there is metabolic failure, such as during MODS, all components of the above metabolic regulators are defective. The pathologic features have been described in cardiomyopathy, but certainly must apply in patients with massive burn injuries. Under the category of substrate utilization, there is decreased fatty acid utilization, initially increased and then decreased glucose utilization, and decreased PPARα activity. For oxidative phosphorylation, metabolic failure includes decreased numbers of respiratory chain complexes, decreased ATP synthase, decreased oxygen consumption, increased expression of uncoupling proteins (thus increased wasting of energy), and decreased PCG-1a activity. Finally, there is an impairment of high-energy phosphate transfer, which includes decreased creatine activity and function, with decreased ATP transfer.

All of the above alterations occur in organ failure and are likely candidates in the development of MODS and ultimately death from major burns. We know that the size of a burn that people can survive depends on their age.[52] For instance, a teenager has a 50% chance of surviving a burn of around 85% TBSA. As one ages, the size burn that leads to a 50% survival drops precipitously. An 80-year-old has a 50% survival chance with a burn of around 10% to 15% TBSA. One hypothesis to explain this disparity could be in the metabolic reserve of the patient. The elderly have less metabolic reserve and thus cannot create the energy to overcome the high caloric demands of a massive burn. The inability to handle metabolic demands leads to increased reactive oxygen species and impaired ability to repair cells. In essence, there is mitochondrial fatigue that must be overcome to survive the burn.

## Managing Metabolic Failure

In simplistic terms, there are 2 ways of preventing or treating metabolic failure. One must supply adequate energy (by supplying nutrition) or reduce or modify metabolic needs.

Both of these strategies need to be utilized in order for a patient to survive a massive burn injury.

## Nutritional Support

One of the great advances in the treatment of burns has been the philosophy of providing aggressive nutrition to burn patients. Before aggressive nutritional support, healthy individuals would waste away and develop diarrhea and pneumonia. In essence, they died deaths similar to those of people dying of starvation. Older studies demonstrated that if relying on oral diet, a patient with massive burns would lose 25% of his or her weight within several weeks.[31,53] Impaired nutritional intake is associated with impaired wound healing, altered immune function, loss of gut mucosal integrity, and increased mortality. Now, nutritional support is routine in the burn unit. We know how to estimate caloric and protein needs in the burn patient. In essence, a formula (such as the Harris-Benedict equation or other formulas) can be used to calculate basal calorie requirements, and that number is multiplied by a factor that estimates the degree of stress. In burns, that multiplier is in the range of 1.4 to 2, dependent on the size of the burn. Proteins should be provided as 1.5 to 2 g/kg body weight/d. The accuracy of feeding calculations can be adjusted on measurements of resting energy expenditures (REE) using a metabolic cart (indirect calorimetry).

In addition, we know that feeding the gut is the best means of providing nutrition to the patient.[54,55] Many centers initiate feedings as part of the routine procedures during admission.[56] Our unit places nasoduodenal feeding tubes under fluoroscopy at the time of admission. Mochizuki's group has shown that there are metabolic and immune benefits to aggressive early feeding.[57] In addition, interruptions of feedings should be kept to a minimum. Jenkins et al. have demonstrated that feedings can safely be given during skin-grafting procedures.[58] Another dilemma is whether special diets such as immune-enhancing diets augment the response to injury.[59] The answer to this question has been debated for years and as of yet has not been resolved. It is clear, however, that no matter in what form, nutritional support is essential for surviving a burn injury.

## Modifying Energy Needs

There are 2 main strategies for modifying energy requirements after a major injury. First, one can reduce energy needs by decreasing hypermetabolism, and second, one can induce anabolism. Both of these strategies are currently being actively pursued. One must ask, however, how aggressively we should try to reduce the hypermetabolic response to injury. Is hypermetabolism necessary for adequate healing? Maybe we need to improve the efficiency of our energy utilization. Does stimulation of anabolism take substrate away from the wound? These questions have not been resolved but are key areas of current research.

There are many extraneous factors that affect the metabolic rates of burn patients.[31,32,53,60] The clinician can at least partially ameliorate the effects of these factors on the metabolic rate. Pain and anxiety increase heart rate and blood pressure, leading to increased metabolic rates. Adequate sedation reduces the energy consumption of any patient. Maintaining a warm ambient temperature is also essential to reduce metabolic needs. If the burn patient is cold, then more energy is required to generate heat to maintain a normal temperature. When a burn patient is asked to adjust the ambient room temperature, he or she always sets the temperature to a warmer level than an uninjured person does. In addition, the hypermetabolism increases the set temperature to around 38.5°C, so more energy is required to reach that temperature. Warming the room reduces extra caloric needs. A clear sign of metabolic failure is present when a patient is unable to maintain his or her temperature (hypothermia).

One of the great advances in burn care occurred when burn surgeons developed the philosophy of early excision and grafting. Since that time, survival after extensive burns has increased greatly.[61-63] Early excision has been shown to reduce metabolic needs by 40%.[60] In addition, any factor that can reduce the incidence of sepsis reduces metabolic requirements. Sepsis has been shown to increase metabolism by 40%.[60] Early excision and wound coverage should decrease the incidence of sepsis to further decrease metabolic needs.

A great deal of research has been dedicated to the pharmacologic manipulation of the metabolic response to injury. The use of β-adrenergic blockers has been the major means of reducing metabolic needs. β-Adrenergic blockers are now routinely used in the perioperative period in general surgery. β-Adrenergic blockers are also prescribed for patients after ischemic cardiac events and appear to improve survival.[64] A recent trial, however, suggests that there may be risks with taking β-adrenergic blockers for noncardiac surgery.[65] Herndon's group in Galveston has performed excellent studies on the use of the nonspecific β-adrenergic blocker propranolol in patients with burns.[66-73] They have found that propranolol decreases thermogenesis, tachycardia, cardiac work, resting energy expenditure, peripheral lipolysis, and muscle wasting (by increasing intracellular amino acid recycling for protein synthesis).

The other means of improving metabolism in burns is to stimulate anabolism or reduce the catabolic response. Herndon and Tompkins have also explored this strategy in great depth.[31] The first strategy was to give growth hormone to children with major burns. They found that growth hormone improved split-thickness skin graft donor-site healing and thus reduced the length of stay in children with burns > 40% TBSA.[74,75] In addition, they found that growth hormone improved protein balance, patient growth, bone formation, and the $T_H1$ lymphocyte immune profile.[76-78] Growth hormone appears to work by increasing IGF-1. Unfortunately, in a large European trial, critically ill adults receiving growth hormone had a higher mortality than controls.[79] These findings led to the disfavor of the use of growth hormone for adult burn patients. The safety profile in children appears to be fine,[80] and many centers use growth hormone for children < 20 kg with major burns.

Since growth hormone appears to work by increasing IGF-1, trials were performed using IGF-1 alone.[26] Unfortunately, despite some benefits, the use of IGF-1 has problems with hypoglycemia and is no longer used. Other trials examined the combination of IGF-1 with its binding protein IGF-1 binding protein 3 (IGF-1/IGF-1 BP3).[27,28] This combination resulted in improved protein balance, less hypoglycemia, and a shift to $T_H2$ lymphocyte response. Again, complications, especially increased peripheral neuropathies, have stopped its use.

Since either IGF-1 or insulin bind to the IGF-1 receptor, many felt that insulin would be another factor that could increase an anabolic response after a major injury. Recent studies suggest that tight glucose control, which provides more insulin, is beneficial in improving survival during sepsis.[81,82] It has been hypothesized that one mechanism of tight glucose control's benefit is through supplying extra insulin to the patient. Insulin has been shown to increase protein synthesis and lean mass and improve donor-site healing.[83-87] It also appears to have immune-enhancing functions such as decreasing acute phase proteins and inflammatory cytokines.[88-90] In addition, metformin may increase the efficacy of the insulin action.[91,92] More studies are needed to prove the efficacy of insulin in treating burn patients. Most burn centers, however, now have a policy of tight glucose control.

Another popular anabolic strategy has been to use anabolic agents such as testosterone or similar agents. Testosterone itself improves protein synthesis[93] and reduces protein breakdown, but its use is obviously not appropriate for women. Fortunately, there are agents that maintain the anabolic effects of testosterone but avoid the androgenic effects. Oxandralone is the agent that currently is popular for treating patients. It has strong anabolic effects with one-sixth of the androgenic effects. Oxandralone has been found to increase net protein synthesis and improve wound healing.[94-98] A current multicenter trial demonstrated that oxandralone reduced the length of stay of burn patients with very few complications.[99] Oxandralone is the current standard of care for patients weighing > 20 kg with massive burns.

An even simpler idea is that muscle may be preserved with simple exercise. It is known that if a limb is immobilized for 3 weeks, it loses about half of its strength. Many critically ill burn patients do not move for weeks. Immobility in itself will lead to the breakdown of muscle. Simple exercise should preserve muscle mass. Herndon's group has also investigated this issue.[17,18] They have found that an aggressive and organized exercise program leads to improved muscle mass, strength, and endurance. These studies have been performed in rehabilitating patients, but they demonstrate the philosophy of using an aggressive exercise program to preserve mass. Maybe we should be exercising our patients while they are in the intensive care unit. Clearly, getting patients out of bed and providing aggressive physical and occupational therapy programs should improve muscle anabolism.

In addition, cardiac studies suggest that conditioning improves mitochondrial function, so exercise appears to improve metabolism at the subcellular level.[40,47,100,101] There are theoretic methods of improving mitochondrial function that could be used to treat burn patients.[47] There are factors that can improve substrate utilization, such as PPARγ agonists (thiazolidinediones), which act as insulin sensitizers, suppress peripheral lipolysis, and redistribute triglycerides to peripheral tissues.[102,103] There are other PPAR agonists

that have the potential for treating metabolic failure.[104,105] Another strategy is to use carnitine palmitoyl transferase-1 inhibitors that lead to partial inhibition of fatty acid oxidation and promote glucose utilization.[106,107] These agents have not been tested in clinical trials, but studies are now being developed.

One can also try to augment oxidative phosphorylation. While no agent is currently available, stimulation of PCG-1a is a potential strategy.[108] Also, altering uncoupling proteins may be another strategy that could be developed.[109] Finally, one could try to manipulate high-energy phosphate metabolites, such as improving cellular stores, increasing availability, improving efficiency of transfer, improving creatine phosphate transfer, or improving myofibrillar efficiency of ATP utilization.[110,111] All of these ideas are currently theoretical, but I would not be surprised that they are tested in the near future.

## CONCLUSION

Burns lead to the greatest increase in metabolic demands that we know of. The mechanisms of how the increase occurs are being discovered. Two areas of treatment are available—providing adequate nutrition and manipulation of the metabolic response are major areas of current investigation. As we learn more about the mechanisms of hypermetabolism, more options will become available for treating these problems.

# TABLE AND FIGURES

## TABLE 1
**American Burn Association consensus conference definitions of sepsis and infection in burn patients.[1]**

**Systemic Inflammatory Response Syndrome (SIRS):** The consensus group felt that all burn patients with extensive burns have some degree of SIRS, so the use of this term in the burn patient is irrelevant and should not be utilized.

**Sepsis:** Sepsis is a change in the burn patient that *triggers* the concern for infection. It is a presumptive diagnosis where antibiotics are usually started, and a search for a cause of infection should be initiated. While there is need for clinical interpretation, the diagnosis needs to be tied to the discovery of an infection (defined below). The definition is age dependent, with adjustments necessary for children.

The trigger includes at least 3 of the following:
Temperature > 39°C or < 36.5°C
Progressive tachycardia
    Adults: > 110 bpm
    Children: > 2 standard deviations (SD) above age-specific norms (85% age-adjusted max heart rate)
Progressive tachypnea
    Adults: > 25 bpm not ventilated
        Minute ventilation > 12 liters/min ventilated
    Children: > 2 SD above age-specific norms (85% age-adjusted max respiratory rate)
Thrombocytopenia (will not apply until 3 days after initial resuscitation)
    Adults: < 100,000/mcl
    Children: < 2 SD below age-specific norms
Hyperglycemia (in the absence of preexisting diabetes mellitus)
    Untreated plasma glucose > 200 mg/dL or equivalent mM/L
    Insulin resistance—examples include:
        > 7 units of insulin/h intravenous drip (adults)
        Significant resistance to insulin (> 25% increase in insulin requirements over 24 h)
Inability to continue enteral feedings > 24 h
    Abdominal distension
    Enteral feeding intolerance (residual > 150 mL/h in children or 2 times feeding rate in adults)
    Uncontrollable diarrhea (> 2500 mL/d for adults or > 400 mL/d in children)

In addition, it is *required* that a documented infection (defined below) is identified as one of the following:
- Culture-positive infection
- Pathologic tissue source identified
- Clinical response to antimicrobials

**Severe Sepsis:**
The term *severe sepsis* is dropped.

**Septic Shock**
Septic shock is sepsis (defined above) in addition to shocklike hemodynamic parameters defined in sepsis "bundles." We will not redefine those parameters.
Septic shock is defined as persistent hypotension despite adequate fluid resuscitation and/or lactate > 4 mmol (36 mg/dL).

FIGURE 1
A cartoon of lipopolysaccharide (LPS) signaling through toll-like receptor-4 (TLR4) reveals
the complexity of the signaling system that regulates the response to gram-negative bacteria.
LPS binds to LPS-binding protein (LBP), which binds to CD14, which interacts with TLR4. Depending
on which adapter protein is present, there are different signaling pathways that lead to
different cellular responses.

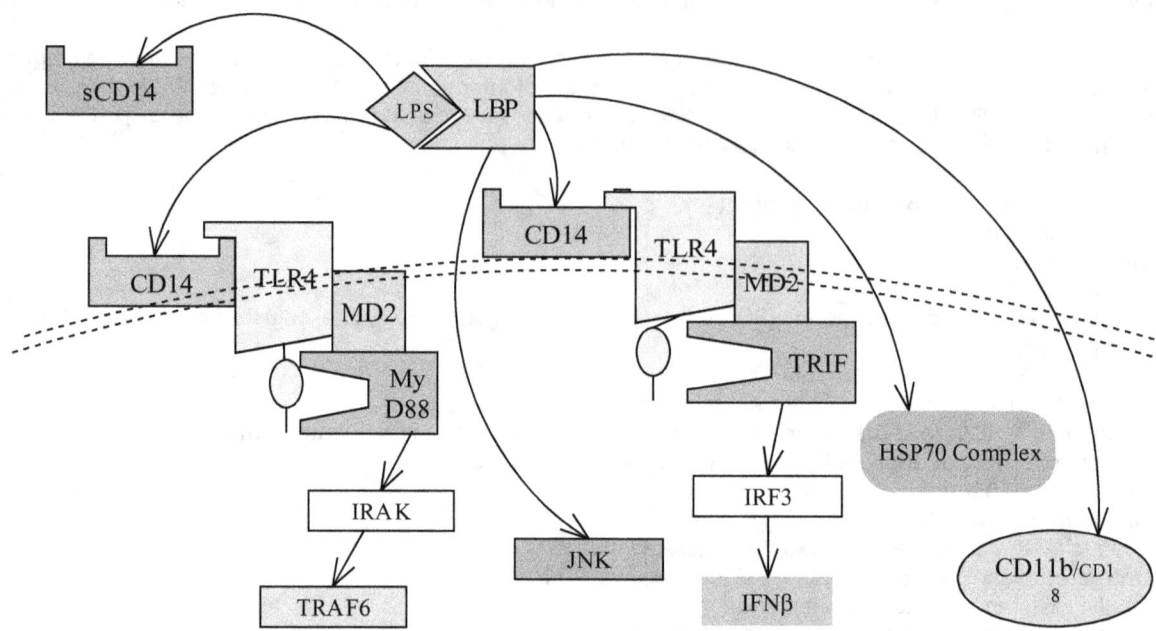

FIGURE 2
The cellular signaling of cortisol is also very complicated. Cortisol binds to the
glucocorticoid receptor (GR), which forms a dimer and binds to the glucocorticoid response element
(GRE) on DNA. The active receptor is the alpha receptor (GR). There are also other inhibitory activities
of the glucocorticoid receptor system. Cortisol may bind to a receptor (GR) which has
no physiologic activity. The receptor complex may also bind to a negative GRE (nGRE) and have no
response. Many of the activities are regulated by the histone acetylation status, which in turn is
regulated by histone deacetylatases (HDAC).

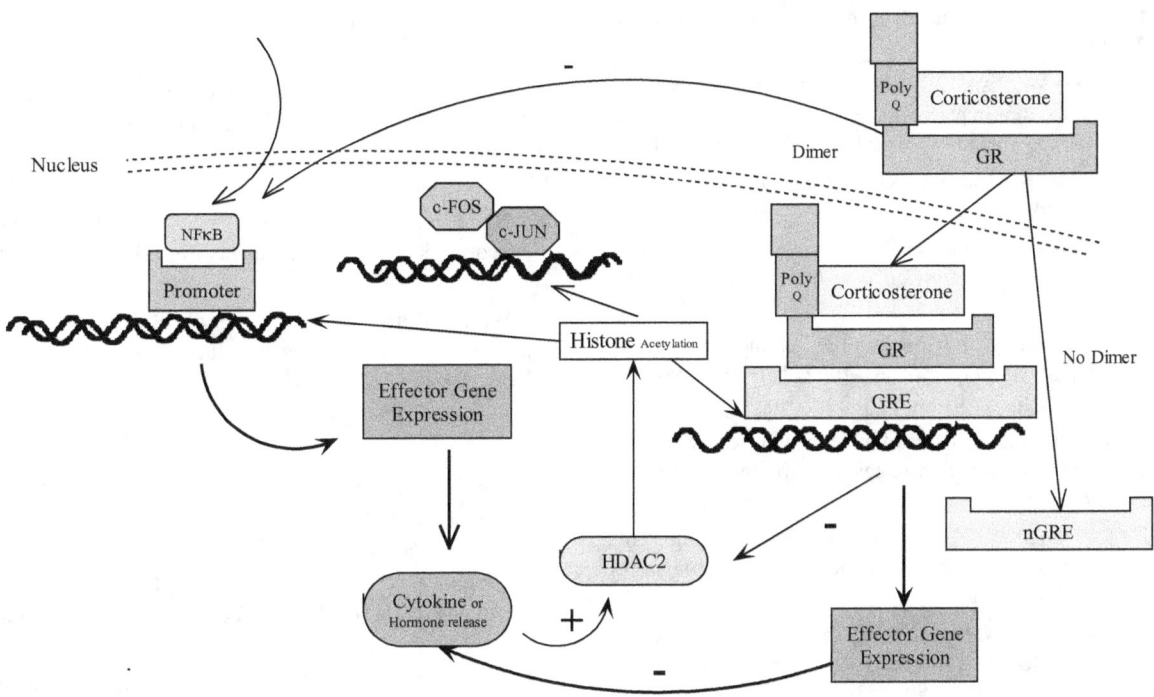

## REFERENCES

1. Greenhalgh DG, Saffle JR, Holmes JH IV, et al. (The American Burn Association Consensus Conference on Burn Sepsis and Infection Group). American Burn Association consensus conference to define sepsis and infection in burns. *J Burn Care Res*. 2007; **28**: 776–790.

2. Cuthbertson D. Post-shock metabolic response. *Lancet*. 1942; **1**: 433–436.

3. Selye H. A syndrome produced by diverse nocuous agents. *Nature*. 1936; **138**: 32–33.

4. Gibran NS, Jang Y-C, Isik FF, et al. Diminished neuropeptide levels contribute to the impaired cutaneous healing response associated with diabetes mellitus. *J Surg Res*. 2002; **108**: 122–128.

5. Akira S, Takeda K. Toll-like receptor signaling. *Nat Rev Immunol*. 2004; **4**: 499–511.

6. West AP, Koblansky AA, Ghosh S. Recognition and signaling by toll-like receptors. *Annu Rev Cell Dev Biol*. 2006; **22**: 409–437.

7. Tracey KJ. Physiology and immunology of the cholinergic antiinflammatory pathway. *J Clin Invest*. 2007; **117**: 289–296.

8. Schroeder S, Wichers M, Klingmuller D, et al. The hypothalamic-pituitary-adrenal axis of patients with severe sepsis: altered response to corticotrophin-releasing hormone. *Crit Care Med*. 2001; **29**: 450–451.

9. Goodall MC, Stone C, Haines BW Jr. Urinary output of adrenalin and/or noradrenaline in severe thermal burns. *Ann Surg*. 1957; **145**: 479–487.

10. Wilmore DW, Long JN, Mason AD Jr, Skreen RW, Pruitt BA Jr. Catecholamines: mediators of the hypermetabolic response to thermal injury. *Ann Surg*. 1974; **180**: 653–669.

11. Becker RA, Vaughan GM, Goodwin CW Jr, et al. Plasma norepinephrine, epinephrine, and thyroid hormone interactions in severely burned patients. *Arch Surg*. 1980; **115**: 439–443.

12. Hume DM, Nelson DH, Miller DW. Blood and urinary 17-hydroxy-corticosteroids in patients with severe burns. *Ann Surg*. 1956; **143**: 316–329.

13. Bane JW, McCaa RE, McCaa CS, et al. The pattern of aldosterone and cortisone blood levels in thermal burn patients. *J Trauma*. 1974; **14**: 605–611.

14. Wise L, Margraf HW, Ballinger WF. Adrenal cortical function in severe burns. *Arch Surg*. 1972; **105**: 213–220.

15. Palmieri TL, Levine S, Schonfeld-Warden N, O'Mara MS, Greenhalgh DG. Hypothalamic-pituitary-adrenal axis response to sustained stress after major burn injury in children. *J Burn Care Res*. 2006; **27**: 742–748.

16. Hasselgren P-O. Molecular regulation of muscle wasting. *Sci Med*. 2002; **8**: 230–239.

17. Suman OE, Spies RJ, Celis MM, Mlcak RP, Herndon DN. Effect of a twelve-week resistance exercise program on skeletal muscle in children with burn injuries. *J Appl Physiol*. 2001; **91**: 1168–1175.

18. Cucuzzo N, Ferrando AA, Herndon DN. The effects of exercise programming versus traditional outpatient therapy and rehabilitation in severely burned patients. *J Burn Care Rehabil*. 2001; **22**: 214–220.

19. Klein GL, Herndon DN, Langman CB, et al. Long-term reduction in bone mass after severe burn injury in children. *J Pediatr*. 1995; **126**: 252–256.

20. Gabay C, Kushner I. Acute-phase proteins and other systemic responses to inflammation. *N Engl J Med*. 1999; **340**: 448–454.

21. Du Clos TW. C-reactive protein and the immune response. *Sci Med*. 2002; **8**: 108–117.

22. Sapolsky RM, Romero L, Munck AU. How do glucocorticoids influence stress responses? Integrating permissive, suppressive, stimulatory, and preparative actions. *Endocr Rev*. 2000; **21**: 55–89.

23. Rhen T, Cidlowski JA. Antiinflammatory action of glucocorticoids—new mechanisms for old drugs. *N Engl J Med*. 2005; **353**: 1711–1723.

24. Wolfe RR, Herndon DN, Jahoor F, et al. Effect of severe burn injury on substrate cycling by glucose and fatty acids. *N Engl J Med*. 1987; **317**: 403–408.

25. Pidcoke HF, Wade CE, Wolf SE. Insulin and the burned patient. *Crit Care Med*. 2007;35(suppl):S524-S530.

26. Cioffi WG, Gore DC, Rue LC, et al. Insulin-like growth factor-1 lowers protein oxidation in patients with thermal injury. *Ann Surg*. 1994; **220**: 310–319.

27. Herndon DN, Ramzy PI, Debroy MA, et al. Muscle protein catabolism after severe burn: effects of IGF-1/IGFBP-3 treatment. *Ann Surg*. 1999; **229**: 713–722.

28. DebRoy MA, Wolf SE, Xhang XJ, et al. Anabolic effects of insulin-like growth factor in combination with insulin-like growth factor binding protein-3 in severely burned adults. *J Trauma*. 1999; **47**: 904–911.

29. Watson RT, Pessin JE. Intracellular organization of insulin signaling and GLUT4 translocation. *Recent Prog Horm Res*. 2001; **56**: 175–193.

30. Kinney JM, Long CL, Gump FE, Duke JH Jr. Tissue comparison of weight loss in surgical patients: I—elective operation. *Am Surg*. 1968; **168**: 459–474.

31. Herndon DN, Tompkins RG. Support of the metabolic response to burn injury. *Lancet*. 2004; **363**: 1895–1902.

32. Wanek S, Wolf SE. Metabolic response to injury and role of anabolic hormones. *Curr Opin Clin Nutr Metab Care*. 2007; **10**: 272–277.

33. Hasselgren P-O, Fischer JE. Muscle cachexia: current concepts of intracellular mechanisms and molecular regulation. *Ann Surg*. 2001; **233**: 9–17.

34. Hotchkiss RS, Karl IE. The pathophysiology and treatment of sepsis. *N Engl J Med*. 2003; **348**: 138–150.

35. Levy RJ, Deutschman CS. Cytochrome c oxidase dysfunction in sepsis. *Crit Care Med*. 2007; **35**(suppl): S468–S475.

36. Elbers FW, Ince C. Mechanisms of critical illness—classifying microcirculatory flow abnormalities in distributive shock. *Crit Care.* 2006;**10**:221.

37. Ince C. The microcirculation is the motor of sepsis. *Crit Care.* 2005; **9**(suppl): S13–S19.

38. Fink MP. Bench-to-bedside review: cytopathic hypoxia. *Crit Care.* 2002; **6**: 491–499.

39. Brealey D, Singer M. Mitochondrial dysfunction in sepsis. *Curr Infect Dis Rep.* 2003; **5**: 365–371.

40. Murphy E, Steenbergen C. Preconditioning: the mitochondrial connection. *Annu Rev Physiol.* 2007; **69**: 51–67.

41. Zeviani M, Lamantea E. Genetic disorders of the mitochondrial OXPHOS system. *Sci Med.* 2005; **10**: 154–167.

42. Singer M. Mitochondrial function in sepsis: acute phase versus multiple organ failure. *Crit Care Med.* 2007; **35**(suppl): S441–S448.

43. Fredriksson K, Rooyackers O. Mitochondrial function in sepsis: respiratory versus leg muscle. *Crit Care Med.* 2007; **35**(suppl): S449–S453.

44. Leverve XM. Mitochondrial function and substrate availability. *Crit Care Med.* 2007; **35**(suppl): S454–S460.

45. Brealey D, Karyampudi S, Jacques TS, et al. Mitochondrial dysfunction in a long-term rodent model of sepsis and organ failure. *Am J Physiol Regul Integr Comp Physiol.* 2004; **286**: R491–R497.

46. Protti A, Singer M. Bench-to-bedside review: potential strategies to protect or reverse mitochondrial dysfunction in sepsis-induced organ failure. *Crit Care.* 2006; **10**: 228.

47. Neubauer S. The failing heart—an engine out of fuel. *N Engl J Med.* 2007; **356**: 1140–1151.

48. Dalgaard LT, Pedersen O. Uncoupling proteins: functional characteristics and the role in the pathogenesis of obesity and type II diabetes. *Diabetologia.* 2001; **44**: 946–965.

49. Dulloo AG, Samec S, Sydoux J. Uncoupling protein 3 and fatty acid metabolism. *Biochem Soc Trans.* 2001; **29**: 785–791.

50. Fink MP, Macias CA, Xiao J, et al. Hemigramicidin-TEMPO conjugates: novel mitochondrial-targeted antioxidants. *Crit Care Med.* 2007; **35**(suppl): S461–S467.

51. Levy RJ, Vijayasarathy C, Raj NR, Avadhani NG, Deutschman CS. Competitive and noncompetitive inhibition of myocardial cytochrome c oxidase in sepsis. *Shock.* 2004; **21**: 110–114.

52. Saffle JR, Davis B, Williams P. Recent outcomes in the treatment of burn injury in the United States: a report from the American Burn Association patient registry. *J Burn Care Rehabil.* 1995; **16**: 219–232.

53. Norbury WB, Herndon DN. Modulation of the hypermetabolic response after burn injury. In: Herndon D, ed. *Total Burn Care.* 3rd ed. Philadelphia: Saunders Elsevier Inc; 2007:420-433.

54. Moore FA, Feliciano DV, Andrassy RJ, et al. Early enteral feeding, compared with parenteral, reduces postoperative septic complications. The results of a meta-analysis. *Ann Surg.* 1992; **216**: 172–182.

55. Herndon DN, Stein MD, Rutan TC, et al. Failure of TPN supplementation to improve liver function, immunity, and mortality in thermally injured patients. *J Trauma.* 1987; **27**: 195–204.

56. McDonald WS, Sharp CW Jr, Deitch EA. Immediate enteral feeding in burn patients is safe and effective. *Ann Surg.* 1991; **213**: 177–183.

57. Mochizuki H, Trocki O, Diminioni L, et al. Reduction of postburn hypermetabolism by early enteral feeding. *Curr Surg.* 1985; **42**: 121–125.

58. Jenkins ME, Gottschlich MM, Warden GD. Enteral feeding during operative procedures in thermal injuries. *J Burn Care Rehabil.* 1994; **15**: 199–205.

59. Todd SR, Kozar RA, Moore FA. Nutritional support in adult trauma patients. *Nutr Clin Pract.* 2006; **21**: 421–429.

60. Hart DW, Wolf SE, Chinkes DL, et al. Determinants of skeletal muscle catabolism after sever burn. *Ann Surg.* 2000; **232**: 455–465.

61. Gray DT, Pine RW, Harnar TJ, et al. Early excision versus conventional therapy in patients with 20 to 40% burns: a comparative study. *Am J Surg.* 1982; **144**: 76–80.

62. Herndon DN, Barrow RE, Rutan RL, et al. A comparison of conservative versus early excision therapies in severely burned patients. *Ann Surg.* 1989; **209**: 547–553.

63. Hart DW, Wolf SE, Chinkes DL, et al. Effects of early excision and aggressive enteral feeding on hypermetabolism, catabolism and sepsis after severe burn. *J Trauma.* 2003; **54**: 755–762.

64. Mangano DT, Layug EL, Wallace A, Tateo I. Effect of atenolol on mortality and cardiovascular morbidity after noncardiac surgery. Multicenter study of perioperative ischemia research group. *N Engl J Med.* 1996; **335**: 1713–1720.

65. POISE Study Group. Effects of extended-release metoprolol succinate in patients undergoing non-cardiac surgery (POISE trial): a randomised controlled trial. *Lancet.* 2008; **371**: 1839–1847.

66. Herndon DN, Barrow RE, Rutan TC, et al. Effect of propranolol administration on human dynamic metabolic response of the burned pediatric patient. *Ann Surg.* 1988; **208**: 484–492.

67. Honeycutt D, Barrow RE, Herndon DN. Cold stress response in patients with severe burns after beta-blockade. *J Burn Care Rehabil.* 1992; **13**: 181–186.

68. Minifee PK, Barrow RE, Abston S, Desai MH, Herndon DN. Improved myocardial oxygen utilization following propranolol in fusion in adolescents with post-burn hypermetabolism. *J Pediatr Surg.* 1989; **24**: 806–810.

69. Baron PW, Barrow RE, Pierre EJ, Herndon DN. Prolonged use of propranolol effectively decreases cardiac work in burned children. *J Burn Care Rehabil.* 1997; **18**: 223–227.

70. Aarsland A, Chinkes DL, Wolfe RR, et al. Beta-blockade lowers peripheral lipolysis in burn patients receiving growth hormone. *Ann Surg.* 1996; **223**: 777–789.

71. Gore DC, Honeycutt E, Jahoor F, et al. Propranolol diminishes extremity blood flow in burn patients. *Ann Surg.* 1991; **213**: 568–574.

72. Morio B, Irtund O, Herndon DN, Wolfe RR. Propranolol decreases splanchnic triaclyglycerol storage in burned patients receiving a high carbohydrate diet. *Ann Surg.* 2002; **236:** 218–225.

73. Herndon DN, Hart DW, Wolf SE, Chinkes DL, Wolfe RR. Reversal of catabolism by beta-blockade after severe burns. *N Engl J Med.* 2001; **345:** 1223–1229.

74. Herndon DN, Barrow RE, Kunkel KR, et al. Effects of recombinant human growth hormone on donor-site healing in severely burned children. *Ann Surg.* 1990; **212:** 424–429.

75. Barret JP, Dziewulski P, Jeschke MG, et al. Effects of recombinant human growth hormone on the development of burn scarring. *Plast Reconstr Surg.* 1999; **104:** 726–729.

76. Aili Low JF, Barrow RE, Mittendorfer B, et al. The effect of short-term growth hormone treatment on growth and energy expenditure in burned children. *Burns.* 2001; **27:** 447–452.

77. Jeschke MG, Herndon DN, Wolf SE, et al. Recombinant human growth hormone alters acute phase reactant proteins, cytokine expression, and liver morphology in burned rats. *J Surg Res.* 1999; **83:** 122–129.

78. Takagi K, Suzuki F, Barrow RE, et al. Recombinant human growth hormone modulates Th1 and Th2 cytokine response in burned mice. *Ann Surg.* 1998; **228:** 106–111.

79. Takala J, Ruokonen E, Webster NR, et al. Increased mortality associated with growth hormone treatment in critically ill adults. *N Engl J Med.* 1999; **341:** 785–792.

80. Ramirez RJ, Wolf SE, Barrow RE, et al. Growth hormone treatment in pediatric burns: a safe therapeutic approach. *Ann Surg.* 1998; **228:** 439–448.

81. Van Den Berghe G, Wouters P, Weekers F, et al. Intensive insulin therapy in the critically ill patient. *N Engl J Med.* 2001; **345:** 1359–1367.

82. Pham TN, Warren AJ, Phan HH, et al. Impact of tight glycemic control in severely burned children. *J Trauma.* 2005; **59:** 1148–1154.

83. Sakurai Y, Aarsland A, Herndon DN, et al. Stimulation of muscle protein synthesis by long-term insulin infusion in severely burned patients *Ann Surg.* 1995; **222:** 283–297.

84. Aarsland A, Chinkes DL, Sakurai Y, et al. Insulin therapy in burn patients does not contribute to hepatic triglyceride production. *J Clin Invest.* 1998; **101:** 2233–2239.

85. Ferrando AA, Chinkes DL, Wolf SE, et al. A submaximal dose of insulin promotes skeletal muscle protein synthesis in patients with severe burns. *Ann Surg.* 1999; **229:** 11–18.

86. Thomas SJ, Morimoto K, Herndon DN, et al. The effect of prolonged euglycemic hyperinsulinemia on lean body mass after severe burn. *Surgery.* 2002; **132:** 341–347.

87. Pierre EJ, Barrow RE, Hawkins HK, et al. Effects of insulin on wound healing. *J Trauma.* 1998; **44:** 342–345.

88. Jeschke MG, Klein D, Herndon DN. Insulin treatment improves the systemic inflammatory reaction to severe trauma. *Ann Surg.* 2004; **239:** 553–560.

89. Wu X, Thomas SJ, Herndon, DN, et al. Insulin decreases hepatic acute phase protein levels in severely burned children. *Surgery.* 2004; **135:** 196–202.

90. Jeschke MG, Klein D, Bolder U, et al. Insulin attenuates the systemic inflammatory response in endotoxemic rats. *Endocrinology.* 2004; **145:** 4084–4093.

91. Gore DC, Wolf SE, Sanford A, et al. Influence of metformin on glucose intolerance and muscle catabolism following severe burn injury. *Ann Surg.* 2005; **241:** 334–342.

92. Gore DC, Wolf Se, Herndon DN, Wolfe RR. Metformin blunts stress-induced hyperglycemia after thermal injury. *J Trauma.* 2003; **54:** 555–561.

93. Ferrando AA, Sheffield-Moore M, Wolf SE, et al. Testosterone administration in severe burns ameliorates muscle catabolism. *Crit Care Med.* 2001; **29:** 1936–1942.

94. Demling RH, DeSanti L. Oxandrolone, an anabolic steroid, significantly increases the rate of weight gain in the recovery phase after major burns. *J Trauma.* 1997; **43:** 47–51.

95. Sheffield-Moore M, Urban RJ, Wolf SE, et al. Short term oxandrolone administration stimulates net muscle protein synthesis in young men. *J Clin Endocrinol Metab.* 1999; **84:** 2705–2711.

96. Demling RH. Comparison of the anabolic effects and complications of human growth hormone and the testosterone analog, oxandrolone, after severe burn injury. *Burns.* 1999; **25:** 215–221.

97. Demling RH, DeSantiL L. The rate of restoration of body weight after burn injury, using the anabolic agent oxandrolone, is not age dependent. *Burns.* 2001; **27:** 46–51.

98. Hart DW, Wolf SE, Ramzy PI, et al. Anabolic effects of oxandrolone following severe burn. *Ann Surg.* 2001; **233:** 556–564.

99. Wolf SE, Edelman LS, Kemalyan N, et al. Effects of oxandrolone on outcome measures in the severely burned: a multicenter prospective randomized double-blind trial. *J Burn Care Res.* 2006; **27:** 131–139.

100. Murry CE, Jennings RB, Reimer KA. Preconditioning with ischemia: a delay of lethal cell injury in ischemic myocardium. *Circulation.* 1986; **74:** 1124–1136.

101. Murry CE, Richard VJ, Reimer KA, Jennings RB. Ischemic preconditioning slows energy metabolism and delays ultrastructural damage during a sustained ischemic episode. *Circ Res.* 1990; **66:** 913–931.

102. Gurnell M. PPARγ and the human metabolic syndrome. *Sci Med.* 2004; **9:** 332–345.

103. Bays H, Mandarino L, DeFronzo. Role of the adipocyte, free fatty acids, and ectopic fat in pathogenesis of type 2 diabetes mellitus: peroxisomal proliferator-activated receptor agonists provide a rational therapeutic approach. *J Clin Endocrinol Metab.* 2004; **89:** 463–478.

104. Shiomi T, Tsutsui H, Hayashidani S, et al. Pioglitazone, a peroxisome proliferator-activated receptor-gamma agonist, attenuates left ventricular remodeling and failure after experimental myocardial infarction. *Circulation.* 2002; **106:** 3126–3132.

105. Frantz S, Hu K, Widder J, et al. Peroxisome proliferator activated-receptor agonism and left ventricular remodeling in mice with chronic myocardial infarction. *Fr J Pharmacol.* 2004; **141:** 9–14.

106. Morrow DA, Fivertz MM. Modulation of myocardial energetics: emerging evidence for a therapeutic target in cardiovascular disease. *Circulation.* 2005; **112:** 3218–3221.

107. Essop MF, Opie LH. Metabolic therapy for heart failure. *Eur Heart J.* 2004; **25:** 1765–1768.

108. Finck BN, Kelly DP. PGC-1 coactivators: inducible regulators of energy metabolism in health and disease. *J Clin Invest.* 2006; **116:** 615–622.

109. Murray AJ, Anderson RE, Watson GC, Radda GK, Clarke K. Uncoupling proteins in the human heart. *Lancet.* 2004; **364:** 1786–1788.

110. Wallis J, Lygate CA, Fischer A, et al. Supranormal myocardial creatine and phosphocreatine concentrations lead to cardiac hypertrophy and heart failure: insights from creatine tranporter-overexpressing transgenic mice. *Circulation.* 2005; **112:** 3131–3139.

111. Ng TM. Levosimendan, a new calcium-sensitizing inotrope for heart failure. *Pharmacotherapy.* 2004; **24:** 1366–1384.

112. Sima AAF, Kamiya H. Insulin, C-peptide, and diabetic neuropathy. Sci Med. 2003; **9:** 308–319.

# CHAPTER SEVENTEEN

# CHANGES TO THE HYPOTHALAMIC-PITUITARY-ADRENAL AXIS IN BURNS AND USE OF STEROIDS

BRADLEY J. PHILLIPS, MD

MARISSA J. CARTER, PhD

## INTRODUCTION

### The Hypothalamic-Pituitary-Adrenal Axis

The hypothalamic-pituitary-adrenal axis (HPA), one of the primary endocrine systems involved in the response to stress, helps maintain hemodynamic stability following major injury or illness. Neuronal input stimulates the release of corticotropin-releasing hormone (CRH) and ADH (antidiuretic hormone, also known as arginine vasopressin) from the paraventricular nucleus of the hypothalamus, which results in corticotrophs in the pituitary gland secreting corticotropin.

When receptors in the adrenal cortex are activated by corticotropin, steroidogenesis occurs, with concurrent production of the glucocorticoids cortisol, cortisone, and aldosterone as well as several androgens. In humans, cortisol is the active hormone, while cortisone is inactive.[1]

Cortisol primarily mobilizes the body's energy reserves by stimulating gluconeogenesis from glycogen, lipids, and proteins. It also exerts several effects in the gastrointestinal (GI) system, reduces bone formation, suppresses the immune system, and causes a generalized movement of potassium ions out of the cell in exchange for sodium. If the stress is transient, the rise in plasma cortisol will provide a feedback loop via the hypothalamus and pituitary, thus removing the stimulus for further corticosteroid secretion. However, if the stress becomes chronic, as is common in critically ill patients, this feedback loop may fail for a variety of reasons. Subsequently, the rise in cortisol becomes sustained and in some cases dangerously high, with adverse consequences.

The HPA axis is fully functional in neonates and is thus developmentally complete. However, the axis is highly susceptible to prenatal and postnatal "programming," (eg, adverse maternal stress, preterm birth, or social deprivation in infants), which may lead to abnormal responses to illness later in life.[2] For example, increased basal levels of cortisol, a shift in the circadian rhythm of cortisol secretion, or hypersensitivity of the HPA axis to stress have been demonstrated in animal and human research as a result of such programming.[3-5] It is interesting to consider whether this programming might constitute a risk factor for adverse outcomes in children with even moderate burn injuries.

In children, cortisol follows a circadian rhythm similar to that in adults, with a nadir around 10 PM and a sharp peak at 8 AM that gradually declines throughout the day.[6] Neonates do not have such a circadian rhythm established until 2 years of age.[7] Corticotropin also follows a diurnal rhythm driven by the suprachiasmatic nucleus, the body's "master clock." Recent research in mice lacking critical "clock genes" demonstrated that the adrenal cortex is subject to a gating mechanism that controls the sensitivity of cortisol-producing cells to corticotropin, depending on the point of time in the diurnal cycle.[8] Loss of this mechanism in burn injuries has implications for subsequent metabolic disturbances.

## Gross Changes in the HPA Axis in Burns

Profound changes in the HPA axis in burn patients are frequently observed. The primary drivers for these changes are cytokines associated with increased inflammation after burn injury, whose sustained elevation can continue for several weeks. Although recent data suggest [BP: suggest; data is always plural] that the inflammatory cytokine profile is not substantially different across the ages of 0 to 18 years, acute phase protein and cortisol levels are significantly lower in younger children (<4 years old), compared to older children (10-18 years old).[9] In addition, increased cardiac work with impaired function has been found to be significantly higher in the younger age group, which may increase the risk of mortality. The most critical factor appears to be the percentage of TBSA (total body surface area) burned. For example, Jeschke et al[10] determined that levels of some proinflammatory cytokines, notably IL-6, IL-8, monocyte chemoattractant protein-1 (MCP-1), and tumor necrosis factor (TNF),

were proportionately related to the percentage of TBSA burned, with burns >80% TBSA eliciting the highest levels.

Serum ADH[11] and corticotropin[12] levels rise sharply after burn injury, in some instances 10 times the upper limit of normal range within the first few days,[13] and remain at persistently high levels for up to 2 months.[13] A correlation between ADH and corticotropin levels has been noted,[12] as well as an association between burn size and ADH levels.[14] The high levels of ADH are sufficient to cause intense vasospasm,[15] which can intensify impaired tissue perfusion, leading to increased burn depth and possible skin graft failure.[12] However, in their study of 25 children with burns greater than 20% TBSAs, Palmieri et al.[13] noted no correlation between corticotropin and cortisol levels, or between cortisol and dehydroepiandrosterone levels. Furthermore, they found that corticotropin levels were lower than predicted, given the level of stress associated with the injury. Their results suggest that dysfunction in the HPA feedback loop occurs at the hypothalamic level, but this interpretation should be tempered by limitations of studies in this area, which include a large variance in levels of measured hormones, considerable variation in regard to the time at which the hormones are measured, and variation in severity of burn injury.

Little is known about the role of CRH in burn injury. Murton et al[12] reported the hormone was transiently increased in the first few hours after a burn. However, this rise might have been missed in many patients due to delayed transfer to the burn unit or the possibility that plasma CRH levels do not reflect hypothalamic secretion activity. Animal studies also indicate that levels of this hormone, measured in the ventromedial region of the hypothalamus, decreased within hours after burn injury, suggesting that CRH itself is not involved. Instead, the CRH type 2 receptor and one of the urocortin peptides (a member of the CRH peptide family) are more likely to be the mediators involved in burn-induced hypermetabolism.[16,17] Which of these peptides is responsible for effects on autonomic functions and acute phase protein synthesis[18] in the liver remains unknown.

Early studies in adults established that cortisol levels become quickly elevated after burn injury, with a response proportional to the percent TBSA burned.[19-22] In most cases, cortisol levels do not significantly decrease until well into the healing phase of the burn wound. The normal range for cortisol is approximately 6.8 to 23.4 µg/dL (190-650 nmol/L)[23] at 8 AM, depending on the analytical method used.[12,24-26] Upon admission to burn units, cortisol levels in the range of 16 to 58 µg/dL (450-1600 nmol/L) have been found in both children and adults, with higher values associated with larger TBSA burned and greater burn depth.

Secretion of other hormones interrelated with the HPA axis system are also greatly perturbed by burn injury. Serum growth hormone (GH) and insulinlike growth factor 1 (IGF-1) are both depressed during burn injury.[26] Moreover, an investigation by Jeschke et al revealed that children with larger burns demonstrated more persistent reductions of GH and slower recovery of IGF-1.[10] Since IGF-1 is involved in cell growth, increasing protein anabolism, attenuating the hepatic acute phase response, and improving dermal and epidermal regeneration,[27,28] a reduction in this factor can have long-term deleterious consequences. While suspicion has fallen on proinflammatory cytokines such as IL-1β as the culprits for reduced GH and IGF-1 secretion,[29] it is unclear what roles the higher levels of catecholamines and cortisol play in this scenario.

## PHYSIOLOGICAL MECHANISMS

### Cytokines, Burns, and the HPA Axis

Questions as to how cytokines raise cortisol levels and about their interaction at all levels of the HPA axis have been studied in both physiological and pathophysiological systems. In particular, data from animal and human burn studies in the last decade are starting to provide insight regarding cytokine involvement following burn injury and their interaction with the HPA axis, which may provide the basis for novel treatment approaches in the future.

There are 6 classes of cytokines, of which the interferons, interleukins, and tumor necrosis factors seem to be the most important. Within the interleukin family, IL-1 (α and β), IL-6, IL-8, IL-11, IL-12, and IL-18 are considered proinflammatory, while IL-10 is considered anti-inflammatory. Many of these entities have overlapping functions, accentuating or mitigating cytokine production under various circumstances.

Although a detailed review of cytokine behavior is beyond the scope of this chapter, it is important for the practicing clinician to understand several concepts. First, cytokines are signaling messengers which possess local as well as systemic effects. Second, following injury, a cascade of proinflammatory as well as some anti-inflammatory cytokines is released at injury sites. Secretion of cytokines at distal sites in response to these initial messengers usually follows. These actions are a normal and necessary response of the body to injury. Finally, of paramount importance, is the overall concentration and balance of these factors. More severe injuries produce higher concentrations and often a major excess of proinflammatory cytokines, whose effects can be lethal if left unchecked. This situation is sometimes referred to as acute hypercytokinemia.

Traditionally, the actions of glucocorticoids (GCs) secreted by the adrenal cortex in response to cytokines and other hormones have been thought of as anti-inflammatory,

but increasing evidence indicates this may not be true. As Yeager et al have eloquently stated, "Varying doses of glucocorticoids do not lead simply to varying degrees of inflammation suppression, but rather GC's can exert a full range of effects from permissive to stimulatory to suppressive."[30] When this concept is better understood, it may become clearer under what conditions steroid administration may be beneficial or detrimental and when blind administration of steroids in the hope of reversing the poor prognosis of a burned patient can be dangerous.

A Turkish study following the course of IL-8 and IL-10 in 36 acutely burned patients demonstrated that IL-8 peaked shortly after burn injury, but that a difference emerged between survivors and nonsurvivors: the IL-8 plasma levels in those who survived were significantly lower.[31] In addition, the concentration of IL-10 peaked between 5 and 9 days postburn, with lower levels in nonseptic survivors, and a second, later peak noted in nonsurvivors. Another study, by Dugan et al,[32] observed a positive correlation between serum IL-8 and mortality in patients with small-to-moderate burns. Furthermore, levels of serum prolactin, IL-6, and IL-1β positively correlated with the percentage of TBSA burned, and increased 2-fold in more severe burns. An additional finding from this study was the association of prolactin with levels of IL-6, IL-8, and IL-10, since prolactin had not previously been suspected of playing a major role in burn injury. A Japanese study of 20 patients with burns exceeding 20% TBSA also suggested a role for leukemia inhibitory factor (LIF) (a cytokine related to IL-6) in burn injury, with a relationship between mortality and elevated IL-6, corticotropin, and cortisol concentrations noted. Significant correlations between serum LIF and plasma corticotropin, as well as serum LIF with urine-free cortisol, were noted, although the strength of the correlation was only poor to fair.[33] Researchers from the Shriners Hospital in Galveston also performed extensive cytokine profiling in severely burned children and discovered maximal cytokine concentrations in the first week postburn. The exception was granulocyte macrophage colony-stimulating factor (GM-CSF), which significantly increased in the second week following burn injury.[34] In a subsequent study at the same facility of 44 children with burns exceeding 40% TBSA, levels of serum IL-6, IL-8, IL-10, IL-12p70 (a subunit of IL-12), GM-CSF, TNF, and IFN-γ (interferon gamma) were found significantly higher in the 15 children who developed sepsis and died compared to nonseptic survivors.[35]

Effector T helper ($T_H$) cells are lymphocytes involved with the immune system which secrete cytokines or proteins that then stimulate or interact with other leukocytes, including other $T_H$ cells. $T_H$ cells are classified into 2 types. Type 1 cells produce IFN-γ and TNF-β, and are thus associated with the cellular immune system. IFN-γ stimulates the production of IL-12, which itself promotes IFN-γ, thus constituting a positive feedback loop. Type 2 $T_H$ cells, associated with the humoral immune system, produce IL-4, IL-5, IL-6, IL-10, and IL-13. IL-4 is a self-promoter of type 2 $T_H$ cells and cytokines produced by these cells, whereas IL-10 inhibits IL-2, IFN-γ, and IL-12. With this background knowledge, the work of Miller et al[36] now comes into focus. By reviewing the literature in regard to the response of $T_H$ cells to burns and trauma, they discovered a greatly diminished $T_H1$ response but an enhanced $T_H2$ response, as evidenced by elevation of IL-4 and IL-10. Furthermore, they suggested the following changes are prognostic for patients at risk of multiple organ failure and sepsis: decreased production of IL-2, IFN-γ, and IL-12 and increased production of IL-10 and IL-18. Of note in this review,[36] and perhaps especially relevant to burn patients, is the significance of the IL-6:IL-10 ratio, which has also been confirmed in other studies. For example, it was observed that a 3-fold increase in this ratio, to 18.7, was fatal in patients with the systematic inflammatory response syndrome, whereas the ratio was stable in survivors.[37] Confirmation of repression of type 1 $T_H$ cells was also demonstrated in a study of mice in which very low levels of IL-12 were measured following burn injury and challenge with lipopolysaccharide. This repression was not ameliorated by prostaglandin $E_2$ ($PGE_2$) or cortisol inhibition, indicating that the HPA axis is not apparently involved.[38] Although cytokines released from burn-injured type 2 $T_H$ cells appear to account for this immunomodulation, studies in mice suggest that the magnitude of immune dysfunction following burn injury also has a substantial genetic component.[39]

Jeschke et al[10] also studied cytokine profiles with regard to burn size in children, noting that levels of 6 out of the 17 cytokines measured were significantly elevated in the highest-burn-size group (>80% TBSA): IL-8, TNF, IL-6, IL-12p70, MCP-1, and GM-CSF. Most importantly, through their ability to increase inflammation, these cytokines have been found to enhance catabolism and hypermetabolism, significant factors involved in children with moderate or large burns.

For many years, it had been known that cytokines affect the highest levels of the HPA axis. For example, intravenous injection of IL-1 had been observed to increase plasma corticotropin levels through release of CRH.[40,41] However, by the 1990s, hypotheses began to emerge regarding the production of cytokines within the adrenal glands. To fully understand the import of research in this area, it is necessary to take a brief detour to discuss the adrenal glands in further detail.

The chromaffin cells in the core of the adrenal gland (the medulla) are responsible for production of catecholamines, while the cortex is the center of mineralocorticoid and glucocorticoid production, as well as a secondary site of androgen synthesis. The *zona glomerulosa*, the outermost layer of the cortex, produces mineralocorticoids, while the *zona fasciculata* is responsible for glucocorticoid production and the *zona reticularis* is the site of weak androgen synthesis. What is rarely appreciated, however, is that chromaffin and cortical cells are intermingled to an astonishing degree, thus setting the stage for intra-adrenal paracrine mechanisms.[42] This is particularly relevant in the transitional zone between the medulla and cortex where macrophages reside.

In 1995, specialized cortical cells in the *zona reticularis* were found to be the principal source of production and expression of IL-1 within the adrenal gland. It was suggested these cells responded to the output of catecholamines from neighboring chromaffin cells.[43] Following this discovery, the secretion of many other cytokines was reported, some in response to stimulation by corticotropin and angiotensin II.[44] Thus, IL-6 significantly increased basal and corticotropin-stimulated cortisol release, whereas TNF-α inhibited such release[45] and LIF significantly enhanced basal and corticotropin-induced production of cortisol and aldosterone in tissue culture.[46]

What, then, is the relevance of intra-adrenal cytokine paracrine mechanisms in burn cases? Under conditions of prolonged or chronic stress, it has been proposed that CRH and corticotropin release are suppressed by feedback inhibition through elevated levels of cortisol. However, IL-6 can maintain elevated cortisol levels by direct stimulation of adrenocortical steroidogenesis via a paracrine mechanism.[47] Here, then, is the foundation of possible HPA axis dysfunction: the basic feedback loop is broken, yet IL-6 or other cytokines (produced in other injured areas of the body) continue to stimulate production of cortisol, which in turn suppresses many immune functions. If we consider this in terms of proinflammatory and anti-inflammatory functions, the situation is analogous to the accelerator of an automobile being jammed to the floor while the brake function is simultaneously inhibited. In order to restore function to the HPA axis, it is necessary to differentiate which burn patients have suffered from this imbalance and then determine those patients who have incurred true adrenal insufficiency.

## Glucocorticoid Binding

Under normal physiological conditions, approximately 80% of circulating cortisol is bound to a monomeric glycoprotein termed corticosteroid-binding globulin (CBG), which has a single binding site.[48] Approximately 10% is bound to albumin,[49] while the remaining unbound fraction of cortisol (5%-10%) is biologically active. Serum CBG levels are affected by a wide variety of factors, including cortisol levels themselves, estrogen levels in pregnant women, and thyroid hormones.[50] Levels are usually low in severely burned adult patients.[50] The finding in 1985 of burn injuries in rats that produced different CBG forms[51] was at first puzzling, but it appears that, as with many other hormone-binding globulins, CBG exists in 2 conformations: a stressed configuration, which is vulnerable to proteolytic cleavage, and a relaxed configuration that is the result of cleavage.[52] The stressed state is the predominant form under normal physiological conditions and is responsible for tight binding of cortisol. However, proteolytic cleavage induced under inflammatory conditions—by neutrophil elastase, for example—produces substantial quantities of the relaxed form and thus constitutes a specific targeted type of cortisol delivery.[49] Moreover, Il-6 was found to decrease CBG production in hepatoma cell culture experiments,[53] and an inverse relationship between serum IL-6 and CBG was noted in severely burned patients.[54] Together, these results suggest that the acute phase response in the liver reduces the total amount of circulating CBG, thus reducing total cortisol and possibly increasing the amount of free cortisol available to cells. At the same time, the burn response causes a targeted increase of cortisol delivery to those cells most in need. Recent CBG gene knockout experiments in mice seem to confirm the "targeted cortisol delivery" theory through the interaction of cell surface receptors in target tissues with CBG-cortisol complexes that initiate cell surface signaling or corticosteroid uptake activities.[55] Interestingly, mice with knocked-out CBG genes were much more vulnerable to septic shock, which might suggest that elevated free cortisol plays less of a role than traditionally advanced in the response to such provocations.

## Cortisol and Cortisone Interconversion: 11-beta-hydroxysteroid Dehydrogenase Activity

Although CBG plays a major role in the delivery of cortisol to cells, another factor that affects cortisol bioavailability is its metabolism. The most important enzyme that controls metabolism is 11β-hydroxysteroid dehydrogenase, which has 2 isoforms: 11β-HSD1, which converts inactive cortisone to cortisol, and 11β-HSD2, which is primarily active in the kidney and inactivates cortisol prior to its binding to the mineralocorticoid receptor.[56,57] The plasma cortisol-cortisone ratio reflects the activities of these enzymes.

Venkatesh et al[58] studied the cortisol-cortisone (F:E) ratio in 3 groups of critically ill patients: (1) sepsis, (2) multitrauma, and (3) burns. Although marked alterations of the ratio occurred in all groups due to proportionately greater increases in 11β-HSD1 versus 11β-HSD2, only the burn group failed to show a significant increase in the F:E ratio,

total plasma cortisol, or cortisone levels. These results may have occurred by activity of 11β-HSD1 in the reverse direction in disrupted cells—that is, catalysis of cortisol to cortisone. Another explanation proposes that the reduction in CBG observed in severe burn cases might have been responsible. Although this was a relatively small study,[58] it provides the first clue that the effect of sepsis and trauma on the HPA axis may be appreciably different compared to burn injuries. It is also known that TNF-α upregulates the activity of 11β-HSD1 while downregulating 11β-HSD2.[59,60] In addition, levels of TNF are proportionately related to the size of a burn.[10] Furthermore, the onset of sepsis in burn injuries raises TNF levels even higher,[35] which suggests the bioavailability of cortisol is vastly enhanced under such conditions. Thus, it might be possible that the immunomodulatory effects of such high glucocorticoid levels are partly responsible for the high mortality rate observed in severe burn injuries with sepsis.

## Glucocorticoid Resistance

Although cortisol can freely cross the cell membrane, it must interact with the glucocorticoid receptor (GR) in order to function as a signal transductor. The number of receptors in the cytosol varies from several thousand to greater than 100000 per cell in every nucleated cell of the body.[61] Under normal physiological conditions, cortisol binds to the GR, which then dissociates from a multiprotein complex, dimerizes, translocates to the nucleus, and binds to specific DNA regions to modulate gene expression.[62] Although this is an oversimplification of the process, it can be understood that during the several consecutive steps that occur, there is the possibility for other biochemical factors to interact. Most of the research to date in this area has involved the inflammatory conditions of shock/sepsis, and although conflicting findings are not uncommon, important results have emerged. First, cytokines (and other factors, such as endotoxin and lipopolysaccharide) are able to modify the affinity of cortisol to its receptor, and second, many cytokines are capable of upregulating or downregulating the receptor itself, thus impacting the number of GRs in a given cell.[62] In sepsis, this accounts for the phenomenon of GC resistance, in which the response of cortisol is vastly diminished due to fewer receptors and/or the reduced ability of cortisol to bind to its receptor. The result is an increasing level of cortisol with progressively less effect, a true dysfunction of the feedback loop that is part of the normal functioning of the HPA axis.

Very few studies of GC resistance in burn injuries have been conducted. In studying rats with a 35% TBSA immersion scald, Liu et al[63] established that the binding capacity of liver GRs was reduced by 32% at 12 hours postburn.

Moreover, the administration of polyclonal antibodies to TNF-α, IL-1β, and IL-10 or the addition of α-melanocyte-stimulating hormone (α-MSH; a broad anti-inflammatory agent) resulted in significant partial recovery of GR binding capacity, a reduction in plasma corticosterone (the active glucocorticoid in rats), and lowering of the cytokines TNF-α, IL-1β, and IL-10. These results indicate that reducing certain cytokine levels may be key to preventing GC resistance and that administration of α-MSH might be a possible treatment in the future.

Currently, it is unknown what role GC resistance plays in the pathology of burn injuries. However, given the associative relationship between burn size and cytokine levels, it is likely that it significantly contributes to the prognosis of severe burn injuries.

## USE OF STEROIDS IN SEVERE BURNS WITH OR WITHOUT SEPSIS

Much of the research with regard to steroid usage originates from the sepsis literature, and since sepsis is a common complication of severe burn injuries, it is a reasonable place to begin examining adrenal insufficiency and the role of steroid administration.

## Definitions of Sepsis

A recent consensus conference to define sepsis in burn injuries began with the statement that patients with large burns are in a state of chronic systemic inflammatory stimulation.[64] Sepsis is a change in a patient's condition that triggers concern for infection and must include 3 of the following:

- Temperature < 36.5°C or > 39°C
- Progressive tachycardia (children 2 SD [standard deviations] above age-specific norms, 85% age-adjusted max heart rate)
- Progressive tachypnea (children 2 SD above age-specific norms, 85% age-adjusted max respiratory rate)
- Thrombocytopenia (3 days after initial resuscitation, children 2 SD below age-specific norms)
- Hyperglycemia or the absence of preexisting diabetes mellitus (untreated plasma glucose > 200 mg/dL or significant resistance to insulin, such as a > 25% increase in insulin requirements over 24 hours)
- Inability to continue enteral feedings for > 24 hours due to abdominal distension, enteral feeding intolerance (such as residual volumes > 150 mL/h), or uncontrollable diarrhea (> 400 mL/day)

In addition, infection needs to be documented by positive cultures, identified pathological tissue source, or clinical response to antimicrobial therapy.

Septic shock is defined as sepsis with persistent hypotension despite adequate fluid resuscitation.[64] The consensus conference also adopted the Marshall MODS Scoring System[65] modified by Cook et al[66] to evaluate multiple organ dysfunction syndrome. This should not be undertaken until initial resuscitation is complete.

The major difference between critically ill patients with sepsis and burn patients with sepsis is the degree of substantial hypercytokinemia already present in patients suffering from large burns. Adding sepsis to a burn patient's profile increases both cytokine levels and the presence of new cytokines, thus threatening to overwhelm an already overburdened HPA axis.

## Inflammatory Markers

Since many different cytokines are elevated in burn injury, questions arise regarding their utility in providing additional information to predict patients' risk of developing sepsis. More specifically, whether there are additional inflammatory markers which may be diagnostic for sepsis and which can improve upon the clinical findings that already define sepsis is subject to debate.[64]

In the majority of burn injuries, provided certain complications are absent, such as inhalation injury, the outcome (mortality versus survival) is dependent on the size and depth of the burn. From the study of Jeschke et al,[10] it would appear that IL-6, IL-8, TNF, and MCP-1 levels rise substantially once the threshold of an 80% TBSA burn is reached. However, the significance of this with regard to mortality is unknown, since this outcome was not analyzed. Another approach could monitor the IL-10:IL-6 ratio[36,37] since IL-6 is proinflammatory and IL-10 anti-inflammatory; a sudden rise in the ratio might herald a deleterious change in condition. An alternative course of action could measure levels of IL-2, IL-12, and IFN-γ,[36,67] which represent the immune suppression that occurs after a burn injury. This concept takes into account immunosuppression that is both glucocorticoid induced and that arises by other mechanisms. Yet another cytokine whose levels have been associated with survival is IL-1β.[67] Furthermore, levels of this cytokine and IL-8 have been associated with infections.[67]

During the 1980s, C-reactive protein (CRP) was developed as an inflammatory marker in a wide variety of conditions, including cardiovascular disease. In burn injury, the results of using this marker have led to conflicting results. Early work suggested CRP levels were proportional to the percent TBSA burned and burn depth, with further increases indicative of infection.[68] In an investigation of 57 children with burn sizes ranging from 3% to 92% TBSA, Neely et al[69] noted CRP levels correctly predicted sepsis in 82% of cases, with an increase detected approximately 2 days before sepsis was clinically determined. On the other hand, nonseptic patients did not generally show increases in CRP. More recent studies of comparable size have reported little change in CRP levels[70] or concluded that CRP has poor predictability with regard to development of sepsis.[71] In conclusion, CRP cannot be advocated as a reliable inflammatory marker at this time.

More recently, procalcitonin (PCT), produced by C-cells of the thyroid gland and the precursor of the hormone calcitonin, has been studied in burn injuries. The first use of this marker in 27 patients with a mean TBSA burn of 51% suggested a positive correlation between the TBSA and mean peak PCT levels during the postburn period.[72] Although the authors reported that using a cut-off value of 3 ng/mL enabled clinicians to reliably confirm severe bacterial or fungal infections, it was also proposed that analyzing values over a prolonged period of time was more important than determining absolute values. In a smaller study, Sachse et al[73] confirmed the utility of serial PCT measurements in diagnosing sepsis, but Neely et al reported that PCT was not as reliable as CRP in their study of 20 children.[74] A similar report of 25 severely burned patients also showed that PCT was not superior to CRP or white blood counts in the diagnosis of sepsis.[75] On the other hand, Lavrentieva et al[71] reported the area under the ROC (receiver operating curve) for PCT was 0.975 with a reasonable discriminative power in a study of 43 critically ill burned adults. In addition, their analysis of absolute PCT levels indicated a clear prediction of survival versus death. These results were subsequently confirmed by Barati et al[70] (N = 60). Although the summation of these results is inconclusive, procalcitonin remains a promising marker for recognizing the onset of sepsis.

Many proposals for inflammatory markers are interesting ideas, but they remain limited in scope until tests to measure these cytokines are widely available at burn centers, ranges have been established with regard to severity of injury, and thresholds or ratios associated with outcomes, such as mortality, have been identified. Hopefully, we will be able to utilize these markers in the near future in order to improve diagnosis and treatment of sepsis.

## Lessons from the General Sepsis/Shock Literature

Throughout the last 3 decades, major studies regarding the use of glucocorticoids in critically ill patients with shock and/or sepsis have produced conflicting results. Annane et al[76] rationalized these results by dividing the studies into

2 groups: (1) those that employed short courses of high doses and (2) those that utilized longer courses of low-dose glucocorticoids. When all trials were considered, there was no difference in mortality at 28 days, but in the latter case (5 trials total), the relative risk (RR) was lower, at 0.80 (95% confidence intervals [CI] 0.67-0.95). It should be noted that although this meta-analytical result was significant ($P < .01$), the effect size was limited, as expressed by the number needed to treat (NNT) parameter. In this case the result was 8.8, which means 8.8 patients would need to be treated in order to save 1 life. Essentially, advocates of steroid therapy were (and still are) proponents of the adrenal insufficiency model, while detractors posited (and still do) that steroid administration increases the risk of oversuppression of the immune system.

Recently, the largest randomized controlled trial (RCT) to date of hydrocortisone therapy in patients with septic shock was published (N = 499).[77] The results appeared to completely contradict the assertion of Annane et al[76] that low doses of glucocorticoids were beneficial, since the trial utilized 200 mg/d of hydrocortisone in the treatment arm and found no statistical difference between treatment and control groups with regard to survival or reversal of shock. To say that clinicians find themselves in a quandary regarding these latest developments would be an understatement, but perhaps further analysis regarding the use of glucocorticoids may place the results in context.

The total number of patients in the original meta-analysis[76] was 465, but the total sample size of the new RCT was 499, which means that a new meta-analysis incorporating these results would weight the trial at 43%. Note that the new RR of 0.83 and NNT of 8.6 are similar to the values for the old meta-analysis, indicating little or no change in the effect size. However, the larger total has changed the precision with a new 95% CI of 0.65 to 1.09. Therefore, the result is no longer significant, suggesting the evidence for steroid use in sepsis/shock is equivocal.

This result is not surprising and should be a salutary lesson to all clinicians who accept meta-analyses at face value. The clue lies in the confidence intervals in the original Annane et al meta-analysis,[76] the upper limit of which is 0.95—not far from 0. Any small shift in this value upward would likely have caused it to cross the 0 line, which is no longer statistically significant. In other words, the analysis should have been greeted with much caution rather than interpreted as a "green light" to treat patients with glucocorticoids. Another important point that is rarely discussed are the actual risks and benefits to patients in the context of the NNT value.[78] For example, not all patients will face the same risks of mortality for a given sepsis/shock situation, and assessment of a patient's risk and possible benefit derived from steroid treatment must be weighed against the

NNT value. For example, if the risk of mortality were substantially less than 10%, then giving glucocorticoids might actually increase the patient's risk of dying.

In order to decide whether these results from the sepsis/shock literature apply to burn injuries, we need to first discuss the adrenal insufficiency model, its merits and deficiencies, and then determine how burn-injured patients differ from critically ill patients without such injuries.

## The Adrenal Insufficiency Model

The adrenal insufficiency model is based on the simple precept that during extreme stress the HPA axis is highly strained and can become incapable of delivering adequate amounts of cortisol demanded by the body's tissues. Essentially, the amount of circulating cortisol is insufficient to meet the needs of the body's tissues due to glucocorticoid resistance. The resultant adrenal insufficiency contributes to increased risk of mortality.[79]

Since not all patients develop adrenal insufficiency, the task is to identify its presence or absence. Once patients have been diagnosed, the protocol then becomes one of remedying the cortisol deficit.

## *Diagnosis*

How does one identify patients with adrenal insufficiency? As already noted, circulating cortisol levels are elevated in burn patients, but the variation in total cortisol values (even in reference to a normal range) is not by itself diagnostic. Annane et al[79] attempted to address this issue by administering the short corticotropin stimulation test to patients with septic shock and then observing the association between cortisol levels and mortality. Three groups were identified:

1. those with a relatively good prognosis (28-day mortality rate 26%; cortisol levels at $T_0$ of ≤34 µg/dL, and a $\Delta_{max}$ of >9 µg/dL; $T_0$ represented the baseline cortisol value prior to the test and $\Delta_{max}$ the difference between cortisol values at 30 or 60 minutes posttest and $T_0$);
2. those with an intermediate prognosis (28-day mortality rate 67%; cortisol levels at $T_0$ of 34 µg/dL, and a $\Delta_{max}$ of ≤9 µg/dL or a $T_0$ of >34 µg/dL and a $\Delta_{max}$ of >9 µg/dL); and
3. those with a poor prognosis (28-day mortality rate 82%; cortisol levels at $T_0$ of >34 µg/dL, and a $\Delta_{max}$ of ≤9 µg/dL).

When examining survival curves, it appears that a baseline cortisol level of > 34 µg/dL may be more predictive of survival rates in comparison to the $\Delta_{max}$ of ≤ 9 µg/dL versus >9 µg/dL.

While the 9 µg/dL increase in total cortisol level (or absolute value of < 18 µg/dL) following the short corticotropin test had been proposed earlier,[80] Marik and Zaloga[81] criticized the test as being too insensitive based upon the 25 µg/dL total cortisol benchmark in critically ill patients and the dosage (250 µg) as being supraphysiological. In essence, the high dosage of corticotropin may override adrenal resistance to corticotropin, or worse, may provoke a "normal" response in some patients in whom the response to current stressors is inadequate.[82] They also believe the $\Delta_{max}$ reflects adrenal reserve[81] rather than adrenal insufficiency.[79,83] The difference can be likened to a factory with finished goods in storage waiting to be delivered versus a factory with the capacity to produce goods upon demand. While low corticotropin dose (1-2 µg) seemed to provide superior results to the high-dose test in septic patients,[80] inferior results in critically ill HIV patients[84] was noted, thus casting doubt on the validity of the test. Moreover, the corticotropin test bypasses the CNS HP (central nervous system hypothalamus pituitary) axis by stimulating the adrenal glands directly and not the entire HPA axis, which is why endogenous stresses, such as hypotension, hypoxemia, fever, and hypoglycemia, are regarded as "gold standards."[80]

In another study by Marik and Zaloga,[85] the authors began administering 100 mg of hydrocortisone every 8 hours to patients with septic shock while awaiting total cortisol measurements after performing the low-dose corticotropin test followed by the high-dose test 1 hour later. Using the diagnostic criterion of 25 µg/dL for adrenal insufficiency, 61% of patients (N = 59) were diagnosed with adrenal insufficiency (22% met the diagnosis of adrenal insufficiency using the low-dose test and only 8% by the high-dose test). However, only 22 patients were responsive to hydrocortisone, which suggests 3 possibilities: (1) far fewer patients had true adrenal insufficiency and so may not have benefited from steroid administration, (2) some patients had severe GC resistance that could not be overcome by steroid administration, and (3) the administered steroids were inactivated by 11β-HSD2.

Considering all these factors, Marik and Zaloga[85] proposed the following approach when assessing patients:

1. Measure the random total cortisol level.
2. For those patients whose values are <25 µg/dL, perform both the low-dose and high-dose corticotropin tests.
3. If the total cortisol level remains below 25 µg/dL following both tests, then primary adrenal insufficiency is present.

4. If the total cortisol level rises above 25 µg/dL in both tests, then adrenal insufficiency is due to HPA axis failure.

5. A total cortisol level that rises above 25 µg/dL with the high-dose test but not the low-dose test suggests corticotropin resistance.

Although Marik and Zaloga[85] espouse a random serum total cortisol of 25 µg/dL as the threshold of an appropriate HPA axis response to critical illness, they do state, "[T]here is no absolute serum cortisol level that distinguishes an adequate from an insufficient adrenal response."

## Free Versus Total Cortisol Considerations

In the preceding section, all diagnostic criteria were based upon measurement of total cortisol. As iterated earlier, free cortisol concentrations normally constitute approximately 10% of total cortisol, although in burn (and critically ill) patients, total cortisol is likely to be lower. However, the fraction of free cortisol may be higher due to lower CBG and albumin levels in the first few days following a burn injury.

In the first investigation of its kind, Hamrahian et al.[86] measured free and total serum cortisol levels in 66 critically ill patients and 33 healthy volunteers. The investigators first analyzed the findings by dividing the critically ill patients into 2 groups: those with serum albumin ≤2.5 g/dL (group 1) and those with values >2.5 g/dL (group 2). As expected, total cortisol concentrations were lower in group 1 compared to group 2 (15.8 µg/dL vs 22.6 µg/dL). After high-dose corticotropin administration, the mean increase in total cortisol in group 1 was 7.6 µg/dL (48%) compared to 11.8 µg/dL (52%) in group 2. However, the mean free cortisol concentrations in plasma (baseline) were nearly identical (5.1 µg/dL in group 1 vs 5.2 µg/dL in group 2), with mean increases in free cortisol after adrenal stimulation of 4.2 (82%) and 4.9 (94%) µg/dL, respectively. These findings confirm that critical illness increases the percentage of free cortisol (it was 8% in the healthy volunteers, but 31% and 23% in groups 1 and 2, respectively) and that hypoproteinemia accompanying critical illness further increases the percentage of free cortisol. The findings also demonstrate that measurement of total cortisol can be highly misleading in cases of hypoproteinemia when attempting to diagnose adrenal insufficiency. Furthermore, based on the overall results and those of a subgroup of 7 patients who had previously documented adrenal insufficiency prior to illness, the authors defined a serum free cortisol of 2.0 µg/dL as a threshold for adrenal insufficiency, or a value of 3.1 µg/dL for corticotropin-stimulated free cortisol levels. It is noteworthy that if the criterion of Marik and Zaloga[85] had been used, all patients in this study would have been classified as having adrenal insufficiency.

In comparison, using the baseline free cortisol 2.0 µg/dL benchmark, with few exceptions, only patients who had previously documented adrenal insufficiency would have been classified as having adrenal insufficiency. However, if the benchmark of an increase of 9 µg/dL (total cortisol) following corticotropin stimulation had been applied, perhaps two-thirds of group 1 patients would have been classified as being adrenal insufficient, whereas approximately one-quarter of group 2 patients would have been so categorized. Finally, no correlation between free cortisol levels and mortality was observed.

Ho et al[87] conducted a similar study, except their groups comprised patients with sepsis and shock (group 1), sepsis alone (group 2), and healthy controls (group 3). Mean free cortisol levels corresponded with severity of illness (6.7 µg/dL for group 1 and 1.1 µg/dL for group 2), while total cortisol levels were 31.9 µg/dL and 15.1 µg/dL for groups 1 and 2, respectively. CBG and albumin levels were lowest in group 1. After corticotropin stimulation, mean free cortisol levels were 7.0 µg/dL (a 4.4 % increase) for group 1 and 2.1 µg/dL (a 91% increase) for group 2. One-third of the patients in group 1 would have thus met the $\Delta_{max}$ of ≤9 µg/dL for adrenal insufficiency following corticotropin stimulation (total cortisol), and a similar number would have been affected using the 3.1 µg/dL benchmark of Hamrahian et al.[86]

Total cortisol benchmarks appear to be in apparent conflict when comparing these 2 studies. However, the explanation might lie in the APACHE scores. The mean score for the septic/shock group in the study of Ho et al[87] was 25 (APACHE II), while it was 42 (APACHE III) in the study of Hamrahian et al.[86] Although the scoring algorithms and ranges are different (0-299 for APACHE III and 0-71 for APACHE II), it can be surmised that patients in the study of Ho et al (group 1) were, on average, sicker than those in the study of Hamrahian et al. This is also reflected in the slightly higher mortality rate of 37% versus 29% for the respective studies. These comparisons illustrate a key point: *Absolute benchmarks, regardless of whether they refer to free or total cortisol levels, must be linked to severity of illness; otherwise they can easily be misinterpreted in the context of the criticality of the illness.*

In summary, while measurement of free cortisol levels offers a more accurate picture compared to measurement of total cortisol levels, it does not entirely solve the diagnostic accuracy problem of adrenal insufficiency.

## Rationale for Cortisol Replacement

If a patient has adrenal insufficiency, the proposed treatment is to replace the cortisol deficit with exogenously administered corticosteroids. The rationale is that the clinician is replacing what the adrenal glands should be producing. There are several assumptions implicit with this supposition. First, the patient has a true adrenal insufficiency. Second, glucocorticoid administration will not place the patient at increased risk of mortality or adverse events. Third, the type and dosage of steroid will improve the patient's condition.

The difficulty in establishing adrenal insufficiency under conditions of severe stress based upon random cortisol level determinations or a corticotropin test has already been described. The decision to administer glucocorticoids must, therefore, be based on other clinical observations, as well as confirmation of adrenal insufficiency when possible. Following the patient's progress with cortisol levels and other inflammatory markers may also provide additional information.

The second assumption, that steroid administration does not increase the risk of mortality, is also important. The meta-analysis of Annane et al[76] suggests this is possible with short courses of high-dose steroids, although the increased risk is probably slight; longer doses of low-dose steroids seemed safe in this regard. However, it should be noted that steroids can be given for a variety of reasons in the ICU (eg, spinal cord injury, septic shock, adrenal insufficiency, optic neuritis, and stridor or airway edema). In a study conducted by Britt et al,[88] steroid use was associated with increased ICU length of stay and ventilator days, secondary to the increased rate of infection. Thus, it is plausible that steroid administration may increase the rate of infection in burn patients as well.

The real issue of whether there is benefit obtained from GC administration remains unproven in critically ill patients with sepsis/shock.

## General Treatment Approaches in Burn Cases

The literature with regard to glucocorticoid usage in burn injury is sparse. The 2 considerations which should be borne in mind during the initial resuscitation phase are (1) development of sudden acute adrenal insufficiency, and (2) patients who have existing adrenal insufficiency or Addison's disease. Acute adrenal insufficiency can develop at any time following a severe burn injury, and although rare, must be treated immediately.

In a patient with preexisting adrenal insufficiency, adequate steroid replacement therapy should be continued with an initial dosage of 75 to 100 mg hydrocortisone every 6 to 8 hours.[89] With this regimen, a target of 18 to 36 µg/dL (500–1000 nmol/L) serum free cortisol can be established. If increased inotropic requirements develop, treatment can be changed to a hydrocortisone infusion at 12 mg/h, with additional increases of 50 or 100 mg for each surgical procedure, or an increase of 10 mg/h during an episode of sepsis.[89] These requirements pertain to adults, so adjustments need to be made for adolescents and younger children. For adolescents, the dosage should be reduced by 15% to 50%, with lower dosages for younger adolescents. In the case of children and infants, initial doses should be 25 to 150 mg/d, given via infusion or divided into 3 or 4 injections.[90] Long-term physiological replacement goals of 12 mg/m$^2$/d can be employed after the patient's condition has stabilized.[90]

Besides acute adrenal insufficiency, another situation which might require an evaluation of the HPA axis and consideration of corticosteroid treatment involves the patient's medication history. The vast majority of studies investigating long-term usage of corticosteroids have focused on asthma in children, where there appears to be no suppression of the HPA axis with newer inhalation medications.[91] However, this is not the case with other GC medications prescribed for a wide variety of conditions, where localized resistance to GCs, suboptimal cortisol secretion, HPA axis suppression, and other adverse events that might affect recovery from burn injuries have been reported.[92-94] Accordingly, any child who has more than a minor burn (eg, >10% TBSA) and has been prescribed long-term GCs for any condition other than asthma in the last year should have his or her HPA axis evaluated following initial resuscitation.

Another question arises concerning the use of steroids in children with moderate or severe burns who exhibit no signs of sepsis. Unfortunately, no studies have been conducted in children, but a single study reported by Fuchs et al[95] in adults with thermal injuries greater than 20% TBSA found disturbances of cortisol secretion in 7 of 20 patients following a corticotropin test performed 1 day after admission; of these 7 patients, 4 appeared to have relative adrenal insufficiency. The risk of developing adrenal insufficiency also appeared to correlate significantly with the abbreviated burn severity index (ABSI).[96] Moreover, a higher mortality rate was observed in patients with adrenal insufficiency.

Although some empirical evidence suggests the nature of the inflammatory process in burn cases is somewhat different compared to shock/sepsis, clinicians should proceed cautiously given the lack of benefit observed from the shock/sepsis literature. Since impending adrenal insufficiency can manifest itself in many ways, there are no clear guidelines regarding clinical parameters. Nevertheless, case reports from the literature[97,98] suggest that hemodynamics need to be monitored closely, and continued hypotension and/or increased need for inotropic support should be sufficient grounds for HPA evaluation. If adrenal insufficiency is diagnosed, empirical GC treatment can then be instituted at the clinician's discretion using the dosages and methods described earlier. If steroid administration appears to be beneficial, hemodynamic improvements within 24 hours should be apparent. Determining the ABSI score after admission may also help in selecting patients for HPA evaluation. In addition, for those burn units with access to measurement of inflammatory markers, screening of more severe cases may assist in selecting patients for further testing.

Most data is available regarding patients with burns who become septic during hospitalization. Winter et al[99] studied 14 adult patients with burn sizes ranging from 10% to 67% TBSA who met the 1992 guidelines for septic shock and were dependent on norepinephrine because of hypotension or high-output circulatory failure. High levels of sustained inotropic support cause impaired microcirculation of burned skin areas[100] and are therefore detrimental to wound healing and regional organ perfusion. All patients were given an intravenous bolus of 100 mg of hydrocortisone 12 hours after developing norepinephrine dependency, followed by continuous infusion at a rate of 0.18 mg/kg/h. For cases in which sepsis resolved or serum sodium concentrations increased to >155 mmol/L, the infusion was tapered in steps of 24 mg/d.

Nonsurvivors required a significant increase in norepinephrine dosage during the initial phase of treatment following steroid administration, whereas it was possible to significantly reduce norepinephrine dosage in survivors. In survivors, the fluid balance was also significantly lower after hydrocortisone administration. Because only 4 patients survived, the authors concluded that steroid administration could not be countenanced in patients with burns and sepsis.

While identical inclusion criteria were utilized by Fuchs et al in their study,[97] different results were observed. In the control group of 9 patients (8 adults and one 15-year-old female) with burn sizes ranging from 20% to 95% who did not receive hydrocortisone, 7 died, compared to only 3 of 10 patients given 200 mg of hydrocortisone daily 24 hours after developing catecholamine dependency. These results, however, need to be cautiously interpreted, since the mean ABSI scores and percent TBSA burned were lower in the steroid group compared to the control group (8.8 vs 9.8 and 40.8 vs 48.8, respectively). However, the contrast in outcomes between the 2 studies requires some comment.

The mean TBSA burned in the study of Winter et al was 38%, which is comparable to the study of Fuchs et al, and ABSI scores were similar (8.3 vs 8.8). If we assume that patients in the study of Winter et al had an average body weight of 75 kg, then the daily hydrocortisone dosage would have been approximately 325 mg versus 200 mg in the study of Fuchs et al. However, it is unclear what this pharmacological difference might represent in terms of physiological

outcome since there are no cortisol data. As we have learned from the general sepsis/shock literature, conflicting results in small studies are not uncommon, so at this point it cannot be determined whether GC administration is beneficial. The report of increased inotropic support in the nonresponders in the study of Winter et al[99] is worrisome, suggesting initiation of steroid therapy was detrimental. The normal response to hydrocortisone administration in septic patients (whether adrenal function is impaired or not) is a *reduced* inotropic requirement, although dose-response curves to norepinephrine suggest that the response is nonlinear and a threshold exists before a response is observed.[101] Therefore, this abnormal response cannot easily be explained. On the other hand, excessively high levels of cortisol are not uncommon in severe burn cases, and sepsis further increases the levels. Another study showed that exogenously added hydrocortisone (240 mg/d) increased free and total cortisol levels in patients with septic shock by 8.5-fold and 4.2-fold, respectively,[102] so it is possible that treatment with hydrocortisone in burn patients with endogenously high cortisol levels will not be beneficial and could even prove deleterious. Indeed, results of a recent study investigating monocyte deactivation in patients with septic shock suggest that this very mechanism could be operative.

Le Tulzo et al[103] investigated the reduced expression of human leukocyte antigen-DR (HLA-DR) as a marker of monocyte deactivation in 23 patients with septic shock and 25 patients with sepsis. Early loss of HLA-DR expression was confirmed in all infected patients, and persistent repression was highly correlated with severity scores, secondary infection, and mortality. Furthermore, these findings were also significantly related to circulating cortisol levels, but not to IL-10 or catecholamines. Finally, in a double-blind randomized crossover trial, Keh et al[104] reported that low-dose hydrocortisone had a small impact on HLA-DR (and other factors) in terms of further suppressing already low levels in septic/shock patients.

What can be done to counter the excessive hypercortisolemia, which may be a factor in risk of mortality in sepsis? Ferrando and Wolfe[105] experimented with ketoconazole, a common antifungal agent that blocks P450-dependent enzyme systems, including the synthesis of 11-deoxycortisol from 17-α-hydroxy-progesterone, the penultimate step of cortisol biosynthesis. A small pilot RCT in which patients were randomized to receive a placebo or 200 mg of ketoconazole prior to elective hip arthroplasty revealed urinary cortisol excretion was normalized with ketoconazole treatment.[105] Furthermore, use of ketoconazole in critically ill patients led to a reduction in acute respiratory failure and shorter length of ICU days.[106] Utilizing this data, Ferrando and Wolfe turned their attention to adult burn patients. Three patients with > 40% TBSA burns were given 200 mg ketoconazole twice daily for 1 week within 2 weeks of sustaining burn injuries. Elevated urinary excretion of cortisol, which was 6-fold to 8-fold above normal, was reduced substantially. Interestingly, protein turnover was also reduced, thus improving muscle balance. Although the numbers in these case studies are small, the results indicate that this treatment might be applicable to septic burn patients as a means of countering the detrimental effects of excess cortisol. In this regard, the findings that early hypercortisolemia in children with severe burns (>40% TBSA) is significantly associated with increased duration of severe infection are important and relevant.[107] Furthermore, persistent hypercortisolemia was associated with increases in both infection rates and duration of severe infection.

The results of these studies have led us to suggest the following protocol when addressing sepsis in burns:

1. Sepsis should be diagnosed according to the 2008 guidelines.[64]
2. Patients requiring increasing inotropic support to maintain sufficient hemodynamics should undergo evaluation of the HPA.
3. Provided that relative adrenal insufficiency is present or cortisol levels are not excessively high, hydrocortisone supplementation can be initiated.
4. If a reduction in inotropic support is not observed within 2 to 5 hours, or if a contrary response is observed (ie, increased catecholamine requirement), steroid therapy should be discontinued.
5. In cases of elevated cortisol levels or a negative response to hydrocortisone, treatment with ketoconazole can be considered (liver function tests should be measured prior to starting treatment and at frequent intervals during treatment to monitor signs of hepatotoxicity; for children, a dosage of 7-10 mg/kg/d divided into at least 2 doses is suggested[108]).

## Acute Adrenal Insufficiency— A Life-Threatening Emergency

Although rare, acute adrenal insufficiency can develop at any time following a severe burn injury. Because its time course is rapid, it will prove fatal unless quickly detected and appropriately treated. Case reports from the literature[90,98,109,110] indicate profound hypotension is common, although sudden tachypnea or dyspnea, oxygen desaturation, delirium, hyponatremia, and hyperkalemia are also frequently encountered. Thus, sudden onset of unexplained hypotension should alert the clinician to the possibility of acute adrenal insufficiency.

A corticotropin test should be immediately performed. A CT scan of the adrenals may be helpful but not necessarily conclusive. In emergent or life-threatening situations, treatment can be initiated with dexamethasone, which does not interfere with cortisol measurements, although electrolytes will need to be followed until hydrocortisone can be administered.[111,112] For children, treatment with cortisol replacement therapy is as described in the preceding section, with inotropic support as needed until the patient's condition stabilizes. Unfortunately, stress imposed by the burn injury can result in cases of permanent loss of the adrenal glands. In this instance, the patient will require lifelong treatment, similar to those with Addison's disease. Destruction of the adrenal glands can result from many factors, but bilateral adrenal hemorrhage, coagulopathy, and ischemia leading to necrosis are common etiologies.[90]

## Bacterial Translocation

Several murine experiments have shown that thermal injury promotes the translocation of viable enteric bacteria from the gut to mesenteric lymph nodes, although in minor burns this process ends within a few days.[113-115] In more severe burns complicated by sepsis, bacterial translocation is more prolonged and widespread, with bacteria spreading to the spleen, liver, and even the circulatory system.[114] Originally it was thought that the burn injury induced an ischemic response in the gut that was responsible for this phenomenon. However, the intestinal atrophy observed in many experiments led researchers to suggest other mechanisms (eg, migration of lymphocytes to injured areas from the gut), which were most likely activated by high, persistent levels of cortisone (the active hormone in rats) observed during burn sepsis models.[115] More recent research has focused on cytokines. For example, administration of IL-1α, a proinflammatory cytokine, ameliorated the reduced mesenteric blood flow following burn and LPS (lipopolysaccharide; also synonymous with bacterial endotoxins) injury in pigs, as well as improving mesenteric oxygen supply and consumption.[116] Furthermore, it also reduced the increase in gut permeability and rates of bacterial translocation following injury. Animal experiments by Jeschke et al[117] and other investigators, however, have centered on the concept of increased small bowel mucosal apoptosis and reduced cell proliferation due to increased cytokine signaling. Thus, administration of IGF-1 bound to its principal binding complex (IGF-1/IGFBP-3) successfully reduced injury-induced apoptosis and increased cell proliferation. Although this recombinant complex has been tested in humans with regard to protein management following burn injury,[118] clinical trials regarding its use in septic burn patients at risk for bacterial translocation have yet to be performed.

## PROTEIN BALANCE AND ANABOLIC STEROIDS

### Adrenal Pathway Switches

Thus far, we have concentrated on the many effects of the adrenal cortex in regard to burn injury and cortisol but have not addressed protein balance and the attenuation of androgens synthesized in the cortex.

It had been observed for many years that while cortisol production was elevated following burn injury, serum levels of dehydroepiandrosterone (DHEA), androstenedione, and testosterone began to fall dramatically within a few days. Additionally, they remained at low levels for many weeks or months, in some instances at levels one-third of normal, depending upon the severity of the burn.[21,22,119] Because urinary 17-ketosteroid excretion was normal or below normal, this led many investigators to propose that a switch occurred following burn injury from adrenal androgen production to glucocorticoid synthesis.

Early animal research suggested the depression of androgen synthesis was detrimental to immune function because DHEA, probably acting through an intracellular receptor, helps boost Il-2 and IFN-γ levels.[120-122] Studies by Araneo and Daynes also revealed that restoration of DHEA levels through exogenous administration, at least in animal models, helped preserve immune function.[122] It is thought that DHEA most likely functions as an antiglucocorticoid through a variety of mechanisms, unlike the classic antiglucocorticoid blockade action of RU486.[122,123] This point should be borne in mind as we discuss protein metabolism.

### Protein Catabolism and Anabolism

By the mid-1990s it had become clear that resting energy expenditure (REE) in burn patients was greatly increased due to changes in protein metabolism induced by the burn injury and in part mediated by the increase in circulating cortisol levels and catecholamines. Moreover, these REE changes were shown to vary by age. According to Jeschke et al,[9] REE is highest in the 10-to-18-year-old group, followed by the 4-to-9.9-year-old group, and lowest in the 0-to-3.9-year-old group. Whereas children younger than 4 years tend to maintain lean body mass and weight, losses in both these parameters are significant in older age groups over a period of months. Profound muscle wasting, decreased bone mineral density, and retarded linear growth in children are also some of the additional consequences that clinicians have sought to counteract for many years.

Considerable research effort has been carried out to understand the biochemical mechanisms in play following burn injury.[105] In brief, under normal circumstances, "old" protein is continually broken down in skeletal muscle and new protein synthesized. These catabolic and anabolic functions are severely disturbed in burn patients, with the former process greatly increased and the latter retarded. In burned rats, lysosomal and energy-dependent components of total calcium-dependent protein breakdown were doubled in muscles and energy-dependent myofibrillar protein breakdown increased almost 7-fold.[124] Further experimentation revealed that the ubiquitin pathway was important (the protein ubiquitin is tagged to any protein marked for degradation by the cell). Later research probed the proteolytic rates and mRNA expression of ubiquitin, determining that muscle wasting after burn injury was mainly due to accelerated breakdown of myofibrils.[125] Another study also determined how proteolysis affected muscles differently, with white fast-twitch muscle being more sensitive to the effects of burn injury than red slow-twitch muscle.[126] Additionally, it was demonstrated that while cortisol levels drove muscle proteolysis, they had no effect on protein synthesis.[126]

Myostatin is a member of the transforming growth factor superfamily and is considered to be a major player in the regulation of protein catabolism in muscle. An investigation into the aspects that influence this growth factor first determined that thermal injury, but not endotoxin or sepsis, increased expression of myostatin, and secondly, that this increase was mediated by the enhanced secretion of endogenous cortisol, but not TNF.[127]

These results, therefore, suggest 2 approaches to the issue of protein metabolism, by finding agents that can counteract the effects of cortisol to minimize protein catabolism, and by searching for ways to enhance protein anabolism.

### Approaches to Prevent Muscle Wasting

Studies in the last 15 years have evaluated many types of approaches. Gore et al[128] explored the effect of metformin, a popular drug used in the treatment of type II diabetes, as well as insulin to reduce the hyperglycemia associated with burn injury. They discovered a significant anabolic effect on muscle protein with metformin and a modest response with insulin. In addition, a synergistic effect was noted when using both to improve muscle protein kinetics. Similar findings also demonstrated an association between hyperglycemia and an increased rate of muscle protein catabolism in severely burned patients, which indicates a possible link between peripheral resistance to insulin in muscle with regard to glucose clearance and muscle protein catabolism.[129] These and other studies provide the foundation for attaining euglycemia in burned children primarily through insulin management. The use of metformin to accomplish this task is not widespread in burn units, since lactic acidosis associated with its use in burn cases has been reported.[130]

Since growth hormone can be adversely affected following burn injury, and because of its anabolic properties, there have been several trials of recombinant human growth hormone to study its effect on protein metabolism and wound healing following thermal injury in children and adults.[105,131,132] In general, the results have been positive in both instances, with increased requirements for insulin needed to manage hyperglycemic episodes. However, such positive experiences have not always been observed in adults.[133]

Testosterone has also been administered in burn patients on the basis that it can increase protein synthesis.[134] However, clinical trials in adults showed that protein synthesis was unchanged although protein synthetic efficiency doubled. Protein degradation was also halved, resulting in an improvement in net amino acid balance that reached approximately zero.[135] In the experience of Ferrando and Wolfe, testosterone administration results in a decrease in protein catabolism in adult burn cases, whereas in children the hormone stimulates protein synthesis.[105] Nevertheless, the use of testosterone is not without risk, principally virilism and hepatotoxicity, and its use has largely been supplanted by oxandrolone.

We have already noted the use of IGF-1/IGFBP-3 in burn patients, and as the effects of growth hormone and perhaps testosterone are mediated through IGF-1, use of this factor has been explored in protein metabolism. Dose studies in both adults and children showed that at rates of 1 to 4 mg/kg daily, IGF-1/IGFBP-3 were effective in improving protein balance, especially in children, due to an increase in muscle protein synthesis.[27] However, its expense and relative effectiveness versus testosterone or insulin likely precludes widespread usage.[105]

Another approach utilizes propanolol, a common beta-blocker. This drug has been used to decrease REE following burn injury, as catecholamines are a primary mediator of hypermetabolism.[136,137] In an RCT involving 25 children with burns <40% TBSA, Herndon et al explored the effect of the drug on muscle protein catabolism and found that net muscle protein balance increased 82% compared to baseline values, whereas it decreased in the control group by 27%.[138] Furthermore, to address concerns in the literature of an adverse effect of propanolol on inflammation and immune function, Jeschke et al[139] demonstrated no significant difference in the rates of infection or sepsis in a large RCT of 245 patients (there was a nonsignificant trend toward higher rates in the control group). Moreover, the experimental group (propanolol) had significantly lower serum levels of TNF and IL-1β. The same group also recently tested the combination of a beta-blocker with recombinant growth hormone (rhGH) in 15 pediatric patients with burn sizes > 40% TBSA who were matched in age, gender, and burn size to a control group.[140] Percent predicted REE was significantly lower in the treatment group compared to the control group, as were levels of serum CRP, cortisone, IL-6, IL-8, MIP-1β, and key amino acid transferases. Thus, hypermetabolism was decreased in the treatment group without the adverse side effects of rhGH therapy alone.

## Oxandrolone

Oxandrolone is a synthetic anabolic steroid used for many decades in a variety of muscle-wasting diseases. Although discontinued in 1989 due to abuse by bodybuilders, it was subsequently rereleased in 1995 by a different pharmaceutical company. Small comparative clinical trials in the late 1990s, one of which was a small RCT, showed promise in severely burned patients by reducing the weight loss associated with burn-induced protein catabolism.[141,142] Relatively low doses (10-20 mg/d) were given to avoid complications, such as interference with testosterone production or hepatotoxicity. A small prospective cohort investigation (N = 14) of critically ill, severely burned children who had suffered long delays in transfer to a burn unit showed that those given oxandrolone (0.1 mg/kg twice daily) versus no steroid for 1 week demonstrated increased protein synthesis using stable isotope methods.[143] Essentially, the steroid increased efficiency of amino acid reuse from the intracellular pool while inward transport of amino acids was unaffected, thus leading to a zero net balance of muscle protein metabolism. An investigation of the gene expression induced by oxandrolone in similarly treated children revealed a dramatic downregulation in the *Adapt 78* gene, which is regarded as an "adaptive response" stress gene whose protein product is a potent inhibitor of calcineurin.[144] Stimulation of gene expression for 2 myosin subtypes as well as other structural proteins was also found. Besides profound differences between genders, further microarray analysis showed that the expression of many genes associated with inflammatory processes was suppressed, indicating that oxandrolone could be beneficial in reducing the burn-induced hyperinflammatory response.[145] Other experiments have also demonstrated that oxandrolone exerts an anticorticosteroid action. However, this action is not mediated through competitive antagonism of the glucocorticoid receptor itself, but rather, the steroid appears to be involved in a form of crosstalk between both androgen and glucocorticoid receptors that involve multiple pathways.[146]

Exercise programs instituted during the recovery phase of severely burned children have demonstrated benefit, and a 3-group RCT conducted by Przkora et al[147] revealed that the combination of oxandrolone and exercise was superior to either alone in improving lean body mass. Improved muscle strength and peak cardiopulmonary capacity were also noted in the combination group as well as in the oxandrolone and exercise groups, with the latter group the most effective. One of the largest RCTs conducted to date of severely burned children (n = 190 for the control group vs 45 for the oxandrolone group) has confirmed the benefits of the anabolic steroid, with preservation of lean body mass and increases in serum prealbumin, total protein, and testosterone, as well as concurrent decreases in acute phase proteins.[148] Although the authors reported that oxandrolone did not significantly affect serum cytokines, there were changes in several cytokines that appeared to vary in a complex manner over a period of weeks that might have been significantly different at specific time points. No hepatotoxicity occurred, although both serum alanine transferase and aspartate transferase levels remained elevated in the oxandrolone group some 4 to 5 weeks postburn. This seems to corroborate previous results that, provided low doses are used, no undue stress is placed upon the liver. It should also be noted that use of oxandrolone has been significantly related to shorter hospital stays.[149]

In summary, the use of oxandrolone is likely to find an increasingly beneficial place in the armamentarium of pediatric burn units treating patients with severe burns.

## SPECIAL TOPICS

### Bone Loss and Glucocorticoids

The adverse effect of high cortisol levels on bone following burn injury has long been noted but little studied. A key study reported by Klein et al[150] established a number of cortisol-related changes that occur in children with burns greater than 40% TBSA. The most important were a major reduction in osteoblasts on the bone surface and decreased biochemical markers of osteoblast differentiation, notably alkaline phosphatase, cbfa1/OSF2 (core-binding factor/ osteoblast stimulating factor), BMP-2 (bone morphogenetic protein), and type I collagen. While GRα mRNA expression was not significantly decreased in the burn group compared to the control group (it decreased approximately 40%), the authors hypothesized that the inflammatory marrow cells proliferated as part of the postburn inflammatory response. In essence, low bone turnover was observed.

Obviously, prolonged suppression of bone growth can have deleterious consequences on the rehabilitation of children if not addressed. Therefore, it seemed logical to determine if oxandrolone treatment could improve the outcome. Several studies in the last few years, most notably the RCT of

Murphy et al,[151] have suggested that bone mineral content and density can be increased using low-dose oxandrolone over a period of several months, either separately or in combination with GH. In a series of osteoblast culture experiments, Bi et al[152] determined that the increase in total body bone mineral was most likely due to the steroid acting directly upon bone. The evidence for this thesis came from the detection of increased nuclear fluorescence of androgen receptors in the nucleus and increased levels of osteomarkers. However, while oxandrolone may have the ability to directly stimulate bone collagen synthesis in addition to its effect on skeletal loading, the mechanisms involved in long-term treatment may not be anabolic in nature in mature bone cells.

### Use of Steroids in Corrosive Burns

Corrosive burns resulting from acid or alkali exposure continue to be a significant source of morbidity, and sometimes mortality. Ingestion remains the most life-threatening type of exposure, and although a variety of treatments are possible depending on the nature of the injury to esophageal and gastrointestinal tissue, steroid application became a common feature in the 1960s to prevent esophageal stricture—collagen production with scar formation.[153] The theory, based on animal experiments, was that steroids would suppress inflammatory and fibroplastic processes and thus prevent stricture formation. Thirty years of research, however, has since demonstrated that steroids are not warranted in grade I burns since patients rarely develop strictures, whereas in grade III burns, strictures develop regardless of therapy.[154] Although several prior analyses produced conflicting results with regard to grade II burns, Fulton and Hoffman[155] concluded that many of the studies included in these analyses did not differentiate the grade of burn sufficiently to infer meaningful outcomes. In their own retrospective analysis, which they admit had some significant limitations, the authors argued that the small benefit obtained with steroids was not clinically or statistically significant. Furthermore, many studies have failed to include the risks inherent with steroid therapy in this context, for example, brain abscess, hemorrhage, pneumonia, severe esophogastric necrosis, osteoporosis, and prepyloric ulcer formation. Consequently, it is recommended that steroids should not be used in the management of corrosive burns.

### Steroid Use in Smoke Inhalation Injuries

Inhalation injury, a significant factor in the mortality of burn patients, has also witnessed the use of steroid therapy in the hope of reversing the extremely poor prognosis. Early studies were inconclusive in terms of affecting outcome, but later evidence began to accrue that steroids were not helpful. Nieman et al[156] studied the use of methylprednisolone given to dogs 2 hours prior to the imposition of smoke inhalation injury and investigated a variety of parameters, including pulmonary compliance, venous admixture blood gases, pH, lung water content, and surface tension of lung tissue. Except for venous admixture, which improved faster in animals treated with steroid versus no steroid and was statistically significant, administration of methylprednisolone did not affect any physiological responses. Most recently, a South Korean study of patients injured in a subway fire provided an opportunity for observational study of inhalation injuries and steroid therapy.[157] Several parameters were evaluated initially and at 3 months in patients who underwent tracheal intubation, including FVC (forced vital capacity), $FEV_1$ (forced expiratory volume in 1 second), $FEV_1/FVC$, and FEF (forced expiratory flow) at 25% to 75% of expiration flow. There were no statistical differences between the steroid-treated group (N = 22) and the nonsteroid-treated group (N = 19).

Accordingly, the sum total of the evidence over the last 20 years, including the 2 studies briefly described here, suggests no role for steroid therapy in the management of inhalation injury with or without thermal burns.

## Prevention of Reintubation by Using Steroids

Burn patients have a high rate of endotracheal intubation because of airway edema, and, once extubated, a significant risk of stridor development exists with a need for reintubation. Although some burn units have developed protocols to administer steroids to prevent stridor and/or the need for reintubation following extubation, there is no study of burn patients to support this protocol. However, a meta-analysis of 6 RCTs that investigated this type of protocol in patients with other critical illnesses (3 studies in neonates and 3 in children) was recently published.[158] One trial examined the use of steroids to treat existing postextubation stridor in children, while the others investigated steroids to prevent reintubation. There was a nonsignificant trend toward a decreased rate of reintubation in all children when prophylactic steroids were used. Furthermore, use of prophylactic steroids reduced postextubation stridor in the pooled studies (n = 325, RR = 0.50, 95% CI = 0.28-0.88). In young children, there were significant reductions of postextubation stridor with preventive treatment (n = 216, RR = 0.53, 95% CI = 0.28-0.97), and a trend toward less stridor in neonates. There was also a nonsignificant trend toward a reduced reintubation rate when steroids were used to treat existing upper airway obstruction requiring reintubation. Overall, these results are sufficiently encouraging that a multicenter prospective RCT to investigate a dexamethasone

protocol in children is currently being conducted by Greenhalgh et al at the Shriners Hospital for Children in Northern California.

## CONCLUSION

Profound disturbances to the HPA axis occur in burned children, especially older children. The most obvious change is higher levels of cortisol, which is correlated with the percent TBSA burned. Most of the changes to the HPA axis result from the burn-induced rise in proinflammatory cytokines as well as the shift in the $T_H1/T_H2$ response. While results from the general sepsis/shock literature indicate that there is no benefit to administering exogenous steroids, there is some evidence that burned patients exhibit a slightly different cytokine response compared to patients with general shock/sepsis. There is also some evidence that a patient with severe burn injury may benefit from steroid use when he or she requires ever-increasing inotropic support. While acute, life-threatening adrenal insufficiency is rare, it must be treated immediately with steroid administration. There are no conclusive guidelines in regard to the diagnosis of relative adrenal insufficiency or its treatment. It is suggested that in conjunction with random cortisol measurements and corticotropin stimulation tests, patients be also evaluated using illness severity algorithms such as APSI or APACHE. If steroid treatment is agreed upon as a course of action, low doses of hydrocortisone should be used, with tapering at the end of treatment. Furthermore, if steroid treatment does not yield hemodynamic benefits within 2 to 5 hours, it should be discontinued. When cortisol levels are excessively high, the use of ketoconazole should be considered. To counter the problem of protein catabolism in patients with more severe burns, long-term administration of oxandrolone is recommended, especially in conjunction with exercise programs. Steroids offer no benefit in cases of esophageal injury due to corrosive materials or in cases of pure smoke inhalation injury. However, they may be of benefit in preventing development of stridor or the need for reintubation following extubation.

## KEY POINTS

- Levels of CRH, corticotropin, and cortisol all dramatically increase after a burn injury. However, these levels do not frequently correlate, suggesting that dysfunction at the hypothalamic level is common.
- Total serum cortisol levels can be extremely high following severe burn injury, although levels in younger children may be slightly lower.

- Cortisol production is under the influence of many different types of cytokines, both within the adrenal cortex and at higher levels.
- The $T_H1$ response is greatly diminished as a result of the increase in cortisol levels, while the $T_H2$ response is enhanced.
- Cortisol-binding globulin (and albumin) levels drop substantially after burn injury.
- The cortisol-cortisone (F:E) ratio does not appear to change much in burn patients, which suggests a difference compared to patients with other types of shock/trauma.
- Little is known about the role of GC resistance in burn injuries, but it is likely to be a factor in severe burns.
- There are no truly reliable inflammatory markers currently available, but this is likely to change within the next few years as cytokine measurement becomes more widely available.
- The general sepsis/shock literature suggests that steroid treatment has no benefit.
- In burn injuries there may be sufficient differences (compared to general shock/sepsis) that there is some benefit to using steroids, particularly in cases where the patient requires ever-increasing inotropic support.
- Acute adrenal insufficiency *must* be treated with steroids as soon as it is diagnosed; diagnosis of "relative" adrenal insufficiency is a more problematic situation. At the very least, cortisol measurements should be undertaken and a corticotropin stimulation test performed. Clinicians should be aware that applying "standard" diagnostic criteria of relative adrenal insufficiency in burn injuries can be misleading; such criteria should be used in conjunction with illness severity algorithms such as APSI or APACHE.
- Burn specialists should be extremely cautious in the use of steroids, especially with septic patients. If corticosteroid administration is decided upon, low doses of hydrocortisone should be used, with tapering at the end of the course. If hemodynamic improvements are not apparent with 2 to 5 hours, GC administration should be discontinued.
- In cases of excessive cortisol levels, the use of ketoconazole may be beneficial.
- To manage the burn-induced protein metabolism imbalance, long-term administration of oxandrolone is recommended in severe burns, especially in combination with exercise programs. Beta-blockers may also be a good alternative.
- Steroids offer no evidence of benefit in cases of esophageal injury due to corrosive agents, nor are they of benefit in cases of smoke inhalation injury.
- Steroids may help prevent stridor or reintubation following extubation.

# REFERENCES

1. Stewart PM, Toogood AA, Tomlinson JW. Growth hormone, insulin-like growth factor-1 and the cortisol-cortisone shuttle. *Horm Res.* 2001; **56**(suppl 1): 1–6.

2. Buske-Kirschbaum A, Krieger S, Wilkes C, Rauh W, Weiss S, Hellhammer DH. Hypothalamic-pituitary-adrenal axis function and the cellular immune response in former preterm children. *J Endocrine Metab.* 2007; **92**: 3429–3435.

3. Matthews SG. Early programming of the hypothalamus-pituitary-adrenal axis. *Trends Endocrinol Metab.* 2002; **13**: 373–380.

4. Sandstrom NJ, Hart SR. Isolation stress during the third postnatal week alters radial arm maze performance and corticosterone levels in adulthood. *Behav Brain Res.* 2005; **30**: 289–296.

5. Levine S, Mody T. The long-term psychobiological consequences of intermittent postnatal separation in the squirrel monkey. *Neurosci Biobehav Rev.* 2003; **27**: 83–89.

6. Knutsson U, Dahlgren J, Marcus C, et al. Circadian cortisol rhythms in healthy boys and girls: relationship with age, growth, body composition, and pubertal development. *J Clin Endocrinol Metab.* 1997; **82**: 536–540.

7. Lewis M, Ramsay DS. Developmental change in infants' responses to stress. In: Lewis M, ed. *Child Development.* Ann Arbor, MI: Society for Research in Child Development; **1995**: 657–670.

8. Oster H, Damerow S, Kiessling S, et al. The circadian rhythm of glucocorticoids is regulated by a gating mechanism residing in the adrenal cortical clock. *Cell Metab.* 2006; **4**: 163–173.

9. Jeschke MG, Norbury WB, Finnerty CC, et al. Age differences in inflammatory and hypermetabolic postburn responses. *Pediatrics.* 2008; **121**: 497–507.

10. Jeschke MG, Mlcak RP, Finnerty CC, et al. Burn size determines the inflammatory and hypermetabolic response. *Crit Care.* 2007; **11**:R90.

11. Crum R, Bobrow B, Shackford S, Hansbrough J, Brown MR. The neurohumoral response to burn injury in patients resuscitated with hypertonic saline. *J Trauma.* 1988; **28**: 1181–1187.

12. Murton SA, Tan ST, Prickett TCR, Frampton C, Donald RA. Hormone responses to stress in patients with major burns. *Br J Plast Surg.* 1998; **51**: 388–392.

13. Palmieri TL, Levine S, Schonfeld-Warden N, O'Mara MS, Greenhalgh DG. Hypothalamic-pituitary-adrenal axis response to sustained stress after major burn injury in children. *J Burn Care Res.* 2006; **27**: 742–748.

14. Smith A, Barclay C, Quaba A, et al. The bigger the burn, the greater the stress. *Burns.* 1997; **23**: 291–294.

15. Hader O, Bähr V, Hensen J, Hofbauer KG, Oelkers WK. Effects of a V1-vasopressin antagonist on ACTH release following vasopressin infusion or insulin-induced hypoglycemia in normal men. *Acta Endocrinol (Copenh).* 1990; **123**: 622–628.

16. Chance WT, Dayal R, Friend LA, Sheriff S. Possible role of CRF peptides in burn-induced hypermetabolism. *Life Sci.* 2006; **78**: 694–703.

17. Chance WT, Dayal R, Friend LA, Thomas I, Sheriff S. Mediation of burn-induced hypermetabolism by CRF receptor-2 activity. *Life Sci.* 2007; **80**: 1064–1072.

18. Hagan PM, Poole S, Bristow AF. Corticotrophin-releasing factor as mediator of the acute-phase response in rats, mice and rabbits. *J Endocrinol.* 1993; **136**: 207–216.

19. Molteni A, Warpeha RL, Brizio-Molteni L, Albertson DF, Kaurs R. Circadian rhythms of serum aldosterone, cortisol and plasma renin activity in burn injuries. *Ann Clin Lab Sci.* 1979; **9**: 518–523.

20. Vaughan GM, Becker RA, Allen JP, Goodwin CW Jr, Pruitt BA Jr, Mason AD Jr. Cortisol and corticotrophin in burned patients. *J Trauma.* 1982; **22**: 263–273.

21. Lephart ED, Baxter CR, Parker CR Jr. Effect of burn trauma on adrenal and testicular steroid hormone production. *J Clin Endocrinol Metab.* 1987; **64**: 842–848.

22. Semple CG, Gray CE, Beastall GH. Adrenal androgens and illness. *Acta Endocrinol (Copenh).* 1987; **116**: 155–160.

23. Woods DR, Arun CS, Corris PA, Perros P. Cushing's syndrome without excess cortisol. *BMJ.* 2006; **332**: 469–470.

24. Sedowofia K, Barclay C, Quaba A, et al. The systemic stress response to thermal injury in children. *Clin Endocrinol (Oxf).* 1998; **49**: 335–341.

25. Hobson KG, Havel PJ, McMurtry AL, Lawless MB, Palmieri TL, Greenhalgh DD. Circulating leptin and cortisol after burn injury: loss of diurnal pattern. *J Burn Care Rehabil.* 2004; **25**: 491–499.

26. Jeffries MK, Vance ML. Growth hormone and cortisol secretion in patients with burn injury. *J Burn Care Rehabil.* 1992; **13**: 391–395.

27. Herndon DN, Ramzy PI, DebRoy MA, et al. Muscle protein catabolism after severe burn: effects of IGF-1/IGFBP-3 treatment. *Ann Surg.* 1999; **229**: 713–722.

28. Jeschke MG, Herndon DN, Vita R, Traber DL, Jauch KW, Barrow RE. IGF-1/BP-3 administration preserves hepatic homeostasis after thermal injury which is associated with increases in NO and hepatic NF-kappa B. *Shock.* 2001; **16**: 373–379.

29. Delhanty PJ. Interleukin-1 beta suppresses growth hormone-induced acid-labile subunit mRNA levels and secretion in primary hepatocytes. *Biochem Biophys Res Commun.* 1998; **243**: 269–272.

30. Yeager MP, Guyre PM, Munck AU. Glucocorticoid regulation of the inflammatory response to injury. *Acta Anaesthesiol Scand.* 2004; **48**: 799–813.

31. Ozbalkan Z, Aslar AK, Yildiz Y, Aksarav S. Investigation of the course of pro-inflammatory and anti-inflammatory cytokines after burn sepsis. *Int J Clin Pract.* 2004; **58**: 125–129.

32. Dugan AL, Malarkey WB, Schwemberger S, Jauch EC, Ogle CK, Horseman ND. Serum levels of prolactin, growth hormone,

and cortisol in burn patients: correlations with severity of burn, serum cytokine levels, and fatality. *J Burn Care Rehabil.* 2004; **25**: 306–313.

**33.** Akita S, Akino K, Ren SG, Melmed S, Imaizumi T, Hirano A. Elevated circulating leukemia inhibitory factor in patients with extensive burns. *J Burn Care Res.* 2006; **27**: 221–225.

**34.** Finnerty CC, Herndon DN, Przkora R, et al. Cytokine expression profile over time in severely burned pediatric patients. *Shock.* 2006; **26**: 13–19.

**35.** Finnerty CC, Herndon DN, Chinkes DL, Jeschke MG. Serum cytokine differences in severely burned children with and without sepsis. *Shock.* 2007; **27**: 4–9.

**36.** Miller AC, Rashid RM, Elamin EM. The "T" in trauma: the helper T-cell response and the role of immunomodulation in trauma and burn patients. *J Trauma.* 2007; **63**: 1407–1417.

**37.** Taniguchi T, Koido Y, Aiboshi J, Yamashita T, Suzaki S, Kurokawa A. Change in the ratio of interleukin-6 to interleukin-10 predicts a poor outcome in patients with systemic inflammatory response syndrome. *Crit Care Med.* 1999; **27**: 1262–1264.

**38.** Utsunomiya T, Kobayashi M, Herndon DN, Pollard RB, Suzuki F. A mechanism of interleukin-12 unresponsiveness associated with thermal injury. *J Surg Res.* 2001; **96**: 211–217.

**39.** Schwacha MG, Holland LT, Chaudry IH, Messina JL. Genetic variability in the immune-inflammatory response after major burn injury. *Shock.* 2005; **23**: 123–128.

**40.** Uehara A, Gottchall PE, Dahl RR, Arimura A. Interleukin-1 stimulates ACTH release by an indirect action which requires endogenous corticotropin releasing factor. *Endocrinology.* 1987; **121**: 1580–1582.

**41.** Bernardini R, Kamilaris TC, Caolgeri AE, et al. Interactions between tumor necrosis factor-alpha, hypothalamic corticotropin-releasing hormone, and adrenocorticotropin secretion in the rat. *Endocrinology.* 1990; **126**: 2876–2881.

**42.** Bornstein SR, Gonzalez-Hernandez JA, Ehrhart-Bornstein M, Adler G, Scherbaum WA. Intimate contact of chromaffin and cortical cells within the human adrenal gland forms the cellular basis for important intraadrenal interactions. *J Clin Endocrinol Metab.* 1994; **78**: 225–232.

**43.** González-Hernández JA, Bornstein SR, Ehrhart-Bornstein M, et al. IL-1 is expressed in human adrenal gland in vivo. Possible role in a local immune-adrenal axis. *Clin Exp Immunol.* 1995; **99**: 137–141.

**44.** Nussdorfer GG, Mazzocchi G. Immune-endocrine interactions in the mammalian adrenal gland: facts and hypotheses. *Int Rev Cytol.* 1998; **183**: 143–184.

**45.** Barney M, Call GB, McIlmoil CJ, et al. Stimulation by interleukin-6 and inhibition by tumor necrosis factor of cortisol release from bovine adrenal zona fasciculata cells through their receptors. *Endocrine.* 2000; **13**: 369–377.

**46.** Bamberger AM, Schulte HM, Wullbrand A, Jung R, Beil FU, Bamberger CM. Expression of leukemia inhibitory factor (LIF) and LIF receptor (LIF-R) in the human adrenal cortex: implications for steroidogenesis. *Mol Cell Endocrinol.* 2000; **162**: 145–149.

**47.** Päth G, Scherbaum WA, Bornstein SR. The role of interleukin-6 in the human adrenal gland. *Eur J Clin Invest.* 2000; **30**(suppl 3):91–95.

**48.** Rosner W. Plasma steroid-binding proteins. *Endocrinol Metab Clin North Am.* 1991; **20**: 697–721.

**49.** D'Elia M, Patenaude J, Hamelin C, Garrel DR, Bernier J. Corticosterone binding globulin regulation and thymus changes after thermal injury in mice. *Am J Physiol Endocrinol Metab.* 2005; **288**:E852-E860.

**50.** Garrel DR. Corticosteroid-binding globulin during inflammation and burn injury: nutritional modulation and clinical implications. *Horm Res.* 1996; **45**: 245–251.

**51.** Hirota T, Hirota K, Sanno Y, Tanaka T. Glucocorticoid binding proteins under various stressful conditions: relation to endogenous glucocorticoid secretion. *J Biochem.* 1985; **97**: 1371–1376.

**52.** Pemberton PA, Stein PE, Pepys MB, Potter JM, Carrell RW. Hormone binding globulins undergo serpin conformational change in inflammation. *Nature.* 1988; **336**: 257–258.

**53.** Bartalena L, Hammond GL, Farsetti A, Flink IL, Robbins J. Interleukin-6 inhibits corticosteroid-binding globulin synthesis by human hepatoblastoma-derived (Hep G20) cells. *Endocrinology.* 1993; **133**: 291–296.

**54.** Bernier J, Jobin N, Emptoz-Bonneton A, Pugeat MM, Garrel DR. Decreased corticosteroid-binding globulin in burn patients: relationship with interleukin-6 and fat in nutritional support. *Crit Care Med.* 1998; **26**: 452–460.

**55.** Petersen HH, Andreassen TK, Breiderhoff T, et al. Hyporesponsiveness to glucocorticoids in mice genetically deficient for the corticosteroid binding globulin. *Mol Cell Biol.* 2006; **26**: 7236–7245.

**56.** Tomlinson JW, Stewart PM. Cortisol metabolism and the role of 11beta-hydroxysteroid dehydrogenase. *Best Pract Res Clin Endocrinol Metab.* 2001; **15**: 61–78.

**57.** Walker EA, Stewart PM. 11beta-hydroxysteroid dehydrogenase: unexpected connections. *Trends Endocrinol Metab.* 2003; **14**: 334–339.

**58.** Venkatesh B, Cohen J, Hickman I, et al. Evidence of altered cortisol metabolism in critically ill patients: a prospective study. *Intensive Care Med.* 2007; **33**: 1746–1753.

**59.** Cooper MS, Bujalska I, Rabbitt E, et al. Modulation of 11β-hydroxysteroid dehydrogenase isozymes by proinflammatory cytokines in osteoblasts: an autocrine switch from glucocorticoid inactivation to activation. *J Bone Miner Res.* 2001; **16**: 1037–1044.

**60.** Heiniger CD, Rochat MK, Frey FJ, Frey BM. TNF-alpha enhances intracellular glucocorticoid availability. *FEBS Lett.* 2001; **507**: 351–356.

**61.** Baxtex JD, Tyrell JB. The adrenal cortex. In: Felig P, Baxter JD, Broadus AE, et al, eds. *Endocrinology and Metabolism.* 2nd ed. New York, NY: McGraw-Hill, **1987**: 511–650.

**62.** Prigent H, Maxime V, Annane D. Science review: mechanisms of impaired adrenal function in sepsis and molecular actions of glucocorticoids. *Crit Care.* 2004; **8**: 243–252.

63. Liu DH, Su YP, Zhang W, et al. Downregulation of glucocorticoid receptors of liver cytosols and the role of the inflammatory cytokines in pathological stress in scalded rats. *Burns*. 2002; **28**: 315–320.

64. Greenhalgh DG, Saffle JR, Holmes JH, et al. American Burn Association consensus conference to define sepsis and infection in burns. *J Burn Care Res*. 2007; **28**: 776–790.

65. Marshall JC, Cook DJ, Christou NV, Bernard GR, Sprung CL, Sibald WJ. Multiple organ dysfunction score: a reliable descriptor of a complex clinical outcome. *Crit Care Med*. 1995; **23**: 1638–1652.

66. Cook R, Cook D, Tilley J, Lee KA, Marshall J. Multiple organ dysfunction: baseline and serial component scores. *Cit Care Med*. 2001; **29**: 2046–2050.

67. Vindenes HA, Ulvestad E, Bjerknes R. Concentrations of cytokines in plasma of patients with large burns: their relation to time after injury, burn size, inflammatory variables, infection, and outcome. *Eur J Surg*. 1998; **164**: 647–656.

68. Pruchniewski D, Pawlowski T, Morkowski J, Mackiewicz S. C-reactive protein in management of children's burns. *Ann Clin Res*. 1987; **19**: 334–338.

69. Neely AN, Smith WL, Warden GD. Efficacy of a rise in C-reactive protein serum levels as an early indicator of sepsis in burned children. *J Burn Care Rehabil*. 1998; **19**: 102–105.

70. Barati M, Alinejad F, Bahar MA, et al. Comparison of WBC, ESR, CRP and PCT serum levels in septic and non-septic burn cases. *Burns*. 2008; **34**: 770–774.

71. Lavrentieva A, Kontakiotis T, Lazaridis L, et al. Inflammatory markers in patients with severe burn injury. What is the best indicator of sepsis? *Burns*. 2007; **33**: 189–194.

72. von Heimburg D, Stieghorst W, Khorram-Sefat R, Pallua N. Procalcitonin—a sepsis parameter in severe burn injuries. *Burns*. 1998; **24**: 745–750.

73. Sachse C, Machens HG, Felmerer G, Berger A, Henkel E. Procalcitonin as a marker for the early diagnosis of severe infection after thermal injury. *J Burn Care Rehabil*. 1999; **20**: 354–360.

74. Neely AN, Fowler LA, Kagan RJ, Warden GD. Procalcitonin in pediatric burn patients: an early indicator of sepsis? *J Burn Care Rehabil*. 2004; **25**: 76–80.

75. Bargues L, Chancerelle Y, Catineau J, Jault P, Carsin H. Evaluation of serum procalcitonin concentration in the ICU following severe burn. *Burns*. 2007; **33**: 860–864.

76. Annane D, Bellisant E, Bollaert PE, Briegel J, Keh D, Kupfer Y. Corticosteroids for severe sepsis and septic shock: a systematic review and meta-analysis. *BMJ*. 2004; **329**: 480.

77. Sprung CL, Annane D, Keh D, et al. Hydrocortisone therapy for patients with septic shock. *New Engl J Med*. 2008; **358**: 111–124.

78. Furukawa TA, Guyatt GH, Griffith LE. Can we individualize the "number needed to treat"? An empirical study of summary effect measures in meta-analyses. *Int J Epidemiol*. 2002; **31**: 72–76.

79. Annane D, Sébille V, Troché G, Raphaël JC, Gajdos P, Bellisant E. A 3-level prognostic classification in septic shock based on cortisol levels and cortisol response to corticotropin. *JAMA*. 2000; **283**: 1038–1045.

80. Streeten DHP. What test for hypothalamic-pituitary adrenocortical insufficiency? *Lancet*. 1999; **354**: 179–180.

81. Marik PE, Zaloga GP. Adrenal insufficiency in the critically ill: A new look at an old problem. *Chest*. 2002; **122**: 1784–1796.

82. Streeten DH, Anderson GH Jr, Bonaventura MM. The potential for serious consequences from misinterpreting normal responses to the rapid adrenocorticotropin test. *J Clin Endocrinol Metab*. 1996; **81**: 285–290.

83. Drucker D, Shandling M. Variable adrenocortical in acute medical illness. *Crit Care Med*. 1985; **13**: 477–479.

84. Marik PE, Kiminyo K, Zaloga GP. Adrenal insufficiency in critically ill HIV infected patients. *Crit Care Med*. 2002; **30**: 1267–1273.

85. Marik PE, Zaloga GP. Adrenal insufficiency during septic shock. *Crit Care Med*. 2003; **31**: 141–145.

86. Hamrahian AH, Oseni TS, Arafah BM. Measurement of serum-free cortisol in critically ill patients. *New Engl J Med*. 2004; **350**: 1629–1638.

87. Ho JT, Al-Musalhi H, Chapman MJ, et al. Septic shock and sepsis: a comparison of total and free plasma cortisol levels. *J Clin Endocrinol Metab*. 2006; **91**: 105–114.

88. Britt RC, Devine A, Swallen KC, et al. Corticosteroid use in the intensive care unit: At what cost? *Arch Surg*. 2006; **141**: 145–149.

89. James SE, Ghosh SJ, Mongomeries J, Philp BM, Dziewulski P. Survival of a 75% burn in a patient with longstanding Addison's disease. *Burns*. 2002; **28**: 391–393.

90. Deeb SA, Rosenberg RB, Wilkerson RJ, Griswold JA. Adrenal hemorrhage in a pediatric burn patient. *Burns*. 2001; **27**: 658–661.

91. Allen DB. Effects of inhaled steroids on growth, bone metabolism, and adrenal function. *Adv Pediatr*. 2006; **53**: 101–110.

92. Ellison JA, Patel L, Ray DW, David TJ, Clayton PE. Hypothalamic-pituitary-adrenal function and glucocorticoid sensitivity to atopic dermatitis. *Pediatrics*. 2000; **105**: 794–799.

93. Abeyagunawardena AS, Hindmarsh P, Trompeter RS. Adrenocortical suppression increases the risk of relapse in nephritic syndrome. *Arch Dis Child*. 2007; **92**: 585–588.

94. McDonough AK, Curtis JR, Saag KG. The epidemiology of glucocorticoid-associated adverse events. *Curr Opin Rheumatol*. 2008; **20**: 131–137.

95. Fuchs P, Groger A, Bozkurt A, Johnen D, Wolter T, Pallua N. Cortisol in severely burned patients: investigations on disturbance of the hypothalamic-pituitary-adrenal axis. *Shock*. 2007; **28**: 662–667.

96. Tobiasen J, Hiebert JM, Edlich RF. The abbreviated burn severity index. *Ann Emerg Med*. 1982; **11**: 260–262.

97. Fuchs P, Bozkurt A, Johnen D, Smeets R, Groger A, Pallua N. Beneficial effects of corticosteroids on catecholamine-dependent patients. *Burns*. 2007; **33**: 306–311.

98. Nácul FE, Jardim A, MacCord F, Penido C, Gomes MV. Hemodynamic instability secondary to adrenal insufficiency in a major burn patient. *Burns*. 2002; **28**: 270–272.

99. Winter W, Kamolz L, Donner A, Hoerauf K, Blaicher A, Andel H. Hydrocortisone improved haemodynamics and fluid requirement in surviving but not non-surviving of severely burned patients. *Burns*. 2003; **29**: 717–720.

100. Knabl JS, Bauer W, Andel H, et al. Progression of burn wound depth by systematic application of a vasoconstrictor: an experimental study with a new rabbit model. *Burns*. 1999; **25**: 715–721.

101. Annane D, Bellisant E, Sebille V, et al. Impaired pressor sensitivity to noradrenaline in septic shock patients with and without impaired adrenal function reserve. *Br J Clin Pharmacol*. 1998; **46**: 589–597.

102. Oppert M, Reinicke A, Gräf KJ, Barckow D, Frei U, Eckardt KU. Plasma cortisol levels before and during "low-dose" hydrocortisone therapy and their relationship to hemodynamic improvement in patients with septic shock. *Intensive Care Med*. 2000; **26**: 1747–1755.

103. Le Tulzo Y, Pangault C, Amiot L, et al. Monocyte human leukocyte antigen-DR transcriptional downregulation by cortisol during septic shock. *Am J Respir Crit Care Med*. 2004; **169**: 1144–1151.

104. Keh D, Boehnke T, Weber-Cartens S, et al. Immunologic and hemodynamic effects of "low-dose" hydrocortisone in septic shock: a double-blind, randomized, placebo-controlled, crossover study. *Am J Respir Crit Care Med*. 2003; **167**: 512–520.

105. Ferrando AA, Wolfe RR. Restoration of hormonal action and muscle protein. *Crit Care Med*. 2007; 35(suppl):S630-S634.

106. Slotman GJ, Burchard KW, D'Arezzo A, et al. Ketoconazole prevents acute respiratory failure in critically ill surgical patients. *J Trauma*. 1988; **28**: 648–654.

107. Norbury WB, Herndon DN, Branski LK, Chinkes DL, Jeschke MG. Urinary cortisol and catecholamine excretion after burn injury in children. *J Clin Endocrinol Metab*. 2008; **93**: 1270–1275.

108. Bardare M, Tortorano AM, Pietrogrande MC, Viviani MA. Pharmacokinetics of ketoconazole and treatment evaluation in candidal infections. *Arch Dis Child*. 1984; **59**: 1068–1071.

109. Sheridan RL, Ryan CM, Tompkins RG. Acute adrenal insufficiency in the burn intensive care unit. *Burns*. 1993; **19**: 63–66.

110. Murphy JF, Purdue GF, Hunt JL. Acute adrenal insufficiency in the patient with burns. *J Burn Care Rehabil*. 1993; **14**: 155–157.

111. Rose LI, Williams GH, Jagger PI, Lauler GP. The 48-hour adrenocorticotrophin infusion test for adrenocortical insufficiency. *Ann Intern Med*. 1970; **73**: 49–54.

112. Axelrod L. Glucocorticoid therapy. *Medicine*. 1976; **55**: 39–65.

113. Maejima K, Deitch EA, Berg RD. Bacterial translocation from the gastrointestinal tracts of rats receiving thermal injury. *Infect Immun*. 1984; **43**: 6–13.

114. Jones WG, Minei JP, Barber AE, et al. Bacterial translocation and intestinal atrophy following thermal injury and burn wound sepsis. *Ann Surg*. 1990; **211**: 399–405.

115. Jones WG II, Minei JP, Richardson RP, et al. Pathophysiologic glucocorticoid elevations promote bacterial translocation after thermal injury. *Infect Immun*. 1990; **58**: 3257–3261.

116. Tadros T, Traber DL, Heggers JP, Herndon DN. Effects of Interleukin-1α administration on intestinal ischemia and reperfusion injury, mucosal permeability, and bacterial translocation in burn and sepsis. *Ann Surg*. 2003; **237**: 101–109.

117. Jeschke MG, Bolder U, Chung DH, et al. Gut mucosal homeostasis and cellular mediators after severe thermal trauma and the effect of insulin-like growth factor-I in combination with insulin-like growth factor binding protein-3. *Endocrinology*. 2007; **148**: 354–362.

118. Debroy MA, Wolf SE, Zhang XJ, et al. Anabolic effects of insulin-like growth factor in combination with insulin-like growth factor binding protein-3 in severely burned adults. *J Trauma*. 1999; **47**: 904–911.

119. Parker CR Jr, Baxter CR. Divergence in adrenal steroid secretory pattern after thermal injury in adult patients. *J Trauma*. 1985; **25**: 508–510.

120. Daynes RA, Dudley DJ, Araneo BA. Regulation of murine lymphokine production in vivo. II. Dehydroepiandrosterone is a natural enhancer of IL-2 synthesis by helper T cells. *Eur J Immunol*. 1990; **20**: 793–801.

121. Suzuki T, Suzuki N, Daynes RA, Engleman EG. Dehydroepiandrosterone enhances IL-2 production and cytotoxic effector function of human T cells. *Clin Immunol Immunopathol*. 1991; **61**: 202–211.

122. Araneo B, Daynes R. Dehydroepiandrosterone functions as more than an antiglucocorticoid in preserving immunocompetence after thermal injury. *Endocrinology*. 1995; **136**: 93–401.

123. Browne ES, Wright BE, Porter JR, Svec F. Dehydroepiandrosterone: antiglucocorticoid action in mice. *Am J Med Sci*. 1992; **303**: 366–371.

124. Fang CH, Tiao G, James H, Ogle C, Fischer JE, Hasselgren PO. Burn injury stimulates multiple proteolytic pathways in skeletal muscle, including the ubiquitin-energy-dependent pathway. *J Am Coll Surg*. 1995; **180**: 161–170.

125. Chai J, Wu Y, Sheng Z. The relationship between skeletal muscle proteolysis and ubiquitin-proteasome proteolytic pathway in burned rats. *Burns*. 2002; **28**: 527–533.

126. Fang CH, James HJ, Ogle C, Fischer JE, Hasselgren PO. Influence of burn injury on protein metabolism in different types of skeletal muscle and the role of glucocorticoids. *J Am Coll Surg*. 1995; **180**: 33–42.

127. Lang CH, Silvis C, Nystrom G, Frost RA. Regulation of myostatin by glucocorticoids after thermal injury. *FASEB J.* 2001; **15**: 1807–1809.

128. Gore DC, Herndon DN, Wolfe RR. Comparison of peripheral metabolic effects of insulin and metformin following severe burn injury. *J Trauma.* 2005; **59**: 316–323.

129. Gore DC, Chinkes DL, Hart DW, Wolf SE, Herndon DN, Sanford AP. Hyperglycemia exacerbates muscle protein catabolism in burn-injured patients. *Crit Care Med.* 2002; **30**: 2438–2442.

130. Riesenman PJ, Braithwaite SS, Cairns BA. Metformin-associated lactic acidosis in a burn patient. *J Burn Care Res.* 2007; **28**: 342–347.

131. Knox J, Demling R, Wilmore D, et al. Increased survival after major thermal injury: the effect of growth hormones in adults. *J Trauma.* 1995; **39**: 526–532.

132. Ramirez RJ, Wolf SE, Barrow RE, Herndon DN. Growth hormone treatment in pediatric burns: A safe therapeutic approach. *Ann Surg.* 1998; **228**: 439–448.

133. Losada F, García-Luna PP, Gómez-Cía T, et al. Effects of human recombinant growth hormone on donor-site healing in burned adults. *World J Surg.* 2002; **26**: 2–8.

134. Ferrando AA, Tipton KD, Doyle D, et al. Testosterone stimulates protein synthesis but not amino acid transport in humans. *Am J Physiol (Endocr Metab).* 1998; **275**:E864-E871.

135. Ferrando AA, Sheffield-Moore M, Wolf SE, et al. Testosterone administration in severe burns ameliorates muscle catabolism. *Crit Care Med.* 2001; **29**: 1936–1942.

136. Wilmore DW, Long JM, Mason AD Jr, Skreen RW, Pruitt BA Jr. Catecholamines: mediator of the hypermetabolic response to thermal injury. *Ann Surg.* 1974; **180**: 653–669.

137. Minifee PK, Barrow RE, Abston S, Desai M, Herndon DN. Improved myocardial oxygen utilization following propranolol infusion in adolescents with postburn hypermetabolism. *J Pediatr Surg.* 1989; **24**: 806–811.

138. Herndon DN, Hart DW, Wolf SE, Chinkes DL, Wolfe RR. Reversal of catabolism by beta-blockade after severe burns. *N Engl J Med.* 2001; **345**: 1223–1239.

139. Jeschke MG, Norbury WB, Finnerty CC, Branski LK, Herndon DN. Propranolol does not increase inflammation, sepsis, or infectious episodes in severely burned children. *J Trauma.* 2007; **62**: 676–681.

140. Jeschke MG, Finnerty CC, Kulp GA, Przkora R, Mlcak RP, Herndon DN. Combination of recombinant human growth hormone and propanolol decreases hypermetabolism and inflammation in severely burned children. *Pediatr Crit Care Med.* 2008; **9**: 209–216.

141. Demling RH, DeSanti L. Oxandrolone, an anabolic steroid, significantly increases the rate of weight gain in the recovery phase after major burns. *J Trauma.* 1997; **43**: 47–51.

142. Demling RH, Orgill RP. The anticatabolic and wound healing effects of the testosterone analog oxandrolone after severe burn injury. *J Crit Care.* 2000; **15**: 12–17.

143. Hart DW, Wolf SE, Ramzy PI, et al. Anabolic effects of oxandrolone after severe burn. *Ann Surg.* 2001; **233**: 556–564.

144. Wolf SE, Thomas SJ, Dasu MR, et al. Improved net protein balance, lean mass, and gene expression changes with oxandrolone treatment in the severely burned. *Ann Surg.* 2003; **237**: 801–811.

145. Barrow RE, Dasu MRK, Ferrando AA, et al. Gene expression patterns in skeletal muscle of thermally injured children treated with oxandrolone. *Ann Surg.* 2003; **237**: 422–428.

146. Zhao J, Bauman WA, Huang R, Caplan AJ, Cardozo C. Oxandrolone blocks glucocorticoid signaling in an androgen receptor-dependent manner. *Steroids.* 2004; **69**: 357–366.

147. Przkora R, Herndon DN, Suman OE. The effects of oxandrolone and exercise on muscle mass and function in children with severe burns. *Pediatrics.* 2007; **119**:e109-e116.

148. Jeschke MG, Finnerty CC, Suman OE, Kulp G, Mlcak RP, Herndon DN. The effect of oxandrolone on the endocrinologic, inflammatory, and hypermetabolic responses during the acute phase postburn. *Ann Surg.* 2007; **246**: 351–362.

149. Wolf SE, Edelman LS, Kemalyan N, et al. Effects of oxandrolone on outcomes measures in the severely burned: a multicenter prospective randomized double-blind trial. *J Burn Care Res.* 2006; **27**: 131–141.

150. Klein GL, Bi LX, Sherrard DJ, et al. Evidence supporting a role of glucocorticoids in short-term bone loss in burned children. *Osteoporos Int.* 2004; **15**: 468–474.

151. Murphy KD, Thomas S, Mlcak RP, Chinkes DL, Klein GL, Herndon DN. Effects of long-term oxandrolone administration in severely burned children. *Surgery.* 2004; **136**;219–224.

152. Bi LX, Wiren KM, Zhang XW, et al. The effect of oxandrolone treatment on human osteoblastic cells. *J Burns Wounds.* 2007; **6**: 53–64.

153. Haller JA Jr, Andrews HG, White JJ, Tamer MA, Cleveland WW. Pathophysiology and management of acute corrosive burns of the esophagus. *J Pediatr Surg.* 1971; **6**: 578–583.

154. Anderson KD, Rouse TM, Randolph KG. A controlled trial of corticosteroids in children with corrosive injury of the esophagus. *N Engl J Med.* 1990; **323**: 637–640.

155. Fulton JA, Hoffman RS. Steroids in second degree caustic burns of the esophagus: a systematic pooled analysis of fifty years of human data: 1956–2006. *Clin Toxicol (Phila).* 2007; **45**: 402–408.

156. Nieman GF, Clark WR, Hakim T. Methylprednisolone does not protect the lung from inhalation injury. *Burns.* 1991; **17**: 384–390.

157. Cha SI, Kim CH, Lee JH, et al. Isolated smoke inhalation injuries: acute respiratory dysfunction, clinical outcomes, and short-term evolution of pulmonary functions with the effects of steroids. *Burns.* 2006; **33**: 200–208.

158. Markovitz BP, Randolph AG. Corticosteroids for the prevention of reintubation and postextubation stridor in pediatric patients: a meta-analysis. *Pediatr Crit Care Med.* 2002; **3**: 223–226.

# CHAPTER EIGHTEEN

# HYPERMETABOLISM AND ANABOLIC AGENT USE IN PEDIATRIC BURN PATIENTS

TODD F. HUZAR, MD, UNITED STATES ARMY INSTITUTE OF SURGICAL RESEARCH; EDWARD MALIN IV, MD, UNITED STATES ARMY INSTITUTE OF SURGICAL RESEARCH; AND STEVEN E. WOLF†, MD, UNIVERSITY OF TEXAS HEALTH SCIENCE CENTER–SAN ANTONIO

## INTRODUCTION

Traumatic injuries are a common cause of morbidity and mortality in the pediatric population, and these injuries lead to major physical, emotional, and metabolic changes. Of the various types of injury, burns induce possibly the greatest physiologic stress on the human body.[1] Increasing energy requirements and varying substrate demands lead to significant alterations in carbohydrate, protein, and fat metabolism. The hypermetabolic state induced by major burns creates a catabolic environment precipitating protein loss and significant reductions in lean body mass.[2]

Burns greater than 20% total body surface area (TBSA) create a physiologic picture similar to that seen in severe systemic inflammatory response syndrome and, at times, septic shock.[1,3] The stress induced by these severe burns leads to release of a variety of hormones from the endocrine system along with cytokines that stimulate and perpetuate this hypermetabolic and catabolic state. There has been extensive research exploring ways to augment the hypermetabolic response, particularly in the pediatric population. Studies examined manipulating the catabolic milieu through the use of anabolic hormones, steroids, and anti-catabolic agents; however, pediatric patients still suffer from severe muscle wasting and growth retardation despite these advances.[4] In general, it was found that use of anabolic agents abates the protein losses associated with injury, but in the state of inflammation does not seem to engender actual anabolism.[5]

## THE PATHOPHYSIOLOGY OF HYPERMETABOLISM

Children are unfortunately prone to suffering from burns, and often, their burns tend to be severe due to thin skin and inability to escape from fire. The injury that is sustained from burns has more effects on the body than what is just seen at skin level. Homeostasis is disrupted as a consequence of inflammatory mediators liberated by the burn, and the changes seen include increases in core body temperature, glycolysis, proteolysis, lipolysis, and futile substrate cycling.[6] In 1930, Cuthbertson characterized the metabolic response to injury as a biphasic response with an early, hypodynamic "ebb" phase and a long-lasting, hyper-metabolic "flow" phase.[7]

After a severe burn, cytokines and other inflammatory mediators are released from injured tissues, propelling the body into a hypodynamic state characterized by generalized depression of metabolic activity. This phase is defined by decreases in blood pressure, cardiac output, body temperature, and oxygen consumption.[8] Surges of catecholamines, vasopressin, and products of the renin-angiotensin system are released in an attempt to regain homeostasis, but they have varying effects on the ensuing hypovolaemic shock.[9] This shock state seen during the resuscitation period is part of the ebb phase and is a consequence of a hypodynamic circulation and intravascular depletion due to fluid loss from the burn wounds and formation of tissue edema.

The ebb phase lasts from 24 hours to 3 days, at which point it transitions into the flow phase around the fifth day after injury. Cuthbertson described this phase as one that consists of both hyperdynamic circulation and hypermetabolism.[7] It is characterized by increased cardiac output (supraphysiologic), body temperature, oxygen, and glucose consumption, with subsequent increases in $CO_2$ production, increased urinary nitrogen losses, altered glucose metabolism, futile substrate cycling, and accelerated tissue catabolism.[10] Metabolic derangements can last for a variable length of time, but are from 9 months to 1 year in severely burned children.[11] The hypermetabolic response is believed to be propagated by catabolic hormones such as catecholamines, glucagon, and cortisol. Many studies show that catecholamines are the primary mediators of hypermetabolism and urinary levels increase in relation to the severity of the burn.[12] Catecholamines are an essential part of the "fight or flight" response, but the quantity secreted after severe burn injury is supranormal. They cause a variety of effects on cellular metabolic capabilities; however, one of the more devastating effects is the ability to decrease and even block the production of anabolic hormones, which tips the scales of the relationship between protein synthesis and breakdown in favor of protein catabolism.[13]

Hypermetabolism in burn patients causes alterations in circulation and substrate cycling in order to keep pace with the new metabolic demands. Burn patients have protein breakdown and loss of amino acids from the cell 2 times greater than that seen in normal nonburned, fasted patients.[14] Cellular synthetic machinery shifts from a balanced anabolic/catabolic state to a hypercatabolic state, requiring increasing quantities of previously unused substrates for energy production. Muscle bears the brunt of the hypermetabolic response and is broken down at a rapid rate in order to keep up with substrate production for the increased metabolic demands due to changes in the resting metabolic rate (RMR). The resting metabolic rate is directly affected by the severity of the patient's burn and increases in a curvilinear fashion (Figure 1). For example, burns less than 40% TBSA can double the RMR; however, burns greater than 40% TBSA have been shown to increase this rate by 180%.[15] The energy requirements needed for this elevated RMR are met by breaking down muscle proteins into amino acids and shunting them to the liver for gluconeogenesis and creation of acute phase proteins.

Nitrogen balance in burn patients tends to be rather distorted, and they will remain in a negative balance until the hypermetabolic state has ceased. Rutan and Herndon demonstrated that skeletal muscle nitrogen loss in burn patients may exceed levels 10 to 15 times greater than those seen in volunteers that had been fasting.[16]

## AUGMENTING ANABOLISM

Given the effects of severe injury to induce skeletal muscle catabolism, investigators noted that many pharmacologic agents are available which induce muscle anabolism through a variety of receptors and signal transduction mechanisms. All of these to date seem to be effective after injury through improving efficiency of muscle protein synthesis of free amino acids within the cells that are available from the increase in protein breakdown associated with the hypermetabolic state (Figure 2). These anabolic agents can be broken roughly into 3 categories: circulating peptides (such as growth hormone and insulin), anabolic steroids (such as testosterone), and inhibitors of hypermetabolism (such as β-adrenergic blockers) (Table 1). In the rest of the chapter, we will discuss each agent that has been used and the data to support its use in severely burned children.

## Recombinant Human Growth Hormone

Anabolic hormone production is diminished as a result of the persistent catabolic state seen after severe burn. Human growth hormone (hGH) was one of the first anabolic agents found to abate the hypermetabolic response seen in burns and nonburn injuries.[17] In fact, Cuthbertson et al studied growth hormone in a leg fracture model before World War II and showed that it improves the net protein balance.[18]

Recombinant human growth hormone (rhGH) has been studied many times in the acutely burned pediatric population. The dose used was 0.2mg/kg given subcutaneously based on preliminary and not conclusive pharmacokinetics.[19] The hormone was found to decrease whole-body catabolism, improve protein synthesis in muscle beds,[20] accelerate donor-site and wound healing,[19] improve the immune response,[21] augment the production of hepatic acute phase proteins,[22] and promote linear growth,[23] all of which are perceived to be beneficial. On the other hand, it had been demonstrated that growth hormone treatment can lead to increases in metabolic rate and thermogenesis due to overstimulation of gluconeogenesis.[24] Growth hormone increases serum levels of insulinlike growth factor

1 (IGF-1), which has also been found to have positive influence on protein metabolism in children.[25] Precocious sexual development, hyperglycemia, insulin resistance, and early growth plate closure are known side effects of growth hormone use,[26] but these seem to be minimized in the doses used in pediatric burns.

In spite of all these beneficial data, growth hormone is not commonly used in severely burned children. This notion arose as a result of a report of increased mortality when hGH was used in a population of nonburned critically ill adults.[27] This was refuted in the pediatric burns shortly after this report became available[28]; in fact, the data, if anything, suggest improved mortality if growth hormone is used in this population. In retrospect, one key difference between these studies and populations was the study design. The study in critically ill adults dosed hGH shortly after arrival to the ICU, while in the pediatric burns, treatment with hGH was withheld until the flow phase of hypermetabolism was firmly established. This brings to mind the notion that perhaps the particular hormonal milieu in which treatment is proffered during critical illness has relevance and should be considered both scientifically and practically. Perhaps hyperglycemia induced by growth hormone is more harmful in the beginning throes of recovery from injury, but is not harmful later and is, in fact, beneficial? Similar changes in fat metabolism may also be at work. Hopefully, these issues will be addressed in future studies. Regardless, because other agents have been discovered with similar beneficial effects and decreased demonstrated risks, most now avoid the use of growth hormone in favor of other agents discussed below.

## Insulinlike Growth Factor

IGF-1 is a small peptide that circulates in the serum, tightly bound to high-affinity proteins. It is synthesized primarily in the liver in response to growth hormone and is released into the circulation. It is also synthesized locally by cells in wounds and such, where it has paracrine effects. Many groups beginning in the 1990s studied this factor and showed it to have potent anabolic effects.[29] IGF-1 has been studied in the pediatric burn population as well, where it was noted to decrease protein oxidation, diminish muscle catabolism, restore gut mucosal integrity, and promote glucose uptake with no changes in resting energy expenditure.[5,29] However, use of IGF-1 in burn patients was found to cause significant hypoglycemia when given in large amounts because of its cross-reactivity with the insulin receptor.[29] However, this is ameliorated by coadministration with its in vivo binding protein, insulinlike growth factor binding protein-3 (IGFBP-3). One side effect which has not received much attention is the reported increase

in neuropathies in burned adults who received IGF-1/IGFBP-3; the etiology is unknown. Currently, no manufacturer exists for the product, so administration of IGF-1 for anabolic effects is not possible. These studies show, however, that promise exists for its use, particularly in association with glucose control, which is now standard of care in most burn ICUs. No direct studies on the use of IGF-1 exist in the era of tight glucose control. Since this agent also has effects in this arena, this should be of interest to burn care practitioners.

## Insulin

Hyperglycemia is a common entity seen in many severely burned patients and has been demonstrated to cause accelerated rates of protein catabolism, reduced graft take, and increases in mortality.[30] Insulin is the most potent anabolic agent known, and its use in burn patients has been well studied. The first of these studies investigated high-dose (> 30 units/h) intravenous infusions for a 3-to-5-day period. This study showed a greater flux of amino acids into cells and an increase in protein synthesis by more than 200%.[31] This has been the only study to show actual increases in inward transport of amino acids into muscle cells in response to an anabolic agent in conjunction with an increase in protein synthesis after injury. However, such large insulin doses required very intensive monitoring and high supplementary glucose intakes, so Ferrando et al infused insulin at a lower rate (7–15 units/h) for 3 to 5 days and found the lower rate to also have a positive effect on protein synthesis, but it no longer improved amino acid influx.[14] This dosing regimen was found to be less labor intensive and did not require any increases in caloric intake. Then, the lower dose (7–15 units/h) intravenous insulin was studied in severely burned children when given throughout the hospitalization and was shown to promote increases in lean body mass and shortened length of hospital stay without increasing caloric requirements.[32] Insulin therapy has also been found to have anti-inflammatory properties. In a study by Jeschke et al, insulin diminished the overall inflammatory response by decreasing the production of proinflammatory mediators and activating propagation of the anti-inflammatory cascade.[33]

These studies were performed shortly before the landmark article by van den Berghe showing the benefit of glucose control with insulin in critically ill patients.[34] Since that time, most have adopted a program of insulin administration to burned children who are hyperglycemic. It serves to reason, then, that perhaps the beneficial effects of insulin seen in other populations are at least partially effective through stimulation of anabolism. The next step is to answer the question whether perhaps more calories (glucose) should be given so that more insulin can be given for maximal anabolic effect; this notion has not been tested to date except in the studies mentioned above and now requires a multicenter controlled randomized trial. Such a trial would be of interest to those treating severely burned children.

## Testosterone

After injury, there are many changes in the hormonal composition of the human body. Various hormones are not produced at the same rate or amount that they were prior to the insult. Testosterone, an androgenic steroid hormone that is secreted from the testes in men and to a lesser extent from the ovaries of women, is one of the hormones found to be decreased in this population, leading to transient hypogonadism.[35] Severe burns, especially large burns (>60% TBSA) will cause significant decreases in total and free testosterone levels.[36] Muscle catabolism can persist unabated due to the diminished levels of testosterone, which normally would prevent muscle catabolism. Ferrando et al demonstrated that testosterone administration in burned adult patients leads to a decline in skeletal muscle decomposition, increased protein synthetic efficiency, and an overall net protein balance of zero, which represents a halt to the process of muscle protein loss.[37] Testosterone functions as a promoter of muscle anabolism by efficiently using free intracellular amino acids, and this in turn increases net protein synthesis.[38,39] There are many benefits to its use; however, testosterone does have its own side effect profile: it can cause virilization and hirsutism in female patients, hepatic toxicity, acne, electrolyte disturbances, and aggressive behavior, and in children, it may lead to accelerated bone maturation and early epiphyseal closure with no further linear growth.[40] For these reasons, it is not surprising that the use of testosterone has not been well studied in the pediatric population after injury. It seems that the side effect profile would not make it the best choice for reversal of hypermetabolism in this population.

## Oxandrolone

Testosterone has been examined as an agent in the anabolic steroid group to be used to augment the hypercatabolic response in adults; however, the long list of side effects has deterred many from using it. Another anabolic steroid that has been well studied is oxandrolone. It is a synthetic, 17 α-methyl derivative of testosterone.[41] It is excreted from the body via the kidneys and does not have the hepatotoxic effects seen in testosterone use.[42]

Initially, it was studied in a variety of adult patient populations that were in sustained catabolic states, and in the pediatric population, it was used in treatment of Turner's syndrome and constitutional growth delay.[43,44] Later, oxandrolone was studied extensively in the severely burned adult

and pediatric populations. Its use is rather appealing because it can be given orally (0.1 mg/kg bid), it is inexpensive, it has fewer side effects than other anabolic agents, and its anabolic effect is 10 times greater than testosterone.[45] Studies have shown that oxandrolone improves muscle synthetic activity, increases expression of anabolic genes in muscle, and increases net muscle protein synthesis, with subsequent improvement in lean body mass composition.[46,47]

The proposed mechanism of action for oxandrolone is an alteration in gene expression and prevention of catabolised muscle amino acid exodus out of the cell, forcing them back into the protein synthetic machinery.[48] The end result is more amino acids remaining within the cell and improved protein synthetic efficiency, allowing for preservation of lean body mass. Wolf et al showed that oxandrolone treatment started 1 week after severe burns in children and continued throughout the hospital stay helped with maintenance of total body weight and lean body mass compared to children in the placebo arm of the study.[48]

Oxandrolone has been proven to be both beneficial in the acute and recovery phases of severe burns. Demling and DeSanti demonstrated that the combination of oxandrolone given 10 mg bid and a high-calorie, high-protein diet given to patients in the recovery phase after burn produced a 4-fold increase in weight gain compared to patients in the retrospective group managed with similar nutrition alone.[49]

It is also effective in expediting healing of donor sites compared to placebo and has been found to have the same degree of wound healing compared to the use of hGH.[50,51] The action of oxandrolone on wound healing is different than that of rhGH. It is believed that skin fibroblasts have androgen receptors that are activated by the binding of oxandrolone, and this in turn leads to the synthesis of local growth factors that increase the rate of wound reepithelialisation.[52] The improvement in wound healing has a dual benefit for the burn population. The use of oxandrolone has been shown to decrease the number of operations needed for burn grafting, and this leads to a decrease in total hospital stay after an acute burn.[53]

Oxandrolone, like any other drug, does have its side effects. It can cause virilization in females, hepatic dysfunction, hirsutism, and other androgenic effects similar to what is seen in patients on testosterone. However, most studies have seen minimal side effects in their study populations compared to historical controls using testosterone. The most commonly seen abnormality is transient increases in liver function tests, which improve with discontinuation. Oxandrolone has been shown to be safe to use in the pediatric population, and its benefits certainly outweigh the risks of its use. Additionally, this drug is much cheaper than using anabolic doses of rhGH, and its oral dosing allows for better compliance in children.

Overall, oxandrolone is a beneficial drug for expediting recovery in children in both the acute and recovery burn phases. Pediatric burn patients on oxandrolone for 1 year showed increases in lean body mass, muscle strength, bone mineral composition, and attenuation of the hypermetabolic response, and these positive effects were noted to continue for up to 1 year after the discontinuation of oxandrolone, with continued weight gain (lean body mass) and linear growth.[54] Oxandrolone is a safe, cheap, and effective drug that should be used in the pediatric burn population to turn the tide on the negative consequences of hypermetabolism and hasten return to school and social environments. To date, this drug has the best combination of demonstrated beneficial effect and limited risk profile, and we recommend its use.

## Beta-Blockers

The hypermetabolic response to burns has been linked to the continuous and persistent release of catecholamines. Therefore, it serves to reason that catecholamine inhibition diminishes these effects on the various body systems and in turn lessens the hypermetabolic response. Beta-blockers were found to have this effect, and propranolol, a nonselective beta-blocker, has been commonly used in this situation. Beta-blockade in severely burned children diminishes supraphysiologic thermogenesis,[55] tachycardia,[56] myocardial oxygen demand/cardiac work,[57] and resting energy expenditure.[58] By decreasing the hypermetabolic response, the deleterious effect of muscle catabolism is also lessened. Herndon et al examined the use of propranolol in children with acute severe burns and found that beta-blockade improves net muscle protein synthesis and increases lean body mass measured with 3 different methods.[59] The dose of propranolol used in these studies was aimed at decreasing the heart rate by 20%. The induced reduction in heart rate was associated with decreased cardiac work and reduced fatty infiltration of the liver. Fatty infiltration of the liver is reduced secondary to decreases in peripheral fat breakdown, diversion of palmitate from the liver, and overall decreases in liver fat uptake.[60,61]

Propranolol has also demonstrated a significant role in substrate recycling. Studies show that it stimulates intracellular recycling of free amino acids released from muscle catabolism and forces these amino acids to be used in protein synthesis within the same myocyte. However, on closer examination, this mechanism is counterintuitive (Figure 3). Since protein synthesis and protein breakdown are both stimulated in critical illness (breakdown more than synthesis, thus catabolism), and this is presumably under some control of catecholamine hypersecretion, the expected effect of catecholamine inhibition might be that of decreased protein breakdown and synthesis, or, in simpler terms, a "cooling off" that favors synthesis over breakdown. However, what we find is that catecholamine inhibition results in even greater protein synthesis without effect on breakdown. This then implies that β-adrenergic stimulation is somehow inhibiting further increases in synthesis in the catabolic milieu, unless the effect is somehow indirect through some other mechanism. One interesting possibility is an indirect effect of propranolol through decreasing fat availability by inhibition of lipolysis.

Propranolol is a promising drug in regards to its use in reversing some of the metabolic effects of burns; however, it is not completely innocuous. Inappropriate dosing can cause diminished cardiac output, causing hypotension and end-organ hypoperfusion. Additionally, care must be taken with use in patients with reactive airway disease due to possible severe bronchospasm as a result of the blockade of $\beta_2$ receptors.[62] There has been some controversy in regards to the relationship of propranolol use and incidence of infections/sepsis. It has been demonstrated in the literature that catecholamines are essential for positive augmentation of the immune response. Jeschke et al examined this relationship in children and determined that the use of nonselective beta-blockade does not increase the incidence of infection and sepsis in pediatric burn patients, nor does it have negative effects on the immune response.[63] Overall, propranolol use in the pediatric burn population is safe and should be considered as part of the regimen to abate the hypermetabolic response.

## CONCLUSION

Anabolic agent use has been investigated heavily in severely ill persons by many groups; pediatric burns are no exception. Several have been tried, each with benefits, but the risk profiles limit use of some of these. At this point, based on the available data, we recommend that glucose in severely burned children should be controlled with continuous insulin infusions, propranolol should be used to decrease heart rate by 20%, and oxandrolone should be given daily in a dose of 0.1 mg/kg. Each of these agents has benefit in terms of metabolism, and some in other areas as well. Further studies are required to find the optimal regimen of anabolic agent use, which also must be considered in relation to nutritional provision.

## FIGURES AND TABLE

### FIGURE 1
**Effect of burn size on protein metabolism. With increasing burn size (% TBSA), net balance of protein across the leg decreases, indicating catabolism with increasing burn size, but when burn size is reaches 40% TBSA, catabolism is maximal and does not consistently increase above this level.**

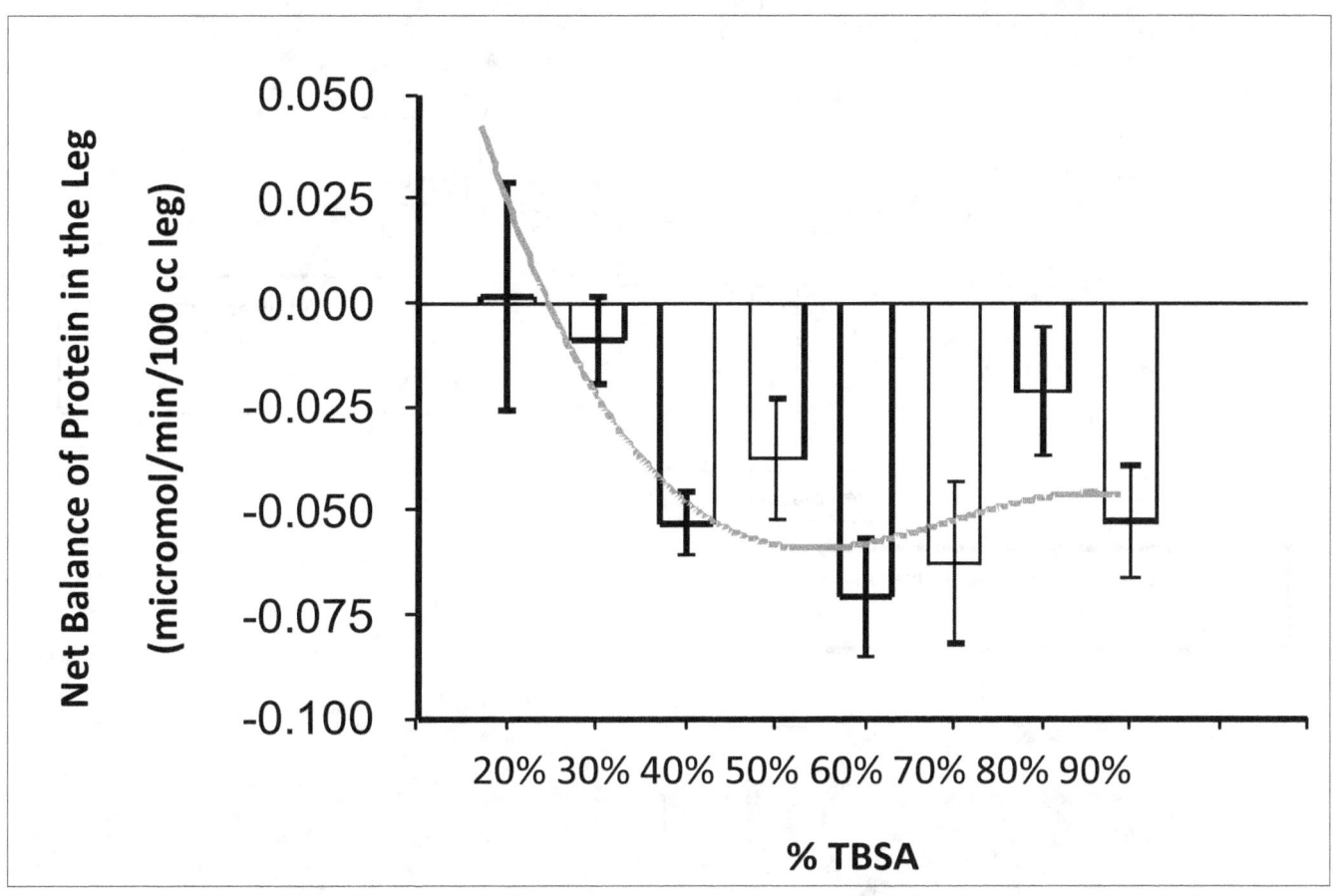

**FIGURE 2**
**Description of amino acid flux within and without the cell after injury.**

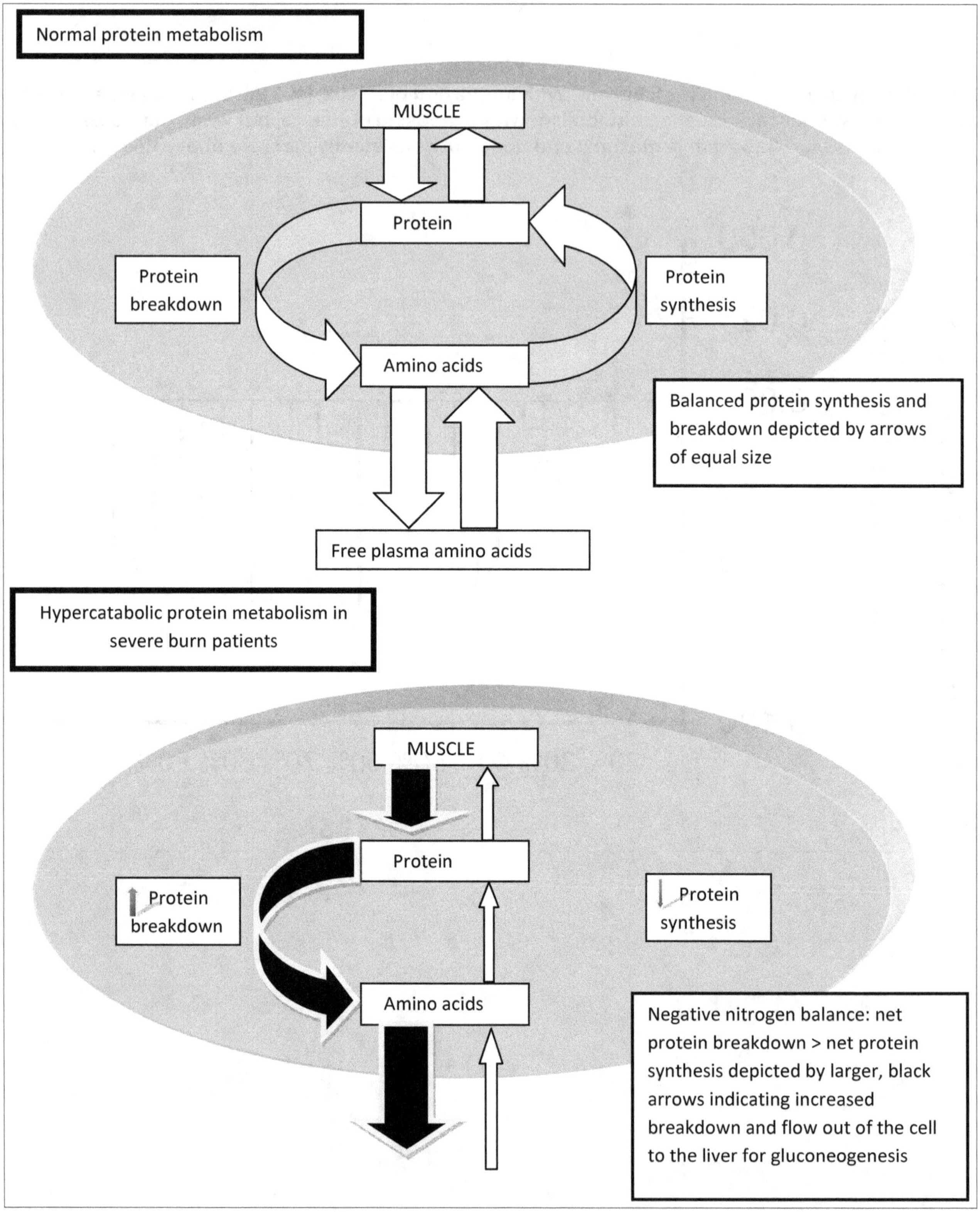

FIGURE 3

Mechanistic effects of propranolol after injury. The white bar represents protein synthesis measured as the rate of disposal of phenylalanine in the leg muscle after burn and before and after treatment with propranolol. The gray bar similarly represents breakdown, and the black bar represents the net balance of the 2. Propranolol induced an increase in protein synthesis without effect on breakdown.

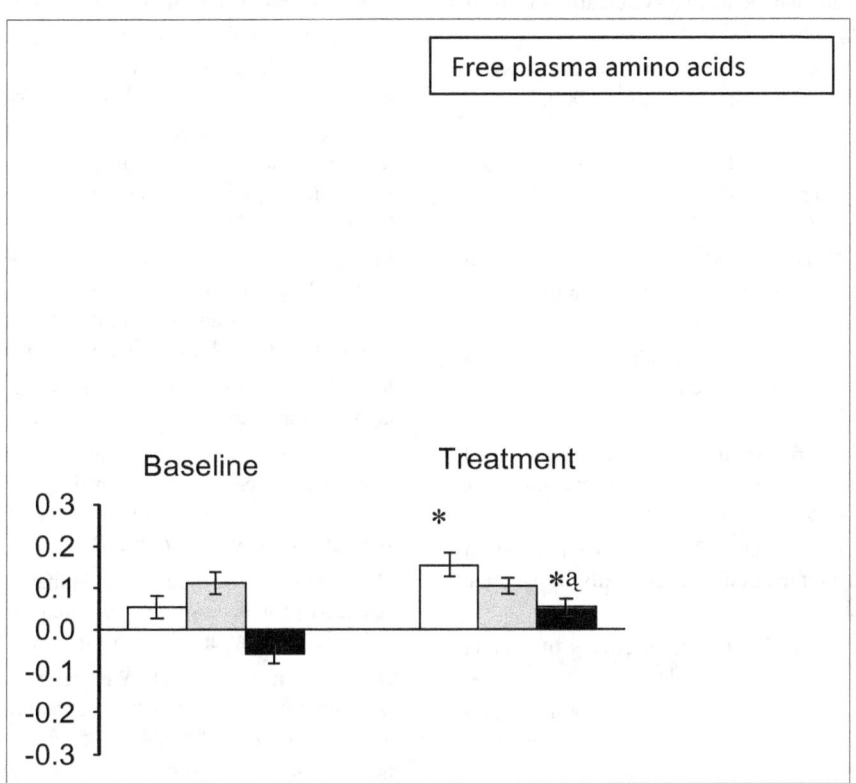

TABLE 1
Anabolic agents by class.

*Peptides*

   Growth hormone

   Insulinlike growth factor

   Insulin

*Steroids*

   Testosterone

   Oxandrolone

*Catabolism Inhibitors*

   Propranolol

# REFERENCES

1. Ipaktchi K, Arbabi S. Advances in burn critical care. *Crit Care Med.* Sep 2006; **34**(suppl 9): S239–S244.

2. Atiyeh BS, Gunn SWA, Dibo SA. Metabolic implications of severe burn injuries and their management: a systematic review of the literature. *World J Surg.* 2008; **32**: 1857–1869.

3. Hart DW, Wolf SE, Chinkes DL, et al. Determinants of skeletal muscle catabolism after severe burn. *Ann Surg.* 2000; **232**(4): 455–465.

4. Fuchs PC, Groger A, Bozkurt A. Cortisol in severely burned patients: investigations on disturbance of the hypothalamic-pituitary-adrenal axis. *Shock.* 2007; **28**(6): 662–667.

5. Herndon DN, Ramzy PI, DebRoy MA, et al. Muscle protein catabolism after severe burn: effects of IGF-1/IGFBP-3 treatment. *Ann Surg.* 1999; **229**(5): 713–720, discussion 720–722.

6. Pereira CT, Murphy K, Jeschke MG, Herndon DN. Post burn muscle wasting and the effects of treatments. *Int J Biochem Cell Biol.* 2005; **37**: 1948–1961.

7. Cuthbertson DP. The disturbance of metabolism pronounced by bony and non-bony injury, with notes on certain abnormal conditions of bone. *Biochem J.* 1930; **24**: 1244–1248.

8. Frankenfield DC, Smith JS, Cooney RN. Relative association of fever and injury with hypermetabolism in critically ill patients. *Injury.* 1997; **28**: 617–625.

9. Stoner HB. Interpretation of the metabolic effects of trauma and sepsis. *J Clin Pathol.* 1987; **40**: 1108–1117.

10. Barret JP, Herndon DN. Modulation of inflammatory and catabolic responses in severely burned children by early burn wound excision in the first 24 hours. *Arch Surg.* 2003; **138**: 127–132.

11. Hart DW, Wolf SE, Mlcak R, et al. Persistence of muscle catabolism after severe burn. *Surgery.* 2000; **128**(2): 312–319.

12. Wilmore DW, Mason AD, Skreen RW, Pruitt BA. Catecholamines: mediator of the hypermetabolic response to thermal injury. *Ann Surg.* 1974; **180**: 653–669.

13. Wang P, Li N, Li JS. The role of endotoxin, TNF-alpha, and IL-6 in inducing the state of growth hormone sensitivity. *World J Gastroenterol.* 2002; **8**: 531–536.

14. Ferrando AA, Chinkes DL, Wolf SE, et al. A submaximal dose of insulin promotes net skeletal muscle protein synthesis in patients with severe burns. *Ann Surg.* 1999; **229**(1): 11–18.

15. Pereira CT, Murphy KD, Herndon DN. Altering metabolism. *J Burn Care Rehabil.* 2005; **26**(3): 194–199.

16. Rutan RL, Herndon DN. Growth delay in postburn pediatric patients. *Arch Surg.* 1990; **125**: 392–395.

17. Wanek S, Wolf SE. Metabolic response to injury and the role of anabolic hormones. *Curr Opin Clin Nutr Metab Care.* 2007; **10**: 272–277.

18. Cuthbertson DP, Webster TA, Young FG. The anterior pituitary gland and protein metabolism: the nitrogen-retaining action of anterior lobe extracts. *J Endocrinol.* 1941; **2**: 459–467.

19. Herndon DN, Barrow RE, Kunkel KR, et al. Effects of recombinant human growth hormone on donor-site healing in severely burned children. *Ann Surg.* 1990; **212**(4): 424–429, discussion 430–431.

20. Gore DC, Honeycutt D, Jahoor F, et al. Effect of exogenous growth hormone on whole-body and isolated limb protein kinetics in burned patients. *Arch Surg.* 1991; **126**: 38–43.

21. Takagi K, Suzuki F, Barrow RE, et al. Growth hormone improves immune function and survival in burned mice infected with herpes simplex virus type 1. *J Surg Res.* 1997; **69**(1): 166–170.

22. Jeschke MG, Barrow RE, Herndon DN. Recombinant human growth hormone treatment in pediatric burn patients and its role during the hepatic acute phase response. *Crit Care Med.* 2000; **28**(5): 1578–1584.

23. Jeschke MG, Finnerty CC, Gabriela AK, et al. Combination of recombinant human growth hormone and propranolol decreases hypermetabolism and inflammation in severely burned children. *Pediatr Crit Care Med.* 2008; **9**(2): 209–216.

24. Zeigler TR. Growth Hormone administration during nutritional support: what is to be gained. *New Horiz.* 1994; **2**(2): 244–256.

25. Jeschke MG, Chrysopoulo MT, Herndon DN, Wolf SE. Increased expression of insulin-like growth factor-I in serum and liver after recombinant human growth hormone administration in thermally-injured rats. *J Surg Res.* 1999; **85**: 171–177.

26. Przkora R, Herndon DN, Suman OE. Beneficial effects of extended growth hormone treatment after hospital discharge in pediatric burn patients. *Ann Surg.* 2006; **243**: 796–803.

27. Takala J, Ruokonen E, Webster NR, et al. Increased mortality associated with growth hormone treatment in critically ill adults. *New Engl J Med.* 1999; **341**: 785–792.

28. Ramirez RJ, Wolf SE, Barrow RE, Herndon DN. Growth hormone treatment in pediatric burns: a safe therapeutic approach. *Ann Surg.* 1998; **228**: 439–448.

29. Cioffi WG, Gore DC, Rue LC. Insulin-like growth factor-1 lowers protein oxidation in patients with thermal injury. *Ann Surg.* 1994; **220**: 310–319.

30. Gore DC, Chinkes DL, Hart DW, et al. Hyperglycemia exacerbates muscle protein catabolism in burn-injured patients. *Crit Care Med.* 2002; **30**(11): 2438–2442.

31. Sakuri Y, Aarsland AA, Chinkes DL, et al. Anabolic effects of insulin in burned patients. *Ann Surg.* 1996; **222**: 283–297.

32. Thomas SJ, Morimoto K, Herndon DN, et al. The effect of prolonged euglycemic hyperinsulinemia on lean body mass after severe burn. *Surgery.* 2002; **132**(2): 341–347.

33. Jeschke MG, Klein D, Bolder U, Herndon DN. Insulin attenuates the systemic inflammatory response in endotoxemic rats. *Endocrinology.* 2004; **145**(9): 4084–4093.

34. van den Berghe G, Wouters P, Weekers F, et al. Intensive insulin therapy in the critically ill patients. *New Engl J Med.* 2001; **345**(19): 1359.

35. Lephart ED, Baxter CR, Parker CR. Effect of burn trauma on adrenal and testicular steroid hormone production. *J Clin Endocrinol Metab.* 1987; **64**: 842–848.

36. Ferrando AA, Wolfe RR. Restoration of hormonal action and muscle protein. *Crit Care Med.* 2007; **35**(9): S630–S634.

37. Ferrando AA, Sheffield-Moore M, Wolf SE, et al. Testosterone administration in severe burns ameliorates muscle catabolism. *Crit Care Med.* 2001; **29**(10): 1936–1942.

38. Ferrando AA, Tipton KD, Doyle D, Wolfe RR. Testosterone injection stimulates net protein synthesis but no tissue amino acid transport. *Am J Physiol.* 1998; **275**(5, pt 1): E864–E871.

39. Sheffield-Moore M, Urban RJ, Wolf SE, et al. Short-term oxandrolone administration stimulates net muscle protein synthesis in young men. *J Clin Endocrinol Metab.* 1999; **84**(8): 2705–2711.

40. Murphy KD, Thomas S, Mlcak RP, et al. Effects of long-term oxandrolone administration in severely burned children. *Surgery.* 2004; **136**: 219–224.

41. Karim A, Ranney RE, Zagarella BA. Oxandrolone disposition and metabolism in man. *Clin Pharmacol Ther.* 1973; **14**: 862–866.

42. Demling RH. Comparison of the anabolic effects and complications of human growth hormone and the testosterone analog, oxandrolone, after severe burn injury. *Burns.* 1999; **25**: 215–221.

43. Wilson DM, McCauley E, Brown DR, Dudley R. Oxandrolone therapy in constitutionally delayed growth and puberty. *Pediatrics.* 1995; **95**: 1095–1100.

44. Rosenfeld RG, Attie KM, Brasel JA, et al. Growth hormone therapy of Turner's syndrome: beneficial effect on adult height. *J Pediatr.* 1998; **132**: 319–324.

45. Fox M, Minor A. Oxandrolone: a potent anabolic steroid. *J Clin Endocrinol Metab.* 1962; **22**: 921–923.

46. Hart DW, Wolf SE, Ramzy PI, et al. Anabolic effects of oxandrolone after severe burn. *Ann Surg.* 2001; **233**(4): 556–564.

47. Barrow RE, Dasu MR, Ferrando AA, Herndon DN. Gene expression patterns in skeletal muscle of thermally injured children treated with oxandrolone. *Ann Surg.* 2003; **237**(3): 422–428.

48. Wolf SE, Thomas SJ, Dasu MR, et al. Improved net protein balance, lean mass, and gene expression changes with oxandrolone treatment in the severely burned. *Ann Surg.* 2003; **237**(6): 801–810, discussion 810–811.

49. Demling RH, DeSanti L. Oxandrolone, an anabolic steroid, significantly increase the rate of weight gain in the recovery phase after major burns. *J Trauma.* 1997; **43**(1): 47–51.

50. Demling RH, Orgill DP. The anticatabolic and wound healing effects of the testosterone analog oxandrolone after severe burn injury. *J Crit Care.* 2000; **15**(1): 12–17.

51. Sherman S, Demling RH. Growth hormone enhances re-epithelialization of human split-thickness skin graft donor sites. *Surg Forum.* 1989; **40**: 37–42.

52. Pitkow H, Labbad Z, Bitgar M. The effects of an anabolic hormone on surgically induced wound healing in lower extremity skeletal muscle in diabetic and normal rats. *Wound Repair Regen.* 1993; **1**: 119.

53. Wolf SE, Edelman LS, Kemalyan N, et al. Effects of oxandrolone on outcome measures in the severely burned: a multicenter prospective randomized double-blind trial. *J Burn Care Res.* 2006; **27**(2): 131–139, discussion 140–141.

54. Przkora R, Jeschke MG, Barrow RE, et al. Metabolic and hormonal changes of severely burned children receiving long-term oxandrolone treatment. *Ann Surg.* 2005; **242**(3): 384–389, discussion 390–391.

55. Herndon DN, Barrow RE, Rutan TC, et al. Effect of propranolol administration on hemodynamic and metabolic responses of burned pediatric patients. *Ann Surg.* 1988; **208**: 484–492.

56. Minifee P, Barrow RE, Abston S, Herndon DN. Improved myocardial oxygen utilization following propranolol infusion in adolescents with postburn hypermetabolism. *J Pediatr Surg.* 1989; **24**: 806–810.

57. Baron PW, Barrow RE, Pierre EJ, Herndon DN. Prolonged use of propranolol effectively decreases cardiac work in burned children. *J Burn Care Rehabil.* 1997; **18**: 223–227.

58. Breitenstein E, Chiolero RL, Jequier E. Effects of beta-blockade on energy metabolism following burns. *Burns.* 1990; **16**: 259–264.

59. Herndon DN, Hart DW, Wolf SE, et al. Reversal of catabolism by beta-blockade after severe burns. *N Engl J Med.* 2001; **345**(17): 1223–1229.

60. Barret JP, Jeschke MG, Herndon DN. Fatty infiltration of the liver in severely burned pediatric patients: autopsy findings and clinical implications. *J Trauma.* 2001; **51**(4): 736–739.

61. Aarsland A, Chinkes D, Wolfe RR, et al. Beta-blockade lowers peripheral lipolysis in burn patients receiving growth hormone. Rate of hepatic very low density lipoprotein triglyceride secretion remains unchanged. *Ann Surg.* 1996; **223**(6): 777–787, discussion 787–789.

62. Dunlop D, Shanks RG. Selective blockade of adrenoceptive beta receptors in the heart. *Br J Pharmacol.* 1968; **32**: 201.

63. Jeschke MG, Norbury WB, Finnerty CC, et al. Propranolol does not increase inflammation, sepsis, or infectious episodes in severely burned children. *J Trauma.* 2007; **62**: 676–681.

# SCALD BURNS

BRADLEY J. PHILLIPS, MD

## INTRODUCTION

### Defining the Scald Injury

Scald burns result when a hot fluid comes into contact with the skin. However, a consensus definition of a scald burn is lacking because there are 2 different methods of classification: (1) by fluidity, and (2) by epidemiology. In the first case, while some substances, such as water, coffee, milk, soup, or radiator fluid, easily meet the definition of a liquid, it is less obvious whether some hot foods, such as mashed potatoes, melted wax, or hot pie filling, should be included. Yamamoto et al[1] suggest that fluidity be divided into 3 broad subcategories: (1) fluid scalds, (2) sludge scalds (such as oatmeal), and (3) solids, such as rice or fries, which are nonscalds and might be better redefined as contact burns. The alternative approach is to classify scald burns by functional epidemiology. Thus, Yamamoto et al[1] suggest (1) bathwater scalds, (2) cleaning/washing scalds (eg, kitchen tap water or dishwater), (3) cooking scalds (any kind of hot food, regardless of viscosity or consistency), (4) other domestic scalds, such as wax or radiator fluid, and (5) industrial scalds, such as steam, tar, or processed foods for canning. Both function and fluidity could also be combined into a third approach that excludes items that are not fluids or sludges at room temperature. As Wibbenmeyer et al[2] point out, the epidemiology of nonfatal burn injuries is still poorly defined, and one can make a case for a simple etiology-based classification in children that can help predict the pattern and severity of the injury and which can be used as the basis for prevention programs.

### Statistics

In young infants (less than 6 months old), where mobility is restricted, scald burns are not overly common and are caused by hot drinks, water, and hot food, in that order.[3] However, as soon as infants learn to crawl, the incidence of scald burns rises significantly. Children in the age group 6 to 24 months are most at risk, which has been attributed to curiosity and exploratory behavior.[4-8] Scald burns are still the most common type of burn injury in children 4 years old or younger, but in older age groups, flame burns tend to predominate.[1,2,4-11] The vast majority of scald burns take place in the home within the kitchen, followed by the bathroom. Based upon Centers for Disease Control and Prevention (CDC) data, the incidence of scald burns that required hospitalization was 40.5 per 100000 children in the Denver metropolitan area during 1989–1990.[12] However, a much larger, more recent study (13453 children younger than 15 years) involving 4 states (California, Florida, New Jersey, and New York) suggests that this figure is much larger, with an estimate of scald injury incidence of 150 per 100000 children aged 0 to 15 years and approximately 210 per 100000 for children aged less than 4 years.[13]

## Outcomes and Mortality

Mortality from scald burns is relatively low. For example, in a sample of 12000 children, 7802 scald injuries were reported. There were 34 fatalities, and 32 of these occurred in children aged 4 years or younger.[6] In this age group, the highest mortality rate occurred for burns ≥ 40% total body surface area (TBSA), which comprised 63% of the case fatalities. Compared to flame burns in this age group, overall mortality rates for scald burns are about 14 times less. However, when the total body surface burn area required for 50% mortality is compared for the types of burn injury, in 2-year-olds to 3.9-year-olds it is much higher for scald injuries, at 97.7%, compared to 89.6% for flame burns.[6] This in part reflects the lack of inhalation injury observed in pediatric patients with scald burns. This data is taken from 1992 through 2002, and the authors of the study comment that recent advances in beta-blockers[14,15] and oxalandrone[16] usage may have led to improved outcomes in the current situation, although the effect on mortality rates is unknown.

## Issues

In brief, children with scald burns, even those with high-percentage TBSA burns, will most likely survive and go on to lead productive lives. Our focus, therefore, in this chapter will be to identify the causes and etiology of scald burns, discuss their pathophysiology, review treatment options, and determine how successful intervention and educational programs have been in regard to preventing injury. Finally, the topics of intentional injury and use of clinical pathways plans and documentation will be touched upon.

## CAUSES OF SCALD INJURY

### General Patterns

Longitudinal studies of scald burn incidence are rare. An interesting investigation in Wales that covered a period of 35 years suggests that while there has been an increase in the overall incidence (in Wales it was 50%), the age distribution of scald injury has not changed, despite the fact that causes of scald burns have changed considerably over the decades.[4,17] For example, in the United Kingdom, the introduction of the tea bag resulted in fewer injuries due to hot teapots, but an increased incidence due to cups containing hot tea.[4] Likewise, in Denmark, the increased popularity of the electric kettle in the 1980s resulted in a surge of scalds caused by children yanking on the electric cord. More recently, the combination of convenience foods designed to be heated in the microwave (with or without the addition of water) has seen the emergence of more scalds induced by hot foods, soups, and noodle-based products.

The prevalence of specific causes of scald injury also varies considerably in different countries due to cultural practices and specific regulations regarding the safety of equipment, as well as awareness of different hazards. Thus, scalds inflicted by hot baths were relatively high in Scotland and Wales during the 1980s and early 1990s compared to the Netherlands, Denmark, and Scandinavian countries due to statutory water temperature control in the latter countries.[17,18]

Patterns of injury also vary considerably, but are consistent when the etiology of the injury is considered (Table 1). In addition to the type of contact, the properties of the causative agent contribute substantially to both the pattern and severity of the injury. For example, hot water has a high heat transfer coefficient and specific heat (heat capacity), but a relatively low viscosity, so the severity of injury depends more on the temperature. In contrast, high-viscosity foods, such as soups or oatmeal, have lower heat transfer coefficients but higher viscosities, which means that they stick to the skin and can cause more partial-thickness or full-thickness skin burns if not quickly removed. Injuries from hot cooking oils can be particularly devastating because of the higher temperatures and viscosity involved compared to boiling water. Immersion in hot bath water tends to produce injuries to the trunk (especially the buttocks) and lower extremities and arms, while spills of hot liquids tend to affect the face, upper torso, and extremities.

In keeping with a simple etiological scheme, the following causes of scald injury will be examined in more detail: (1) baths and hot tap water scalds and the spilling of hot liquids, (2) hot soups and more viscous foods and materials, and (3) cooking oils.

## Baths

If a child's skin comes into contact with water at a temperature of 60°C to 65°C, a full-thickness burn can occur in as little as 2 to 5 seconds.[19] Reducing the water temperature to 54°C raises the required exposure time for the same degree of injury to 30 seconds, and further lowering to 49°C requires a 5-minute exposure for a full-thickness skin burn. To prevent any injury at all, children should not be exposed to bath water temperatures exceeding 37°C to 38°C.

Unintentional scald injuries due to children being immersed in bath water that is too hot are, unfortunately, still common. The primary reason is that many hot water thermostats are set at high temperatures. Awareness and bathing practices are contributory factors, and these will be discussed in more detail in a later section.

No reliable recent statistics in the United States have been published regarding the incidence of hot tap water scald burns, although older reports suggested that 7% to 17% of all childhood scald burns were due to such injuries.[19] Similar data from other countries vary considerably: Scotland (10%–13%),[18] Wales (10%),[20] United Kingdom (12%–16%),[17,21] the Netherlands (4%),[22] and Denmark (0%).[23] A longitudinal Australian study demonstrated, however, an 83% reduction in hot bath and tap water scald admissions from 1973 to 1994, largely as a result of legislation and educational campaigns.[24]

Burns resulting from hot bath immersion tend to show a much different pattern compared to other scald burns. If the child is sitting in the bath, the buttocks, legs, and hands are likely to be affected,[17] whereas if the child adopts an "all fours" position, the hands and legs will receive burns.[18] When running water is involved, splash injuries are usually present, but this is predicated on the temperature of the water.[25] "Stocking" patterns (a pattern showing a circumferential scald around the leg, thigh, or torso) tend to be more common in intentional injury cases. Injuries resulting from hot bath water are usually more extensive in terms of TBSA burned compared to other scald burns when hospitalization is required, and extensive autografting is needed in many cases.[17] Hypertrophic scarring in these instances is, unfortunately, also common. Mortality rates in hospitalized cases can be relatively high, as exemplified in an analysis of Brooke Army Hospital cases (34%).[17]

In cases of unintentional injuries, analysis has shown that many causes exist. For example, carelessness is a major factor, particularly in stressed families in which chronic neglect or financial, employment, divorce, or other problems are apparent.[17] In some cases, older siblings or inexperienced caretakers who have no knowledge of scalding or safe bathing procedures may be the primary cause. In older-style tubs where separate faucets exist, the practice of running hot water first followed by cold water may lead to excessively high temperatures, or the hot water faucet in a sink may be accidentally selected instead of the cold water faucet. Lack of vigilance, as a factor, is also a contributory cause, as children can quickly get themselves into trouble by turning on faucets[25] or even climbing into tubs, as was elegantly demonstrated in a recent video study of children.[26]

## Spilling of Hot Liquids

The spilling of containers of hot water or beverages is probably the single largest component of scald injuries in children, although such injuries most commonly occur in very young children (6 months to 2 years old).[3,4,8,12,17] Older children tend to acquire a rudimentary appreciation of the hazards of hot liquids and thus are injured less frequently. There is evidence from the last 2 decades that the incidence of scalds due to hot water or beverages has increased substantially,[17] perhaps due to the introduction of the microwave in most households. A large study conducted by Drago[4] of 17237 emergency department–treated burns found that in cases of incidents that involved cookware, hot water accounted for 48.5% of all scalds, while only 3.9% of scalds were accounted for by hot beverages. The 3 most common modes of accident were "reached up and pulled down pot from stove or other elevated surface;" "grabbed, overturned, or spilled pot onto self;" and "pot contents splashed onto child." The most common age at which children were involved in these accidents was 12 months, which suggests that parents and caretakers do not always appreciate the reach of toddlers or their creativity in grabbing pans. In this study, nearly 25% of the scald injuries resulted in hospitalization or transfer to a burn unit, compared to 0.1% of thermal burns, which emphasizes both the larger TBSA affected as well as deeper tissue injury. The head, neck, upper torso, and upper limbs are typically the areas of the body injured, although when a child pulls a pot containing hot water down from a stove, burns to the lower extremities are also common due to the cascade of water. It should be also noted that in all cases, injuries to boys are far more common than to girls.

## Soups and Viscous Foods

Although soups have been a traditional source of scald burns, the popularity of "instant" soups, most of which require heating with water on the stove or in a microwave in the original container, has caused a surge of injuries. For example, Greenhalgh et al[27] reported that soup burns constituted 8% of their pediatric burn admissions, while Ray[28] reported that in a burn trauma unit in Ontario, Canada, 44% of food preparation burns were associated with soup, and Lin et al stated that 32% of scald burns in pediatric patients admitted to a Taiwanese burn center were due to soup.[29] Results from a survey conducted by Palmieri et al[30] indicate that the majority of accidents occurred when adults or siblings were heating the soup with the child in close proximity, in low-income families with multiple children and low educational status. While all parts of the body were involved, injuries to the trunk and upper extremities were more common.[27,30] The mean age of the children in the latter 2 studies was 3.7 to 4.8 years, with no significant difference in regard to gender. Although the burn size was usually small, Greenhalgh et al noted that 13% of patients required grafting procedures, and the authors of both studies observed that long-term scarring was a possibility in highly visible areas.

The problem with the soup containers appears to be that they are tall with a narrow base, making them prone to tipping over. According to the survey of Palmieri et al,[30] 74% of respondents had read the instructions, but instructions are often inconsistent, and many users do not transfer the contents of instant soup packages to safer containers.

## Cooking Oils

Although the least common of accidents in the kitchen, the spilling of hot cooking oil onto a child is perhaps one of the most potentially dangerous situations because the oil is typically much hotter than boiling water, is more viscous (Table 1), and has a higher specific heat compared to water.[31] This is exemplified in a recent study which demonstrated that while hot oil burns constituted only 28% of incidents in which children pulled a container of hot liquid onto themselves, the TBSA burned was slightly higher compared to other hot liquids (18.3% vs 14.4%) and the extent of full-thickness injury was 8.1% vs 4.5%.[32] In addition, 56% of the children with oil burns required skin grafting compared to 34% of children burned by other hot liquids. Furthermore, 22% of the children with oil-caused burns required intensive care, compared to 6% in the other group, and required significantly more ventilatory support (20% vs 6%, $P < .01$), all of which required nearly twice as many days' stay in the hospital.

Relatively small TBSA burns due to oil can be fatal in extremely young patients. For example, a 7-month-old infant with a hot grease scald to the neck and head that constituted an 18% TBSA burn required intubation, and

he quickly developed respiratory distress syndrome with barotrauma that proved fatal secondary to multisystem organ failure.[7]

## PATHOPHYSIOLOGY OF SCALD BURNS

### Mechanics

In general, the severity of the scald injury and its percent TBSA dictate the type of treatment, as do gross features of the burn and the underlying pathophysiology. The older literature refers to first-degree, second-degree, and third-degree burns as a means of differentiating the burn severity, but it is being gradually superseded by a more functional, descriptive approach that includes superficial, partial-thickness, and full-thickness burns.

Superficial burns only involve the outermost layer of the skin—the epidermis. Swelling may occur, but redness, tenderness, and pain without the presence of blisters characterize this type of injury.[11,33] These types of injuries heal in 3 to 7 days and leave no scarring. Superficial partial-thickness burns, common in splash injuries, extend the damage to a portion of the underlying dermis and produce a soft, red, and moist skin with frequent blistering. Although very painful, healing typically takes 2 to 3 weeks, usually without scarring. Deep partial-thickness burns affect most of the dermis, which causes variable destruction of the reticular layer, although it usually leaves the sweat glands and hair follicles intact. The skin color is often a mixture of red and blanched white with slow capillary refill. Thick-walled blisters that frequently rupture are also common. Although most of these deeper injuries will heal in about 3 weeks, because of scarring potential, consideration of grafting must be part of the assessment.

Full-thickness injury that results from immersion-type scald burns or hot oil includes destruction of the entire epidermis and dermis. The burn itself may be colored white, red, brown, or black and have a leathery or charred appearance. There is usually little or no sensation and therefore minimal pain. When the burn extends to muscle and/or bone, which also includes destruction of the subcutaneous tissue and underlying fascia, extensive debridement and grafting will be necessary.

### Temperatures

Scald injuries in children can induce a rapid rise in temperature that, in our experience, can last several days postburn. This can be seen in either a continuous hyperthermic manner or in an intermittent "spiking" fashion. This burn-induced temperature elevation has been studied in animals for many decades in an attempt to understand its cause and to develop countermeasures that will aid the patient. Strome et al,[34] for example, developed a rat model to mimic observation of their patients and found that a 50% TBSA scald burn increased body temperature several degrees and basal metabolism by 12%. However, experiments conducted by Rothwell et al[35] in rats suggest that the rise in metabolic rate is preceded by a fall in temperature, metabolic rate, and oxygen consumption; to date, these effects have not been observed in humans, thus raising the possibility that this model is far from ideal. Nevertheless, these experiments indicate that sympathetic activation of brown adipose tissue (BAT) may be responsible in part for the changes in metabolism. For example, 2-fold increases in BAT activity have been demonstrated in children with major burns compared to noninjured children.[36]

Caldwell et al[37] attempted to discover whether the signal for the increased metabolism was mediated by the afferent vagal fibers and concluded that a "signal" to the central nervous system (CNS) as proposed was not the major pathway. The same group then conducted a series of experiments with indomethacin (a cyclooxygenase inhibitor) in rats and established that the drug could prevent the postburn increase in temperature and that the pyrogenic cytokines responsible were likely to be interleukin 1 alpha (IL-1α) and IL-6, but not IL-1β, tumor necrosis factor α, or lipopolysaccharide.[38-40]

## Circulatory and Other Changes

Major changes in the microcirculation occur following severe burn scalds. For example, movement of water, protein, and other plasma constituents into the extracellular spaces quickly occurs due to changes in the net fluid filtration rate, interstitial compliance (a measure of how much pressure is required to change the volume of the interstitial space), and the inability of the lymphatic system to drain the excess fluid from the interstitium.[41] The mechanism of edema development and necessity for fluid resuscitation in these cases is described in more detail in other chapters.

Experiments in which hamsters had dorsal skin flap windows surgically created to monitor the peripheral microvasculatory response following scald burns of 17% to 55% TBSA from boiling water showed that both the incidence and magnitude of the response in tissue adjacent to the burned area was proportional to the percentage TBSA burned.[42] In general, vasomotion was suppressed for several hours postburn. These and other studies[43-45] in which methysergide, a serotinergic receptor blocking agent, was administered following scald burns have led to an understanding that serotonin effectively reduces nutritive flow

to muscle following scald burns by inducing arteriovenous shunting as well as by increasing vascular permeability, which increases edema formation. In addition to interference with protein anabolism, scald burn injuries also activate apoptosis in muscle cells—even in muscle quite distal to the site of injury—via caspases 1, 3, 9, and ceramide.[46] The effects of other sympathomimetic agents, vasoactive entities, and cytokine cascades are also widespread and lead to such diverse problems as liver dysfunction,[47] increases in gut permeability,[48] and migration of neutrophils to the lungs at the expense of the gut.[49]

It should be emphasized that the majority of changes described here only occur with severe burns of 10% to 20% TBSA or more.

## Wound Progression and Stages

There are 4 stages of wound healing: inflammation, destruction, proliferation, and maturation.[11] Inflammation starts within minutes of injury and persists for 2 to 3 days. Heat and redness result from the increased blood flow to the area and activity of mast cells as well as the arrival of macrophages. Edema is common in more severe injuries. Each burned area is associated with 3 distinct concentric zones.[33] The innermost zone, the zone of coagulation, which was in direct contact with the hot liquid, consists of dead or dying cells, while the zone of stasis surrounding it will typically turn from red to white as the capillary network feeding it collapses and the tissue becomes necrotic due to action of histamine and cytokines as vaso-occlusive agents. The outermost zone of hyperemia, which is red and blanches upon pressure, will usually become redder. In severe cases of scald burns, the associated hemodynamic changes in the body will usually start to disappear by the third day, although some of the metabolic changes are long-term and persist beyond healing (up to 2 years in some studies).

By the end of the third day, the destruction phase usually begins, which lasts some 2 to 5 days. During this process, cellular debris and bacteria are removed by macrophages and polymorphs, aided by numerous enzymes, such as the metalloproteinases. Unless there are indications to the contrary, minor wounds should be undisturbed until this phase has ended, as the presence of macrophages triggers the development of fibroblasts and the production of collagen fibers.

The third phase, proliferation, can last up to 3 weeks and is the process in which epithelialization takes place, the migration of epithelial cells from the wound margins toward its center. Epithelialization is dependent on angiogenesis, the creation of new blood vessels. The network of new blood vessels and collagen creates a matrix in which granulation tissue can start to grow. The maturation phase begins as soon as the wound is covered by epithelial cells and continues for several weeks or months until the tensile strength of the new skin is nearly equal to that of the surrounding (noninjured) skin. During this phase the red appearance of the skin will gradually diminish.

The first 3 phases can be interrupted by other events, such as infection, and so must be closely monitored. In addition, for deep partial-thickness or full-thickness injuries, debridement, excision, and skin grafting procedures are often needed to ensure proper healing without excessive scar tissue formation.

## TREATING THE SCALD INJURY

### Assessment

Assessment of the scald burn is carried out to (1) estimate the TBSA affected, (2) determine what areas are deep partial-thickness or full-thickness that might require skin grafting, (3) locate and study burned areas that might require specialized treatment, such as fasciotomy because of possible compartment syndrome development, (4) determine the agent that caused the burn, (5) determine any other burn-related injuries that require immediate treatment, and (6) determine the presence of other coexisting injuries or conditions that might interfere with treatment.

The American Burn Association defines 3 classifications of burns: major, moderate, and minor.[50] Major burn injury is categorized as > 20% TBSA (partial-thickness burns), full-thickness burns exceeding 10% TBSA, and burns involving the face, ears, eyes, hands, feet, or perineum that have the potential to cause functional impairment and/or disfigurement. The moderate burn category includes partial-thickness burns 10% to 20% TBSA or full-thickness burns involving 2% to 10% TBSA that do not include the problems specified in the major burn category. A minor burn injury is categorized as involving partial-thickness burns < 10% TBSA or full-thickness burns of < 2% TBSA with no high-risk potential for functional impairment or disfigurement. In general, major burns should be treated in a specialized burn center, while moderate burns can initially be treated in a local hospital with an optional transfer to a burn unit at a later date. Most minor burns can be treated on an outpatient basis.

In calculating the burn's percentage TBSA, whether used in initial assessment or later in fluid resuscitation, it is important to be cognizant of the fact that body proportions change in children as they age, as illustrated by modification of the rule of nines for adults. Thus, a child-specific nomogram should be employed when calculating TBSA. Most physicians tend to overestimate burns' percent TBSA in adults,[51] which can significantly affect burn management, although error in this direction is preferable to underestimation of burned surface area.

Although inhalation injuries are rarely associated with scald burns, a few types of injury may present with acute respiratory failure, and these will take priority. When burns are extensive, the most important parameter is to accurately define the TBSA burned and start fluid resuscitation.

## Resuscitation

Because the majority of scald burns are classified as minor, most patients will not require aggressive resuscitation. However, children with a TBSA burn > 10% should be resuscitated.[52] This lower figure, in comparison to the requirements for adults, results in part from higher maintenance volumes due to a higher surface to weight ratio.[4,53,54] Moreover, resuscitation must not be delayed, as sepsis, renal failure, and mortality rise significantly after a delay of 2 hours or more.[55]

Since this subject is covered in more detail in another chapter, only the highlights of resuscitation will be touched upon. There is no consensus regarding the formula for resuscitation since correct use of all formulas leads to successful resuscitation after a period of 24 to 48 hours. In the United States, the Parkland formula is the most popular; it uses lactated Ringer's solution infused at a rate of 4 mL/kg/percent of burn area for the first 24 hours of resuscitation, with one-half administered in the first 8 hours.[56] Maintenance fluids to replace insensible losses of water and salts can be estimated via use of the 4:2:1 approach: 4 mL/kg for the first 10 kg of body weight; 2 mL/kg for the next 11 to 20 kg; and 1 mL/kg for weight above 20 kg. Many burn centers use colloids in varying amounts and at different times during resuscitation to help reverse the burn-associated edema and loss of proteins in the plasma, but there is no universal agreement on whether colloids make a difference. A recent systematic review and meta-analysis indicates that the use of plasma or albumin appears not to substantially increase mortality, but that use of other colloids can adversely affect this parameter.[57] Based upon these findings, the best options appear to be plasma, albumin, or modified gelatin.

The use of advanced goals and endpoints that involve invasive monitoring should be reserved for the most serious cases, as evidence suggests that benefits are limited.[58-61] Classic endpoints for children weighing < 30 kg are still a urine output of 1 mL/kg/h, reiterated at the State of the Science meeting in 2006,[62] although a range of 1.0 to 1.5 mL/kg/h is acceptable for the first 24 hours, provided that under-resuscitation or overresuscitation does not occur.[63] Children approaching 50 kg in weight are better served using adult endpoints.

The investigation of inotropic support in human burn patients has been little studied, but evidence-based reviews suggest that norepinephrine or dopamine can be used to maintain an initial target of mean arterial pressure $\geq$ 65 mm Hg.[64,65] Dobutamine therapy is also useful when cardiac output is low during fluid resuscitation. Likewise, although ketanserin, a serotonin antagonist, has been applied in animals with scald burns with good success[66] and the drug has been studied in wound healing with some positive results, trials in humans with burns are lacking.

## Acute Respiratory Failure

In a few cases, acute respiratory failure will occur following a scald injury. Occasionally this can be attributed to the aspiration of hot liquid in conjunction with upper-body skin injuries and may be apparent from burns in or around the mouth.[67] However, often the development of respiratory complications is insidious and may be related to (1) the result of fluid overresuscitation, (2) decreased pulmonary compliance associated with alveolar flooding, or (3) an aggressive systemic inflammatory response.[68] Under the ages of 5 or 6 years, the risk of airway compromise is higher, as peripheral airway resistance can make up 50% of total airway resistance. Results from a study conducted by Zak et al[68] led the authors to suggest that the presence of 1 or more of 3 risk factors (age < 2 years, burn size > 20% TBSA, and need for large volumes of fluid resuscitation) merit increased vigilance. Blot[69] also suggests that the development of intra-abdominal hypertension may be responsible for progressive respiratory distress; this can be verified by attaching a pressure monitor to the Foley catheter[70] (checking to see if bladder pressure is $\geq$ 30 mm Hg), and if measurements show these values are present, a laparotomy should be immediately considered. Although we may not understand the exact mechanism of respiratory distress in these young children, the important point is that emergency personnel, who may be less familiar with these patients, understand the possibilities and be proactive, ensuring that the patient is sitting upright and considering endotracheal intubation if airway compromise is suspected at any time.

When aggressive ventilatory support is insufficient, early institution of extracorporeal life support (ECLS) can save at least two-thirds of such children before irreversible lung damage occurs.[71] Unfortunately, indications for such treatment are difficult to formulate. Kane et al[71] suggest that peak inspiratory pressure, positive end-expiratory pressure (PEEP), mean arterial pressure, and oxygen index are useful parameters upon which to make a decision. For example, in an analysis of survivors versus nonsurvivors, the pre-ELCS values for these parameters were 52.5 cm $H_2O$ vs 69.5 cm $H_2O$; 7.8 cm $H_2O$ vs 16 cm $H_2O$; 33.1 mm Hg vs 58 mm Hg; and 53.3 mmHg vs 119 mmHg.[71] PEEP is probably the most important parameter to monitor. If ECLS is undertaken, these authors also recommend that excision and autografting or allografting of burn wounds be carried out prior to ECLS to prevent life-threatening bleeding at the margins of the unexcised wounds.

Our own experience in a recent case of a 2-year-old child who sustained a 60% TBSA partial-thickness burn involving bilateral lower extremities and most other parts of the torso and arms following an abusive hot water tub immersion was also positive. After being placed on mechanical ventilation, the child required extracorporeal membrane oxygenation (ECMO) 8 days postburn as a result of progressive hypoxemia. After 9 days of ECMO support and several transfusions of packed red blood cells, platelets, fresh frozen plasma, and factor VII, the child was transferred to standard mechanical ventilation; he then underwent staged grafting with wound closure and has done well with physical therapy.

## Wound Care: Preparation, Infection Prevention, and Dressings

It has long been known that cooling burn wounds immediately after injury is beneficial, although application of ice is detrimental and contraindicated.[72] Recent data suggest, however, that the temperature of the water should be 12°C to 18°C rather than cold (ie, 1-8°C).[73] In addition, while it was thought that a short window of up to 30 minutes postburn existed, newer data indicate that cooling for 30 minutes, even a half hour after injury, can still be beneficial. Further, running water is superior to water sprays or wet towels.[74] Cooling the scald injury quickly improves hemodynamics by decreasing histamine release.[75]

Cleansing the burned areas thoroughly with the goal of infection prevention is important. Warm, sterile, normal saline[76] or a nontoxic surfactant, such as poloxamer 188 applied with a fine-pore cell-size sponge, have been shown to be successful.[33] Although no consensus has been reached regarding blisters overlying partial-thickness burns, one approach is to remove ruptured blisters but aspirate existing blisters and leave the skin as a protective agent if the capillary refill response is present.[77] Blisters can be debrided in order to assess an underlying area, but suitable dressings must be applied. Two trials suggest that infection is far less when blisters are left intact[78] and that more pain is experienced when blisters are deroofed,[79] but these results need to be confirmed before consistent changes are likely to be applied by burn specialists. One advantage to removing blistered tissue is that it allows a proper assessment of the underlying wound bed.

A variety of dressings and topical antibacterial agents are available. For minor burns, soft dressings that maintain a warm, moist environment while allowing exudates to drain into a top nonadherent layer secured with absorbent padding are preferable.[11] These basic dressings follow the principle of moist wound care treatment. Silver sulfadiazine cream is a popular antibacterial agent used for partial-thickness burns, provided the child is not allergic to sulfa drugs; mafenide can be applied if the child is allergic to sulfa or if the wound becomes infected. However, mafenide should be used cautiously, as it can cause metabolic acidosis.[33] Poloxamer 188, which contains bactricin and polymyxin, is another alternative. Topical nystatin can be added to such a gel if fungal colonization starts to occur. Unless infection occurs, for minor partial-thickness burns, silver-containing creams should be discontinued after about 3 days, as there is no strong evidence that they are useful after this period. It should also be noted that silver ions might eventually interfere with wound healing if they have contact with the wound in the final stage of healing, due to possible cytotoxicity issues, although this may be a function of silver ion concentration.[80] Daily dressing changes (or twice-daily dressings with hydrotherapy) are normally instituted until the wound starts to epithelialize.

In high-risk patients or patients that have critical bacterial colonization of burn wounds, the relatively new silver-impregnated dressings present another viable option to prevent or lower bacterial colonization and improve wound healing rates as a result. Both Acticoat and Aquacel Ag have been assessed in a variety of clinical trials, such as randomized control trials, cohort studies, and case-control studies, as well as cost-effectiveness studies.[81-87] Although from an evidence-based standpoint the efficacy of such types of dressings can be classified only as fair, in one particular area their applications are starting to make inroads: allowing children to spend more time at home instead of being hospitalized, and allowing fewer dressing changes, which is both cost-effective and easier on the children and families in terms of quality of life.

Occlusive dressings (air-tight and water-tight) can also be used for superficial partial-thickness burns that are clean, provided they are applied within 24 hours.[34] The 2 most commonly used occlusive dressings are Biobrane and TransCyte (although the latter is no longer commercially available). Biobrane is a biosynthetic dressing composed of a 6-μm-thick silicone membrane bonded to a 360-μm-thick 3-dimensional nylon fabric mesh to which porcine type I collagen has been chemically bound. This construction allows for fibrin ingrowth, causing firm adhesion to the nylon portion until epithelialization occurs, at which point gradual separation occurs.[88] TransCyte uses a similar construction, except human dermal fibroblasts are cultured onto the nylon. Proliferation of the fibroblasts causes secretion of structural proteins and growth factors that assist in developing a 3-dimensional dermal matrix, essentially a synthetic skin.[89] A systematic review of bioengineered skin substitutes suggests that they are at least as efficacious as topical agents/wound dressings or allografts,[90] although the evidence base for this type of technology is hampered by outcome parameters, such as long-term follow-up. Whether these types of more advanced dressings will prove efficacious in deep partial-thickness burns remains to be seen.

Two final items are noteworthy, particularly in the case of patients with moderate or major burns: creams containing polyethylene glycol should be avoided as they are toxic, and latex gloves without powder should be used (the powder should not come into contact with fresh wounds).[34]

## Treating Deeper Wounds

Traditionally, deep partial-thickness and full-thickness burns have been debrided and/or excised to prevent hypertrophic scar formation and wound contraction, as well as to improve the rate of healing. However, when and how to proceed with these procedures is still the subject of vigorous debate. Because of the difficulty in determining burn depth, one school of thought advocates using cultured epidermal allografts without escharectomy to promote rapid regeneration of partial-thickness burns.[91] In fact, a nonrandomized study conducted by Rose et al in 1997,[92] which involved comparing allografts from cadavers versus topical antimicrobial therapy in children with 20% to 75% TBSA partial-thickness burns (undetermined depth), demonstrated that healing time, as well as pain control, was significantly better in the allograft group, thus supporting this approach. On the other hand, the Viennese approach promotes early excision followed by coverage of allogeneic keratinocytes in lieu of autologous skin grafts.[93] A small randomized controlled trial (N = 24) conducted by Desai et al[94] on patients with scald burns who were randomized to early versus late excision suggested a benefit from delayed excision, but this trial was too small to deduce strong conclusions. Irei et al carried out a retrospective study of children under the age of 4 years who were admitted to their burn unit within 3 days of injury. Their results suggested that excision within 5 days or fewer was counterproductive, but that excision should be conducted within 20 days.[95] A more recent study reported by Barett and Herndon indicated that early excision (within 24 hours postburn) was associated with significantly less bacterial colonization ($P = .001$), and infection/graft loss ($P < .05$) compared to delayed excision (6 days postburn).[96] A rabbit model that examined the survival of skin grafts based on excision times varying from 3 hours to 5 days postburn demonstrated that graft survival was inversely associated with the degree of tissue edema in the graft bed, which suggests, based upon their results[97] and a general consideration of the course of edema in burn patients, that the ideal time to excise is in the 1-to-3-day range postburn.

Clearly, the decision to excise early depends on many factors. Although there is some evidence to suggest that relatively early excision (1-3 days postburn) is of benefit, against this must be weighed potential blood loss[98] and resulting trauma in very large wounds. One way to better evaluate potential wounds for early excision is the use of indocyanine green video angiography, which essentially allows better determination of vascular patency instead of 1 or 2 more subjective assessments.[99]

## Avoiding Scars

Although the subject of grafting itself is covered in another chapter, it is worth briefly discussing the subject of avoidance of scars in general. Children are more prone to hypertrophic scars compared to adults,[100] in part because of thinner skin, higher growth rates, and differences in biochemistry compared to adults. Furthermore, a multivariate regression model (703 patients) showed that females, burn sites on the neck and/or upper limbs, multiple surgical procedures, and meshed skin grafts were the principal independent risk factors for postburn pathological scarring.

One cause of scarring is delayed wound healing, which can be addressed through the application of growth factors such as basic fibroblast growth factor (bFGF).[101] However, the modern mainstay of scar prevention is the pressure garment, which has long been known to accentuate the hypoxemic wound environment, resulting in the degeneration of fibroblasts and the favoring of collagen degradation over synthesis.[102] In addition, the induced mechanical compression appears to disrupt the endothelial cell cytoplasm and help disintegrate perivascular satellite cells.[103] Recent data suggest that pressure garments should provide a compression pressure of at least 10 mm Hg, but that garments exerting a pressure of 15 mm Hg may be beneficial when worn for the first month because of an acceleration in scar maturation.[104] One study assessing scar minimization via compression garments using ultrasound measurements concluded that for effective treatment, a period of 18 to 24 months is required.[105] Excessive compression should not be used, as children are more susceptible to pressure ulcers compared to adults.

## Physical Therapy: Splinting and Range of Motion

When wounds are grafted, they must be then immobilized to prevent shear forces from disturbing the grafts. Normally, this is achieved by splinting, assuring that joints are placed at maximum stretch. In fact, many practitioners advocate splinting 24 to 48 hours after injury, during the resuscitation phase, prior to any grafting or excision.[106] In the case of the axilla, this should be 90° to the horizontal with respect to

bedside troughs; for wrists, slightly extended by 10° to 30°; for the metatarsophalangeal joints of the fingers, flexed, 70° to 90°; for interphalangeal joints, fully extended; and 40° to 50° of abduction for the thumb. Using this kind of splinting, with an intensive physiotherapy program instituted 5 days after grafting, the mean abduction obtained for 17 patients with 23 axillary burns was 152°.[107] Another study utilizing this approach of 495 children with 698 acutely burned hands carried out over 10 years demonstrated normal functional results in 97% and 85% of moderate and major burns, respectively.[106] These authors also stress the importance of physiotherapy. For example, even during periods of critical illness, twice-daily range of motion was performed by occupational therapists, except for periods following grafting. Physical therapy, in the form of continuous passive motion followed by progressively active therapy and compression, is increasingly key as different surgeries and grafting procedures continue and burns heal.

Some burn centers use plaster casts instead of splints for severe cases. For example, in extensive below-the-knee burns, one center showed that this technique produced superior results (more rapid wound closure, fewer therapy treatments, more complete graft take) in comparison to conventional posterior splinting.[108] Another alternative is to use dynamic splints, which are spring-loaded, adjustable devices designed to provide low-load prolonged stretch while patients are asleep or at rest, but which also provide increasing resistance against muscle flexure, thus allowing for exercise. Comparing static versus dynamic splints in burns to the hand, Tan et al reported superior outcomes using the dynamic splints.[109]

## SPECIAL TOPICS

### Safety Awareness and Interventions to Lower Accidental Scalds

Many public awareness campaigns and individual studies that involved surveying selected groups before and after educational interventions have demonstrated that awareness of the potential for hot water to cause scald burns is generally good. However, all these studies have also noted that such awareness rarely changes behavior, and thus the risk of children being scalded in households does not diminish.[110,111] Most investigators argue that if the temperature of hot water heaters is lowered or suitable safety devices are installed to prevent excessive temperatures at the faucet, this risk will be lowered.

An experiment conducted by Katcher et al in 1989 showed that giving households a means to demonstrate the actual hot water temperature may help make a behavioral modification.[112] Consecutive pediatric clinic clients were randomized to 1 of 2 groups: the first group received an informational pamphlet, a 1-minute discussion on tap water safety, and a baseline questionnaire, while the second group received in addition a liquid crystal thermometer for testing maximum hot water temperature. A follow-up survey 1 month later demonstrated that while approximately 80% of both groups had read the pamphlet, twice as many households in the second group had tested their hot water compared to the first group. However, the difference between the groups regarding the percentages that had lowered the thermostats of their heaters was not significant. An attempt by investigators to take this one step further was to install 20 antiscald devices in the bathroom faucets, which were randomly assigned out of the 80 participating families in a large rental property. Although the devices worked, 9 months later virtually all had been removed due to sediment build-up.[113] These studies demonstrate that more aggressive action is necessary to produce effective results.

The approach taken by most countries and some municipal bodies is to enact legislation mandating lower thermostat settings by either changing factory settings or changing temperature settings of installed water heaters, or both. In one New York City study, no patients were admitted for scald burns in the covered structures during the study period (5 years).[114] However, 281 patients were admitted from structures exempt from the enacted law. This study clearly demonstrated the value of such a law and highlights the fact that injuries will continue to come from households dwelling in exempted structures. In Ontario, Canada, the cost-effectiveness of an intervention that would mandate new maximum hot water settings of 49°C was estimated to save approximately 531 Canadian dollars per scald averted.[115] Sensitivity analyses also demonstrated that the legislation would still be cost-effective through wide ranges of the variables studied. In the United States, some states have been successful in lowering scald injuries through legislation, notably Washington state, which in 1983 mandated preset hot water heater temperatures of 130°F, but much more effort both at the federal and state level will be required to impact injuries due to hot water. For injuries due to other causes—typically accidents in the kitchen—safer container designs would help, but changes in household practice are likely to come only through intensive interventions rather than public awareness campaigns.

## Intentional Scalding and Abuse

Since this subject is thoroughly covered in another chapter, only some simple facts will be highlighted. While the true incidence of intentional scalds remains unknown, on average it appears about 10% of all pediatric burn admission are due to intentional abuse.[116] Abusive burns tend to be more severe, deeper, and larger than accidental burns. Although intentional scalds often present with a pattern that is distinctive, particularly in bath immersions, some patterns may be similar to accidental scalds, and in such cases, investigators should proceed cautiously, checking the parent's or caregiver's story against the evidence presented by the child in the form of type of injury, extent of injury, body locations injured, and depth of burn. Often, inappropriate responses by the parent/caretaker following injury will occur, such as delays in getting the child to the hospital. The typical profile of the abuser is a young, single, uneducated parent with more than 2 children or a parent in a severe marital conflict.

## Use of Clinical Pathway Plans and Documentation

In many hospitals and burn centers, consistent management of the acute phase of the burn injury is a major goal. When properly implemented, clinical pathways or guidelines can help meet that goal by requiring staff members to follow checklists of key items, such as assessment aspects, analgesia considerations, obtaining blood samples, and documenting that they have addressed each point. Thus the pathway not only assists the staff member in covering all the bases but provides an audit trail. Pathways are particularly important in calculating, monitoring, and assessing fluids given for resuscitation, as mistakes can be made when documentation is not used. Further, if a mistake is subsequently discovered, knowing what the mistake was can result in more accurate corrective action.

Implementation of a pediatric scald burn system at a New Zealand hospital in 1999 demonstrated that over the first 6 months of its operation, the percentage of pathway goals achieved rose significantly in many categories. Although 100% compliance was not expected since staff members were free to exercise judgment regarding the guidelines, 70% to 80% compliance was still achieved 12 months later.[117]

Although long-term outcomes are mostly absent in the literature regarding these types of programs, it is hoped that more widespread application will lead to reductions in mortality and increases in favorable healing.

## KEY POINTS

- Scald burns are the most common form of burn injury in children aged 4 years and younger.
- While the majority of scald burns are minor and can be treated on an outpatient basis, some can be severe and life-threatening.

- Hot bath water and cooking oil burns give rise to the most serious injuries.
- Children with a burn > 10% TBSA will require fluid resuscitation.
- Hyperthermia and temperature spikes are common following scald burns, yet the mechanisms responsible for such clinical phenomena are unclear.
- Deep partial-thickness and full-thickness burns will require grafting.
- The treatment of blisters remains controversial.
- Aspirating blisters and minimizing deroofing are one option; active debridement to ensure adequate assessment and treatment is another.
- Many second-generation types of dressing are cost-effective in the treatment of superficial partial-thickness burns, but there is insufficient evidence to know how effective they are in deeper burns.
- The use of growth and healing factors is becoming more common, and there is some evidence that they are useful adjunct therapies for serious burns.
- Preventing infection is important at all stages of healing.
- There is evidence that early excision can lead to better outcomes; however, this must be balanced against bleeding complications.
- Splinting is essential prior to or immediately after grafting.

TABLE 1

**Examples of etiological agents, their associated properties, and resultant patterns of injury.**

| Agent | Location | Contact Type | Heat Transfer | Viscosity | Temperature (°C) | Injury Pattern |
|---|---|---|---|---|---|---|
| Hot water | Bath | Immersion | High | Low | 45–65 | Trunk/both legs & feet or both arms |
| Hot beverages | Kitchen/living rooms | Spill | High | Low | 45–95 | Face, torso, and extremities |
| Hot soups | Kitchen/living rooms | Spill | Medium | Medium | 45–95 | Mainly upper extremities/ anterior trunk |
| Boiling cooking oils | Kitchen | Spill | Medium | Medium | 150–200 | Face, upper torso, & extremities |
| Hot viscous foods | Kitchen/living rooms | Spill | Low | High | 45–95 | Upper body |

# REFERENCES

1. Yamamoto LG, Wiebe RA, Matthews WJ Jr. A one-year prospective ED cohort of pediatric burns: a proposal for standardizing scald burns. *Pediatr Emerg Care*. 1991; **7**: 80–84.

2. Wibbenmeyer LA, Amelon MJ, Torner JC, et al. Population-based assessment of burn injury in southern Iowa: identification of children and young-adult at-risk groups and behaviors. *J Burn Care Rehabil*. 2003; **24**: 192–202.

3. Warrington SA, Wright CM. Accidents and resulting injuries in premobile infants: data from the ALSPAC study. *Arch Dis Child*. 2001; **85**: 104–107.

4. Drago DA. Kitchen scalds and thermal burns in children five years and younger. *Pediatrics*. 2005; **115**: 10–16.

5. Silfen R, Chemo-Lotan M, Amir A, Hauben DJ. Profile of the pediatric burn patient at the Schneider Children's Medical Center of Israel. *Isr Med Assoc J*. 2000; **2**: 138–141.

6. Thombs BD, Singh VA, Milner SM. Children under 4 years are at greater risk of mortality following acute burn injury: evidence from a national sample of 12,902 pediatric admissions. *Shock*. 2006; **26**: 358–352.

7. Morrow SE, Smith DL, Cairns BA, Howell PD, Nakayama DK, Peterson HD. Etiology and outcome of pediatric burns. *J Pediatr Surg*. 1996; **31**: 329–333.

8. Carlsson A, Udén G, Håkansson A, Karlsson ED. Burn injuries in small children: a population-based study in Sweden. *J Clin Nurs*. 2006; **15**(2): 129–134.

9. Ryan CA, Shankowsky HA, Tredget EE. Profile of the paediatric burn patient in a Canadian burn centre. *Burns*. 1997; **18**: 267–272.

10. Mercier C, Blond MH. Epidemiological survey of childhood burn injuries in France. *Burns*. 1996; **22**: 29–34.

11. Taylor K. The management of minor burns and scalds in children. *Nurs Stand*. 2001; **16**: 45–52, 54.

12. Simon PA, Baron RC. Age as a risk factor for burn injury requiring hospitalization during early childhood. *Arch Pediatr Adolesc Med*. 1994; **148**: 394–397.

13. Bessey PQ, Arons RR, DiMaggio CJ, Yurt RW. The vulnerabilities of age: burns in children and older adults. *Surgery*. 2006; **140**: 705–717.

14. Herndon DN, Dasu MRK, Wolfe RR, Barrow RE. Gene expression profiles and protein balance in skeletal muscle of burned children after β-adrenergic blockage. *Am J Physiol Endocrinol Metab*. 2003; **285**: E783–E789.

15. Arbabi S, Ahrns KS, Wahl WL, et al. Beta-blocker use is associated with improved outcomes in adult burn patients. *J Trauma*. 2004; **56**: 265–271.

16. Przkora R, Jeschke MG, Barrow RE, et al. Metabolic and hormonal changes of severely burned children receiving long-term oxandrolone treatment. *Ann Surg*. 2005; **242**: 384–389.

17. Eadie PA, Williams R, Dickson WA. Thirty-five years of paediatric scalds: are lessons being learned? *Br J Plast Surg*. 1995; **48**: 103–105.

18. Tennant WG, Davison PM. Bath scalds in children in the south-east of Scotland. *J R Coll Surg Edinb*. 1991; **36**: 319–322.

19. Feldman KW, Schaller RT, Feldman JA, McMillon M. Tap water scald burns in children. *Pediatrics*. 1977; **62**: 1–7.

20. Green AR, Fairclough J, Sykes PJ. Epidemiology of burns in childhood. *Burns*. 1984; **10**: 368–371.

21. Smith RW, O'Neill TJ. An analysis into childhood burns. *Burns*. 1984; **11**: 117–124.

22. Klasen HJ, ten Duis HJ. Changing patterns in the causes of scalds in young Dutch children. *Burns*. 1986; **12**: 563–566.

23. Lyngdorf P. Epidemiology of scalds in small children. *Burns*. 1986; **12**: 250–253.

24. Streeton C, Nolan T. Reduction in paediatric burn admissions over 25 years, 1970–94. *Inj Prev*. 1997; **3**: 104–109.

25. Titus MO, Baxter AL, Starling SP. Accidental scald burns in sinks. *Pediatrics*. 2003; **111**: e191–e194.

26. Allasio D, Fischer H. Immersion scald burns and the ability of young children to climb into a bath tub. *Pediatrics*. 2005; **115**: 1419–1421.

27. Greenhalgh DG, Bridges P, Coombs E, et al. Instant cup of soup: design flaws increase risk of burns. *J Burn Care Res*. 2006; **27**: 476–481.

28. Ray JG. Burns in young children: a study of the mechanism of burns in children aged 5 years and under in the Hamilton, Ontario burn unit. *Burns*. 1995; **21**: 463–466.

29. Lin TM, Wang KH, Lai CS, Lin SD. Epidemiology of pediatric burn in southern Taiwan. *Burns*. 2005; **31**: 182–187.

30. Palmieri TL, Alderson TS, Ison D, et al. Pediatric soup scald burn injury: etiology and prevention. *J Burn Care Res*. 2008; **29**: 114–118.

31. Schubert W, Ahrenholz DH, Solem LD. Burns from hot oil and grease: a public health hazard. *J Burn Care Rehabil*. 1990; **11**: 558–562.

32. Allen SR, Kagan RJ. Grease fryers: a significant danger to children. *J Burn Care Rehabil*. 2004; 25; 456–460.

33. Edlich RF. Burns, thermal. eMedicine from WebMD Web site. http: //www.emedicine.com/plastic/TOPIC518.HTM. Published 2007. Accessed April 28, 2008.

34. Strome DR, Aulick LH, Mason AD Jr, Pruitt BA Jr. Thermoregulatory and nonthermoregulatory heat production in burned rats. *J Appl Physiol*. 1986; **61**: 688–693.

35. Rothwell NJ, Little RA, Rose JG. Brown adipose tissue activity and oxygen consumption after scald injury in the rat. *Circ Shock*. 1991; **33**: 33–36.

36. Bianchi A, Bruce J, Cooper AL, et al. Increased brown adipose tissue activity in children with malignant disease. *Horm Metab Res*. 1989; **21**: 640–641.

**37.** Caldwell FT Jr, Graves DB, Wallace BH. Vagotomy modifies but does not eliminate the increase in body temperature following burn injury in rats. *Burns.* 1999; **25:** 295–305.

**38.** Caldwell FT Jr, Graves DB, Wallace BH. Pathogenesis of fever in a rat burn model: the role of cytokines and lipopolysaccharide. *J Burn Care Rehabil.* 1997; **18:** 525–530.

**39.** Caldwell FT Jr, Graves DB, Wallace BH. The effect of indomethacin on the cytokine cascade and body temperature following burn injury in rats. *Burns.* 1999; **25:** 283–294.

**40.** Caldwell FT Jr, Graves DB, Wallace BH. Chronic indomethacin administration blocks increased body temperature after burn injury in rats. *J Burn Care Rehabil.* 1998; **19:** 501–511.

**41.** Demling RH. The burn edema process: current concepts. *J Burn Care Rehabil.* 2005; **26:** 207–227.

**42.** Aggarwal SJ, Diller KR, Blake GK, Baxter CR. Burn-induced alterations in vasoactive function of the peripheral cutaneous microcirculation. *J Burn Care Rehabil.* 1994; **15:** 1–12.

**43.** Ferrara JJ, Westervelt CL, Kukuy EL, et al. Burn edema reduction by methysergide is not due to control of regional vasodilation. *J Surg Res.* 1996; **61:** 11–16.

**44.** Rippe B, Folkow B. Simultaneous measurements of capillary filtration and diffusion capacities during graded infusions of noradrenaline (NA) and 5-hydroxytryptamine (5-HT) into the rat hindquarter vascular bed. *Acta Physiol Scand.* 1980; **109:** 265–273.

**45.** Zhang XJ, Irtun O, Zheng Y, Wolfe RR. Methysergide reduces nonnutritive blood flow in normal and scalded skin. *Am J Physiol Endocrinol Metab.* 2000; **278:** E452–E461.

**46.** Yasuhara S, Kanakubo E, Perez ME, et al. The 1999 Moyer award. Burn injury induces skeletal muscle apoptosis and the activation of caspase pathways in rats. *J Burn Care Rehabil.* 1999; **20:** 462–470.

**47.** Rink RD, Dew KD, Campbell FR. Effects of scald injury on hepatic PO2, blood flow, and ultrastructure in the rat. *Circ Shock.* 1985; **17:** 73–84.

**48.** Ryan CM, Bailey SH, Carter EA, Schoenfeld DA, Tompkins RG. Additive effects of thermal injury and infection on gut permeability. *Arch Surg.* 1994; **129:** 325–328.

**49.** Dries DJ, Lorenz K, Kovacs EJ. Differential neutophil traffic in gut and lung after scald injury. *J Burn Care Rehabil.* 2001; **22:** 203–209.

**50.** National Safety Council. *Accident Facts 1992 Edition.* Chicago, IL: National Safety Council; 1992: 22, 96.

**51.** Nichter LS, Bryant CA, Edlich RF. Efficacy of burned surface area estimates calculated from charts—the need for a computer-based model. *J Trauma.* 1985; **25:** 477–481.

**52.** Warden GD. Burn shock resuscitation. *World J Surg.* 1992; **16:** 16–23.

**53.** Ahrns KS, Harkins DR. Initial resuscitation after burn injury: therapies, strategies, and controversies. *AACN Clin Issues.* 1999; **10:** 46–60.

**54.** Diller KR. Adapting adult scald safety standards to children. *J Burn Care Res.* 2006; **27:** 314–324.

**55.** Barrow RE, Jeschke MG, Herndon DN. Early fluid resuscitation improves outcomes in severely burned children. *Resuscitation.* 2000; **45:** 91–96.

**56.** Merrell SW, Saffle JR, Sullivan JJ, Navar PD, Kravtiz M, Warden GD. Fluid resuscitation in thermally injured children. *Am J Surg.* 1986; **152:** 664–669.

**57.** Perel P, Roberts I. Colloids versus crystalloids for fluid resuscitation in critically ill patients. *Cochrane Database Syst Rev.* 2007; CD000567.

**58.** Connors AF, Speroff T, Dawson NV, et al. The effectiveness of right heart catheterization in the initial care of critically ill patients. *JAMA.* 1996; **276:** 889–897.

**59.** Gattinoni L, Brazzi L, Pelosi P, et al. A trial of goal-oriented hemodynamic therapy in critically ill patients. *N Engl J Med.* 1995; **333:** 1025–1032.

**60.** Ahrns KS. Trends in burn resuscitation: shifting the focus from fluids to adequate endpoint monitoring, edema control, and adjuvant therapies. *Crit Care Nurs Clin North Am.* 2004; **16:** 75–98.

**61.** Pham TN, Ciancio LC, Gibran NS. American Burn Association practice guidelines burn shock resuscitation. *J Burn Care Res.* 2008; **29:** 257–266.

**62.** Greenhalgh DG. Burn resuscitation. *J Burn Care Res.* 2007; **28:** 555–565.

**63.** Graves TA, Cioffi WG, McManus WF, Mason AD, Pruitt BA. Fluid resuscitation of infants and children with massive thermal injury. *J Trauma.* 1988; **28:** 1656–1659.

**64.** Beale RJ, Hollenberg SM, Vincent JL, Parrillo JE. Vasopressor and inotropic support in septic shock: an evidence-based review. *Crit Care Med.* 2004; **32**(11): S455–S465.

**65.** Dellinger RP, Levy MM, Carlet JM, et al. Surviving Sepsis Campaign: international guidelines for management of severe sepsis and septic shock: 2008. *Crit Care Med.* 2008; **36:** 296–327.

**66.** Holliman CJ, Meuleman TR, Larsen KR, et al. The effect of ketanserin, a specific serotonin antagonist, on burn shock hemodynamic parameters in a porcine burn model. *J Trauma.* 1983; **23:** 867–871.

**67.** Sheridan RL. Recognition and management of hot liquid aspiration in children. *Ann Emerg Med.* 1996; **28:** 246–247.

**68.** Zak AL, Harrington DT, Barillo DJ, Lawlor DF, Shirani KZ, Goodwin CW. Acute respiratory failure that complicates the resuscitation of pediatric patients with scald injuries. *J Burn Care Rehabil.* 1999; **20:** 391–399.

**69.** Blot S. Acute respiratory failure that complicates the resuscitation of pediatric patients with scald injuries. *J Burn Care Rehabil.* 2000; **21:** 289–290.

**70.** Greenhalgh DG, Warden GD. The importance of intra-abdominal pressure measurements in burned children. *J Trauma.* 1995; **36:** 685–690.

71. Kane TD, Greenhalgh DG, Warden GD, Goretsky MJ, Ryckman FC, Warner BW. Pediatric burn patients with respiratory failure: predictors of outcome with the use of extracorporeal life support. *J Burn Care Rehabil.* 1999; **20:** 145–150.

72. Sawada Y, Urushidate S, Yotsuyanagi T, Ishita K. Is prolonged and excessive cooling of a scalded wound effective? *Burns.* 1997; **23:** 55–58.

73. Venter TH, Karpelowsky JS, Rode H. Cooling of the burn wound: the ideal temperature of the coolant. *Burns.* 2007; **33:** 917–922.

74. Yuan J, Wu C, Holland AJ, et al. Assessment of cooling on an acute scald burn injury in a porcine model. *J Burn Care Res.* 2007; **28:** 514–520.

75. Boykin JV Jr, Crute SL. Mechanism of burn shock protection after severe scald injury by cold-water treatment. *J Trauma.* 1982; **22:** 859–866.

76. Gowar J, Lawrence J. The incidence, causes and treatment of minor burns. *J Wound Care.* 1995; **4:** 71–74.

77. Sargent R. Management of blisters in the partial-thickness burn: an integrative research review. *J Burn Care Res.* 2006; **27:** 66–81.

78. Swain AH, Azadian BS, Wakeley CJ, et al. Management of blisters in minor burns. *BMJ.* 1987; **295:** 81.

79. Singer AJ, Thode HC Jr, McClain SA. The effects of epidermal debridement of partial-thickness burns on infection and reepithelialisation in swine. *Acad Emerg Med.* 2000; **7:** 114–119.

80. Leaper DJ. Silver dressings: their role in wound management. *Int Wound J.* 2006; **3:** 282–294.

81. Cuttle L, Naidu S, Mill J, Hoskins W, Das K, Kimble RM. A retrospective cohort study of Acticoat versus Silvazine in a paediatric population. *Burns.* 2007; **33:** 701–707.

82. Argirova M, Hadjiski O, Victorova A. Acticoat versus Allevyn as a split-thickness skin graft donor-site dressing: a prospective comparative study. *Ann Plast Surg.* 2007; **59:** 415–422.

83. Huang Y, Li X, Liao Z, et al. A randomized comparative trial between Acticoat and SD-Ag in the treatment of residual burn wounds, including safety analysis. *Burns.* 2007; **33:** 161–166.

84. Peters DA, Verchere C. Healing at home: comparing cohorts of children with medium-sized burns treated as outpatients with in-hospital applied Acticoat to those children treated as inpatients with silver sulfadiazine. *J Burn Care Res.* 2006; **27:** 198–201.

85. Fong J, Wood F, Fowler B. A silver coated dressing reduces the incidence of early burn wound cellulitis and associated costs of inpatient treatment: comparative patient care audits. *Burns.* 2005; **31:** 562–567.

86. Paddock HN, Fabia R, Giles S, Hayes J, Lowell W, Besner GE. A silver impregnated antimicrobial dressing reduces hospital length of stay for pediatric patients with burns. *J Burn Care Res.* 2007; **28:** 409–411.

87. Caruso DM, Foster KN, Blome-Eberwein SA, et al. Randomized clinical study of Hydrofiber dressing with silver or silver sulfadiazine in the management of partial-thickness burns. *J Burn Care Res.* 2006; **27:** 298–309.

88. Ou LF, Lee SY, Chen YC, Yang RS, Tang YW. Use of Biobrane in pediatric scald burns—experience in 106 children. *Burns.* 1998; **24:** 49–53.

89. Noordenbos J, Doré C, Hansbrough JF. Safety and efficacy of TransCyte for the treatment of partial-thickness burns. *J Burn Care Rehabil.* 1999; **20:** 275–281.

90. Pham C, Greenwood J, Cleland H, Woodruff P, Maddern G. Bioengineered skin substitutes for the management of burns: a systematic review. *Burns.* 2007; **33:** 946–957.

91. Soeda J, Inokuchi S, Ueno S, et al. Use of cultured human epidermal allografts for the treatment of extensive partial thickness scald burn in children. *Tokai J Exp Clin Med.* 1993; **18:** 65–70.

92. Rose JK, Desai MH, Mlakar JM, Herndon DN. Allograft is superior to topical antimicrobial therapy in the treatment of partial-thickness scald burns in children. *J Burn Care Rehabil.* 1997; **18:** 338–341.

93. Rab M, Koller R, Ruzicka, et al. Should dermal scald burns in children be covered with autologous skin grafts or with allogeneic cultivated keratinocytes?—"The Viennese concept." *Burns.* 2005; **31:** 578–586.

94. Desai MH, Rutan RL, Herndon DN. Conservative treatment of scald burns is superior to early excision. *J Burn Care Rehabil.* 1991; **12:** 482–484.

95. Irei M, Abston S, Bonds E, Rutan T, Desai M, Herndon DN. The optimal time for excision of scald burns in toddlers. *J Burn Care Rehabil.* 1986; **7:** 508–510.

96. Barett JP, Herndon DN. Effects of burn wound excision on bacterial colonization and invasion. *Plast Reconstr Surg.* 2003; **111:** 744–752.

97. Wang YB, Ogawa Y, Kakudo N, Kusumoto K. Survival and wound contraction of full-thickness skin grafts are associated with the degree of tissue edema of the graft bed in immediate excision and early wound excision and grafting in a rabbit model. *J Burn Care Res.* 2007; **28:** 182–186.

98. Ong YS, Samuel M, Song C. Meta-analysis of early excision of burns. *Burns.* 2006; **32:** 145–150.

99. Kamolz LP, Andel H, Haslik W, et al. Indocyanine green video angiographies help to identify burns requiring operation. *Burns.* 2003; **29:** 785–791.

100. Herndon DN, Pierre EJ. Treatment of burns. In: O'Neill JA, Rowe MI, Gorsfield JL, et al, eds. *Pediatric Surgery.* 5th ed. St Louis, MO: Mosby; 1998: 343–358.

101. Gangemi EN, Gregori D, Berchialla P, et al. Epidemiology and risk factors for pathologic scarring after burn wounds. *Arch Facial Plast Surg.* 2008; **10:** 93–102.

102. Kischer CW, Shetlar MR, Shetlar CL. Alteration of hypertrophic scars induced by mechanical pressure. *Arch Dermatol.* 1975; **111:** 60–64.

103. Kischer CW, Shetlar MR. Microvasculature in hypertrophic scars and the effects of pressure. *J Trauma.* 1979; **19:** 757–764.

104. Van den Kerckhove E, Stappaerts K, Fieuws S, et al. The assessment of erythema and thickness on burn related scars during pressure garment therapy as a preventive measure for hypertrophic scarring. *Burns*. 2005; **31**: 696–702.

105. Cheng W, Saing H, Zhou H, Han Y, Peh W, Tam PKH. Ultrasound assessment of scald scars in Asian children receiving pressure garment therapy. *J Pediatr Surg*. 2001; **36**: 466–469.

106. Sheridan RL, Baryza MJ, Pessina MA, et al. Acute hand burns in children: management and long-term outcome based on a 10-year experience with 698 injured hands. *Ann Surg*. 1999; **229**: 558–564.

107. Vehmeyer-Heeman M, Lommers B, Van den Kerckhove E, Boeckx W. Axillary burns: extended grafting and early splinting prevents contractures. *J Burn Care Rehabil*. 2005; **26**: 539–542.

108. Ricks NR, Meagher DP Jr. The benefits of plaster casting for lower-extremity burns after grafting in children. *J Burn Care Rehabil*. 1992; **13**: 465–468.

109. Tan O, Atik B, Dogan A, Uslu M, Alpaslan S. Postoperative dynamic extension splinting compared with fixation with Kirschner wires and static splinting in contractures of burned hands: a comparative study of 57 cases in 9 years. *Scand J Plast Reconstr Surg Hand Surg*. 2007; **41**: 197–202.

110. Katcher ML. Prevention of tap water scald burns: evaluation of a multi-media injury control program. *Am J Public Health*. 1987; **77**: 1195–1197.

111. Adams LE, Purdue GF, Hunt JL. Tap-water scald burns: Awareness is not the problem. *J Burn Care Rehabil*. 1991; **12**: 91–95.

112. Katcher ML, Landry GL, Shapiro MM. Liquid-crystal thermometer use in pediatric office counseling about tap water burn prevention. *Pediatrics*. 1989; **83**: 766–771.

113. Fallat ME, Rengers SJ. The effect of education and safety devices on scald burn prevention. *J Trauma*. 1993; **34**: 560–564.

114. Leahy NE, Hyden PJ, Bessey PQ, Rabbitts A, Freudenberg N, Yurt RW. The impact of a legislative intervention to reduce tap water scald burns in an urban community. *J Burn Care Res*. 2007; **28**: 805–810.

115. Han RK, Ungar WJ, Macarthur C. Cost-effectiveness analysis of a proposed public health legislative/educational strategy to reduce tap water scald injuries in children. *Inj Prev*. 2007; **13**: 248–253.

116. Renz BM, Sherman R. Child abuse by scalding. *J Med Assoc Ga*. 1992; **81**: 574–578.

117. Taylor KO, Goudie CM, Muller MJ. Evaluation of a pediatric scald burn clinical pathway. *J Burn Care Rehabil*. 2004; **25**: 256–261.

# CHAPTER TWENTY

# ELECTRICAL BURNS AND RHABDOMYOLYSIS

LENA PERGER, MD

BRADLEY J. PHILLIPS, MD

## INTRODUCTION

Since the beginning of mankind, humans have been exposed to the threat of lightning strikes. Harnessing of electrical energy is a relatively recent invention, which drove the second industrial revolution during the latter part of the 19th century. Since then, electricity has become ubiquitous in our everyday environment and, as a result, electrical injury is now a recognized clinical entity. Most electrical injuries in children occur at home and fortunately do not result in tissue damage, disability, or death. Even though electrical burns account for a minority of pediatric thermal injuries, significant electrical injury can result in substantial morbidity, mortality, and long-term disability. In general, electrical injuries represent 3% to 5% of admissions to burn units. As in other areas of pediatric trauma, prevention is a key factor, and simple safety measures can avert most electrical injuries.

## DEFINITIONS

Electrical injuries are broadly divided into low-voltage (< 1000 V), high-voltage (> 1000 V), and lightning injuries (> 1000000 V). Technically, electrocution is defined as death due to electrical injury.

## SOURCES OF ELECTRICITY

Electric current can either run in one direction (direct current—DC) or oscillate (alternating current—AC). In the 1880s, both forms competed for dominance. Thomas Edison and his company, General Electric, attempted to popularize the use of DC, claiming it was less dangerous. However, the industry shifted towards the use of AC, provided by the Westinghouse Company, after it was originally invented by Nikola Tesla. AC is far superior to DC in terms of range and efficiency of distribution of electrical power.

Electric current is a flow of charged particles (electrons) through a conductor between 2 points of different electric potential. Electric current (I) is measured in amperes, resistance (R) of a conductor in ohms, and difference in electric potential (U) in volts. This relationship is expressed in the equation $I = \Delta U/R$. Thermal energy is released when current passes through the conductor according to Joule's first law, $Q = R^2 \times I \times t$, where $Q$ represents heat and $t$ is time.

In today's world, electricity is produced in power plants and transmitted to substations through power lines, which are made of noninsulated aluminum alloy.[1] After passing through substation transformers, electricity is delivered via subtransmission (33–115 kV) and distribution lines (3.3–25 kV) to consumers in the form of monophasic AC with a frequency of 60 Hz and voltage of 120 V in the US, Canada, and Mexico. High-tension appliances in North America are supplied by outlets delivering 240 V.[1] In Europe, Australia, and Asia, household outlets provide 220 V. Electric power (P) constitutes the product of current and voltage, according to the equation $P = I \times U$. To minimize dissipation of electric power as heat, current in power lines is minimized while voltage is maximized.

Lightning is an instantaneous surge of massive electrical discharge that occurs when the electric potential between a charged storm cloud and the earth overcomes the resistance of intervening air. Lightning acts as an ideal source of direct current because it delivers a constant amount of amperage without being dependent on resistance. The voltage of a lightning strike usually exceeds 1000000 V, with a median peak current of 30000 A. Current rises to a peak in 2 microseconds and then decreases to half in 40 microseconds, with a duration of 1 to 2 milliseconds. Although large amounts of heat can be generated at the interface with a conductor, melting does not occur due to the event's short duration.[1]

## DEMOGRAPHICS

In the general population, electrical injury accounts for the sixth-leading cause of injury-related occupational death.[2] Between 1992 and 2002, 3378 US workers died of electrocution and 46598 were nonfatally injured.[2] In 2002, there were 432 reported deaths by electrocution in the United States, of which 22 occurred in children younger than 15 years old. In children, more than half of the accidents occurred in the home environment, with the remainder happening in the street or a public setting, on a farm, or in industrial environments.[3] Overall, there has been a decrease of 18% in electrocution-related deaths since 1992.[3]

In 2006, there were more than 3500 emergency room visits in the United States for electrical injuries affecting children below 15 years of age. A large majority of these injuries were low voltage, occurred at home, and did not require hospitalization. In toddlers, low-voltage injuries usually occur in the home environment; in older children, outdoor exposure becomes a more important factor. In Canada, 22 electrocution deaths were reported over 5 years (1991–1996) in patients younger than 19 years, with a quarter of them attributed to lightning strikes. The annual death rate from electrocution is much lower in Canada (0.045/100000) than in the United States (0.73/100000) for those 0 to 19 years of age.[4]

## MECHANISMS OF ELECTRICAL INJURY

Electricity can be harmful via several different mechanisms:

- thermal injury
- direct effects of electrical current
- electroporation
- indirect injuries

## Thermal Injury

Heat is generated when electric current passes through a conductor and causes collisions of particles. It can be quantified according to Joule's first law, $Q = R^2 \times I \times t$. Thermal injury results from the effects of heat on tissues and therefore depends on the resistance of tissue, the amount of current, and the time of exposure. Skin acts as an insulator which determines the amount of current passing through internal tissues. Skin resistance is variable depending on its thickness and decreases tremendously if wet. In infants and small children, the skin layer is thinner, with higher water content, and therefore presents less resistance to electrical current. Even if no skin marks are visible, as is the case with low-resistance contact (ie, bathtub electrocution), current can still be lethal. Although the resistance of individual internal tissues differs, they function as a single unit with a total internal resistance between 500 and 1000 Ω.[1] Resistance to electrical current varies among different tissues, with the highest resistance in bones, tendons, and fat and the lowest in nerves, blood, and muscular tissue. This is clinically important because damage to deep muscles and other tissues can be much more severe than is apparent on the skin's surface.[5]

An arc injury is a burn caused when electrical current passes through the air without direct contact between the patient and the source of electricity. It occurs with high-voltage sources (> 1000 V) and can generate temperatures 5000°C or higher. The most important determinants of injury severity are arc power and duration rather than temperature.[1] Resulting burns are usually full thickness with extensive tissue damage.

An unfortunate complication of thermal injury is the development of cataracts. They form due to overheating of lenses by radiant energy produced by high voltages. Cataracts can develop immediately after electrical injury or after a delay of weeks or even years.[6] Occasional cases of spontaneous resolution of cataracts have been reported.[7]

## Direct Effects of Electric Current

Severity of tissue injury depends primarily on the amount of current. However, if contact is prolonged (ie, if a child is unable to release his or her grip), current can increase over time due to perspiration causing a drop in resistance. In these instances, even low-voltage electricity can become very damaging or even deadly.

The effect of electrical current on an individual depends on the type of current along with its wave form. Household AC with a frequency of 60 Hz and 0.5 mA will cause a person to startle. At 5 mA, muscle tetany is induced, preventing release of the source of current. Ventricular fibrillation can result from 50 mA of at least 2 seconds' duration or 500 mA of more than 0.2 seconds' duration. At currents above 1 A, asystole occurs.[1]

Another important determinant of electric injury is the pathway of the current through the victim. Current travels between points of contact connecting the victim to the electrical circuit. Therefore, all organs lying in the path will be affected. Points of contact can be determined from the mechanism of injury and are marked by burns, particularly in high-voltage injuries.

Cell membrane properties change depending on electric potential across the membrane. Small amounts of current in the form of ions are tightly regulated by ionic channels to preserve electrical homeostasis. The function of some cells, most notably muscle fibers and neurons, relies on electrical processes. Action potential is a membrane-based process tightly coupled to muscle contraction and interneuronal conduction. These are therefore most sensitive to externally applied electric current.

A variety of cardiac arrhythmias can result after electrical injury, with the most common including benign nonspecific ST and T wave changes, premature contractions, and sinus tachycardia.[8] Supraventricular tachycardia, atrial fibrillation, heart blocks, bundle branch blocks, and QT prolongation have also been reported.[9] The most serious dysrhythmias are asystole and ventricular fibrillation. Asystole can result from a lightning strike or high-voltage exposure. Ventricular fibrillation is possible after high-voltage or low-voltage exposure. Low-voltage exposure is more dangerous when AC is involved because multiple discharges of oscillating current are more likely to affect the heart in the vulnerable phase of repolarization.[10] In cases of ventricular fibrillation, immediate defibrillation can be life-saving. With asystole, innate automaticity of the myocardium will restore the rhythm in most cases while cardiopulmonary resuscitation is performed. Arrhythmias can also occur due to necrotic foci in the myocardium from thermal or electroporation injury of cardiomyocytes, as well as from ischemia due to vascular spasm/ischemic injury.

Direct current causes muscle contraction only at initial contact and for the second time when the electric circuit is disrupted. In contrast, alternating current causes muscle tetany, which causes inability of the victim to release his or her grip on the source of electricity, prolonging the exposure time. Tetany of respiratory muscles can result in respiratory arrest. In addition, passage of electrical current through the central nervous system can interrupt the automaticity of the respiratory center and result in central apnea. Immediate respiratory support is crucial until spontaneous breathing is restored. Spasm of vascular smooth muscles can cause ischemia in affected organs.

A variety of central and peripheral neurological deficits have been described, most commonly transient loss of consciousness and headaches.[11] Although most neurologic symptoms are temporary, long-lasting or even delayed presentations have been described.[12] Additional reported abnormalities include homonymous hemianopia (visual defect involving either the 2 left or 2 right halves of the visual field in both eyes), seizures, muteness, quadriplegia, hemiplegia, hemiparesis, general motor weakness, urinary incontinence, total body paresthesias, and reflex sympathetic dystrophy.[13] Long-lasting and chronic sequelae such as amyotrophic lateral sclerosis[14] and carpal tunnel syndrome[15] have been attributed to low-voltage exposure in rare cases. Movement disorders, most commonly segmental or focal dystonia, as well as tremors, athetosis, parkinsonism, and segmental myoclonus have all been reported after electrical injury.[12] Exact mechanisms are unclear, but numerous factors are likely involved.[16] Myelin damage, as well as transient deafness and blindness, has been described after lightning strike.[17,18] Vascular injury can result in thrombosis or hemorrhage, with the severity of consequences depending on the body region. Delayed hemorrhage has also been reported.[19] Other complications, such as delayed pneumothorax (without rib fractures) and development of a colonic fistula, both resulting from high-voltage injuries, have been described in children.[20,21]

## Electroporation

Electroporation, or electropermeabilization, results when an electric field pulse is applied to cell membranes, resulting in microperforations in the plasma membrane without generation of heat.[22] Reversible electroporation technology is widely used in laboratories for introduction of viruses, DNA particles, or drugs into cells.[12] Irreversible electroporation results in permanent membrane damage that leads to cellular apoptosis. The extent of tissue damage from electroporation is proportional to the strength of the electrical field and the duration and number of pulses, and is usually disproportionate to the extent of thermal injury. It can occur anywhere along the pathway of electric current, even at sites distant to the point of contact.

## Indirect Injuries

Blunt trauma can result from a fall associated with electric shock, a blast injury, or collision with an object. A comprehensive trauma evaluation is necessary for all high-voltage and lightning injuries as well as for low-voltage injuries associated with a fall, an unclear mechanism, or loss of consciousness.

In addition to electrical burns, flash burns can be caused by ignition of clothing. Spinal and long bone fractures as well as joint (primarily shoulder) dislocations can result from forceful muscle contractions due to electric shock. Therefore, a thorough physical exam and appropriate radiological studies should be performed when a patient presents with blunt trauma, particularly if he or she is unconscious or has distracting injuries. Compartment syndrome can occur in extremities exposed to electric current, where tissue damage is more severe due to the extremities' small diameter and therefore higher current density as compared to the torso.

Brain damage is generally not a direct result of electric current effect on neural tissue. Rather, neurological injury occurs indirectly as a consequence of anoxia due to respiratory and/or cardiac arrest. The possibility of intracranial hemorrhage as a complication of high-voltage injuries should be considered in patients with decreased level of consciousness. Brain death resulting from electrocution is not a contraindication for organ donation.[24] Blast effect can result in rupture of the tympanic membrane as well as hemorrhage in the inner or middle ear. Possible infectious complications of hemorrhage in the auditory system include mastoiditis, brain abscess, sinus thrombosis, and meningitis.[25] Careful examination of the auditory system and documentation of hearing at initial exam is important.

## LIGHTNING STRIKES

Lightning strikes kill approximately a hundred people each year in the United States, with the number of lightning victims remaining stable despite the rise in population. This is likely due to population expansion in urban rather than rural areas, where lightning occurs more often.[1] Common scenarios for victims of lightning are standing under a tree, participating in water sports, working on a farm or in construction, playing golf, or using a telephone or similar device. Approximately 20% to 32% of people struck by lightning die,[26] primarily from sudden cardiac arrest at the scene. Delayed death is less common and usually occurs from sepsis or multiple organ system failure in patients with extensive tissue damage. During the mid-20th century, deaths due to lightning markedly decreased due to the advent of defibrillators as well as other improvements in emergency and critical care medicine.[27] Lightning accounted for 2% of electrical

injuries in a major US children's hospital over 25 years.[8] Lightning injuries are caused not only by electrical current but also by the mechanical force of the blast or a fall or collision with another object. Mechanical force causes blunt trauma, which can be present in 32% of lightning injuries.[28] Three main mechanisms of electrical injury by lightning[26,29] are direct strike, splash or side flash, and ground current or stride potential. Direct strike is the most dangerous type, in which current travels through the victim from head to feet or strikes a metal object a victim is holding. The most common type of lightning injury, however, is splash, which occurs when a nearby object is struck by lightning, with secondary arcing of current between the object and the victim. Stride potential occurs when lightning strikes the ground and the current travels to the person, enters through one foot, and exits through the other foot. This commonly happens when multiple people are injured by one lightning strike.

Current travels by the path of least resistance, which can be either through the body or across a wet body surface, causing a flash-over phenomenon with vaporization of surface water and a blast effect on clothing and shoes.[30] Flash-over injury is more common, although current will travel through the body if a person is grounded (ie, standing in the water).[31]

Quick initiation of advanced cardiac life support (ACLS) protocols with the ABCs of trauma and cardiac care is of crucial importance. No danger to the rescuer is present since the victim is no longer electrically charged. Hence, he or she can be approached and touched immediately. Triage differs from other trauma situations since victims without signs of life should receive help first. Cardiorespiratory arrest in lightning victims is reversible, with successful resuscitation possible in up to 50% of victims. Therefore, resuscitation should be continued for a prolonged period even if initiated after a delay.[26] Indications for endotracheal intubation include decreased level of consciousness as well as seizures. Signs of brain death, such as fixed or dilated pupils or loss of brainstem reflexes, may be transient and warrant aggressive resuscitation. Blunt trauma should be assumed in every lightning victim, and strict spinal precautions should be maintained. In cases of unwitnessed injury, skin changes described by multiple names, such as *arborization*, *keraunographic markings*, *ferning*, and *feathering*, can provide clues characteristic of lightning injury. These unique findings usually spontaneously resolve in a few days. In addition, burns may be noted at points of contact and where metal objects (ie, watches, jewelry) are in contact with skin.

Upon arrival to the hospital, a thorough secondary survey should be performed, looking for signs of blunt trauma and burns. This includes full ophthalmologic and auditory exams, with particular attention to testing of hearing and vision in conscious patients. A detailed baseline neurological exam should be documented. A baseline ECG and chest X-ray should be obtained. Laboratory investigations should include a basic metabolic profile as well as serum creatine kinase (CK) and urine myoglobin levels to determine the presence of rhabdomyolysis. Depending on the severity of the patient's condition, additional studies to consider include arterial blood gas and serum lactate measurements. If the patient is unconscious, uncooperative, or has distracting injuries, radiographs of suspicious extremities are needed to rule out fractures and dislocations. Spinal clearance is performed per institutional protocol for blunt trauma. CT of the head is indicated for prolonged loss of consciousness or external signs of blunt head trauma. An abdominal scan may be necessary if the patient is symptomatic or has extensive abdominal wall burns.

## LOW-VOLTAGE INJURIES

Low-voltage exposure inside the home is the most common source of pediatric electric injury. Toddlers tend to get injured by inserting objects or fingers into outlets, biting an electrical cord, or contacting an exposed wire. Adults and older children usually sustain injuries from the use of electrically powered devices such as computers, audio/video media equipment, and other household appliances. Faulty appliances and electrical installations become an important source of injury in this population. In 2007, the Consumer Product Safety Commission, responsible for overseeing the safety of electrical products and investigation of related injuries, recalled 19 products due to the risk of electrocution or electric shock.

Voltage in household injuries is 120 V to 240 V depending on the country and type of outlet/appliance. For triage and clinical purposes, low-voltage injuries can be divided into minor and major events depending on the amount of current passing through the victim.[32] Tissue injury occurs due to the electrical current, with even low voltage causing severe injuries if resistance is low or contact is prolonged. Examples of major events include water contact (ie, bathtub exposure or contact with wet hands) or prolonged contact due to muscle tetany. All other events are regarded as minor.

When electrical injury to a child is witnessed, the responder's first action should be to safely break the circuit and turn off the source of electricity. Victims of major events are treated along the same lines as patients receiving high-voltage injuries. The vast majority of patients present with minor events. Although these patients may complain of pain, numbness, and tingling, the majority are asymptomatic. On physical exam, sensation may be decreased at

the injury site and superficial or partial-thickness burns may be present.[32] Laboratory investigations are unnecessary in this group of patients since a published series revealed that of the 4% to 5% of patients with elevated CK levels, none had myoglobinuria and laboratory values did not influence clinical management.[8,32] A baseline ECG should be obtained and if abnormal, the patient should be monitored for 24 hours prior to discharge. In asymptomatic patients with a normal ECG, severity of the burn should determine the need for admission. If the home environment is deemed safe with reliable caregivers, the child can be discharged with instructions on wound care after 4 hours of normal cardiac monitoring.[33,34,35,36] Any doubts or concerns regarding the child's home environment or safety should warrant admission for wound care. Close outpatient follow-up is necessary to monitor wound healing and assess for the necessity of delayed surgical procedures for debridement of wound infections and excision of cosmetically bothersome or hypertrophic scars.[8]

## Oral Injuries

Oral electrical injuries are common in toddlers, occurring when a child places an exposed wire into the mouth or bites through the insulation of a protected wire. The oral commissure is involved in most cases, with injury extending into the upper, lower, or both lips. Electrical current can arc through the saliva and generate temperatures up to 3000°F, causing a full-thickness burn. Current may then travel through the body between the mouth and another point of contact where the child is grounded. In most cases, however, oral injuries are localized to the burned area of the mouth with no systemic effects. Fatalities have been noted, with cardiac and/or respiratory arrest reported in 5% of cases in an older series.[37,38,39] Determination of CK and urine myoglobin levels is not required unless exposure was prolonged.[8] Cardiac monitoring is indicated if the initial ECG is abnormal or in cases of loss of consciousness.

Electrical burns appear as a grayish area of necrosis surrounded by a thin rim of erythema due to hyperemia. Initially it is well demarcated, but over several hours the area becomes edematous with irregular margins. Labial incompetence occurs, with drooling and feeding difficulties. Feeding may need to be assisted with a catheter-tipped syringe or with tube feeds via nasal feeding tube. Lesions are mainly painless from nerve damage caused by electrical current. The eschar demarcates over time and usually sloughs 2 weeks after the injury. At that time, there is a risk of bleeding from the labial artery, which can be profuse and occasionally requires a blood transfusion.[8] Healing occurs by secondary intention via epithelialization from the wound edges. Extensive scarring and contracture of the wound can result in disfigurement and microstomia. Developing dental arches and teeth can suffer a variety of long-term consequences, including dental dysplasia, abnormal development of dental arches, malocclusion, and sequestration.[40,41,42,43]

Initial management and treatment begins with gentle cleansing and irrigating the wound bed with saline, then applying topical ointment to keep the area moist. Systemic antibiotic prophylaxis is generally not recommended.[44] Different approaches to surgical treatment include immediate excision within 12 hours of injury,[45] delayed primary reconstruction in 2 to 3 weeks,[46] and delayed reconstruction following complete healing of the wound.[47] Invasive early surgical treatment is now of historical interest only and has not remained part of modern practice. Immediate splinting of the commissure with an intraoral or extraoral appliance can help prevent contractures and possibly obviate the need for surgery. This is the least invasive approach for the young patient and therefore recommended as first-line therapy. Patients should return the day after injury in order to be fitted with an oral splint. Oral appliances can be intraoral or extraoral and need to be

- simple and inexpensive to fabricate, modify, and adjust
- easily inserted with minimal discomfort to the patient
- well tolerated, nontraumatic, and comfortable to wear
- retentive and well adapted to the site of injury
- aesthetically acceptable[44]

A child with an oral electrical burn does not necessarily require admission unless there is a concern about care at home, or in cases of loss of consciousness or an abnormal ECG. Arm splints can be placed to prevent the child from exploration of the burned area.[48] Otherwise, close follow-up is needed in the burn clinic and with a pediatric dentist/prosthodontist.

Parents need to be warned about the possibility of delayed bleeding from the labial artery 2 to 3 weeks after injury. If bleeding does occur, parents are instructed to apply pressure and bring the child to an emergency room. If bleeding does not stop after application of pressure, the labial artery may require ligation. When granulation tissue sets in, the wound can be massaged on a daily basis to keep the scar soft and promote perfusion.[49] Complete healing usually takes in 6 to 12 months. Success of oral splint therapy is usually successful, with reports of up to 100% of patients not requiring surgical reconstruction.[50] Once the wound is healed and the splint removed, the child should be evaluated by a plastic surgeon to assess whether reconstructive surgery is needed.

## HIGH-VOLTAGE INJURIES

High-voltage injuries result from exposure to greater than 1000 V, as is present in power lines. Children are typically injured in their teens, especially by climbing trees or flying a kite into power lines. Pediatric high-voltage injury is more common in developing countries, where climbing of power line posts to collect bird eggs and balcony injury are important risk factors. Balcony injury occurs in urban areas where power lines run in close proximity to residential buildings and children contact them with metal objects during play.[51,52]

Initial evaluation and management in the field and upon arrival to the hospital are the same as for lightning injuries. A fall from a tree or power line post requires a thorough trauma work-up.

Firm evidence-based guidelines for cardiac monitoring in patients who have experienced high-voltage exposure without loss of consciousness or ECG abnormalities do not exist. Monitoring for 24 hours is appropriate since patients are generally admitted for other reasons. All patients with loss of consciousness and/or ECG evidence of dysrhythmia or myocardial ischemia require cardiac monitoring. Since the myocardial (MB) fraction of CK isoenzyme is usually elevated due to high levels of total CK, it is not reliable for diagnosis of myocardial ischemia. A troponin level may be a better alternative, but not enough evidence exists to formulate guidelines at this time.[36]

A major complication of high-voltage injury is compartment syndrome, which requires immediate fasciotomies in affected limb. Serial clinical exams every 4 hours, along with adjunctive use of compartment pressure measurements and duplex sonography, are used for monitoring and early detection of compartment syndrome. There is no evidence that immediate nonselective escharotomy or fasciotomy improves outcome or reduces the number of amputations.[36] Indications for surgical decompression include increasing pain disproportionate to physical findings, progressive neurologic dysfunction, vascular compromise, increased compartment pressures, and systemic deterioration from suspected ongoing myonecrosis. Rates of amputation in high-voltage injuries range from 20% to 40%, including the digits.[36]

Burns on points of contact should be debrided of necrotic tissue and dressed with cadaveric skin or skin substitutes. As with other types of burns, early debridement and coverage is essential, as it decreases the systemic inflammatory and hypermetabolic responses as well as the risk of burn wound sepsis. Multiple debridements over several days after the injury may be necessary if necrosis progresses. Coverage with flaps and skin autografts should be performed once the wound bed is ready.

# Rhabdomyolysis and Fluid Resuscitation

Rhabdomyolysis is necrosis of skeletal muscle cells; in electrical injury it results from heating and electroporation. The common pathophysiological pathway is an increase in intracellular calcium concentration, which causes maximal contraction of myofibrils with resulting depletion of adenosine triphosphate (ATP) stores. Without ATP, more calcium enters the sarcolemma, resulting in failure of the sarcoplasmic reticulum and further increase in intracellular calcium. This causes oxidative-phosphorylation uncoupling and failure to generate ATP. Myofibrils remain in a state of maximal contraction from the lack of ATP. Disintegration of membranes with release of lysosomal enzymes follows, with release of cell contents into the bloodstream. This results in an increase of serum CK, potassium, phosphorus, and myoglobin. Levels of CK peak in 24 hours after an injury and can rise dramatically; destruction of just 2 grams of skeletal muscle can result in a 10-fold increase in CK. Levels subsequently decrease consistent with a half-life of 20 hours. Hyperkalemia can cause cardiac rhythm disturbances, while hyperphosphatemia can exacerbate hypocalcemia.[53] Myoglobin is excreted renally and can therefore precipitate in the glomerular filtrate and cause acute tubular necrosis and renal failure. This is more likely to occur in hypovolemic patients with decreased urine flow and concentrated urine. Myoglobinuria is associated with high-voltage exposure, prehospital cardiac arrest, full-thickness burns, and compartment syndrome.[54] It results in dark brown urine and is suspected when urine is positive for hemoglobin on dipstick but negative for red blood cells. Spectroscopic analysis can confirm the diagnosis. If myoglobinuria is present, aggressive crystalloid fluid resuscitation is initiated to maintain a urine output of at least 2 mL kg/h. Older studies recommended the addition of sodium bicarbonate to IV fluids in order to alkalinize the urine; this has subsequently fallen out of favor. If urine output does not promptly respond to fluids, mannitol can be given starting with an initial dose of 1 g/kg, followed by an infusion 0.5 g/kg/h with monitoring of serum osmolarity and renal function. Mannitol not only acts as an osmotic diuretic but also as a free radical scavenger.

## Wound Care and Rehabilitation

Electrical burns are treated in the same way as other thermal injuries. Early excision and grafting are essential to remove necrotic tissue, which represents a focus of infection, as well as to provide coverage. In addition, removal of burned tissues decreases the systemic inflammatory and hypermetabolic responses. Early coverage with autologous grafts/flaps, cadaveric skin, or biologic skin substitutes provides a barrier to microbial invasion and diminishes evaporative losses. As for all extensive burns, multiple operative procedures may be needed throughout the acute and recovery phases. Rehabilitation focuses on prevention and management of contractures.

Nutritional support is crucial to provide substrates for healing as well as to augment the immune system. Caloric needs in pediatric burn patients may be doubled or tripled compared to baseline and are difficult to reliably calculate. Use of a metabolic cart may aid in obtaining a more accurate assessment of a patient's energy expenditure and guide dietary decisions.

Neurological sequelae of high-voltage exposure can be long lasting and sometimes permanent. Follow-up with a neurologist is necessary for patients with neurological deficits.

Children recovering from a significant electrical injury need to be managed in specialized burn centers by a multidisciplinary team of surgeons, pediatricians, nutritionists, physical therapists, psychologists, and social workers.

## Prevention

As with all other pediatric injuries, prevention of electrical burns is crucial. Most injuries occur at home and result from low-voltage exposure. Outlet protectors should be placed on all unused outlets. However, not all outlet protectors currently on the market are appropriately designed and may offer false security to parents.[55] Manufacturers and consumer safety agencies have yet to agree on industry standards to assure safe and effective outlet protectors that would be age-labeled. An outlet protector should be designed to be difficult and time-consuming for a toddler to remove while easy and quick for an adult to remove. All outlets in the vicinity of water need to have a ground fault circuit interrupter (GFCI), which needs to be tested on a regular basis.

In the toddler age group, factors associated with injuries are sensation seeking, risk taking, and difficulty of behavior management; parental factors are lack of protectiveness and supervision. Boys tend to get injured more often than girls, with injuries occurring in designated play areas and often resulting from misbehavior. On the other hand, girls obtain injuries during play activities in nonplay areas of a home. Most injuries occur in the morning hours and during meal preparation times, when lapses in parental supervision are more common.[56] Successful prevention focuses on both parental and environmentally based strategies. These include controlling access to hazards, increased supervision, and proper education of parents. Child strategies based on education and rule implementation are usually unsuccessful in the toddler age group (2–3 years) and may actually increase the risk of injury at home.[57]

Increased supervision during play time would probably be successful in the prevention of high-voltage injury in older children and teenagers. However, this measure is hard to implement in the general population. This is because high-voltage injuries are so rare to begin with that it is virtually impossible to measure a decrease after the implementation of parental education. Close supervision of power lines by utility companies is important to prevent trees growing into and around power lines. Urban planning with sufficient distance between housing and power lines is important in developing countries to help prevent balcony injury.

## CONCLUSION

Electrical injury in children is most commonly seen in toddlers and usually occurs from low-voltage exposure at home. Fortunately, most patients do not require hospital admission and suffer no long-term consequences. Although major low-voltage events, high-voltage exposure, and lightning strikes are uncommon in this age group, they convey significant morbidity and mortality. When presented with patients with these injuries, it is important to remember that internal tissue damage can be much more extensive than external burns would suggest. Significant complications, such as cardiac and neurologic abnormalities, compartment syndrome, and rhabdomyolysis, can occur, and a high index of suspicion is important for early diagnosis and treatment.

Children with significant electrical injuries and tissue damage should be treated in a specialized burn center by a multidisciplinary team and followed long-term to achieve maximal recovery. Prevention is a key factor, with parental education, increased supervision of children, and minimized access to sources of electricity being the most important strategies.

## KEY POINTS

- Electrical injury in children is rare but can result in significant morbidity and long-term disability.
- Lightning strike victims are not electrically charged—immediate cardiopulmonary resuscitation should be initiated as needed.
- Disruption of electric circuit should be the first action in a witnessed electrical exposure.
- Injury to deep tissues can be a lot more extensive than skin burns would suggest.
- A high index of suspicion is needed for early diagnosis and treatment of cardiac and neurologic abnormalities, compartment syndrome, and rhabdomyolysis.
- Early excision and grafting are the cornerstone of local treatment, along the same lines as for thermal burns.
- Significant electrical burns should be treated in a specialized burn center by a multidisciplinary team.

# REFERENCES

1. Bernstein T. Electrical injury: electrical engineer's perspective and a historical review. *Ann N Y Acad Sci.* 1994; **720:** 1–10.

2. Cawley JC, Homce GT. *Trends in Electrical Injury, 1992–2002. Proceedings of the IEEE Petroleum and Chemical Industry Committee Annual Conference, Philadelphia, PA, September 11–13, 2006.* Philadelphia: National Institute for Occupational Safety and Health; 2006: 325–338.

3. Chowdhury RT. 2003 electrocutions associated with consumer products, Consumer Product Safety Commission. htp: //www. cpsc.gov/library/foia/foia07/os/2003electrocutions.pdf. 2006.

4. Nguyen BH, MacKay M, Bailey B, Klassen TP. Epidemiology of electrical and lightning related deaths and injuries among Canadian children and youth. *Inj Prev.* 2004; **10**(2): 122–124.

5. Ofer N, Baumeister S, Megerle K, Germann G, Sauerbier M. Current concepts of microvascular reconstruction for limb salvage in electrical burn injuries. *J Plast Reconstr Aesthet Surg.* 2007; **60**(7): 724–730.

6. Saffle JR, Crandall A, Warden GD. Cataracts: a long-term complication of electrical injury. *J Trauma.* 1985; **25:** 17–21.

7. Craig SR. When lightning strikes. Pathophysiology and treatment of lightning injuries. *Postgrad Med.* 1986; **79:** 109–112, 121–124.

8. Zubair M, Bessner GE. Pediatric electrical burns: management strategies. *Burns.* 1997; **23**(5): 413–420.

9. Arrowsmith J, Usgaocar RP, Dickson WA. Electrical injury and the frequency of cardiac complications. *Burns.* 1997; **23**(7–8): 576–578.

10. Geddes LA, Bourland JD, Ford G. The mechanism underlying sudden death from electric shock. *Med Instrum.* 1986; **20:** 303–315.

11. Grube BJ, Heimbach DM, Engrav LH, et al. Neurologic consequences of electrical burns. *J Trauma.* 1990; **30:** 254–258.

12. Lim ECH, Seet RC. Segmental dystonia following electrocution in childhood. *Neurol Sci.* 2007; **28:** 38–41.

13. Baskerville JR, McAninch SA. Focal lingual dystonia, urinary incontinence, and sensory deficits secondary to low voltage electrocution: case report and literature review. *Emerg Med J.* 2002; **19:** 386–371.

14. Sirdofsky MD, Hawley RJ, Manz H. Progressive motor neuron disease associated with electrical injury. *Muscle Nerve.* 1991; **14:** 977–980.

15. Rosenberg DB. Neurologic sequelae of minor electric burns. *Arch Phys Med Rehabil.* 1989; **70:** 914–915.

16. Jankovic J. Post-traumatic movement disorder: central and peripheral mechanisms. *Neurology.* 1994; **44:** 2006–2014.

17. Kleinschmidt-DeMasters BK. Neuropathology of lightning-strike injuries. *Semin Neurol.* 1995; **15:** 323–328.

18. Fish RM. Electric injury, part II: specific injuries. *J Emerg Med.* 2000; **18**(1): 27–34.

19. Chuang SS, Yu CC. Delayed obturator artery rupture: a complication of high-voltage electrical injury. *Burns.* 2003; **29**(4): 395–398.

20. Rijhwani A, Sunil I. Colonic fistula complicating electric burns—a case report. *J Pediatr Surg.* 2003; **38**(8): 1232–1233.

21. Ceber M, Ozturk C, Baghaki S, Cinar C. Pneumothorax due to electrical burn injury. *Emerg Med J.* 2007; **24**(5): 371–372.

22. Bhatt DL, Gaylor DC, Lee RC. Rhabdomyolysis due to pulsed electric fields. *Plast Reconstr Surg.* 1990; **86**(1): 1–11.

23. Isaka Y, Imai E. Electroporation-mediated gene therapy. *Expert Opin Drug Deliv.* 2007; **4**(5): 561–571.

24. Todeschini DP, Maito ED, Maldotti ALM, et al. Brain death caused by electric shock and organ donation in children. *Transplant Proc.* 2007; **39:** 399–400.

25. Somogyi E, Tedeschi CG. Injury by electrical force. In: Eckert WG, Tedeschi CG, Tedeschi LG, eds. *Forensic Medicine: a Study in Trauma and Environmental Hazards.* Philadelphia, PA: WB Saunders; 1977: 661.

26. Blount BW. Lightning injuries. *Am Fam Physician.* 1990; **42**(2): 405–415.

27. Hansen J. National summary of lightning. *Storm Data.* 1989; **31**(12): 11–12.

28. Cooper MA. Lightning injuries. *Emerg Med Clin North Am.* 1983; **1:** 639–641.

29. Fahmy SF, Brinsden MD, Smith J, et al. Lightning: the multisystem group injuries. *J Trauma.* 1999; **46:** 937–940.

30. Jain S, Bandi V. Electrical and lightning injuries. *Crit Care Clin.* 1999; **15:** 319–331.

31. Peters WJ. Lightning injuries. *Can Med Assoc J.* 1983; **128:** 148–150.

32. Garcia CT, Smith GA, Cohen DM, Fernandez K. Electrical injuries in a pediatric emergency department. *Ann Emerg Med.* 1995; **26**(5): 604–608.

33. Cunningham PA. The need for cardiac monitoring after electrical injury. *Med J Aust.* 1991; **154**(11): 765–766.

34. Bailey B, Gaudreault P, Thivierge RL, Turgeon JP. Cardiac monitoring of children with household electrical injuries. *Ann Emerg Med.* 1995; **25**(5): 612–617.

35. Wilson CM, Fatovich DM. Do children need to be monitored after electric shocks? *J Paediatr Child Health.* 1998; **34**(5): 474–476.

36. Arnoldo B, Klein M, Gibran NS. Practice guidelines for the management of electrical injuries. *J Burn Care Res.* 2006; **27**(4): 439–447.

37. Kazanjian VH, Roopenian A. The treatment of lip deformities resulting from electrical burns. *Am J Surg.* 1954; **88:** 884–890.

38. Oeconomopoulos CT. Electrical burns in infancy and early childhood. A review of the current literature. *Am J Dis Child.* 1962; **103:** 35–38.

39. Thomson HG, Juckes AW, Farmer AW. Electrical burns to mouth in children. *Plast Reconstr Surg.* 1965; **35:** 466–477.

40. Alexander WN. Composite dysplasia of a single tooth as a result of electrical burn damage: report of a case. *J Am Dent Assoc.* 1964; **69:** 589–591.

41. Gormley MB. Electrical trauma to the oral cavity. *J Oral Surg.* 1969; **27:** 190–193.

42. Pitts W, Pickrell K. Electrical burns of lips and mouth in infants and children. *Plast Reconstr Surg.* 1969; **44:** 471–479.

43. Dahl E, Fogh-Andersen P. Electric burns of the mouth: long-term effects on the dentition: surgical and orthodontic considerations. *Eur J Orthod.* 1980; **2:** 207–217.

44. Linebaugh ML, Koka S. Oral electrical burns: etiology, histopathology, and prosthodontic treatment. *J Prosthodont.* 1993; **2(2):** 136–141.

45. Hyslop VB. Treatment of electrical burns to the lips. *Plast Reconstr Surg.* 1957; **20:** 315–317.

46. Ortiz-Monasterio F, Facter R. Early definitive treatment of electrical burns of the mouth. *Plast Reconstr Surg.* 1980; **65:** 169–176.

47. Edlich RF, Nichter LS, Morgan RF, et al. Burns of the head and neck. *Otolaryngeal Clin North Am.* 1984; **17:** 361–388.

48. Nichter LS, Morgan RF, Bryant CF, et al. Electric burns of the oral cavity. *Compr Ther.* 1985; **11:** 65–71.

49. Hirschfeld JJ, Assael LA. Conservative management of electric burns to the lips of children. *J Oral Surg.* 1984; **42:** 197–202.

50. Silverglade D. Splinting electrical burns utilizing fixed splint technique: a report of 48 cases. *J Dent Child.* 1983; **50:** 455–458.

51. Celik A, Ergun O, Ozok G. Pediatric electrical injuries: a review of 38 consecutive patients. *J Pediatr Surg.* 2004; **39(8):** 1233–1237.

52. Maghsoudi H, Adyani Y, Ahmadian N. Electrical and lightning injuries. *J Burn Care Res.* 2007; **28(2):** 255–261.

53. Brumback RA, Feedback DL, Leech RW. Rhabdomyolysis following electrical injury. *Semin Neurol.* 1995; **15(4):** 329–334.

54. Rosen CL, Adler JN, Rabban JT, et al. Early predictors of myoglobinuria and acute renal failure following electrical injury. *J Emerg Med.* 1999; **17(5):** 783–789.

55. Ridenour MV. Age appropriateness and safety of electric outlet protectors for children. *Percept Mot Skills.* 1997; **84(2):** 387–392.

56. Morrongiello BA, Ondejko L, Littlejohn A. Understanding toddlers' in-home injuries: I. Context, correlates, and determinants. *J Pediatr Psychol.* 2004; **29(6):** 415–431.

57. Morrongiello BA, Ondejko L, Littlejohn A. Understanding toddlers' in-home injuries: II. Examining parental strategies, and their efficacy, for managing child injury risk. *J Pediatr Psychol.* 2004; **29(6):** 433–446.

# CAUSTIC INGESTIONS

NAVEED U. SAQIB, MD

TISHA K. FUJII, DO

BRADLEY J. PHILLIPS, MD

## INTRODUCTION

A caustic, also referred to as corrosive, is a chemical which is capable of causing injury upon tissue contact. Generally, strong acids having a pH of less than 3.0 and strong alkalis with a pH above 11.0 are of greatest concern in regard to human exposure. Hydrofluoric acid is a unique weak acid which can cause extensive damage due to the formation of a strong alkali in the form of fluoride ions.[1] Caustic agent ingestion may produce corrosive lesions that extend beyond adjacent organs. The spectrum of injuries may range from local oral cavity trauma to extensive upper gastrointestinal or severe tracheal and airway injuries. These injuries have been categorized as oropharyngeal, tracheal and respiratory, esophageal, and upper gastrointestinal for description in this chapter.

The severity of the inflicted injury is related to multiple factors, most notably pH, titratable acid or alkaline reserve, physical state, and tissue contact time, as well as the quantity and concentration of the agent.[2] Subsequent to corrosive ingestion, contact tissue undergoes 3 distinct phases. The clinical presentation depends on the phase of injury. Patients may present with or without symptoms. However, symptoms may not be the best indicator of severity or extent of injury caused by caustic ingestion. Although investigators have attempted to correlate laboratory values with injury severity and outcomes following caustic ingestion, they have not conclusively been shown to predict morbidity or mortality. Radiological studies are not a reliable means to identify the presence of early esophageal injury, but are considered beneficial for surveillance purposes. Rather, early esophagogastroduodenoscopy (EGD) has been advocated to identify the presence of esophageal caustic injury.

Although the most commonly affected body areas from exposure are the face, eyes, and extremities, most fatalities result from aerodigestive injuries. Extensive necrosis of the esophagus frequently leads to perforation and is best managed by resection. Only a small percentage of caustic ingestions lead to esophageal perforation. Caustic-induced esophageal stricture is a major morbid consequence of corrosive ingestion. Recent clinical and basic science research has been aimed at predicting stricture formation, devising invasive and pharmacological interventions to prevent strictures, and developing minimally invasive procedures to treat established strictures.

Little controversy exists in the management of dermal and ocular caustic exposure injuries. Immediate water irrigation at the site of exposure followed by routine burn care with analgesia, fluids, and electrolyte replacement is considered the standard of care.[2] Because of the high morbidity and mortality associated with aerodigestive tract injuries from caustic exposure, as well as the current controversy regarding appropriate management, this chapter will review the pertinent factors involved in caustic injuries, with particular attention to the pediatric population.

## EPIDEMIOLOGY

Accidental ingestion of caustic materials is common in children. In teenagers and adults, however, ingestion is usually deliberate, during suicidal attempts. The exact incidence of accidental and suicidal caustic ingestions is unclear because the percentage of ingestions reported to poison centers is unknown.[1,3] Toxic Exposure Surveillance System (TESS) data are compiled by the American Association of Poison Control Centers[4] (AAPCC) on behalf of US poison centers. The cumulative AAPCC database now contains 43.4 million human poison exposure cases since 1983.[4] In 2004, AAPCC reported 2438644 human exposure cases in serving a population of 293.7 million (0.83%) in the United States.[1] Consequently, the AAPCC reported 2403539 human exposures in serving a population of 299.4 million (0.80%) in 2006.[4] The vast majority of exposures were unintentional (83.4%); suicidal intent was present in 12.8% . Of the reported human exposures, 92% to 93% occurred at a residence. Otherwise, exposures occurred in schools, health care facilities, or public areas most frequently, followed by the workplace and restaurants or food services.[1,3-5] Ingestion was the route of exposure in 77.1% of cases, followed in frequency by dermal, inhalational, and ocular routes. Of the 1221 fatalities in 2006, the inhalational route was predominant (75.3%) as compared to 1883 fatalities in 2004.[1,4]

Children younger than 3 years were involved in 45.3% of cases, and 50.9% occurred in children younger than 6 years. A male predominance is found among exposure victims in patients younger than 13 years, but the sex distribution is reversed in teenagers and adults. Although

responsible for a large proportion of exposures, children younger than 6 years comprised just 2.4% of deaths[4].

The majority of cases reported to poison centers were managed in a non health care facility (72.9%), usually at the site of exposure. Treatment in a health care facility was rendered in 23.5% of cases. The percentage of patients treated in a health care facility varied considerably with age. Only 10.2% of children younger than 6 years and only 13.4% of children between 6 and 12 years were managed in a health care facility as compared to 48.5% of teenagers and 36.7% of adults. Of patients evaluated at a health care facility, 11.9% were treated and released without admission, 3.5% were admitted for critical care, and 2% were admitted to a noncritical ward[4].

## TYPES OF AGENTS

Caustic agents ingested by children which lead to aerodigestive tract injuries can be broadly categorized into (1) household cleaning agents, (2) industrial caustic agents, (3) pharmacological agents, and (4) nonpharmacological agents.

Common household cleaning products such as oven and drain cleaners are strong lyes that contain sodium and potassium hydroxides.[6,7] Laundry detergents and cleaning agents contain sodium phosphate, sodium carbonate, and ammonia.[8-10] Cosmetic products such as hair relaxants also contain caustic agents. They are accidentally ingested commonly in the pediatric population, but appear to be rare causes of severe esophageal injury.[11,12] Common acid household products include toilet cleaners, battery fluids, and muriatic (hydrochloric) acid used in cleaning swimming pools.[8,13,14] Children living on farms may be at particularly high risk for incurring serious burns because of the presence of industrial-strength agents commonly used in this setting.[15] Due to their relatively neutral pH, mild caustic burns have rarely been reported with household bleaches (sodium hypochlorite).[16-19] Industrial-strength or household bleaches in other countries may be more corrosive because of higher concentrations of sodium hypochlorite. Fortunately, industrial bleach exposure in children is low in developed countries.[19]

The 2006 annual report of AAPCC showed considerable differences between pediatric and adult ingestions in regard to the type of substance. In the pediatric population, cosmetic and personal care products were the most commonly ingested substances (13.3%), followed by cleaning substances (9.8%), analgesics (8.4%), topical preparations (7.0%), and pharmacological agents[4]. In comparison, the most frequently ingested substances in adults included analgesics (11.9%), cosmetic/personal care products and cleaning substances (8.9% each), and pharmacological substances (5.9%) .

# PATHOPHYSIOLOGY

Acid and alkaline agents are known to produce tissue damage by different mechanisms. Acids cause coagulation necrosis with eschar formation which may limit tissue penetration and subsequently injury depth.[20] In contrast, alkalis combine with tissue proteins and produce liquefactive necrosis and saponification. Alkalis are thus thought to penetrate the tissues deeper as compared to acids. Absorption of alkaline agents into the circulation leads to microcirculatory thrombosis, impeding flow to already damaged tissue and mucosa.[20,21] Consequently, more serious injuries and complications are expected from alkaline ingestion. However, this distinction is not clinically relevant in the setting of strong acid and alkali ingestions because both are able to rapidly penetrate the esophageal wall, potentially leading to full-thickness esophageal wall necrosis.

Poley et al performed a retrospective review of 179 hospitalized patients with a history of caustic ingestion. Outcomes were compared between 85 patients in the acid ingestion group and 94 in the alkaline ingestion group. Outcomes were found to be less favorable in those ingesting acids compared to alkaline substances in regards to mucosal injury, hospital and ICU stay, systemic complications, esophageal perforation, and mortality. There was no difference in stricture formation. Patients who ingested acids were hospitalized for a longer period of time (9.9 days compared to 7.2 days in patients who ingested alkalis; $P = .01$). Intensive care was required for 44% of the acid-ingested patients as compared to 22% of alkali-ingested patients ($P = .002$). Mucosal damage identified by EGD to the upper gastrointestinal tract was median grade 2 in the acid group versus grade 1 in the alkaline group ($P = .013$). Seventy-one percent of the patients in the acid group had at least grade 2 mucosal damage compared to 49% of patients in the alkali group. The overall mortality rate in the acid group was 14% vs 2% in the alkali group ($P = .003$). Most of the deaths occurred as a consequence of systemic complications such as intractable bleeding, multiorgan failure, sepsis, or a combination of these complications[22].

Strong acids have been associated with a greater frequency of gastric complications in relation to alkaline agents. Kaushik and Bawaet al reported hydrochloric acid as the most common corrosive causing gastric outlet obstruction and diffuse gastric scarring in a retrospective review of all patients with caustic-induced gastric complications.[23] However, there are retrospective studies showing a higher incidence of gastric outlet obstruction in the pediatric population with alkaline ingestion as compared to acid ingestion.[24]

Although coagulative necrosis induced by acids limits the depth of penetration, the inability of gastric secretions to neutralize acidic agents contributes to the onset of lesions and necrosis in the gastric mucosa, duodenum, intestines, and esophagus. This might explain the development of more severe gastric lesions, particularly in the antrum and pyloric regions, after acid ingestion. Suppression of gastric acid production or achlorhydria can lead to extensive gastric necrosis. On the other hand, since alkalis can be partially neutralized by gastric secretions, their exposure to gastric mucosa is reduced.

## Phases of Injury

The lesions caused by lye ingestion occur in 3 phases: acute necrotic phase, ulceration-granulation phase, and cicatrization-scarring phase. Each will be discussed in further detail, beginning with the acute necrotic phase, which is initiated by coagulation of intracellular proteins occurring immediately after caustic exposure. This ultimately leads to cell necrosis, with the surrounding viable tissue consequently developing an intense inflammatory reaction. This acute phase lasts between 1 and 4 days post–caustic injury[2] and is characterized by decreased perfusion of affected tissue and increased breakdown of cellular membranes by lipid peroxidation and hydrolysis at the injury site. Reactive oxygen radicals, especially hydroxyl radicals, react directly with polyunsaturated fatty acids, leading to lipid peroxidation within the cell membranes. Indirectly, reactive oxygen radicals trigger the accumulation of neutrophils within the affected tissue, initiating an inflammatory process that leads to severe mucosal lesions. Generation of reactive oxygen species with subsequent lipid peroxidation has been implicated as contributing to initial esophageal injury and subsequent stricture formation commonly seen after caustic ingestion.[25] During this phase, esophageal injury may begin within minutes after corrosive ingestion and persist for hours thereafter.[26]

Malondialdehyde (MDA) is an end product of lipid peroxidation, and glutathione (GSH) is an important antioxidant substance that augments glutathione peroxidase activity. GSH functions by scavenging free oxygen radicals and protecting thiol groups against oxidation, thereby maintaining cellular integrity. GSH also restores other free radical scavengers and antioxidants to their reduced state.[25,27] Studies have shown significantly higher MDA levels at 24, 48, and 72 hours after caustic injury. Moreover, tissue GSH levels at 48 and 72 hours were found to be significantly lower in injured patients.

The ulceration and granulation phase starts 3 to 5 days after injury and lasts 10 to 12 days. Initially, sloughing of superficial necrotic tissue occurs, leaving an ulcerated, acutely inflamed base.[21] Granulation tissue then fills the defect left by the sloughed mucosa. Around day 4, fibroblasts appear at the injury site, followed by formation of an esophageal mould consisting of dead cells, secretions, and possibly food particles.[21,28] It is during this phase that the esophageal wall is weakest,[7] and perforation may occur if ulceration extends beyond muscle planes.

The third phase begins during the third week post-exposure. During this period, previously formed connective tissue begins to contract, resulting in narrowing of the esophagus. In addition, adhesions between granulating areas results in the formation of pockets and bands. Due to the long-term consequences and morbidity resulting from stricture bands, efforts to reduce stricture formation occur during this phase. Early bougienage dilatation during this phase has been shown to reduce stricture formation.[29] Clinical studies using mitomycin C after dilatation have also reported favorable outcomes.[30-32] The effect of steroids on prevention of caustic esophageal stricture formation has been controversial. More recent studies suggest that systemic corticosteroids are not beneficial for second-degree and third-degree burns of the esophagus.[33] Animal studies have shown that use of a new class of intracellular secondary messengers, sphigosyl-phosphoryl-choline, to prevent stricture formation after caustic ingestion has a wide spectrum of activity in cell growth regulation and signal transduction. Yagmurlu et al concluded that SPC improved healing following caustic ingestion in rats and was effective in preventing caustic esophageal strictures.[34]

## Factors Affecting Severity of Injury

The severity of esophageal and related aerodigestive tract injuries in patients with caustic exposure is related to the following factors:

- pH of the agent/titratable acid or alkali
- duration of contact and concentration of the agent
- acid or alkali
- physical state of the agent
- mode of ingestion: accidental vs intentional
- patient age
- socioeconomic factors

Even with ingestion of small amounts, alkaline agents with a pH of greater than 11.0 are associated with severe burn injuries. Substances with a pH between 9 and 11, such as household detergents, rarely cause serious injury unless large amounts are ingested. In the emergency department, the pH of an ingested agent can be determined by either litmus paper testing (if the agent is available) or by locating its material safety data sheet online at http://www.msdsonline.com. Hoffman et al have reported that a better predictor of esophageal injury is the amount of acid or base required to titrate a chemical's pH to 8.0 (ie, titratable acid or base), rather than the pH of the agent.[35] However, information concerning the titratability of the agent may not be as readily available as other chemical properties, such as pH and concentration.

In a rat model, the effect of caustic soda was studied by Mattos et al in order to demonstrate the interdependence of contact time and concentration of caustic soda in causing caustic esophageal injury. Macroscopic and microscopic evaluations of affected and distant organs were performed after 1 mL of caustic soda at concentrations between 1.83% and 73.3% was applied to the esophagus for 10 to 120 minutes. The investigators found epithelial necrosis at all concentrations: at 7.33%, necrosis involved the submucosa; at 14.66%, damage to the muscular layer and adventitia were noted; at 33.66%, pulmonary parenchymal and tracheal damage were encountered after 10 minutes of exposure. Esophageal perforation was noted to be time dependent, occurring 120 minutes following exposure.[28]

Upper airway injuries are more common with acids. This association may perhaps be related to the bad taste which tends to stimulate gagging, choking, and attempts to expel the substance.[16] Theoretically, the alkaline pH of the epithelium and squamous epithelium of the esophagus helps limit the severity of esophageal injury from acids. However, the esophagus is not spared from such trauma, as severe injuries occur after 6% to 20% of acid ingestions.[17,36-38] Typically, alkali exposure produces more intense esophageal injuries. Acids have been shown to cause more severe gastric complications compared to alkalis, presumably because of the ability of acidic gastric secretions to neutralize alkaline agents.

The physical state of the agent influences the tissue contact time, which in turn has been shown to influence the severity of injury. Solid granules are more likely to adhere to the mucous membranes of the gastrointestinal tract as compared to liquids. This increased adherence results in prolonged duration of contact. Therefore, while solid caustic materials can produce deep burns of the oral cavity and esophagus, they are less likely to reach the stomach. The immediate and severe pain produced by ingestion of these substances may limit the amount ingested and thus reduce the extent of injury. Powdered or granular detergents tend to injure the upper airway, resulting in stridor and epiglottitis, while esophageal injury is less common.[2,17,39,40]

Most ingestions by children are accidental, and the amounts ingested tend to be minimal. However, cases of alkali ingestion as a result of child abuse have been reported.[41] On the other hand, ingestion in adults is often deliberate and related to attempted suicide.[42] In cases of suicide, the amount ingested is larger and related esophageal and gastric injuries are severe.[43] Patient age and socioeconomic factors have been previously discussed (under "Epidemiology" and "Types of Agents").

## SPECTRUM OF INJURIES AND NATURAL HISTORY

Ingestion of caustic agents may produce corrosive lesions that extend beyond adjacent organs of exposure.[44] Patients with caustic ingestion may experience a varied spectrum of injuries, ranging from local oral cavity injury to extensive upper gastrointestinal necrosis. This damage may begin within minutes of ingestion and persist for several hours.

Corrosives produce partial-thickness to deep-thickness burns to the oral mucosa and proximal pharynx. Stricture and scar formation resulting from the healing process can subsequently lead to microstomia, shallow vestibule, ankyloglossia, speech impairments, loss of teeth, impediment of facial expressions, and stricture of salivary ducts.[45]

Aspiration of ingested caustic substances or inhalation of vapors results in injuries to the upper and lower respiratory systems. Reaction to caustic injury by formation of edema may result in upper respiratory obstruction. In a retrospective study of pediatric patients with caustic ingestions and concomitant airway lesions, it was found that 14 of the 33 patients admitted to the hospital had evidence of upper airway lesions on direct laryngoscopy. Three patients required endotracheal intubation for severe airway obstruction, 4 patients had severe dyspnea, and 7 experienced mild respiratory distress.[46] Aspiration pneumonitis and pneumonia as well as acute respiratory distress syndrome (ARDS) have been reported from caustic injuries. Tseng et al retrospectively reviewed the medical records of patients admitted to a tertiary medical center during a 12-year period. Of 370 patients, 15 (4.2%) developed aspiration pneumonia related to intentional ingestion of hydrochloric acid (pH < 1). These patients had a higher incidence of requiring intubation (50% vs 0.3%). Furthermore, aspiration pneumonia was found to significantly increase mortality in acid-injured patients who required emergency abdominal surgery (87.5% vs 32%), as well as in those who did not undergo surgery (28.5% vs 5.1%). Of the 15 patients who developed aspiration pneumonia, 6 survived, of whom 2 later developed laryngeal complications.[47]

Injuries to the esophagus and distal pharynx following caustic ingestion are associated with high morbidity and mortality. Corrosive injuries range from acute esophagitis to esophageal perforation leading to mediastinitis. The incidence of esophageal perforation during the necrotic and ulcerative phases is relatively high. During the cicatrisation or scarring phase, scar formation can lead to the development of esophageal strictures.[50] The incidence of esophageal stricture increases as lesion severity increases.[2] Formation of strictures following a grade 2b burn is as high as 71%, and up to 100% after a grade 3 burn.[51,52] Esophageal stric-

tures can occur randomly throughout the esophagus, and multiple lesions are frequently seen.[53] The extent of narrowing can vary from 1 cm to involvement of the entire length of the esophagus. Intramural pseudodiverticula, often associated with reflux and *Candida* esophagitis, have also been described with corrosive injury. Barrett's esophagus associated with caustic stenosis and stricture has been reported. Andreollo et al reviewed 120 patients with esophageal stenosis from 1981 to 2000. All patients experienced gastroesophageal reflux disease (GERD), and 9 were found to have Barrett's esophagus (7.5%). Three of these 9 patients had disease proximal to the stricture, whereas the other 6 had Barrett's distal to the stricture.[54]

Esophageal carcinoma is a well-known sequela of lye ingestion.[55] The incidence of such cancer in patients with chronic caustic esophageal strictures is reported to be significantly higher than in the general population.[56] In one study, 2 patients had been diagnosed with esophageal carcinoma 25 and 40 years after the corrosive injury occurred.[57] Kim et al reported that during a 12-year period between 1988 and 1999, 54 patients with caustic esophageal strictures were treated at their facility. Esophageal cancer was diagnosed in 7 patients. Due to the high incidence of cicatrix carcinoma, simultaneous resection of the esophagus with reconstruction was recommended for patients with chronic intractable caustic strictures.[58] Often a fatal complication, aortoesophageal fistula after caustic ingestion has been seen, and was diagnosed at autopsy in 3 of the reported cases.[44] Tracheoesophageal fistula is an uncommon clinical entity but has been reported in the literature.[48,49,59-62]

In the stomach, the pylorus and antrum are the most common sites of corrosive injuries.[53,63,64] Corrosive material can cause intense pylorospasm, which results in retention of the substance in the antral area. The resultant fibrosis produces a narrow, nondistensible antrum which resembles carcinoma. Late sequelas of gastric injuries include antral stenosis, hourglass deformity, and a linitis plastica pattern. Currently, there is no evidence to support an increased risk of gastric carcinoma after corrosive gastric injury, unlike esophageal cancer. However, a few case reports of gastric cancer and squamous metaplasia in patients with corrosive injury exist, although the etiological relationship is not well established.[65] Other gastric complications which have been reported include gastric erosions and perforation (during the acute necrotic and ulceration phase), gastric fibrosis (from scar formation during the cicatrisation phase), and gastric outlet obstruction (due to scar and stricture formation in the pylorus). Gastric scarring may be isolated or related with esophageal strictures.[47]

Caustic ingestion may produce injuries and lesions which extend beyond the exposed organs. Acute gastric, jejunal, and ileal necrosis noted on exploratory laparotomy have been reported following caustic ingestion. Guth et al presented 2 cases of liquid caustic ingestion that resulted in gangrene of the duodenum and adjacent colon, along with severe esophageal, gastric, and pancreatic injury.[66] Acute pancreatitis is an unusual complication of corrosive ingestion.[67] Gastrobronchial and gastropericardial fistulas following caustic ingestion have been reported as well.[68,69] Scarring of the lower part of the esophagus from corrosive injury can entrap vagal fibers in the process of fibrosis and lead to motility disorders. Henry et al studied the morphological and functional alterations of the esophagus in rabbits submitted to infusion of caustic soda. Exposure to 4% and 6% sodium hydroxide resulted in lower esophageal sphincter spasm and reduced both the amplitude and number of contractions in the distal esophagus.[70] In patients with a history of lye ingestion, gallbladder dysfunction as a consequence of vagal damage was studied by Khan et al. The study concluded that patients with corrosive-induced strictures, particularly in the distal third of the esophagus, demonstrated increased fasting gallbladder volume and reduced cephalic phase emptying. These findings suggest that impaired vagal cholinergic transmission, possibly due to vagal entrapment during the cicatrisation phase, occurred.[71]

## CLINICAL PRESENTATION

Patients with mild caustic exposure may not present for medical care. Those who do seek medical attention following caustic ingestion may exhibit a wide range of signs and symptoms. However, they can also be asymptomatic. Depending on the severity and phase of injury, patients can present with obstructive airway symptoms, drooling, nausea, vomiting, dysphagia, upper gastrointestinal bleeding, or acute abdomen.

In the acute presentation following caustic ingestion, the patient may complain of oropharyngeal pain due to partial-thickness or deep-thickness burns to the oral mucosa and pharynx. Scar formation in previously injured mucosa can lead to microstomia, speech impairments, dysphagia, difficulty chewing, dry mouth, or oropharyngeal tumors. Direct inspection of the oral cavity and pharynx may indicate ingestion of caustic substances but does not rule out esophageal injury. Conversely, esophageal burns can be present without apparent oral injuries.[72,73]

Laryngeal or epiglottic involvement may be suggested by hoarseness and stridor after caustic ingestion. Other reported complications include laryngeal edema, laryngospasm, pulmonary edema, aspiration pneumonia, and ARDS. Over a 9-year period, 362 tracheostomies in the pediatric population were reviewed. This large series showed an increased frequency of such procedures in cases of subglottic and tracheal stenosis, respiratory papillomatosis, caustic alkali ingestion, and craniofacial syndromes.[74]

The clinical presentation in patients presenting with esophageal injury following caustic ingestion can be subdivided as follows:

1. Asymptomatic

2. Symptomatic
   A. Acute necrotic phase
      i. Pain in the oral cavity
      ii. Substernal pain
      iii. Hypersalivation
      iv. Odynophagia, dysphagia
      v. Fever, nausea
      vi. Hemetemesis
      vii. Respiratory distress
   B. Ulcerative phase
      i. Hemetemesis
   C. Cicatrization phase
      i. Dysphagia
      ii. Heartburn
      iii. Intractable strictures

3. Systemic complications
   A. Dehydration
   B. Renal damage
   C. Multiple organ failure

Prediction of the severity of esophageal injury following ingestion of caustic substances is a challenge for physicians. Although attempts have been made to correlate symptoms and physical findings with the presence and severity of injury, the literature remains inconclusive. Crain et al found that the presence of 2 or more symptoms and signs predicted serious esophageal injury.[75] A retrospective review of 98 pediatric patients under the age of 15 years who were treated for caustic injury between 1976 and 1990 revealed that drooling and dysphagia independently correlated with the presence of esophageal injury.[6] Chen et al reported that the frequency of symptoms and signs in serious esophageal injury was higher compared to patients with low-grade injury. The presence of more than 3 of these correlated with severe injury. Similarly, patients with more severe injury were more inclined to develop future esophageal strictures. Furthermore, the characteristics of the ingested material were associated with esophageal strictures but not with the severity of injury on presentation.[72] Other studies, however, have not supported the above conclusions and suggest that clinical findings do not correlate with the presence or severity of esophageal injury.[36,76] It has been demonstrated that the absence of oropharyngeal injuries does not exclude esophageal or gastric lesions.[77] Gaudreault et al performed a retrospective review of 378 asymptomatic children who were subsequently found to have a 12% incidence of grade 2 esophageal lesions.[36]

Caustic esophageal strictures[50] are a long-term complication of caustic ingestions, which present with dysphagia, malnutrition, and, in severe cases, aversion to oral intake. The incidence of strictures from mild esophagitis after corrosive ingestion has been reported at 5% and reaches 47% in severe esophagitis.[78] The presence of intractable strictures or an acute worsening of dysphagia in patients known to have an existing stricture is concerning for the development of esophageal carcinoma.[53]

Acute gastric perforation can present as peritonitis, whereas acute gastric erosions may lead to upper gastrointestinal bleeding. Gastric fibrosis usually occurs in the antrum because of pooling of acidic agents in this area. Antral strictures present with symptoms of progressive outlet obstruction, which may not become clinically apparent for up to 3 years.[79] Between 1996 and 2001, Tekant et al reported on 6 pediatric patients with caustic-induced gastric outlet obstruction. Two had ingested acidic agents, while the other 4 had ingested alkaline substances. The mean age of patients was 2.9 years (range 1.5 to 3 years). The most common complaint was postprandial vomiting which had begun an average of 3 weeks after the event (range 1-10 weeks). Endoscopic and barium studies revealed 4 patients with pyloric strictures, 1 with an antral stricture, and 1 with an antropyloric stricture.[24]

Ingestion of caustic substances can cause systemic damage which requires treatment in an acute care setting. Disseminated intravascular coagulation (DIC) leading to multiple organ failure occurred in a patient who ingested 60% hydrochloric acid.[80] Such complications can occur due to the direct toxic effects of a substance or from the systemic inflammatory response elicited by aerodigestive tract necrosis. As would be expected, the risk of mortality is even higher in patients exposed to caustic ingestion when such complications arise. Dehydration and renal failure can result from caustic ingestion as well. Renal failure in particular increases mortality in patients. Special care is particularly required when these complications are seen in patients at the extremes of age.

## DIAGNOSTIC MODALITIES

1. Laboratory studies
   A. CBC
   B. Electrolytes, liver function tests
   C. ABG
   D. C-reactive protein

2. Radiological studies
   A. Plain X-rays
   B. Gastrograffin and barium swallow, & upper gastrointestinal (UGI) studies

   C. Esophageal Tc 99m sulfur colloid scintigraphy
   D. CT scan

3. Endoscopic studies
   A. Esophagogastroduodenoscopy (EGD)
   B. Endoscopic ultrasonography (EUS)
   C. Bronchoscopy and laryngoscopy

In severe cases of caustic ingestion, laboratory findings of hemolysis, severe acidosis, DIC, and liver and renal failure have been reported. Although this suggests that laboratory studies may help guide patient management, studies have, however, not shown these values to be able to predict morbidity or mortality. Investigators have attempted to correlate laboratory values with injury severity and outcomes following caustic ingestion.[2] Rigo et al analyzed clinical and endoscopic parameters obtained from patients admitted to their facility between 1982 and 1999. Their multivariate review identified age, ingestion of strong acid, leukocytosis (defined as WBC > 20K at admission), deep gastric ulcers, and gastric necrosis as independent predictors of death after caustic ingestion.[81] In a subsequent study by Chen et al, leukocytosis and C-reactive protein (CRP) levels were not found to be useful parameters for predicting severity of esophageal injury or occurrence of stricture formation in the pediatric population.[73] Acidosis has been implicated with severity of injury following caustic ingestion. The retrospective study by Cheng et al of 129 patients with caustic injury revealed that patients requiring salvage surgery (exploration) had a mean pH of 7.22 +/- 0.12 and base excess of -12 +/- 5.2. Patients who survived surgery were found to have a mean pH of 7.27 +/- 0.09 and base excess of -10.3 +/- 4.7, whereas those who died after surgery had a mean pH of 7.11 +/- 0.11 and base excess of -16.1 +/- 4.6. The mean pH in patients treated conservatively was 7.38 +/- 0.06 with a base excess -1.8 +/- 3.7. Therefore, the authors concluded that an arterial pH lower than 7.22 and base excess below -12.0 indicated severe injury requiring consideration of emergent salvage surgery.[82]

A prospective clinical study was conducted between 1994 and 2000 to evaluate whether there was any biochemical predictor of caustic ingestion and complicated esophageal injury. Seventy-eight children who were admitted to the hospital within 24 hours of caustic ingestion were evaluated. The ingested substance and complaints upon admission were recorded. Groups were created according to the type of ingested agent, such as household bleach (group 1), acid (group 2), or alkali (group 3). Full biochemical analysis, chest X-ray, blood gas estimations, and endoscopy were performed. There were 19, 20, and 39 children in groups 1, 2, and 3, respectively. No sex or age differences were noted among the groups. Esophagogastric injury was not found in the first group of patients. Second-degree injury was present in 12 and 11 children in group 2 and group 3, respectively. Blood pH was decreased in group 1 ($P = .013$) but similar in groups 2 and 3 ($P > .05$); nor did pH differ in patients with or without esophageal injury ($P > .05$). While serum uric acid values were significantly increased in children with an esophageal burn ($P = .001$), phosphorous and alkaline phosphatase levels were significantly decreased in those with esophageal injury ($P = .01$ and $P = .019$, respectively). Other parameters which were similar between the groups ($P > .05$) or between patients with or without complicated esophageal injury ($P > .05$) included serum bicarbonate, potassium, chloride, urea nitrogen, creatinine, glutamine-oxaloacetic transaminase, glutamic pyruvic transaminase, lactic dehydrogenase, calcium, glucose, protein, albumin, and bilirubin levels.[83] The study concluded that a low serum pH is an indicator of ingestion of household bleach and that routine endoscopy may not be necessary in children with normal pH levels following caustic ingestion. Although normal values of pH, uric acid, phosphorous, or alkaline phosphatase do not rule out ingestion of an acid or alkali substance other than bleach, increased uric acid and decreased phosphorus and alkaline phosphatase levels point to the presence of an esophageal injury.[83]

Radiographic studies are not a reliable means to exclude the presence of early esophageal injury. Although they may show features suggestive of perforation, radiological evaluation is most useful in later stages to identify strictures. Patients who present with chest or abdominal pain and peritoneal findings should have corresponding radiographs to determine the presence of intraperitoneal air, pleural effusions, or mediastinal air.[20] Chest X-rays have been useful in children with a history of caustic ingestion in diagnosing aspiration pneumonia by confirming the presence of pulmonary infiltrates. Essentially, we recommend routine chest and abdominal radiographs upon arrival to the hospital. Besides the above-mentioned findings, pneumatosis and benign portal air have also been reported following caustic ingestion.[84]

Further radiographic studies which may be useful in diagnosing and managing caustic injuries include gastrograffin, barium swallow, and an upper gastrointestinal series. Ramasamy et al have stated that if necessary to confirm perforation, a water-soluble agent such as hypaque or gastrograffin should be used, as they are less irritating to the mediastinum and peritoneum compared to barium sulfate. However, some investigators believe that both agents are equally irritating. Nevertheless, these authors recommend barium sulfate as the preferred contrast agent for an anatomically intact but scarred gastrointestinal tract. Furthermore, it has been noted that barium studies may be helpful as a follow-up measure to evaluate complications because they provide better radiographic details compared to water-soluble contrast agents and are also relatively nonirritating to pulmonary tissues if aspirated.[85]

The majority of patients with endoscopic grade 1 and 2a esophageal injuries recover without sequela, while most patients with grade 2b and 3 injuries develop strictures.[51,86] The best method by which to demonstrate the presence, number, length, and location of esophageal strictures (and associated gastric abnormalities) is by a barium contrast study.[53] Ideally, a barium study should be obtained approximately 3 weeks after corrosive injury.

Esophageal scintigraphy using radiolabeled sucralfate has been used to reveal the extent and severity of reflux esophagitis, peptic ulceration, and inflammatory bowel disease. Millar et al evaluated the superiority of sucralfate in diagnosing the presence and extent of esophageal injury by comparing it to endoscopy under anesthesia. Within 24 hours of admission, a sucralfate-labeled scan followed by endoscopy of the upper GI tract with documentation of the extent and grade of injury was performed in all patients (except for 6 patients who underwent scan after endoscopy). Sucralfate was labeled by the direct stannous reduction method, and esophageal transit was studied by recording 120 images at 1 image per second while the patient swallowed 5 mL of labeled sucralfate containing 2 to 3 MBq technetium 99m. Retention of radiolabeled sucralfate was considered abnormal. Of the 22 children, 11 scans showed residual activity in the esophagus, which correlated with endoscopic findings. The other 11 patients had normal esophageal mucosa, although 2 were found to be false positives. In these 2 cases, a repeat scan correlated well with the healing process as assessed endoscopically. The study concluded that technetium 99m sucralfate scanning is an accurate technique for assessing esophageal injury after ingestion of caustic substances. In addition, it may be useful to document healing.[87] However, esophageal scintigraphy is not commonly used.

Due to the poor correlation of signs, symptoms, laboratory findings, and physical examination findings to establish the presence of esophageal injury, early endoscopy (EGD) has been advocated.[22,26,29,37,88-91] Even though data suggest that the decision to perform endoscopy should be made on a case-by-case basis, typical indications include the following:

- visible posterior pharyngeal burn
- stridor
- vomiting
- chest or abdominal pain without radiological evidence of perforation
- inability or refusal of oral intake
- suicide attempt

Clinical and radiological suspicion for a perforated viscous is a contraindication to EGD.[51] In addition, Ramasamy et al emphasize that a third-degree hypopharyngeal burn is also a contraindication for endoscopy.[85] When caustic ingestion occurs, prompt and accurate assessment of the location, extent, and severity of the injury will define optimal treatment and predict long-term outcome.[88] The necessity of early endoscopic evaluation has been challenged due to the previously reported risk of perforation. In order to reduce the danger of this complication, the endoscope should not be passed beyond the proximal esophageal lesion.[85,86,91] As the first endoscopes were rigid, there existed an increased incidence of esophageal perforation. However, flexible EGD has since been established as a safe and reliable tool for assessing esophageal damage for up to 96 hours after caustic ingestion.[51] Zargar et al prospectively evaluated the role of fiberoptic EGD in the management of 81 patients with corrosive ingestion. A total of 381 endoscopic examinations were performed: 88 within 96 hours of corrosive ingestion, 108 between the third and ninth week, and 185 during the follow-up period after bougie dilation of esophageal strictures. The customary endoscopic classification of esophageal burns (grades 0-3) was modified by the authors for prognostic and therapeutic purposes as follows:

## Modified Di Costanzo Classification:

| Grade | Endoscopic findings |
|-------|---------------------|
| Grade 0 | No mucosal injury |
| Grade 1 | Edema, erythema, and/or exudates |
| Grade 2 | Moderate ulceration and/or hemorrhage |
| Grade 3 | Extensive ulceration and/or hemorrhage |

## Zargar's Classification:

| Grade | Endoscopic findings |
|-------|---------------------|
| Grade 0 | Normal esophagus |
| Grade 1 | Mucosal edema and hyperemia |
| Grade 2a | Friability, hemorrhages, erosion, blisters, whitish membranes, exudates, superficial ulcerations |
| Grade 2b | Deep or circumferential ulcers in addition to 2a lesions |
| Grade 3a | Small, scattered areas of necrosis |
| Grade 3b | Extensive esophageal necrosis |

There was no significant correlation between oropharyngeal and upper gastrointestinal tract injury. Early major complications and deaths were confined to patients with

grade 3 burns. All patients with grade 0, 1, and 2a burns recovered without sequela. The majority of patients (71.4%) with grade 2b injury and all survivors with grade 3 injury developed esophageal and/or gastric cicatrisation which required endoscopic or surgical treatment. There were no complications related to endoscopy. The study concluded that early endoscopy is not only a safe, reliable, and accurate diagnostic tool in such patients, but is also of crucial importance in management and prognosis.[51]

EGD has been established as the best diagnostic tool for evaluation of the oropharyngeal and upper gastrointestinal tract. In addition, EGD findings have the best predictive value in determining formation of strictures. In a study to evaluate the diagnostic yield of EGD in children with esophageal disease from caustic injuries, the yield was 86%.[88] Over the past 20 years, dramatic improvements in fiberoptic and video technology, conscious sedation, nursing support, and physicians' experience have enhanced the field of pediatric endoscopy. Diagnostic and therapeutic endoscopic procedures, including EGD, colonoscopy, ligation, variceal sclerotherapy or banding, polypectomy, and percutaneous endoscopic gastrostomy, are performed annually in thousands of infants, children, and adolescents. Pediatric endoscopy has become a valuable tool in the evaluation of gastrointestinal bleeding, dysphagia, severe pain disorders, inflammatory bowel disease, and radiographic abnormalities, as well as for tissue diagnosis, removal of foreign bodies, and other clinical situations.[91]

Genc[92] and Mutaf[51] retrospectively reviewed patients with caustic injury over a span of 28 years after implementing an early EGD protocol at their institution. They reported that patients with grade 1 injury healed spontaneously. Those with grade 2 injuries could be managed conservatively, but repeat EGD was needed to help define when intervention was necessary, as 6 of the 25 patients in this group required operative intervention. Grade 3 injuries ultimately required surgical intervention. One death was reported in their study in a patient with grade 3 injury.[92] A retrospective review of clinical and endoscopic parameters found after caustic ingestion was performed by Rigo et al. A multivariate logistic model identified age (10-year intervals; odds ratio [OR] 2.4; 95% confidence interval 1.4–4.1), ingestion of strong acids (OR 7.9; 1.8–35.3), white blood cell count at admission > or = 20 000 units/mm3 (OR 6.0; 1.3–28), deep gastric ulcers (OR 9.7; 1.4–66.8), and gastric necrosis (OR 20.9; 4.7–91.8). The values of the risk score system devised from the results of the multivariate analysis ranged from 1 to 16. No patient scoring < 10 points died and just one of the patients scoring > 14 points survived. The study identified ingestion of a strong acid, leukocytosis, and deep gastric ulcers or necrosis on EGD as independent predictors of mortality.[81] Poley et al evaluated the prognostic value of

EGD by studying outcomes in acid and alkaline ingestions. The study demonstrated that the grade of mucosal injury identified by EGD possessed the strongest predictive value for the occurrence of gastrointestinal and systemic complications as well as death.[22]

Despite the evidence in favor of EGD, attempts have been made to determine which patients should undergo endoscopy after caustic or corrosive ingestion. Some authors[75,91,93] recommend all patients who have ingested a corrosive agent undergo EGD, given the fact that studies have shown that patients who are asymptomatic may still have significant esophageal or gastric injury. A retrospective study, however, found that all asymptomatic patients who had accidentally ingested caustic substances were unlikely to have clinically significant findings on EGD, whereas those with clinically significant injury (grades 2 and 3) were symptomatic at initial presentation.[90] Another retrospective review of children who had ingested hair relaxant (often containing sodium or lithium hydroxide with a pH > 11) found that despite the presence of lip and oropharyngeal injuries, none who underwent EGD had greater than grade 1 esophageal or gastric injury. In addition, no clinically adverse outcomes were noted. Their findings suggest that in patients with confirmed ingestion of such a substance, careful observation without routine EGD is an acceptable plan of management.[12] Since the conflicting data do not provide a solid set of guidelines regarding this difficult dilemma, the clinician should use his or her best judgment in such situations and strongly consider the indications as previously mentioned. In addition, further guidance concerning endoscopic management of patients who experience caustic injury can be sought from the following recommendations published by Ramasamy et al[85]:

1. Initial endoscopy should be performed as soon as possible, as long as the patient is stable and there is no evidence of perforation.
2. Third-degree burns of the hypopharynx are a contraindication to endoscopy.
3. A complete but careful examination of the esophagus and stomach must be attempted.
4. The endoscope can be safely advanced until a circumferential burn is seen.
5. It is prudent to avoid endoscopy between days 5 to 15, as tissue softening increases the danger of perforation.
6. The risk of procedure-related perforation is low.

High-resolution ultrasonography (endoscopic ultrasonography, or EUS) using a 20-MHz miniprobe (which is smaller than a traditional transesophageal echocardiogram probe) can be performed concomitantly with EGD.[20] While standard endoscopy in patients with corrosive esophagitis can visualize mucosal lesions, the extent of injury involving the deeper layers of the esophagus cannot be determined. A CT scan can grossly depict thickening of the esophageal wall but cannot identify the extent to which various anatomic layers contribute to this finding. This modality, therefore, has limited ability to assess the extent of damage or predict the likelihood of stricture formation.[94] Berhardt et al were the first clinical investigators to evaluate the utility of EUS using a 12-MHz miniprobe for assessment of caustic esophageal injuries. The affected wall sections with macroscopic necrosis consistently displayed a richer echo, broader first layer, and low echo wall edema which had developed beneath the necrosis. Differences existed between the width of the first echo-rich layer and the one below. The indiscriminate nature of single wall layers correlated with intensity of the edema. This study proposed that injury depth could be correctly estimated earlier with EUS compared to EGD and thus help to direct therapy.[95]

EUS allows a detailed study of the esophageal wall, normally displayed as a 5-layered structure, to be seen. The first layer is hyperechogenic and corresponds to the interface between ultrasonographic jelly and mucosa; the second layer is the mucosa, which is hypoechogenic; the third is submucosa (hyperechogenic); the fourth is the muscularis propria (hypoechogenic, but this layer can be separated into an inner circular muscle layer and outer longitudinal muscle layer by intervening hyperechogenic connective tissue); and the fifth layer is the adventitia (hyperechogenic).

EUS carries no additional risks other than those inherent to standard endoscopy.[94] Since EUS requires the use of jelly for ultrasonography, Yamada et al evaluated its use and reported the jelly infusion method.[146] They performed EUS with ultrasonographic jelly in 100 duodenal ulcer lesions and obtained high-resolution images. No adverse effects were noted. The same jelly was studied by Kamijo et al, who dissolved 20 to 40 mL of jelly in water and consequently aspirated as much as possible after obtaining ultrasonographic images. This jelly has a high enough viscosity to remain in the esophagus during imaging, thus constantly providing high-resolution images. Water (70%–80%), glycerin (<15%), and propylene glycol (<15%) comprise the main ingredients of jelly. Every lot of jelly undergoes bacteriological testing to ensure the number of bacteria and fungi is less than 300/g. Furthermore, mass ingestion by animals have demonstrated no adverse effects, such as diarrhea and vomiting, as previously reported.[94]

Kamijo et al devised the following classification of esophageal injury depending on EUS images[94]:

| Grade | Findings |
|-------|----------|
| O | Distinct muscular layers without thickening |
| I | Distinct muscular layers without thickening |
| II | Obscured muscular layers with indistinct margins |
| III | Muscular layers could not be differentiated |

Depending on the most damaged area, lesions were either labeled *a* (partly circumferential) or *b* (completely circumferential). According to the study by Kamijo, stricture formation does not occur with grade O or grade I esophageal injury. Formation of transient strictures was seen in grade IIa injuries. Patients with grade IIIb injuries required repeated bougienage for their strictures.[94] Chiu et al devised the following classification based on EUS images[29]:

| Grade | Findings |
|-------|----------|
| O | Normal sonographic appearance |
| M | Thickening of first and second sonographic layer (mucosa) |
| SM | Involvement of third sonographic layer (submucosa) |
| MP | Involvement of fourth sonographic layer (muscularis propria) |
| SS | Involvement of all layers (includes sub-adventitia/subserosa) |

In order to compare the accuracy of predicting bleeding and stricture formation after caustic ingestion, Chiu et al performed EUS and EGD concurrently in 16 patients. The accuracy of EGD for predicting such occurrences was 100% when grade IIIa injuries were used as an endpoint. For EUS, the highest accuracy was observed in predicting bleeding (75%) and strictures (100%) when EUS grade MP was used. The authors concluded that concomitant EUS along with EGD did not increase the accuracy in predicting early or late complications. These findings are contrary to the theoretical benefit of EUS over EGD.[29] Despite the enhanced visualization of the esophageal wall with EUS, there are limitations with this procedure, which include scarce experience with this modality, limited trained personnel, no added benefit compared to EGD, and a complication rate similar to EGD.

Finally, Ramasamy et al have recommended performing laryngoscopy and bronchoscopy prior to endoscopy since a supraglottic or epiglottic burn with erythema and edema formation may indicate the need for early endotracheal intubation or tracheostomy.[85]

## TREATMENT AND MANAGEMENT

## Initial Evaluation and Management

In the emergency department, any patient suspected of ingesting a caustic substance must be managed in a serious manner. If possible, patients should be asked about the type and quantity of agent ingested. Initial evaluation should focus on the airway and circulatory status, with particular attention to respiratory distress, signs or symptoms of shock, or impending perforation. If any evidence of airway compromise is present, intubation or surgical airway management should be performed without delay. A comprehensive physical examination should be performed, bearing in mind that lack of oropharyngeal involvement or other symptoms does not rule out the possibility of esophageal injury. Although administration of activated charcoal is common after toxic ingestion, this practice is contraindicated after caustic ingestion because of its inability to adsorb such agents and interfere with endoscopic evaluation.[2] Patients with a known history of caustic ingestion require admission to the hospital.

A potential early intervention to consider is pH neutralization by having the patient consume either a weak acid or base. This practice is generally not recommended due to the fear of compounding injury by inducing an exothermic reaction. This concern, however, has not been borne out in animal studies, which demonstrate that intraluminal temperatures do not increase to dangerous levels with neutralization therapy and there is no additive damage from an exothermic reaction.[96,97] Furthermore, Homan and colleagues revealed reduced esophageal injury on a histopathologic level from neutralization therapy in a rat model. Delayed therapy was found to increase esophageal damage.[98] However, there are no data to support this practice in humans, and therefore neutralization therapy is not currently recommended.

In addition to pH neutralization, dilution has been suggested as a possible method of mediating esophageal injury after caustic ingestion. One study in rats investigated the effects of dilution with milk and water after exposing the esophagus to 50% sodium hydroxide. The investigators concluded that this resulted in decreased esophageal injury from alkali exposure.[99] Once again, no clinical data in humans exist to support this practice, and as such it is currently not recommended routinely due to concerns over the potential for emesis, which can obscure EGD evaluation and increase intraluminal pressure, possibly leading to perforation.

Other strategies that have been suggested immediately following corrosive ingestion include enteral or parenteral H2 blockers or proton pump inhibitors. These medications are used to suppress reflux of gastric contents back into the esophagus, thereby minimizing esophageal injury.[93]

However, one study found increased gastric injury when H2 blockers were administered immediately following corrosive ingestion.[21] The authors of this study postulated that this was the result of gastric acid suppression and decreased caustic neutralization; this led them to recommend starting treatment 24 hours after caustic ingestion. At this time, however, human clinical studies demonstrating efficacy of gastric acid suppression are lacking.

Once the patient's condition has been stabilized, further management considerations should include a chest and/or abdominal X-ray, CT scan, laryngoscopy and/or bronchoscopy, and endoscopy. Details regarding these diagnostic tests have been discussed earlier in the chapter. All patients with a completely normal EGD evaluation, and in whom additional hazards have been ruled out, can be safely discharged home. Patients not meeting these criteria should be observed in a hospital setting. Patients with grade 1 or 2a corrosive injuries can usually resume oral intake and be discharged home with antacid therapy within days. On the other hand, patients with grade 2b or 3 corrosive injuries require appropriate fluid resuscitation, nutritional support, and observation in an intensive care unit.

## Considerations and Options for Surgical Intervention

Adult patients who have signs of a perforated viscus or hemodynamic instability may require prompt surgical evaluation and intervention, including exploratory laparotomy or laparoscopy, necrotic tissue resection, or esophagectomy with delayed colonic interposition.[16] Indications for emergent surgery include acute peritonitis, mediastinitis, irreversible shock, severe acidosis, DIC, massive caustic ingestion, or endoscopic grade IIIb injury. Criteria for emergent surgery have been proposed, such as the presence of shock or DIC, the need for hemodialysis, acidosis, and the degree of injury seen on endoscopic evaluation.[100] One study found that following caustic ingestion, an arterial pH < 7.22 or base excess < –12 indicated severe esophageal injury and the need for consideration of emergency surgery.[82] Some suggest that the presence of grade 3 lesions alone mandates immediate exploratory laparoscopy with removal of necrotic tissue because this approach has been associated with improved outcomes and decreased mortality.[20,101,102] These criteria, however, have been reported only in the adult literature. In the pediatric population, these findings have not been studied, and some authors recommend exhausting all resources in order to preserve the child's native esophagus.[103]

Early surgical interventions include esophagectomy alone or with near-total gastrectomy, diversion and jejunostomy, and debridement of adjacent necrotic viscera.

Other options to consider include esophageal stenting, early bougienage, and mitomycin or steroid therapy. Extensive necrosis of the esophagus frequently leads to perforation and is best managed by esophagectomy and diversion or primary reconstruction. When significant gastric involvement is present, the esophagus is nearly always necrotic or severely burned, and total gastrectomy and near-total esophagectomy with diversion are necessary. Some authors have recommended placing an intraluminal esophageal stent in patients who are found to have no operative evidence of esophageal or gastric necrosis.[104] In these patients, a biopsy of the posterior gastric wall should be performed to exclude occult injury. If the histological examination reveals a question of viability, a second-look operation should be performed within 36 hours. If a stent is placed, it should be kept in position for 21 days and removed only after a satisfactory barium esophagogram has been completed. If strictures are seen on the esophagogram, endoscopy with dilatation should be performed.[105-107] In the past, such patients required open laparotomy or thoracotomy. With advances in laparoscopic procedures and reported comparable success rates in the literature, these operations are not performed as frequently.

## Approach to and Management of Esophageal Strictures

The most concerning chronic complications from caustic ingestion include stricture formation and esophageal malignant transformation. Since strictures may develop in 26% to 55% of patients who ingest caustic substances, early interventions are aimed at preventing or minimizing this complication.[101,108] Prevention of stricture formation includes the following: (1) corticosteroids, (2) antibiotics, (3) vitamin E, (4) mitomycin, (5) ketotifen, and (6) phosphatidylcholine.

The most common, and perhaps most controversial, treatments used to prevent stricture formation are parenteral corticosteroids and antibiotics. Corticosteroids are believed to attenuate inflammation, granulation, and fibrous tissue formation.[109] One prospective study found no benefit from systemic steroid administration in children who had ingested caustic substances and that development of strictures was related only to severity of the esophageal injury.[110] A subsequent study found that high doses of methylprednisolone were beneficial in patients who had grade 2b esophageal lesions, with a decreased incidence of stricture formation and reduced need for bougienage after stricture formation.[78] However, some animal studies have demonstrated increased morbidity and mortality associated with corticosteroid use. In addition, a meta-analysis of studies published between 1991 and 2004 ultimately found that corticosteroids are of no benefit and do not significantly decrease the incidence of strictures after corrosive ingestion.[111] Therefore, abandonment of this practice is advocated by many investigators.[112] In conclusion, systemic steroid treatment appears to have no beneficial effect on esophageal wound healing following caustic esophageal burns. There have been no prospective clinical trials evaluating the utility of antibiotics alone. Therefore, their value in the setting of caustic ingestion without signs of concomitant infection, such as peritonitis or mediastinitis, is unknown.

Because of the reactive oxygen species generated after caustic ingestion, investigators have been focusing on antioxidant therapy to prevent formation of esophageal strictures. In a rat model, treatment with vitamin E resulted in decreased collagen synthesis and stricture formation.[25] Additionally, ketotifen, an H1 blocker and mast cell stabilizer, decreased stricture formation and fibrosis when given either orally or intraperitoneally to rats with caustic ingestion.[113] Further, phosphatidylcholine, which stimulates collagenase activity and prevents excessive collagen accumulation, also prevented strictures when given to rats after caustic ingestion.[114] Currently, data regarding antioxidant treatment in humans are lacking. However, further investigation may reveal this unique therapy to be considered in the future.

Other treatment modalities which exist for the prevention and treatment of strictures include bougienage, esophageal stent placement, intralesional corticosteroid injection, and endoscopic dilatation. Instrumentation of the esophagus can lead to perforation, particularly 7 to 21 days after ingestion, during which time the area of injury is weakest as necrotic tissue begins to slough.[93] Treatment of symptomatic esophageal strictures often requires (1) bougienage and dilatation, (2) stent placement, or (3) esophageal reconstruction.

Hypopharyngeal and proximal esophageal strictures have been reported to be repaired with the methods depicted in. Esophageal stents have been shown to reduce the incidence of stricture formation.[104,115,116] In fact, intraluminal esophageal stenting has been used to decrease the likelihood of stricture formation in patients with corrosive esophageal burns for several decades.[117] Fell et al had initially established the experimental foundation for stenting in the treatment of caustic esophageal injury.[118] Reyes and Hill subsequently attempted this technique in cats with considerable success.[119] Based on their study, Wang et al modified the technique of esophageal intraluminal stenting by custom building a stent constructed of medical silicone rubber tubing in the range of 40 to 60 cm in length, with an inside diameter of 1.0 to 1.2 cm and an outside diameter of 1.4 to 1.6 cm. A 12F catheter was affixed to the proximal end of the stent with transfixion ligature to suspend the stent. The distal end of the stent was tailored into the shape of a duck's beak and transfixed with a pair of 10-0 thread (to pull the stent). The procedure began with creation of a midline laparotomy under general anesthesia. The abdominal esophagus, serosal surface of the stomach, and pylorus were then evaluated, especially in patients with ingestion of acidic agents. A pyloroplasty was performed if a pyloric stricture was present; otherwise, a gastrotomy of the anterior gastric wall was created. Three patients with associated gastric injury underwent concomitant pyloroplasty. The proximal end of a nasogastric tube (which had been placed over a guide wire preoperatively) was pulled out of the mouth, and the distal end was brought out of the stomach via the gastrotomy. If the nasogastric tube could not be successfully inserted because of strictures, esophageal dilation was performed under endoscopy. Two strings of 10-0 filament were tied to the distal end of the nasogastric tube, which was then pulled out of the oral cavity in order to free the knot of the 10-0 filament while the other end remained in the abdomen. The nasogastric tube was then removed. One string of the filament from the mouth was connected with the thread attached to the distal end of the stent. The other string of the filament was attached to another nasogastric tube, which was sheathed in the stent earlier in order to guide the stent and prevent its diversion. The stent was then inserted in an antegrade fashion, followed by removal of the nasogastric tube from the oral cavity. The upper end of the stent was positioned 2 cm below the esophageal orifice by direct laryngoscopy. A side core with a diameter larger than half of the stent's circumference was cut at the intragastric wall of the stent. Finally, the catheter that suspended the upper end of the stent was fastened through the nostril. Its lower end was fixed on the abdominal wall and used as a feeding gastrostomy. The esophageal stent remained in place for 4 to 6 months, as most of the scar had stabilized by that period. The stent was subsequently removed without need for anesthesia. Afterwards, the stent was replaced with a piece of thread from the nostril to the gastrostomy orifice and remained for 2 to 3 months in the event of future esophageal stricture development requiring dilatation. Of all patients in this study, 2 with esophageal perforation were able to resume oral intake of solids. Barium swallow studies in all patients showed decreased esophageal peristalsis but no evidence of strictures or perforation. Esophageal manometric examination in 5 patients revealed reduced lower esophageal sphincter pressures, which were still within normal limits. A 24-hour pH study demonstrated DeMeester scores less than 14.72 with no evidence of reflux.[120] Follow-up was completed in all 33 patients, with a median follow-up period of 36.5 months (range 1–60). Twenty-eight patients tolerated a full diet without dysphagia. Of the 5 patients who developed esophageal strictures 2 to 3 months after stent removal, 1 patient responded to esophageal dilatation and the remaining 4 underwent esophageal replacement. The time interval from withdrawal of the stent to esophageal reconstruction ranged from 9 to 44 months (average 18 months). Colonic interposition was performed in 2 patients; the other 2 underwent gastric transposition. Consequently, all 4 patients resumed a normal diet following surgery. No deaths occurred in this series, and overall, excellent results were achieved in patients with corrosive esophageal burns.[104]

Multiple dilatations may be required long term in order to resolve strictures. In addition, some authors advocate intralesional corticosteroid injections as an augmentation to stricture dilation, since use of this technique, though technically difficult, reduces the number of dilatations required for stricture resolution.[121] Tiryaki and colleagues found early, prophylactic dilatation with bougienage to be safe and effective and to reduce the time required for stricture resolution.[108] Surgical intervention may be necessary if these treatments fail, for lengthy or narrow strictures, or in the presence of malignant transformation. Once the acute phase has passed, attention is turned to the prevention and management of strictures. Both antegrade dilation with a Hurst or Maloney bougie and retrograde dilation with a Tucker bougie have provided satisfactory results. Occasionally, the patient is instructed to swallow a string over which metal sippy dilators are passed until an adequate lumen can be obtained for passage of a mercury bougie. In a series of 1079 patients, early dilations initiated during the acute phase produced excellent results in 78% of patients, good results in 13%, and poor results in 2%. Fifty-five patients died during treatment. Of the 333 patients who underwent dilatation when their strictures became symptomatic, only 21% had excellent results, 46% had good results, and 6% had poor results, with 3 deaths.[122]

The length of time in which a surgeon should persist with dilatation is unpredictable. An adequate lumen should be reestablished within 6 months to a year, with progressively longer intervals between dilatations. If during the course of treatment an adequate lumen cannot be established or maintained (ie, smaller bougies must be used), then operative intervention should be considered.

## Indications for Surgical Intervention in Corrosive Stricture Management

1. complete stenosis in which all attempts above and below have failed to establish a lumen
2. marked irregularity and pocketing on barium swallow
3. development of a severe periesophageal reaction or mediastinitis with dilatation
4. fistula formation
5. inability to dilate or maintain the lumen above a 40F bougie or width of patient's thumb
6. patient unable or unwilling to undergo prolonged periods of dilation

Surgical options include colonic or small bowel interposition and gastric transposition.[116] Although these procedures are highly invasive, a minimally invasive approach has been described using thorascopic and laparoscopic techniques.[123] Controversy exists about whether to use the colon, stomach, jejunum, or a myocutaneous flap to reconstruct the esophagus.[116] Treatment of an undilatable cervical esophageal or anastomatic stenosis has not been well established. Zhou et al reviewed their experience with 149 adult patients who were treated for corrosive esophageal injuries at their institution between 1976 and 2003. They described prevention of stenosis with a modified technique of intraluminal esophageal stenting with a silicone stent and repair of severe cervical esophageal or anastomatic strictures resistant to dilation with a platysma myocutaneous flap. Of the patients included, modified intraluminal stenting was performed in 28 patients, colon interposition in 71, gastric transposition in 25, repair of cervical stricture with myocutaneous flap in 17, and miscellaneous procedures occurred in the remaining 11 patients. Twenty-three of the corrosive ingestion patients underwent successful intraluminal stent placement without subsequent development of stricture reformation. Five patients developed strictures after stent removal, of which 1 responded to esophageal dilation and the other 4 ultimately required esophageal reconstruction. Of the 71 patients undergoing colon interposition, 5 died postoperatively. Postoperative complications in this group of patients included proximal anastomatic fistula (17 patients), anastomatic stenosis (6 patients), and abdominal incision dehiscence (2 patients). Postoperative complications in the 25 patients who underwent gastric transposition consisted of anastomatic stricture in 2 patients and empyema in 1 patient. Cervical leak occurred in 1 of 17 patients who underwent repair of cervical esophageal or anastomatic stricture with platysma myocutaneous flap. All of the survivors were able to eventually resume a regular diet.[116]

Esophageal intraluminal stents have been used by Broto and associates in the treatment of severe esophageal strictures by conventional dilatation and placement of silicone stents. However, since several months are required for esophageal scars to stabilize, strictures soon reformed because stents were removed too early.[124] In contrast, Zhou and his colleagues placed stents in their patients 2 to 3 weeks after ingestion of caustic agents and kept them in place for 4 to 6 months. Consequently, 23 of their 28 patients were able to resume a normal diet. Of note, at the time of admission, 1 of these 23 patients had developed perforation of the esophagus into the right hemithorax and became critically ill. This patient immediately underwent thoracotomy, jejunostomy, esophageal stenting, and ligation of the abdominal esophagus with adsorbable suture to prevent regurgitation of gastric contents into the thorax. A barium esophagogram at the time of stent removal revealed free passage of contrast medium without evidence of stricture or perforation.[116]

## Advantages of Modified Intraluminal Esophageal Silicone Stents[104,116]

1. maintenance of both oral and gastrostomy feeding
2. less irritation of the nose because the stent is fastened at both the nostril and abdominal wall to prevent migration, thus allowing the patient to tolerate the stent for several months
3. the ability to readily adjust the stent if displaced
4. decreasing thoracic contamination from a perforated esophagus
5. convenient removal of stent

Management of the diseased esophagus is problematic because the extensive dissection necessary to remove the esophagus, particularly in the presence of marked periesophagitis, is associated with significant morbidity. While leaving the esophagus in place preserves vagal nerve function (and therefore stomach function), it can result in multiple blind sacs and subsequent development of mediastinal abscesses years later. In addition, ulceration from gastroesophageal reflux or development of carcinoma must be considered.[58] Despite the 1000 times greater incidence of esophageal cancer in patients who have ingested caustics, routine screening is not currently recommended. Most surgeons recommend removal of the esophagus unless the operative risk is unduly high. Kim et al and Csikos et al recommend resection, rather than bypass, of the damaged esophagus during esophageal reconstruction.[58,125] Among 54 patients with corrosive esophageal burns, Kim et al found 7 with cicatrix carcinoma. The interval between injury and development of cancer ranged from 29 to 46 years. Csikos and associates also reported 36 patients with scar cancer after corrosive agent ingestion, with an interval of 46.1 years between the time of the caustic injury and diagnosis of cancer. Therefore, they suggested that esophagectomy, instead of bypass, should be performed in all patients with severe corrosive esophageal strictures.[125] Zhou et al, however, believe that esophagectomy is indicated only in patients with strictures caudal to the carina because the procedure is easier due to the distance between the damaged esophagus

and contiguous mediastinal structures. In addition, morbidity and mortality rates are lower in these patients.[116]

As for selection of a substitute organ for the damaged esophagus, colon or jejunum interposition can be performed, but they are fraught with major complications and conduit loss.[126] Some investigators have advocated using the stomach to reconstruct the esophagus because of its length, dependable blood supply, and vast submucosal vascular network. "Using the stomach as an esophageal substitute only requires 1 anastamosis." Zhou et al advocate using the stomach to replace the resected or diseased esophagus.[116] In the majority of their patients with caustic ingestion who underwent esophagectomy, gastric transposition was performed. The mean operating time was 4 hours, with a mean volume of 400 mL of packed red blood cells transfused intraoperatively. All but 2 patients underwent intrathoracic anastomosis. In another study from the author's (Zhou et al) institution, the DeMeester score was 89.2 +/− 109 in 12 patients who underwent intrathoracic anastomosis, with only 3 scores within the normal range. Therefore, asymptomatic patients may still experience reflux. Reflux was managed by elevating the head of the bed and avoiding recumbency for 3 hours after meals. In addition, H2 blockers or proton pump inhibitors can be prescribed.

When a severe and extensive stricture is proximal to the carina, colon interposition is indicated. Raffensperger and colleagues reported 30 patients with caustic strictures who underwent colon interposition with no cases of cicatrix cancer noted on follow-up.[129] Zhou et al note that even though the stomach, jejunum, and colon can be used to replace the resected esophagus after corrosive ingestion, they preferred the colon as an esophageal substitute in the majority of their patients who had strictures proximal to the carina. The left colon, supplied by the middle colic artery, was primarily used (97%), and is generally preferred for colon interposition for the following reasons: (1) it has the most constant and reliable arterial supply and venous drainage, and (2) the left colon and esophagus have similar diameters.[116]

A cervical esophageal or anastamotic stricture which cannot be dilated requires surgical treatment. Free jejunal and myocutaneous flaps can be used to repair such severe abnormalities. However, the use of jejunum to treat cervical esophageal strictures requires a technically demanding microvascular anastamosis. In contrast, the platysma myocutaneous flap is thin, broad, and possesses a rich blood supply. Zhou et al successfully used these flaps to repair 17 cervical esophageal or anastamotic strictures. Since preoperative CT scans or barium contrast studies were not predictive of the distal extent of the stricture, the authors performed myocutaneous flaps or colon interposition, depending on intraoperative findings. If the distal end of the stricture was proximal to the thoracic inlet, then a platysma flap repair was performed. Otherwise, a colon interposition was done if the distal end extended into the chest. Zhou and his colleagues emphasize that utilizing the thin, well-vascularized platysma myocutaneous flap is a simple, relatively atraumatic procedure associated with low mortality, and is therefore suitable for repair of undilatable cervical esophageal or anastamotic strictures caused by caustic exposure.[116]

Critical in the operative planning for esophageal reconstruction is the selection of cervical esophagus, pyriform sinus, or posterior pharynx as the site for proximal anastamosis. The location of the upper anastamosis depends on the extent of the pharyngeal and cervical esophageal damage. When the cervical esophagus is destroyed and a pyriform sinus remains open, the anastamosis can be made to the hypopharynx.[130] When the pyriform sinuses are completely stenosed, a transglottic approach is used to perform an anastamosis to the posterior oropharyngeal wall. This allows excision of the supraglottic structures as well as elevation and anterior tilting of the larynx.[130,131] In both of these situations, the patient must relearn to swallow. Recovery is long and difficult and may often require several endoscopic dilatations and possibly reoperations.

## Gastric Complications

Gastric cicatrisation and gastric outlet obstruction are unfortunate consequences of caustic ingestion. Augmentation gastroplasty, Y-V advancement antropyloroplasty, Bilroth I, and laparoscopic distal Bilroth I have all been reported to alleviate symptoms after gastric cicatrisation. Although the oropharynx and esophagus are usually involved in corrosive ingestions, the true incidence of associated gastric injury is unknown, but may be as high as 5%.[132] Furthermore, the diagnosis may be delayed unless early endoscopy has alerted the physician to such a possibility. Ingested acids may pass rapidly through the esophagus and pool in the antrum because acid tends to follow the natural curve of the lesser curvature of the stomach formed by the magenstrasse. This is further aggravated by pylorospasm which confines the acid in the antrum where maximal injury is exerted. The severity of injury is dependent on the volume and concentration of the acid and is worsened if the stomach is empty at the time of exposure.[110] Alkali ingestion may also cause antral damage, and in one series, the overall incidence of antral strictures was greater with alkali (5.3%) compared to acid (3.8%) ingestion.[132]

The development of gastric outlet obstruction (GOO) can be anticipated by inspection of the antrum if routine complete upper gastrointestinal fiberoptic endoscopy is performed at initial presentation. An assessment of the extent of injury at this stage can predict the likely long-term outcome.[110] If the antrum is not inspected endoscopically,

a delay in the diagnosis of an antral stricture is inevitable, and symptoms of GOO usually commence subtly a few weeks later, once the outlet narrowing becomes significant. Presentation and diagnosis of GOO have been delayed for up to 3 years post-ingestion.[79] Confirmatory investigations include a contrast meal, which often shows GERD due to gastric outlet obstruction. Brown et al reported that this finding may distract the radiologist from the true cause, as occurred twice in their study. A distorted narrow antrum with minimal flow of barium into the duodenum is typically seen. A radioisotope scan to assess gastric emptying may show marked delay; 87% of ingested isotope was still present in the stomach at 2 hours in one of their cases (with normal being less than 40% residual activity at 2 hours).[79] At endoscopy, an abnormal, erythematous antral mucosa may be seen, with the familiar circular pylorus obscured by the distorted, narrowed antrum.

Once an antral stricture has developed, surgery is indicated to bypass the obstruction, which will increase further with progressive fibrosis. Prior to surgery, nutritional parameters should be restored to normal, preferably using the enteral route. Several surgical procedures, including a partial Bilroth I gastrectomy, excision of the stricture, or a Bilroth II with a gastroenterostomy, have been proposed for corrosive strictures of the antrum.[133] The optimal timing for these procedures has not been established, as healing fibrosis and contraction may further alter the anatomy following surgery if the strictured area is not completely excised or if the procedure is performed too soon after ingestion. This has led some surgeons to delay surgery until the stricture has matured.[133] Dilatation of the stricture is difficult as the anatomy at the entrance to the stricture is distorted. Perforation or rupture may occur with minimal luminal dilatation, which works against attempts at repeated dilatation.[79]

In milder cases of antral strictures, a pyloroplasty may bypass the obstruction, with the Finney procedure possibly offering better relief of the obstruction than the Heineke-Mikulicz. Randolph et al first proposed using a pedicle pyloroplasty for treatment of antral strictures,[134] which was initially introduced by Moschel et al for peptic ulcer disease in adults.[135] Animal studies have shown up to a 30% increase in luminal diameter with this procedure.[134] Furthermore, Hall and Lilly confirmed its efficacy in children with corrosive antral strictures.[136] The procedure is easy to perform and requires minimal dissection, and adequate widening of the lumen can be achieved with minimal anatomical or physiological disruption. A single layer of interrupted absorbable sutures contributes to a maximal luminal diameter without infolding of the fibrosed wall. A further advantage of the procedure is that it can be performed early in the evolution of the stricture, as any further fibrosis that may occur in the residual stricture tends to increase the contribution of normal tissue, thus expanding the luminal opening further. Since the stomach wall, which is advanced through the stricture, is not actually a pedicle but rather the normal gastric wall interposed into the longitudinal incision through the strictured antrum onto the normal pylorus and first part of the duodenum, the procedure was renamed advancement antroplasty (AAP).

Y-V advancement antroplasty (Y-V AAP) offers a simple surgical option for corrosive antral strictures in children. It can be performed soon after injury with effective opening of the narrowed antrum. The procedure is performed through a midline abdominal incision, which also facilitates creation of a gastrostomy required for management of an esophageal stricture. At laparotomy, an inflamed gastric wall with adherent omentum can usually be seen; on closer inspection, there is evidence of fibrosis and scarring in the distorted region of the antrum/pylorus, which is contracted and rigid. Palpation of the area reveals underlying thickening in the gastric outlet region. The duodenum is kocherised and the affected area mobilized into the wound for easier access. The stricture is then clearly visualized and palpated, and a point $Y$ is identified on the normal antrum proximal to the stricture. A second point, $V$, is marked on the normal duodenum 1 to 2 cm distal to the pylorus. A broad-based, U-shaped flap of the normal anterior stomach wall with the apex at $Y$ is fashioned. A linear incision is then made through the stricture from $Y$, ending the normal duodenum at point $V$. The U-shaped antral flap of normal stomach is advanced into the duodenum, approximating $Y$ to $V$ and completing the advancement with a single layer of interrupted absorbable sutures. A gastrostomy tube is inserted for feeding and to assist string-guided esophageal dilatation if necessary. Gradual reintroduction of oral or gastrostomy feeds can usually be commenced on the fifth or sixth day following surgery.[79]

Long-term sequela of leaving the damaged antrum in situ are unknown.[132] This statement may reflect a relatively short follow-up period, as long-term complications such as achlorhydria, duodenal atonicity, and mucosal metaplasia with carcinoma have been reported in adults.[137] Thus, careful endoscopic follow-up for a prolonged period is advisable.

## PREVENTATIVE MEASURES

Injuries occurring from caustic ingestion result in major morbidity and mortality. The majority of these exposures occur at home or school. The prevention of such incidents would translate into the well-being of a healthy and productive section of the community. Preventative measures revolve around implementing safety regulations,

instruction of safety-related behavior, education on how to limit exposure, and compliance.

Caustic ingestion initially emerged as a significant concern in the 1800s when lye products became available as household cleaners. Accidental ingestion of these products led to serious upper aerodigestive and esophageal injuries in children. Because of this growing problem, Chevalier Jackson became a pioneer against caustic ingestion, and his efforts resulted in the Federal Caustic Act of 1929, which mandated basic labeling of toxic substances. Further advances in the campaign against caustic ingestion included the creation of the Poison Control Center (1953), which provided a central source of information about product contents, toxicity, and treatment of poisoning. In addition, the Poison Prevention Packaging Act (PPPA) was passed in 1970 and required toxic products to be packaged in "childproof" containers. Similarly, toxic substance regulations control the concentrations of toxic agents.[138] The effects of these legislative efforts were quite dramatic, as evidenced by the reduced incidence of caustic ingestions.

There is good evidence of the effectiveness of multiple interventions in reducing pediatric injuries. Such examples include bicycle helmet legislation to prevent head injuries, area-wide traffic-relieving measures to avoid pedestrian and cyclist injuries, child safety restraint legislation to reduce motor vehicle occupant injuries, window bars to stop falls, domestic swimming pool fencing, and standards for playground equipment. International experience indicates that use of child-resistant packaging has led to a decline in the number of childhood poisonings. Although there are data for various other preventative measures, the actual evidence whether this necessarily translates into fewer incidents is less clear, as in cases of education aimed at children and parents, provision of smoke detectors, and education of parents on reduction of home hazards.[139]

The United States Preventative Services Task Force (USPSTF) reported that the most effective measures for controlling unintentional poison ingestions are structural or passive interventions which do not rely on the potential victim to adopt protective behaviors. As a case in point, health promotion and counseling have limitations in the time requirements and necessity of active cooperation from caregivers. Nevertheless, such approaches are most likely an important complement to structural changes.[140]

There is strong evidence for the effectiveness of home-visiting interventions in reducing pediatric trauma and poison exposures. A systematic review of 11 randomized controlled trials showed a significant preventative result of home visitations on the occurrence of such injuries.[141] A review of 20 studies concluded that evidence supports childhood injury prevention counseling as part of routine health supervision.[142] In particular, one RCT has demonstrated a reduction in home health hazards associated with providing an individualized course on child safety during well-baby visits.[143] The USPSTF considers good evidence exists from controlled trials for counseling parents of young children on safety-related behaviors. Studies have shown counseling to be effective, particularly when combined with safety regulations and other measures which promote compliance.[144] While the overall evidence supports a beneficial effect of counseling on safety-related knowledge and behavior, it is less clear whether such information actually lowers rates of ingestion. Moreover, some promising results have been seen from school-based programs teaching safety skills.

## CONCLUSION

Strong acids having a pH of less than 3.0 and strong alkalis with a pH above 11.0 are of greatest concern regarding human exposure and subsequent tissue damage. Caustic ingestion may produce corrosive lesions that extend far beyond adjacent organs, and injuries can range from local oral cavity trauma to extensive upper gastrointestinal or severe airway destruction. Severity of injury is related to multiple factors, most notably, pH, titratable acid or alkaline reserve, physical state, and tissue contact time, as well as the quantity and concentration of the agent.[2] As described, patients may present with or without symptoms. However, symptoms may not be the best indicator of severity or extent of injury caused by caustic ingestion. Although investigators have attempted to correlate laboratory values with injury severity and outcomes following caustic ingestion, they have not conclusively been shown to predict morbidity or mortality. Radiological studies are not a reliable means to identify the presence of early esophageal injury but are considered beneficial for surveillance purposes. Rather, early EGD has been advocated to identify the presence of esophageal caustic injury.

Little controversy exists in the management of dermal and ocular caustic exposure injuries. Immediate water irrigation at the site of exposure followed by routine burn care with analgesia, fluids, and electrolyte replacement is considered the standard of care.[2] Because of the high morbidity and mortality associated with aerodigestive tract injuries from caustic exposure, as well as the current controversy regarding appropriate management, this chapter has reviewed the pertinent factors involved in caustic injuries, with particular attention to the pediatric population.

## KEY POINTS

- Caustic or corrosive substances produce injury upon contact with tissue, which can be localized or can extend beyond adjacent organs.
- The most commonly affected areas from caustic ingestion include the oral cavity, pharynx, gastrointestinal tract, and trachea/upper airway.
- The severity of injury is related to multiple factors, most importantly pH, contact time, quantity and concentration of the agent, physical state, and titratable acid or alkaline reserve.
- The clinical presentation of caustic injury is variable, and patients can be asymptomatic.
- No specific laboratory test predicts the severity of injury or outcome from caustic injury; however, routine laboratory work should be part of the workup of any patient with such an injury.
- Radiological studies have limited value in the initial assessment of caustic injury but may be valuable in later stages to identify strictures.
- EGD has largely supplanted other modalities as the primary diagnostic procedure for evaluating and grading oropharyngeal and upper gastrointestinal tract caustic injury.
- Esophageal strictures are a chronic complication of caustic ingestion, with a variety of management options in both areas of prevention and treatment.
- Gastric complications include scarring, gastric outlet obstruction, and antral strictures.
- Treatment includes supportive measures, appropriate resuscitation, medical therapy, and surgical interventions when necessary.

# REFERENCES

1. Watson WA, Litovitz TL, Rodgers GC Jr, Klein-Schwartz W, Reid N, Youniss J, Flanagan A, Wruk KM. 2004 annual report of the American Association of Poison Control Centers Toxic Exposure Surveillance System. *Am J Emerg Med.* 2005; **23**(5): 589–666.

2. Salzman M, O'Malley RN. Updates on the evaluation and management of caustic exposures. *Emerg Med Clin North Am.* 2007; **25**(2): 459–476, abstract x.

3. Watson WA, Litovitz TL, Klein-Schwartz W, Rodgers GC Jr, Youniss J, Reid N, Rouse WG, Rembert RS, Borys D. 2003 annual report of the American Association of Poison Control Centers Toxic Exposure Surveillance System. *Am J Emerg Med.* 2004; **22**(5): 335–404.

4. Bronstein AC, Spyker DA, Cantilena LR Jr, Green J, Rumack BH, Heard SE. 2006 annual report of the American Association of Poison Control Centers' National Poison Data System (NPDS). *Clin Toxicol (Phila).* 2007; **45**(8): 815–917.

5. Watson WA, Litovitz TL, Rodgers GC Jr, Klein-Schwartz W, Youniss J, Rose SR, Borys D, May ME. 2002 annual report of the American Association of Poison Control Centers Toxic Exposure Surveillance System. *Am J Emerg Med.* 2003; **21**(5): 353–421.

6. Nuutinen M, Uhari M, Karvali T, Kouvalainen K. Consequences of caustic ingestions in children. *Acta Paediatr.* 1994; **83**(11): 1200–1205.

7. Adam JS, Birck HG. Pediatric caustic ingestion. *Ann Otol Rhinol Laryngol.* 1982; **91**(6, pt 1): 656–658.

8. Byrne WJ. Foreign bodies, bezoars, and caustic ingestion. *Gastrointest Endosc Clin N Am.* 1994; **4**(1): 99–119.

9. Wasserman RL, Ginsburg CM. Caustic substance injuries. *J Pediatr.* 1985; **107**(2): 169–174.

10. Moore WR. Caustic ingestions. Pathophysiology, diagnosis, and treatment. *Clin Pediatr (Phila).* 1986; **25**(4): 192–196.

11. Stenson K, Gruber B. Ingestion of caustic cosmetic products. *Otolaryngol Head Neck Surg.* 1993; **109**(5): 821–825.

12. Aronow SP, Aronow HD, Blanchard T, Czinn S, Chelimsky G. Hair relaxers: a benign caustic ingestion? *J Pediatr Gastroenterol Nutr.* 2003; **36**(1): 120–125.

13. Zargar SA, Kochhar R, Nagi B, Mehta S, Mehta SK. Ingestion of corrosive acids. Spectrum of injury to upper gastrointestinal tract and natural history. *Gastroenterology.* 1989; **97**(3): 702–707.

14. Nunes AC, Romãozinho JM, Pontes JM, Rodrigues V, Ferreira M, Gomes D, Freitas D. Risk factors for stricture development after caustic ingestion. *Hepatogastroenterology.* 2002; **49**(48): 1563–1566.

15. Edmonson MB. Caustic alkali ingestions by farm children. *Pediatrics.* 1987; **79**(3): 413–416.

16. Friedman EM. Caustic ingestions and foreign bodies in the aerodigestive tract of children. *Pediatr Clin North Am.* 1989; **36**(6): 1403–1410.

17. Hawkins DB, Demeter MJ, Barnett TE. Caustic ingestion: controversies in management. A review of 214 cases. *Laryngoscope.* 1980; **90**(1): 98–109.

18. Wason S. The emergency management of caustic ingestions. *J Emerg Med.* 1985; **2**(3): 175–182.

19. Harley EH, Collins MD. Liquid household bleach ingestion in children: a retrospective review. *Laryngoscope.* 1997; **107**(1): 122–125.

20. Havanond C. Is there a difference between the management of grade 2b and 3 corrosive gastric injuries? *J Med Assoc Thai.* 2002; **85**(3): 340–344.

21. Mamede RC, de Mello Filho FV. Ingestion of caustic substances and its complications. *Sao Paulo Med J.* 2001; **119**(1): 10–15.

22. Poley JW, Steyerberg EW, Kuipers EJ, Dees J, Hartmans R, Tilanus HW, Siersema PD. Ingestion of acid and alkaline agents: outcome and prognostic value of early upper endoscopy. *Gastrointest Endosc.* 2004; **60**(3): 372–377.

23. Kaushik R, Singh R, Sharma R, Attri AK, Bawa AS. Corrosive-induced gastric outlet obstruction. *Yonsei Med J.* 2003; **44**(6): 991–994.

24. Tekant G, Eroğlu E, Erdoğan E, Yeşildağ E, Emir H, Büyükünal C, Yeker D. Corrosive injury-induced gastric outlet obstruction: a changing spectrum of agents and treatment. *J Pediatr Surg.* 2001; **36**(7): 1004–1007.

25. Günel E, Cağlayan F, Cağlayan O, Akillioğlu I. Reactive oxygen radical levels in caustic esophageal burns. *J Pediatr Surg.* 1999; **34**(3): 405–407.

26. Satar S, Topal M, Kozaci N. Ingestion of caustic substances by adults. *Am J Ther.* 2004; **11**(4): 258–261.

27. Topaloglu B, Bicakci U, Tander B, Ariturk E, Kilicoglu-Aydin B, Aydin O, Rizalar R, Ayyildiz SH, Bernay F. Biochemical and histopathologic effects of omeprazole and vitamin E in rats with corrosive esophageal burns. *Pediatr Surg Int.* 2008; **24**(5): 555–560.

28. Mattos GM, Lopes DD, Mamede RC, Ricz H, Mello-Filho FV, Neto JB. Effects of time of contact and concentration of caustic agent on generation of injuries. *Laryngoscope.* 2006; **116**(3): 456–460.

29. Chiu HM, Lin JT, Huang SP, Chen CH, Yang CS, Wang HP. Prediction of bleeding and stricture formation after corrosive ingestion by EUS concurrent with upper endoscopy. *Gastrointest Endosc.* 2004; **60**(5): 827–833.

30. Rosseneu S, Afzal N, Yerushalmi B, Ibarguen-Secchia E, Lewindon P, Cameron D, Mahler T, Schwagten K, Köhler H, Lindley KJ, Thomson M. Topical application of mitomycin-C in oesophageal strictures. *J Pediatr Gastroenterol Nutr.* 2007; **44**(3): 336–341.

31. Uhlen S, Fayoux P, Vachin F, Guimber D, Gottrand F, Turck D, Michaud L. Mitomycin C: an alternative conservative treatment for refractory esophageal stricture in children? *Endoscopy.* 2006; **38**(4): 404–407.

32. Olutoye OO, Shulman RJ, Cotton RT. Mitomycin C in the management of pediatric caustic esophageal strictures: a case report. *J Pediatr Surg*. 2006; **41**(5): e1–e3.

33. Howell JM, Dalsey WC, Hartsell FW, Butzin CA. Steroids for the treatment of corrosive esophageal injury: a statistical analysis of past studies. *Am J Emerg Med*. 1992; **10**(5): 421–425.

34. Yagmurlu A, Aksu B, Bingol-Kologlu M, Renda N, Altinok G, Fitoz S, Gokcora IH, Dindar H. A novel approach for preventing esophageal stricture formation: sphingosylphosphoryl-choline-enhanced tissue remodeling. *Pediatr Surg Int*. 2004; **20**(10): 778–782.

35. Hoffman RS, Howland MA, Kamerow HN, Goldfrank LR. Comparison of titratable acid/alkaline reserve and pH in potentially caustic household products. *J Toxicol Clin Toxicol*. 1989; **27**(4-5): 241–246.

36. Gaudreault P, Parent M, McGuigan MA, Chicoine L, Lovejoy FH Jr. Predictability of esophageal injury from signs and symptoms: a study of caustic ingestion in 378 children. *Pediatrics*. 1983; **71**(5): 767–770.

37. Lamireau T, Rebouissoux L, Denis D, Lancelin F, Vergnes P, Fayon M. Accidental caustic ingestion in children: is endoscopy always mandatory? *J Pediatr Gastroenterol Nutr*. 2001; **33**(1): 81–84.

38. Maull KI, Osmand AP, Maull CD. Liquid caustic ingestions: an in vitro study of the effects of buffer, neutralization, and dilution. *Ann Emerg Med*. 1985; **14**(12): p1160–1162.

39. Kirsh MM, Ritter F. Caustic ingestion and subsequent damage to the oropharyngeal and digestive passages. *Ann Thorac Surg*. 1976; **21**(1): 74–82.

40. Einhorn A, Horton L, Altieri M, Ochsenschlager D, Klein B. Serious respiratory consequences of detergent ingestions in children. *Pediatrics*. 1989; **84**(3): p472–474.

41. Friedman EM. Caustic ingestions and foreign body aspirations: an overlooked form of child abuse. *Ann Otol Rhinol Laryngol*. 1987; **96**(6): 709–712.

42. Arevalo-Silva C, Eliashar R, Wohlgelernter J, Elidan J, Gross M. Ingestion of caustic substances: a 15-year experience. *Laryngoscope*. 2006; **116**(8): 1422–1426.

43. Cello JP, Fogel RP, Boland CR. Liquid caustic ingestion. Spectrum of injury. *Arch Intern Med*. 1980; **140**(4): 501–504.

44. Yegane RA, Bashtar R, Bashashati M. Aortoesophageal fistula due to caustic ingestion. *Eur J Vasc Endovasc Surg*. 2008; **35**(2): 187–189.

45. Hashem FK, Al Khayal Z. Oral burn contractures in children. *Ann Plast Surg*. 2003; **51**(5): 468–471.

46. Moulin D, Bertrand JM, Buts JP, Nyakabasa M, Otte JB. Upper airway lesions in children after accidental ingestion of caustic substances. *J Pediatr*. 1985; **106**(3): 408–410.

47. Tseng YL, Wu MH, Lin MY, Lai WW. Early surgical correction for isolated gastric stricture following acid corrosion injury. *Dig Surg*. 2002; **19**(4): 276–280.

48. Crema E, Fatureto MC, Gonzaga MN, Pastore R, da Silva AA. Tracheoesophageal fistula after caustic ingestion. *J Bras Pneumol*. 2007; **33**(1): 105–108.

49. Restrepo S, Mastrogiovanni L, Kaplan J, Gordillo H, Palacios E. Tracheoesophageal fistula caused by ingestion of a caustic substance. *Ear Nose Throat J*. 2003; **82**(5): 349–350.

50. Schutte H, Nava O, Yarmuch J, Csendes A, Braghetto I, Sepulveda A, Wünkhaus R. Early complications of caustic injuries of the digestive tract (Article in Spanish). *Rev Med Chil*. 1989; **117**(9): 1006–1011.

51. Zargar SA, Kochhar R, Mehta S, Mehta SK. The role of fiberoptic endoscopy in the management of corrosive ingestion and modified endoscopic classification of burns. *Gastrointest Endosc*. 1991; **37**(2): 165–169.

52. Baskin D, Urganci N, Abbasoğlu L, Alkim C, Yalçin M, Karadağ C, Sever N. A standardised protocol for the acute management of corrosive ingestion in children. *Pediatr Surg Int*. 2004; **20**(11-12): 824–828.

53. Nagi B, Kochhar R, Thapa BR, Singh K. Radiological spectrum of late sequelae of corrosive injury to upper gastrointestinal tract. A pictorial review. *Acta Radiol*. 2004; **45**(1): 7–12.

54. Andreollo NA, Lopes LR, Tercioti V Jr, Brandalise NA, Leonardi LS. Barrett's esophagus associated to caustic stenosis of the esophagus (Article in Portuguese). *Arq Gastroenterol*. 2003; **40**(3): 148–151.

55. Hopkins RA, Postlethwait RW. Caustic burns and carcinoma of the esophagus. *Ann Surg*. 1981; **194**(2): 146–148.

56. Ben Temime L, Marrakchi M, Moussi A, Abdesselem Mel M, Ferjaoui M, Zaouche A.. Two cases of cancerization of esophageal stenosis due to a caustic burn (Article in French). *Tunis Med*. 2004; **82**(11): 1038–1043.

57. Isolauri J, Markkula H. Lye ingestion and carcinoma of the esophagus. *Acta Chir Scand*. 1989; **155**(4-5): 269–271.

58. Kim YT, Sung SW, Kim JH. Is it necessary to resect the diseased esophagus in performing reconstruction for corrosive esophageal stricture? *Eur J Cardiothorac Surg*. 2001; **20**(1): 1–6.

59. Shaw A. Tracheoesophageal fistula following caustic ingestion. *Surgery*. 1979; **85**(3): 360.

60. Scala G, Chiummariello A, Palumbo U. Neoplastic tracheoesophageal fistula in a patient with esophageal stenosis caused by caustic substances (Article in French). *Bronches*. 1975; **25**(4): 256–260.

61. Mutaf O, Avanoğlu A, Mevsim A, Ozok G. Management of tracheoesophageal fistula as a complication of esophageal dilatations in caustic esophageal burns. *J Pediatr Surg*. 1995; **30**(6): 823–826.

62. Kaya M, Inan M, Bedel D. Detection of tracheoesophageal fistula caused by ingestion of a caustic substance by esophageal scintigraphy. *Clin Nucl Med*. 2005; **30**(5): 365–366.

63. Rana SV, Kochhar R, Pal R, Nagi B, Singh K. Orocecal transit time in patients in the chronic phase of corrosive injury. *Dig Dis Sci*. 2008; **53**(7): 1797–1800.

64. Kujawska-Danecka H, Sein Anand J, Chodorowski Z, Ciechanowicz R. Acute oral double intoxication with caustic substance—a case report (Article in Polish). *Przegl Lek.* 2007; **64**(4-5): 334–335.

65. Eaton H, Tennekoon GE. Squamous carcinoma of the stomach following corrosive acid burns. *Br J Surg.* 1972; **59**(5): 382–387.

66. Guth AA, Pachter HL, Albanese C, Kim U. Combined duodenal and colonic necrosis. An unusual sequela of caustic ingestion. *J Clin Gastroenterol.* 1994; **19**(4): 303–305.

67. Nijhawan S, Jain P. Acute pancreatitis as an unusual complication of corrosive ingestion. *J Gastrointestin Liver Dis.* 2007; **16**(3): 345–346.

68. Purucker EA, Sudfeld S, Matern S. Gastrobronchial fistula after caustic injury due to lye ingestion. *Endoscopy.* 2003; **35**(3): 252.

69. Susarla S, Khouzam RN, Lowell D, Marshall T. Gastropericardial fistula presenting 22 years after lye ingestion. *Can J Cardiol.* 2005; **21**(4): 371–372.

70. Henry MA, Pelissari CE, Carvalho LR. Morphological and functional evaluation of distal esophagus of rabbits submitted to esophageal infusion with caustic soda. *Acta Cir Bras.* 2008; **23**(1): 16–21.

71. Khan BA, Kochhar R, Nagi B, Raja K, Singh K. Gall bladder emptying in patients with corrosive-induced esophageal strictures. *Dig Dis Sci.* 2005; **50**(1): 111–115.

72. Chen YM, Ott DJ, Thompson JN, Gelfand DW. Progressive roentgenographic appearance of caustic esophagitis. *South Med J.* 1988; **81**(6): 724–728, 744.

73. Chen TY, Ko SF, Chuang JH, Kuo HW, Tiao MM. Predictors of esophageal stricture in children with unintentional ingestion of caustic agents. *Chang Gung Med J.* 2003; **26**(4): 233–239.

74. Hadfield PJ, Lloyd-Faulconbridge RV, Almeyda J, Albert DM, Bailey CM. The changing indications for paediatric tracheostomy. *Int J Pediatr Otorhinolaryngol.* 2003; **67**(1): 7–10.

75. Crain EF, Gershel JC, Mezey AP. Caustic ingestions. Symptoms as predictors of esophageal injury. *Am J Dis Child.* 1984; **138**(9): 863–865.

76. Gorman RL, Khin-Maung-Gyi MT, Klein-Schwartz W, Oderda GM, Benson B, Litovitz T, McCormick M, McElwee N, Spiller H, Krenzelok E. Initial symptoms as predictors of esophageal injury in alkaline corrosive ingestions. *Am J Emerg Med.* 1992; **10**(3): 189–194.

77. Previtera C, Giusti F, Guglielmi M. Predictive value of visible lesions (cheeks, lips, oropharynx) in suspected caustic ingestion: may endoscopy reasonably be omitted in completely negative pediatric patients? *Pediatr Emerg Care.* 1990; **6**(3): 176–178.

78. Boukthir S, Fetni I, Mrad SM, Mongalgi MA, Debbabi A, Barsaoui S. High doses of steroids in the management of caustic esophageal burns in children (Article in French). *Arch Pediatr.* 2004; **11**(1): 13–17.

79. Brown RA, Millar AJ, Numanoglu A, Rode H. Y-V advancement antropyloroplasty for corrosive antral strictures. *Pediatr Surg Int.* 2002; **18**(4): 252–254.

80. Riffat F, Cheng A. Pediatric caustic ingestion: 50 consecutive cases and a review of the literature. *Dis Esophagus.* 2009; **22**(1): 89–94. Epub 2008 Oct 1.

81. Rigo GP, Camellini L, Azzolini F, Guazzetti S, Bedogni G, Merighi A, Bellis L, Scarcelli A, Manenti F. What is the utility of selected clinical and endoscopic parameters in predicting the risk of death after caustic ingestion? *Endoscopy.* 2002; **34**(4): 304–310.

82. Cheng YJ, Kao EL. Arterial blood gas analysis in acute caustic ingestion injuries. *Surg Today.* 2003; **33**(7): 483–485.

83. Otçu S, Karnak I, Tanyel FC, Senocak ME, Büyükpamukçu N.. Biochemical indicators of caustic ingestion and/or accompanying esophageal injury in children. *Turk J Pediatr.* 2003; **45**(1): 21–25.

84. Lewin M, Pocard M, Caplin S, Blain A, Tubiana JM, Parc R. Benign hepatic portal venous gas following caustic ingestion. *Eur Radiol.* 2002; **12**(supplement 3): S59–S61.

85. Ramasamy K, Gumaste VV. Corrosive ingestion in adults. *J Clin Gastroenterol.* 2003; **37**(2): 119–124.

86. Zargar SA, Kochhar R, Nagi B, Mehta S, Mehta SK. Ingestion of strong corrosive alkalis: spectrum of injury to upper gastrointestinal tract and natural history. *Am J Gastroenterol.* 1992; **87**(3): 337–341.

87. Millar AJ, Numanoglu A, Mann M, Marven S, Rode H. Detection of caustic oesophageal injury with technetium 99m-labelled sucralfate. *J Pediatr Surg.* 2001; **36**(2): 262–265.

88. Tohda G, Sugawa C, Gayer C, Chino A, McGuire TW, Lucas CE. Clinical evaluation and management of caustic injury in the upper gastrointestinal tract in 95 adult patients in an urban medical center. *Surg Endosc.* 2008; **22**(4): 1119–1125.

89. Wilsey MJ Jr, Scheimann AO, Gilger MA. The role of upper gastrointestinal endoscopy in the diagnosis and treatment of caustic ingestion, esophageal strictures, and achalasia in children. *Gastrointest Endosc Clin N Am.* 2001; **11**(4): 767–787, vii-viii.

90. Gupta SK, Croffie JM, Fitzgerald JF. Is esophagogastroduodenoscopy necessary in all caustic ingestions? *J Pediatr Gastroenterol Nutr.* 2001; **32**(1): 50–53.

91. Squires RH Jr, Colletti RB. Indications for pediatric gastrointestinal endoscopy: a medical position statement of the North American Society for Pediatric Gastroenterology and Nutrition. *J Pediatr Gastroenterol Nutr.* 1996; **23**(2): 107–110.

92. Genc A, Mutaf O. Esophageal motility changes in acute and late periods of caustic esophageal burns and their relation to prognosis in children. *J Pediatr Surg.* 2002; **37**(11): 1526–1528.

93. Katzka DA. Caustic injury to the esophagus. *Curr Treat Options Gastroenterol.* 2001; **4**(1): 59–66.

94. Kamijo Y, Kondo I, Kokuto M, Kataoka Y, Soma K. Miniprobe ultrasonography for determining prognosis in corrosive esophagitis. *Am J Gastroenterol* 2004; **99**(5): 851–854.

95. Bernhardt J, Ptok H, Wilhelm L, Ludwig K. Caustic acid burn of the upper gastrointestinal tract: first use of endosonography to evaluate the severity of the injury. *Surg Endosc.* 2002; **16**(6): 1004.

96. Homan CS, Singer AJ, Henry MC, Thode HC Jr. Thermal effects of neutralization therapy and water dilution for acute alkali exposure in canines. *Acad Emerg Med.* 1997; **4**(1): 27–32.

97. Homan CS, Singer AJ, Thomajan C, Henry MC, Thode HC Jr. Thermal characteristics of neutralization therapy and water dilution for strong acid ingestion: an in-vivo canine model. *Acad Emerg Med.* 1998; **5**(4): 286–292.

98. Homan CS, Maitra SR, Lane BP, Thode HC Jr, Davidson L. Histopathologic evaluation of the therapeutic efficacy of water and milk dilution for esophageal acid injury. *Acad Emerg Med.* 1995; **2**(7): 587–591.

99. Homan CS, Maitra SR, Lane BP, Thode HC, Sable M. Therapeutic effects of water and milk for acute alkali injury of the esophagus. *Ann Emerg Med.* 1994; **24**(1): 14–20.

100. Brun JG, Celerier M, Koskas F, Dubost C. Blunt thorax oesophageal stripping: an emergency procedure for caustic ingestion. *Br J Surg.* 1984; **71**(9): 698–700.

101. Estrera A, Taylor W, Mills LJ, Platt MR. Corrosive burns of the esophagus and stomach: a recommendation for an aggressive surgical approach. *Ann Thorac Surg.* 1986; **41**(3): 276–283.

102. Cattan P, Munoz-Bongrand N, Berney T, Halimi B, Sarfati E, Celerier M. Extensive abdominal surgery after caustic ingestion. *Ann Surg.* 2000; **231**(4): 519–523.

103. Erdoğan E, Eroğlu E, Tekant G, Yeker Y, Emir H, Sarimurat N, Yeker D. Management of esophagogastric corrosive injuries in children. *Eur J Pediatr Surg.* 2003k; **13**(5): 289–293.

104. Wang RW, Zhou JH, Jiang YG, Fan SZ, Gong TQ, Zhao YP, Tan QY, Lin YD. Prevention of stricture with intraluminal stenting through laparotomy after corrosive esophageal burns. *Eur J Cardiothorac Surg.* 2006; **30**(2): 207–211.

105. Ferguson MK, Migliore M, Staszak VM, Little AG. Early evaluation and therapy for caustic esophageal injury. *Am J Surg.* 1989; **157**(1): 116–120.

106. Middelkamp JN, Ferguson TB, Roper CL, Hoffman FD. The management and problems of caustic burns in children. *J Thorac Cardiovasc Surg.* 1969; **57**(3): 341–347.

107. Wu MH, Lai WW. Surgical management of extensive corrosive injuries of the alimentary tract. *Surg Gynecol Obstet.* 1993; **177**(1): 12–16.

108. Tiryaki T, Livanelioglu Z, Atayurt H. Early bougienage for relief of stricture formation following caustic esophageal burns. *Pediatr Surg Int.* 2005; **21**(2): 78–80.

109. Jain AL, Robertson GJ, Rudis MI. Surgical issues in the poisoned patient. *Emerg Med Clin North Am.* 2003; **21**(4): 1117–1144.

110. Anderson KD, Rouse TM, Randolph JG. A controlled trial of corticosteroids in children with corrosive injury of the esophagus. *N Engl J Med.* 1990; **323**(10): 637–640.

111. Pelclova D, Navratil T. Do corticosteroids prevent oesophageal stricture after corrosive ingestion? *Toxicol Rev.* 2005; **24**(2): 125–129.

112. Ulman I, Mutaf O. A critique of systemic steroids in the management of caustic esophageal burns in children. *Eur J Pediatr Surg.* 1998; **8**(2): 71–74.

113. Yukselen V, Karaoglu AO, Ozutemiz O, Yenisey C, Tuncyurek M. Ketotifen ameliorates development of fibrosis in alkali burns of the esophagus. *Pediatr Surg Int.* 2004; **20**(6): 429–433.

114. Demirbilek S, Aydin G, Yücesan S, Vural H, Bitiren M. Polyunsaturated phosphatidylcholine lowers collagen deposition in a rat model of corrosive esophageal burn. *Eur J Pediatr Surg.* 2002; **12**(1): 8–12.

115. Berkovits RN, Bos CE, Wijburg FA, Holzki J. Caustic injury of the oesophagus. Sixteen years experience, and introduction of a new model oesophageal stent. *J Laryngol Otol.* 1996; **110**(11): 1041–1045.

116. Zhou JH, Jiang YG, Wang RW, Lin YD, Gong TQ, Zhao YP, Ma Z, Tan QY. Management of corrosive esophageal burns in 149 cases. *J Thorac Cardiovasc Surg.* 2005; **130**(2): 449–455.

117. Mills LJ, Estrera AS, Platt MR. Avoidance of esophageal stricture following severe caustic burns by the use of an intraluminal stent. *Ann Thorac Surg.* 1979; **28**(1): 60–65.

118. Fell SC, Denize A, Becker NH, Hurwitt ES. The effect of intraluminal splinting in the prevention of caustic stricture of the esophagus. *J Thorac Cardiovasc Surg.* 1966; **52**(5): 675–681.

119. Reyes HM, Lin CY, Schlunk FF, Replogle RL. Experimental treatment of corrosive esophageal burns. *J Pediatr Surg.* 1974; **9**(3): 317–327.

120. Khajanchee, YS, Hong D, Hansen PD, Swanström LL. Outcomes of antireflux surgery in patients with normal preoperative 24–hour pH test results. *Am J Surg.* 2004; **187**(5): 599–603.

121. Kochhar R, Ray JD, Sriram PV, Kumar S, Singh K. Intralesional steroids augment the effects of endoscopic dilation in corrosive esophageal strictures. *Gastrointest Endosc.* 1999; **49**(4, pt 1): 509–513.

122. Lahoti D, Broor SL. Corrosive injury to the upper gastrointestinal tract. *Indian J Gastroenterol.* 1993; **12**(4): 135–141.

123. Nwomeh BC, Luketich JD, Kane TD. Minimally invasive esophagectomy for caustic esophageal stricture in children. *J Pediatr Surg.* 2004; **39**(7): e1–e6.

124. Broto J, Asensio M, Marhuenda C, Gil Vernet JM, Acosta D, Boix Ochoa J. Intraesophageal stent in the prevention of stenosis caused by caustic ingestion (Article in Spanish). *Cir Pediatr.* 1999; **12**(3): 107–109.

125. Csíkos M, Horváth O, Petri A, Petri I, Imre J. Late malignant transformation of chronic corrosive oesophageal strictures. *Langenbecks Arch Chir.* 1985; **365**(4): 231–238.

126. Hirschl RB, Yardeni D, Oldham K, Sherman N, Siplovich L, Gross E, Udassin R, Cohen Z, Nagar H, Geiger JD, Coran AG. Gastric transposition for esophageal replacement in children: experience with 41 consecutive cases with special emphasis on esophageal atresia. *Ann Surg.* 2002; **236**(4): 531-539, discussion 539–541.

127. Ein SH. Gastric tubes in children with caustic esophageal injury: a 32–year review. *J Pediatr Surg*. 1998; **33**(9): 1363–1365.

128. de Jong AL, Macdonald R, Ein S, Forte V, Turner A. Corrosive esophagitis in children: a 30-year review. *Int J Pediatr Otorhinolaryngol*. 2001; **57**(3): 203–211.

129. Raffensperger JG, Luck SR, Reynolds M, Schwartz D. Intestinal bypass of the esophagus. *J Pediatr Surg*. 1996; **31**(1): 38-46, discussion 46–47.

130. Tran Ba Huy P, Celerier M. Management of severe caustic stenosis of the hypopharynx and esophagus by ileocolic transposition via suprahyoid or transepiglottic approach. Analysis of 18 cases. *Ann Surg*. 1988; **207**(4): 439–445.

131. Tran Ba Huy P, Assens P, Mislawski R, Brun JG, Frachet B, Beutter P, Brasnu D, Celerier M. Esophagopharyngoplasty by transplantation of a right ileocolic graft in the treatment of sequelae of esophageal and hypopharyngeal caustic stenosis (Article in French). *Ann Otolaryngol Chir Cervicofac*. 1982; **99**(10-11): 489–495.

132. Ciftci AO, Senocak ME, Büyükpamukçu N, Hiçsönmez A. Gastric outlet obstruction due to corrosive ingestion: incidence and outcome. *Pediatr Surg Int*. 1999; **15**(2): 88–91.

133. Chaudhary A, Puri AS, Dhar P, Reddy P, Sachdev A, Lahoti D, Kumar N, Broor SL. Elective surgery for corrosive-induced gastric injury. *World J Surg*. 1996; **20**(6): 703–706, discussion 706.

134. Randolph JG. Pedicle pyloroplasty. *J Pediatr Surg*. 1971; **6**(3): 388–392.

135. Moschel DM, Walske BR, Neumayer F. A new technique for pyloroplasty. *Surgery*. 1958; **44**(5): 813–816.

136. Hall RJ, Lilly JR. Treatment of acid burns of the stomach in children by pedicle pyloroplasty. *Surg Gynecol Obstet*. 1988; **167**(2): 152–154.

137. McAuley CE, Steed DL, Webster MW. Late sequelae of gastric acid injury. *Am J Surg*. 1985; **149**(3): 412–415.

138. Rogers RG. The effects of family composition, health, and social support linkages on mortality. *J Health Soc Behav*. 1996; **37**(4): 326–338.

139. Dowswell T, Towner EM, Simpson G, Jarvis SN. Preventing childhood unintentional injuries—what works? A literature review. *Inj Prev*. 1996; **2**(2): 140–149.

140. Runyan CW. Progress and potential in injury control. *Am J Public Health*. 1993; **83**(5): 637–639.

141. Roberts I, Kramer MS, Suissa S. Does home visiting prevent childhood injury? A systematic review of randomised controlled trials. *BMJ*. 1996; **312**(7022): 29–33.

142. Bass LW, Wolfson JH, Breck JM. Patient and parent education, office laboratory procedures, and urinary tract infections. *Curr Opin Pediatr*. 1993; **5**(6): 733–747.

143. Kelly B, Sein C, McCarthy PL. Safety education in a pediatric primary care setting. *Pediatrics*. 1987; **79**(5): 818–824.

144. Gallagher SS, Hunter P, Guyer B. A home injury prevention program for children. *Pediatr Clin North Am*. 1985; **32**(1): 95–112.

145. Luedtke P, Levine MS, Rubesin SE, Weinstein DS, Laufer I. Radiologic diagnosis of benign esophageal strictures: a pattern approach. *Radiographics*. 2003; **23**(4): 897–909.

146. Yamada, Y, Sakaguchi, T, Kida, M, et al. A study of duodenal ulcers by utrasonic probe: Application of jelly infusion method. Gastroenterol Endosc 1994; **36**: 499–508.

# BURN-RELATED CHILD ABUSE

DAVID G. GREENHALGH, MD, FACS, SHRINERS HOSPITALS FOR CHILDREN,
NORTHERN CALIFORNIA AND DEPARTMENT OF SURGERY,
UNIVERSITY OF CALIFORNIA, DAVIS

## INTRODUCTION

Child abuse is an unfortunate reality in the treatment of burns. Since a sizeable percentage of pediatric burn admissions are caused by abuse or neglect, the burn caregiver must be able to recognize suspicious burn injuries. If suspected, the caregiver must then know how to manage not only the medical problems but also the social dilemma of these unfortunate patients. The goal of this chapter is to acquaint the caregiver with the signs and symptoms of abuse, discuss mechanisms of injuries related to abuse, and provide treatment options for the burn team.

It is best to start with definitions. *Child abuse or maltreatment* is described as intentional harm or threat of harm to a child by someone acting in the role of caregiver, even if for a short time.[1,2] In general, there are 4 types of child abuse:

- *Physical abuse*: inflicting bodily injury by force or by forcing physically harmful activity. For the most part, burn-related child abuse fits into this category. Other, nonburn abuse will be mentioned but not emphasized.
- *Sexual abuse*: exposing a child to sexual acts or materials, passively using a child for sexual stimuli, or engaging in actual sexual contact with a child. Although this chapter will not cover this form of abuse, the burn team must always check for sexual abuse when performing their evaluations.

- *Emotional abuse*: coercive, demeaning, overly distant behavior by the caregiver that interferes with the child's normal psychosocial development. While this form of maltreatment will not be covered in detail, emotional abuse is a likely component of all forms of abuse.
- *Neglect*: failure to provide basic shelter, supervision, medical care, or support. While neglect may not be an active form of maltreatment, it is the most common and life-threatening type of abuse. Neglect is often associated with physical abuse.

While the focus of this chapter is to describe abuse in children, it must be remembered that abuse also occurs in at-risk adult groups such as the disabled, elderly, and intimate partners.

## BURN-RELATED CHILD ABUSE

Burn maltreatment comprises around 10% (6% to 25%) of all forms of abuse.[3-6] Many of these statistics are based on suspected abuse, with proven abuse cases making up a much lower percentage. Although legal proof of abuse is often difficult and not a direct responsibility of the burn team, cooperation with investigators is one of their obligations. Since statistics are only derived from documented cases, it is likely that many incidents are never entered into burn unit databases.

Child abuse comprises between 4% and 10% of pediatric burn unit admissions.[7-12] As described below, the at-risk population is the child at toilet-training age in lower socioeconomic situations. By far, scalds are the most common type of burn, and many preventative efforts, such as lowering temperatures of hot water heaters, would circumvent many of these injuries. Contact burns are also found as a form of burn-related abuse but tend to cover smaller areas and are more commonly seen in emergency departments or burn clinics. The major role of the burn caregiver is to learn to recognize intentionally committed burns.

## RECOGNITION OF INTENTIONAL BURNS

All members of the burn team are obligated to report any suspicious burn which may have been committed intentionally or as a form of punishment or retaliation. In many cases, my impression is that it is not the intent of the perpetrator to actually burn the child, but rather to "teach the child a lesson" by exposing him or her to some source of heat. Most of the community does not understand the potential for an agent such as hot water to cause a life-threatening injury. Our task, then, is to attempt to correlate the burn pattern with the story. If there is any concern about matching the history with the injury, caregivers are obligated *by law* to report it to the appropriate authorities (frequently Child Protective Services [CPS]).

In order to understand whether the burn pattern correlates with the story, one must be familiar with the mechanisms of burn injuries as well as factors that can increase the depth of such injuries. For instance, it is known that a first-degree burn remains above the epidermis and is thus red, dry, and painful. A second-degree (or partial-thickness) burn enters the dermis but leaves the epidermal appendages so the wound is able to reepithelialize on its own. Since the epidermis is gone but the dermal plexus of vessels and nerves remain, the burn is moist, red, blanches, and is extremely painful. One of the principles of burn healing is that a wound which heals within 2 weeks rarely develops hypertrophic scarring. If, however, it takes longer to heal, then such scarring is fairly common. This fact is particularly relevant for investigators who examine wounds months to years after the original injury. Once the burn is full thickness (through the dermis) or third degree, the wound may be multiple colors (white, black, red, yellow), does not blanch, and is dry and less painful since the dermal plexus of vessels and nerves are destroyed. These wounds usually require grafting for expeditious closure. Fourth-degree burns involve the bone, tendon, muscle, or other underlying structures below the layer of subcutaneous fat.

Scald burn patterns follow 2 basic principles:

- The burn occurs where the hot liquid touches the skin (contrary to areas that are not exposed, such as folds of opposing skin).
- Water follows the law of gravity. In a spill, water goes towards the floor. When in a container (such as the tub), water forms a flat, horizontal surface.

Utilizing these 2 principles, the mechanisms of most scalds can usually be determined. The first rule, the burn will only occur where the hot liquid touches the skin, assists with understanding the position of the child when the burn occurred. Skin folds are often spared as the juxtaposition of the skin surfaces prevents hot liquid from contacting that area. For instance, if the legs are involved but there is sparing behind the knees, then it is likely that the child had his or her legs bent. Occasionally, the entire lower legs are involved except for the soles of the feet. This pattern is explained by the fact that the feet were pushed against the bottom of the tub, which is not as hot as the water. When combining both rules, one can formulate a good idea of how the liquid caused a burn. For classic spill scalds, such as a child pulling a container of hot liquid on himself or herself, the water strikes the child near the top of the body and then moves down the body. As the volume decreases, the burn area narrows so that the patient develops a classic V-shaped injury. Frequently, narrow streaks are also seen as the water drips off the person. If the child is standing, then the V shape is seen on the chest or back. If the body part is horizontal, such as a hand being exposed to hot water from a faucet, then the burn occurs on top and drips off before touching the bottom.

If the child is placed into a container (tub, sink) with hot liquids, then a burn with a linear demarcation at the top of the body where the child was dipped will be evident. This classic dip burn is of uniform depth with a clearly demarcated line, typically at the top of the knees, abdomen, and back. Combining this burn with the first principle, the backs of the knees are spared as the legs are bent, as are the soles of the feet since they are in contact with the tub. In addition, a doughnut sparing of the buttocks is frequently seen since it also contacts the bottom of the tub. It is essential to remember that the position of the child can change as he or she is dipped in hot water. For instance, I treated one child whose mother confessed to dipping his head in hot water. This patient had an *upside-down* version of the classic dip burn. To assist with the investigation, pictures should be taken with the child in the position of injury so that the horizontal line of liquid is clearly visible.

A few comments regarding contact burns should be mentioned. Most accidental contact burns have different patterns than those which are inflicted. An experienced burn team member should recognize common accidental contact burns. Since toddlers explore their environments with their hands or mouths, they often grab hot items such as stoves or irons and sustain demarcated burns on their palms and fingertips. They also chew on electric cords and thus develop classic oral commissure burns. When a hot item such as an iron is pulled down by its cord, the glancing contact leads to varying depth burns as it falls against the skin. Usually, only parts of the iron pattern will mark the child's skin since it is rare for the entire surface to contact the skin. Intentional injuries leave a more demarcated and deeper burn as the item is held against the skin, with the burn reflecting the size and pattern of the inflicting device. By examining the pattern on the skin, the size of the contacting item can sometimes be determined. For instance, cigarette burns are approximately the size of the cigarette. Another important factor to remember is that intentional burns tend to occur in areas the child does not normally use for contacting the environment. Recently, we saw a patient who had spotty and superficial burns on his thighs but a well-demarcated burn on his penis. This pattern is highly suspicious for abuse, with an intentional burn on the genitalia while the thigh burns would occur from fighting to escape.

By understanding the factors that influence the depth of burn injuries, a better assessment as to the cause of injury can be made. Four main factors that determine the depth of burn injury and contribute to the ultimate ability for a burn wound to heal are

- temperature of the contacting agent
- duration of contact
- thickness of the skin
- blood supply to the skin

The role of temperature of the contacting agent in determining depth of injury is quite obvious: the hotter the agent, the deeper the burn. For example, exposure to molten steel will tend to leave a deeper burn than hot wax. Prevention strategies utilize this principle when recommending lowering water heaters to 120°F.

Duration of contact is directly related to temperature of the contacting agent when determining depth of injury. This principle is also obvious: the longer the duration of contact, the deeper the burn. This is why we do not suffer burns when testing the temperature of hot surfaces, since we pull away rapidly as the hot surface is sensed. Unfortunately, young children have not learned this reflex, and so it is not uncommon for them to freeze when touching a hot surface such as a stove or iron. Subsequently, this freezing reflex results in a deeper burn. This principle also applies to low-temperature devices such as heating pads. Even though it may require hours for a burn to occur with heating pads, deep burns are not uncommon in an insensate part of the body or an infirm person. The threshold temperature for a burn to occur after several hours is around 43.5°C (around 109°F).[13]

The same principle applies to hot water and the common dip burn. In the 1940s, Moritz and Henriques documented the time required in order to sustain a full-thickness burn from hot water.[14] Their classic plot demonstrates this relationship for an adult suffering a third-degree burn. This study continues to be the hallmark utilized in investigations of burn-related child abuse. At 160°F, a third-degree burn occurs in less than 1 second; at 150°F, in 2 seconds; and at 140°F, in 5 seconds. At 130°F, 30 seconds are required for a third-degree burn to develop, whereas 10 minutes are necessary for the same depth burn at a temperature of 120°F. Since young children have thinner skin than adults, the time to develop a full-thickness burn is shorter for this at-risk population. It is my hypothesis that many dip burns result from stressful situations or occur without the intention of creating third-degree burns. For instance, when a toddler has several accidents during toilet training and the caregiver is stressed, the child might be dipped in a tub of hot water in order to clean or teach him or her a lesson. Water heaters set at 150°F produce damage quickly. If all water heaters were set at 120°F, the number of dip burns would greatly decrease. Clothing may also prolong exposure to liquids. When clothing becomes soaked with a hot liquid, the tighter-fitting areas allow longer contact than other areas where the liquid falls off the body. As an example, we commonly see accidental scalds that leave hypertrophic scars at the collar and nowhere else. This occurs because the collar maintains the hot water against the skin longer, resulting in a deeper burn which heals after a 2-week period into a hypertrophic scar. Other areas which are more superficial heal faster and do not scar.

The third principle for determining burn depth is skin thickness. The depth of burn penetration is relatively constant. For example, a burn may cause damage to a skin depth of 1 mm. A partial-thickness burn will result if the skin is 2 mm thick, whereas a full-thickness burn occurs if the skin is 0.7 mm deep. The classic example of this principle is when examining burns of the hand and distal forearm. Although the burn injury is of equal depth, the skin is thickest on the palm, intermediate on the dorsal hand, and thinnest along the distal volar forearm. Thus, healing time correlates with skin depth, with the palm healing more quickly and the distal volar forearm requiring the longest time to heal. Along the same lines, back donor sites tend to scar less than other areas simply because this is where some of the thickest skin in the body is located.[15]

The final principle involves the blood supply influencing the depth of injury. Areas with an excellent blood supply dissipate heat and lessen the severity of injury. The face has an excellent blood supply and tends to suffer from more superficial burns compared to other areas of the body that are similarly exposed. On the other extreme, areas with poor blood supply tend to sustain deeper burns and heal poorly. We evaluated a patient who had forced-air heating around his legs while undergoing aortic surgery. Since the aorta was clamped during the procedure, there was no blood supply to the lower extremities. At the end of the operation, third-degree burns were noted. It is well known that an adequate blood supply is required for healing, so even relatively superficial wounds will have difficulty healing in areas of poor perfusion. One must also remember that the blood supply becomes impaired, the skin thins, and the adnexa (hair follicles, oil glands) tend to disappear in the elderly. Subsequently, this fragile, thin, hairless skin may not heal from even a very superficial burn due to an inadequate blood supply and adnexa. (It does not convert to third degree as commonly stated, but instead lacks the tools to heal.)

## BURN PATTERN AND THE STORY

Obtaining a history about the circumstances of the burn is essential in order to ascertain if there are clues which may lead one to suspect burn-related abuse. The caregiver must try to correlate the history with the burn pattern. Is the burn consistent with the story? Using the above principles of how burn patterns are created will assist with judging whether the story is appropriate. One method is to imagine where the water or hot item would contact the child and then determine if the burn pattern matches the injury. If not, one is obligated to report his or her suspicions. Other clues from the history which lead to concerns of abuse include a changing history, inconsistent reports from different people at the scene, and whether the perpetrator alters the story to explain the burn. I once dealt with a father who kept changing his story in order to convince the staff of his explanations. He would say, "How about if the baby did this and the faucet was like this..." He ultimately confessed to burning the child.

It is also important to determine who was supervising the child at the time of the injury. Frequently, one can discern whether there was adequate supervision or if a boyfriend, girlfriend, or friend was present. Another warning sign is when a young sibling is blamed for the accident. Even if the sibling was present, it leads to a question of neglect due to poor supervision (e.g., an 18-month-old sibling placing a 4-month-old child in the tub). One must remember that

although small children might be able to lift infants, they are not strong enough to hold them at arm's length or place them in a tub without dropping them.

Another factor to consider is the typical activities of a child at his or her developmental age. What position can the child hold himself or herself in? Can he or she sit up, roll over, or walk? Does he or she have the dexterity to turn on the faucet? Can he or she lift a heavy item? For instance, if a 2-month-old cannot sit up, it is unlikely that he or she would have a burn pattern consistent with this position. Also, can the child climb into the tub or sink? Can he or she get out? It is important to match the capabilities of a child with his or her developmental milestones.

The other factor to consider is the response of the responsible party, especially the parent. Classic signs of abuse have been well documented. Was there a delay in seeking treatment? Most parents of burned children will seek immediate care, whereas abused children will often not be brought to the hospital for hours to days. The perpetrator will claim that he or she did not notice any problem until later. Frequently, a person other than the perpetrator (a grandmother or neighbor, for example) will bring the child to the hospital for care. Another scenario is a mother who returns from work to find the babysitter ignored the child. The mother discovers the problem and seeks care herself, instead of the person responsible at the time doing so. Although it seems as though a boyfriend or babysitter is frequently involved, all members of the family may be responsible. Another sign to watch for is a parent who seems to lack concern for his or her child. Most parents are extremely upset when their child sustains a burn. If they are not worried, then concern is warranted. Another classic reaction for abusive parents is to display anger about the whole affair, appear bothered by the inconvenience of the situation, or want to leave as soon as possible.

The family dynamics should also be observed. Abuse is more likely in a "broken" home.[3,7,9,12,16,17] It is also not uncommon for a parent to support the perpetrator instead of the child. After treating a severely abused child, I once had a mother abandon her child and leave with the convicted abuser. Another issue to be alert for is a parent's fear of the perpetrator. I am certain that some mothers have taken the blame for abuse when the real concern is for their boyfriend. This situation may suggest fear of retribution and an abusive relationship between the parent and perpetrator. It is also common that another family member (classically the grandmother) dislikes the perpetrator and voices concern as to his or her role. Several studies have demonstrated that the incidence of abuse is increased in a single-parent, low-income family.[3,7,9,12,16,17] Although abuse is more common in minority groups, this increase in risk seems to be related to a higher incidence of poor socioeconomic status. Additional risk factors for abuse include parents with a very low or no income, as well as those with lower educational levels. A significant drug or alcohol history increases concern for abuse as well. If a parent was abused, then his or her child is at increased risk since it is well documented that abuse is an "inherited" disease. Clearly, abuse is a social problem that would improve with better support of the socioeconomically deprived. Moreover, most of the above patterns can also be applied to physical abuse. Sexual abuse, however, occurs with all socioeconomic groups.[1]

The response of the child is just as important a factor to consider when evaluating abuse. Abused children frequently seem to have an abnormal response to painful procedures. For example, placing intravenous lines, cleaning or dressing wounds, or participating in therapy may not elicit a normal response such as wincing, fear, or crying. It is sad to observe this, since it suggests that the child has found such responses have no effect to repeated painful abuse. Abused children will frequently demonstrate passive acknowledgment or be developmentally delayed (due to neglect). Knowing how a child normally reacts to separation from his or her parents is helpful, since separation anxiety is pronounced during the toddler years. Therefore, when a child does not seem to care about being separated from his or her caregivers, one must take note. One should also be concerned if the child shows signs of fear or a different behavior when near the perpetrator. Another warning sign occurs when the child seems to bond to the burn team more than to his or her parents. Finally, unusually promiscuous behavior is a warning sign of a child who has been sexually abused. If a child knows more about sexual issues than appropriate for his or her age, then sexual abuse should also be suspected.

A focused physical examination with appropriate documentation is very important. The report should remain objective rather than subjective or biased. In addition, pictures should be taken to substantiate the documented findings. The child should be placed in the position in which the burn occurred when taking photographs, since these images may assist future investigations. Occasionally, the device involved in creating the burn can be placed on the child (when no longer hot) to demonstrate how the injury occurred. If one is uncomfortable with any part of the physical, then consultants should be invited to assist with the examination. This is particularly true when examining the genitalia for signs of sexual abuse. While burn doctors are experts at evaluating burn injuries, they frequently lack the training regarding the subtle findings of sexual abuse.

The goal of the physical examination is to determine whether other injuries in addition to the one bringing the child to the hospital exist. Burns should be inspected to determine their suspected age. Concern is warranted if the burn appears older than described. Burns of different ages or those that have healed should be evaluated. Multiple burns of different ages likely point to repeated abuse over a period of time. Other signs of physical abuse, such as bruises, abrasions, or lacerations in unusual areas, should be sought. Children will normally have bruises on their shins from falling or on their foreheads from bumping into tables. Bruises on the upper arms suggest someone has been grabbing and shaking the child. Abrasions that fit the pattern of restraining a child during an incident or tying a child occur on obvious sites such as the wrists or ankles. One commonly mistaken bruiselike mark is the Mongolian spot. My recollection from the first time that I saw these spots was that it looked as though the child had been beaten. These marks are bluish in color but have subtle differences from an ecchymosis.

Other signs of physical abuse can include loss of hair from forced rubbing or being pulled. Damage to teeth may also occur. Occasionally, a child may accidentally chip a tooth but should not lose several teeth. A subtle sign of head trauma is retinal hemorrhage. If there are significant concerns for abuse, the child should be examined by an ophthalmologist. As fractures occurring from abuse are well documented, a complete radiological examination is an essential component of the child abuse workup. If the child is grabbed and shaken by the upper arms, then humeral fractures may occur. As for burn wounds, concomitant multiple fractures of different age are clearly a sign of abuse. Another sign of concern is with fractures exhibiting periosteal elevation. Subgaleal hematomas or skull fractures may occur from striking the head. In addition, head-computed tomography should be considered to investigate possible traumatic brain injury.

Another important consideration during the physical examination is seeking signs of neglect. Is the child filthy? Have the clothes or diapers been changed recently? One needs to assess the nutritional status of the child as well. Has he or she reached an appropriate weight for his or her age? Is he or she extremely thin or wasted? Has the child received the appropriate nurturing? Has he or she reached appropriate developmental milestones? Are there other children with similar injuries? For instance, I once saw a child who sustained a perioral burn from a vaporizer. Abuse was suspected and subsequently proven when his sibling arrived with an identical burn. If previous CPS reports have been filed, then suspicions about repeated abuse are justified.

## ASSISTANCE WITH THE INVESTIGATION

All caregivers are obligated by law to report any suspicious injury, which is not superseded by professional-patient confidentiality. In fact, penalties exist for those who do not comply. Every team member has the obligation to report a concern, even if he or she is uncertain about abuse. It is not his or her responsibility to judge the person but rather to report findings and assist investigators. In addition, the team member should document his or her observations related to the interactions between the patient and other people. While the team member may question the patient about the circumstances of injury, he or she should not try to coerce information from the child. For instance, one time I simply asked a suspected abused child what happened, and she stated that her "uncle burned her." Although it was the only time she named an assailant, it nonetheless assisted with the investigation. It is always the best policy to be honest with families and express concern to parents, since most appropriate caregivers will understand our obligations to report abuse. It is our duty to remain objective and unbiased towards the patient as well as the family, even if abuse is suspected. If concerns arise regarding risks to the patient, then CPS will dictate visiting rights.

Although it is not our role to investigate the scene of the crime, we should be available to assist investigators. At the scene, the temperature of the water should be determined in order to match the potential duration of contact with the depth of burn. What is the temperature of the water running out of the faucet, and how long did it take to reach that temperature? At what temperature is the hot water heater set? The distance from the child's buttocks to the top of the dip burn should be measured to acquire an idea of the water depth in the tub or sink at the time of injury. How high are the sides of the tub, since it might influence whether a child could climb into a tub or whether a sibling could lift a child into the tub? The size of any potential items that caused contact should also be measured to determine whether they match the burn pattern. For instance, inspecting a curling iron which might match a corresponding contact burn could clarify the story of a suspicious burn.

## THE BURDEN OF ABUSE

The cost of child abuse is quite significant and cannot always be measured in actual dollars. Our impression is that patients who suffer child abuse have higher complication rates and increased mortality compared to children sustaining accidental scalds. To address this issue, we performed 2 studies where we analyzed the outcomes of children suspected of scald-related child abuse against age-matched and burn-matched children with accidental scald burns (Table). Information over 2 time periods (1986–1991 and 1991–1995) consisting of 52 abused versus 50 controls for the first period and 54 abused and 52 controls during the second period were collected.[7,18] The incidence of suspected abuse was 4.3% during the first review and 5.7% in the second

period. No differences in nutritional parameters were found during either period. The mean age was less than 2 years old, with a burn size of approximately 20% total body surface area (TBSA). Full-thickness burns ranged between 8 and 14% TBSA. While trends towards increased morbidity and mortality were observed, there were no significant differences. Overall, our findings confirmed those of previous and later studies. There was approximately a doubling in the length of stay (11–14 days vs 23–26 days), as well as far more minorities, single-parent families, broken homes, and unemployed parents represented in the group of children with suspected abuse burns. Approximately two-thirds of abused families had an income of less than $20,000 per year. These findings exemplify the costs of caring for these patients, since the length of stay was prolonged and there were frequent problems returning the child to his or her original parent.

## CASE REPORT

I will finish the chapter with a case that demonstrates many of the issues discussed above. A 2-month-old child was transferred to our unit with 44% TBSA burns to the legs, back, perineum, and left arm. The burns were asymmetric but well demarcated. The emergency department physician from the transferring hospital expressed concern that the child was intentionally burned. The pediatric intensivist, however, disagreed and documented that he felt the burn was an accidental injury. The father, who had 3 previous neglect complaints filed with CPS, stated that he had placed the baby in the tub and then left the room. He claimed that the 2-year-old sibling had turned on the water and he had returned to find the child exposed to hot water. Examination revealed well-demarcated burns extending up the left side of the back and involving the left arm and both legs. There was sparing of the right knee extending to the right thigh, as well as of the left hand and shoulder. As for most small children with extensive burns, the child had a rocky course, with significant airway compromise requiring intubation and eventual tracheostomy. There was one bout of *Pseudomonas* sepsis that resulted in septic shock. He required extensive grafting and was eventually discharged from the hospital.

At the criminal case which was brought against the father, I was asked to testify and explain why I felt this was an intentionally committed act. Questions regarding the asymmetry of the burns and the reason why I felt that the child had been dipped into hot water arose. The keys to this case were the child's capabilities for his developmental age and the pattern of the burn. At 2 months of age, children cannot sit up by themselves, nor can they roll over or support their heads. In essence, the only position they can maintain when in a tub is lying on their back. The description of the bathtub was a typical, relatively flat tub. The depth of the water that the child was placed into would have to have been approximately 20 cm deep. If the child was placed in the tub and the water was then turned on, he would have sustained symmetric burns on the legs, back, and head since he would be unable to raise his head. In addition, there would have been sparing of the sites touching the tub, such as the buttocks, scapular region, and occiput. Subsequently, the father inquired if the burn injury was consistent with the child being placed on his side. Firstly, it is unlikely that a 2-month-old could remain in this position. For the sake of argument, if he was on his side, the pattern would have been more symmetric on that side, with the entire arm being under, and, again, the head would have been burned. In my opinion, essentially the only action which could explain the burn pattern for a child of his age was being held and dangled by his right arm while being placed into the hot tub.

During the trial, the father confessed to dipping the child into the water. Despite this confession, the judge freed him. The child was returned to his biologic mother, who abandoned the child approximately 2 weeks after discharge and left him with his aunt (who had spent the entire duration of the hospital stay with the baby). Eventually, the aunt adopted him and the biologic parents completely abandoned the child. This case demonstrates many of the classic signs of abuse. It also stresses the difficult future that still remains for a child who has been abandoned by his or her biologic parents. Fortunately, this child was rescued by a loving aunt who has greatly improved his life. All of these cases are distressing, but this case exemplifies the long-term problems of abuse.

## CONCLUSION

Burn-related child abuse is a significant burden to society that is tied to families who are stressed and broken. The most common form of burn-related abuse is a scald injury. My conviction is that perpetrators do not fully understand the consequences of hot water quickly resulting in full-thickness burns. Preventative measures, such as lowering water heaters to 120oF, would reduce many of these injuries. Such simple prevention could make a notable difference in a child's life. These injuries can have profound physical and cognitive impacts on children, even leading to their deaths. Oftentimes, it is not only the visual scars of a deep burn which are always permanent, but the psychological and social wounds also remain throughout a child's life.

TABLE 1

Results of 2 comparisons between children suffering from suspected scald burn abuse versus children suffering from similarly sized accidental scalds. The first study period included 52 abused (first abused) and 50 control (first controls) between 1/1/86 and 6/30/91 (4.3% of admissions). The second study period included 54 abused (second abused) and 52 controls (second controls) between 7/1/91 and 12/31/95 (5.7% of admissions).[7,18] Abused children had significantly prolonged lengths of stay, tended to be a minority, had younger parents, were more often in single-parent or broken homes, were less likely to have working parents, and had lower family incomes than the nonabused control groups.

| Group | Age (years) | % Burn | % Full-Thickness |
|---|---|---|---|
| 1st abused | $2.0 \pm 0.1$ | $22 \pm 2$ | $14 \pm 2$ |
| 1st controls | $1.8 \pm 0.1$ | $20 \pm 2$ | $12 \pm 2$ |
| 2nd abused | $1.7 \pm 0.1$ | $19 \pm 3$ | $11 \pm 2$ |
| 2nd controls | $1.6 \pm 0.1$ | $18 \pm 2$ | $8 \pm 2$ |

| Group | Length of Stay | Black/White | |
|---|---|---|---|
| 1st abused | $26 \pm 3$ | 27/25 | |
| 1st controls | $14 \pm 2$* | 8/41* | |
| 2nd abused | $23 \pm 3$ | 26/28 | |
| 2nd controls | $11 \pm 2$* | 10/42* | |

| Group | Mother's Age (Years) | Father's Age (Years) | |
|---|---|---|---|
| 1st abused | $23.9 + 0.8$ | $27.6 + 1.1$ | |
| 1st controls | $26.3 + 0.9$* | $29.3 + 1.0$ | |
| 2nd abused | $23.1 + 0.7$ | $25.8 + 0.9$ | |
| 2nd controls | $25.9 + 0.9$* | $28.3 + 1.1$ | |

| Group | % With Single Parent | % With Intact Family | |
|---|---|---|---|
| 1st abused | 71.7 | 26.5 | |
| 1st controls | 22.9* | 71.4* | |
| 2nd abused | 64.7 | 38.5 | |
| 2nd controls | 34.0* | 71.4* | |

| Group | % Employed | % With Income < $20,000/y | |
|---|---|---|---|
| 1st abused | 47.8 | 95.6 | |
| 1st controls | 84.4* | 66.7* | |
| 2nd abused | 48.2 | 92.0 | |
| 2nd controls | 82.7* | 71.7* | |

Values are expressed as mean ± standard error of the mean or percentage. An asterisk (*) indicates significant differences between controls and abused for the same periods.

## REFERENCES

**1.** Wissow LS. Child abuse and neglect. *N Engl J Med.* 1995; **332:** 1425–1431.

**2.** Dubowitz H, Bennett S. Physical abuse and neglect of children. *Lancet.* 2007; **369:** 1891–1899.

**3.** Feldman KW, Schaller RT, Feldman JA, McMillon M. Tap water burns in handicapped children. *Pediatrics.* 1978; **62:** 1–7.

**4.** Caniano DS, Beaver BL, Boles ET. Child abuse: an update on surgical management in 256 cases. *Ann Surg.* 1986; **203:** 219–224.

**5.** Scalzo AJ. Burns and child maltreatment. In: Monteleone JA, Brodeur AE, eds. *Child Maltreatment: A Clinical Guide and Reference.* St. Louis, MO: GW Medical Publishing Inc; **1994:** 89–111.

**6.** Hight DW, Bakalar HR, Lloyd JR. Inflicted burns in children. Recognition and treatment. *JAMA.* 1979; **242:** 517–520.

**7.** Hummel RP III, Greenhalgh DG, Barthel PP, et al. Outcome and socioeconomic aspects of suspected child abuse scald burns. *J Burn Care Rehabil.* 1993; **14:** 121–126.

**8.** Peck MD, Priolo-Kapel D. Child abuse by burning: a review of the literature and an algorithm for medical investigations. *J Trauma.* 2002; **53:** 1013–1022.

**9.** Chester DL, Jose RM, Aldlyami E, King H, Moiemen NS. Non-accidental burns in children—are we neglecting neglect? *Burns.* 2006; **32:** 222–228.

**10.** Deitch EA, Staats M. Child abuse through burning. *J Burn Care Rehabil.* 1982; **3:** 89–94.

**11.** Keen JH, Lendrum J, Wolman B. Inflicted burns and scalds in children. *BMJ.* 1975; **4:** 268–269.

**12.** Purdue GF, Hunt JL, Prescott PR. Child abuse by burning—an index of suspicion. *J Trauma.* 1988; **28:** 221–224.

**13.** Greenhalgh DG, Lawless MB, Chew BB, et al. Temperature threshold for burn injury: an oximeter safety study. *J Burn Care Rehabil.* 2004; **25:** 411–415.

**14.** Moritz AR, Henriques FC. Studies of thermal injury: II. The relative importance of time and surface temperature in the causation of cutaneous burns. *Am J Pathol.* 1947; **23:** 695–720.

**15.** Greenhalgh DG, Barthel PP, Warden GD. Comparison of back versus thigh donor sites in pediatric burn patients. *J Burn Care Rehabil.* 1993; **14:** 21–25.

**16.** Carrigan L, Heimbach DM, Marvin JA. Risk management in children with burn injuries. *J Burn Care Rehabil.* 1988; **9:** 75–78.

**17.** Fuchs VR, Reklis DM. America's children: economic perspectives and policy opinions. *Science.* 1992; **255:** 41–46.

**18.** Brown DL, Greenhalgh DG, DeSerna SM, et al. Outcome and socioeconomic aspects of suspected child abuse scald burns. *J Burn Care Rehabil.* 1997; **17**(suppl): S167.

# PEDIATRIC BURN INJURY: A NEUROSURGERY PERSPECTIVE

ANDREW P. CARLSON, MD, DEPARTMENT OF NEUROSURGERY, UNIVERSITY OF NEW MEXICO

ERICH MARCHAND, MD, ASSOCIATE PROFESSOR, DIRECTOR OF PEDIATRIC NEUROSURGERY, DEPARTMENT OF NEUROSURGERY, UNIVERSITY OF NEW MEXICO

## INTRODUCTION

Though neurosurgical involvement in burn injury is rare, there are several situations where a neurosurgical perspective may be of benefit to the patient. In addition, there may be neurosurgical or neurological implications in management that may be under-recognized. One situation where neurosurgical intervention in burn injury is required is with severe, full-thickness burns of the calvarium or skull base. These injuries may require multiple specialties to address complex management and reconstruction needs. The neurosurgeon may aid in surgical handling of burned brain tissue and with coverage of the remaining defect. Another scenario is the burned patient with a coexisting traumatic brain injury. In general, the management of these patients should follow existing guidelines for pediatric traumatic brain injury; however, it is important for the burn physician to take into consideration the needs of the vulnerable brain, particularly with regard to hypotension, fluid shifts, and electrolyte balance. Finally, it has become recognized that there are myriad neurologic complications in patients with burn injury; future investigations may clarify potential factors where interventions and monitoring techniques may identify and potentially mitigate some of this morbidity and improve outcomes.

## CLINICAL PROBLEMS REQUIRING NEUROSURGICAL INVOLVEMENT

### Calvarial Burns

Burns to the calvarium are graded by depth; full-thickness burns involving the outer and inner table of the skull are classified as grade IV. The etiology of calvarial burns in children is typically related to flame or electrical burns, leading to increased morbidity in terms of hospital stay and operative procedures.[1] Full-thickness calvarial burns can leave the vulnerable dura mater and brain parenchyma open to infection or further damage during the healing process. Computed tomography (CT) remains the most important tool to assess the extent of damage preoperatively. However, various nuclear imaging techniques such as 99mTc MDP bone SPECT and 99mTc sestamibi muscle SPECT have also been used both to assess bony viability and to monitor healing after flap coverage.[2,3,4] As with other burns, debridement is a major step during the first stages of injury. Removal of necrotic bone may also be necessary, and familiarity with the underlying structures, especially the venous sinuses and cortical structures, is important in order to avoid massive hemorrhage or further neurologic deficit. Once the bone has been debrided to vascularized margins, the extent of dural damage should be assessed. Necrotic brain tissue should then be carefully excised using suction and Malis bipolar electrocautery. If there is associated hematoma or large infarct, further debridement may be necessary, depending on the comfort of the surgeon. The need for evacuation of hematoma or removal of nonviable tissue is controversial in the neurosurgical literature; considerations of size, location, and clinical condition of the patient need to be taken into account.

Wound closure can be obtained in a number of ways, depending on the depth of the burn. When tissue permits, local flap coverage is most desirable.[5,6] Usually electrical burns are focal enough to allow such a strategy. Staged or immediate autograft coverage after bone debridement is an option for larger wounds, provided there is a vascular base such as viable inner cortical bone.[1,5] Alternatively, the wound may be allowed to granulate with allograft coverage and delayed autografting.

When the burn is full thickness and involves a dural opening, often the dura cannot be repaired primarily, and a different closure strategy must be explored. It is of key importance to avoid cerebrospinal fluid (CSF) leak postoperatively in order to decrease the risk of infection. There are many dural substitutes available, including autografts such as fascia lata, biological substitutes such as collagen matrix (DuraGen: Integra, Plainsboro, NJ), and synthetic products (Gore Preclude MVP: Gore Medical, Flagstaff, AZ). Fibrin glue–based sealants such as Tisseal (Baxter Healthcare, Deerfield, IL) and more recently the synthetic DuraSeal (Confluent Surgical, Waltham, MA) may further reinforce the closure. Burn surgeons have described the use of omentum or AlloDerm (LifeCell, Branchburg, NJ) as a dural substitute as well, though this is uncommon in neurosurgical practice.[1,7,8] Selecting the ideal dural substitute involves considering the properties of the material, the type of wound being closed, and the surgeon's familiarity with the graft. Whichever method is employed, a dural substitute should be placed over the wound and sutured with a watertight closure to avoid CSF leak, particularly for burns involving the skull base. Origitano et al[9] have reported several severe skull-base injuries due to firework penetration and stress the importance of adequate debridement and watertight dural closure with cosmetic reconstruction of the skull base. Techniques including vascularized periosteal flaps and fascia lata or temporalis muscle grafts are used commonly. In these cases, it is important to involve an experienced surgical team comfortable in skull-base surgery and closure.

Once the dura has been satisfactorily closed, skin coverage can be obtained with several techniques. Standard wet-to-dry dressings may be used, although vacuum-assisted systems at low suction can also be used over exposed dura if the surgeon is comfortable with the security of the watertight closure. Otherwise, the dural substitute itself can be allowed to granulate, followed by delayed autograft.[8,10] Care must be taken when the autograft is applied to the granulation tissue to avoid violating the dura. The disadvantage of this technique is the long period of recovery and the challenges with later cranioplasty. Another option is transfer of a vascularized pedicle flap such as the trapezius for coverage. Many types of vascular flaps have been described in these patients,[11,12] with the goal of providing adequate vascular supply to the healing tissue.[13] The vascularized flap offers earlier coverage and more protection for the fragile dura and typically requires involvement of a plastic surgeon.

As implied above, after debridement, the skull is typically not reconstructed immediately. This is partly due to concern of potential infection which would require removal of the plate, as well as the inability to establish skin coverage over the plate. The exception is when a myocutaneous, vascularized pedicle is transferred onto necrosed skull. Some authors have reported adequate healing rates using this technique, while avoiding a cranial defect.[11,14] When there is a bony defect, care must be taken during the rehabilitation period to avoid injury to the underlying brain. Therefore, all patients with a cranial defect should be fit with a protective helmet for 2 to 6 months, until they can be evaluated for cranioplasty for cosmesis as well as protection of the underlying brain. There are many products, from molded methylmethacrylate to custom-made plates, which all serve well for cranioplasty. These procedures are often more complex than standard neurosurgical cranioplasty due to the fragile nature of the skin coverage. Therefore, plastic surgery may need to be involved in the reconstruction as well.

## Patients with Coexistent Burn Injury and Traumatic Brain Injury

Patients with burn injuries coincident with moderate or severe traumatic brain injury may present with various difficult management issues. The primary concern from a neurosurgical point of view is with regard to fluid management. The injured brain frequently behaves differently from the normal brain in terms of blood flow, metabolism, and other parameters. This makes it sensitive to physiologic changes which might not otherwise be problematic. It is clear that secondary insults to the injured brain, such as hypoxia and hypotension, are detrimental in terms of outcomes. The goals of neurocritical care, therefore, are to diligently recognize and prevent these insults as much as possible.

Burned patients are particularly prone to hypotension due to hypovolemia as well as to massive fluid shifts in the course of resuscitation. Hemodynamic indices of perfusion must be followed closely in the patient with coexisting traumatic brain injury. In addition, serum sodium should be carefully monitored, as severe hyponatremia can lead to significant and/or irreversible neurological damage. Regarding correction of hyponatremia, it is recommended that sodium levels not be allowed to rise more than 0.5 mEq/L/h (or ≤ 12 mEq/L/d) in order to avoid such complications as osmotic demyelination or central pontine myelinolysis. This is particularly relevant since some data suggest increased sensitivity to osmotic changes in the brain during burn injury.[15]

General management decisions for pediatric traumatic brain injury should proceed in cooperation with the burn team. Indications for invasive monitoring, treatment of increased intracranial pressure, and surgical decompression of the brain are guided by consensus guidelines based on the available neurosurgical evidence.[16]

Other than the issues discussed above, very little evidence exists to guide practice in this specific situation. One series from Taiwan describes patients with electrical burn associated with brain injury. The incidence of brain injury in the electrical burn group was 3%, and the authors argue that early aggressive intervention for the brain injury is indicated, even with severe burn injury.[17]

## NEUROLOGICAL COMPLICATIONS OF BURN INJURY

Historically, it has been recognized that there are many neurologic complications in severely burned children which often occur in a delayed fashion. This concept was vaguely characterized and often generically described as "burn encephalopathy." As diagnostic and therapeutic technology has advanced, the understanding of the varied processes which can occur after burn injury has been better elucidated. Though many of the described complications are somewhat sporadic and lack clear definitions of underlying mechanisms, others are better characterized. Overall, though neurologic complications after burn injury are common, there is a scarcity of therapeutic or diagnostic recognition of this in clinical practice.

The concept of burn encephalopathy was used initially to describe general neurologic deterioration after burn injury in children, typically manifested by coma or seizures.[18,19] Though the etiology was initially thought to be obscure,

large series of patients have confirmed that a clear precipitating factor can usually be identified. The most common factors include hypoxia, either from the initial injury or from delayed pulmonary edema or pneumonia, and hypovolemia due to shock and inadequate resuscitation.[18,19] Complex metabolic abnormalities related to fluid management and shifts have also been identified in these patients, most commonly hyponatremia and hypocalcemia. Other complications, such as infection (meningitis, meningoencephalitis, or abscess), cortical vein thrombosis, or various types of cerebral infarct, have also been described.[18]

The frequency of neurological complications in pediatric burn patients varies from 5% to 15%.[18,19] Nearly all patients show electroencephalogram (EEG) abnormalities, usually slow waves and epileptiform activity, which is thought to correlate with metabolic and electrolyte disturbances.[20] In autopsy series, the frequency of neurologic complications is 53%.[21] Major complications include infections (abscess, infarction), hemorrhage, metabolism-related problems such as central pontine myelinolysis, and trauma.[15] Other reported problems include transient parkinsonism,[22] nonspecific leukoencephalopathy,[23,24] septic venous thrombosis,[25,26] cerebral edema,[27,28] and diffuse delayed cerebral atrophy.[29]

Many endocrine abnormalities have also been described in burned patients, suggesting the presence of intrinsic pituitary dysfunction in this population.[30] In men, testosterone levels may be greatly decreased,[31] while in women, ovulation and menstruation may be disrupted.[32] These changes likely are related to the shift in endocrine priorities during the period of catabolism and stress of burn injury.[31] In children specifically, corticotropin and cortical feedback loops are disrupted due to systemic stress. For this reason, it is controversial whether an isolated total cortisol level is an accurate predictor of adrenocortical insufficiency in burned children. Rather, a free cortisol level or corticotropin stimulation test may be necessary to determine the need for exogenous steroid replacement.[33]

Neuropsychological complications are also becoming more recognized in these patients. Likely multifactorial in etiology, they include impaired memory and recall tasks[34] as well as attention and other cognitive slowing.[35] Hypoxia during the burn episode has been implicated as resulting in even more pronounced long-term cognitive problems.[36]

## FUTURE DIRECTIONS IN NEUROMONITORING IN PEDIATRIC BURN INJURY

Tools for monitoring neurologic function during burn injury have not been extensively studied, though general advances in neurologic monitoring in critical care are becoming more sophisticated. There are many situations where some of the technology discussed below may be applicable in burn injury to aid in determining treatment strategies which may minimize secondary injury to the brain. First and foremost, attention to changes in the clinical exam should initiate further investigation regarding pulmonary status, electrolyte balance, or other neurologic insults. There are many cases, however, where the clinical exam may not be reliable due to the age of the patient, administration of sedative or pain medications, or other factors. In these situations, additional technology may be employed. EEG may be a useful tool for detecting epileptic tendencies, especially in heavily sedated patients.[20] This is also becoming a more widely used modality in critical care to monitor for nonconvulsive status epilepticus, which may be a more common cause of depressed mental status than widely recognized.[37] One German article describes the use of brainstem auditory evoked potentials to monitor for neurologic deterioration.[38] This technology, along with somatosensory evoked potentials, may be of some utility in cases of severe deficit in order to help prognosticate outcome. Bilateral absence of the cortical N20 response has been shown to be a strong predictor of poor outcome and may be the best overall tool for predicting outcome in children, particularly those with anoxic-type injury.[39]

Though not widely practiced, monitoring of cerebral blood flow (CBF) may be useful in certain cases. The only published data regarding this involve nuclear imaging to detect abnormalities.[40] Other potential technologies include positron emission tomography (PET) using labeled oxygen or xenon-enhanced CT,[41] which are the most accurate methods for obtaining quantitative measurements of CBF. Both of these approaches are noninvasive, allowing for tomographic analysis of CBF in order to determine tissue which may be at risk for infarction. Currently, both technologies have limitations in terms of general availability, though they may offer additional options for the future.

Another noninvasive monitoring technique commonly used in neurointensive care is near infrared scalp oximetry, which detects oxygenation of the outer layers of cortical tissue. The INVOS device (Somanetics, Troy, MI) consists of pads generally applied to the forehead bilaterally, similar to a finger oximeter. These are connected to a monitor which displays cortical oxygenation and trends. The device is used commonly in neurosurgery, neurocritical care, and pediatric cardiac surgery[42] and may provide additional information regarding adequacy of cerebral oxygenation in selected patients.

In cases where imaging or clinical deterioration suggests a severe or malignant problem such as worsening cerebral edema, more invasive monitoring may be indicated, though there are no data specifically addressing indications or results in pediatric burn injury. Being invasive, they carry some chance of infection or hematoma, so the risks and benefits to a patient must be weighed. Simple intracranial pressure monitoring may be obtained with the use of an external ventricular drain or a brain parenchymal monitor. These devices are often utilized when there is concern of adequate cerebral perfusion pressure during relative hypotension or to assess for intracranial hypertension. Invasive technology is becoming more refined and provides the intensivist with detailed information regarding cerebral physiology to help guide treatment. Brain tissue oxygenation monitors such as the Licox (Integra, Plainboro, NJ) may give early information regarding adequacy of brain oxygenation and have been used in pediatric traumatic brain injury with some utility.[43] These devices can also measure cerebral temperature, which can vary widely from systemic temperature. Hyperthermia has been shown in many situations, particularly traumatic brain injury, to decrease seizure threshold and have deleterious effects on outcome.[44] For this reason, monitoring cerebral temperature and aggressive maintenance of normothermia are likely beneficial in this population. Intraparenchymal CBF monitors measure blood flow by thermal diffusion, and there are several commercially available models. These devices provide focal, real-time data regarding changes in CBF and may be used with tomographic techniques described above to determine parameters to optimize CBF. Finally, cerebral tissue microdialysis provides intriguing data regarding brain metabolism. This information may then be used in conjunction with other technologies to determine the specific needs of a patient.[45] For example; a patient with a globally decreased cerebral metabolic rate may tolerate much lower blood flow or cerebral perfusion pressures than a patient with a normal or hypermetabolic state. These technologies are being adopted by many neuroscience ICUs and may be an additional parameter which can aid in patient care in other critical care situations, such as severe burn injury, if a thoughtful, physiologic, patient-based approach is used.

## CONCLUSION

Neurosurgical involvement in pediatric burn injury is rarely necessary. Nonetheless, there are situations where neurosurgeons' perspective may be of utility in patient management. The complex management of patients with large full-thickness scalp burns requires a multidisciplinary approach to care and treatment. Patients with coexistent traumatic brain injury may be at even more risk of neurologic complications, warranting careful monitoring of neurologic status. Unfortunately, though there are many complications affecting the brain, very little guidance or data exists to direct physicians in the most effective monitoring and management of neurocritical care issues. At this time, it would seem most prudent to consider aggressive neurologic monitoring in burned patients, whether it is through frequent examinations, EEG monitoring, or other technologies. Hopefully, implementation of such a strategy will detect changes in oxygenation, hypoperfusion, neurologic status, or other developing abnormalities before potentially devastating complications happen. This should occur both in terms of individual care of the burned patient as well as through further research directed at better understanding how to assess and decrease neurologic morbidity and mortality in burned children.

## KEY POINTS

- Neurosurgical involvement in pediatric burn injury is rarely needed.
- Repair of full-thickness calvarial and skull-base burns requires a team approach to treatment and reconstruction.
- Watertight dural closure is important to avoid infection.
- Patients with burns and traumatic brain injury should have careful attention paid to fluid shifts and electrolyte balance.
- Neurologic complications are fairly common in burn injury, and further research is needed to improve treatment strategies.
- Many neuromonitoring technologies are available which may provide important information to assist with management decisions in appropriately selected burn patients.

## REFERENCES

1. Spies M, McCauley RL, Mudge BP, Herndon DN. Management of acute calvarial burns in children. *J Trauma*. 2003; **54**: 765–769.

2. Pegg SP, Jenkins AM. Deep electrical burns to the scalp. *Burns Incl Therm Inj*. 1987; **13**: 62–65.

3. Fried M, Rosenberg B, Tuchman I, et al. Electrical burn injury of the scalp—bone regrowth following application of latissimus dorsi free flap to the area. *Burns*. 1991; **17**: 338–339.

4. Sarikaya A, Aygit AC. Combined 99mTc MDP bone SPECT and 99mTc sestamibi muscle SPECT for assessment of bone regrowth and free muscle flap viability in an electrical burn of scalp. *Burns*. 2003; **29**: 385–388.

5. Hunt J, Purdue G, Spicer T. Management of full-thickness burns of the scalp and skull. *Arch Surg*. 1983; **118**: 621–625.

6. Bizhko IP, Slesarenko SV. Operative treatment of deep burns of the scalp and skull. *Burns*. 1992; **18**: 220–223.

7. Caffee HH. Scalp and skull reconstruction after electrical burn. *J Trauma*. 1980; **20**: 87–89.

8. Barret JP, Dziewulski P, McCauley RL, Herndon DN, Desai MH. Dural reconstruction of a class IV calvarial burn with decellularized human dermis. *Burns*. 1999; **25**: 459–462.

9. Origitano TC, Miller CJ, Izquierdo R, Hubbard T, Morris R. Complex cranial base trauma resulting from recreational fireworks injury: case reports and review of the literature. *Neurosurgery*. 1992; **30**: 570–576.

10. Yeong EK, Huang HF, Chen YB, Chen MT. The use of artificial dermis for reconstruction of full thickness scalp burn involving the calvaria. *Burns*. 2006; **32**: 375–379.

11. Shen Z. Reconstruction of refractory defect of scalp and skull using microsurgical free flap transfer. *Microsurgery*. 1994; **15**: 633–638.

12. Chavoin JP, Gigaud M, Clouet M, Laffitte F, Costagliola M. The reconstruction of cranial defects involving scalp, bone and dura following electrical injury: report of two cases treated by homograft, free groin flap and cranioplasty. *Br J Plast Surg*. 1980; **33**: 311–317.

13. Dalay C, Kesiktas E, Yavuz M, Ozerdem G, Acarturk S. Coverage of scalp defects following contact electrical burns to the head: a clinical series. *Burns*. 2006; **32**: 201–207.

14. Shen Z, Wang N, Ma C. Treatment of extensive deep burn of scalp with full-thickness necrosis of calvarial bone [Article in Chinese]. *Zhonghua Zheng Xing Shao Shang Wai Ke Za Zhi*. 1995; **11**: 10–12.

15. McKee AC, Winkelman MD, Banker BQ. Central pontine myelinolysis in severely burned patients: relationship to serum hyperosmolality. *Neurology*. 1988; **38**: 1211–1217.

16. Adelson PD, Bratton SL, Carney NA, et al. Guidelines for the acute medical management of severe traumatic brain injury in infants, children, and adolescents. Chapter 1: Introduction *Pediatr Crit Care Med*. 2003; **4**: S2–S4.

17. Chen CT, Yang JY. Electrical burns associated with head injuries. *J Trauma*. 1994; **37**: 195–199.

18. Antoon AY, Volpe JJ, Crawford JD. Burn encephalopathy in children. *Pediatrics*. 1972; **50**: 609–616.

19. Mohnot D, Snead OC III, Benton JW Jr. Burn encephalopathy in children. *Ann Neurol*. 1982; **12**: 42–47.

20. Hughes JR, Cayaffa JJ, Boswick JA Jr. Seizures following burns of the skin. III. Electroencephalographic recordings. *Dis Nerv Syst*. 1975; **36**: 443–447.

21. Winkelman MD, Galloway PG. Central nervous system complications of thermal burns. A postmortem study of 139 patients. *Medicine (Baltimore)*. 1992; **71**: 271–283.

22. Shahar E, Keidan I, Brand N, Frand M, Barzilay Z. Uncommon neurologic complications of burns in infants: a parkinsonian extrapyramidal disorder and massive cerebral infarction. *J Burn Care Rehabil*. 1991; **12**: 54–57.

23. Gregorios JB. Leukoencephalopathy associated with extensive burns. *J Neurol Neurosurg Psychiatry*. 1982; **45**: 898–904.

24. Eldad A, Neuman A, Weinberg A, et al. Late onset of extensive brain damage and hypertension in a patient with high-voltage electrical burns. *J Burn Care Rehabil*. 1992; **13**: 214–217.

25. Reper P, Van Der Rest P, Creemers A, Vandenen D, Vanderkelen A. Medical treatment of a central vein suppurative thrombosis with cerebral metastatic abscesses in a burned child. *Burns*. 2001; **27**: 662–663.

26. Arseni C, Horvath L, Carp N. Thrombophlebitis of the cerebral cortex in children. *Rom Med Rev*. 1971; **15**: 33–40.

27. Emery JL, Campbell Reid DA. Cerebral oedema and spastic hemiplegia following minor burns in young children. *Br J Surg*. 1962; **50**: 53–56.

28. Prekop R, Bardosova G, Simko S, Varady L. Brain oedema in burned children. *Acta Chir Plast*. 1984; **26**: 184–192.

29. Isao T, Masaki F, Riko N, Seiichi H. Delayed brain atrophy after electrical injury. *J Burn Care Rehabil*. 2005; **26**: 456–458.

30. Da M, Ma K, Duan T. Clinical studies on the effects of burn trauma on pituitary-testis axis [Article in Chinese]. *Zhonghua Zheng Xing Shao Shang Wai Ke Za Zhi*. 1999; **15**: 373–375.

31. Dolecek R, Dvoracek C, Jezek M, Kubis M, Sajnar J, Zavada M. Very low serum testosterone levels and severe impairment of spermatogenesis in burned male patients. Correlations with basal levels and levels of FSH, LH and PRL after LHRH + TRH. *Endocrinol Exp*. 1983; **17**: 33–45.

32. Diem E, Schmid R, Schneider WH, Spona J. The influence of burn trauma on the hypothalamus-pituitary axis in normal female subjects. *Scand J Plast Reconstr Surg*. 1979; **13**: 17–20.

33. Palmieri TL, Levine S, Schonfeld-Warden N, O'Mara MS, Greenhalgh DG. Hypothalamic-pituitary-adrenal axis response to sustained stress after major burn injury in children. *J Burn Care Res*. 2006; **27**: 742–748.

34. Stokes DJ, Dritschel BH, Bekerian DA. The effect of burn injury on adolescents autobiographical memory. *Behav Res Ther*. 2004; **42**: 1357–1365.

35. Willebrand M, Norlund F, Kildal M, Gerdin B, Ekselius L, Andersson G. Cognitive distortions in recovered burn patients: the emotional Stroop task and autobiographical memory test. *Burns*. 2002; **28**: 465–471.

36. Rosenberg M, Robertson C, Murphy KD, et al. Neuropsychological outcomes of pediatric burn patients who sustained hypoxic episodes. *Burns*. 2005; **31**: 883–889.

37. Claassen J, Mayer SA. Continuous electroencephalographic monitoring in neurocritical care. *Curr Neurol Neurosci Rep*. 2002; **2**: 534–540.

38. Tegenthoff M, Waskonig MT, Buttemeyer R. Assessment of central nervous system functional disorders in severely burned patients by auditory evoked brain stem potentials [Article in German]. *Handchir Mikrochir Plast Chir*. 1994; **26**: 232–236.

39. Carter BG, Butt W. A prospective study of outcome predictors after severe brain injury in children. *Intensive Care Med*. 2005; **31**: 840–845.

40. Deveci M, Bozkurt M, Arslan N, Sengezer M. Nuclear imaging of the brain in electrical burn patients. *Burns*. 2002; **28**: 591–594.

41. Wintermark M, Sesay M, Barbier E, et al. Comparative overview of brain perfusion imaging techniques. *Stroke*. 2005; **36**: e83–e99.

42. Tortoriello TA, Stayer SA, Mott AR, et al. A noninvasive estimation of mixed venous oxygen saturation using near-infrared spectroscopy by cerebral oximetry in pediatric cardiac surgery patients. *Paediatr Anaesth*. 2005; **15**: 495–503.

43. Narotam PK, Burjonrappa SC, Raynor SC, Rao M, Taylon C. Cerebral oxygenation in major pediatric trauma: its relevance to trauma severity and outcome. *J Pediatr Surg*. 2006; **41**: 505–513.

44. Suz P, Vavilala MS, Souter M, Muangman S, Lam AM. Clinical features of fever associated with poor outcome in severe pediatric traumatic brain injury. *J Neurosurg Anesthesiol*. 2006; **18**: 5–10.

45. Poca MA, Sahuquillo J, Vilalta A, de los Rios J, Robles A, Exposito L. Percutaneous implantation of cerebral microdialysis catheters by twist-drill craniostomy in neurocritical patients: description of the technique and results of a feasibility study in 97 patients. *J Neurotrauma*. 2006; **23**: 1510–1517.

# CHAPTER TWENTY-FOUR

# REHABILITATION OF THE PEDIATRIC BURN PATIENT

Kevin L. LaPratt, MS, OTR/L

David Lorello, PT, DPT

Anne M. Tiernan, MS, OTR/L, CEES, CKTP

Bradley J. Phillips, MD

## INTRODUCTION

The multidisciplinary burn team involved in the care of pediatric patients typically consists of physicians, physician assistants, nurses, nurse practitioners, clinical nutritionists, occupational therapists, physical therapists, social workers, child-life specialists, psychologists, and psychiatrists.[1,2] In addition, speech-language pathologists, orthotists, prosthetists, recreation therapists, music therapists, and clergy often provide specialty services.[3,4,5] Group support is provided to the patient and his or her family throughout the entire process of resuscitation, acute care, rehabilitation, and reconstruction. Although individual team members play varying roles, the collective goal is the optimal physical, emotional, and psychological recovery of the child or adolescent during what could otherwise be a dehumanizing experience.[4] Patience, compassion, empathy, consistency, and a positive approach are needed from each team member.

Occupational and physical therapists provide rehabilitation treatment and care throughout the patient's recovery. Academic preparation of therapists can be supplemented by completion of internships in burn care in order to provide the specialized experiences needed by this unique patient population.[6] Therapists maintain high standards of care through continual professional development and postgraduate education.[5]

This chapter focuses on the rehabilitative efforts by occupational therapists and physical therapists from the acute period through the grafting stage and, finally, to the outpatient and reconstructive surgery phases in the treatment of children and adolescents with burns.

## PREVENTING POSTURAL AND POSITIONAL DEFORMITIES

Occupational and physical therapists utilize many types of positioning, including splinting, casting, traction, and the use of soft materials in order to prevent postural and positional deformities in children and adolescents with burns. The initial needs assessment of the patient should be done within the first 24 hours of hospitalization. Burns crossing joints can lead to deformities if not treated promptly and correctly, but initiation of an early treatment protocol and continued positioning can decrease the likelihood of contractures.[7]

The goals of positioning in the acute phase are to prevent joint contracture formation, provide proper joint alignment, control edema, and maintain soft tissue elongation.[4] Practitioners and nursing staff are relied upon to maintain the wearing schedule of positioning devices for children (Table 1). Ongoing reevaluation to assess the appropriate positioning needs should be done throughout the child's hospitalization and subsequent outpatient therapy. Modifications are expected on a weekly basis.

Children often have significant difficulty understanding the need for positioning. Increased fear and/or anxiety related to being away from family members and the pain experienced during dressing changes may result in poor compliance with positioning programs.[8] Treatment and dressing changes should be done in a room other than the child's in order to allow him or her to feel safe. Since children may also display decreases in attention span, cooperation, and understanding,[7] distraction therapy may be beneficial during procedures and therapies.[9]

Children are likely to experience less stiffness in response to immobilization but more scar tissue formation compared to adults.[10] There are a variety of items that can be used for positioning a child, including pillows, towel rolls, elastic wraps, foam materials, low-heat thermoplastic materials, fiberglass, and plaster. Soft materials are preferable for shoulders, elbows, and hands of infants and toddlers. Practitioners determine the items best suited to support the limbs.

Splints are the modality of choice for protecting joints, deep wounds, and skin grafts.[7] The 3 types of splints used for positioning are static, dynamic, and serial splints.[7] A static splint maintains the affected body part in a functional position to maintain range of motion. Use of a dynamic splint may substitute for weak or nonfunctional muscles, with a low-load stretch to the soft tissues.[11] When a low-force splint cannot be fabricated to fit the child, or if a child is uncooperative, serial casting may be an option.[4] Serial casts, which gradually increase the stretching of tissue, can be used to prevent contractures. All splints and casts should be monitored closely to prevent pressure on bony prominences, tissue maceration, sensory disturbances, and pain. To avoid poor alignment, bulky dressings should be minimized when splints are used.[12] The surgeon may place Kirschner wires (K-wires) to position fingers with severe burns in order to prevent rotation and flexion contractures as well as to provide alignment to open joints. An external fixator can also be used to position the fingers to prevent contractures and ensure proper joint alignment. Upon application of an allograft or autograft, the patient is accordingly positioned and immobilized following specific burn center guidelines. Generally, splints are used to immobilize autografted sites for 5 to 7 days.

When applying a splint on children, considerations may include the anxiety of the child, location of pressure areas, decreased cooperation, diminished understanding, limited verbal communication, and inability to don splints independently. A child who is active during the day may be better suited to use of nighttime positioning. The importance of education of family members and caregivers is also significant.

## Serial Casting

Casts are especially effective for pediatric patients since they cannot be removed and do not slip. They can be applied over dressings or inserts and feature excellent conformability with minimal shear forces.[13] In 1992, Ricks and Meagher demonstrated serial casting was useful for immobilization after acute grafting for burns below the knee.[14] Early serial casting of palmar burns was found by Knutsen et al[15] to prevent contractures and minimize the need for contracture release in children. A specific casting procedure has been outlined.[16]

There are 3 materials used in serial casting: plaster, fiberglass, and nonlatex polyester (such as Delta-Cast™). Plaster casting utilizes bandages which are economical, lightweight, and easy to use while allowing ventilation of the tissue surface. Fiberglass casts are also lightweight but tend to be stronger and set more quickly than plaster casts. Delta-Cast™ is a recent option with the unique properties of elasticity, flexibility, and conformity to the patient's extremities. All casts can be bivalved to allow easy removal for cleaning and exercise. Before application of the cast, stretching exercises of the joint and/or soft tissue massage should be performed. It is important to place a light dressing and padding on bony prominences to avoid any complications. The initial cast is removed within 24 hours to assess the patient's tolerance.

## Skeletal Suspension and Traction

Skeletal suspension and traction systems may also be used to facilitate proper positioning and prevent contractures. In addition, suspension can prevent excessive pressure on wounds and grafts, thereby promoting proper wound healing.[17] The surgeon inserts pins into the lower and upper extremities for attachment to the suspension apparatus. Suspension is then managed by burn staff, who adjust the tension in order to maintain the desired position. Suspension can be removed to assist the child with therapeutic exercises and gait training. Larson et al[18] described the successful use of more than 350 Steinmann pins for skeletal suspension and traction, allowing exposure of skin grafts and correction of contractures. Because of the considerable time and effort involved in setting the mechanism, the team should rule out any alternative techniques before skeletal suspension and traction are implemented.

## Positioning of the Neck

Children who sustain anterior neck burns should be positioned with the neck in an extended or hyperextended position while maintaining the head midline. This can be accomplished with a soft towel roll placed between the scapulae at the level of the spine of the scapulae. Types of splints which promote good neck positioning include both prefabricated (soft cervical collars and neck conformers) and custom semirigid thermoplastic neck splints. They are worn over topical dressings and should not add pressure to the ears. Following autografting, the wearing schedule is 24 hours a day except for dressing changes.[10] Upon healing, neck conformers are worn except for dressing changes and when exercising. Significant neck burns to the lateral and anterior aspect of the neck may lead to torticollis. A splint that incorporates both thermoplastic splinting and strapping to gently maintain midline positioning during the day (splint only) and night (splint plus strapping attached to the side of the bed) has been reported.[19] Other options include foam conformers, Wastusi splints made with plastic tubing, and clear plastic, silicone-lined neck splints.[20] Due to the risk of mandibular retraction in children, thermoplastic splints involving the lower edge of the mandible are not recommended.[21] Nakamura et al[22] advocate utilization of a gel-laden elastic neck wrap as an alternative for patients with normal range of motion.

X-rays of the cervical spine should be performed prior to positioning the neck in hyperextension. Atlantoaxial instability can be present in 20% of children with Down syndrome, so hyperextension may not be appropriate for these children with anterior neck burns.[23] Older children can be encouraged to lie prone while reading and during other play activities to further optimize positioning of the neck in extension. Foley et al[24] describe use of an inverted television and video games to facilitate neck immobility after anterior neck grafting. In order to increase neck flexion, children with posterior neck burns can be positioned in a seated position with functional and play activities placed at waist level.

## Ears

The area around the ear should be free and clear in order to prevent pressure necrosis and folding of the helix. Pressure can impair circulation to ear cartilage, resulting in development of chondritis.[25] Since a pillow may increase the potential for this complication, a foam ring or gel pad may be used to lift the head off the bed. Use of a respiratory mask or thermoplastic cups placed over the ears may also be beneficial.

## Nose

A burn involving the nose may develop microstomia contractures if untreated. Loss of function may cause difficulties with breathing by mouth and/or nose and mucosal crusting. Application of a nasal obturator with serial splinting can be initiated in the acute phase of rehabilitation to open nostrils. In addition, manual therapy for stretching the nostrils as well as employment of nasal dilators are often used in order to maintain patency and prevent occlusion by scarring. Materials utilized for the production of nasal dilators include acrylic, soft plastic, or rubber tubing.[23]

## Face

Facial burns are one of the most challenging types of injury since complications due to involvement of the eyes, ears, nose, and mouth can occur.[26] If left untreated, resultant scars may impair basic functions of eating, talking, and swallowing. Soft tissue defects can include alar retraction, nostril stenosis, columellae contractures, scar bands, and asymmetry of the nose. Knowledge of head and face development is necessary in order to provide appropriate positioning. Head circumference of a normally developing infant increases approximately 12 cm during the first 12 months of life.[23] By 2 to 3 years, 85% of cranium growth is achieved,[23] and by 5 to 7 years, the cranium reaches 90% of its full size.[23] The mandible is not completely developed in an infant. Although the temporomandibular articulation has developed many of its adult traits by 4 years, jaw growth continues to develop until approximately 16 to 17 years of age for girls and 19 to 20 years for boys.[23] Due to the possibility of distorted facial features or changes in facial bony structures during this period of physical development, infants and children require more consistent clinical observation than adolescents.[23] Once wound healing is complete, the child may be measured for a custom face mask.

## Eyes

Serious injury and visual disorders can result from eye burns. Patients may complain of eye irritation, dryness, tearing, or the inability to properly close their eyes. Deep burns of the eyelid margin may lead to scarring, resulting in entropion or ectropion disorders requiring surgery.[27] Still et al[28] reported grafts to the eyelids, tarsorrhaphies, enucleation, corneal transplants, and lid reconstruction are all possible interventions. Passive stretching of the skin, active stretching exercises, and adequate facial pressure are also part of the treatment plan.[29]

## Mouth

Mouth burns require special attention. Commissure contractures and dental conditions such as crossbite, crowding, lower lip eversion, loss of lip competence, and exposure of mandibular dentition have often been linked to such injuries.[30] Facial growth deficits and poor teeth position can be caused by excessive facial pressure.[31] Electrical burns account for 4% of mouth burns.[32] If destruction occurs to 1 or both oral commissures, scar contractures with an asymmetrical opening may result if untreated. A mouth splint is required if the child is unable to follow through with self–range of motion exercises. Family and caregivers need instruction regarding the wearing schedule and manual mouth stretches. Mouth splints ranging from simple to complex can be used for compliant and noncompliant children. Cooperative children benefit most from mouth appliances. Custom mouth splints can be made from low-heat thermoplastic materials or by using 2 conformers that fit the commissures and are applied with elastic bands. Splints must be monitored to prevent skin breakdown. A commercially available microstomia prevention appliance (MPA), which has an adjustable metal bar and plastic conformers that fit the commissures, can be used. This splint can provide an objective measurement for determining the width of the mouth by noting the distance at which the adjustable screw is set. An MPA must be worn at all times except

when eating, talking, providing oral care, and exercising. Furthermore, an MPA can be applied alternately with use of a face mask.[23] More cosmetically appealing, but difficult to create, are custom static acrylic conformers. A dentist fabricates the conformer, fitting the palate after making an impression of the child's mouth. More than 20 different mouth appliances to prevent microstomia have been described by Staley et al,[23] with the majority intended for horizontal mouth opening. Davis et al[33] described a cost-effective, comfortable, and easy-to-use mouth orthosis for the treatment of vertical microstomia which can be used by children and adolescents. The Therabite appliance (Therabite Corporation, Newton Square, PA) was created to provide vertical stretching.[32] Taquino et al[34] developed a dynamic vertical and horizontal mouth splint utilizing thermoplastic materials found in a typical clinic.

## Axilla/Shoulder

Many burns of the upper extremities involve the shoulders and axillary areas. A common complication is limitation in all planes of shoulder movement. The position of comfort is when the shoulders are adducted and internally rotated. The axilla is one of the most difficult areas to successfully treat,[7] as scar band formation usually prevents full range of motion. The shoulder should be placed at 90 degrees of abduction and 15 to 20 degrees in the plane of the scapula.[10] Arms can be placed on pillows (or other supports) on bedside tables, with care taken to avoid undue pressure on elbows. The type of splint used for positioning the shoulder and axilla is often referred to as an *airplane splint*. Manigandan et al[35] used an airplane splint for axillary burns, positioning the shoulder as far as 150 to 160 degrees of abduction. A papoose splint places the child's shoulders in 90 to 160 degrees of abduction and 20 degrees in the plane of the scapula.[36] Darton, Templeton, and Mcinnes utilized splinting intermittently at 150 to 170 degrees abduction and unstated degrees of forward flexion without any vascular or neuropathic complications.[37] Abhyankar[38] described a splint with the hand resting on the forehead and the shoulder positioned at greater than 90 degrees of abduction in order to increase shoulder abduction after grafting and/or contracture release surgeries. Chown[39] reported modified use of the high-density foam airplane splint as an effective treatment modality and approach. Another type of commercially made abductor brace has the capability of increasing or decreasing the angle of the shoulder for abduction. A figure-of-8 axillary wrap to provide pressure and stretch the axillary skin has also been used.[12–40] Use of a soft clavicle brace can facilitate scapular retraction.

## Elbow and Forearm

Assessing the location of a burn on the elbow and forearm areas will determine what type of splint best counteracts the potential contracture. A child typically holds the elbow in flexion, which is a position of comfort. If a significant burn is located on the antecubital fossa, an elbow extension splint or cast should be fabricated to prevent a flexion contracture. For infants or toddlers, tongue depressors wrapped in gauze have been used after skin grafting in order to place the elbow in extension.[41] The forearm is placed in neutral until healing has occurred and the child is actively using the elbow fully. If a contracture develops, a 3-point splint or serial bivalve casting may be required to facilitate stretching of the soft tissue. A dynamic elbow extension splint can be used for contracture correction with both children and adolescents.[42] A supination/pronation splint may be needed if forearm contractures develop. Lastly, Cantrill et al[43] suggest use of a serpentine splint, which facilitates forearm supination and improved overall upper body posture.

## Wrist and Hand

Functional use of the hands is an important aspect of a child's ability to participate in daily activities at home, in school, and during play time. Losing this capacity can result in emotional and psychological distress. Therapists carefully assess wrist and hand burns before deciding the positioning needs. Goals are to place the wrist and hand in antideformity postures and to minimize contracture development of soft tissues.[21]

Generally, the wrist is placed in the functional position of 0 to 15 degrees extension,[12] which is also the position used after volar wrist burns. If dorsal burns are present, however, the wrist is splinted in neutral or up to 35 degrees of extension.[10] Wrists burned on either the radial or ulnar aspect require placement in neutral in order to prevent deviation deformities.

The antideformity position for dorsal hand burns is the intrinsic-plus posture, with the metacarpalphalangeal (MP) joints in 60 to 90 degrees of flexion and interphalangeal (IP) joints in full extension.[16,44,45] If edema is pronounced, 60 to 70 degrees of MP flexion may be advisable in order to avoid ischemia secondary to loss of capillary integrity.[37] Burn injuries to the dorsum of the fingers should be evaluated for joint integrity. If the child is unable to actively extend his or her fingers, an extensor hood mechanism injury is suspected. Involved proximal interphalangeal (PIP) joints are then splinted in full extension for 6 weeks.[25] The antideformity position for the thumb is in between palmar and radial abduction with 10 degrees metacarpalphalangeal flexion and full interphalangeal extension.[16]

Burns to the first web space require a thumb abduction splint.

Hands volarly burned are splinted with the goal of preserving expansion of palmar creases: the hand is placed with the digits hyperextended and abducted. Regardless of the location of the burns, or in the presence of edema, a splint should conform to the child's hand and wrist rather than being forced to fit the splint.[16] Soft materials such as pieces of foam may be used for positioning an infant's wrist and hand in a functional posture. A dynamic MP flexion splint may be fabricated for adolescents who develop MP tightness and intrinsic-minus (MP extension or hyperextension with IP flexion) posturing.[25] This splint can be combined with use of individual finger extension gutter splints to place the IP joints in full extension. The small size of a child's hands makes fabrication of dynamic splints difficult; in addition, tolerance is typically poor.

Children and adolescents with circumferential hand burns need 2 types of splints, 1 to place the hand in the intrinsic-plus position and the other to position the digits in hyperextension and abduction. These splints can be alternately worn throughout the day and night. Composite extensor shortening and/or joint stiffness can be addressed by utilizing elastic wrap to place the fingers in composite flexion for short periods of time.

As with all splints, consistent monitoring for areas of pressure is needed. Children benefit from prolonged splinting regimens without developing the joint stiffness so commonly seen in adults.[10] If poor compliance is encountered, a bivalve splint can be fabricated to prohibit removal by the child. Patient and family education, including wound healing, exercise programs, and positioning/splint schedules, is stressed.

## Trunk/Hips

A trunk-splinting protocol with good alignment of the shoulders and hips is necessary to prevent scoliosis and kyphosis. Towel rolls can be placed along the spine to assist with alignment and increase expansion of the trunk. Common positions after surgery with autografts may include, but are not limited to, any of the following: side-lying, prone, trendelenburg, and reverse trendelenburg. Additional devices to assist with appropriate positioning include bolsters, beanbags, jellyrolls, and foam.

When burns affect the anterior abdomen, the hips need to be positioned appropriately to avoid hip flexion causing lumbar lordosis and/or knee flexion. Asymmetric contractures can cause an oblique pelvis and scoliosis. Preambulatory children with thigh burns can develop contractures in abduction. Hip position should be in full extension (0 degrees rotation) with symmetric abduction of 15 to

20 degrees.[12,46] If the child is not positioned correctly, contractures in flexion, rotation, or adduction can occur. Long-term effects can cause postural and functional leg-length discrepancy. Ways to prevent hip contractures are to avoid use of soft mattresses, position in reverse trendelenburg, use abduction wedges, place towel rolls under hips, and fabricate or use an extension spica splint with the hip positioned in neutral. If burns cross the anterior pelvis, prolonged sitting positions should be avoided.[46] Surgical intervention may be required to prevent or correct scoliosis or lordosis.

## Knee

Positioning of the knee should be in extension, even while sitting. Burns to the lateral/medial aspect of the knee or popliteal area are at high risk for contractures. Knee external rotation or flexion should be avoided. Commercially available adjustable knee splints are superior to in-house fabrications but are more expensive. The knee can be positioned with a conforming thermoplastic splint, a 3-point brace, or a knee immobilizer.[12,46] If contractures occur, the child may have instability of gait stance or loss of ambulatory ability.

## Foot/Ankle

An ankle burn can develop into equinovarus, foot plantar flexion, and inversion.[46] Knees should be supported at 0 degrees of extension and feet positioned at 0 degrees (neutral) to assist with preservation of the Achilles tendon. The ideal position of the ankle is 5 to 10 degrees of dorsiflexion to maintain Achilles tendon length and allow for a normal gait pattern.[10] Positioning devices such as footboards and foam blocks at the end of a mattress can be used. Foot splints are commercially available or custom-made with thermoplastic splint materials. Use of elastic wraps in a figure-8 pattern can assist in alleviating edema and maintaining neutral positioning of the ankle. The foot should be positioned to prevent any pressure areas along the lateral and medial borders and heel. Deep and superficial peroneal nerve damage can cause the foot to assume nonfunctional postures.[47] Circumferential foot and ankle burns should be managed by using anterior/posterior foot splints with alternating schedules. Surgical intervention for releases may involve pinning or traction to prevent contractures of the ankle and/or toes. The first and fifth toes may be displaced due to scar band formation on the medial and lateral aspects. Since toes have a tendency to hyperextend with dorsal burns, use of toe plate splints may be necessary to maintain proper alignment. Serial casting of the ankle may be an option to gradually stretch soft tissue and prevent foot contractures.

## Edema Management

Edema following burn injury requires prompt attention in order to reduce subsequent pain, contractures, and soft tissue adhesions.[48] Elevation with the use of elastic and compressive wraps such as Coban™ is utilized during healing to promote reduction of edema and therefore increase range of motion. Elevation of the hands above the heart assists in reducing overall swelling.[49,50] Persistent swelling may adversely affect joints, tendons, and ligaments, resulting in reduced mobility.[49] Once the child initiates active range of motion, compression wraps may be eliminated. In circumferential burns, severe edema can cause compartment syndrome, with decreased blood flow to muscles causing significant damage, ischemia, and decreased neurovascular function. If tissue pressures become elevated, escharotomies and/or fasciotomies may be necessary.[50,51]

## Pain Management

A child experiencing inadequate pain management will often exhibit nervousness, agitation, or apprehension towards staff and required interventions such as dressing changes. Practitioners need to be knowledgeable about the types of pain and be able to quantify a patient's perception of pain by utilizing readily available instruments.[52]

During acute hospitalization, most pediatric patients with burn injuries demonstrate 2 types of pain. The first is procedural pain, also labeled as acute or short-term pain. Procedural pain occurs with wound care, dressing changes, staple removal, or venipuncture. The second type of pain is background or ongoing acute pain. Background pain occurs when distressing feelings are experienced during rest or activities (such as therapies) in the absence of procedures.[53] Both types of pain require objective and subjective evaluation to facilitate appropriate overall care of the patient. Ongoing assessment of pain management is critical throughout the child's hospital stay and subsequent participation in outpatient therapies, focusing on the effectiveness of both pharmacologic and nonpharmacologic treatment.[52]

Three methods of pain measurement in children have been identified as useful: physiologic, behavioral, and self-reported. All are part of the total patient care plan. Physiologic methods easily quantified include heart rate, blood pressure, respiratory rate, and oxygen saturation. These are especially useful when a patient is unable to communicate due to such limitations as present injuries, developmental disabilities, and cultural or language differences. Behavioral methods of pain management include use of keen observation by staff and parents. Behaviors of very young patients or those with cognitive challenges often depict whether they are experiencing pain or discomfort. Self-reports by children are those who can express, through words or use of pictorial stimuli, how they feel. Pain measurement tools commonly used in clinical settings are shown in Table 2.

Sleep and emotional adjustment problems often coexist with pain. Relaxation can reduce anxiety, nervousness, and pain and may be useful for children in improving their sleep patterns and coping abilities. Children reportedly as young as 1 year old have been trained in relaxation techniques.[54] In addition, appropriate play activities may decrease the perception of pain and enhance self-esteem.[55]

Practitioners have an important role in providing therapeutic activities which allow children experiencing pain to develop both coping strategies and skills essential for optimal functional performance. Treatment interventions may include communication of pain,[56] physical activity,[56] relaxation training,[53] cognitive restructuring,[56] distraction,[53] art therapy,[57] music therapy,[58] and social support.[56] Communication of pain may include training which emphasizes how, when, and with whom the child will discuss his or her pain. Social skill training with focus on expression of feelings has also been found to be beneficial. When a patient demonstrates pain behaviors, incorporating activities to promote progressive mobility, endurance, and strengthening may be helpful. Relaxation training often includes progressive muscle relaxation, autogenic training, and guided imagery.[56] Pereyra et al[57] concluded that art therapy provided a constructive means of expression in their study of 21 children who participated in art therapy during their inpatient hospitalization. Similarly, Tan et al.[58] found that music therapy during daily burn debridement significantly reduced pain, anxiety, and muscle tension levels in 29 children and adult inpatients. A social support group can be an especially valuable therapeutic medium for helping children with burns learn to express emotions, share coping skills, and make new friends.[54]

## PRESERVING JOINT INTEGRITY AND MUSCULOSKELETAL FUNCTION

Burn injuries can be particularly devastating for children who are in the midst of growing and developing. It is beyond the scope of this chapter to review the typical motor development of a child. Although a figure of typical motor milestones is included (Table 2),[59,60] it is recommended that therapists treating a child with burns review a book on pediatric motor development.[59,60]

The extent of the burn injury will dictate treatment. As the total body surface area (TBSA) of a burn injury increases, the chance for greater loss of function leading to disability increases. Burns cause a hypermetabolic response coupled with increased resting energy expenditure which leads to loss of lean body mass from protein catabolism.[61,62,63] This catabolic response can last up to 2 years postinjury.[61,62,63] Furthermore, studies have shown that prolonged bed rest or immobilization results in loss of muscle mass, decreased bone mineral density, and an increased risk for fractures, joint contractures, and deconditioning.[64,65,66] During this period, the child should continue to develop functional movement, motor control, and musculoskeletal abilities. The therapist's responsibility includes ensuring the maintenance of such abilities while assisting children in reaching their future developmental milestones.

Studies dealing with the effects of prolonged immobility have shown inability of the body to regain strength once bed rest ends.[64] Studies have also demonstrated exercise performed during bed rest can help reverse some of the effects of deconditioning.[64]

Therapy should be initiated the day the child arrives in the burn center. During the first 24 to 72 hours, when the inflammatory phase is predominant, edema reduction through patient positioning is the primary goal of the therapist. Once the patient is medically stable, the role of the therapist expands from positioning and splinting to preserving soft tissue mobility through range of motion (ROM) and exercise. As children are at increased risk for hypertrophic scarring that leads to contractures, therapy must focus on maintaining ROM long after their initial hospitalization. This can become a prolonged process which is not completed until scars have fully matured and the child has stopped growing. In addition to ROM, the therapist must include strengthening and endurance activities, which can be accomplished through an exercise program, play, and activities of daily living (ADLs).

Throughout the rehabilitative process, the foremost goal of the therapist is to preserve range of motion. Although it is always best for the patient to actively participate in exercises, the child is often unable to because of sedation, pain, or decreased strength and endurance. Range of motion can therefore be performed passively (PROM) until the patient can either assist the therapist or fully participate himself or herself.

The primary goal of PROM is to maintain mobility of soft tissue. Secondary goals include decreasing the potential for contractures, enhancing synovial function of cartilage nutrition through diffusion into joints, decreasing/inhibiting pain, and assisting circulation and vascular dynamics.[67] When performing range of motion on a child, it is important to keep the movements within a pain-free range and not use a stretch force. All movements should be done smoothly and slowly. When performed correctly, PROM should not cause pain or agitation for the child. In most circumstances, PROM is contraindicated for patients with exposed tendons. However, in our center we continue to perform PROM despite exposed tendons in order to prevent the tendon from adhering to surrounding tissue. Typically during tendon gliding, the exposed tendon is covered in petroleum-impregnated gauze, which prevents desiccation and possible dehiscence.

If a child begins to lose range of motion, manual stretching techniques should be utilized to regain lost range. During passive stretching, movement is carried just beyond the point of pain. If a child is unable to communicate his or her pain, movement is carried just past the point of tension.[67] It is often helpful to have the child participate in an active-assistive stretch. As the child uses the agonist muscle to complete the movement, a reciprocal relaxation of the antagonist muscle occurs.[67] When stretching, it is important to be mindful of the grip on the child. Pressure should be exerted evenly, as uneven pressure may cause pain. Caution with hand placement on bony prominences such as the epicondyles or the malleoli is warranted, since excessive pressure may be more painful than the stretch itself.[67] Once the origin of the muscle being stretched is firmly stabilized, the therapist should ease into the stretch and then slowly release. Although PROM can help maintain soft tissue mobility and stretching and can assist with maintaining ROM, these techniques cannot prevent muscle atrophy, nor increase strength or endurance. Therefore, it is extremely crucial for children to participate in therapy sessions and become an active part of their rehabilitation as soon as possible.

Exercise benefits healthy children in many ways, such as improving cardiorespiratory endurance, providing a pathway toward optimal growth and development, and reducing the risk of diabetes and coronary artery disease.[68] For the child who has suffered a burn injury, exercise has been shown to improve muscle strength and lean body mass, reduce the risk for future surgical intervention, and provide beneficial effects on overall quality of life.[69-73]

Many authors have designed exercise programs for patients with burn injuries.[71-75] Since each child's injury is unique, it is dependent upon the creativity of the therapist to decide which exercises will achieve the best outcome and promote the greatest healing. Oftentimes the initial goal is getting the child to move, since he or she may be in pain or frightened. Since exercises should correspond with the goals for a patient, it may be most effective to introduce playing as a therapeutic exercise, as opposed to a regimented series of active extremity exercises. Having the child actively participate in his or her ADLs, such as dressing and eating, can also help accomplish full, active range of motion not achieved with a specific exercise. Dressing changes can be an excellent time to promote range of motion of an affected joint as well as help alleviate fears regarding the procedure by allowing the child to assist with removal of dressings and washing of wounds.

Parental or caregiver involvement during the entire rehabilitation process is vital to ensure success. As the family will also be experiencing tremendous stress, it is important for the therapist to maintain a good rapport with both the child and his or her family. This allows the therapist to more readily identify problems and assist parents in obtaining appropriate support.[76] The therapist's responsibilities include furnishing appropriate attention to the child as well as providing interventions to the parents to assist them in optimizing the child's abilities.[77] Rone-Adams et al[78] found that a family's problems and the physical limitations of a child predicted compliance with a home exercise program. The ongoing interaction and involvement between the therapist and child's family may help lessen stress on the family and increase compliance with the child's therapy.

Another important component to a child's recovery, besides play activities and ADLs, is ambulation. In our center, gait training begins once the child is medically stable, unless he or she has severe burns to the plantar surface of the foot or the medical team determines that ambulation is unwarranted. For younger children who are not yet ambulating, crawling is initiated once medically stable. To help prevent venous stasis and pain that can occur from having the lower extremities in a dependent position, compression wraps or stockings are donned from the distal feet to the proximal thighs. Assistive devices are generally discouraged except when necessary to allow a child to accept weight through the lower extremities. Once the patient is comfortable with weight bearing, the assistive device is replaced with a handhold assist. With younger children, a toy tricycle, such as a Big Wheel™, can be used to achieve AROM of the lower extremities. It also allows the child to achieve some weight bearing through the lower extremities.

For children who are having an extremely difficult time standing—either due to pain, fear, or in some instances, extreme deconditioning—a tilt table can be used to initiate weight bearing. A tilt table is also effective at reducing orthostatic hypotension, which occasionally occurs with patients who have experienced prolonged bed rest.[79] A tilt table, however, does not typically allow movement of the lower extremities required to alleviate venous pooling and associated dependent pain.[79]

For grafted lower extremities, ambulation is dependent upon the protocols established by the burn center. Typically, therapy can begin the next day on an extremity with an allograft (homograft) or xenograft. For an extremity with an autograft, therapy is withheld for 3 to 5 days, during which time exercise continues with the nongrafted extremities.

Once the medical team determines the child has healed enough to be discharged from the acute hospital setting, the rehabilitation process must continue. As the scar maturation process continues for up to 18 months and muscle catabolism and resting energy expenditure last for up to 2 years, the child must remain involved in an outpatient therapy setting coupled with a home exercise program.

Once a child has reached the outpatient setting, more emphasis can be placed on resistance training to increase strength and muscle mass, as well as on aerobic activity to help increase endurance. Studies have found resistance training to be a safe and effective way of conditioning children.[80-83] Both the American Academy of Pediatrics and the Department of Human Performance and Fitness have stated that resistance training is safe and effective.[82,83] Exercise can also have positive effects on self-esteem, self-confidence, and self-perception in children with disabilities.[81,82] Many different authors have shown promising research regarding exercise programs for children with burns and/or disabilities.[70-73,78,80,81] Higher repetition exercises with moderate weight are favored over lower repetitions with high weight for children. Any exercise program should begin with a warm-up, after which periods of aerobic activity and strength training can begin. Every session should conclude with a cool-down period.

## MINIMIZING SCAR EFFECTS

Almost as immediately as there are goals to prevent joint contractures, therapists working with children and adolescents who have been burned formulate goals to minimize scar contractures. The stages of wound healing and subsequent scar formation are carefully considered and reconsidered throughout inpatient, outpatient, and reconstruction phases. Each surgical procedure results in both new wounds and potential future contractures.

During every phase of rehabilitation, therapy goals related to scar management include promotion of optimal wound healing; minimization of hypertrophic and keloid scar formation; minimization of pain, pruritis, hyperesthesia, and overall discomfort caused by scars; optimization of functional performance, endurance, and independence in ADLs and instrumental activities of daily living (IADLs); provision of psychosocial support to the patient and family members/support system; and completion of patient and family education on topics of wound healing, scar management, splint usage, home exercises, and skin protection.[7]

Wound healing is generally divided into 3 stages or phases. The first stage is an inflammatory phase which is marked by local cellular and vascular responses resulting in clearing the wound of devitalized tissue, debris, and foreign materials. Initially, clotting and vasoconstriction occur in order to decrease blood loss. Platelet aggregation along the endothelium of injured blood vessels occurs with vasocon-

striction (hemostasis).[84] The platelets release vasoconstrictive, chemotactic, and growth-producing substances which facilitate fibrin clot formation for hemorrhage control.[84,85] Subsequent release of vasoactive substances such as histamine and prostaglandins, as well as stimulation of local sensory nerve endings, causes local reflex action with resultant vasodilation and increased permeability.[7,86] Research has shown that edema is caused by interstitial components generating strong negative tissue pressure.[87,88]

At this stage, excessive swelling must be avoided.[89] Use of edema management techniques and devices is indicated as part of the therapeutic intervention. It has been suggested that increased and/or chronic inflammation may result in decreased quality and quantity of cellular activity and, subsequently, excessive scar formation[50,86,90]; decreasing inflammation and edema may therefore assist in achieving less scarring. Care is taken with passive range of motion in order to minimize additional tissue damage and concomitant further inflammation. If possible, active range of motion is encouraged. Splints may be introduced if atraumatic and desired for advantageous positioning.

Following vasodilation, vasocongestion and leakage of serous fluids into the wound bed occurs. White blood cells (leukocytes) migrate towards the wound while neutrophils move through the blood vessel walls in order to phagocytize bacteria and foreign contaminants. By day 2, monocytes are converted into macrophages, which are critical for cleaning the wound and breaking down necrotic tissue. Cellular repair has thus begun.[7] The duration of this phase lasts from a few days to 2 weeks, depending on such factors as presence of a dirty wound, severe tissue trauma at the time of injury, rough handling during surgery, overly aggressive therapy, and inappropriate, damaging dressings.[4,7,91]

The next phase is the proliferative or fibroplastic phase, which includes granulation and epithelialization processes.[92] Epithelialization occurs as a result of mobilization, migration, proliferation, and differentiation. New collagen and blood vessels form red granulation tissue and facilitate wound contraction. Myofibroblasts connect to the wound margins and pull the epidermal layer inward. This produces the characteristic picture frame beneath the skin.[93] Contraction decreases the size of the affected area, which is then repaired by scar formation. As such, the goal of therapy is to inhibit wound contraction.[7] If contraction occurs, centripetal force will pull all structures towards the wound. Joint contractures, as sometimes seen in full-thickness burns, are often the result of uncontrolled wound contraction.[86] The deeper the wound, the longer it takes to heal, resulting in increased risk of pain, infection, and ultimately, scar formation.[94-96] Early administration of basic fibroblast growth factor has been shown to improve the quality of pediatric burn scars.[97]

Use of skin grafts can diminish wound contraction,[98] with the thickness of the graft correlating to the degree of wound suppression. Split-thickness grafts diminish contraction of the wound by 31%, full-thickness grafts diminish contraction by 55%, and early combined use of full-thickness grafts with splinting inhibits contraction by 77%.[86,99,100] During the proliferative phase, splinting the wound areas is an important element of ultimate scar management. Externally applied splints can provide stress to desirably orient the deposited collagen as well as provide appropriate joint alignment positioning.[16] If the wound has been recently grafted, consideration of inosculation of the blood vessels will be essential. Cells of the new graft are nourished by tissue fluid until inosculation between the graft and wound is established in 1 to 3 days.[4]

Immobilization of the graft is imperative until take of the graft is seen.[4] Therapists are often called upon to apply cohesive wrap over primary dressings after autografts have been placed on hand burns in order to minimize edema development and facilitate graft take.[16] After graft adherence has been achieved, pressure can be applied to inhibit scar contraction and hypertrophy, decrease vascular and lymphatic pooling, and avert hypersensitive, fragile skin.[101] Examples of uses of pressure are tubular bandages applied over primary dressings, conforming splints applied over dressings (especially at palmar and thenar web spaces), and elastic bandages to secure splints worn over dressings.[12,16] Elastic wraps can be used for both providing gentle retrograde edema control and adhering finger splints. Lowell et al[102] found that Coban™ wrapping reduced edema in a case study of 2 skin-grafted hands.

The tensile strength and durability of remodeled skin arises from new collagen formed after fibroblasts synthesize collagen and undergo cross-linkage. This strength is, however, less than the original skin: it will never exceed 75% to 80%.[103] Following grafting, there is generally enough tensile strength between the graft and the wound to permit active range of motion on the fourth day and at least by the sixth day.[4] Gentle passive range of motion can be added after 6 to 7 days.[4]

The proliferative phase is completed when epithelialization has resurfaced the wound, a collagen layer has been formed, and initial remodeling is complete[84]; this phase generally lasts 2 weeks. Appropriate wound care and edema management are paramount burn team concerns, with proper positioning and maintenance of functional range of motion (both active and passive now) as primary therapy goals. If possible, participation in light ADLs and limited ambulation is encouraged.[104] Strengthening exercises can be introduced during the proliferative phase.[7] Positioning, splinting, range of motion, functional and strengthening exercises, gait training, and patient education are important in preventing or minimizing both cosmetic and performance impacts of scar formation.[105]

The final phase of wound healing is referred to as the maturation or remodeling phase and generally lasts a year or longer.[21] Its hallmark is the relative balance of collagen synthesis and lysis, that is, the formation and breakdown of collagen.[16] Scar formed during fibroplasia is dense, disorganized, and different from surrounding tissue. As maturation occurs, collagen lysis increases and scar tissue becomes smoother, more elastic, and stronger. If synthesis exceeds lysis, hypertrophic scarring or keloid formation may occur.[16] Keloid scars extend beyond the boundary of the wound and appear raised. On the other hand, hypertrophic scars occur within the area of the wound and may eventually decrease in both size and shape.[16]

During the remodeling phase, use of pressure is emphasized. There are 2 primary theories which explain how collagen fibers become aligned: induction theory and tension theory.[86] Induction theory purports that scar tissue attempts to mimic characteristics of the tissue it is healing, while tension theory proposes that the internal and external stresses applied on the wound affect and align the fibers during remodeling. Using principles of induction theory, the surgeon attempts to design the repair field by separating dense and soft tissues. The latter theory is partially supported by many studies which have suggested that adding tension during healing increases tensile strength of soft tissue and bone. These same studies have noted that immobilizing an area results in decreased strength and collagen fiber organization.[106-109] Tension theory, at least in part, supports the use of compression garments, silicone inserts, dynamic splinting, serial casting, continuous passive motion (CPM), positional heat and stretching techniques, neuromuscular electrical stimulation (NMES), and functional electrical stimulation (FES) in order to optimize wound healing and minimize hypertrophic scar formation.[86]

The remodeling phase can last up to 2 years.[46] As long as the scar exhibits a rosier appearance than normal, remodeling is underway.[86] Mitigating factors include presence of foreign objects or microorganisms (infections), repeated surgical procedures, inadequate nutrition (including comorbidities such as diabetes mellitus, atherosclerosis, and acquired immune deficiency syndrome),[84] use of systemic medications (such as steroids, nonsteroidal anti-inflammatory drugs, chemotherapeutic agents, antibiotics, and anticoagulants),[110] burn depth,[111,112] type of graft,[113] and burn size.[114] Dark-skinned individuals appear to have a higher likelihood of experiencing hypertrophic scarring or keloid formation.[94,111] True partial-thickness wounds do not predictably scar, as opposed to full-thickness injuries.[7]

Typically, use of a meshed but not expanded sheet graft results in less scarring and contraction than use of an expanded meshed graft.[16] Schwanholt et al[115] found that use of full-thickness skin grafts for deep palmar burns in pediatric patients resulted in better range of motion and required less reconstructive surgery than palms covered with split-thickness skin grafts. The total percentage of dermis grafted is more critical than the thickness of the graft, according to McDonald and Deitch[111]; in their prospective study of 70 patients, the presence of dermal elements in the recipient graft bed was associated with less scarring than those on beds without dermal elements. Deitch et al[94] reported in their study of 59 pediatric and 41 adult patients that hypertrophic scarring was 3 times more likely to occur if healing took longer than 21 days. Pediatric patients demonstrate a greater propensity to scar than adults.[94,111,114,116] Deitch et al[94] listed the feet, perineum/buttocks, chest, back, head/neck, and upper extremities (in descending order) as most likely to develop hypertrophic scars in their prospective study of 59 pediatric patients, while Kraemer et al[114] stated that the majority of contractures occurred at the hands, axillae, head, and antecubital fossae (again, in descending order) in their retrospective study of 64 pediatric patients. During the maturation wound-healing phase, therapy goals include all those previously mentioned, and scar management becomes a primary focus.

Prevention of raised hypertrophic scars and/or formation of keloid scars extending beyond wound boundaries can be at least partially achieved by use of pressure.[117-119] Prolonged pressure creates an ischemic condition whereby blood flow (and oxygen) is decreased in the wound tissue. With less oxygen, synthesis is curtailed while lysis is unaffected; tissue balance is achieved when scar bulk is flattened to approximate normal tissue.[86] Mechanical compression controls the release of cytokines in a hypertrophic scar and reduces the binding of collagen fibers.[118-120]

Fitting of interim pressure garments is started as soon as the remodeling phase has become evident; patients are measured for custom garments once grafts are healed and can tolerate shearing forces.[119] Small open and granulating areas can be covered with dressings.[16,21] It has been recommended that all patients whose wounds require longer than 14 days to heal and those with split-thickness grafts receive prophylactic pressure therapy.[4,94,121] Generally, pressures ranging from 20 to 30 mmHg are needed for effective treatment.[122,123] Appropriate pressure produces results within a few days and notably after a few weeks of implementation.[4,124] Decreased overall edema with concomitantly reduced redness, increased pliability, increased softness, and flattening of scar tissue has been noted.[125,126] Garments should be worn at all times (except during bathing and skin care) until scar maturation is achieved. Glove removal is occasionally specified for a home exercise program or particular sensory or motor experiences.[16] Machine washing garments (versus hand washing) may be surprisingly superior for maintaining optimal pressure.[127] Macintyre et al[127] also recommend prestressing powernet fabrics (ie, those fabric structures most commonly used in the construction of garments) prior to designing or constructing particular pieces. Interim pressure gloves and custom pressure gloves are shown in photos 21 and 22, respectively.

Garments generally last 3 months before skin blanching is no longer noted and replacements are necessary.[128] Application of interim garments may need to be postponed if skin appears too fragile.[16] Grigsby deLinde and Knothe[16] outline many custom and commercially available options for both interim and permanent garment selection. Considerations include whether to use open fingertip gloves during the day (recommended) versus closed fingertip ones (nighttime use recommended), if dart closures (eg, in the area of the thenar eminence, in order to pull the thumb into opposition) are needed, and whether to request zippers. Although zippers facilitate independent donning, they also contribute to a youngster's impulsive removal of the garment. In addition, they can disrupt pressure because they take the place of elastic material, are immobile, and ripple.

Recently, O'Brien et al[129] and Dewey et al[130] evaluated the effects of modifying gloves in order to increase grip, dexterity, and ADL function. Although further studies are needed, they found that adding suede or silicone (respectively) improved performance in functional tasks. Moore and Robinson[4] describe a custom garment designed for diaper-wearing children that provides pressure on buttock scars and enables less traumatic diaper changes. Similarly, Serghiou et al[131] provide specific guidelines for garment-fitting children younger than 3 years. Although garments may partially protect vulnerable skin from harmful ultraviolet sun rays, application of total sunblock lotion is advised for patients when outdoors.[16]

Pediatric patients require special consideration during compressive garment selection and fitting because of decreased understanding and reasoning, potential fear and anxiety, and decreased attention span.[7] Repeated fittings may be needed as the child grows. Placement of fasteners away from a child's grasp may increase wearing time as she or he accommodates to wearing the garment, and use of bright colors[132] may aid in a child's acceptance. Ultimately, family support of garment wearing is critical to successful compliance.

Silastic™ and elastomer conformers as well as other types of padding can supplement pressure garments for use over scars with irregular or concave surfaces.[4,16,21] Web spacers may be sewn into a glove to prevent syndactyly.[16] A bivalve approach for nighttime splinting, including elastomer inserts, can be used to provide sufficient pressure for circumferential burns.[16] Long-term longitudinally applied paper tape application can prevent or lessen hypertrophic scarring by preventing longitudinal stretching.[119,133] Coban™ wrapping of the hand and wrist can be alternately utilized if discomfort or poor compliance is reported with glove use.[12] Similarly, Kealey et al[134] found that use of elasticized cotton pressure garments resulted in significantly better patient compliance, lower cost, and equivocally equal efficacy compared with use of elasticized nylon pressure garments.

Use of silicone gel sheeting (SGS) has been shown to be a safe and effective management tool for treatment of hypertrophic scars and keloids; results from randomized, controlled trials and a meta-analysis demonstrate good evidence of its efficacy.[135-138] The exact mechanism is unknown. It has been shown that the surface temperature of scar tissue increases significantly following application of SGS, raising the possibility that temperature alteration is involved in the mechanism of action.[139,140] Alternately, friction on the silicone surface may create a static electrical field with a resultant inhibitory effect on scar tissue.[141] Lastly, increased hydration[142] and hydration with occlusion[143] have been posited as the most likely factors of the mechanism of action. Mustoe et al[137] reported that use of totally occlusive dressings (eg, polyethylene films) or semiocclusive dressings (eg, polyurethane films) did not demonstrate efficacy, and results using glycerin or other non-silicone-based dressings were mixed. Klopp[144] obtained his best results from use of compression therapy with SGS or polyurethane dressing. SGS may be especially helpful for use with children because of the relative ease and painlessness of its application. Garments can be lined with a silicone coating in order to provide more uniform pressure.[113] Silicone elastomer can be used to fashion a custom splint, for example, a web-space elastomer splint. Finally, silicone products appear to reduce chronic hypertrophy as well.[145] Typical complications encountered are petechial rash and skin maceration, but these are easily resolved by temporarily stopping use.[135,146] Van den Kerckhove et al[147] feel the key to success with pressure therapy is ensuring hygienic precautions are taken, especially regarding possible maceration of adjacent healthy tissue.

Providing adequate pressure to facial areas can be achieved with use of a custom or commercially available, frequently monitored face mask.[21] Studies have found, however, that close attention to facial and dental development during the use of masks is needed in order to avoid complications; referral to an orthodontist is recommended.[31,148] Excessive mandibular pressure can also occur, resulting in obstructive sleep apnea.[4] Wearing a transparent mask may seem less offensive and enable visible facial expressions, thereby increasing compliance.[29,149]

Scar management includes treating both raising forces and contractile forces.[84] While application of pressure is a broadly accepted method for addressing raising forces, use of low-load, prolonged stress and other methods of supplying internal and external forces can also positively affect contractile properties. Examples of forces acting on the collagen array in order to facilitate permanent elongation of the scar are muscle tension, joint movement, passive gliding of fascial planes, soft tissue loading and unloading, temperature changes, mobilization, and splinting.[86,150] Sustained stretching is one of the most effective exercises for lengthening scar bands and increasing range of motion[4]; blanching of the scar represents appropriate stretch.[4,7,16] Progressive, judicious massage may release scar tissue from adjacent tissue and increase range of motion as well.[7]

Recently, use of low-level laser therapy was shown to soften burn scars and increase pliability.[151] Moist heat packs and paraffin have been used for treatment of scar contractures; using subsequent sustained stretches, Head and Helm[152] stated that increased collagen extensibility, skin pliability, and joint range of motion, as well as decreased joint pain, were seen in the 20 adult and pediatric patients they treated. Paraffin is the most consistently effective modality for use with pediatric patients, according to Moore and Robinson.[4] Johnson[153] demonstrated trunk and shoulder scar contracture correction following use of paraffin and manual therapy in her case study of a 6-year-old boy. Fluidotherapy is another treatment option.[4] Ultrasound has been utilized for increasing range of motion and decreasing pain, with equivocal results reported thus far[154]; in addition, use over growing epiphyseal plates is controversial.[155] Functional electrical stimulation has been successfully used with adult patients,[156] and the combination of iontophoresis (utilizing iodine), manual therapy, and exercises was reported to correct scar contracture following a bunionectomy.[157]

Application of physical agents can be contraindicated if impaired sensation or cognition prevents the patient from accurately and consistently reporting response to the modality.[155] Precautions to consider are the fragility of newly resurfaced skin and inadequate overall tolerance. Furthermore, since young children often appear fearful of heat, gradual introduction and possible temperature reduction of hydrocollator water, paraffin wax, or fluidotherapy particles is recommended. Lastly, continuous passive motion has been shown to be effective for restoring range of motion in adult patients with hand burns.[158] Contractures, however, were not studied. Research reporting the utilization of electrical stimulation or CPM with children or adolescents with scar contractures was not found.

The goal during the remodeling phase is to influence scar formation by applying controlled stress as the scar matures. Ultimately, achieving a dense, parallel union of scar tissue to surrounding tissue is the preferred outcome.[86]

Besides those mentioned above, methods to provide tension to scars include static, static-progressive, and dynamic splinting,[16,21] serial casts,[4,12-14,159] and traction.[12,16,160]

There are many subjective and objective assessments of scars. These include visual inspection and use of photographs,[161] numeric scales,[162] patient rating scales,[163] the visual analog scale,[161] the facial cosmetic disfigurement scale,[164] the Vancouver burn scar assessment scale (VBSAS),[165] the modified Vancouver scar scale (mVSS),[166] the matching assessment of scars and photographs,[167] oximetry,[168] laser Doppler flowmetry,[169] tonometry,[170,171] colorimetry,[172] histology with digital image analysis,[173] elastometers,[174] cutometers,[175] quasi-static extensometers,[176] dermal torque meters,[177] durometers,[178,179] and ultrasound.[180]

Recently, Nedelec et al[181] found that the Mexameter®, DermaScan C®, and the Cutometer® demonstrated greater reliability and validity than the mVSS. The most conveniently and commonly utilized assessment tools are visual inspection, use of photographs, and VBSAS or mVSS[7,16,165,166,182,183]. It has also been suggested that functional limitations incurred as a result of scarring be assessed.[184] Lastly, evaluating donor sites for development of hypertrophic scarring, as well as assessing levels of pain and pruritis, is recommended.[16,179,185-187]

Scars can be painful[188]; rest, massage, compression garment use, and elevation have been found to be helpful.[189,190] Transcutaneous electrical nerve stimulation (TENS) has also been used successfully for pain control.[191] Low-level laser therapy has shown promising results for decreasing the pain as well as pruritis of burn scars in 12 of 13 adults.[151] Scars also itch. Although pruritis is commonly reported by patients, medications do not appear to provide satisfactory control[98]; however, wearing compression garments may help.[189,192] In her individual case report, Whitaker[193] used TENS successfully to significantly decrease pruritis in an adult patient. Patino et al[194] found massage reduced pruritis in pediatric burn patients. Field et al[195] noted that adult patients receiving massage reported significantly decreased pruritis, pain, and anxiety as well as improved mood. Partial-thickness wounds without grafts but with hypertrophic scarring can demonstrate higher evaporative water loss and resultant extreme dryness and pruritis.[196] Hypertrophic scars have also been shown to demonstrate increased nerve density; Liang et al[197] proposed that the debilitating itching and pain associated with hypertrophic scars implicates injured sensory nerves within the aberrant healing process. Grigsby deLinde and Knothe[16] have recommended massaging at least twice daily, and up to 4 times a day, using non-water-based creams. Lubricants should not contain perfume or other skin irritants. Patients who require extensive grafting, with loss of hair follicles, sebaceous glands, and sweat glands, should avoid high environmental heat and humidity.[4]

Sensory disturbances, including hypoesthesia, sensory loss, and hyperesthesia, are not uncommon.[4,96,198] Ward et al[198] studied loss of cutaneous sensibility in 60 patients with skin grafts and found a decrease in sensation of all grafted areas with no predictable recovery. Other problems with sensory awareness were noted, including increased sensitivity to ambient temperatures, chronic itching, and pain. Regeneration of nerve endings into burned areas may cause altered sensations.[4] Neuromas are reported as well, with associated hypersensitivity.[4] Massage and use of modalities may assist with desensitization.[4,12] Children are often unable to accurately describe impairments, so extra care is needed with any sensory input. Family teaching should emphasize safety and protection. Moore and Robinson[4] report peripheral nerve damage occurs in 15% to 29% of burn patients, but it is estimated that children and adolescents sustain a lower percentage given the typical causes of burns in these age groups. Using sural nerve grafts to reconstruct the median and ulnar nerves, McCauley[199] restored sensation in 8 children who had sustained electrical burns to their hands. Neurotized flaps placed for sensate plantar reconstruction in weight-bearing feet, however, have yielded unsatisfactory results.[200]

Scars can cause significant disfigurement, pain, pruritis, and functional impairment as well as associated emotional distress.[201] Therapists need to be keenly aware of their patients' responses to therapeutic interventions in order to subsequently provide appropriate feedback, realistic goal-setting, thorough education on relevant topics, and both patient and family psychosocial support.

## RESTORING ACTIVITIES OF DAILY LIVING/INSTRUMENTAL ACTIVITIES OF DAILY LIVING INDEPENDENCE

Throughout childhood, functional demands of children consist of participating in school, play, and daily activities. As a result of being hospitalized, children with burns may experience delays in their developmental milestones as well as their ability to participate in age-appropriate functional activities. To encourage optimal performance in these areas, occupational and physical therapists need to be astute observers and carefully select activities in which the child can be successful. The goal is for the child or adolescent to functionally improve, first during the acute care phase and then throughout the discharge, outpatient rehabilitation, school reentry, and subsequent reconstructive surgery phases, in order to achieve optimal functioning in all areas of life.

The occupational therapist develops a needs assessment based on the child's performance in ADLs and IADLs[202]; ADLs include eating/feeding, bathing/showering, hygiene and grooming, dressing, toilet hygiene, functional mobility, personal device care, sexual activity, and sleep/rest, while IADLs include care of pets, use of communication devices, ability to follow safety/emergency procedures, and the areas of education, play, leisure, and social participation.

A child may be unable to perform certain tasks independently due to a burn injury. He or she may need adaptive equipment for feeding, dressing, or toileting. Adaptive clothing can facilitate independence in dressing if decreased ability to button, zip, or fasten clothing is noted. Simple to complex aids, ranging from built-up or extended handles to environmental control units, may be required as well. ADL retraining can assist in the prevention of joint contractures and facilitate increased strength and endurance.[203]

Adaptive equipment use should be eliminated as soon as the child becomes functionally proficient in an activity. A young child often totally depends on his or her caregiver to assist with self-care tasks. The caregiver should be advised to provide additional time for the child to achieve task completion and positively support the child's personal autonomy and independence. Since children who have sustained large burns often exhibit low frustration tolerance and demanding behavior,[204] activities can be divided into smaller tasks to emphasize graded achievements. Successful functional outcomes in most ADLs/IADLs for children after a burn injury have been documented, including areas of school, sports, self-care, and rest/sleep.[205]

## DISCHARGE PLANNING

The rehabilitation team focuses on the development and implementation of programs that will assist the pediatric burn survivor as she or he transitions through the various phases of burn recovery. Once the child is discharged from acute hospitalization, transfer to a rehabilitation facility is typical. If possible, both family education and communication with the rehabilitation facility's therapists are completed prior to discharge from the burn center. Danowski et al[206] found that increased parent knowledge and compliance occurred when written pediatric educational materials were provided (versus verbal instruction) prior to discharge. Returning home is the ultimate goal, including reentry into school and community activities. School reentry programs have been remarkably successful, whether using individualized videotapes or school visits by hospital staff, in facilitating acceptance and preventing teasing.[207,208] Follow-up outpatient therapy and reconstructive surgery are planned as needed. Practitioners communicate with social workers as well as case managers

to ensure that continued care is arranged. If the burn center has an outpatient burn clinic, it can be a good avenue for patient follow-up. Local burn support groups can be invaluable resources for emotional and psychological issues ranging from self-image to sexuality. Via interviews, Forbes-Duchart et al[209] qualitatively studied the experiences of 9 adults who had been burned as children. Participant advice included discussing sexuality as children mature, having a trusted person raise the issue, using a flexible approach, and encouraging participation in survivor support groups early in recovery. Lastly, urging children and adolescents with burns to attend a regional burn camp is recommended as another opportunity for building self-esteem.[210]

## CONTRACTURE CORRECTION WITH RECONSTRUCTIVE SURGERY

Despite appropriate initial management, reconstruction is commonly required after deep partial-thickness and full-thickness burns.[211] Large wounds and skin grafts crossing joints, as well as spontaneously healing burns, are factors associated with increased need for contracture release. In addition, contractures tend to develop in areas under minimal stretch when at rest, for example, axillae, antecubital fossae, web spaces, and wrists.[212] Children are almost 4 times more likely to require reconstructive surgery than adults.[114] Spurr and Shakespeare[116] reported greater than 50% of children under the age of 5, and Bombaro et al[213] found 84% of children under the age of 15 required hypertrophic scar treatment post-discharge. Sheridan et al[214] studied 698 acutely burned hands in 495 children; 32% of those who had received acute skin grafting and 65% of the hands with injuries involving underlying bone and tendon required reconstructive surgery. The number of areas addressed by surgeons is extensive: Moore and Robinson[4] list over 30 potential impairments of the body that can be reconstructed.

Schneider et al[215] examined 4 joints (shoulder, elbow, hip, and knee) in their study of 985 patients and found shoulders (38%), elbows (34%), and knees (22%) were most frequently contracted; Kraemer et al[114] listed the 4 most commonly contracted areas in pediatric patients as the hands (42%), axillae (17%), head (13%), and antecubital fossae (11%). When considering the hand, the PIP joint is especially vulnerable. Rupture of the central slip of the extensor tendon or attenuation-laxity of the extensor hood will lead to a boutonniere deformity.[16] Pseudoboutonniere deformity occurs when the MCP hyperextension deformity does not involve central slip injury.[21] Also commonly seen and difficult to remedy are burns involving the fifth digit.[216] With grafting often needed both volarly and dorsally, contractures can result which limit finger extension and concomitantly turn the tip outward so that functional activities, such as putting the hand in a pants pocket, are limited and painful.[212] Amputation can also change the mechanics of the developing hand; therapists need to monitor functional deficits and provide adaptive equipment and teaching as needed prior to and following reconstructive procedures. Lastly, burn syndactyly (interdigital contracture) is common; unless involving the first web space, however, it rarely causes significant functional deficits in children.[199]

Full-thickness skin grafts are generally better than split-thickness grafts in producing less scarring.[115] Early grafting (ie, fewer than 15 days postburn) was described by Tambuscio et al[217] as significantly reducing need for reconstruction in their study of 191 hands with deep burns. Data from van Zuijlen et al,[218,219] however, revealed no significant influence of the timing of surgery on long-term hand function. While hands are one of the most common anatomic sites requiring surgical release, according to Kraemer et al,[114] central body regions such as the head, neck, and axillae were found to have the highest incidence of unsatisfactory postoperative results. This may be due to difficulty providing adequate postoperative pressure and splinting/positioning.[114] Children are often unable to resist contractile forces with sufficient strength, which further increases the risk of contracture development.[212]

Heterotopic ossification (HO) is rare in children but may be evident in the adolescent population.[4] The most common site for burn patients is the elbow; Klein et al[220] found that time to wound closure significantly increased risk of HO in their study of 45 adult patients who developed HO at the elbow. Surgical excision is generally advised after 12 months.[221] Gaur et al[222] reported excellent results years following excision of HO in 7 children (9 elbows). Static or dynamic extension splinting is implemented immediately. Postoperative use of continuous passive motion has been recommended,[221] but units are currently only adult-sized; they may fit larger adolescents but not smaller children.

All regions of the body experience potential impairments, and reconstruction surgery options include procedures for every area from the face to the feet. As Bjarnason et al[223] and, more recently, Rea et al[224] found in their surveys with patients, however, goals may differ between patients and their parents or surgeons. Consultation with patients (and/or parents, in the case of young children) is therefore strongly advised before proceeding with a reconstruction plan.

Therapists utilize many nonoperative or minimally invasive approaches in order to attempt to correct scar contractures and contracted or stiff joints. Use of static, static-progressive, and dynamic splints can decrease the need for reconstructive surgery, especially if provided to prevent contracture or scar bands at areas such as the volar aspect of the hand, wrist, elbow, posterior knee, or dorsum of the ankle and foot.[4] The constant tension produces elongated tissue.[4,225] Both custom and commercially available splints can be used for progressive stretching of the neck, axilla, elbow, forearm, knee, ankle, and foot, whereas custom wrist and hand splints are needed for ideal fit and expected revisions.

Huang et al[226] found 93% of patients who did not use splints required reconstructive surgery versus 26% of those who did. According to Richard et al,[225] splinting and casting corrected contractures faster than massage, exercises, or pressure. Adding conforming pressure inserts increases overall comfort and compliance as well as facilitates increased tension on targeted tissues.[16] Vehmeyer-Heeman et al[227] noted that extended grafting and early custom splinting prevented axillary contractures. Meanwhile, in a study by Scott et al[228] of 194 pediatric palmar burns, aggressive hand therapy, conservative surgical management, and splinting resulted in 85% healing without need for surgery. Serial casting has been useful for correction of joint contractures at the wrist, elbow, knee, and ankle following burn injury.[13] Bennett et al,[13] who applied casts to 35 joints in 15 pediatric and adult burn patients, found that casts delayed or eliminated the need for reconstruction.

Earlier sections in this chapter have included a comprehensive review of splints and positioning devices for upper and lower extremities as well as for central region positioning. Jordan et al[21] also provide a thorough discussion of upper and lower extremity splints used during the acute, rehabilitative, and reconstructive burn care phases. Achieving adequate wearing time of any splint can be especially challenging with the pediatric population. Having a splint schedule that is consistently enforced by all staff and family members can be pivotally helpful in this endeavor postreconstruction.

Reconstructive surgery has been defined as surgery which attempts to change an abnormality into something as normal as possible; this is in contrast to aesthetic surgery, which tries to improve upon something that is already "normal."[229] Children can undergo reconstruction surgery at the end of their inpatient stay or, more typically, during subsequent visits to the burn center. Besides previously identified factors, other issues which can result in a need for reconstruction include noncompliance (including language barriers and inadequate family support),[216,227,230-232] growth plate disturbances,[212,233] depression,[234] and learning disabilities/behavioral issues.[235] In addition, weight gain and/or growth can cause circumferential bands that require excision and resurfacing with grafts.[16,212] A recent study demonstrated that most young children 12 to 48 months of age admitted to an acute burn center manifested multiple symptoms of post-traumatic stress disorder,[236] which can affect a child's ability to participate in therapy. Relaxation training, hypnosis, guided imagery, music therapy, massage, and therapeutic touch have been used as complimentary techniques to reduce anxiety.[58,237-240]

Although surgery is generally not attempted until at least 6 months postburn in order to ensure full wound maturation, reconstructive surgery is sometimes necessary to allow a patient to perform critical functions.[114] Examples include eyelid releases to protect exposed corneas and releases of severe contractures and microstomias. Greenhalgh[212] and Greenhalgh et al[242] have also demonstrated that early surgical releases can be performed during active scar maturation. In general, it is best to perform as many procedures as possible during a child's preschool years. This approach can maximize use of time, effort, and finances.

Klein et al[229] stress the effective management of a scar and its sequelae as priorities in reconstructive burn surgery. Young and Burd[231] found good results were obtained in children undergoing release surgeries for axilla, elbow, and wrist contractures regardless of whether local flaps, Integra™, or free tissue transfers were used; they recommended consideration of these options rather than use of skin grafting when appropriate follow-up care is provided. Excellent recovery of shoulder range of motion was reported following use of scapular island flaps, splinting, and therapy in 13 children with axillary scar contractures.[243] Figus et al[244] also demonstrated excellent results utilizing total scar tissue excision and resurfacing with Integra™ for a case of severe multiple contracture reconstruction. Emsen[245] presented good results utilizing the cross-incision plasty combined with releases and flaps for the correction of 35 cases of dorsal and volar neosyndactyly in 15 children and adults. Tissue expanders with subsequent flaps are increasingly used for hypertrophic scar repair.[246,247] Positioning the hand in a fist for skin grafting a postdorsal hand burn has resulted in excellent functional and cosmetic results.[248] External fixation has been used following grafting and reconstruction for knees,[249] hands,[250] and upper extremities.[251] Bar-Meir et al[249] used a combination of free muscle flap, Iliazarov external fixation, and therapy for the successful correction in 1 child, 1 adolescent, and 2 adults who demonstrated previously failed knee flexion contracture reconstruction.

Following reconstructive surgery, the therapist may follow the same protocols as when dealing with newly grafted areas and donor sites, albeit in smaller areas. Goals of therapy are to promote optimal wound healing; minimize hypertrophic and keloid scar formation; minimize pain, pruritis, hyperesthesia, and overall discomfort caused by scars; maximize range of motion, strength, and endur-

ance; optimize functional performance and independence in ADLs and IADLs; provide psychosocial support to the patient and family members/support system; and offer patient and family education.[7]

Therapeutic interventions encompass all those previously reviewed in this chapter. Edema management is initially emphasized and can include the use of elevation, pressure wrapping, intermittent vasopneumatic compression, exercise, and manual therapy. Positioning devices, including custom or prefabricated static, static-progressive, and dynamic splints,[16,19,21,35,36,38-40,42,252-255] casts,[13,14] and traction,[12,18] are commonly used following reconstruction.

Following release and grafting for severe burn microstomia, Al-Qattan et al[254] reported successfully using silicone oral splints rather than standard acrylic splints for children. Simplicity, ease of fabrication, availability, and suitability (especially for young children without teeth) were noted. Davis et al[33] also presented a prototype for an economical vertical microstomia orthosis. For palmar burns postreconstruction, Schwanholt et al[256] found 90% improvement using volar and dorsal splints that positioned the wrist in 30 to 40 degrees of extension and MCP joints in approximately 30 degrees of hyperextension. Pain management is also as previously outlined; therapists may find it useful to measure pain levels preoperatively and postoperatively.[257,258] Patient and family education, community referrals, and school reentry are revisited upon each reconstructive procedure.

Reconstruction can be a lengthy process. A child may undergo various procedures during most of his or her childhood, with expected intermittent surgeries throughout adulthood as well. Developing a good rapport with the child and his or her family is very important, especially if the same therapist will be treating the child for the bulk of the procedures done during formative years. Therapy visits should include both routine and spontaneity, with the child being able to choose most of the activities planned for the visit.[2] Involving family members will help ensure carryover of new splint regimens, exercise programs, massage techniques, and play activities designed to facilitate specific movement patterns or muscle activity.

Tyack and Ziviani[259] found that premorbid factors (eg, behavioral or psychological problems, learning difficulties, or developmental delays) and parent factors (eg, anxiety, depression, or poor coping skills) but not injury factors (eg, TBSA burned, number of operative procedures, or source of burn) had a significant impact on functional outcomes of children aged 5 to 14 years with burns of less than 35% TBSA at 6 months postburn. Their findings suggest placing more emphasis on premorbid and parent factors in the first 6 months postinjury in order to enhance functional outcomes in these children.

Typical therapy visits might include use of physical agents or massage, specific manual therapy and exercises, gross and fine motor games or activities, splint and positioning device fabrication and adjustment, home exercise program review, and family teaching. As always, customizing splints, casts, and any other type of positioning equipment may facilitate patient acceptance and compliance. Ending a session with a fun game[28] or including an occasional "prize" can help maintain motivation and good morale. Helm et al[260] reported that exercises incorporated into movement to music improved range of motion in children younger than 7 years. As the child or adolescent reenters school, communication with teachers before and after procedures promotes a smooth transition.[16] If splints are to be worn, a written schedule for both home and school may prove vital to a successful surgical outcome.

## SUMMARY AND RESEARCH CONSIDERATIONS

According to Sheridan et al,[261] "[t]he successful treatment of massive burns is one of the major advances in trauma care in the last 20 years." As more people survive what was once thought of as a fatal injury, it ultimately falls upon physical and occupational therapists to help restore burn survivors' function. This daunting task takes both dedication and creativity. Both disciplines continue to move towards evidence-based practice which allows our professions to improve patient care. There exists an incredible wealth of research regarding therapeutic exercise, with promising research specifically targeting the pediatric burn population.[72,262,263] However, much is still unknown. Prospective studies which define the duration and content of exercise programs are needed that specify age, gender, and severity of injury.[260] As health care becomes increasingly more managed and patients lose the ability to receive long-term therapy, it will become necessary to know which treatments are effective, with the greatest carryover effect down the road.[260] As discussed, both positioning and exercise are 2 important modalities in the treatment of burns. However, there is little research exploring the balance between the 2. For example, knowing the optimal time to maintain joint immobility and when to begin exercises would be of value when treating burns of the hand.[216] Finally, we need to assess the successful transition and application of exercise-based rehabilitation programs into community-based rehabilitation programs.[260]

## KEY POINTS

- Appropriate positioning, including use of static and dynamic splints, prevents joint contracture formation and provides joint alignment.
- Each burn-injured body part requires specialized assessment and individualized treatment in order to enhance healing and regain functional use.
- Edema management is essential for reduction of pain, contractures, and soft tissue adhesions.
- Understanding pain management is an important part of the rehabilitation process.
- Serial casting is used to rectify significant contractures in all phases of burn rehabilitation.
- Skeletal suspension and traction systems may be used to facilitate proper positioning.
- Therapeutic exercise helps to prevent loss of strength and preserves range of motion.
- Physical and occupational therapy helps to ensure children continue to achieve motor milestones throughout their development.
- Management of edema during the inflammatory wound healing phase may assist in minimizing hypertrophic scarring.
- Splinting during the fibroplastic wound-healing phase can facilitate collagen alignment.
- Pressure is used on raising forces to facilitate lysis during the maturation wound-healing phase.
- Sustained stretching is used on contractile forces to facilitate scar band lengthening during the maturation wound-healing phase.
- Assessment and treatment are required for any loss of independence in activities of daily living and instrumental activities of daily living, since they are important aspects of pediatric patients' lives and vital links to successful reentry into home, school, and community participation.
- Reconstructive surgery is often needed for children and adolescents; identifying the patient's, parents', and surgeon's goals is important for a successful outcome.

# TABLES

### TABLE 1
### Positioning, splinting, and exercises.

| Area(s) of Concern | Positioning | Splints | Exercises |
|---|---|---|---|
| **Head** | | | Facial exercises |
| Eyes | Symmetrical | | A/PROM stretches |
| Nose | Symmetrical | Nasal dilator | A/PROM stretches |
| Mouth | Vertical, horizontal lengthening | Microstomia prevention appliance (MPA) | A/PROM oral stretches, massage |
| Ear | No pillow | Ear protector | Massage |
| **Neck** | | | |
| **Anterior** | No pillow, place towel roll under scapulae | Soft cervical collar, neck conformer, semirigid thermoplastic neck splint | A/AA/PROM with prolonged stretches |
| Posterior | Pillow to support in neck flexion | Soft cervical collar, neck conformer, semirigid thermoplastic neck splint | A/AA/PROM with prolonged stretches |
| **Shoulder/Axilla** | 90 degrees abduction with forward flexion, shoulder in retraction | Hard/soft airplane splint, axillary conformer, shoulder soft clavicle brace | A/AA/PROM with prolonged stretches Overhead pulleys, dowel, wall exercises, shoulder CPM, BTE |
| **Elbow/Forearm** | Extension, flexion, supination, and pronation | Extension, flexion splint, dynamic, 3-point, cast, and serial splint | Elbow CPM, A/AA/PROM, weights, overhead pulleys, supination/ pronation exercises |
| Wrist/Hand | Volar<br>Wrist/hand elevated above level of heart, wrist in extension, digits in extension, abduction<br>Dorsal<br>Wrist/hand elevated above level of heart, wrist in neutral or extension, fingers in intrinsic-plus, thumb in midabduction | Volar<br>Extension, abduction, dynamic, 3-point, serial splint, cast<br>Dorsal<br>Neutral or extension, intrinsic-plus, dynamic, 3-point, serial splint, cast | Volar<br>A/AA/PROM, tendon glides, intrinsic & composite extension stretching, strengthening, CPM, PNF<br>Dorsal<br>A/AA/PROM, tendon glides, extrinsic and composite flexion stretching, intrinsic strengthening, CPM, PNF |
| **Trunk/Hip** | Side-lying, prone, Trendelenburg, bolsters, foam, bean bags, and so on, hip in neutral | Hip spica splints, cast, abductor wedges, knee immobilizer to prevent knee/hip flexion | Exercises in prone to stretch anterior trunk and anterior hip, reaching exercises to facilitate trunk, PNF, bridging exercises |
| **Knee** | Knee in full extension, no pillow, no "frog-leg" positioning | Knee immobilizer including gutter, dynamic brace | Gait training and weight-bearing exercises (depending upon child's age), prolonged stretches, AA/A/PROM |

(continued on next page)

TABLE 1 (*continued*)

| Area(s) of Concern | Positioning | Splints | Exercises |
|---|---|---|---|
| **Ankle** | Ankle in neutral position | Foot board, foam wedges, dynamic foot plate, foot drop splint, ie, AFO (ankle foot orthosis), cast | Gait training and weight-bearing exercises (depending upon child's age), prolonged stretches, AA/A/PROM |
| **Foot** | Foot in neutral, foam heel protectors, egg crate foam | Foot drop splint, splint to prevent plantar and inversion, cast | Gait training and weight-bearing exercises (depending upon child's age), prolonged stretches, AA/A/PROM |
| **Toe** | Toe in neutral | Toe plate static or dynamic to prevent hyperextension of toes | Tendon glides, stretching |

TABLE 2
**Typical motor development.**

| Age | Motor Tasks | | |
|---|---|---|---|
| 3 months | Lift head to 45°–90° in prone | Accepts weight in standing | |
| 4 months | Rolls supine to side-lying | Bilateral reaching | Trunk and LE extension in prone |
| 6 months | Full head control in supine and prone | Rolling supine to prone | Prone pivoting |
| 8 months | Crawls on hands and knees | Stands independently at furniture | Bangs 2 toys together in midline |
| 10 months | Begins walking with 1 handhold assist | Two-handed play activities | |
| 12 months | Walks independently with foot flat | Can perform bimanual tasks | |
| 1-2 years | Able to stand with only use of legs | Heel strike by 24 months | Can catch a ball with arms and body |
| 3-5 years | Increased control, stability, and velocity with gait | Can feed themselves | Independent dressing by age 5 |
| 6-10 years | Mature gait pattern | Good eating skills | Coordination continues to mature |

# REFERENCES

1. Duncan CE, Cathcart ME. A multi-disciplinary model for burn rehabilitation. *J Burn Care Rehabil.* 1988; **9**: 191–192.

2. Smith M, Doctor M, Boulter T. Unique considerations in caring for a pediatric burn patient: a developmental approach. *Crit Care Nurs Clin North Am.* 2004; **16**: 99–108.

3. Williams AI, Baker BM. Advances in burn care management: role of the speech-language pathologist. *J Burn Care Rehabil.* 1992; **13**: 642–649.

4. Moore ML, Robinson CA. The burn unit. In: Campbell SK, Vander Linden DW, Palisano RJ, eds. *Physical Therapy for Children.* St Louis, MO: Saunders Elsevier; 2006: 1025–1051.

5. Simons M, King S, Edgar D. Occupational therapy and physiotherapy for the patient with burns: principles and management. *J Burn Care Rehabil.* 2003; **24**: 323–335.

6. Keller C, Ward RS. Educational preparedness for physical therapists and occupational therapists in burn care. *J Burn Care Rehabil.* 2002; **23**: 67–73.

7. Ward RS. Physical rehabilitation. In: Carrougher GJ, ed. *Burn Care and Therapy.* St Louis, MO: Mosby; 1998: 293–327.

8. Apfel LM, Irwin CP, Staley MJ, Richard RL. In: Richard RL, Staley MJ, eds. *Burn Care and Rehabilitation: Principles and Practice.* Philadelphia, PA: FA Davis Co; 1994: 235.

9. Martin-Herz SP, Thurber CA, Patterson, DR. Psychological principles of burn wound pain in children. II: Treatment applications. *J Burn Care Rehabil.* 2000; **21**: 458–471.

10. Willis BA, Larson DL, Abston S. Positioning and splinting the burned patient. *Heart Lung.* 1973; **2**: 696–700.

11. Duncan RM. Basic principles of splinting the hand. *Phys Ther.* 1989; **69**: 1104–1116.

12. Serghiou MA, Ott S, Farmer S, Morgan D, Gibson P, Suman OE. Comprehensive rehabilitation of the burn patient. In: Herndon DN, ed. *Total Burn Care.* Philadelphia, PA: Elsevier; 2007: 620–651.

13. Bennett GB, Helm P, Purdue GF, Hunt JL. Serial casting: a method of treating burn contractures. *J Burn Care Rehabil.* 1989; **10**: 543–545.

14. Ricks NR, Meagher DP Jr. The benefits of plaster casting for lower-extremity burns after grafting in children. *J Burn Care Rehabil.* 1992; **13**: 465–468.

15. Knutsen AC, Franzen B, Solem LD. Early casting for palmar burns to prevent contractures. *J Burn Care Res.* 2006; **27**: S146.

16. Grigsby deLinde L, Knothe B. Therapist's management of the burned hand. In: Mackin E, ed. *Rehabilitation of the Hand and Upper Extremity.* St Louis, MO: Mosby; 2002: 1492–1526.

17. Youel L, Evans EB, Heare TC, Herndon DN, Larson DL, Abston S. Skeletal suspension in the management of severe burns in children. A sixteen year experience. *J Bone Joint Surg Am.* 1986: **68**: 1375–1379.

18. Larson DL, Evans EB, Abston S, Lewis SR. Skeletal suspension and traction in the treatment of burns. *Ann Surg.* 1968; **6**: 981–985.

19. Serghiou MA, McLaughlin A, Herndon DN. Alternative splinting methods for the prevention and correction of burn care torticollis. *J Burn Care Rehabil.* 2003; **24**: 336–340.

20. Rivers EA. Skin dysfunction: burns. In: Willard HS, Crepeau EB, Cohn ES, Schell BAB, eds. *Willard & Spackman's Occupational Therapy.* Philadelphia, PA: Lippincott Williams & Wilkins; 2003: 867–883.

21. Jordan RB, Daher J, Wasil K. Splints and scar management for acute and reconstructive burn care. *Clin Plast Surg.* 2000; **27**: 71–85.

22. Nakamura DY, Costa BA, Mann R, Engrav LH. Silipos neck wraps. *J Burn Care Rehabil.* 1998; **19**: 181–182.

23. Staley M, Richard R, Billmire D, Warden G. Head/face/neck burns: therapist considerations for the pediatric patient. *J Burn Care Rehabil.* 1997; **18**: 164–171.

24. Foley KH, Kaulkin C, Palmieri TL, Greenhalgh DG. Inverted television and video games to maintain neck extension. *J Burn Care Rehabil.* 2001; **22**: 366–368.

25. Fader P. Preserving function and minimizing deformity: the role of the occupational therapist. In: Carvajal HF, Parks DH, eds. *Burns in Children: Pediatric Burn Management.* Chicago, IL: Year Book Medical Publishers; 1988: 324–344.

26. Lin JT, Nagler W. Use of surface scanning for creation of transparent facial orthoses. A report of two cases. *Burns.* 2003; **29**: 599–602.

27. Wardrope J, Edhouse JA. *The Management of Wounds and Burns.* New York, NY: Oxford University Press; 1999.

28. Still JM Jr, Law EJ, Belcher KE, Moses KC, Gleitsmann KY. Experience with burns of the eyes and lids in a regional burn unit. *J Burn Care Rehabil.* 1995; **16**: 248–252.

29. Groce A, Meyers-Paal R, Herndon DN, McCauley RL. Are your thoughts of facial pressure transparent? *J Burn Care Rehabil.* 1999; **20**: 478–481.

30. Nahlieli O, Kelly JP, Baruchin AM, Ben-Meir O, Shapira Y. Oro-maxillofacial skeletal deformities resulting from burn scar contractures of the face and neck. *Burns.* 1995; **21**: 65–69.

31. Fricke NB, Omnell ML, Dutcher KD, Hollender LG, Engrav LH. Skeletal and dental disturbances after facial burns and pressure garments. *J Burn Care Rehabil.* 1996; **17**: 338–345.

32. Colcleugh RG, Ryan JE. Splinting electrical burns of the mouth in children. *Plast Reconstr Surg.* 1976; **58**: 239–241.

33. Davis S, Thompson JG, Clark J, Kowal-Vern A, Latenser BA. A prototype for an economical vertical microstomia orthosis. *J Burn Care Res.* 2006; **27**: 352–356.

34. Taquino LM, Clayton RJ, Mayemura L, Mann R. Quick and easy dynamic mouth splint. *J Burn Care Res.* 2007; **28**: S151.

35. Manigandan C, Bedford E, Ninan S, Gupta AK, Padankatti SM, Paul K. Adjustable aesthetic aeroplane splint for axillary burn contractures. *Burns.* 2005; **31**: 502–504.

36. Macdonald LB, Covey MH, Marvin JA. The papoose: device for positioning the burn child's axilla. *J Burn Care Rehabil.* 1985; **6**(1): 62–63.

37. Darton A, Templeton C, Mcinnes G. Axillary splinting. From: Clinical audits—The Children's Hospital at Westmean Web site. Available at: http: //www.chw.edu.au/research/groups/chbri/05_clinical_audits.htm. Accessed April 13, 2006.

38. Abhyankar SV. The salute splint for axillary contractures. *Br J Plast Surg.* 2001; **54**: 213–215.

39. Chown GA. The high-density foam areoplane splint: a modified approach to the treatment of axilla burns. *Burns.* 2006: **32**: 916–919.

40. Obaidullah, Ullah H, Aslam M. Figure-of-8 sling for prevention of recurrent axillary contracture after release and skin grafting. *Burns.* 2005; **31**: 283–289.

41. Kaufman T, Newman RA, Weinberg A, Wexler MR. The Kerlix tongue-depressor splint for skin-grafted areas in burned children. *J Burn Care Rehabil.* 1989; **10**: 462–463.

42. Richard R, Shanesy CP, Miller SF. Dynamic versus static splints: a prospective case for sustained stress. *J Burn Care Rehabil.* 1995; **16**: 284–287.

43. Cantrill K, Parry I, O'Mara M, Palmieri TL, Greenhalgh DG. Serpentine splint for improving posture in burned children. *J Burn Care Res.* 2008; **29**: S139.

44. Simpson RL, Gartner MC. Management of burns of the upper extremity. In: Mackin E, ed. *Rehabilitation of the Hand and Upper Extremity.* St Louis, MO: Mosby; 2002: 1475–1491.

45. Nakamura D. Occupational therapy principles for the burn patient. In: Sood R, Achauer BM, eds. *Achauer and Sood's Burn Surgery Reconstruction and Rehabilitation.* Philadelphia, PA: Saunders Elsevier; 2006: 371–387.

46. Alvadro MI. Burns. In: Trombly CA, ed. *Occupational Therapy for Physical Dysfunction.* Baltimore, MD: Williams & Wilkins; 1995: 831–848.

47. Framer S, Rogers S, Serghiou M, Evans E, Herndon DN. Providing an anchored calcaneal strap to maintain ankle mobility following peroneal nerve injury [presentation]. Miami, FL: American Burn Association 35th Annual Meeting; Apr 2006.

48. Pasquinelli S. Lower extremity amputations and prosthetics. In: Pedretti LW, ed. *Occupational Therapy: Practice Skills for Physical Dysfunction.* St Louis, MO: Mosby-Year Book; 1996: 599–612.

49. Villeco P, Mackin E, Hunter J. Edema: therapist's management. In: Mackin E, ed. *Rehabilitation of the Hand and Upper Extremity.* St Louis, MO: Mosby; 2002: 183–193.

50. Gaspard DJ, Kohl RD Jr. Compartmental syndromes in which the skin is the limiting boundary. *Clin Orthop Relat Res.* 1975; **113**: 65–68.

51. Zuker RM. Initial management of the burn wound. In: Carvajal HF, Parks DH, eds. *Burns in Children: Pediatric Burn Management.* Chicago, IL: Year Book Medical Publishers; 1988: 99–105.

52. Marvin JA. Pain assessment versus measurement. *J Burn Care Rehabil.* 1995; **16**: 348–357.

53. Martin-Herz SP, Thurber CA, Patterson DR. Psychological principles of burn wound pain in children. II: Treatment applications. *J Burn Care Rehabil.* 2000; **21**: 458–472.

54. Kuttner L. Methods to help relieve pain. In: Kuttner L, ed. *A Child in Pain: How to Help, What to Do.* Point Roberts, WA: Hartley & Marks; 1996: 90–132.

55. Melzack R, Wall PD. Pain mechanisms: a new theory. *Science.* 1965; **150**: 971–978.

56. Engel JM. Pain management. In: Willard HS, Crepeau EB, Cohn ES, Schell BAB, eds. *Willard & Spackman's Occupational Therapy.* Philadelphia, PA: Lippincott Williams & Wilkins; 2003: 634–637.

57. Pereyra R, Rimmer R, Strawn M, Drachman D, Davidson M, Foster K. Art therapy: an effective means of expression for burn-injured children. *J Burn Care Res.* 2008; **29**: S81.

58. Tan X, Yowler C, Super D, Fratianne R. Music therapy significantly reduces pain, anxiety, and muscle tension involved with burn debridement. *J Burn Care Res.* 2008; **29**: S83.

59. Chech D, Martin S. *Functional Movement and Development Across the Life Span.* Philadelphia, PA: WB Saunders Co; 1995.

60. Bly L. *Motor Acquisition Checklist.* San Antonio, TX: Therapy Skill Builders; 2000.

61. Hart DW, Wolf SE, Chinkes DL, et al. Determinants of skeletal muscle catabolism after severe burn. *Ann Surg.* 2000; **232**(4): 455–465.

62. Przkora R, Barrow RE, Jeschke MG, et al. Body composition changes with time in pediatric burn patients. *J Trauma.* 2006; **60**: 968–971.

63. Mlcak RP, Jeschke MG, Barrow RE, Herndon DN. The influence of age and gender on resting energy expenditure in severely burned children. *Ann Surg.* 2006; **244**: 121–130.

64. Convertino VA, Bloomfield SA, Greenleaf JE. An overview of the issues: physiological effects of bed rest and restricted physical activity. *Med Sci Sports Exerc.* 1997; **29**(2): 187–190.

65. Bloomfield SA. Changes in musculoskeletal structure and function with prolonged bed rest. *Med Sci Sports Exerc.* 1997; **29**(2): 197–206.

66. Timmerman RA. A mobility protocol for critically ill adults. *Dimens Crit Care Nurs.* 2007; **26**(5): 175–179.

67. Scudder G. PT 6280, Clinical Assessment: Passive Range of Motion and Manual Stretching [lecture]. Minneapolis, MN: University of Minnesota; 9 Oct 2002.

68. Stout JL. Physical fitness during childhood and adolescence. In: Campbell SK, Vander Linden DW, Palisano RJ, eds. *Physical Therapy for Children.* Philadelphia, PA: WB Saunders Co; 2000: 141–169.

69. Mayes T, Gottschlich M, Scanlon J, Warden GD. Four-year review of burns as an etiologic factor in the development of long bone fractures in pediatric patients. *J Burn Care Rehabil.* 2003; **24**(5): 279–284.

70. Przkora R, Herndon DN, Suman OE. The effects of oxandrolone and exercise on muscle mass and function in children with severe burns. *Pediatrics*. 2007; **119**(1): e109–e116.

71. Suman OE, Spies RJ, Celis MM, Mlcak RP, Herndon DN. Effects of a 12-wk resistance exercise program on skeletal muscle strength in children with burn injuries. *J Appl Physiol*. 2001; **91**(3): 1168–1175.

72. Celis MM, Suman OE, Huang TT, Yen P, Herndon DN. Effect of a supervised exercise and physiotherapy program on surgical interventions in children with thermal injury. *J Burn Care Rehabil*. 2003; **24**(1): 57–61.

73. Cucuzzo NA, Ferrando A, Herndon DN. The effects of exercise programming vs traditional outpatient therapy in the rehabilitation of severely burned children. *J Burn Care Rehabil*. 2001; **22**(3): 214–220.

74. McElroy K, Alvarado MI, Hayward PG, Desai MH, Herndon DN, Robson MC. Exercise stress testing for the pediatric patient with burns: a preliminary report. *J Burn Care Rehabil*. 1992; **13**: 236–238.

75. Richard RL, Staley M. *Burn Care and Rehabilitation Principles and Practice*. Philadelphia, PA: FA Davis; 1994.

76. Moore ML. The burn unit. In: Campbell SK, Vander Linden DW, Palisano RJ, eds. *Physical Therapy for Children*. Philadelphia, PA: WB Saunders Co; 2000: 813–839.

77. Chiarello LA, Palisano RJ. Investigation of the effects of a model of physical therapy on mother-child interactions and the motor behaviors of children with motor delay. *Phys Ther*. 1998; **78**(2): 180–194.

78. Rone-Adams SA, Stern DF, Walker V. Stress and compliance with a home exercise program among caregivers of children with disabilities. *Pediatr Phys Ther*. 2004; **6**: 140–148.

79. Trees DW, Ketelsen CA, Hobbs JA. Use of a modified tilt table for perambulation strength training as an adjunct to burn rehabilitation: a case series. *J Burn Care Rehabil*. 2003; **24**: 97–103.

80. Schreiber J, Marchetti G, Crytzer T. The implementation of a fitness program for children with disabilities: a clinical case report. *Pediatr Phys Ther*. 2004; **16**(3): 173–179.

81. Fragala-Pinkham MA, Haley SM, Rabin J, Kharasch VS. A fitness program for children with disabilities. *Phys Ther*. 2005; **85**: 1182–1200.

82. Faigenbaum AD, Westcott WL, Loud RL, Long C. The effects of different resistance training protocols on muscular strength and endurance development in children. *Pediatrics*. 1999; **104**(1): e5.

83. Bernhardt DT, Gomez J, Johnson MD, et al; Committee on Sports Medicine and Fitness. Strength training by children and adolescents. *Pediatrics*. 2001; **107**(6): 1470–1472.

84. Bracciano AG. *Physical Agent Modalities: Theory and Application for the Occupational Therapist*. New Jersey, NJ: Slack Inc; 2000.

85. Davidson JM. Wound repair. *J Hand Ther*. Apr-Jun 1998; **11**(2): 80–94.

86. Hardy MA. The biology of scar formation. *Phys Ther*. 1989; **69**: 1014–1024.

87. Lund T. The 1999 Everett Idris Evans memorial lecture. Edema generation following thermal injury: an update. *J Burn Care Rehabil*. 1999; **20**: 445–452.

88. Demling RH. The burn edema process: current concepts. *J Burn Care Rehabil*. 2005; **26**: 207–227.

89. Su CW, Alizadeh K, Boddie A, Lee RC. The problem scar. *Clin Plast Surg*. 1998; **25**: 451–465.

90. Robson MC. Disturbances of wound healing. *Ann Emerg Med*. 1988; **17**: 1274–1278.

91. Smith KL, Price JL. Care of the hand wound. In: Mackin E, ed. *Rehabilitation of the Hand and Upper Extremity*. 5th ed. St Louis, MO: Mosby; 2002: 331–343.

92. Su CW, Alizadeh K, Boddie A, Lee RC. The problem scar. *Clin Plast Surg*. 1998; **25**: 451–465.

93. Watts GT, Grillo HC, Gross J. Studies in wound healing: II. The role of granulation tissue in contraction. *Ann Surg*. 1958; **148**: 153–160.

94. Deitch EA, Wheelahan TM, Rose MP, Clothier J, Cotter J. Hypertrophic burn scars: analysis of variables. *J Trauma*. 1983; **23**: 895–898.

95. Richard RL, Staley MJ. Biophysical aspects of normal skin and burn scar. In: Richard RL, Staley MJ, eds. *Burn Care and Rehabilitation: Principles and Practice*. Philadelphia, PA: FA Davis; 1994: 49–69.

96. Gibran NS, Boyce S, Greenhalgh DG. Cutaneous wound healing. *J Burn Care Res*. 2007; **28**: 577–579.

97. Akita S, Akino K, Imaizumi T, et al. The quality of pediatric burn scars is improved by early administration of basic fibroblast growth factor. *J Burn Care Res*. 2006; **27**: 333–338.

98. Nedelec B, Gharary A, Scott PG, Tredget EE. Control of wound contraction. *Hand Clin*. 2000; **16**: 289–302.

99. Sawhey CP, Monga HL. Wound contraction in rabbits and the effectiveness of skin grafts in preventing it. *Br J Plast Surg*. 1970; **23**: 318–321.

100. Stone PA, Madden JW. Biological factors affecting wound contraction. *Surg Forum*. 1975; **26**: 547–548.

101. Bruster JM, Pullium G. Gradient pressure. *Am J Occup Ther*. 1983; **37**: 485–488.

102. Lowell M, Pirc P, Ward RS, et al. Effect of 3M Coban™ self-adherent wraps on edema and function of the burned hand: a case study. *J Burn Care Rehabil*. 2003; **24**: 253–258.

103. Dunphy JE, Jackson DS. Practical applications of experimental studies in the care of the primarily closed wound. *Am J Surg*. 1962; **104**: 273–282.

104. Burnsworth B, Krob MJ, Langer-Schnepp M. Immediate ambulation of patients with lower-extremity grafts. *J Burn Care Rehabil*. 1992; **13**: 89–92.

105. Ward RS. Pressure therapy for the control of hypertrophic scar formation after burn injury: a history and review. *J Burn Care Rehabil*. 1991; **12**: 257–262.

106. Arem AJ, Madden JW. Effects of stress on healing wounds: I. Intermittent noncyclical tension. *J Surg Res.* 1976; **20**: 93–102.

107. Gelberman RH, Woo SL-Y, Lothringer K, Akeson WH, Amiel D. Effects of early intermittent passive mobilization on healing canine flexor tendons. *J Hand Surg.* 1982; **7**: 170–175.

108. Akeson WH, Amiel D, Abel MF, Garfin SR, Woo SL-Y. Effects of immobilization on joints. *Clin Orthop Relat Res.* 1987; **219**: 22–37.

109. Costa AMA, Peyrol S, Porto LC, Comparin J-P, Foyatier J-L, Desmoulière A. Mechanical forces induce scar remodeling: Study in Non-Pressure-Treated versus Pressure-Treated Hypertrophic Scars. *Am J Pathol.* 1999; **155**(5): 1671–1679.

110. Hunt TK. Disorders of wound healing. *World J Surg.* 1980; **4**: 271–277.

111. McDonald WS, Deitch EA. Hypertrophic skin grafts in burned patients: a prospective analysis of variables. *J Trauma.* 1987; **27**: 147–150.

112. Sheridan R. Burns at the extremes of age. *J Burn Care Res.* 2007; **28**: 580–585.

113. Spence RJ, Ware LC. Clinical management of burn scars. In: Sood R, Achauer BM, eds. *Achauer and Sood's Burn Surgery: Reconstruction and Rehabilitation.* Philadelphia, PA: Saunders Elsevier; 2006: 124–145.

114. Kraemer MD, Jones T, Deitch EA. Burn contractures: incidence, predisposing factors, and results of surgical therapy. *J Burn Care Rehabil.* 1988; **9**: 261–265.

115. Schwanholt C, Greenhalgh DG, Warden GD. A comparison of full-thickness versus split-thickness autografts for the coverage of deep burns in the very young pediatric patient. *J Burn Care Rehabil.* 1993; **14**: 29–33.

116. Spurr ED, Shakespeare PG. Incidence of hypertrophic scarring in burn-injured children. *Burns.* 1990; **16**: 179–181.

117. Sproat JE, Dalcin A, Weitauer N, Roberts RS. Hypertrophic sterna scars: silicone gel sheet versus Kenalog injection treatment. *Plast Reconstr Surg.* 1992; **90**: 988–992.

118. Atiyeh BS. Nonsurgical management of hypertrophic scars: evidence-based therapies, standard practices, and emerging methods. *Aesthetic Plast Surg.* 2007; **31**: 468–492.

119. Linares HA, Larson DL, Willis-Galstaun BA. Historical notes on the use of pressure in the treatment of hypertrophic scars or keloids. *Burns.* 1993; **19**: 17–21.

120. Rayner K. The use of pressure therapy to treat hypertrophic scarring. *J Wound Care.* 2000; **9**: 151–153.

121. Ward RS. Pressure therapy for the control of hypertrophic scar formation after burn injury: a history and review. *J Burn Care Rehabil.* 1991; **12**: 257–262.

122. van den Kerckhove E, Stappaerts K, Fieuws S, et al. The assessment of erythema and thickness on burn related scars during pressure garment therapy as a preventive measure for hypertrophic scarring. *Burns.* 2005; **31**: 696–702.

123. Macintyre K, Baird M. Pressure garments for use in the treatment of hypertrophic scars—a review of the problems associated with their use. *Burns.* 2006; **32**: 10–15.

124. Garcia-Velasco M, Ley R, Mutch D, Surkes N, Williams HB. Compression treatment of hypertrophic scars in burned children. *Can J Surg.* 1978; **21**: 450–452.

125. Kloti J, Pochon JP. Long-term therapy of second and third degree burns in children using Jobst-compression suits. *Scand J Plast Reconstr Surg.* 1979; **13**: 163–166.

126. Fournier R, Piérard GE. Skin tensile strength modulation by compressive garments in burn patients: a pilot study. *J Med Eng Technol.* 2000; **24**: 277–280.

127. Macintyre L, Gilmartin S, Rae M. The impact of design variables and aftercare regime on the long-term performance of pressure garments. *J Burn Care Res.* 2008; **28**: 725–733.

128. Tilley W, McMahon S, Shukalak B. Rehabilitation of the burned upper extremity. *Hand Clin.* 2000; **16**: 303–318.

129. O'Brien KA, Weinstock-Zlotnick G, Hunter H, Yurt RW. Comparison of positive pressure gloves on hand function in adults with burns. *J Burn Care Res.* 2006; **27**: 339–344.

130. Dewey WS, Richard RL, Hedman TL, et al. A review of compression glove modifications to enhance functional grip: a case series. *J Burn Care Res.* 2007; **28**: 888–891.

131. Serghiou M, Farmer S, Coleman L, Herndon DN. Optimal pressure therapy for the toddler burn survivor. *J Burn Care Res.* 2007; **28**: S203.

132. Thompson R, Summers S, Rampey-Dobbs R, Wheeler T. Color pressure garments versus traditional beige pressure garments: perceptions from the public. *J Burn Care Rehabil.* 1992; **13**: 590–596.

133. Reiffel RS. Prevention of hypertrophic scars by long-term paper tape application. *Plast Reconstr Surg.* 1995; **96**: 1715–1718.

134. Kealey GP, Jensen KL, Laubenthal KN, Lewis RW. Prospective randomized comparison of two types of pressure therapy garments. *J Burn Care Rehabil.* 1990; **11**: 334–336.

135. Ahn ST, Monafo WM, Mustoe TA. Topical silicone gel: a new treatment for hypertrophic scars. *Surgery.* 1989; **106**: 781–787.

136. Poston J. The use of silicone gel sheeting in the management of hypertrophic and keloid scars. *J Wound Care.* 2000; **9**: 10–16.

137. Mustoe TA, Cooter RD, Gold MH, et al. International clinical recommendations on scar management. *Plast Reconstr Surg.* 2002; **110**: 560–571.

138. Li-Tsang CW, Lau JC, Choi J, Chan CC, Jianan L. A prospective randomized clinical trial to investigate the effect of silicone gel sheeting (Cica-Care) on post-traumatic hypertrophic scar among the Chinese population. *Burns.* 2006; **32**: 678–683.

139. Krieger LM, Pan F, Doong H, Lee RC. Thermal response of the epidermis to surface gels. *Surg Forum.* 1993; **44**: 738–739.

140. Musgrave MA, Umraw N, Fish JS, Gomez M, Cartotto RC. The effect of silicone gel sheets on perfusion of hypertrophic burn scars. *J Burn Care Rehabil.* 2002; **23**: 208–214.

141. Hirschowitz B, Lindenbaum E, Har-Shai Y, Feitelberg L, Tendler M, Katz D. Static-electric field induction by a silicone cushion for the treatment of hypertrophic and keloid scars. *Plast Reconstr Surg.* 1998; **101**: 1173–1183.

142. Quinn KJ, Evans JH, Courtney JM, Gaylor JD. Non-pressure treatment of hypertrophic scars. *Burns.* 1985; **12**: 102–108.

143. Sawada Y, Sone K. Hydration and occlusion treatment for hypertrophic scars and keloids. *Br J Plast Surg.* 1992; **45**: 599–603.

144. Klopp R. Effect of four treatment variants on the functional and cosmetic state of mature scars. *J Wound Care.* 2000; **9**: 319–324.

145. Katz BE. Silastic gel sheeting is found to be effective in scar therapy. *Cosmet Dermatol.* 1992; **6**: 32–34.

146. Argirova M, Hadjiski O, Victorova A. Non-operative treatment of hypertrophic scars and keloids after burns in children. *Ann Burns Fire Disasters.* 2006; 19(2): 80. http: www.medbc.com/annals/review/vol_19/num_2/text/vol19n2p80.asp. Accessed March 28, 2007.

147. van den Kerckhove E, Stappaerts K, Boeckx W, et al. Silicones in the rehabilitation of burns: a review and overview. *Burns.* 2001; **27**: 205–214.

148. Rappoport K, Muller R, Flores-Mir C. Dental and skeletal changes during pressure garment use in facial burns: a systemic review. *Burns.* 2008; **34**: 18–23.

149. Weber-Robertson K. Physical therapy principles for the burn patient. In: Sood R, Achauer BM, eds. *Achauer and Sood's Burn Surgery, Reconstruction and Rehabilitation.* Philadelphia, PA: Saunders Elsevier; 2006: 357–370.

150. Rudolf R. Contraction and the control of contraction. *World J Surg.* 1980; **4**: 279–287.

151. Gaida K, Koller R, Isler C, et al. Low level laser therapy—a conservative approach to the burn scar? *Burns.* 2004; **30**: 362–367.

152. Head MD, Helm PA. Paraffin and sustained stretching in the treatment of burn contractures. *Burns.* 1977; **4**: 136–139.

153. Johnson CL. Physical therapists as scar modifiers. *Phys Ther.* 1984; **64**: 1381–1387.

154. Ward RS, Hayes-Lundy C, Reddy R, Brockway C, Mills P, Saffle JR. Evaluation of topical therapeutic ultrasound to improve response to physical therapy and lessen scar contracture after burn injury. *J Burn Care Rehabil.* 1994; **15**: 74–79.

155. Cameron MH. *Physical Agents in Rehabilitation: From Research to Rehabilitation.* Philadelphia, PA: WB Saunders; 1999.

156. Apfel LM, Wachtel TL, Frank DH, Frank HA, Hansbrough JF. Functional electrical stimulation in intrinsic/extrinsic imbalanced burned hands. *J Burn Care Rehabil.* 1987; **8**: 97–102.

157. Tannenbaum M. Iodine iontophoresis in reducing scar tissue. *Phys Ther.* 1980; **60**: 792.

158. Covey MH, Dutcher K, Marvin JA, Heimbach DM. Efficacy of continuous passive motion (CPM) devices with hand burns. *J Burn Care Rehabil.* 1988; **9**: 397–400.

159. Ridgeway CL, Daughtery MB, Warden GD. Serial casting as a technique to correct burn scar contractures: a case report. *J Burn Care Rehabil.* 1991; **12**: 67–72.

160. Evans EB, Larson DL, Abston S, Willis B. Prevention and correction of deformity after severe burns. *Surg Clin North Am.* 1979; **50**: 1361–1375.

161. Oliveira GV, Chinkes D, Mitchell C, Oliveras G, Hawkins HD, Herndon DN. Objective assessment of burn scar vascularity, erythema, pliability, thickness, and planimetry. *Am Soc Derm Surg.* 2005; **31**: 48–58.

162. Yeong EK, Mann R, Engrav LH, et al. Improved burn scar assessment with use of a new scar-rating scale. *J Burn Care Rehabil.* 1997; **18**: 353–355.

163. Martin D, Umraw N, Gomez M, Cartotto R. Changes in subjective vs objective burn scar assessment over time: does the patient agree with what we think? *J Burn Care Rehabil.* 2003; **24**: 239–244.

164. Smith GM, Tompkins DM, Bigelow ME, Antoon AY. Burn-induced cosmetic disfigurement: can it be measured reliably? *J Burn Care Rehabil.* 1988; **9**: 371–375.

165. Sullivan T, Smith J, Kermode J, McIver E, Courtemanche DJ. Rating the burn scar. *J Burn Care Rehabil.* 1990; **11**: 256–260.

166. Forbes-Duchart L, Marshall S, Strock A, Cooper JE. Determination of inter-rater reliability in pediatric burn scar assessment using a modified version of the Vancouver scar scale. *J Burn Care Res.* 2007; **28**: 460–467.

167. Masters M, McMahon M, Svens B. Reliability testing of a new scar assessment tool, matching assessment of scars and photographs (MAPS). *J Burn Care Rehabil.* 2005; **26**: 273–284.

168. Berry RB, Tan OT, Cooke ED, et al. Transcutaneous oxygen tension as an index of maturity in hypertrophic scars treated by compression. *Br J Plast Surg.* 1985; **38**: 163–173.

169. Leung KS, Sher A, Clark JA, Cheng JC, Leung PC. Microcirculation in hypertrophic scars after burn injury. *J Burn Care Rehabil.* 1989; **10**: 436–444.

170. Lye I, Edgar DW, Wood FM, Carroll S. Tissue tonometry is a simple, objective measure for pliability of burn scar: is it reliable? *J Burn Care Res.* 2006; **1**: 82–85.

171. Corica GF, Wigger NC, Edgar DW, Wood FM, Carroll S. Objective measurement of scarring by multiple assessors: is the tissue tonometer a reliable option? *J Burn Care Rehabil.* 2006; **27**: 520–523.

172. Gorissen KJ, Boeckx WD, Van den Kerckhove E, Colla C. The effect of pressure therapy on hypertrophic (burn) scar: objective assessment by colorimetry. *J Burn Care Res.* 2006; **27**: S138.

173. Rawlins JM, Lam WL, Karoo RO, Naylor IL, Sharpe DT. Quantifying collagen type in mature burn scars: a novel approach

using histology and digital image analysis. *J Burn Care Res.* 2006; **1**: 60–65.

**174.** Bartell TH, Monafo WM, Mustoe TA. A new instrument for serial measurements of elasticity in hypertrophic scar. *J Burn Care Rehabil.* 1988; **9**: 657–660.

**175.** Rennekampff H-O, Rabbels J, Reinhard V, Becker ST, Schaller H-E. Comparing the Vancouver scar scale with the cutometer in the assessment of donor site wounds treated with various dressings in a randomized trial. *J Burn Care Res.* 2006; **27**: 345–351.

**176.** Clark JA, Cheng JC, Leung KS. Mechanical properties of normal skin and hypertrophic scars. *Burns.* 1996; **22**: 443–446.

**177.** Boyce ST, Supp AP, Wickett RR, Hoath SB, Warden GD. Assessment with the dermal torque meter of skin pliability after treatment of burns with cultured skin substitutes. *J Burn Care Rehabil.* 2000; **21**: 55–63.

**178.** Cartotto R, Shortt R, Gomez M, Musgrave M, Umraw N. Measuring change in burn scar hardness over time with the durometer. *J Burn Care Rehabil.* 2003; **24**: S87.

**179.** Oliveira GV. Objective scar evaluation: a prospective study. *J Burn Care Rehabil.* 2004; **25**: S234.

**180.** Hambleton J, Shakespeare PG, Pratt BJ. The progress of hypertrophic scars monitored by ultrasound measurements of thickness. *Burns.* 1992; **18**: 301–307.

**181.** Nedelec B, Correa JA, Rachelska GR, Armour A, LaSalle L. Quantitative measurement of hypertrophic scar: interrater reliability and concurrent validity. *J Burn Care Res.* 2008; **29**: 501–511.

**182.** Nedelec B, Correa JA, Rachelska G, Armour A, LaSalle L. Quantitative measurement of hypertrophic scar: intrarater reliability, sensitivity, and specificity. *J Burn Care Res.* 2008; **29**: 489–500.

**183.** Baryza MJ, Baryza GA. The Vancouver scar scale: an administration tool and its interrater reliability. *J Burn Care Rehabil.* 1995; **16**: 535–538.

**184.** Powers PS, Sarkar S, Goldgof DB, Cruse CW, Tsap LV. Scar assessment: current problems and future solutions. *J Burn Care Rehabil.* 1999; **20**: 54–60.

**185.** von Baeyer CL, Spagrud LJ. Systemic review of observational (behavioral) measures of pain for children and adolescents aged 3 to 18 years. *Pain.* 2007; **127**: 140–150.

**186.** Elman S, Gabriel VA, Chouteau W, Mayo MJ. The 5-D itch scale, a new tool to measure post burn pruritus. *J Burn Care Res.* 2007; **29**: S146.

**187.** Parent-Vachon M, Parnell LK, Rachelska G, LaSalle L, Nedelec B. Cross-cultural adaptation and validation of the questionnaire for pruritis assessment for use in the French Canadian burn survivor population. *Burns.* 2008; **34**: 71–92.

**188.** Nedelec B, Shankowsky HA, Tredget EE. Rating the resolving hypertropic scar: comparison of the Vancouver scar scale and scar volume. *J Burn Care Rehabil.* 2000; **21**: 205–212.

**189.** Schneider JC, Harris NL, Shami AE, et al. A descriptive review of neuropathic-like pain after burn injury. *J Burn Care Res.* 2006; **27**: 524–528.

**190.** Leung PC, Ng M. Pressure treatment for hypertrophic scars resulting from burns. *Burns.* 1980; **6**: 244–250.

**191.** Kimball KL, Drews JE, Walker S, Dimick AR. Use of TENS for pain reduction in burn patients receiving Travase. *J Burn Care Rehabil.* 1987; **8**: 28–31.

**192.** Kloti J, Pochon JP. Conservative treatment using compression suits for second and third degree burns in children. *Burns.* 1982; **8**: 180–187.

**193.** Whitaker C. The use of TENS for pruritis relief in the burns patient: an individual case report. *J Burn Care Rehabil.* 2001; **22**: 274–276.

**194.** Patino O, Novick C, Merlo A, Benaim F. Massage in hypertrophic scars. *J Burn Care Rehabil.* 1998; **19**: 268–271.

**195.** Field T, Peck M, Hernandez-Reif M, Krugman S, Burman I, Ozment-Schenck L. Postburn itching, pain, and psychological symptoms are reduced with massage therapy. *J Burn Care Rehabil.* 2000; **21**: 189–193.

**196.** Carnes RW, Sollecito WA, Salisbury RE. Evaporative water loss from healed burn wounds. *J Burn Care Rehabil.* 1981; **2**: 239–245.

**197.** Liang Z, Engrav LH, Muangman P, et al. Nerve quantification in female red Duroc pig (FRDP) scar compared to human hypertrophic scar. *Burns.* 2004; **30**: 57–64.

**198.** Ward RS, Saffle JR, Schnebly WA, Hayes-Lundy C, Reddy R. Sensory loss over grafted areas in patients with burns. *J Burn Care Rehabil.* 1989; **10**: 536–538.

**199.** McCauley RL. Reconstruction of the pediatric burned hand. *Hand Clinics.* 2000; **16**: 249–259.

**200.** Goldberg DP, Kucan JO, Bash D. Reconstruction of the burned foot. *Clin Plast Surg.* 2000; **27**: 145–161.

**201.** Esselman PC, Thombs BD, Magyar-Russell G, Fauerbach JA. Burn rehabilitation: state of the science. *Am J Phys Med Rehabil.* 2006; **85**: 383–413.

**202.** American Occupational Therapy Association. Occupational therapy practice framework: domain and process. *Am J Occup Ther.* 2002; **56**: 609–639.

**203.** Yeakel M. Occupational therapy. In: Arts CP, Moncrief JA, Pruitt BA, eds. *Burns: A Team Approach.* Philadelphia, PA: WB Saunders; 1979: 500–511.

**204.** Simons RD, McFadd A, Frank HA, Green LC, Malin RM, Morris JL. Behavioral contracting in a burn care facility: a strategy for patient participation. *J Trauma.* 1978; **18**: 257–260.

**205.** Tyack ZF, Ziviani J, Pegg S. The functional outcome of children after a burn injury: a pilot study. *J Burn Care Rehabil.* 1999; **20**: 367–373.

**206.** Danowski P, O'Brien KA, Yurt RW. Efficacy of education provided to parents by rehabilitation therapists. *J Burn Care Res.* 2007; **28**: S151.

207. Tran K, Anderson L, Kagan R. School reentry: the school's perspective. *J Burn Care Res.* 2006; **27**: S157.

208. Rosenberg L, Rosenberg M, Perez A, et al. Benefits of school reentry for children with burns. *J Burn Care Res.* 2006; **27**: S157.

209. Forbes-Duchart L, McMillan-Law G, Nicholson D. Using the experiences of adults burned as children to address sexuality in pediatric burns. *J Burn Care Res.* 2006; **27**: S121.

210. Rimmer RB, Fornaciari GM, Foster KN, et al. Impact of a pediatric residential burn camp experience on burn survivors' perception of self and attitudes regarding the camp community. *J Burn Care Rehabil.* 2007; **28**: 334–341.

211. Engrav LH, Garner WL, Tredget EE. Hypertrophic scar, wound contraction and hyper-hypopigmentation. *J Burn Care Res.* 2007; **28**: 593–597.

212. Greenhalgh DG. Management of acute burn injuries of the upper extremity in the pediatric population. *Hand Clin.* 2000; **16**: 175–186.

213. Bombaro KM, Engrav LH, Carrougher GJ, et al. What is the prevalence of hypertrophic scarring following burns? *Burns.* 2003; **29**: 299–302.

214. Sheridan RL, Baryza MJ, Pessina MA, et al. Acute hand burns in children: management and long-term outcome based on a 10-year experience with 698 injured hands. *Ann Surg.* 1999; **229**: 558–564.

215. Schneider JC, Holavanahalli R, Helm P, Goldstein R, Kowalske K. Contractures in burn injury: defining the problem. *J Burn Care Res.* 2006; **27**: 508–514.

216. Kowalske KJ, Greenhalgh DG, Ward SR. Hand burns. *J Burn Care Res.* 2007; **28**: 607–610.

217. Tambuscio A, Governa M, Caputo G, Barisoni D. Deep burn of the hands: early surgical treatment avoids the need for late revisions? *Burns.* 2006; **32**: 1000–1004.

218. van Zuijlen PP, Kreis RW, Vloemans AF, Groenevelt F, Mackie DP. Prognostic factors regarding long-term functional outcome of full-thickness hand burns. *Burns.* 1999; **25**: 709–714.

219. van Zuijlen PP, Vloemans AF, Tempelman FR, Kreis RW. The timing of surgery for deep burns of the hands: early versus delayed surgery [letter to the editor]. *Burns.* Sep 2007; **33**(6): 807.

220. Klein MB, Logsetty S, Costa B, et al. Extended time to wound closure is associated with increased risk of heterotopic ossification of the elbow. *J Burn Care Res.* 2007; **28**: 447–450.

221. Hunt JL, Arnoldo BD, Kowalske K, Helm P, Purdue GF. Heterotopic ossification revisited: a 21-year surgical experience. *J Burn Care Res.* 2006; **27**: 535–540.

222. Gaur A, Sinclair M, Caruso E, Peretti G, Zaleske D. Heterotopic ossification around the elbow following burns in children: results after excision. *J Bone Joint Surg.* 2003; **85A**: 1538–1543.

223. Bjarnason D, Phillips LG, McCoy B, et al. Reconstructive goals for children with burns: are our goals the same? *J Burn Care Rehabil.* 1992; **13**: 389–390.

224. Rea SM, Goodwin-Walters A, Wood FM. Surgeons and scar: differences between patients and surgeons in the perceived requirement for reconstructive surgery following burn injury. *Burns.* 2006; **32**: 276–283.

225. Richard R, Miller S, Staley M, Johnson RM. Multimodal versus progressive treatment techniques to correct burn scar contractures. *J Burn Care Rehabil.* 2000; **21**: 506–512.

226. Huang T, Blackwell SJ, Lewis SR. Ten years of experience in managing patients with burn contractures of axilla, elbow, wrist, and knee joints. *Plast Reconstr Surg.* 1978; **61**: 70–76.

227. Vehmeyer-Heeman M, Lommers B, Van den Kerckhove E, Boeckx W. Axillary burns: extended grafting and early splinting prevents contractures. *J Burn Care Rehabil.* 2005; **26**: 539–542.

228. Scott JR, Costa BA, Gibran NS, Engrav LH, Heimbach DH, Klein MB. Pediatric palm contact burns: a ten-year review. *J Burn Care Res.* 2008; **29**: 614–618.

229. Klein MB, Donelan MB, Spence RJ. Reconstructive surgery. *J Burn Care Res.* 2007; **28**: 602–606.

230. Pidcock FS, Fauerbach JA, Ober M, Carney J. The rehabilitation/school matrix: a model for accommodating the noncompliant child with severe burns. *J Burn Care Rehabil.* 2003; **24**: 342–346.

231. Young RC, Burd A. Paediatric upper limb contracture release following burn injury. *Burns.* 2004; **30**: 723–728.

232. Chaudhari S, Roggy D, Zieger M, Sood R. Use of AlloDerm to prevent recontracture following burn scar contracture release. *J Burn Care Res.* 2007; **28**: S73.

233. Goldberg DP, Kucan JO, Bash D. Reconstruction of the burned foot. *Clin Plast Surg.* 2000; **27**: 145–161.

234. Fauerbach JA, Pruzinsky T, Saxe GN. Psychological health and function after burn injury: setting research priorities. *J Burn Care Res.* 2007; **28**: 587–592.

235. Sheridan R. Burns at the extremes of age. *J Burn Care Res.* 2007; **28**: 580–585.

236. Drake JE, Stoddard FJ, Murphy M, et al. Trauma severity influences acute stress in young burned children. *J Burn Care Res.* 2006; **27**: 174–182.

237. Field T, Morrow C, Valdeon C, Larson S, Kuhn C, Schanberg S. Massage reduces anxiety in child and adolescent psychiatric patients. *J Am Acad Child Adolesc Psychiatry.* 1992; **31**: 125–131.

238. Patterson DR. Non-opioid-based approaches to burn pain. *J Burn Care Rehabil.* 1995; **16**: 372–376.

239. Hernandez-Reif M, Field T, Largie S, et al. Childrens' distress during burn treatment is reduced by massage therapy. *J Burn Care Rehabil.* 2001; **22**: 191–195.

240. Harandi AA, Esfandani A, Shakibaei F. The effect of hypnotherapy on procedural pain and state anxiety related to physiotherapy in women hospitalized in a burn unit. *Contemp Hypnosis.* 2004; **21**: 28–34.

241. McCall JE, Lloyd S, Smith R, Carbis CR. Virtual reality hypnosis reduces preoperative anxiety in pediatric reconstructive burn patients. *J Burn Care Res.* 2008; **29**: S78.

242. Greenhalgh DG, Gaboury T, Warden GD. The early release of axillary contractures in pediatric patients with burns. *J Burn Care Rehabil.* 1993; **14**: 39–42.

243. Turkaslan T, Turan A, Dayicioglu D, Ozsoy Z. Uses of scapular island flap in pediatric axillary burn contractures. *Burns.* 2006; **32**: 885–890.

244. Figus A, Leon-Villapalos J, Philp B, Dziewulski P. Severe multiple extensive postburn contractures: a simultaneous approach with total scar tissue excision and resurfacing with dermal regeneration template. *J Burn Care Res.* 2007; **28**: 913–917.

245. Emsen IM. The cross incision plasty for reconstruction of the burned web space: introduction of an alternative technique for the correction of dorsal and volar neosyndactyly. *J Burn Care Res.* 2008; **29**: 378–385.

246. Filho JM, Belerique M, Franco D, Porchat CA, Franco T. Tissue expansion in burn sequelae repair. *Burns.* 2007; **33**: 246–251.

247. Gousheh J, Arasteh E, Mafi P. Super-thin abdominal skin pedicle flap for the reconstruction of hypertrophic and contracted dorsal hand burn scars. *Burns.* 2008; **34**: 400–405.

248. Burm JS, Oh SJ. Fist position for skin grafting on the dorsal hand: II. Clinical use in deep burns and burn scar contractures. *Plast Reconstr Surg.* 2000; **105**: 581–588.

249. Bar-Meir E, Yaffe B, Winkler E, Sher N, Berenstein M, Schindler A. Combined Iliazarov and free flap for severe recurrent flexion-contracture release. *J Burn Care Res.* 2006; **27**: 529–534.

250. Ilhami K, Safak O, Orhan G. Specifically designed external fixators in treatment of complex postburn hand contractures. *Burns.* 2003; **29**: 609–612.

251. Konstantakos EK, Miller SF, Dalstrom DJ, Shapiro ML, Laughlin RT. Uniplanar external fixation for care of circumferential extremity burn wounds in adults. *J Burn Care Res.* 2007; **28**: 892–896.

252. Manigandan C, Gupta AK, Venugopal K, Ninan S, Cherian RE. A multi-purpose, self-adjustable aeroplane splint for the splinting of axillary burns. *Burns.* 2003; **29**: 276–279.

253. Kumar P, Manova H. A multi purpose, self-adjustable aeroplane splint for the splinting of axillary burns [letter to the editor]. *Burns.* 2004; **30**: 204–205.

254. Al-Qattan MM, Rasool M, Al-Kattan W. Fabrication of silicone oral splints for severe burn microstomia in children. *Burns.* 2005; **31**: 217–219.

255. Manigandan C, Gupta AK, Ninan S, Padankatti SM. Re-emphasizing the efficacy of the multi-purpose, self-adjustable, aeroplane splint for the splinting of axillary burns. *Burns.* 2005; **31**: 500–501.

256. Schwanholt C, Daugherty MB, Gaboury T, Warden GD. Splinting the pediatric palmar burn. *J Burn Care Rehabil.* 1992; **13**: 460–464.

257. O'Rourke D. The measurement of pain in infants, children and adolescents: from policy to practice. *Phys Ther.* 2004; **84**: 560–570.

258. von Baeyer CL, Spagrud LJ. Systemic review of observational (behavioral) measures of pain for children and adolescents aged 3 to 18 years. *Pain.* 2007; **127**: 140–150.

259. Tyack ZF, Ziviani J. What influences the functional outcome of children at 6 months post-burn? *Burns.* 2003; **29**: 433–444.

260. Helm P, Herndon DN, deLateur B. Restoration of function. *J Burn Care Res.* 2007; **28**: 611–614.

261. Sheridan RL, Hinson MI, Liang MH, et al. Long-term outcome of children surviving massive burns. *JAMA.* 2000; **283**: 69–73.

262. Suman OE, Thomas SJ, Wilkins JP, Mlcak RP, Herndon DN. Effect of exogenous growth hormone and exercise on lean mass and muscle function in children with burns. *J Appl Physiol.* 2003; **94**(6): 2273–2281.

263. Suman OE, Herndon DN. Effects of cessation of a structured and supervised exercise conditioning program on lean mass and muscle strength in severely burned children. *Arch Phys Med Rehabil.* 2007; **88**(12)(suppl 2): S24–S29.

# CHAPTER TWENTY-FIVE

# PAIN MANAGEMENT IN THE BURNED CHILD

HERNANDO OLIVAR, MD, CLINICAL ASSISTANT PROFESSOR,
DEPARTMENT OF ANESTHESIOLOGY AND PAIN MEDICINE,
UNIVERSITY OF WASHINGTON SCHOOL OF MEDICINE,
SEATTLE, WA

SAM R. SHARAR, MD, PROFESSOR, DEPARTMENT OF ANESTHESIOLOGY AND PAIN MEDICINE,
UNIVERSITY OF WASHINGTON SCHOOL OF MEDICINE,
SEATTLE, WA

NICOLE S. GIBRAN, MD, DIRECTOR, UW REGIONAL BURN CENTER,
PROFESSOR, DEPARTMENT OF SURGERY,
UNIVERSITY OF WASHINGTON SCHOOL OF MEDICINE,
HARBORVIEW MEDICAL CENTER

*Pain: An unpleasant sensory and emotional experience associated with actual or potential tissue damage, or described in terms of such damage. The inability to communicate verbally does not negate the possibility that an individual is experiencing pain and is in need of appropriate pain-relieving treatment.*
International Association for the Study of Pain, 1994

## INTRODUCTION

Burn injuries are accompanied by severe pain and significant physiologic and emotional stress. Burn pain starts with the injury itself and varies throughout a long healing process that includes frequent painful procedures. These factors make analgesic treatment plans complex and unpredictable and often require a multidisciplinary approach that involves both pharmacological and nonpharmacological interventions.

Historically, children's pain has been underestimated and therefore undertreated.[1-4] Fortunately, in the past few decades a trend in providing adequate pain relief to this vulnerable population is encouraging,[5-8] but pediatric burn pain treatment remains a particular challenge. Unwarranted fear of harmful opioid side effects (eg, respiratory depression, addiction), difficulty with pain assessment in young children, and absence of standardized pain management protocols (particularly in hospitals with high health care staff turnover) all contribute to this poor pain management.[9]

Burn pain itself and the pain associated with therapeutic procedures have been described as the most intense types of human suffering, so their relief is paramount for several reasons. Inadequate pain management can initiate conflicts between patients and burn care staff (eg, doctors, nurses, and therapists), thus complicating the normal course of burn treatment.[11] Inadequate pain control in the initial stage of burn care likely decreases effective adequate analgesia in subsequent procedures.[11] Burned patients who report worse pain scores during hospitalization also report poorer emotional adjustment up to 2 years after discharge.[12] Up to 50% of severely burned children eventually develop post-traumatic stress disorder (PTSD) symptoms at some time after a burn injury.[13] Activation of inflammatory cytokines and expansion of the stress response to trauma and surgery and its consequences can be ameliorated with the use of appropriate analgesic regimens.[14] Each of these observations argues for careful attention to good pain control both immediately after injury and throughout the postburn period.

Treatment of burn pain in the pediatric population must take into account maturational variables such as age, cognitive stage, personality, and emotional states and patient interpersonal interactions in order to offer an effective multidisciplinary therapeutic approach. Although ethical, methodological, and economical considerations make pain research in children challenging, investigations involving treatment of chronic pain and behavioral responses have been increasing in an effort to provide better understanding of pediatric pain pathophysiology as well as the foundation for its treatment.[6]

## NEUROANATOMY OF PAIN

Thermal, mechanical, or chemical stimuli cause activation of peripheral sensory neuron axonal endings (nociceptors), initiating the pain response. Tissue injury promotes release of inflammatory mediators (Table 1), leading to conformational changes of ion channels and G protein-coupled receptors in the nerve terminals. These changes translate into action potentials and ultimately into transmission of painful information to the central nervous system. Pain signaling from the nociceptors enters the spinal cord through the ventrolateral part of the dorsal root, connecting with a second-order neuron in the dorsal horn. Many ascending paths transfer the information to the brain. The spinothalamic tract is the most important of these paths, projecting to the thalamus, periaqueductal gray matter, reticular formation, and hypothalamus. Once the afferent information is

processed in the central nervous system, efferent pathways carry the responses to the periphery, elucidating pain behaviors (Figure 1). Pain responses are modulated at different levels of the pain pathway, including the nociceptors themselves, the substantia gelatinosa, and descending supraspinal paths. Excitatory or inhibitory neurotransmitters like glutamate and aspartate or glycine and γ-aminobutyric acid (GABA), respectively, are involved in this process.[15,16]

Under normal conditions, nociceptors are in a resting state, with variable rates of activation depending on the type and intensity of stimuli and the degree of specialization of the nociceptor[15,17,18] (Table 2). Pain associated with burn injuries results from thermal damage of nociceptive receptors and inflammation of the burned site. Initial repair of the tissue damaged from heat injuries includes activation of coagulation pathways and liberation of inflammatory mediators, including substance P and calcitonin gene-related protein, which activate nociceptors and initiate the pain response. Inflammatory cell migration into the wound and activation of keratinocytes and endothelial cells increase local concentrations of inflammatory mediators such as IL-6,[19] which has been identified as a major contributor to burn-induced hyperalgesia (increased sensitivity in damaged tissue or surrounding inflamed tissue).[20] Other mechanisms for hyperalgesia include sensitization of cutaneous heat nociceptors and recruitment of mechanical or chemical receptors due to changes in their responsiveness to heat.[21]

## DEVELOPMENTAL BIOLOGY OF PAIN

Previous dogmas that young children's memory to pain is limited or that incomplete myelinization in young children prevents pain perception[22] have been successfully refuted. Recent studies suggest that pain and distress in children have persisting negative effects on physiological parameters such as eating and sleep/arousal patterns.[23,24]

At birth, fully functional C-polymodal sensory nerve fibers and almost fully functional Aδ and Aβ nociceptors can be found in the skin. Although the transmission of the afferent impulse in the spinal cord is somewhat immature, painful stimuli can evoke central responses via spinothalamic tracts. These tracts activate areas in the brain stem, limbic system, and cerebral cortex, generating autonomic and motor responses to pain. Thalamocortical axons can be found at 22 weeks of gestation in the human cortex, but somatosensory-evoked potentials can be recorded only as early as 27 weeks of gestation, suggesting an ongoing process of neurophysiologic maturation.[25]

At birth, efferent pathways in the pain modulating system are less developed, but the presence of pain responses in

353

the form of reflexes (eg, flexion withdrawal reflex) suggests that the pain system is fully functional at this stage of development.[26] Early experiences of pain may produce permanent structural and functional reorganization of developing nociceptive pathways, which may influence future experiences of pain perception.[27] This response was demonstrated by Ruda et al when continuous inflammation of newborn rat pup paws produced increases in the density of dorsal horn primary afferent neurons. Furthermore, eventual adult behavioral responses to painful stimuli were increased in the neonatal treated rats.[28]

## PSYCHOLOGICAL, FAMILIAL, CULTURAL, AND RELIGIOUS FACTORS THAT AFFECT PAIN

Psychological factors such as operant learning mechanisms (differing pain behavior depending on negative or positive reinforcements), respondent learning mechanisms (anticipated uncomfortable experiences even in the absence of the noxious stimulus), and social learning mechanisms (pain experienced as it is observed) can all influence the pain experience.[29] Children's response to pain differs with age. Whereas infants and toddlers usually react to pain with crying, preschool-age children are more likely to exhibit regressive behaviors. In contrast, older children may display symptoms of depression or anxiety manifested by verbal and physical expressions of anger.[30] Pediatric burn pain management is further complicated by interindividual differences, temporal changes in intensity or quality of pain as the wounds heal, and the presence of previous or concomitant emotional and behavioral problems.[31] Anxiety, fear, and depression frequently accompany burn pain problems[32] and therefore should be addressed in the comprehensive treatment plan.

As a result of their burn injuries, previously active and independently functioning children and their families are suddenly exposed to an unfamiliar hospital environment, rigid therapy schedules, complicated medical care routines, and uncertainty about the future (ie, fear of physical disfiguration). These factors lead to feelings of helplessness and a decreased sense of control that can exacerbate the pain experience.[31] Adequate education about the goals and details of painful procedures, using honest communication, age-appropriate language, or playacting, can decrease a child's anxiety level, improve the sense of control, and contribute to analgesic effect.

Among families, particular pain behaviors are expected and modeled. These behaviors are positively reinforced and are valued by family members, exerting a strong modifying effect on how children interpret and express their pain.

Ethnic and religious groups may have common ways of perceiving, responding to, and communicating cultural beliefs about pain. For example, Lipton and Marbach studied facial pain in patients from 5 different ethnicities. They found no significant interethnic differences in the intensity of reported pain experiences, but identified differences in emotionality (stoicism vs expressiveness), which influenced response to pain.[33] The impact of ethnicity and religion on children's pain behavior has not been widely studied, and further research is needed in this area.

## ASSESSMENT OF PEDIATRIC PAIN

As stated in the definition of pain presented at the beginning of the chapter, the emotional component of pain makes it a subjective experience that does not always correlate with extent of tissue damage. Suffering, as a component of pain, is manifested by fear, frustration, and nonverbal actions such as grimacing, moaning, or crying. These pain behaviors, in addition to physiologic responses (ie, increase in heart rate, hypertension), should be included in attempts to quantify a patient's pain level.[34]

Assessment of pain in children is challenging due to the inability of children to

fully communicate feelings, the plasticity and complexity of children's pain perception, and the influence of psychological and developmental factors.[35]

Newborns express their pain automatically in the form of physiological or behavioral changes (variations in respiratory rate, oxygen saturation, withdrawal, crying, or facial expressions). Infants and toddlers (ages 1-2 years) start to experience emotions manifesting anger or sadness to pain. They can identify painful situations as well as attach pain to an external cause. Preschoolers (ages 3-5 years) start to give indications of pain intensity. They learn from daily painful events (bruises and bumps) how to interpret and modify their pain. At this age, children can simulate, exaggerate, or suppress signs of pain, altering in this way adults' emotional response to their pain.[36] Older children (ages 6-12 years) clearly differentiate levels of pain intensity and attach more elaborate feelings to painful situations. Adolescents are able to self-report pain intensity and quality as well as pain-related emotions, including fear, disability, and disfigurement (Table 3).

### Pain Assessment Scales

Multiple pain assessment scales have been designed in attempts to objectively measure children's pain, but no single tool is applicable to all children and all painful circumstances.[22,37] There are 3 dimensions typically assessed: behavioral reactions, self-reports of pain intensity, and physiologic reactions.

Behavioral pain assessment scales measure pain-related behaviors such as crying, facial expressions, body position, and nonverbal expressions different from crying. Behavioral scales have proven to be useful to assess acute, time-limited pain of preverbal children (Table 4). All behavioral scales provide a systematic approach for assessment and documentation of pain in infants and preschoolers, but some are complex and difficult to apply in busy clinical settings.[38]

Once the child matures and acquires communication skills, subjective measures are appropriate. These include verbal self-report forms, questionnaires, pain drawings, and rating scales. The main limitation of these subjective measures is that the scores provided may be affected by different factors, including family pressure, pain modulating strategies, fear, or the chance of secondary gain[36,39] (Table 5). Physiologic changes that are helpful in assessment of pain include heart rate, mean arterial pressure, and pulse rate variability.[40] As with adults, the interpretation of pain scores from these pain-measuring tools should account for patients' cognitive, emotional, and physical conditions at the time they are applied.

## TYPES OF BURN PAIN

The size and depth of the burn wound are important factors to consider in the initial clinical assessment of burn pain. Epidermal first-degree burns (eg, sunburns) generally are painful to the touch due to sensitization of sensory fibers. Superficial partial-thickness (second-degree) dermal burns (eg, scald burns) cause significant hyperalgesia and moderate to severe pain due to the presence of marked inflammatory response and sensitization of the nerve terminals. Deep partial-thickness dermal burns (eg, grease burns) may have damaged sensory receptors and lead to a less predictable presentation. Full-thickness (third-degree) burns (eg, flame or prolonged contact burns) completely destroy the dermis, including the resident sensory terminals and blood vessels, making the burn relatively painless. Regardless of these generalities, concomitant first-degree or second-degree burns within or surrounding a third-degree burn can produce painful areas and mislead the clinician in the initial assessment of burn depth[41] (Table 6).

Burn pain is classically described in 5 categories: background, breakthrough, procedural, postoperative, and chronic. Background pain is due to burn-associated tissue injury and is characterized by a persistent low-intensity to moderate-intensity pain when the patient is at rest. Breakthrough pain represents acutely increased pain occurring spontaneously or with movement, often due to inadequate background pain treatment. Procedural pain represents the intense pain during and immediately after therapeutic treatments such as wound care or physical therapy. Postoperative pain occurs after surgical procedures, including extensive debridements, donor site harvesting, and grafting, and may last for 2 to 4 days[31] (Figure 2). Chronic pain symptoms such as hyperalgesia, painful paresthesias, or neuropathic pain (tingling, warmth, shooting pains, pins and needles) frequently are present after burn injuries but are poorly characterized or understood, particularly in children. Choiniere et al reported the presence of pain and paresthetic sensations in fully healed burn wounds up to 1 year after the injury. The mechanism of this painful sensation seems to be related to abnormal or deficient reinervation of the scar tissue.[42] Sensations such as pruritus and phantom limb pain may replace background pain as significant chronic sources of anxiety and distress. Itching is particularly problematic in the pediatric burn population; the scratching causes recurrent breakdown in the newly healed skin and delays recovery and rehabilitation. Additionally, itching may interfere with recovery by causing agitation, leading to frustration and impaired sleep and or eating. The "itch man" scale created by Blakeney and Marvin is a 0-4 scale that rates the intensity of itching and can be used to guide pharmacologic therapies (Figure 3).

Anxiety deserves special attention in the pediatric burned population. Signs of anxiety are prevalent in burn patients, probably due to the thermal injury itself, fear of painful procedures, long hospitalization, separation from parents, and fear of disfiguration.[43] Anxiety often precedes painful therapeutic procedures as a conditioned response to such frightening and repetitive pain experiences (ie, anticipatory anxiety). Often mistaken for pain during procedures, it is occasionally mistreated with opioids rather than anxiolytics, leading to an unsatisfactory analgesia outcome.

## PHARMACOKINETICS

The goal of pharmacologic analgesic therapy is to deliver an effective concentration of a drug to its site of action and obtain a desired therapeutic effect without toxicity.[44] Because the use of pharmacologic analgesics is a pillar of burn pain treatment, a sound understanding of basic pharmacology and its variations in early stages of life is imperative.[44-46] Unfortunately, approximately 80% of the medications used in children have never been formally tested or approved by the United States Food and Drug Administration (FDA) for use in children. In response to this problem, the American Academy of Pediatrics (AAP) has requested formal FDA approval and labeling of essential drugs for pediatric patients, including morphine, naloxone, and dopamine.[47]

## Pediatric Pharmacokinetics

Drug absorption of enterally administered drugs from the gastrointestinal tract of neonates and young infants may be prolonged by diminished intestinal motility, delayed gastric emptying, different gastric pH, and limited gastrointestinal flora. In addition, practical issues such as medication presentations in tablets or as sustained release compounds make them either impossible to administer to young children or release toxic doses of the medication if the tablet is bitten or crushed.[48]

Intravenous (IV) drug administration provides more predictable blood levels since portal circulation is bypassed, but it is limited in the need for closer observation and the difficulty to transition to oral formulations for postdischarge outpatient care. Intramuscular (IM) injections in children should be avoided to prevent the psychological connection between complaining of pain and receiving more pain as a result (ie, punishment for a pain complaint). Additionally, absorption from intramuscular injections is unpredictable. Transdermal medication administration in neonates increases the risk of systemic toxicity due to the fact that neonatal skin is relatively thin and more permeable, increasing drug absorption.[45]

Drug distribution depends in part on protein binding (eg, albumin and $\alpha$1-acid glycoproteins), chemical properties of the drug (eg, liposolubility and degree of ionization), and total body water. Concentrations of proteins in neonates and children younger than 1 year are decreased, leading to elevated concentrations of free drug and greater pharmacologic effect. Patients with burns larger than 20% of the total body surface commonly have hypoalbuminemia that may alter clearance of drugs that are usually protein-bound. Other pathological states such as malnourishment, protein-losing renal diseases, or chronic inflammation also alter plasma protein concentrations and affect free drug availability. Children have increased total body water compared with adults, thus affecting volumes of distribution of water-soluble drugs. As a result, larger doses (normalized to body weight) of drugs may be necessary to obtain similar plasma concentrations[44,45,48,49] despite the potential for elevated concentrations of free drug, as noted above.

Children have altered metabolism and excretion of analgesics compared to adults. Both hepatic and plasma enzymatic systems are immature at birth. However, rapid maturation in the first year of life allows infants and young children to have higher metabolic capacity than adults. By puberty, hepatic metabolic activity decreases to adult levels. Newborn renal function is about 40% that of the adult. Children younger than 1 year have decreased glomerular filtration and tubular secretion, delaying excretion of active by-products and increasing risk of drug toxicity. Therefore,

in the first months of life, increased pharmacologic doses used to compensate for the higher volume of distribution should be administered with longer dosing intervals in order to prevent drug accumulation.[49]

In summary, differences in organ development, body composition, physiologic states, and pathologic states of the pediatric population affect drug pharmacology and clinical response in varying ways, requiring careful administration and monitoring of clinical effects.

## Pharmacokinetic Changes in Burns

Choosing the ideal analgesic medication for burn pain must account for potential pharmacokinetic changes present in this setting. During the resuscitative phase (first 72 hours after burn injury) patients present with decreased protein plasma concentration due to a plasma leak from increased vascular permeability and aggressive crystalloid resuscitation. These low plasma protein levels reduce drug-protein binding and potentially increase free drug availability. Reduced cardiac output during the very initial phase of a severe burn injury may alter absorption of medication administered by nonintravenous routes. Clinical effects of this altered pharmacology include a reduced therapeutic index of drugs with high protein binding (eg, benzodiazepines) and altered effectiveness of regular doses of analgesic drugs due to the increase in volume of distribution.[50] Furman et al reported reduced morphine clearance, longer terminal half-life, and a smaller volume of distribution in adult burned patients during anesthesia. Interestingly, these results contradict the hypothesis that burned patients may have larger volumes of distribution, but the small sample size (14 subjects in total) and poor criteria for matching subjects (only by age and not by burn size) decrease the value of this study.[51] In contrast, Herman et al found an increased terminal half-life for controlled-release morphine administered to adult burned patients.[52]

Within 72 hours of injury, patients with major burns develop a hypermetabolic and high cardiac output state that also alters drug pharmacology. Medications administered intravenously during this period typically have quicker onset and shorter half-life, clinically manifested by the necessity to increase the dose or decrease the interval of drug administration to achieve therapeutic levels.[53,54] Because patients with major burn injuries have long hospitalizations, drug tolerance frequently develops. Tolerance is characterized by increasingly poor response to standard doses of analgesics. Opioid tolerance may be apparent after as little as 1 week of uninterrupted opioid use or in patients with a history of preexisting drug abuse. It is important to note that the opioid dosing necessary to provide adequate pain relief in patients with major burns often exceeds common textbook recommendations. Equally important is to prevent opioid withdrawal by careful, tapered reduction of opioid analgesics in these patients as wounds heal and analgesic needs decrease.[31,55] Anticipating changes in treatment location is paramount; if a patient is being discharged home, transition to medication that can be distributed on an outpatient basis must be anticipated before the day of discharge.

## MANAGEMENT OF PAIN IN BURNED CHILDREN

An ideal burn analgesic plan should include age-appropriate pain assessment followed by pharmacological and nonpharmacological modalities individualized to patient needs and institutional capabilities. Specific to the case of the burned pediatric patient, unique pain issues such as separation anxiety, the patient's fear of the hospital environment, previous pain experiences, and the family's influence on the patient's pain behaviors should be addressed and modified if necessary. Pain management for the burned child is based on the presence of different types of pain depending on the stage of burn recovery and the clinical setting in which this pain occurs.

## Treatment of Background Pain

The goal of background analgesia is to provide patients with sufficient comfort to allow daily activities such as adjusting their position in bed or ambulating.[56] To date, opioids are the foundation of burn pain treatment. These medications provide excellent pain relief and dose-dependent sedation. Additionally, their use is flexible as they are available in different routes of administration, potencies, and durations of action. Other nonopioid medications and nonpharmacologic approaches also should be introduced as soon as possible in order to achieve an effective, multimodal analgesic approach.[57]

Important factors to consider in choosing the route of administration of pain medications in burned children are the presence of IV access, enteral function status, and safety associated with the physical location where the patient is receiving care (intensive care unit versus hospital ward).

A reasonable approach for background pain therapy in the very initial stage of thermal injuries (less than 72 hours) is the administration of escalating doses of IV short-acting intravenous opioids (fentanyl, morphine, hydromorphone)[58] in 30% dose increments until pain is under control.[59] If intolerable side effects appear, an alternative opioid should be established at equianalgesic dose.[60] *Equianalgesia* refers to the relative doses of 2 different opioids required to produce the same analgesic effect. The amount of drug that

produces analgesia equivalent to 10 mg of parenteral morphine is routinely referred to as an *opioid equivalent*. When changing drugs, the initial calculated equivalent dose of the alternative opioid should be reduced by 25% to 50% since tolerance to the previous opioid often is incomplete[59,60] (Table 7). Once pain control is achieved, the goal for treating background pain must be to transition to a long-acting opioid.

In order to provide uniform and effective pain management for hospitalized patients, many burn centers have developed guidelines to help the clinical staff choose an appropriate analgesic regimen according to patient needs.[58] The simplicity, effectiveness, and safety over a broad range of ages and clinical stages of the burn injury make these guidelines an invaluable tool in the analgesic treatment of pediatric burned patients[61] (Table 8).

A variety of nonopioid medications are worth considering as adjuvants in the treatment of burn pain symptoms. Acetaminophen or nonsteroidal anti-inflammatory drugs (NSAIDs) are useful adjuncts to opioids and can be the first line of treatment in minor burns.[62] NSAIDs should not be used in patients who are likely to need excision and grafting due to their association with bleeding complications during surgery. It has been reported that NSAIDs can decrease opioid requirements and hence indirectly reduce their side effects. Use of NSAIDs in children appears to be safe, but in hypovolemic patients, administration should be carefully implemented due to the risk of potential renal dysfunction.

Acetaminophen is safe if administered in recommended doses. Oral or rectal administration offers flexibility with minimal side effects. It has no anti-inflammatory effects and does not alter platelet function. Appropriate interval dosing for acetaminophen is crucial in order to prevent toxicity, manifested by signs of liver dysfunction, malaise, nausea, and vomiting.[63] (Table 9).

Gabapentin has been shown to be effective in alleviating acute burn pain in adults when combined with opioids[64] and could prove effective in the prevention of chronic pain due to the suppression of development of hyperalgesia.[65] Further research is necessary to determine the proper application of gabapentin in the management of background pain in burned children.

Children as young as 6 years or who are able to understand the concept of patient-controlled analgesia (PCA) can potentially use this technique safely.[66,67] PCA is an effective and efficient method for controlling procedural or postoperative burn pain. Serious adverse events (respiratory depression) can result, however, when family members, caregivers, or clinicians administer the analgesia for the patient by proxy.[68] In the setting of long-term pain treatment of a burned child, other routes of analgesic administration should be considered before PCA since IV access limits patient mobility and interferes with physical therapy.

## Treatment of Breakthrough Pain

Breakthrough pain usually relates to precipitants such as moving in bed, coughing, sitting, and touching.[69] Episodes of breakthrough burn pain may last seconds to minutes and may occur 3 to 4 times per day.[70] Effective treatment of breakthrough pain is based on continual reassessment of pain and its triggers, with adjustment of background analgesic doses when appropriate. Tight adherence to scheduled analgesics or IV infusions is imperative in order to maintain relatively constant therapeutic drug levels and avoid end-of-dose exacerbation of pain.

Because of the short duration of breakthrough pain episodes, a rapid-onset and short-acting medication such as immediate-release morphine or oxycodone or a dose of IV fentanyl is recommended. Children with breakthrough pain may also benefit from nonpharmacological treatments and psychological support that target predictable episodes of such pain (eg, pain occurring with activity).

## Treatment of Procedural Pain

Procedural pain associated with burn wound care or therapy is described as sharp, excruciating, of short duration, and charged with significant emotional distress, such as anticipatory anxiety. Procedures such as daily wound care, dressing changes, and staple removal may predispose to development of hyperalgesia. The goals of procedural analgesia/sedation should be to blunt physiological responses to pain, prevent psychological distress, provide amnesia, control patient behavior through the provision of comfort, and increase safety during the procedure.[71]

For an adequate planning of the pharmacologic management of procedural pain, it is ideal to establish beforehand the extent of the procedure to be performed and to determine the level of analgesia/sedation required to safely and humanely complete the procedure. The American Society of Anesthesiologists (ASA) has defined the continuum of depth of sedation, summarized in Table 10.[72] Sedatives and analgesic drugs used for procedural pain with a target level of moderate/deep sedation should be easy to administer, be well tolerated by the child, and have rapid onset of action, short duration, and few side effects (Table 11).

Most limited procedures in burned children (eg, dressing changes without significant debridement) can be performed with minimal sedation after a dose of opioid alone. More extensive procedures may require deeper states of sedation that can be achieved with the addition of a benzodiazepine or with anesthetic drugs such as ketamine.[73]

In some cases (eg, extensive removal of skin staples or delicate wound care procedures on the face), general anesthesia may be required. At least 1 report suggests that operating room facilities are appropriate for only a small fraction (2.5%) of all wound debridements and that daily wound care can be effectively performed under adequate analgesia/sedation on the ward.[73] Unfortunately, complications can occur with moderate or deep sedation performed in these settings. In a prospective descriptive study of complications during procedural sedation in 1244 pediatric procedural sedations performed by pediatric emergency physicians in the emergency department of a tertiary care pediatric hospital, procedural sedation was successful in 98% of the cases but was accompanied by an 18% overall complication rate, with hypoxia being the most common complication. Although none of the patients required endotracheal intubation or had adverse outcomes, these data suggest that pediatric procedural sedation should be performed by personnel appropriately trained to treat potential serious complications.[74]

Because procedural analgesia in burned patients frequently requires high doses of opioids, institutional policies regarding appropriate monitoring in settings where high doses of opioids or sedatives are administered should be very explicit and should follow the guidelines of the Joint Commission on Accreditation of Healthcare Organizations (JCAHO)[75] regarding monitoring during sedation.[9,76] These guidelines should be complemented by the recommendations on monitoring published by the American Society of Anesthesia[77] and the American Academy of Pediatrics.[71,78,79] One provision is that a trained provider be dedicated to administer and monitor the analgesia/sedation while others perform the procedure. The use of such a provider may not be practical in every case of procedural analgesia but is most critical for problematic painful procedures that require deeper sedation, very young children, or children with concurrent medical issues.

## Pharmacological Agents

Opioids are the most commonly used analgesics for all types of postburn pain. Opioid medictions are available in multiple formulations and routes of administration that allow therapeutic flexibility in the burn setting (Table 7). Transmucosal administration of fentanyl has a more rapid onset of action than orally administered opioids, is well tolerated by children, and is particularly attractive for procedural analgesia/sedation in alert, cooperative patients[80–83]

Benzodiazepines have hypnotic, amnesic, anxiolytic, and sedative effects. They also potentiate the analgesic effects of opioids and can be used as adjuvants in the treatment of burn pain. Midazolam is a short-acting benzodiazepine with high lipid solubility which avidly binds plasma proteins. It can be administered by IV, oral, intranasal, IM, and rectal routes. Lorazepam is also a commonly used benzodiazepine that has similar anxiolytic effects as midazolam, but with a longer duration. Lorazepam is not recommended for children younger than 12 years (Table 11).

Ketamine has been used effectively as an analgesic for wound care. Ketamine is a unique anesthetic in that it produces cognitive dissociation from the immediate environment, providing sedation, amnesia, and analgesia (N-methyl-D-aspartate [NMDA] receptor antagonist) while maintaining protective airway reflexes. It has a rapid onset of action (3-5 min) and short duration (15 min) when administered intravenously and can produce both moderate sedation and deep sedation in a dose-dependent fashion.[84] Side effects of ketamine include tachycardia, hypertension, increased oral secretions, airway obstruction, and visual/aural hallucinations. Ketamine is reported to be a safe agent for pediatric procedural sedation in selected settings when administered by nonanesthesiology personnel who are specifically trained in its use[85–88] and to patients who are adequately assessed and monitored for moderate or deep sedation (Table 11).

Other potent anesthetic agents such as propofol and dexmedetomidine have been used for moderate sedation in pediatric burn patients, but their administration may be limited to intubated patients in the intensive care unit due to the significant anesthetic potency of these drugs, which can quickly result in potential life-threatening situations related to airway management and cardiovascular changes.[89–92]

Dexmedetomidine is a newer ɑ2-agonist with a more selective action on the ɑ2-adrenoceptor, and a shorter half-life than Clonidine. It has been frequently used for sedation in adult burn care units. When used intranasally, dexmedetomidine has a bioavailability of 80% and has been reported to produce adequate preoperative and procedural sedation in children and adults.[93,94] Experience with its use in burn-injured children is limited, however.

Propofol (2,6 di-isopropylphenol) is classified as a nonopioid, nonbarbiturate, sedative-hypnotic agent with sympatholytic and vagotonic effects. Its rapid onset of action, short duration, and rapid recovery are ideal for procedural sedation. Although commonly used for sedation in some intensive care units, its use for deep procedural sedation requires comprehensive and vigilant monitoring by trained providers (ie, anesthesiologists) due to its potential for profound cardiovascular and respiratory effects. Its use in children as a prolonged infusion (18-115 hours) for sedation may be associated with metabolic acidosis, bradyarrhythmias, and myocardial failure.[95]

An inhaled mixture of 50% oxygen and 50% nitrous oxide (Entonox®) has been used in treating procedural burn pain.[96] Self-administered mask inhalation produces analgesia within 20 seconds that peaks at 2 minutes and rapidly dissipates upon discontinuation. Advantages of using this mixture include the absence of cardiovascular side effects and the ability to self-administer. Side effects include possible development of megaloblastic anemia and leukopenia following 2 to 6 hours of exposure to nitrous oxide. It is not clear whether shorter duration but repeated daily exposure to nitrous oxide during burn procedures will potentiate hematologic abnormalities that are already present in burned patients.[96]

The use of local anesthetics in topical application or regional nerve blocks may have selective analgesic benefit. One important source of postoperative pain is skin graft donor sites. Topical local anesthetic mixtures of prilocaine and lidocaine have been shown effective in providing analgesia/anesthesia of donor sites following skin harvesting for up to 90 minutes.[97] Subcutaneous infiltration of bupivacaine with epinephrine at doses less than 1.9 mg/kg have been shown to be safe (blood concentration below the potential toxic threshold of 4 µg/mL) and effective in reducing donor site pain for approximately 12 to 24 hours after surgery.[98,99] Unfortunately, its use is not feasible in large donor sites requiring large injection volumes that increase the risk for systemic bupivacaine toxicity.

Regional nerve blocks can provide adequate pain control of longer duration. A single-shot fascia iliaca compartment block targeting the anterolateral thigh donor site reportedly reduces pain for up to 74 hours in adult burn patients.[100] Regional analgesia techniques have limited use in burned patients because large injured skin areas are unlikely to be controlled by blockade of a single sensory nerve distribution but may still be useful if limited skin areas are affected. A major concern of continuous regional analgesia in children is the possibility of local anesthetic toxicity due to systemic absorption of the drug. However, a cohort study to determine plasma concentrations of bupivacaine and its main metabolite after 48 hours of continuous fascia iliaca compartment blockade showed both safety and adequate pain relief in children with traumatic injuries to the knee and thigh, offering encouragement for this technique in burn-injured children.[101]

Range-of-motion exercises are essential in preventing contractures and promoting functional use of the involved extremities.[102] Furthermore, more stretching and exercise often reduce edema and decrease pain symptoms. Unfortunately, pain during therapy may jeopardize a child's ability or willingness to engage in exercise.[103] Although opioid analgesics provide ideal pharmacological treatment for procedural pain when a patient has open wounds, their sedative and gastrointestinal side effects limit patient ability to participate fully in occupational and physical therapy treatments or return to activities of daily living. Therefore, once the wounds are healed, NSAIDs usually provide the level of comfort necessary to perform such activities.

## NONPHARMACOLOGICAL APPROACHES

Nonpharmacological interventions may supplement pharmacologic treatment of pain and anxiety in burned children and should be implemented early in the treatment course to avoid the anxiety-pain cycle.[31] Multiple nonpharmacological approaches are available, including avoidance techniques (distraction, imagery, hypnosis, virtual reality), relaxation (breathing techniques, muscle relaxation), operant techniques (positive reinforcement, information), cognitive restructuring (thought stopping, reappraisal), and participation (setting schedules, self-wound care) and are reviewed in detail elsewhere.[31] Typically, children and adolescents respond well to distraction techniques, including play, listening to music, or playing a video game.[9,30,31] This multimodal analgesic approach can facilitate background analgesia as well as procedural analgesia for wound care, physical therapy, and occupational therapy. Ideally, such interventions should be simple, easy to learn and use, and should provide minimal expenditure of time and effort by patients and caregivers.[104] The analgesic effectiveness of nonpharmacological techniques likely relates to reduction in the affective components of pain as supported by Melzack's gate control theory, which suggests that sensory, affective, and cognitive systems modify the neurophysiologic pain process, the reaction to pain, and the evaluation of past pain experiences.

Determining a child's coping style by observing his or her response to stressful procedures provides insight into which nonpharmacologic approach may be more effective. Children who have an avoidance coping style (do not want information and give up control to health care providers) may benefit from distraction, imagery, hypnosis, or virtual reality techniques. On the other hand, patients with an approach coping style (want procedure-related information, participate in the procedure) are more likely to benefit from active involvement in their own care.[31]

Immersive virtual reality (VR) is an extension of video game technology that isolates patients from the sights and sounds of the outside world, including painful stimuli associated with wound care. The patient view of the real world is blocked by a head-mounted display that presents an interactive, computer-generated 3-dimensional virtual environment and provides the illusion of being immersed ("present") in that location. The theory of the VR analgesia mechanism posits that the level of painful experience in response to a given noxious stimulus can be interpreted differently depending on what patients are thinking at the time

and where they focus their attention. VR efficiently captures the patient's attention, leaving little conscious attention available to process pain.[31] Clinical trials in children using VR during burn wound care[105–107] and burn-related physical therapy[108,109] have demonstrated its effectiveness as an adjunct to pharmacologic analgesia. In one such application, a virtual environment specifically designed for burn patients ("SnowWorld") depicts an icy, 3-dimensional arctic canyon with a river and waterfalls. Patients interact with the environment by shooting virtual snowballs at snowmen and igloos by aiming with their gaze (head position) and pressing the space bar on a keyboard.[108] Figure 4 shows a burn-injured adolescent undergoing wound care in the hydrotank while experiencing VR using a water-safe system. A variation of this software was tested in a crossover controlled trial during wound care procedures of burned children and found that VR is useful in relieving both procedural pain and anticipatory anxiety.[110] Potential limitations of this technology include the initial acquisition cost of such a system, logistic challenges of the equipment in the wound care environment, and adaptation of the equipment to fit smaller pediatric users.

## KEY POINTS

- Treatment of burn pain in the pediatric population must take into account maturational variables such as age, cognitive stage, personality, and emotional states as well as patient's interpersonal interactions in order to offer an effective multidisciplinary therapeutic approach.

- No single tool for measuring children's pain is applicable to all children and all painful circumstances consequently age appropriate pain assessment scales should be applied. Assessing pain in children should include 3 dimensions: behavioral reactions, self-report of pain intensity and physiologic reactions. Interpretation of pain scores should account for patient's cognitive, emotional and physical conditions at the time that are applied.

- Pain management for the burned child is based on the presence of different types of pain depending on the stage of burn recovery and the clinical setting in which this pain occurs. This goal can be achieved using guidelines to help clinical staff choose an appropriate analgesic regimen according to patient needs. These guidelines should include opioid and non-opioid analgesics, anesthetic medications, sedatives and local anesthetics.

- Severe burn injuries alter physiologic and pharmacologic states prompting to a judicious dosing of pain and anxiolytic medications.
- Procedural analgesia/sedation in burned patients should follow the JCAHO guidelines regarding monitoring during sedation. These guidelines should be complemented by recommendations on monitoring published by the ASA and the AAP.
- Anxiety should be treated early in the clinical course of the burn injury with benzodiazepines and non-pharmacological approaches in order to reduce the anxiety-pain cycle.

## TABLES AND FIGURES

### TABLE 1

**Tissue injury produces local inflammatory response releasing multiple molecules that have direct action or facilitate activation of nerve endings. PGE$_2$ prostaglandin E$_2$; PGI$_2$ prostaglandin I$_2$.**

Molecules that are released after tissue damage and their action on the afferent fibers.

| Molecule | Action |
|---|---|
| Bradykinin | Acts in specific receptors (B1/B2) activating free nerve endings. |
| Prostaglandins | PGE$_2$ directly activate C fibers. PGI$_2$ facilitates excitability of C fibers. |
| Histamine | Activates local inflammatory cells sustaining the inflammatory response. |
| Calcitonine gene related peptide (CGRP) | Released from distal terminals of C fibers. Produce stimulation and sensitization of free nerve endings. |
| Substance P | Released from terminals of C fibers. Produce stimulation and sensitization of free nerve endings. |
| High H$^+$ (low pHd) and high K$^+$ | Directly stimulate C fibers. |

### TABLE 2

**Classification of primary afferents according to conduction velocity and nature of stimuli.**

Classification of primary afferent nerve fibers.

| Fiber Class | Conduction Velocity (m/sec) | Nature of Stimuli |
|---|---|---|
| Aβ fibers | 30-70 | Low threshold mechanoreceptor. Encapsulated endings (Meissner, Ruffini, Pacinian corpuscles) |
| Aδ fibers | 5-30 | Low or high threshold mechano or thermal receptors. |
| C fibers | 0.5-2 | High threshold Polymodal (mechano, thermal and chemical) receptors. |

TABLE 3

### Characteristics of pain expressions according to biological age.

| Newborn | Physiological or behavioral changes (variations in respiratory rate, oxygen saturation, withdrawal, crying or facial expressions) |
|---|---|
| Infants and toddlers (2months-2 years) | Expression of anger or sadness associated to pain. Can identify painful situations leading to anxiety. |
| Preschoolers (3-5 years) | Initial manifestation of pain intensity. |
| Schoolers (6-12 years) | Clearly differentiate levels of pain intensity Attach more elaborate feelings to pain |
| Adolescents | Able to report pain intensity and quality as well as pain related affects (fear, anxiety, depression) |

TABLE 4
### Pain measuring scales used in preverbal ages.

### Behavioral pain assessment scales used in non-communicating children.

| Measure | Description | Indication | Pros | Cons |
|---|---|---|---|---|
| Premature Infant Pain Profile (PIPP) | Assessment of 15 indicators of distress. 2 physiologic (changes in the heart rate, oxygen saturation). 11 behavioral (facial expressions, crying, and body movements). 2 modifiers (gestational age and behavioral state). | Neonates and preterm babies. | good inter-rater reliability* | |
| Observational Scale of Behavioral Distress | Assessment of 11 behaviors associated with pediatric procedure-related distress, anxiety and pain. | Young Children | useful to assess acute, time limited pain | Clinically relevant data about the type of distress being exhibited is lost |
| Children's Hospital of Eastern Ontario Pain Scale (CHEOPS) | Assessment of distress behaviors in 6 categories. (Crying, facial expression, verbal expression, torso position, touching, and leg position) | Young children | Comprehensive | Complex and difficult to apply in busy clinical settings |
| FLACC (face, legs, activity, cry and consolability) scale | Assessment of distress behaviors in 5 categories. (face, legs, activity, cry and consolability) | Validated in children 2 months -7 years** | useful to assess acute, time limited pain | Easy to apply |

TABLE 5

Pain measuring scales used in verbal ages.

| Measure | Description | Indication | Pros | Cons |
|---|---|---|---|---|
| Bieri Faces scale | Represents a series of facial expressions illustrating different degrees of discomfort | Validated in children as young of 4 years old* | Easy to apply | Non-numeric score. The Faces Pain Scale - Revised (FPS-R) was adapted from this in order to score on 0-10 scale ** |
| Oucher scale *** | Six color photos of a child's face showing different intensities of pain, and a numerical scale of scores ranging from 0 (no pain) to100 (worst pain ever). | Children of 7 years or older who can use numbers as abstraction of pain intensity | Two separate scales. Only one is used to assess pain intensity at one time. Variations are available in different languages | Possibility of mixing scales at one time thus altering the score. |
| Visual Analogue Scale (VAS). | A line without markers with end points of least or greatest value for intensity of pain, | School age and older | Easy to apply | Not applicable in young children. |
| Numerical Rating Scale (NRS) | Variation of VAS. Uses numbers to rate the pain | Children of 7 years or older who can use numbers as abstraction of pain intensity | Easy to apply. | Not applicable in young children |

TABLE 6

**Types of burn wounds and their clinical manifestation. Concomitant partial thickness or first-degree burns within or surrounding third-degree burns can produce painful areas in this type of burn.**

Types of burn wounds and clinical sensory manifestation

| | |
|---|---|
| Epidermal first degree burns (e.g. sunburns) | Painful to touch due to sensitization of sensory fibers |
| Superficial second degree partial thickness dermal burns (e.g. scald burn) | Moderate/severe pain due to presence of marked inflammatory response and sensitization of the nerve terminals. |
| Deep second degree partial thickness dermal burns (e.g. grease burn) | Moderate to mild pain due to partial damage of nerve endings |
| Full thickness subdermal third degree burns like flame or contact burns | Painless due to complete damage of nerve endings |

TABLE 7

Recommended intravenous opioid pediatric dosing guidelines. NA: Not available. NR: Not recommended

| Agent | Dose IV | Peak (hrs) | IV/PO ratio | Dose PO | Duration (hrs) | Equianalgesic Dose | Side Effects |
|---|---|---|---|---|---|---|---|
| Morphine | >2 years: Bolus: 0.1 mg/Kg every 2–3 hrs; Infusion: 0.03 mg/Kg/hr; <2 years: Bolus 0.025–0.05 mg/Kg every 2–3 hrs; Infusion 0.015 mg/kg/h | IV: 0.25; PO: 1–1.5 | 1:3 | Immediate Release: 0.3 mg/Kg every 3–4 hrs; Sustained Release: (every 8–12 hrs) 20–35 Kg: 10–15 mg; 35–50 Kg: 15–30 mg; >50 Kg: 30–45 mg | 1.5–3 | Parenteral: 10 mg; Oral: 30 mg | Respiratory depression, nausea, constipation, bronchial constriction, histamine release, seizures at high doses |
| Hydromorphone | >2 years: Bolus: 0.02 mg/Kg every 2–3 hrs. <2 years: Bolus: 0.005–0.01 mg/Kg every 2–3 hrs | IV: 0.25; PO: 1.5–2 | 1:4 | 0.04–0.08 mg/Kg every 3–4 hrs | 3–4 | Parenteral: 1.5–2.0 mg; Oral: 6–8 mg | Like Morphine |
| Fentanyl | >2 years: Bolus: 0.5–1 Mcg/Kg every 1–2 hrs; Infusion: 0.5–1.5 Mcg/Kg/hr; <2 years: Bolus: 0.25–0.5 Mcg/Kg every 1–2 hrs; Infusion: 0.25–0.5 Mcg/Kg/hr | IV: 0.025–0.05; Transmucosal: 0.3–0.5 | NA | Transmucosal: 10–20 Mcg/Kg | 1 | 0.1 mg | Respiratory depression, chest wall rigidity (>5 Mcg/Kg rapid IV bolus) |
| Oxycodone | NA | 1 | NA | <50 Kg: 0.1–0.2mg/Kg every 3–4 hr; >50 Kg: 5–10 mg every 3–4 hr. | 4–6 | Oral: 15–20 mg | Like Morphine |
| Methadone | >2 years: Bolus: 0.1 mg/Kg every 4–8 hr; <2 years: Bolus: 0.025–0.05 mg/Kg every 4–12 hr. | IV: 0.25; PO: 1.5–2 | 1:2 | 0.2 mg/Kg every 4–8 hr | 4–12 | Parenteral: 10 mg; Oral: 10–20 mg | Deep sedation, respiratory depression. Accumulates with repeated doses |
| Codeine | NR | 0.5–1 | NA | <50 Kg: 0.5–1 mg/Kg every 3–4 hr; >50 Kg: 30–60 mg every 3–4 hr. | 3–4 | 20 mg | Allergic reactions, constipation, itching. |

TABLE 8

UW Regional Burn Center analgesic guidelines for the pediatric (<40 Kg) burned patient.

| | ICU<br>No PO intake | ICU<br>Taking PO | Acute Care Ward<br>Large Open Areas/<br>Long Stay | Acute Care Ward<br>Small Open Areas/<br>Pre Discharge |
|---|---|---|---|---|
| Background Pain | Continous Morphine<br>IV infusion | Scheduled<br>Oxycodone or<br>Methadone | Scheduled<br>Acetaminophen,<br>Ibuprofen or<br>Oxycodone | Scheduled<br>Acetaminophen or<br>Ibuprofen |
| Procedural Pain | Morphine IV or<br>Fentanyl IV | Transmucosal<br>Fentanyl<br>Citrate (TMF)<br>or Hydromorphone | Hydromorphone<br>or TMF | Acetaminophen<br>with Codeine or<br>Oxycodone |
| Breakthrough Pain<br>(PRN dosing) | Morphine IV | Oxycodone | Codeine,<br>Acetaminophen or<br>Oxycodone | Codeine,<br>Acetaminophen or<br>Oxycodone |
| Background<br>anxiolysis | Continous<br>Lorazepam or<br>Midazolam | Lorazepam (PO) | Discuss with Burn<br>Team | None |
| Procedural Anxiolysis | Midazolam IV or<br>Lorazepam | Midazolam (PO) | Midazolam (PO) | None |
| Discharge or Transfer<br>Pain Drugs | NA | For transfer to ward<br>(wean drips and<br>establish PO pain<br>meds early) | Acetaminophen<br>with Codeine or<br>Acetaminophen | Acetaminophen<br>with Codeine or<br>Acetaminophen |

Note. PO, per oral; ICU, intensive care unit.

TABLE 9

Recommended non-opioid medication pediatric dosing.

| Medication | Dose |
|---|---|
| Acetaminophen | Neonates: PO: 10–15 mg/kg every 4 hr<br>≤ 50 mg/kg/24hr<br>< 2 yo: ≤ 75 mg/kg/24 hr<br>> 2 yo: ≤ 100 mg/kg/24/hr<br>PR: 30–40 mg/kg every 6 hr.* |
| Ibuprofen | PO: 8–10 mg/Kg every 6 hr<br>≤ 40 mg/kg/24hr |
| Naproxen | PO: 6–8mg/kg every 8–12 hr<br>≤ 20 mg/Kg/24hr |

* Notice maximum dose as PO

TABLE 10

**Continuum of depth of sedation.**

| Minimal Sedation (Anxiolysis) | Moderate Sedation/Analgesia (Conscious Sedation) | Deep Sedation/Analgesia |
|---|---|---|
| Drug-induced state during which patients respond normally to verbal commands. Ventilatory and cardiovascular functions are unaffected. | Drug-induced depression of consciousness during which patients respond to verbal commands, either alone or with light tactile stimulation. Airway is patent and no interventions are required. Ventilation and cardiovascular function is usually maintained. | Drug-induced depression of consciousness during which patients cannot be easily aroused. Patients may respond after repeated or painful stimulation. Ventilatory function may be impaired. Assistance may be required to maintain a patent airway. Cardiovascular function is usually maintained. |

TABLE 11

**Common drugs used in procedural sedation.**

| Drug | Dose | Onset of Action | Duration | Side Effects |
|---|---|---|---|---|
| Lorazepam | PO: 2–4 mg every 6–8 hrs | 20–30 min | 6–8 hr | Not recommended for young children (<12 yo) |
| Midazolam | Sedation for intubated patients: Infusion: 0.06–0.12 mg/Kg/Hr IV<br><br>Procedural sedation: 6 months to 5 years: 0.05–0.1 mg/Kg up to 0.6 mg/Kg IV every 2–3 min; ≤ 6 mg total.<br><br>> 5 yo: 0.025–0.05 up to 0.4 mg/Kg IV every 3–5 min; ≤ 10 mg total.<br><br>Oral and rectal: 0.25–0.5 mg/Kg; ≤ 20 mg total<br><br>Intranasal: 0.2 to 0.6 mg/kg | IV: 3 min<br><br>Transmucosal: 10–15 min | 2–3 hr | Respiratory depression, hypotension, nausea and vomiting. |
| Ketamine | Procedural sedation: 0.5–1 mg/Kg IV followed by infusion of 10–15 Mcg/Kg/min or repeated bolus dose (half of the initial dose)<br><br>Oral: 3–6 mg/kg | IV: 1 min<br>Oral: 15–30 min | IV 5–10 min<br><br>Oral: 30–45 min | Hypertension, tachycardia, hallucinations, delirium, flashbacks |

*(continued on next page)*

TABLE 11 (*continued*)

| Drug | Dose | Onset of Action | Duration | Side Effects |
|------|------|-----------------|----------|--------------|
| Propofol | Procedural sedation: 1 mg/kg IV followed by 0.5 mg/kg every 3 to 5 min as needed for sedation | 15–50 sec | 3–10 min upon discontinuation | Contraindicated in patients allergic to egg and soy products. Cardiac depressor (hypotension, bradycardia, asystole) Respiratory depression Propofol Infusion Syndrome |
| Dexmedetomidine | IV: 1 Mcg/kg over 10 min; followed by 0.2 to 0.7 mcg/kg/hr in intubated patients<br><br>Intranasal: 1 Mcg/Kg | IV: 20- 30 min Intranasal: 45–60 min | 2 hr | Long onset time Hypotension |

FIGURE 1

**Pain information from the nociceptors enters the spinal cord through the ventrolateral part of the dorsal root connecting with a second order neuron in the dorsal horn. The spinothalamic tract projects to the thalamus, periaquedultal gray matter, reticular formation and hypothalamus. Thalamocortical tracts carry the information to the cortex producing the somatic representation of pain.**

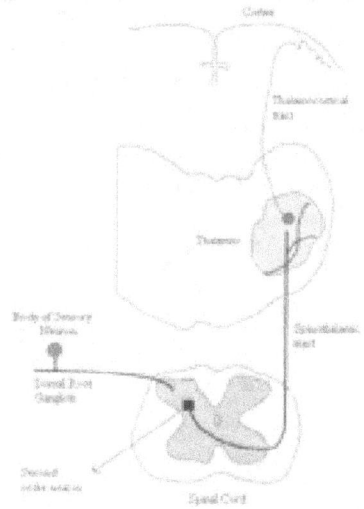

FIGURE 2
Graphic representations of the pain intensity during time at different painful clinical settings.
Time (X axis), pain intensity (Y axis). (A) Background pain, (B) breakthrough pain, (C) procedural pain.

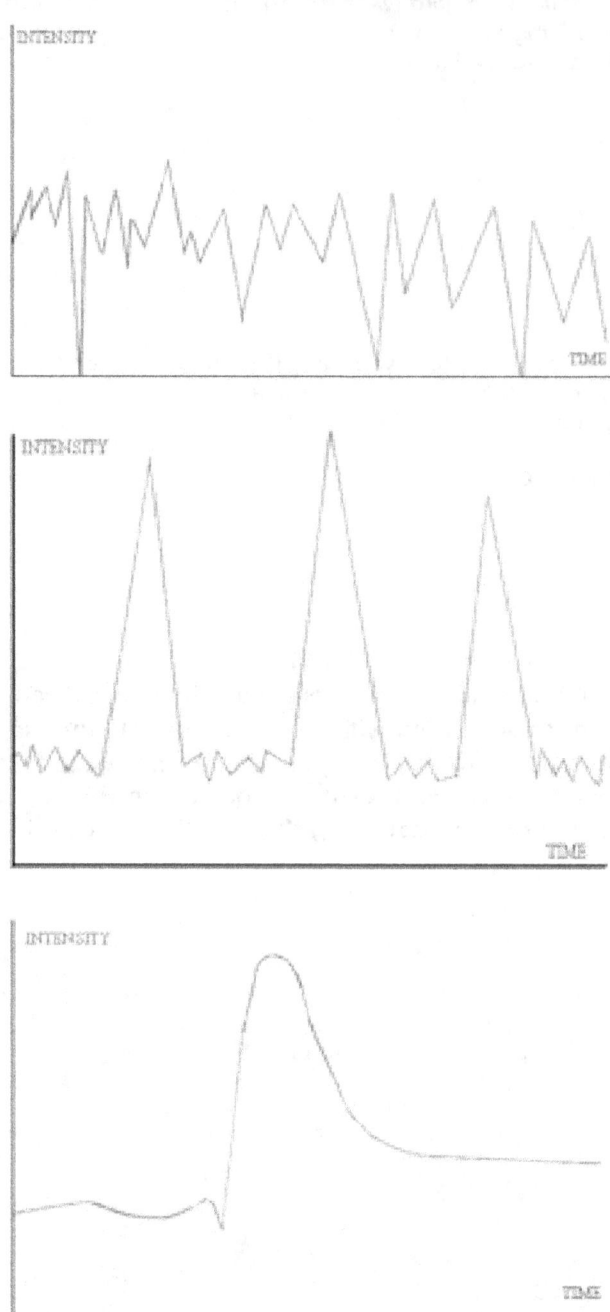

FIGURE 3
**The itch man. Rates intensity of pruritus in a scale from 0-4.**

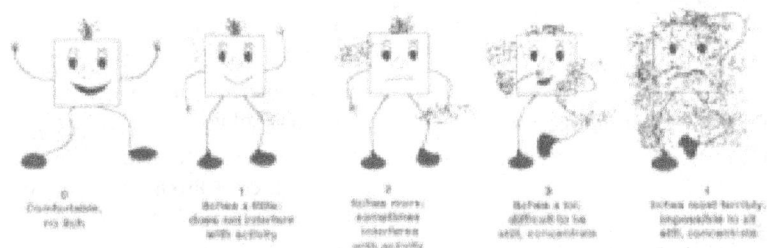

*Source.* Shriners Hospitals for children, 2000.

FIGURE 4
**Burn patient undergoing wound care using virtual reality as an adjuvant of analgesic therapy.**

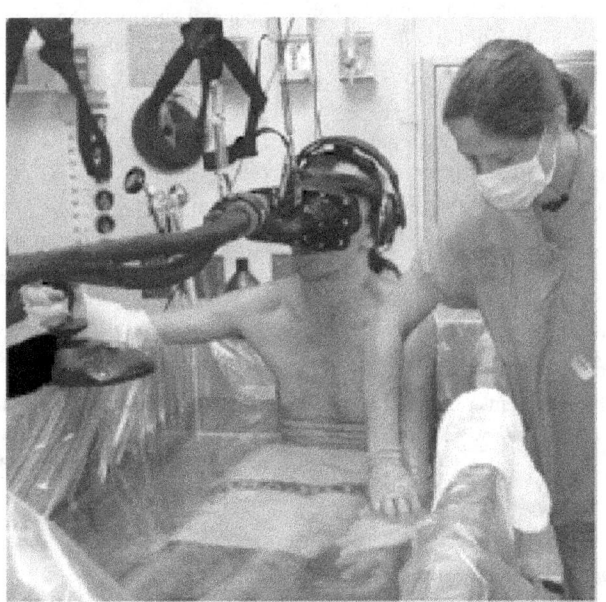

# REFERENCES

1. Petrack EM, Christopher NC, Kriwinsky J. Pain management in the emergency department: patterns of analgesic utilization. *Pediatrics*. 1997; **99**(5): 711–714.

2. Simons SHP, van Dijk M, Anand KS, Roofthooft D, van Lingen RA, Tibboel D, et al. Do we still hurt newborn babies? A prospective study of procedural pain and analgesia in neonates. *Arch Pediatr Adolesc Med*. 2003; **157**(11): 1058–1064.

3. Perry S, Heidrich G. Management of pain during debridement: a survey of U.S. burn units. *Pain*. 1982; **13**(3): 267–280.

4. Schechter NL, Allen DA, Hanson K. Status of pediatric pain control: a comparison of hospital analgesic usage in children and adults. *Pediatrics*. 1986; **77**(1): 11–15.

5. McGrath PA. Children—not simply "little adults." In: Merskey H, Loeser JD, Dubner R, eds. *The Paths of Pain 1975–2005*. Seattle, WA: IASP Press; 2005: 433–446.

6. Howard RF. Current status of pain management in children. *JAMA*. 2003; **290**(18): 2464–2469.

7. Khan AN, Sachdeva S. Current trends in the management of common painful conditions of preschool children in United States pediatric emergency departments. *Clin Pediatr (Phila)*. 2007; **46**(7): 626–631.

8. Martin-Herz SP, Pelley Martin-Herz S, Patterson D, Honari S, Gibbons J, Gibran N, Heimbach D, et al. Pediatric pain control practices of North American Burn Centers. *J Burn Care Rehabil*. 2003; **24**(1): 26–36.

9. Patterson DR, Sharar SR. Burn pain. In: Loesler JD, Butler SH, Chapman CR, Turk DC, eds. *Bonica's Management of Pain*. Philadelphia, PA: Lippincott Williams & Wilkins; 2001: 780–793.

10. Latarjet J, Choinere M. Pain in burn patients. *Burns*. 1995; **21**(5): 344–348.

11. Weisman SJ, Bernstein B, Schechter NL. Consequences of inadequate analgesia during painful procedures in children. *Arch Pediatr Adolesc Med*. 1998; **152**(2): 147–149.

12. Patterson DR, Tininenko J, Ptacek JT. Pain during burn hospitalization predicts long-term outcome. *J Burn Care Res*. 2006; **27**(5): 719–726.

13. Stoddard FJ, Norman DK, Murphy JM. A diagnostic outcome study of children and adolescents with severe burns. *J Trauma*. 1989; **29**(4): 471–477.

14. Desborough JP. The stress response to trauma and surgery. *Br J Anaesth*. 2000; **85**(1): 109–117.

15. Bond M, Simpson KH. Basic Mechanisms of Pain In: Parkinson M, Kenner H, eds. *Pain Its Nature and Treatment*. Edinburg, NY: Elsevier-Churchill Livingstone; 2006: 43–56.

16. Cohen SA. Pathophysiology of pain. In: Warfield CA, Bajwa ZH, eds. *Principles and Practice of Pain Medicine*. New York, NY: McGraw-Hill; 2004: 35–48.

17. Yaksh TL. Molecular biology of pain. In: Warfield CA, Bajwa ZH, eds. *Principles and Practice of Pain Medicine*. New York, NY: McGraw-Hill; 2004: 13–27.

18. Waldman SD, ed. *Pain Management*. Philadelphia, PA: Saunders/Elsevier; 2007.

19. Gibran NS, Heimbach DM. Current status of burn wound pathophysiology. *Clin Plast Surg*. 2000; **27**(1): 11–22.

20. Summer G, Romero-Sandoval E, Bogen O, Dina O, Khasar S, Levine J, et al. Proinflammatory cytokines mediating burn-injury pain. *Pain*. 2007; **135**(1): 98–107 (March 2008).

21. LaMotte RH, Thalhammer JG, Torebjörk, HE, Robinson CJ, et al. Peripheral neural mechanisms of cutaneous hyperalgesia following mild injury by heat. *J Neurosci*. 1982; **2**(6): 765–781.

22. Ross DM, Ross SA. Pain: an overview. In: Mitchell CW, ed. *Childhood Pain : Current Issues, Research, and Management*. Baltimore, MD: Urban & Schwarzenberg; 1988: 1–33.

23. Marshall RE, Stratton WC, Moore JA, Boxerman SB. Circumcision. I. Effects upon newborn behavior. *Infant Behav Dev*. 1980; **3**: 1–14.

24. Taddio A, Katz J, Ilersich AL, Koren G, et al. Effect of neonatal circumcision on pain response during subsequent routine vaccination. *Lancet*. 1997; **349**(9052): 599–603.

25. Fitzgerald M, Howard RF. The neurobiologic basis of pediatric pain. In: Schechter NL, Berde CB, Yaster M, eds. *Pain in Infants, Children, and Adolescents*. Philadelphia, PA: Lippincott Williams & Wilkins; 2003: 19–42.

26. Goldschneider KR, Mancuso TJ, Berde CB. Pain and its management in children. In: Loesler JD, Bonica JJ, eds. *Bonica's Management of Pain*. Philadelphia, PA: Lippincott Williams & Wilkins; 2001: 797–812.

27. Fitzgerald M, Beggs S. The neurobiology of pain: developmental aspects. *Neuroscientist*. 2001; **7**(3): 246–257.

28. Ruda MA, Ling QD, Hohmann AG, Peng YB, Tachibana T, et al. Altered nociceptive neuronal circuits after neonatal peripheral inflammation. *Science*. 2000; **289**(5479): 628–631.

29. Turk DC, Okifuji A. Psychological aspects of pain. In: Warfield CA, Bajwa ZH, eds. *Principles and Practice of Pain Medicine*. New York, NY: McGraw-Hill; 2004: 139–147.

30. Stoddard FJ, Sheridan RL, Saxe GN, King BS, King BH, Chedekel DS Schnitzer JJ, Martyn JAJ, et al. Treatment of pain in acutely burned children. *J Burn Care Rehabil*. 2002; **23**(2): 135–156.

31. Sharar SR, Patterson DR. Burn pain. In: Waldman SD, ed. *Pain Management*. Philadelphia, PA: Saunders/Elsevier; 2007: 240–256.

32. Craig KD. Emotional aspects of pain. In: Wall PD, Melzack R, eds. *Textbook of Pain*. New York, NY: Churchill Livingstone; 1994: 261–274.

33. Lipton JA, Marbach JJ. Ethnicity and the pain experience. *Soc Sci Med*. 1984; **19**(12): 1279–1298.

34. Loeser JD. The current issues in pain management. In: Von Roenn J, Preodor ME, Paice JE, eds. *Current Diagnosis and*

*Treatment of Pain.* New York, N.Y: Lange Medical Books/ McGraw-Hill Medical Publishing Division; 2006: 1–9.

35. American Academy of Pediatrics Committee on Psychosocial Aspects of Child and Family Health, The assessment and management of acute pain in infants, children, and adolescents. *Pediatrics.* 2001; **108**(3): 793–797.

36. von Baeyer CL, Spagrud LJ. Social development and pain in children. In: McGrath PJ, Finley GA, eds. *Pediatric Pain: Biological And Social Context.* Seattle, WA: IASP Press; 2003: 81–97.

37. Finley GA, McGrath PJ, eds. *Measurement of Pain in Infants and Children Progress in Pain Research and Management.* Vol 10. Seattle, WA: IASP Press; 1998.

38. Merkel SI, Shayevitz JR, Voepel-Lewis T, Malviya S, et al. The FLACC: a behavioral scale for scoring postoperative pain in young children. *Pediatr Nurs.* 1997; **23**(3): 293–297.

39. Scott PJ, Ansell BM, Huskisson EC. Measurement of pain in juvenile chronic polyarthritis. *Ann Rheum Dis.* 1977; **36**(2): 186–187.

40. Young K. Pediatric procedural pain. *Ann Emerg Med.* 2005; **45**(2): 160–171.

41. Heimbach D, Engrav L, Grube B, Marvin J, et al. Burn depth: a review. *World J Surg.* 1992; **16**(1): 10–15.

42. Choiniere M, Melzack R, Papillon J. Pain and paresthesia in patients with healed burns: an exploratory study. *J Pain Symptom Manage.* 1991; **6**(7): 437–444.

43. Pardo G, Moreno I, Miralles F, Gomez T, et al. Psychological impact of burns on children treated in a severe burns unit. *Burns.* 2008; **34**(7): 986–93.

44. Wood M, Wood AJ. *Drugs and Anesthesia: Pharmacology for Anesthesiologists.* 2nd ed.: Williams & Wilkins; Baltimore, MD; 1990.

45. Bartelink IH, Rademaker C, Schobben A, van den Anker JN, et al. Guidelines on paediatric dosing on the basis of developmental physiology and pharmacokinetic considerations. *Clin Pharmacokinet.* 2006; **45**(11): 1077–1097.

46. Bouwmeester NJ, Anderson BJ, Tibboel D, Holford NHG, et al. Developmental pharmacokinetics of morphine and its metabolites in neonates, infants and young children. *Br J Anaesth.* 2004; **92**(2): 208–217.

47. Kauffman RE. Essential drugs for infants and children: North American perspective. *Pediatrics.* 1999; **104**(3, pt 2): 603–605.

48. Yaster M. Clinical pharmacology. In: Schechter NL, Berde CB, Yaster M, eds. *Pain in Infants, Children, and Adolescents.* Philadelphia, PA: Lippincott Williams & Wilkins; 2003: 71–84.

49. Cote CJ, Lugo RA, Ward RM Pharmacokinetics and Pharmacology of Drugs in Children. In: Cote CJ, Lerman J, Todres DI, eds. *A Practice of Anesthesia for Infants and Children*: Philadelphia, PA: Saunders/Elsevier; 2009 4th edition: 121–171.

50. MacLennan N, Heimbach DM, Cullen BF. Anesthesia for major thermal injury. *Anesthesiology.* 1998; **89**(3): 749–770.

51. Furman WR, Munster AM, Cone EJ. Morphine pharmacokinetics during anesthesia and surgery in patients with burns. *J Burn Care Rehabil.* 1990; **11**(5): 391–394.

52. Herman RA, Veng-Pedersen P, Miotto J, Komorowski J, Kealey GP, et al. Pharmacokinetics of morphine sulfate in patients with burns. *J Burn Care Rehabil.* 1994; **15**(2): 95–103.

53. Bonate PL. Pathophysiology and pharmacokinetics following burn injury. *Clin Pharmacokinet.* 1990; **18**(2): 118–130.

54. Jaehde U, Sorgel F. Clinical pharmacokinetics in patients with burns. *Clin Pharmacokinet.* 1995; **29**(1): 15–28.

55. Summer GJ, Puntillo KA, Miaskowski C, Green PG, Levine JD, et al. Burn injury pain: the continuing challenge. *J Pain.* 2007; **8**(7): 533–548.

56. Ulmer JF. Burn pain management: a guideline-based approach. *J Burn Care Rehabil.* 1998; **19**(2): 151–159.

57. Ballantyne J, Mao J. Opioid therapy for chronic pain. *N Engl J Med.* 2003; **349**(20): 1943–1953.

58. Faucher L, Furukawa K. Practice guidelines for the management of pain. *J Burn Care Res.* 2006; **27**(5): 659–668.

59. Cherny N, Foley K. Nonopioid and opioid analgesic pharmacotherapy of cancer pain. *Hematol Oncol Clin North Am.* 1996; **10**(1): 79–102.

60. Collins JJ, Weisman SJ. Management of pain in childhood cancer. In: Schechter NL, Berde CB, Yaster M, eds. *Pain in Infants, Children, and Adolescents.* Philadelphia, PA: Lippincott Williams & Wilkins; 2003: 517–538.

61. Sheridan RL, Hinson M, Nackel A, Blaquiere M, Daley W, Queszoli B, Spezzafar J, Lybarger, Martyn J, et al. Development of a pediatric burn pain and anxiety management program. *J Burn Care Rehabil.* 1997; **18**(5): 455–459, discussion 453–454.

62. Patel SI, Bhananker SM. Anesthesia and analgesia for pediatric burns. *Curr Rev Clin Anesth.* 2007; **28**(3): 25–40.

63. American Academy of Pediatrics: Committee in Drugs, Acetaminophen toxicity in children. *Pediatrics.* 2001; **108**(4): 1020–1024.

64. Cuignet O, Pirson J, Soudon O, Zizi M, et al. Effects of gabapentin on morphine consumption and pain in severely burned patients. *Burns.* 2007; **33**(1): 81–86.

65. Dirks J, Petersen KL, Rowbotham MC, Dahl JB, et al. Gabapentin suppresses cutaneous hyperalgesia following heat-capsaicin sensitization. *Anesthesiology.* 2002; **97**(1): 102–107.

66. McDonald AJ, Cooper MG. Patient-controlled analgesia: an appropriate method of pain control in children. *Paediatr Drugs.* 2001; **3**(4): 273–284.

67. Gaukroger PB, Tomkins DP, van der Walt JH. Patient-controlled analgesia in children. *Anaesth Intensive Care.* 1989; **17**(3): 264–268.

68. Joint Commission. Patient controlled analgesia by proxy. Sentinel Event 2004; (33) Dec 20 2004. http://www.jointcommission.org/SentinelEvents/SentinelEventAlert/sea_33.htm. Accessed May 15, 2010.

69. Portenoy RK, Hagen NA. Breakthrough pain: definition, prevalence and characteristics. *Pain*. 1990; **41**(3): 273–281.

70. Friedrichsdorf S, Finney D, Bergin M, Stevens M, Collins JJ, et al. Breakthrough pain in children with cancer. *J Pain Symptom Manage*. 2007; **34**(2): 209–216.

71. American Academy of Pediatrics, American Academy of Pediatric Dentistry, Coté CJ, Wilson S, Work Group on Sedation American Academy of Pediatrics Committee on Drugs. Guidelines for monitoring and management of pediatric patients during and after sedation for diagnostic and therapeutic procedures. *Pediatrics*. 1992; **89**(6, pt 1): 1110–1115.

72. American Association of Anesthesiologists (ASA) Committee for Quality Management and Departmental Administration. Continuum of depth of sedation; definition of general anesthesia and levels of sedation/analgesia. Oct 27 2009. http://www.asahq.org/publicationsAndServices/standards/20.pdf. Accessed 5/16/2010.

73. Ebach DR, Foglia RP, Jones MB, Langer JC, Skinner MA, Moushey R, Meadows L, et al. Experience with procedural sedation in a pediatric burn center. *J Pediatr Surg*. 1999; **34**(6): 955–958.

74. Pitetti RD, Singh S, Pierce MC. Safe and efficacious use of procedural sedation and analgesia by nonanesthesiologists in a pediatric emergency department. *Arch Pediatr Adolesc Med*. 2003; **157**(11): 1090–1096.

75. Joint Commission on Accreditation of Healthcare Organizations. http://www.jointcommission.org/AccreditationPrograms/AmbulatoryCare/Standards/09_FAQs/PC/Moderate_Sedation_Medication.htm. Accessed 5/16/2010.

76. Kelly JS. *Sedation by Non-Anesthesia Personnel Provokes Safety Concerns; Anesthesiologists Must Balance JCAHO Standards, Politics, & Safety*. Anesthesia Patient Safety Foundation Newsletter Fall 2001: (16)2. http://www.apsf.org/resource_center/newsletter/2001/fall/07personnel.htm. Accessed 5/16/2010.

77. American Society of Anesthesiologists (ASA). Standards for Basic Anesthetic Monitoring. http://www.asahq.org/publicationsAndServices/standards/02.pdfhttp://www.asahq.org/publicationsAndServices/standards/20.pdf. Oct 25, 2005. Accessed May 16, 2010.

78. American Society of Anesthesiologists. Practice guidelines for sedation and analgesia by non-anesthesiologists. *Anesthesiology*. 2002; **96**(4): 1004–1017.

79. Cote CJ, Wilson S. Guidelines for monitoring and management of pediatric patients during and after sedation for diagnostic and therapeutic procedures: an update. *Pediatrics*. 2006; **118**(6): 2587–2602.

80. Robert R, Brack A, Blakeney P, Villareal C, Rosenberg L, Thomas C, Meyer WJ, et al. A double-blind study of the analgesic efficacy of oral transmucosal fentanyl citrate and oral morphine in pediatric patients undergoing burn dressing change and tubbing. *J Burn Care Rehabil*. 2003; **24**(6): 351–355.

81. Sharar SR, Bratton SL, Carrougher GJ, Edwards WT, Summer G, Levy FH, Cortiella J, et al. A comparison of oral transmucosal fentanyl citrate and oral hydromorphone for inpatient pediatric burn wound care analgesia. *J Burn Care Rehabil*. 1998; **19**(6): 516–521.

82. Sharar SR, Carrogher GJ, Selzer K, O'Donnell F, Vavilala MS, Lee LA, et al. A comparison of oral transmucosal fentanyl citrate and oral oxycodone for pediatric outpatient wound care. *J Burn Care Rehabil*. 2002; **23**(1): 27–31.

83. Borland ML, Bergesio R, Pascoe EM, Turner S, Woodger S, et al. Intranasal fentanyl is an equivalent analgesic to oral morphine in paediatric burns patients for dressing changes: a randomised double blind crossover study. *Burns*. 2005; **31**(7): 831–837.

84. Montgomery RK. Pain management in burn injury. *Crit Care Nurs Clin North Am*. 2004; **16**(1): 39–49.

85. Owens VF, Palmieri TL, Comroe CM, Conroy JM, Scavone JA, Greenhalgh DG, et al. Ketamine: a safe and effective agent for painful procedures in the pediatric burn patient. *J Burn Care Res*. 2006; **27**(2): 211–216, discussion 217.

86. Heinrich M, Wetztein V, Muensterer OJ, Till H. Conscious sedation: off-label use of rectal S(+)-ketamine and midazolam for wound dressing changes in paediatric heat injuries. *Eur J Pediatr Surg*. 2004; **14**(4): 235–239.

87. Acworth JP, Purdie D, Clark RC. Intravenous ketamine plus midazolam is superior to intranasal midazolam for emergency paediatric procedural sedation. *Emerg Med J*. 2001; **18**(1): 39–45.

88. Karapinar B, Yilmaz D, Demirag, Kantar M. Sedation with intravenous ketamine and midazolam for painful procedures in children. *Pediatr Int*. 2006; **48**(2): 146–151.

89. Barbi E, Gerarduzzi T, Marchetti F, Neri E, Verucci E, Bruno I, Martelossi S, Zanazzo G, Sarti A, Ventura A. Deep sedation with propofol by nonanesthesiologists: a prospective pediatric experience. *Arch Pediatr Adolesc Med*. 2003; **157**(11): 1097–1103.

90. Walker J, MacCallum M, Fischer C, Kopcha R, Saylors R, McCall J. Sedation using dexmedetomidine in pediatric burn patients. *J Burn Care Res*. 2006; **27**(2): 206–210.

91. Bassett KE, Anderson JL, Pribble CG, Guenther E. Propofol for procedural sedation in children in the emergency department. *Ann Emerg Med*. 2003; **42**(6): 773–782.

92. Guenther E, Pribble CG, Junkins EP, Kadish HA, Basset KE, Nelson DS. Propofol sedation by emergency physicians for elective pediatric outpatient procedures. *Ann Emerg Med*. 2003; **42**(6): 783–791.

93. Yuen VM, Hui TW, Irwin MG, Yuen MK. A comparison of intranasal dexmedetomidine and oral midazolam for premedication in pediatric anesthesia: a double-blinded randomized controlled trial. *Anesth Analg*. 2008; **106**(6): 1715–1721.

94. Carollo D, Nossaman B, Ramadhyani U. Dexmedetomidine: a review of clinical applications. *Curr Opin Anaesthesiol*. 2008; **21**(4): 457–461.

95. Fodale V, La Monaca E. Propofol infusion syndrome: an overview of a perplexing disease. *Drug Saf*. 2008; **31**(4): 293–303.

**96.** Pal S, Cortiella J, Herndon D. Adjunctive methods of pain control in burns. *Burns*. 1997; **23**(5): 404–412.

**97.** Gupta A, Bhandari PS, Shrivastava P. A study of regional nerve blocks and local anesthetic creams (Prilox) for donor sites in burn patients. *Burns*. 2007; **33**(1): 87–91.

**98.** Fischer CG, Lloyd S, Kopcha R, Warden GD, McCall JE. The safety of adding bupivacaine to the subcutaneous infiltration solution used for donor site harvest. *J Burn Care Rehabil*. 2003; **24**(6): 361–364.

**99.** Bussolin L, Busoni P, Giergi L, Crescioli M, Messeri A. Tumescent local anesthesia for the surgical treatment of burns and postburn sequelae in pediatric patients. *Anesthesiology*. 2003; **99**(6): 1371–1375.

**100.** Cuignet O, Mbuyamba J, Pirson J. The long-term analgesic efficacy of a single-shot fascia iliaca compartment block in burn patients undergoing skin-grafting procedures. *J Burn Care Rehabil*. 2005; **26**(5): 409–415.

**101.** Paut O, Sallabery M, Schreiber-Deturmeny E, Remond C, Bruguerolle B, Camboulives J. Continuous fascia iliaca compartment block in children: a prospective evaluation of plasma bupivacaine concentrations, pain scores, and side effects. *Anesth Analg*. 2001; **92**(5): 1159–1163.

**102.** Ferguson SL, Voll KV. Burn pain and anxiety: the use of music relaxation during rehabilitation. *J Burn Care Rehabil*. 2004; **25**(1): 8–14.

**103.** Melchert-McKearnan K, Deitz J, Engel JM, White O. Children with burn injuries: purposeful activity versus rote exercise. *Am J Occup Ther*. 2000; **54**(4): 381–390.

**104.** de Jong AEE, Middelkoop E, Faber AW, Van Loey NEE. Non-pharmacological nursing interventions for procedural pain relief in adults with burns: a systematic literature review. *Burns*. 2007; **33**(7): 811–827.

**105.** Hoffman HG, Patterson DR, Magula J, Carrougher GJ, Zeltzer K, Dagadakis S, Sharar SR. Water-friendly virtual reality pain control during wound care. *J Clin Psychol*. 2004; **60**(2): 189–195.

**106.** Hoffman HG, Doctor JN, Patterson DR, Carrougher GJ, Furness TA. Virtual reality as an adjunctive pain control during burn wound care in adolescent patients. *Pain*. 2000; **85**(1-2): 305–309.

**107.** van Twillert B, Bremer M, Faber AW. Computer-generated virtual reality to control pain and anxiety in pediatric and adult burn patients during wound dressing changes. *J Burn Care Res*. 2007; **28**(5): 694–702.

**108.** Hoffman HG, Patterson DR, Carrougher GJ, Sharar SR. Effectiveness of virtual reality–based pain control with multiple treatments. *Clin J Pain*. 2001; **17**(3): 229–235.

**109.** Sharar SR, Carrougher GJ, Nakamura D, Hoffman HG, Blough DK, Patterson DR. Factors influencing the efficacy of virtual reality distraction analgesia during postburn physical therapy: preliminary results from 3 ongoing studies. *Arch Phys Med Rehabil*. 2007; **88**(12)(suppl 2): S43–S49.

**110.** Chan EA, Chung JW, Wong TK, Lien AS, Yang JY. Application of a virtual reality prototype for pain relief of pediatric burn in Taiwan. *J Clin Nurs*. 2007; **16**(4): 786–793.

# CHAPTER TWENTY-SIX

# The Psychology of Pediatric Burn Pain

Shawn T. Mason, PhD

Lisa L. Arceneaux, PsyD

James A. Fauerbach, PhD

## Overview

Among the 500000 US burns each year requiring medical care, approximately 88000 are emergency room visits from children under 14 years of age.[1] Scald burns account for 25000 of these admissions and commonly occur in the 0-to-5-year age range.[1] Thermal burns account for 62000 admissions and commonly occur in children from 5 to 15 years old.[2] These injuries are associated with significant pain from the time of injury through recovery. Although analgesic opioids are the essential front-line treatment, they are not 100% effective for all patients. Psychological principles of pain management and intervention have been useful in filling this void in the past, and these methods continue to contribute to overall pain management in burn patients. Consequently, this chapter will include theories of pain, psychological principles of pain and behavior, pediatric developmental stages, and burn pain treatment. It is hoped that in reading this chapter, 2 major themes will become abundantly clear. First, burn pain management begins with the initial contact from medical personnel and continues throughout the entire treatment and recovery phases.

Second, everyone involved in the burn patient's treatment plays a role in the management of burn pain.

## What Is Pain and Why Treat It?

"Pain is an unpleasant sensory and emotional experience associated with the actual or potential tissue damage, or described in terms of such damage," according to the International Association for the Study of Pain.[3] The severity of pain in the burn care setting is intense, and pediatric burn patients have described their burn pain as unparalleled and not easily forgotten.[4] Memories of burn pain occurring in patients as young as 5 years are present in adults recalling burn pain.[5] Pain control is desired beyond the obvious reason of alleviating suffering. Negative psychological and physiological outcomes from the trauma and severe burn pain have been well documented.[6] In the burn care setting, pain interferes with comfort, sleep, wound healing, participation in occupational and physical therapy, and emotional stability.[7]

Physiological stress responses from the body are directly related to the severity of the injury[8] and are inherently related to the severity of pain. Physiological activity includes a host of neurohormonal and endocrine responses that serve as markers for altered autonomic nervous system processes, including amygdala and limbic system functioning.[8,9] Substantial numbers of children with burn injuries report long-term psychological difficulties.[10,11] Pain in particular has been associated with the onset of acute traumatic stress reactions.[12–14] Although some work has been conducted on the long-term outcomes associated with pediatric burn pain, more research is needed.

Pharmacological agents, mainly opioids, are the foundation for pain management and provide pain relief for most patients. However, for a variety of reasons, many patients continue to report significant pain. It has been suggested that this may be due to inadequate dosing attributable to a number of concerns, including fears about suppressed respiration, side effects, interactions effects, and addiction, the belief that infants do not register pain experience, or physician discomfort with prescribing high doses of pain medicines.[15–17] Underprescribing has also been a consequence of believing myths that pain medication will lead to addiction or that the infant nervous system cannot experience pain—even though these have been empirically refuted.[10,18] Substantial data also undermine another notable misconception, that burn size and depth are always correlated with the severity of pain.[19] As such, providers may not understand the disproportionate relationship and react accordingly. This misconception is particularly pernicious in those who treat pain in pediatric patients. For example, it has been reported that inadequate analgesia has resulted from antiquated knowledge of pain assessment and pain management implementation.[19] One of the primary tenets of pain management in the Shriners Burn Center in Galveston, Texas, is if a patient reports pain, he or she is in pain, and it should be treated. As will be discussed later, the pain experience is affected significantly by psychological and environmental variables beyond tissue damage.

## Burn Injury Characteristics

In the burn care setting, burns are described according to size, depth, and location. Size is indicated by the percentage of total body surface area (TBSA) burned. Roughly 1% of an individual's TBSA is equal to the surface of his or her palm and fingers together. Burn severities are commonly referred to as *first degree*, *second degree*, and *third degree*. However, burn-specific descriptions include *superficial*, *superficial partial thickness*, *deep partial thickness*, and *full thickness*. These terms coincide with layers of the skin, the epidermis and dermis. Superficial burns only affect the thin outer epidermis and are typically caused by radiation (eg, sunburn). Partial-thickness burns can be either superficial

or deep, each term describing how far into the dermis the damage has penetrated. These types commonly show blistering or skin sloughing. Full-thickness burns have damaged both skin layers beyond repair and have insensate properties, but often remain painful. Depending on the severity of the injury, extent and duration of treatment and recovery varies widely. Burns are considered more severe when they occur in body locations that serve important functional and cosmetic roles. For example, physical impairment may be greater among those with hand and foot burns, while psychological and social impairment may be greater among those with face/head/neck or genitalia burns.

## Context of Burn Care

For hospitalized burn patients, treatment and recovery includes 4 stages.[20] The first stage involves initial evaluation and resuscitation, which occurs within the first 72 hours. Communication during this period may be difficult, but an adequate pain assessment is desired after survival is established. Proper attention to pain in the initial phases obviates many problems. For example, patients develop a repertoire of fear responses to pain (behavioral, cognitive, emotional), and studies have shown that inadequate pain control in the first wound care procedure can diminish the effectiveness of later interventions.[21] The second stage consists of initial excision and wound closure, where patients are under general anesthesia during procedures but can develop significant pain after or between surgeries. This period is particularly challenging because pain needs can change dramatically over time and frequent assessment is important. During the third stage, definitive wound closure and final operative procedures are concluded, often resulting in painful donor sites. The combination of the initial injury and surgical creation of new wounds (ie, donor sites) is typically associated with a significant increase in pain. After discharge from the burn intensive care unit, patients begin the rehabilitation, reconstruction, and reintegration phase, where pain-related problems such as ranging contracted burn scars arise and make activities such as physical therapy extremely challenging. Every treatment and recovery phase has pain-related aspects, and the pain experience can change rapidly.

## Pain

### Types of Pain

Categorizations of pain include transient, acute, and chronic pain.[23] Transient pain is by definition very brief and not associated with significant tissue damage (eg, needle injection). Acute pain may last up to 6 weeks and is usually associated with injuries that require medical attention and significant time to heal (eg, burn injury and surgical procedures). Chronic pain typically lasts more than 3 months beyond the time required for healing the wound. Transient and acute pain are associated with observable tissue damage (eg, nociceptive sensory stimulation). In contrast, chronic pain is not always associated with continued tissue damage and neuropathic pain is not associated with new damage. Chronic pain can result from a chronic disease state that causes continued tissue damage or may last well beyond wound healing and have no apparent physiological cause. Neuropathic pain is associated with neuronal damage or dysfunction in the nervous system but does not necessarily indicate ongoing tissue damage.[23] In general, children are less likely to develop neuropathic pain than adults.[24] However, amputations are the most common source of neuropathic pain for children, and they are sometimes necessary in the context of a major burn.[25]

Given the specificity of pain issues in burn care, burn pain has been described in 3 general types or contexts.[26] The burn-specific concepts are compatible with the general pain definitions provided above. Transient pain and acute pain are typically observed during inpatient care or the early phases of recovery, and chronic pain occurs much later. The contextual terms for burn pain include *background, breakthrough*, and *procedural pain*. Background pain describes the continuous, resting, or basal rate of pain over the period of 24 hours or more. Breakthrough pain describes sudden increases in pain that can result from movement, wound healing, fluctuations in pain thresholds, and so on. The onset of breakthrough pain is typically sudden, and it can last for a few hours. Procedural pain occurs in the context of wound care or scar management activities. Burn wound care, for example, involves multiple procedures for excision and debridement of the injury site as well as dressing changes that occur daily. These 3 concepts of burn pain result directly from the context of multiple surgical procedures, fluctuations in wound healing, necessary physical and occupational therapy (eg, ranging skin contractures), and the multitude of factors in burn care. The 3 burn-specific distinctions are primarily useful for medication management. Analgesic agents are selected to match the duration of pain. For example, background pain would be best treated with long-acting analgesic agents (eg, 12 hours) and procedural pain with short-acting analgesic agents (eg, 2–3 hours). The reader is directed elsewhere for detailed pharmacological interventions.[27]

There exist a number of methods for describing pain, depending on the context. In experimental studies, 3 primary variables are assessed. They are pain threshold, pain tolerance, and pain intensity. *Pain threshold* refers to the point where intensity of sensation is experienced as painful. *Pain tolerance* refers to the amount of time an individual can bear a painful stimulus. *Pain intensity* refers to the overall

evaluative rating of the pain experience. As discussed below in regards to theories of pain, pain ratings are a combination of sensory, affective, and cognitive dimensions. These pain characteristics have not been routinely reported in previous pediatric burn pain studies but are used extensively in pediatric pain studies that employ laboratory-induced pain in nonclinical samples. The pain literature is rapidly evolving to include and understand distinctions and nuances in the pain experience to test and develop pain theory.

## Pain Theory

Theories of pain have evolved from initial 1-dimensional models to integrative models.[28,29] One-dimensional models were based on writings from 15th-century philosopher Renee Descartes, whose theory suggested that sensory pathways carried information from parts of the body to the brain. In his conceptualization, the brain is passive and merely accepts messages from the damaged site. Accordingly, tissue damage and the pain experience should be proportional.[30] However, clinical and empirical observations demonstrate that pain cannot be wholly explained in these terms. Historical accounts and the pain literature at large have demonstrated that pain reporting and severity of tissue damage are not always equivalent. In 1956 Henry Beecher conducted a seminal study on pain-reporting differences[31] and noted that surgical patients and combat soldiers with similar wounds reported pain very differently, with surgical patients reporting much higher pain levels. He suspected that soldiers viewed the pain as a reprieve from combat; perhaps the injury was reason to be sent home. This seminal work implied that factors beyond tissue damage affected the pain experience. Hence, theories evolved to include psychogenic factors to explain why physiological damage can be disproportional to the experience of pain.[32] Originally, psychiatric disorder and variants in emotional processing were used to explain the differences. In other attempts, malingering for secondary gains (eg, disability benefits) was proposed. Although some individuals may be prone to report pain for such gains, this phenomena is context specific and does not necessarily apply elsewhere. As such, early models of pain were significantly limited.

The gate control theory was proposed by Melzack in 1965[33] and had significant explanatory power, enduring copious pain research that followed. This theory was the first to challenge popular mind-body dualism and introduced the brain as an active agent in the experience and modulation of pain. The theory postulated that the dorsal horn of the spine served as a hypothetical gate. In this model, nerve transmissions sent from both the injured site and the brain communicated with each other in the dorsal horn. During this communication process, signals from the brain modulate the pain experience by either facilitating or muting the sensory pain signals traveling to the spine. In order to account for these additional factors in the pain experience, a tripartite model was developed that consisted of the following factors: (1) nociceptive-sensory, (2) motivational-affective, and (3) cognitive-evaluative. This theoretical factor structure was used to create the McGill pain questionnaire,[34] which has received extensive empirical support. In contrast, one primary shortcoming of the gate control theory was highlighted by observations of phantom limb pain in patients with high spinal breaks, where sensory inputs do not result from or cannot be transmitted from an injured site.

In response to this shortcoming of the gate control theory,[35,36] Melzack revised his theory and further emphasized the role of the brain. Neuromatrix theory posits that the brain has a genetically predisposed synaptic architecture that represents the body-self as a whole and develops in concert with learning inputs, or experience. Gate control theory components remain central to this theory and are linked to neuroanatomic structure and function: nociceptive-sensory (somatosensory), affective-motivational (limbic), and cognitive-affective modulators (thalamocortical). Parallel processing of neural circuits, or loops, between the thalamus and cortex and the limbic system and cortex are continuous and create a neurosignature that influences nerve impulses of the neuromatrix. Neuromatrix outputs include pain perception, involuntary and voluntary actions, and stress regulation systems (eg, immune, cortisol, norepinephrine, and endorphin systems). The neurosignature purportedly affects the neurological pain experience and can maintain the representation of an intact physiological body-whole despite amputation. Although this concept is very similar to the gate control theory, the primary difference is that brain structure and function play a more central role in the pain experience, thus identifying the important roles of cognition and affect in the pain experience. These 2 factors combined with basic knowledge of animal conditioning provide the rationale for conducting psychological interventions with people who have pain problems. The reader is referred elsewhere for a more detailed review of pain theories.[37,38]

## DEVELOPMENTAL CONSIDERATIONS

## Stages of Development

### Psychological Response to Burn Injuries

The events surrounding a burn injury can vary widely but are never pleasant. In some instances, the events are extremely aversive and may qualify as traumatic events. Features that distinguish traumatic events are sudden or unexpected events, the shocking nature of the events, death or threat to life or body integrity, and subjective feelings of intense terror, horror, or helplessness.[39] Not all children are traumatized after burn events. Several factors influence a child's response: developmental level, inherent or learned resiliency, and external sources of support. For example, younger children rely on their parents' reaction to the burn event more than their older counterparts do, regardless of injury severity. If parents cope well, their children are less likely to develop long-lasting trauma symptoms.[40]

Pain management is one of the most difficult aspects of pediatric burn care and can exacerbate traumatic symptoms and responses. Children have distinctive ways of coping and understanding their burn injuries and subsequent painful treatment procedures. They utilize a variety of skills at different stages of development to understand and cope. Children will often seek out new information to aid in their ability to cope and adapt to the treatment experiences.[41] It is important for the burn care team to have a clear understanding of development and a patient's ability to cope with the burn injury in an effort to prevent retraumatizing the child.

The treatment of pediatric burn pain requires understanding developmental differences among children. Piagetian theory[42] of development provides a useful 4-stage framework. The stages of development include sensorimotor (birth to 2 years), preoperational (2–7 years), concrete operational (7 years to adolescence), and formal operational (adolescence). In the sensorimotor stage, infants use a function simply because it exists (eg, grasping), and they later demonstrate effortful physical behaviors with intention (eg, playing with a toy). The beginnings of stranger anxiety are also observed just before age 1. By the end of this period, the 2-year-old does not rely on concrete trial and error; he or she now uses forms of mental trials that promote efficiency. Near the end of this stage is when children are more aware of their environment and more interactive forms of distraction can be introduced during painful procedures.[42] Their increased awareness also highlights discrepancies between their home environment and the burn unit. The consequent deviation from norms is challenging and may incite a variety of fears.[42]

Piaget's preoperational stage consists of a few major features that include symbolic reasoning and decentration.[42] Language and imagination become more well developed, and over the course of the stage, children start to appreciate their own minds as distinct from others (ie, decentration). Despite significant developments during this period, initial limitations for children up to 7 years old include a lack of differentiation between themselves and the world, a limited concept of time, and a tendency to use alogical reasoning where cause and effect relationships are mysterious. These characteristics can make painful procedures fantastical and scary for the child who has very little sense of time and reason. Over the course of this stage, intervention techniques can become more interactive for either distraction or the introduction of child-mediated control methods. In the concrete operational stage, children begin to understand the difference between fantasy and reality and are able to apply basic principles of logic. Explanations can be provided for the necessity of wound care, and plans can be made with the child for appropriate interventions.

Piaget's formal operational stage is characterized by a significant increase in mental abilities that include a shift from rudimentary deductive methods to inductive reasoning that constitutes a type of theory development and manipulation of ideas.[42] This period includes development of moral characteristics such as understanding the nature of motives and special circumstance. At this point the youth has developed many adult characteristics and is more appropriate for intervention methods that use reasoning and evidence-based thinking (ie, cognitive-behavioral methods). For more details on child development and burn care, the reader is referred to a review by Dise-Lewis.[41]

Across these developmental stages, there are also differences in abilities to perceive pain, understand pain, and communicate meaningful information about pain. Choosing appropriate treatment requires knowledge of the child's ability to cope during painful procedures and his or her behavioral responses to pain depending on his or her developmental age. See Table 1 for age-related developmental issues and descriptions of the child's burn injury experience at different ages. Interventions that are appropriate to the developmental capacities of children in different age groups are also provided. Understanding the psychological ability of a pediatric burn patient to cope based on his or her developmental level is of particular value for pain management.

# PSYCHOLOGICAL PRINCIPLES OF HUMAN BEHAVIOR

## Learning Theory and Practice

### Psychological Principles

Both simple and complex psychological principles underlie the experience of pain and associated anxiety. For example, behavioral conditioning has long been understood as one of the basic rules of human functioning, while more recent studies have examined details of cognitive functioning and attention in experiments conducted using laboratory-induced pain. Before discussing specific pediatric burn issues, a review of foundational principles and theories is provided.

### Classical Conditioning

Classical, or Pavlovian, conditioning established that a neutral stimulus could take on reflexive response properties after associative conditioning with a reflex-inducing stimulus. In his famous experiments, Pavlov induced a reflexive salivary response in dogs by using a neutral stimulus with no inherent salivation-inducing property. The conditioning procedures consisted of an unconditioned stimulus (ie, food) that naturally produced an unconditioned response (ie, salivation). After repeatedly presenting a neutral stimulus (ie, a bell tone) prior to presenting the food, the bell tone became a conditioned stimulus that was able to elicit salivation even when food was not present. This can be understood in the context of burn care. For example, a needle stick would naturally produce an unconditioned response in children to tense, move away, cry, or withdraw. After repeated pairings of a person wearing a neutral white lab coat with needle sticks, the white lab coat can become the conditioned stimulus that produces the conditioned response of tension, movement, or crying. Children are especially susceptible to this kind of conditioning in the burn unit,[43] and associations can be formed very quickly when the stimulus is extremely aversive.[44,45] This process is quite clear with individual and explicit examples such as these. In the context of usual care on a busy burn unit, these processes are occurring continuously for many reflexive responses. As such, thoughtful planning of daily activities is important for pain management and overall care. While this principle of animal learning is important, its explanatory power does not cover all aspects of psychological burn care.

### Operant Conditioning

Although operant conditioning has been loosely described for over a century, BF Skinner[46] identified many of the processes by which these basic levels of behavioral learning operate. Most people are familiar with the concepts of positive reinforcement and punishment, but are less so with the concepts of negative reinforcement or schedules of reinforcement. In brief, positive reinforcement is used to increase a particular behavior. In this process, a reward is provided after the desired behavior to increase its frequency (eg, praise is given after the child takes his or her medicine). Punishment is used to decrease a behavior. In this process, an aversive stimulus is applied after the behavior to decrease its frequency (eg, the child is reprimanded for throwing food on the floor). Negative reinforcement is used to increase behavior by removing an aversive stimulus. For example, if the child experiences the wound care hospital room as aversive, time away from the room could be provided after good behavior. Science has clearly shown that the type of reinforcement and the schedule of reinforcement have a substantial impact on learning.[47] It is also fairly common knowledge that rewards and punishments should be given consistently and immediately in order to be most effective. In this process, the primary issues are timing (ie, actual time elapsed since the behavior) and consistency. Reinforcers can be applied on a fixed ratio or variable ratio schedule. A description of each schedule type is beyond the scope of this paper, but a few important examples will be discussed.

The definition of a fixed schedule is when response or consequence is provided reliably after any set number of behaviors. For example, a vending machine is on a particular type of fixed ratio schedule, called continuous ratio, because it provides a response every time the behavior is performed (eg, paying and selecting equals product each time). Consistency is the main feature of this schedule. When the behavior is performed without the desired response, significant frustration follows that may include aggression. This is called an *extinction burst*, which precedes discontinuance of the behavior. For example, people do not typically insert more money into the vending machine if it did not perform the first time.

The purpose of this example is to highlight the importance of maintaining continuity of care and reliable administration of psychological rewards, tangible reinforcers (eg, candy), and pain medications. In the context of burn care, let's look at the case of a child who performs a desired behavior during wound care (eg, sitting still during washing) because that behavior has been consistently rewarded (eg, with praise, empathy, or gentleness). Since this behavior is difficult for the child (ie, it takes effort to sit still when pain is being experienced), the child's motivation to continue that good behavior can be seriously compromised after the first time the reward is not provided. Per the vending machine example, if a product costs 10 dollars (ie, equating expense with difficulty), one trial with no product might be enough for most to discontinue trying. This principle is applicable for the administration of pain medications as well.

Reinforcement can also be delivered in a variable ratio schedule. Here, a powerful reinforcement is delivered after an unknown number of behavioral responses. For example, gambling slot machines are on a variable ratio schedule. Players have been conditioned to expect that after enough attempts, they will eventually win something. Extinguishing behaviors on this reinforcement schedule is very difficult. In burn terms, this can be discussed in the context of wound care and escape behaviors. Thurber et al nicely described the difficulty with escape behaviors and the need to maintain structure in wound care.[48] In this context, escape from wound care pain is a powerful

negative reinforcement. If crying, screaming, or tantrums provide the child with escape on an inconsistent basis, the behaviors will likely continue throughout care. Alternatively, time can be used to determine breaks in wound care. For example, nurses can instruct the child that each wound care segment lasts a given period of time (eg, 30 seconds), after which they can break for another block of time. This particular type of intervention can be delicate and should be coordinated with the psychological services available to the burn unit. Although this case in particular was identified, it is useful to consult with psychological services before implementing many of these conditioning procedures.

Principles of classical and operant conditioning were highlighted in a series of papers on pediatric burn pain management.[47-50] These papers also discuss characteristics of the burn care setting by their conditioning properties and their effect on pain and discuss reasons why long-acting analgesic medications are well preferred over short-acting agents. Untreated pain creates a repertoire of pain behaviors used to get analgesic pain control. In effect, pain is reinforced by providing relief only after a high intensity of pain has been reached. Optimally, patients should need to make few requests for pain medication. The reader is referred elsewhere for more detail and a useful outline of theory and practical applications.[48-50]

## Social Learning Theory

Social learning theory posits that learning does not require firsthand experience, as do the ones discussed above.[51] In Bandura's original studies, children merely observed aggressive behaviors and imitated them with ease. In short, humans learn from others by example and modeling. In the burn context, even verbal reports from other children can change patient expectations, anxiety, and pain behaviors,[45] all of which have a significant effect on the pain experience. Also consistent with the theory is that if staff and parents demonstrate maladaptive responses to pain, the child will learn and reproduce those behaviors. This has been well demonstrated in parent-child dyads with acute laboratory pain. This also occurs in the realm of chronic pain, where children of parents with chronic pain report higher rates of pain and appear to imitate their pain behaviors. This topic will be particularly relevant when family issues and parent-mediated wound care are discussed later. Social learning theory highlights the importance of setting appropriate examples in the burn care setting. Children easily learn from others how to interpret, experience, and respond to pain. Additional models of learning that make meaningful contributions with relevance to pediatric pain management have been researched.[52-55]

## Cognitive-Behavioral Models

One further theory with relevance to burn care that must be highlighted is cognitive-behavioral theory. This model presents an exceptionally broad integrative model that has demonstrated effectiveness across psychological conditions. As such, a general overview will be followed by pain-specific examples. Components of the approach include thoughts, feelings, and behaviors of the person. Each component is assessed for both conceptualization and intervention purposes. The cognitive component is not appropriate for younger children in early stages of development. In these cases, reliance on behavioral and emotional components consistent with classical and operant conditioning should be used. However, once children reach a developmental level where language and reasoning abilities are appropriate, cognitive and behavioral strategies should be used in concert.[56]

Cognitive strategies can be adaptive or maladaptive and can influence the severity of pain experiences.[57] They are based on individuals' beliefs, appraisals of meaning, expectations, problem-solving abilities, automatic thoughts, and self-coping thoughts. Adaptive cognitive strategies include using accurate information to derive an evidence-based assessment and evaluation of the situation which can lead to the use of effective strategies for dealing with distress. Maladaptive strategies include inflexible styles of thinking that can include preoccupation with inaccurate, aversive, or insignificant information. Interventions are designed to transform maladaptive strategies into adaptive strategies, produce concurrent modifications in behaviors and emotions, and promote change.[57]

Cognitive approaches are inherently collaborative because participation is required from the patient. Patients must be willing to engage in the process and provide necessary information with which to work. Particularly with children, many behaviors based on cognitive variables are automatic and make it necessary to examine the underlying reasons for their reactions. For example, if a child believes that pain during a dressing change means he or she is getting worse, his or her automatic reaction may be physical resistance. The provider must elicit this belief from the child in order to make modifications with accurate information. A common approach is to have patients treat their thoughts as hypotheses or guesses, and encourage them to acquire the information necessary to refute or support their original belief. In pediatric patients, significant assistance is required from the provider to facilitate this process.

Expectations are an important feature of children's pain-related distress. Even before children come to the hospital, many have preconditioned fears to medical staff clothing.[58] In addition, initial experiences are powerful (eg, primacy effects) and can serve to create expectations for the remainder of care. Providers can make a difference through their interactions with the patient. In a seminal study,[59] the effects of providing individuals with different kinds of information before a painful medical procedure were addressed. Study participants were more amenable to the procedure if given accurate information regarding the physical sensations they could expect and specific instructions for what to do or how to behave during the procedure. This was only effective in making the experience more tolerable when using sensory and behavioral preparation in combination. This work has been extrapolated to the burn care context and is a recommended approach for good care.[60] It is important to consider individual characteristics of the child and the family. Common language used with the family and developmentally appropriate language for the child are most suitable. Providing preparatory information is one component of the care plan and may help reduce distress, but it is not nearly exhaustive. Children are still forced to cope with noxious wound care procedures.

Individuals engage in coping behaviors when faced with a situation that makes or appears to make demands in excess of their available resources[61] (stress coping). Coping strategies are numerous and include information seeking, problem solving, support seeking, acceptance, distraction, and so on. Higher-order coping strategies have been identified that capture clusters of essential features.[62] For example, dichotomous coping strategies include approach coping versus avoidance coping or active coping versus passive coping, and some include distraction as a third higher-order category. In a study of coping strategies used by multiple pediatric samples with chronic abdominal pain, cluster analysis identified groups characterized hierarchically by attachment styles and mastery efforts.[62] Attachment (quality of interpersonal relationships) and mastery efforts were identified as positive or negative. The combination of positive or negative scores on the higher-order factors determined their assignment to 1 of the 4 subgroups described by the following coping styles: engaged, self-reliant, dependent, and avoidant. Engaged copers were identified by positive interpersonal relationships and mastery efforts. Self-reliant copers were identified by negative interpersonal relationships and positive mastery efforts. Dependent copers were identified by positive relationships and negative mastery efforts. And avoidant copers were identified by negative relationships and mastery efforts. This study nicely complements previous work highlighting the importance of matching the intervention to patient characteristics. The results from this study could help direct selection of intervention. For example, if a burned child has distant or poor relationships with caregivers and does not appear to strive for mastery in his or her environment, he or she could be characterized as an avoidant coper. Hence, a distraction technique is most appropriate. In laboratory-induced pain studies with children, the interaction between preferred coping styles and cognitive interventions has demonstrated higher pain thresholds and tolerance are associated with appropriate matching.[63] For example, children with active coping styles performed better when directed to focus on the sensations of the pain experience, and children with avoidance coping performed better when provided with distraction techniques. Interestingly, studies using adults with chronic pain suggest the use of active coping methods provides individuals a sense of control over the pain experience,[64] an important variable in pain reporting. Many pediatric burn patients are unable to perform cognitive coping strategies due to their level of development. Despite the fact that active coping may enhance a sense of control, distraction may be the only realistic approach for younger children.

Martin and colleagues applied the concepts of control and coping to treatment selection in pediatric burns.[65] The child's preferred coping style was first identified (eg, avoidance vs approach). That is, staff members identified patient preferences to be very little or very much involved in their burn care. The terms *psychologically distant* and *psychologically close* were used as anchors on a continuum. The two-process theory of control is used in conjunction with coping style. Primary and secondary control processes each have a unique focus. *Primary control* indicates making changes directly with the source of the pain (eg, self-mediated dressing change), and *secondary control* indicates that an individual changes himself or herself to adapt (eg, reappraisal of the meaning of the pain). The absence of either would indicate helplessness or "giving up." Children's preferred coping styles and ability to engage in control processes can help select the type of interventions most appropriate. This approach is supported by principles based on the pediatric pain literature at large and should be considered as guidelines. The full parameters of this approach have not been demonstrated in pediatric burn patients in acutely painful procedures.

Catastrophizing is a cognitive style characterized by an exaggeration of pain-related symptoms, pessimism, and perseverance about the pain. Catastrophizing is related to negative pain-related outcomes in multiple samples,[66] but it has not been researched in pediatric burn samples. Some authors have interpreted pediatric catastrophizing as a response to feelings of helplessness or lack of control over the pain experience.[67] As a result, catastrophizing is described as a communication mechanism requesting help from others for control over the pain, typically parents or caregivers. Nonclinical samples show more verbal communication, while clinical samples demonstrate more protective pain-related behaviors and experience more

pain.[68] Using a sample of adult burn patients,[69] researchers examined the effects of suppression-based (avoidant) coping versus processing-based (active) methods. Results suggested relative equivalence between suppression and active coping during wound care, but noted that pre–wound care suppression (ignoring) strategies were associated with higher distress during and after the procedure. Findings are discussed in the context of a rebound theory of cognition.

Beliefs about helplessness and perceived control have been demonstrated as important in the pain literature.[70] Control is mediated by the use of coping strategies[71] and is the conceptual opposite of helplessness, which is associated with more distress and pain intensity. While coping is one example of exercising control, burn wound care allows for a more hands-on experience during dressing changes and debridement. Some evidence suggests a positive effect when wound debridement is mediated by the burned child.[72] Another component of control is predictability, which has also been studied in burn patients.[73] In this case, predictability and control had a positive effect for a small sample of burned children when compared to controls. Even outside burns, it has been established that increased control has positive effects on the pain experience, but notably, the meaning of the pain is a significant component.[74]

Physiological sensations aside from the wound site are also important. The relationship between anxiety and pain is partially mediated by anxiety sensitivity, which involves the interpretation of physiological symptoms of anxious arousal such as heart rate, respiratory rate, sweating, and so on. *Anxiety sensitivity* specifically refers to a fear of bodily sensations related to anxiety and shows predictive power in nonpediatric samples.[75] Together, anxiety sensitivity and anticipatory anxiety accounted for over half of the pain-reporting variance in at least one laboratory-induced pain study. When evaluating the mediational effects of heart rate in nonclinical pediatric samples, it was found that children in early puberty had a higher heart rate and lower pain tolerance than their older counterparts. Together, these results highlight the importance of how one experiences and interprets sensations of heart rate and physiological symptoms of increased arousal. Findings such as these suggest that managing anxiety and arousal throughout burn care is important, especially in younger children.

Taken together, the psychological conditioning and cognitive aspect of the burn care setting are vast. The focus has traditionally been on the actual procedure of wound care, but nearly everyone appears to have a potential role in mediating the anxiety and associated pain in the pediatric patient. In the sections above, principles and theories have been discussed to provide context with some interwoven examples. In the following sections, topics address actual practices in pediatric burn units and interventions used during wound care. These sections also provide a more detailed review of the evidence for nonpharmacological pain intervention.

## CURRENT PRACTICES IN PEDIATRIC BURN CARE

Martin-Herz et al[76] conducted a recent survey of pediatric pain control practices in North American burn centers. Of the 155 burn centers selected for participation, 85 responded with information from one or more of the following specialists: surgeons, anesthesiologists, pharmacists, or various staff. Across all age groups, anxiolytics were commonly used, and the frequency of use increased with age group (17%–39%). Seventy-seven percent reported using nonpharmacological adjuncts to medication during burn care. In the youngest children, many centers used distraction (62%) and music/art therapy (27%). Fewer used relaxation (13%) and massage (11%). Among preschoolers, many still used distraction (67%), music/art therapy (37%), and relaxation (19%), while few used massage (9%) and nearly none used hypnosis or imagery. In the school-age and adolescent groups, nearly half of centers endorsed using distraction, music/art therapy, and relaxation to an equitable degree. Less than 10% of responders endorsed using massage or hypnosis, and almost none used imagery-based techniques. The authors cogently argue that pediatric pain control interventions are seriously underutilized, especially regarding the use of adjunctive pharmacological and nonpharmacological interventions. It was beyond the scope of this investigation to discuss the depth and breadth of psychological principles employed at each of these centers. Further, the quality of the interventions was not addressed. It is likely a high degree of variability exists across centers. Although interventions are a core feature of pain control, proper assessments are necessary to rate, understand, and monitor patient needs.

## Assessment

### Assessment of Pediatric Burn Pain

Primary goals in the emergency room are to remove the source of tissue damage (eg, heat, chemicals) from the injured child and provide first-aid procedures, including clearing the airway, evaluating breathing, stabilizing respiration, managing bleeding and shock, conducting minor debridement, providing a tetanus toxoid injection, and splinting injured extremities. As all of these procedures are being performed, the child's level of consciousness is constantly being monitored. The level of consciousness is

extremely important in burn injuries as patients are alert, oriented, and verbal, even with severe burn injuries. Assessment of pain during this phase of burn care consists mainly of physiological and observational assessments.

Once patients are stabilized, the acute phase of treatment begins. This phase is considered the most painful phase the pediatric patient endures as intensive effort is given toward wound care and medical procedures, including aversive procedures, frequent IV placements, dressing changes 1 to 2 times daily with vigorous debridement (cleansing) of wounds, and multiple surgical procedures. Fear, anxiety, and pain often have similar symptoms, perhaps especially in younger patients: feelings of fear or dread, trembling, restlessness, muscle tension, rapid heart rate, lightheadedness or dizziness, perspiration, cold hands/feet, shortness of breath, worrying excessively, difficulty falling asleep, and nightmares.

The inescapable and unavoidable daily burn wound dressing changes are aversive and can be critical in determining the patient's fear and anticipatory anxiety. These medical procedures are done in a sterile environment (hats, gloves, gowns, and mask must be worn). As children observe staff in these garments, they learn that painful procedures will follow. This is one of the many factors that make assessing pain difficult. As a clinician, it is important to discern pain versus anxiety. Assessment of pain becomes intricately intermingled with symptoms of anxiety, fear, and depression. Depending upon developmental level and understanding, children will report pain when actually experiencing anxiety or fear. Another confounding issue is pruritis and itching. During later stages of wound healing, children may also equate itching with pain. As such, special attention should be paid to this distinction to direct assessment; itch-specific scales have been developed for this reason.

A Joint Commission on Accreditation of Healthcare Organizations (JCAHO) initiative to improve the assessment base for pediatric burn pain has prompted a number of systematic reviews and evidence-based papers.[76-79] Studies have investigated both observational and self-reporting methods of assessment. Among the observational methods, only 6 of the 30-plus available instruments were identified as suitable for use. That is, only 6 instruments demonstrated adequate reliability and validity. Among the self-report studies, 7 could be evaluated for psychometric properties, use, and feasibility. Studies agreed that no instrument was appropriate for all age groups or developmental stages, and they identified a significant gap for instruments in the preschool-age group. Three general methods of assessment are used with children, including observational or behavioral, self-report, and physiological assessments. General recommendations are to use self-reporting whenever possible and to avoid physiological methods, as they are often unreliable.

Of note, careful attention should be paid to instrument selection, as age groups do not always coincide with developmental stages. For excellent reviews and detailed recommendations, please see von Baeyer and Spragrud (2007) which includes 6 observational instruments described according to age group, setting, characteristics, and level of evidence[80] and Stinson et al. (2006) which includes seven self-report instruments are described similarly.[78]

## Treatment of Pediatric Burn Pain

### Pharmacological Intervention: A Brief Synopsis

Pharmacologic management of burn pain includes opioids, nonsteroidal anti-inflammatory drugs (NSAIDs), mild analgesics, parenteral agents (opioid patches), inhaled anesthetic agents, and anxiolytics. Opioids act by attaching to specific proteins called *opioid receptors*, which are found in neurons in the neural networks throughout the brain, spinal cord, and gastrointestinal tract. When these compounds attach to certain opioid receptors in the brain and spinal cord, they can effectively change the way a person experiences pain. The most common pharmacological management of pain during this emergency phase is morphine (an opioid). Depending on age and burn injury, a large percentage of children are also given lorazepam (Ativan) for symptoms of anxiety and to assist with calming. Anesthetics such as ketamine and propofol are used when performing emergency medical procedures to stabilize the child. Although propofol is a newer sedative that has a rapid onset and a short half-life, it and other similar drugs are advantageous for treating pediatric burns during this phase because they can be titrated to level of consciousness and duration of action.

### Nonpharmacological Intervention

The pain experienced with a burn injury event as well as during the treatment of burn injuries can produce severe psychological distress in pediatric burn survivors. Although pharmacological interventions are the foundation of pediatric pain management, pain perception has a strong psychological component that has proven difficult to manage solely with pharmacological agents.

Procedural pain management for children during wound dressing changes is often excruciating. Measurement and treatment of pain in the pediatric population can be both complicated and frustrating for burn center staff. Ratcliff et al[81] conducted a retrospective review of 286 acute pediatric burn survivors treated in 2001 with a pharmacologic analgesia protocol for pain, anxiety, and itching. He documented an increasing trend towards using stronger analgesia in the treatment of pediatric burns in an attempt to reduce pain.

Further progress in pain management may benefit from knowledge of the many variables that influence pain.

Schecter et al[82] conducted a study in 2002 which concluded that age, gender, and ethnicity influence perception of pain. Meyer et al[83] found that the status of wound closure and familial traditions have an impact on a child's perception of pain. Zeitlin[84] and Meyer et al[85] found that interpersonal interactions as well as the patient's ability to control the situation greatly influenced the perception of pain. Although all of the factors may impact the perception of pain, they are factors that are not easily manipulated.

While opioids work well for controlling tonic pain for many burn patients, they tend to be inadequate for controlling the severe phasic pain associated with the daily wound care and physical therapy sessions. Even with aggressive use of opioid pain medication, most burn patients report severe to excruciating pain during these events.[86-88] Hoffman et al [89] reported data on physical therapy sessions of burn patients in which the average pain level in the standard treatment condition over the course of 3 days ranged from 67 to 78 on a 100-mm visual analog scale. In sum, pain varies widely by type and intensity of the course of recovery from a burn injury, and nearly every burn care professional involved in the patient's care is involved to some degree.

Psychological interventions to manage pain during the initial phase are limited due to the chaotic nature of emergency departments and the limited availability of trained psychologists. Several of the Shriners burn hospitals for children have trained psychologists on call, while other hospitals may have child life specialists available to provide psychological interventions for pain management. The primary interventions utilized are cognitive-behavioral interventions and hypnosis.[90]

### Psychological Interventions for Pain During the Acute Phase

There are several techniques that are essential when enhancing pain control during the acute phase of burn care. The most useful time for a psychologist to become involved is during dressing changes and physical therapy; for example, preparing a child for procedures can reduce anticipatory anxiety. Preparation can be done with a child life specialist and/or a psychologist. It is useful for a psychologist and child life specialist to use developmentally appropriate distraction techniques (ie, blowing bubbles, reading, music therapy, aromatherapy, games, storytelling, and so on). Psychologists and other interventionists should also teach developmentally appropriate relaxation skills to the burn patient. Psychoeducation for anxiety and pain prior to a dressing change or after a painful procedure is also helpful.

Dolls used to demonstrate or describe procedures can also be helpful when preparing a child for wound care. The child changes dressings on the doll in the same locations as his or her own burns, and the exact materials for actual care should be used in the practice session (ie, xeroform bacitracin, chlorapactin, biobrane, adaptic, silvadine, water, and gauze). Another helpful technique is to prepare the child with pictures. The pictures should include images of the treatment room and the materials that will be utilized for his or her wound care as well as distraction tools that will be in the room to help him or her.

## Psychological Interventions for Pain During the Rehabilitation Phase

During the rehabilitation phase, pain management has a different purpose than during the acute phase. During the rehabilitation phase of treatment, pharmacological interventions are titrated and psychological interventions become the primary form of treatment for pain. Often, patients' perceived pain is just as difficult to manage as real pain. Patients often become irritable, depressed, and frustrated during this phase. They also develop fears and anxiety about treatment progress as well as returning home. Teaching effective coping strategies and cognitive-behavioral interventions are beneficial in treating these symptoms. The goal of this stage is reintegration to family, school, and community. It is important to develop a safety zone at home so that the child may use the safety zone when he or she is afraid or anxious. It is important that no wound care, physical therapy, or painful procedures occur in the safety zone. As with each stage, it is important to continue to use age-appropriate language with children to ensure they have a clear understanding of goals.

## Overall Management

The overall management requires a multidisciplinary team approach. This team should include a surgeon, psychologist, anesthesiologist, psychiatrist, child life specialist, intensivist, social worker, nurse, nutritionist, physical therapist, and occupational therapist. Each of the members of the burn team has a significant impact on and role in the treatment. There are several important tasks that should be conducted by the multidisciplinary team to ensure that wound care and dressing changes flow smoothly. In order to provide appropriate pharmacological dosing for the procedure, the anesthesiologist must have precise information regarding the patient's wounds from nursing and surgical members of the team and then must accurately assess the level of pain himself or herself. The psychologist should complete a detailed daily assessment of the patient's pain and anxiety level. This is an essential component for long-term treatment.

Due to the extensive pain involved in burn wound care, patients will develop anticipatory anxiety before it is time for dressing changes. As patients begin to heal, the initial doses of strong narcotic medications to treat pain are titrated. Patients will often report experiencing the same level of pain when they are really experiencing anxiety triggered by previous pain and the anticipation that the pain will return with the same intensity. Distinguishing the difference at times is difficult but should be done on a daily basis, with subsequent treatment that is reflective of the symptoms. If the anxiety level warrants pharmacological intervention, then an anxiolytic such as a benzodiazepine should be initiated. A child life specialist should discuss with the child his or her preferences, likes, and dislikes prior to wound care to aid in determining the appropriate distraction techniques.

Time management and coordination are other key features for wound care. The nursing team is responsible for administering medications in a timely fashion to ensure that medication will last throughout the entire treatment procedure. The nursing team is also responsible for conducting the wound care; the child life specialist is responsible for providing distraction during wound care. When a parent is present, the child life specialist and psychologist will work together to ensure that the parent is able to provide the necessary comfort to the child. This is achieved by coaching the parent to utilize breathing techniques taught prior to wound care in order to remain calm. It also involves coordinating with nursing staff signals for when to take planned and strategic breaks during wound care. As wound care involves many team members in the treatment room, coordination is important for each step, from the beginning of preparing for wound care to administering medication, transporting the patient from his or her room to the treatment room, completing wound care, returning the patient to his or her room, and completing documentation.

Consistency is essential in burn care as there are numerous members of the treatment team, which at times may make it difficult to arrive at consensus. It is imperative the team meets several times per week to communicate and share information on the progress of the patient in each discipline. Each team member should clearly understand his or her role, in particular who is responsible for disclosing to the parents and child and what information he or she is to convey. It is also important for team members to communicate about the time of day for various treatment procedures and communicate this to the child. Instituting a schedule and posting the schedule in the child's room not only prevents various treatments from being scheduled at the same time, it also establishes a daily routine for the patient.

## Cognitive-Behavioral Therapy

Nearly all of the empirical nonpharmacological studies for treating pediatric burn pain consist of cognitive-behavioral techniques. The most common is distraction, but techniques also include relaxation, variations of patient-centered control, and parent-mediated methods.[91–99] In a recent systematic review of the acute burn pain intervention literature, only 12 studies were identified as meeting the US Preventive Task Force criteria for methodological rigor.[100] Seven of these studies were identified as "good" and 5 were "poor." The authors conceptually divided studies into 3 categories: health care provider–mediated treatment, child-mediated treatment, and parent-mediated treatment. Provider-mediated studies included massage therapy, increased procedural predictability, music distraction, and mediated debridement. Child-mediated interventions included virtual reality (VR), a stress management program, imagery-based hypnosis, and cartoon viewing. Parent-mediated treatments included parent presence in a supportive capacity during procedures. Although results were generally optimistic, these studies reflected the difficulties of researching pediatric burn pain. There is a myriad factors affecting intervention and obtaining adequate sample sizes to interpret results.

Since this systematic review was compiled, a handful of additional intervention studies have been published. Nearly all had small sample sizes (ie, < 10 per group), and some included adults and children together.[101-106] The topic areas included VR, music therapy, and hypnosis. The music study and one VR study included pediatric-only samples and demonstrated moderately optimistic results. Interestingly, the VR study did not demonstrate a statistically significant increase over the distraction condition of watching television. Altogether, the paucity of studies points to a need for future interventions with larger sample sizes and increased methodological rigor.

## Distraction

Distraction techniques are very suitable for all age groups but are clearly indicated for younger children. The primary target is the focus of the patient's attention. As described in the theories reviewed above, when less attention is available for evaluation of nociceptive input, for example, patients are expected to experience and report less pain. Distraction-based cognitive-behavioral interventions have been developed for burn care,[111] but evidence on their efficacy has been mixed.[107,108] The most common distraction interventions are playing, listening to music, cartoon or television viewing, various visual distractions, conversing with the wound care nurse, and using video format tools. It has been argued that ignoring sensations through distraction may work well for milder, shorter pain stimuli, but less so with the intensity and duration of pain encountered in clinical settings.[109] It has also been suggested that a common shortcoming of previous work in this area is the relatively low salience of the distractors used in the interventions.[110] In order to use distraction as an intervention, a user-friendly method of capturing attention must be used that is sufficiently powerful to override the noxious physical sensation.

## Virtual Reality

Virtual reality is essentially a distraction intervention. The underlying principle of distraction treatment proposes that the more attention demanded by the distracting task, the less attention is available for processing painful signals. Numerous studies support the effectiveness of distraction for procedural pain during pediatric burn procedures.[111–114] Dahlquist et al[113] conducted a trial that demonstrated that although any distraction technique is better than none, interactive VR distraction was far more effective in the management of acute pediatric pain than passive distraction. The theoretical basis for this enhanced effect of VR is Wickens'[114] multiple sensory theory. This theory suggests that tasks involving 1 sensory modality (visual, auditory, tactile, or kinesthetic) do not absorb the individual's attentional resources available in the other sensory modalities. Interactive VR involves all 4 senses and potentially blocks more of the sensory modalities associated with acute pain.[115-117]

Preliminary work using VR in treating burn pain has been conducted by Hoffman et al at the University of Washington.[118–121] In a case report, they initially measured pain levels of 2 adolescents undergoing staple removal from skin grafts while being distracted with VR.[118] Results revealed 3 minutes of immersive VR to be more effective in reducing pain than playing a Nintendo game for 3 minutes.[119] Hoffman et al[120] also conducted a crossover design study with 12 adult burn patients performing their physical therapy while immersed in VR. Results indicated significant reductions in the time they spent thinking about their pain during a VR session compared to physical therapy sessions without VR.[121] Hoffman et al conducted a follow-up study in which they found that VR can be used over several physical therapy sessions without losing its analgesic effectiveness. Hoffman et al have also successfully reduced pain utilizing VR with a 40-year-old 19% TBSA patient undergoing wound care in a hydrotherapy tub.[122] Of greatest relevance to this chapter, researchers in Australia[95] conducted a pilot crossover study (n = 7) evaluating the efficacy of usual care (pharmacological analgesia alone) versus a VR game plus usual care in decreasing procedural pain in children ages 5 to 18 years with acute burn injuries. The average pain score on the faces scale for usual care was 4.1. VR, when used in conjunction with usual care, reduced the average pain score to 1.8.

Immersive VR is a powerful, technology-driven distraction technique that has been developed for use as an adjunctive nonpharmacologic analgesic with burn patients during wound care and rehabilitation. Hoffman and colleagues[120–123,125] have tested the multiple-sensory assertion that by drawing large amounts of attention into the virtual world, burn patients are left with substantially reduced conscious attention available to process incoming pain signals generated during wound care or physical therapy. Large drops in pain (eg, averaging 50% lower pain reports in VR compared to the usual care/no distraction control condition) have been achieved when burn patients were distracted with immersive VR during a single therapy session.[121] In another study, therapists conducted nearly identical active range-of-motion exercises with patients for 3 minutes with VR and 3 minutes with no VR (control condition). The therapist held the patient's injured limb (eg, arm) and moved the patient's limb through a predetermined sequence of active-assistive exercises while the patient was in VR. Each patient also participated in the control condition, during which he or she performed active-assistive physical therapy exercises with no distraction for the same amount of time he or she spent performing exercises in VR. By design, maximum active range of motion, measured using a standard goniometer, was held constant in both conditions.

Thus, the VR distraction paradigm developed by Hoffman and colleagues has demonstrated unprecedented reductions in acute pain for nonpharmacological methods in patients with burn injuries during physical therapy when range of motion is held constant. Until now, this has only been tested in various experimental frameworks, but it is expected that this will translate into a powerful pain-reduction technique that can be incorporated over the normal course of treatment for burn injuries.

### Hypnosis

Hypnosis, as it is applied in clinical/medical settings, allows patients to focus intently on a specific problem and its resolution while maintaining a comfortable state of physical relaxation. It also helps patients to enhance control over their body responses. Hypnosis is a normal state of aroused, attentive, and highly focused concentration—comparable to being so absorbed in a movie or novel that one loses awareness of his or her surroundings.[123]

In 1992 Patterson et al completed a study on rapid-induction analgesia.[90] This study revealed a reduction in both patient and staff reports of baseline pain. This intervention also impacted pain perception and anticipatory anxiety during and after burn care. There is a rich and still evolving body of evidence supporting the efficacy of hypnosis in reducing pain and anxiety related to burn care procedures.[124] Unfortunately, there are few studies using pediatric burn samples.

The earliest reports of hypnosis in burn patients noted that it must be altered as appropriate to the developmental abilities and needs of infants, children, and adolescents. Labaw,[125] in a small study of hospitalized children with burn injury (N = 23, ages 6 months to 16 years), described "trance therapy" and reported good results for the targeted problematic or disruptive behaviors. Another study described a case series of burn patients aged 10 to 62 years where a 3-step process was used in managing procedural pain and anxiety.[126] First, patients were trained in progressive muscle relaxation; then, if successful, they were trained in guided imagery; and finally, if judged likely to benefit from a deeper level of suggestion, posthypnotic suggestions were provided to induce self-hypnosis. Of concern, only 10% "achieved self-hypnosis," 27% "entered a state of hypnosis that enabled them to cope with their pain," while 82% "enjoyed some relaxation".[127(p42)] The adult studies and these early pediatric studies provided evidence that hypnosis may be a promising technique for pediatric burn patients during painful procedures.

The only controlled study of hypnosis to date conducted exclusively among pediatric burn patients (N = 23, ages 3–12 years) was conducted by Foertsch and colleagues.[99] Their multicenter controlled study used a suggestion approach, "familiar imagery treatment," versus social support in managing procedural pain during dressing changes. However, there were no group differences in pain or distress.

There have been 2 randomized controlled trials (RCTs) of hypnosis involving pediatric and adult burn patients, but they do not separately examine the effect of hypnosis in different age/developmental groups. In the first RCT, Shakebaie and his colleagues[127] conducted a randomized controlled trial of hypnotherapy versus usual care in managing burn pain. Standard trance-induction methods were used across 5 sessions, and posthypnotic suggestions targeted pain and reexperiencing. The hypnotherapy group, but not the control group, reported significant change in pain from the baseline to the fifth session and significant change in reexperiencing symptoms from the baseline to the third session and from the baseline to the fifth session. In the second RCT, Wiechman and colleagues conducted an RCT testing the efficacy of rapid-induction analgesia relative to an attention-control condition in reducing pain related to burn wound debridement.[128] Notably, relative to control, hypnotherapy significantly improved change in the affect dimension of pain from the baseline to later sessions. Taken together, the 2 RCT studies involving pediatric and adult patients indicate that hypnosis may be a viable adjunct to pharmacologic approaches. However, there were null findings from the single study of hypnosis for burn-related procedural pain conducted exclusively in children and adolescents.

## CLOSING SUMMARY

The empirical investigation of pediatric burn pain is gaining momentum. However, given the severity of pain experienced and the vulnerability of children, more attention is warranted. With knowledge from pain theories and empirical studies identifying the important role of psychological variables, opportunities for improvement are abundant. The vast scope of psychological factors implicates the entire team in the management and treatment of burn pain. From the initial contact of emergency personnel to outpatient physical therapy follow-up, each provider can have an impact. The complex interaction between developmental levels and conditioning and cognitive factors makes assessment and intervention with this population particularly challenging. Extant studies have not reliably used adequate methods of assessment and rely mainly on distraction intervention techniques and hypnosis. However, the need for a comprehensive approach has been identified in the literature. Though significantly more complicated, studies that attend to conditioning, social learning, attention, and anxiety variables in the delivery of care from start to finish may be necessary. Pain is such a powerful aversive stimulus; one or a few bad experiences can incite uncontrolled pain throughout treatment. Some important information missing from the literature includes measures typical to laboratories such as pain sensitivity, tolerance, pain threshold, and sensitivity threshold. This additional information may serve to better clarify the fluctuations in pain experienced and highlight the role of contextual as well as psychological variables. The complexity of implementing hypnosis and virtual reality is meaningful and may not be readily available to many burn centers. However, investigations utilizing these methods lie in the forefront of interventions for procedural burn pain.

## Closing Comments

Pain management remains an insidious problem in pediatric patients with burn injuries. The experience and report of pain is affected by a plethora of factors across domains, such as physical (eg, nociception), psychological (eg, developmental stage, emotional reactivity), and social (eg, attachment, support). Similarly, the burn injury and the acute, rehabilitation, and recovery phases of burn care each provide a complex psychosocial environment. For example, some patients and families may respond best to a team with an adaptable and nurturing style, while others may respond best to a regimented and reserved style. This chapter suggests some development, psychological, and social considerations to be taken into account in assessment and intervening. There are 2 other lines of research that may further enlighten future directions. First, in addition to managing the affective and sensory aspects of pain, pediatric pain management must involve managing both pain behavior in child and family and responses to pain and pain behavior in team members. Second, as a result of this, it is important when designing a burn care environment and burn care team culture that certain factors be taken into account. Key factors include the different attachment styles in their patients and the systemic dynamics of various families with various needs and strengths, and both attachment issues and system dynamics must necessarily include the members of the burn care team.

TABLE 1

Developmental considerations in the attachment, behaviors, and pain management of burned children.

| | Cognitive Abilities | Attachment | Emotional Behaviors Associated with Pain | Pain Management |
|---|---|---|---|---|
| Newborn | 1 to 4 months development of coordination between vision and prehension (hand-eye coordination) Sensorimotor stage initiates | Will look at attached parent, will turn toward attached parent's voice | Withdrawal Crying Facial expressions | **Relaxation:** Soothing voice **Distraction:** Singing, changing colors or lights on wall, mother nursing during procedures when possible **Psychoeducation:** Prepare parent and explain to parent that infant will respond in similar manner to parent's reaction |
| 6 months to 2 years | Sensorimotor experience continues and the development of essential spatial abilities and understanding of the world Can identify painful situations | Will look for attached parent for comfort and security Will reach for attached parent for comfort and security | Crying Anger Sadness Anxiety | **Relaxation:** Blowing bubbles, comfort object (teddy bear, blanket) **Distraction:** Music, singing, cartoons **Psychoeducation:** Burn doll to explain procedures |
| 3 to 5 years | Symbolic thinking (child learns to use and represent objects by images and words) Initial manifestation of pain intensity Will use intuitive rather than logical reasoning | Will ask for attached parent for comfort and security: "I want mommy first" | Crying Screaming Avoiding treatment room | **Relaxation:** Blowing bubbles to promote slow, deep breathing **Distraction:** Singing, pictures of loved ones, playing with a toy **Psychoeducation:** Burn doll to explain procedures |
| 6 to 12 years | Develops skills to think logically about events and will use multiple aspects of a problem to solve it Can clearly differentiate levels of pain intensity | Will seek attached parent for comfort but will also accept others' comfort and support during painful procedures if parents not available | Attach feelings to pain | **Relaxation:** Deep breathing **Distraction:** Virtual reality, playing video games, watching DVDs, hearing stories **Psychoeducation:** Verbally explain as requested and child's ability to tolerate details of medical procedures. Should remain concrete in description |
| Adolescents | Able to think logically and able to reason Will report pain intensity and quality of pain and pain-related affects | Will consult and collaborate with parents about treatment decisions | Fear Anxiety Depression | **Relaxation:** Deep breathing **Distraction:** Virtual reality, joking, guided imagery, pleasant imagery, playing video games **Psychoeducation:** Verbally explain as requested details of medical procedures; explain role of medication to control pain and how relaxation enhances effects |

# REFERENCES

1. McCaig L, Nawar E. National Hospital Ambulatory Medical Care Survey; National Ambulatory Medical Care Survey; Medical Expenditure Panel; CPSC/NEISS National Electronic Injury Surveillance System, 2000-2004 data. *Advance Data* 2006 (372).

2. Latenser B, Miller S, Bessey P, Browning S, et al. National Burn Repository 2006: A Ten Year Review. 2007 (28) 5.

3. International Association for the Study of Pain Web site. http://www.iasp-pain.org/AM/Template.cfm?Section=Pain_ Definitions&Template=/CM/HTMLDisplay.cfm&ContentID= 1728#Pain. Accessed February 10, 2009. It is a particular page within the site that identifies itself as "Part III: Pain Terms, A Current List with Definitions and Notes on Usage" (pp 209-214) Classification of Chronic Pain, Second Edition, IASP Task Force on Taxonomy, edited by H. Merskey and N. Bogduk, IASP Press, Seattle, © 1994.

4. Spence NA, Miller M, Hendricks L. Perception of burn injury pain in relation to other painful experiences of the pediatric burn patient: a descriptive study. *Child Health Care*. 1991; 21 3: 163–167.

5. Zeitlin REK. Long-term psychosocial sequelae of paediatric burns. *Burns*. 1997; **23**: 467–472.

6. Stoddard FJ, Ronfeldt H, Kagan J, et al. Young burn children; the course of acute stress and physiological and behavioral responses. *Am J Psychiatry*. 2006; **163**: 1084–1090.

7. Rose M, Sanford A, Thomas C, Opp MR. Factors altering the sleep of burned children. *Sleep*. 2001; **23**: 45–51.

8. Treede RD, Kenshalo DR, Gracely RH, Jones AKP. The cortical representation of pain. *Pain*. 1999; **79**: 105–111.

9. Schaible HG. The neurophysiology of pain. In: Isenberg D, Maddison P, Glass D, Breedveld F, eds. *The Oxford Textbook of Rheumatology*. 3rd ed. New York, NY: Oxford University Press; 2005.

10. Chambliss CR, Anand KJ. Pain management in the pediatric intensive unit. *Curr Opin Pediatr*. 1997; **9**: 246–253.

11. Ptacek J, Patterson D, Montgomery K, Heimbach D. Pain, coping and adjustment in patients with burns: preliminary findings from a prospective study. *J Pain Symptom Manage*. 1995; 10: 446–455.

12. Shalev AY, Peri T, Canetti L, Schreiber S. Predictors of PTSD in injured trauma survivors: a prospective study. *Am J Psychiatry*. 1996; **153**: 219–225.

13. Stoddard FJ, Ronfeldt H, Kagan J, et al. Young burned children: the course of acute stress and physiological and behavioral responses. *Am J Psychiatry*. 2006; **163**: 1084–1090.

14. Saxe GN, Stoddard F, Hall E, et al. Pathways to PTSD, part 1: children with burns. *Am J Psychiatry*. 2005; **162**: 1299–1304.

15. Brill JE. Control of pain. *Critical Care Clin*. 1992; **8**: 203–218.

16. Latarjet J, Choinere M. Pain in burn patients. *Burns*. 1995; 21: 344–348.

17. Anand KJ, Craig KD. New perspectives on the definition of pain. *Pain*. 1996; **67**: 3–6.

18. Patterson D. Practical applications of psychological techniques in controlling burn pain. *J Burn Care Rehabil* 1992; **13**: 13–18.

19. Hennes H, Kim MK, Pirrallo RG. Prehospital pain management: a comparison of providers' perceptions and practices. *Prehosp Emerg Care*. 2005; **9**: 32–39.

20. Sheridan RL. Burn care: results of technical and organizational progress. *JAMA*. 2003; **290**: 719–722.

21. Weisman SJ, Bernstein B, Schechter NL. Consequences of inadequate analgesia during painful procedures in children. *Arch Pediatr Adolesc Med*. 1998; **152**: 147–149.

22. Loeser JD, Melzack R. Pain: an overview. *Lancet*. 1999; **353**: 1607–1609.

23. Schaible H, Richter F. Pathophysiology of pain. *Langenbecks Arch Surg*. 2004; **389**: 237–243.

24. Ingelmo PM, Fumagalli R. Neuropathic pain in children. *Minerva Anestesiol*. 2004; **70**: 393–398.

25. Melzack R, Isreal R, Lacroix R, Schultz G. Phantom limbs in people with congenital limb deficiency or amputation in early childhood. *Brain*. 1997; **120**: 1603–1620.

26. Patterson DR, Ptacek JT, Corrougher G, Heimbach DM, Sharar SR, Norari S. PRN vs regularly scheduled opioid analgesics in pediatric burn patients. *J Burn Care Rehabil*. 2002; **23**: 424–430.

27. Olivar H, Sharar S, Gibran N. Pain management in the burned child. In: Phillips B, ed. *Pediatric Burns*. Amherst, NY: Cambria Press; forthcoming.

28. Turk D. Physiological and psychological bases of pain. In: Baum A, Revenson T, Singer J, eds. *Handbook of Health Psychology*. Mahwah, NJ: Lawrence Erlbaum & Associates; 2001,

29. Melzack R, Wall PD. *The Challenge of Pain*. New York, NY: Basic Books; 1982.

30. Melzack R, Wall PD, Ty TC. Acute pain in an emergency clinic: latency of onset and descriptor patterns related to different injuries. *Pain*. 1982; **14**: 33–43.

31. Beecher HK. Limiting factors in experimental pain. *J Chronic Dis*. 1956; **4**: 11–21.

32. Beutler LE, Engle D, Oro'-Beutler ME, Daldrup R, Meredith K. Inability to express intense affect: a common link between depression and pain? *J Consult Clin Psychol*. 1986; **54**: 752–759.

33. Melzack R, Wall P. Pain mechanisms: a new theory. *Science*. 1965; **150**: 971–979.

34. Melzack R. The McGill pain questionnaire; major properties and scoring methods. *Pain*. 1975; **1**: 277–299.

35. Melzack R. Phantom limbs and the concept of a neuromatrix. *Trends Neurosci*. 1990; **13**: 88–92.

36. Melzack R. The McGill pain questionnaire: from description to measurement. *Anesthesiology*. 2005; **103**: 199–202.

37. Turk D, Melzack R, eds. *Handbook of Pain Assessment*. New York, NY: Guilford Publications; 2001.

38. Wall P, Melzack R, eds. *Textbook of Pain*. Edinburgh, Scotland: Churchill Livingston Publishers; 1999.

39. American Psychological Association. *Diagnostic and Statistical Manual of Mental Disorders IV Text Revision*. Washington, DC: American Psychiatric Association; 2000.

40. Laor N, Wolmer L, Cohen DJ. Mothers' functioning and children's functioning 5 years after a SCUD missile attack. *Am J Psychiatry*. 2001; **158**: 1020–1026.

41. Dise-Lewis JE. A developmental perspective on psychological principles of burn care. *J Burn Care Rehabil*. 2001; **22**: 255–260.

42. Piaget J. The development of time concepts in the child. Proceedings of the Annual Meeting of the American Psychopathology Association. This was the best I could get. 1954: 34–55.

43. Patterson D. Non-opioid-based approaches to burn pain. *J Burn Care Rehabil*. 1995; **16**: 372–376.

44. Rescorla RA. Pavlovian conditioning: It's not what you think. *Am Psychol*. 1988; **43**: 151–161.

45. Beales JG. Factors influencing the expectation of pain among patients in a children's burn unit. *Burns*. 1983; **9**: 187–192.

46. Skinner BF. *The Behavior of Organisms*. New York, NY: Appelton-Century Crofts; 1938.

47. Skinner BF, Morse WH. Fixed interval reinforcement of running in a wheel. *J Exp Analysis Behavior*. 1958; **1**: 371–379.

48. Thurber CA, Martin-Herz SP, Patterson DR. Psychological principles of burn wound pain in children. 1: Theoretical framework. *J Burn Care Rehabil*. 2000; **21**: 376–387.

49. Patterson D. Non-opioid based approaches to burn pain. *J Burn Care Rehabil*. 1995; **16**: 372–376.

50. Martin-Herz SP, Patterson DR, Honari S, Gibbons J, Gibran N, Heimbach DM. Pediatric pain control practice of North American burn centers. *J Burn Care Rehabil*. 2003; **24**: 26–36.

51. Bandura A. Social learning of moral judgments. *J Pers Soc Psychol*. 1969; **11**: 275–279.

52. Mowrer OH. *Learning Theory and Behavior*. New York, NY: Wiley; 1960.

53. Delprato DJ, McGlynn FD. Behavioral theories of anxiety disorders. In: Turner SM, ed. *Behavioral Treatment of Anxiety Disorders*. New York, NY: Plenum; 1984: 63–122.

54. Lang PJ. A bio-informational theory of emotional imagery. *Psychophysiology*. 1971; **16**: 495–512.

55. Barlow DH. *Anxiety and Its Disorders: The Nature and Treatment of Anxiety and Panic*. New York, NY: Guilford Press; 1988.

56. Mash EJ, Barkley RA, eds. *Treatment of Childhood Disorders*. New York, NY: Guilford; 1998.

57. Turk D, Meichenbaum D, Genest M. *Pain and Behavioral Medicine*. New York, NY: Guilford; 1983.

58. Meyer D. Children's responses to nursing attire. *Pediatr Nursing*. 1992; **18**: 157–160.

59. Johnson JE, Leventhal H. Effects of accurate expectations and behavioral instructions on reactions during a noxious medical examination. *J Pers Soc Psychol*. 1974; **29**: 710–718.

60. Everett JJ, Patterson DR, Chen AC. Cognitive and behavioral treatment for burn pain. *Pain Clin*. 1990; **3**: 133–135.

61. Lu Q, Tsao JI, Myers CD, Kim SC, Zeltzer LK. Coping predictors of children's laboratory induced pain tolerance, intensity, and unpleasantness. *J Pain*. 2007; **8**: 708–717.

62. Walter LS, Baber KF, Garber J, Smith CA. A typology of coping strategies in pediatric patients with chronic abdominal pain. *Pain*. 2008; **137**: 266–275.

63. Forys KL, Dahlquist LM. The influence of preferred coping style and cognitive strategy on laboratory induced pain. *Health Psychol*. 2007; **26**: 22–29.

64. Haythornthwaite JA, Menefee LA, Heinberg LJ, Clark MR. Pain coping strategies predict perceived control over pain. *Pain*. 1988; **77**: 33–39.

65. Martin-Herz SP, Thurber CA, Patterson DR. Psychological principles of burn wound pain in children. II: Treatment applications. *J Burn Care Rehabil*. 2000; **21**: 458–472.

66. Edwards RR, Haythornthwaite JA, Sullivan MJ, Fillingim RB. Catastrophizing as a mediator of sex differences in pain: differential effects for daily pain versus laboratory-induced pain. *Pain*. 2004; **111**: 335–341.

67. Sullivan MJ, Martel MO, Tripp DA, Crombez G. Catastrophic thinking and heightened perception of pain in others. *Pain*. 2006; **123**: 37–44.

68. Vervoort T, Goubert L, Eccleston C, et al. The effects of parental presence upon the facial expression of pain: the moderating role of child pain catastrophizing. *Pain*. 2008; **138**: 277–285.

69. Haythornthwaite JA, Menefee LA, Heinberg LJ, Clark MR. Pain coping strategies predict perceived control over pain. *Pain*. 1998; **77**: 33.

70. Fauerbach JA, Engrav L, Kowalske K, et al. Barriers to employment among working-aged patients with major burn injury. *J Burn Care Rehabil*. 2001; **22**: 26–32.

71. Tarnowski KJ, McGrath ML, Calhoun MB, Drabman RS. Pediatric burn injury: self- versus therapist-mediated debridement. *J Pediatr Psychol*. 1987; **12**: 567–579.

72. Kavanagh C. Alternative approach to burned children. *Am J Psychiatry*. 1983; **140**: 268–269.

73. Thompson SC. Will it hurt less if I can control it? A complex answer to a simple question. *Psychol Bull*. 1981; **90**: 89–101.

74. Zeltzer LK, Tsao JC. What's in a face: can parents "read pain" in their children's faces? *Pain*. 2006; **126**: 64–71.

75. Lu Q, Zeltzer LK, Tsao JC, Kim SC, Turk N, Naliboff BD. Heart rate mediation of sex differences in pain tolerance in children. *Pain*. 2005; **118**: 185–193.

76. Martin-Herz SP, Patterson DR, Honadi S, Gibbons J, Gibran N, Heimbach DM. Pediatric pain control practices of North American burn centers. *J Burn Care Rehabil*. 2003; **24**: 26–36.

77. Cohen LL, Lemanek K, Blount RL, Dahlquist LM. Evidence-based assessment of pediatric pain. *J Pediatr Psychol*. 2008; **33**: 939–955.

78. Stinson JN, Kavanagh T, Yamada J, Gill N, Stevens B. Systematic review of the psychometric properties interpretability measures for use in clinical trials in children and adolescents. *Pain.* 2006; **125:** 143–157.

79. von Baeyer CL. Understanding and managing children's recurrent pain in primary care: a biopsychosocial perspective. *Paediatric Child Health.* 2007; **12:** 121–150.

80. von Baeyer CL, Spragrud LJ. Systematic review of observational (behavioral) measures of pain for children and adolescents aged 3 to 18 years. *Pain.* 2007; **127:** 140–150.

81. Ratcliff SL, Brown A, Rosenburg L, et al. The effectiveness of a pain and anxiety protocol to treat the acute pediatric burn patient. *J Burns.* 2006; **32:** 554–562.

82. Schechter NL, Berde CB, Yaster M. Pain in infants, children and adolescents: an overview. In: Schechter NL, Berde CB, Yaster M, eds. *Pain in Infants, Children and Adolescents.* 2nd ed. Philadelphia, PA: Lippincott, Williams, & Wilkins; 2002: 3–18.

83. Meyer WJ III, Brown A, Villarreal C, et al. Reduction in acute stress disorder incidence in acute burn survivors after more intense pain and anxiety management. In: *2001 Proceedings of the 9th Congress of the European Burn Association.*

84. Zeitlin R. Long-term psychosocial sequelae of pediatric burns. *Burns.* 1997; **23:** 467–472.

85. Meyer WJ III, Marvin JA, Patterson DR, Thomas C, Blakeney PE. Management of pain and other discomforts in burned patients. In: Herndon DN, ed. *Total Burn Care.* 2nd ed. New York, NY: WB Saunders; 2002: 747–765.

86. Carrougher GJ, Ptacek JT, Sharar SR, et al. A comparison of patient satisfaction and self-reports of pain in adult burn-injured patients. *J Burn Care Rehabil.* 2003; **24:** 1–8.

87. Choiniere M, Melzack R, Rondeau J, Girard N, Paquin MJ. The pain burns: characteristics and correlates. *J Trauma.* 1989; **29:** 1531–1539.

88. Perry S, Heidrich G, Ramos E. Assessment of pain by burn patients. *J Burn Care Rehabil.* 1981; **2:** 322–327.

89. Hoffman HG, Patterson DR, Carrougher GJ, Sharar SR. Effectiveness of virtual reality-based pain control with multiple treatments. *Clin J Pain.* 2001; **17:** 229–235.

90. Patterson DR, Everett JJ, Burns GL, Marvin JA. Hypnosis for the treatment of burn pain. *J Consult Clin Psychol.* 1992; **60:** 713–717.

91. Hernandez-Reif M, Field T, Largie S, et al. Children's distress during burn treatment is reduced by massage therapy. *J Burn Care Rehabil.* 2001; **22:** 191–195.

92. Kavanagh C. Psychological intervention with the severely burned child: report of an experimental comparison of two approaches and their effects on psychological sequelae. *J Am Acad Child Psychiatry.* 1983; **22:** 145–156.

93. Whitehead-Pleaux AM, Baryza MJ, Sheridan RL. The effects of music therapy on pediatric patient's pain and anxiety during donor site dressing change. *J Music Ther.* 2006; **43:** 136–153.

94. Das DA, Grimmer KA, Sparnon AL, McRae SE, Thomas BH. The efficacy of playing virtual reality game in modulating pain for children with acute burn injuries: a randomized controlled trial. *BMC Pediatr.* 2005; **5:** 1–10.

95. Foertsch CE, O'Hara MW, Stoddard FJ, Kealey GP. Treatment of resistant pain and distress during pediatric burn dressing changes. *J Burn Care Rehabil.* 1998; **19:** 219–224.

96. Landolt MA, Marti MD, Widmer MA, Meuli M. Does cartoon movie distraction decrease burned children's pain behavior? *J Burn Care Rehabil.* 2002; **23:** 61–65.

97. Kelley ML, Jarvie GJ, Middlebrook JL, McNeer MF, Drabman RS. Decreasing burned children's pain behavior: impacting the trauma of hydrotherapy. *J Appl Behav Anal.* 1984; **17:** 147–158.

98. Doctor ME. Parent participation during painful wound care procedures. *J Burn Care Rehabil.* 1994; **15:** 288–292.

99. Foertsch CE, O'Hara MW, Stoddard FJ, Kealey GP. Parent participation during burn debridement in relation to behavioral distress. *J Burn Care Rehabil.* 1996; **17:** 372–377.

100. Hanson MD, Gauld M, Wathen CN, MacMillan HL. Nonpharmacological interventions for acute wound care distress in pediatric patients with burn injury: a systematic review. *J Burn Care Res.* 2008; **29:** 730–741.

101. Whitehead-Pleaux AM, Zebrowski N, Baryza MJ, Sheridan RL. Exploring the effects of music therapy on pediatric pain: phase 1. *J Music Ther.* 2007; **44:** 217–241.

102. Sharar SR, Carrougher GJ, Nakamura D, Hoffman HG, Blough DK, Patterson, DR. Factors influencing the efficacy of virtual reality distraction analgesia during postburn physical therapy: preliminary results from 3 ongoing studies. *Arch Phys Med Rehabil.* 2007; **88:** S43–S49.

103. Van Twillert B, Bremen M, Faber AW. Computer generated virtual reality to control pain and anxiety in pediatric and adult burn patients during wound dressing changes. *J Burn Care Res.* 2007; **28:** 694–702.

104. Chan EA, Cheng JWY, Wong TKS, Lein ASY, Yang JY. Application of a virtual reality prototype for pain relief of pediatric burn in Taiwan. *J Clin Nurs.* 2007; **16:** 786–793.

105. Patterson, D. Non-opioid-based approaches to burn pain. *J Burn Care Rehabil.* 1995; **16:** 372–376.

106. Haythornthwaite JA, Lawrence JW, Fauerbach JA. Brief cognitive interventions for burn pain. *Ann Behav Med.* 2001; **23:** 42–49.

107. Miller AC, Hickman LC, Lemasters GK. A distraction technique for control of burn pain. *J Burn Care Rehabil.* 1992; **13:** 576–580.

108. McCaul KD, Malott JM. Distraction and coping with pain. *Psychol Bull.* 1984; **95:** 516–533.

109. Bonham A. Managing procedural pain in children with burns. Part 1: assessment of pain in children. *Int J Trauma Nurs.* 1996; **2:** 68–73.

110. Kelly M, Jarvie G, Middlebrook J, McNeer M, Drabman R. Decreasing burned children's pain behavior: impacting the trauma of hydrotherapy. 1984 (17)2: 147–158.

111. Landolt MA, Marti D, Widmer J, Meuli M. Does cartoon distraction decrease burned children's pain behavior? *J Burn Care Rehabil*. 2002; **23:** 61–65.

112. Dise-Lewis JE. A developmental perspective on psychological principles of burn care. *J Burn Care Rehabil*. 2001; **22:** 255–260.

113. Dahlquist LM, McKenna KD, Jones KK, Dillinger L, Weiss KE, Ackerman C. Active and passive distraction using head-mounted display helmet effects on cold pressor pain in children. *Health Psychol*. 2007; **26:** 794–801.

114. Wickens CD. Multiple resources and performance prediction. *Theor Issues Ergonom Sci*. 2002; **3:** 150–177.

115. Dahlquist LM, Busby SM, Slifer KJ, et al. Distraction for children of different ages who undergo repeated needle sticks. *J Pediatr Oncol Nurs*. 2002; **19:** 22–34.

116. Dahlquist LM, Pendley J, Landthrip D, Jones C, Steuber CP. Distraction intervention for preschoolers undergoing intramuscular injections and subcutaneous port access. *Health Psychol*. 2002; **21:** 94–99.

117. Pringle B, Hilley L, Gelfand K, et al. Decreasing child distress during needle sticks and maintaining treatment gains over time. *J Clin Psychol Med Settings*. 2001; **8:** 119–130.

118. Hoffman HG, Doctor JN, Patterson DR, Carrougher GJ, Furness TA III. Virtual reality as an adjunctive pain control during burn wound care in adolescent patients. *J Pain*. 2000; **85:** 305–309.

119. Hoffman HG, Patterson DR, Carrougher GJ. Use of virtual reality for adjunctive treatment of adult burn pain during physical therapy: a controlled study. *Clin J Pain*. 2000; **16:** 244–250.

120. Hoffman HG, Patterson DR, Carrougher GJ, Sharar SR. Effectiveness of virtual reality-based pain control with multiple treatments. *Clin J Pain*. 2001; **17:** 229–235.

121. Hoffman HG, Patterson DR, Carrougher GJ, Sharar SR. Water-friendly virtual reality pain control during wound care. *J Clin Psychol*. 2004; **60:** 189–195.

122. Hoffman HG, Sharar SR, Coda B, et al. Manipulating presence influences the magnitude of virtual reality analgesia. *Pain*. 2004; **111:** 162–168.

123. Stanford Center for Integrative Medicine of the Stanford Hospital and Clinics Web site. http://www.stanfordhospital.com/clinicsmedServices/clinics/complementaryMedicine/hypnosis.html. Accessed January 20, 2009.

124. deJong AE, Middelkoop E, Faber AW, Van Lowy NE. Non-pharmacological nursing interventions for procedural pain relief in adults with burns: a systematic literature review. *Burns*. 2007; **33**(7): 811–827.

125. Labaw WL. Adjunctive trance therapy with severely burned children. *Int J Child Psychiatry*. 1973; (2): 80–92.

126. Gilboa D, Borenstein A, Seidman DS, Tsur H. Burn patients' use of autohypnosis: making a painful experience bearable. *Burns*. 1990; **16**(6): 441–444.

127. Shakebaie F, Barandi AA, Gholamrezai A, Samoei R, Salehi P. Hypnotherapy in management of pain and reexperiencing of trauma in burn patients. *Int J Clin Exp Hypn*. 2008; **56**(2): 185–197.

128. Askay SW, Patterson D, Jensen M, Sharar S. A randomized controlled trial of hypnosis for burn wound care. *Rehab Psychol*. 2007; **52**(3): 247–253.

# CHAPTER TWENTY-SEVEN

# PSYCHOSOCIAL ASPECTS OF PEDIATRIC BURN CARE

JENNIFER L. PERRY, PhD, INSTRUCTOR (PSYCHOLOGY), DEPARTMENT OF SURGERY*

SHERRI A. SHARP, PhD, PSYCHOLOGIST, DEPARTMENT OF PSYCHOLOGICAL AND PSYCHIATRIC SERVICES+
CLINICAL INSTRUCTOR, DEPARTMENT OF PSYCHIATRY AND BEHAVIORAL SCIENCES*

MARTA A. ROSENBERG, PhD, PSYCHOLOGIST, DEPARTMENT OF PSYCHOLOGICAL AND PSYCHIATRIC SERVICES+
CLINICAL ASSISTANT PROFESSOR, DEPARTMENT OF PSYCHIATRY AND BEHAVIORAL SCIENCES*

LAURA E. ROSENBERG, PhD, CHIEF PSYCHOLOGIST, DEPARTMENT OF PSYCHOLOGICAL AND PSYCHIATRIC SERVICES+
CLINICAL ASSISTANT PROFESSOR, DEPARTMENT OF PSYCHIATRY AND BEHAVIORAL SCIENCES*

WALTER J. MEYER III, MD, GLADYS KEMPNER AND R. LEE KEMPNER PROFESSOR OF CHILD PSYCHIATRY,
DEPARTMENT OF PSYCHIATRY AND BEHAVIORAL SCIENCES*
DIRECTOR, DEPARTMENT OF PSYCHOLOGICAL AND PSYCHIATRIC SERVICES+

* THE UNIVERSITY OF TEXAS MEDICAL BRANCH (UTMB)
+ SHRINERS HOSPITALS FOR CHILDREN–GALVESTON (SHC-G)

## INTRODUCTION

Suffering a burn injury can be a frightening and overwhelming experience for both a child and his or her family. The role of mental health staff in a pediatric burn unit is ongoing, with the goal of easing the discomfort and assisting in the psychosocial recovery of the patient and his or her family. Services these professionals provide include supportive counseling, interventions for anxiety, depression, grief and loss, and community reentry.

## INITIAL CLINICAL INTERVIEW

The first step for mental health professionals is to conduct a clinical interview with the caregiver upon the patient's initial acute admission. The primary objective during this interview is to gather pertinent information about the burn incident, assess the needs of the patient and family, provide support, and plan interventions. If abuse and/or neglect are suspected by hospital staff or from the referring hospital, a report to the state's Child Protective Services (CPS) or an equivalently named state agency may be warranted in some cases.

Vital information to be collected during this interview includes family constellation and dynamics, coping resources, and recent environmental stress as well as the patient's preinjury development and mental health status. Of note, preburn behavioral problems have been found in pediatric burn patients.[1-3] The child's current psychological functioning also needs to be assessed, specifically, symptoms of delirium, psychosis, anxiety, depression, and general discomfort. In addition, a detailed history of the burn injury needs to be obtained, which can be particularly important if there is a reason to suspect abuse or neglect. Based on the information gathered, a plan of care for both the patient and family should be developed and agreed upon, and all relevant parties should be informed of this plan.

## Abuse and/or Neglect

The federal definition of child abuse and neglect is described as

> at a minimum, any recent act or failure to act on the part of a parent or caretaker, which results in death, serious physical or emotional harm, sexual abuse or exploitation, or an act or failure to act which presents an imminent risk of serious harm.[4]

Documented prevalence rates for pediatric burn injuries caused by abuse or neglect vary, as there are different methods used by hospitals to classify cases. In a study conducted in the United Kingdom, 40.5% of persons aged 16 years and younger suffered burn injuries with a cause that generated "concern" by medical staff. Of these children, 0.9% and 9.3% were found to have sustained their injuries as a consequence of abuse or neglect, respectively.[5] In a US sample of children aged 12 years and younger, nearly 6% were suspected by medical staff to have received their burn injuries as a result of abuse.[6]

### Risk Factor Assessment

As part of the intake process, mental health professionals should gather information from the family about the nature of the burn injury and, in consultation with physicians, consider the plausibility and consistency of the story. In addition, behavioral observations, such as caregiver-child interactions, as well as the presence of any risk factors for abuse or neglect should be noted. However, the presence of a risk factor is not evidence of abuse or neglect, and it is important that any assessment be evaluated in the context of the family's culture and environmental circumstances. An example of a risk factor checklist, developed by Rhonda Robert, PhD, can be found in the book *Total Burn Care*.[7]

### Reporting Process

Every state mandates reporting of suspected child abuse and neglect, and nearly all states identify persons in certain professional classes who are required to report (eg, physicians, teachers, mental health professionals).[8] The Childhelp USA National Child Abuse Hotline can be contacted at 1-800-4-A-CHILD (1-800-422-4453) for information and guidance on the reporting process. The obligation to report suspicion of abuse or neglect in other countries may vary (eg, in Mexico, the appropriate agency is Desarrollo Integral de la Familia [DIF]).

Although not required, mental health professionals may chose to inform families that a report will be (or has been) made, explaining the reason and legal mandate. Moreover, in the case of neglect (or accidents), it is helpful to provide home safety information to families, including a handout listing products (eg, cabinet door locks, outlet covers, and so on). A request for a home visit and/or parenting training can also be made to the appropriate state agency at the time a report is made.

## PATIENT ASSESSMENT

From the time of admission to the inpatient unit, patients should be assessed daily for symptoms of psychological distress. In particular, signs of the following conditions should be considered: sleep disturbance, delirium, and psychosis as well as anxiety and depressive symptoms. Particular attention should also be paid to any losses the patient has suffered. When completing an assessment, patients are the ideal respondents; however, because patients may be asleep, sedated, and/or involved in a medical procedure, parents, caregivers, physicians, nurses, and other staff members should also be utilized as informants for the patient's possible symptoms.

## Sleep Disturbance

Sleep disturbance is a common phenomenon among adult[9] and pediatric burn patients.[10] Sleep disruption can be due to a multitude of factors, such as continuous light in the patient's room, numerous noises, and the performance of various medical procedures during nighttime (eg, changing dressings, cleaning wounds, drawing blood, giving medications, and taking vital signs). In addition, a patient's sleep can be disturbed due to inadequate pain and/or anxiety management.

Treatment for sleep disturbance should begin with an assessment of the patient's experience of pain and anxiety, and if warranted, medication should be given for these conditions (treatment for anxiety will be discussed later in this chapter). In addition, good sleep hygiene should be established in order to reinstitute the patient's normal circadian wake/sleep cycle, which will also help in the outpatient phase of recovery. Sleep hygiene can be established by creating bedtime routines (eg, turning off the TV at a certain hour or reading a bedtime story) as well as by turning out the lights in the patient's room during nighttime. At our hospital, we have found sleep aids such as diphenhydramine (Benadryl[Rx]) 1.25 mg/kg helpful and our first choice during the first few nights. If this medication fails, benzodiazepines can be considered. Recently, Armour et al[11] also found haloperidol to be efficacious in improving sleep in pediatric burn patients, although Ratcliff et al[12] found a high incidence of side effects with haloperidol.

## Delirium and Psychosis

An evaluation should begin with the determination of the patient's mental status and orientation to person, place, time, and condition. If the patient is not oriented, is confused, and/or has deficits with mental status, delirium should be suspected. Delirium is a condition in which there is (1) a reduced awareness of the environment, with a diminished ability to focus, sustain, or shift attention, and (2) a change in cognition (eg, deficits of memory, language, or orientation). These symptoms tend to fluctuate throughout the day.[13]

If symptoms of delirium are present, it is important to first consider metabolic disorders (eg, abnormalities in blood sugar, electrolytes, and calcium), blood pressure abnormalities (too high or too low), drug reactions or withdrawal, and sepsis. There may be other causes of delirium, including severe pain, anoxia, fever, intracranial problems (eg, increased intracranial pressure), and acute renal or liver failure.

Once these medical conditions are treated and/or ruled out, if the patient is experiencing hallucinations, it can be helpful to uncover the content of the hallucinations. This can inform and guide diagnosis and treatment. For example, if the hallucinations are very bizarre or persecutory in nature, an acute brief reactive psychosis should be considered.

If the hallucinations (and possible nightmares) are related to the burn injury, acute stress disorder (ASD) may be the culprit. On the other hand, if the hallucinations are rather depressing in nature, the onset of depression may be the source (ASD and depressive symptoms and their treatments will be discussed in more detail later in the chapter).

Nonetheless, medical treatment for delirium and psychosis are similar. At our hospital, we have noted that benzodiazepines, such as lorazepam at 0.05 mg/kg every 4 hours or more often as needed, are helpful if the patient's respirations are not being suppressed. We have found lorazepam has the advantage of not severely suppressing respirations; it usually seems effective in sedating the patient to some extent. If benzodiazepines fail to sedate the individual, we consider clonidine at 3 to 5 $\propto$g/kg every 6 hours or its more active cousin, dexmedetomidine, at 0.5 $\propto$g/kg every 30 minutes (in a drip format). In extreme cases, ketamine is used at our hospital.

If the patient is experiencing psychosis and is belligerent, we might consider an antipsychotic. For children, risperidone now seems to be the drug of first choice. Traditionally, phenothiazines such as haldoperidol were used; however, we have found haldoperidol often causes dystonic reactions and can cause malignant hyperthermia.[12] If one of these reactions occurs, the diphenhydramine (Benadryl[Rx]) 50 mg IV can be given, followed by a scheduled dose of benztropine or trihexyphendyl (Artane[Rx]). If hyperthermia occurs, rapid aggressive cooling can be done and dantrolene can be given.

In addition to medical management of delirium and psychosis, we have observed that environmental manipulation can promote a calm and soothing atmosphere and reduce the patient's agitation. Examples include controlling noise and lighting as well as limiting the disruptions in the intensive care room. In addition, providing clear and simple communication, orienting the patient to reality, displaying a clock, and allowing for the presence of familiar people and objects can help.

## Anxiety

Anxiety can be a common phenomenon in pediatric burn patients, both during the acute and outpatient phases of recovery.[2,14,15] A patient may suffer symptoms of ASD or post-traumatic stress disorder (PTSD). Moreover, patients may experience anxiety that does not meet diagnostic criteria for a disorder but is nonetheless distressing to the patient and can be treated or managed. Examples include anticipatory, procedural, separation, and general anxiety, particularly as they relate to medical procedures and being in a hospital setting. In addition, anxiety surrounding social situations may occur (this topic will be discussed later in the chapter, under "Community Reentry").

## ASD/PTSD

With respect to ASD/PTSD, signs of ASD include (1) dissociation (eg, feeling numb, detached, or "in a daze"), (2) reexperiencing the trauma (eg, nightmares, flashbacks), (3) avoidance of trauma-related reminders, and (4) marked anxiety or arousal.[13] Signs of PTSD also involve reexperiencing, avoidance, and marked anxiety. In children, reexperiencing symptoms may take the form of repetitive play, reenacting the trauma, and/or experiencing frightening dreams with unrecognizable content.[13] Symptoms that present in the first month following an event are referred to as ASD, whereas those that appear or persist beyond this time period are labeled PTSD.[13]

The incidence of ASD in burn patients has been noted to range from 10% to 23% in adults[16–18] and from 8% to 31% in children.[19–21] The prevalence of PTSD in adult burn survivors has been reported to be 24% to 40%[18,22–24] at 4 to 6 months, 15% to 45% at 12 months,[18,24,25] and 25% at 2 years[18] postinjury. Moreover, in a study in which the average time since burn was 8 years, chronic PTSD was found in 36% of the adult participants.[17] The variability in prevalence rates in these studies may be a result of the assessment tool used (self-report versus clinical interview), sample characteristics and size, study design (retrospective versus prospective), and presence or absence of treatment interventions.

With respect to pediatric burn survivors, the current and lifetime rate of PTSD has been noted to be nearly 7% and 30%, respectively, for those who were children at follow-up.[14] For pediatric burn survivors who were young adults at follow-up, the current and lifetime rates of PTSD were nearly 9% and 21%, respectively, with both rates higher than those found in epidemiological samples.[15]

Predictors of ASD in adults have been noted to involve preburn mental health treatment and a burn to the head or neck, but not burn size.[18] In addition, ASD has proven to be a robust predictor of subsequent PTSD in adults,[17,18,26,27] particularly dissociative[25] and avoidant[26] symptoms. Also, the personality trait of neuroticism has been associated with PTSD.[28] However, apart from one study,[25] burn size has not been shown to be a predictor of PTSD in adults.[18,24,27,29]

Risk factors for the development of acute stress symptoms in children with burns include physiological arousal and parents' level of stress,[19,20,30] with the additional risk factors of burn size and pain in preschool age[19] and body image in school-age[20] children. Moreover, in preschool-age children, several in-hospital trauma symptoms were related to behavioral observations of concern (less smiling and vocalizations) at a 1-month follow-up.[31] Predictors of PTSD in school-age children also include burn size and pain as well as acute-phase separation anxiety and dissociative symptoms.[32]

ASD in children can be assessed with a clinical interview and/or with 1 of a number of instruments. Examples include the child stress reaction checklist, burn version (CSRS), which is a version of the child stress disorder checklist[33]; the acute stress disorder symptom checklist[34]; and the Stanford acute stress reaction questionnaire.[35] When choosing an assessment, it is important to consider the age of the child.

Concerning ASD interventions, if the patient is experiencing distressing sleep (ie, having nightmares or night terrors), he or she should not be awakened, as this may exacerbate the patient's anxiety and disrupt the sleep/wake cycle.[36] At our hospital, we have found early treatment of ASD symptoms to be efficacious in ameliorating symptoms, particularly with the use of tricyclic antidepressants (TCAs) such as imipramine[37] or amitriptyline or selective serotonin reuptake inhibitors (SSRIs) such as fluoxetine[37] or sertraline. Recently, Meighan et al[38] described the use of risperidone for these symptoms in preschoolers.

PTSD in children can also be assessed with a general clinical interview or with structured measures such as the CSRS[33]; the Missouri assessment of genetics interview for children (MAGIC)[39]; the University of California at Los Angeles post-traumatic stress disorder reaction index (UCLA-PTSD RI)[40]; or the diagnostic interview for children and adolescents (DICA).[41,42]

In terms of interventions, psychoeducation about trauma symptoms, their course, and treatment options can be provided to both the caregiver and child (if appropriate). Cognitive-behavioral therapy (CBT) is considered the standard of care for treatment of PTSD, and in review analyses, CBT has been shown to be efficacious with adults who have suffered a variety of traumas.[43–45] However, authors of a review article on psychosocial treatment for children who experienced a single-incident trauma noted it is a neglected area of research.[46] Nonetheless, CBT has demonstrated success with children who have experienced a single-incident trauma,[47,48] although it does not appear to have been studied with pediatric burn survivors. CBT can involve a number of components, such as exposure (talking or writing about the trauma) accompanied by relaxation and anxiety management techniques, cognitive restructuring of distorted thoughts (eg, "I will never be safe"), and/or desensitization.

With young children, who tend to have limited verbal skills, play therapy can be utilized. This type of intervention can involve games, dolls and other toys, music, and artwork. At our hospital, we have also found TCAs and SSRIs helpful as an adjunctive treatment for symptoms of PTSD.[37] We have found this useful, for example, in situations in which the procedure (eg, debridement/tubbing) may be similar to the original injury (eg, a scald injury in a bathtub).

### Anticipatory and Procedural Anxiety

Anticipatory anxiety refers to a fear of an upcoming event, either because the aspects of the event are unknown or because it is expected that the event will be unpleasant or painful. Procedural anxiety is fear experienced while involved in a procedure such as bathing or physical therapy.

To assess for the presence and severity of anticipatory and procedural anxiety, one can use a visual rating scale such as the fear thermometer.[49] The fear thermometer is used to have patients (or their caregivers and nurses) rate the extent of the patient's anxiety by viewing a 5-point Likert scale in the shape of thermometers. For example, to assess for anticipatory anxiety, one could ask the child, "When you are not touched and your wounds are bandaged, are you afraid? If yes, how much?" For procedural anxiety, an example question would be "When you are exercising, are you afraid? If so, how much?" Behavioral signs of possible anxiety may involve crying, clinging, and shaking.

There are different types of interventions that can help lower the patient's anticipatory or procedural anxiety, and caregivers can be encouraged to participate in these efforts. One of the more basic ways to lower anxiety is to provide the child with information about the procedure and/or surgery. This can be achieved through medical play and pre-operative education using visual aids such as medical dolls, pictures, and storybooks. Child life specialists and other mental health professionals have expertise in using these interventions.

For procedural anxiety, the child can be given some measure of control by giving him or her choices (eg, the order of procedures to be done) and/or by allowing him or her to help with some aspect of the process (eg, holding a small instrument). In addition, distraction techniques can be employed, such as engaging the child in a discussion of an interesting topic to him or her, listening to music, or participating in play. Moreover, the patient can be taught relaxation and visual imagery exercises. For example, while a child is being bathed, he or she can be guided to imagine being in a favorite vacation spot or a peaceful place. A patient experiencing procedural anxiety can also be taught positive self-talk (eg, "I can handle this") and can

be given positive reinforcement statements by caregivers and hospital staff.

At our hospital, we have also noticed that benzodiazepines can be useful in reducing anticipatory and procedural anxiety. For example, diazepam (0.1 mg/kg can be given the night before and the morning of the procedure. Alternatively, lorazepam (0.05 mg/kg/os) can be used approximately 30 to 60 minutes prior to a procedure, sometimes in combination with pain medication (eg, fentanyl, transmucosal, at 10-15 $\propto$g/kg).

### General and Separation Anxiety

Symptoms of general anxiety may also be present in the acute or outpatient phases, even if they do not meet the diagnostic threshold. In children, generalized anxiety disorder (GAD) is defined as (1) excessive worry about a number of events or activities, (2) difficulty controlling the worry, and (3) the presence of 1 or more of the following 6 symptoms: restlessness or feeling on edge, fatiguing easily, irritability, muscle tension, sleep difficulties, and difficulty concentrating. GAD must be present for at least 6 months and cause clinically significant distress.[13]

The current and lifetime incidences of GAD in pediatric burn survivors have been noted to be approximately 30% in a study in which the individual was a child or adolescent at follow-up; rates which were statistically higher than the nonburned, matched control group.[14] However, in another study in which the person was a young adult when assessed, the current and lifetime rates of GAD were both 7%, with the current rate statistically higher than found in an epidemiological sample.[15]

Separation anxiety disorder is defined as anxiety concerning separation from home or loved ones that is excessive and inappropriate and that meets the *DSM-IV* diagnostic criteria for the disorder.[13] The symptoms must be present for a month or more and cause clinically significant impairment to meet criteria. Again, subthreshold separation anxiety may be present. The lifetime prevalence rate for separation anxiety disorder in children with burns has been observed to be nearly 7% at follow-up, which was not statistically different from a nonburned, matched control group.[14]

Symptoms of general anxiety and/or separation anxiety can be assessed with a general clinical interview. CBT has proven to be helpful in treating adults with GAD[50] and children with anxiety disorders.[51] At our hospital, we have found education and reassurance helpful, as well as allowing the child to have a personal item of comfort with him or her. We have also found scheduled diazepam (0.1 mg/kg every 8 hours) given over the weeks and months following the injury to be beneficial with symptoms of general anxiety.[21] In addition, medications such as fluoxetine (an SSRI) can be useful for both general and separation anxiety.

## Depressive Symptoms

Depressive symptoms can be common in pediatric burn patients, either during the acute or outpatient phases of recovery.[2,14,15] These symptoms may meet the diagnostic criteria for major depressive disorder or dysthymic disorder, or the symptoms may be subthreshold. Regardless, depressive symptoms can be addressed with counseling and/or medications.

Signs of major depressive disorder include 5 or more of the following: (1) depressed mood, (2) diminished interest in usual activities, (3) significant weight changes, (4) sleep difficulties, (5) restlessness or lethargy, (6) low energy, (7) excessive guilt, (8) difficulty concentrating, and (9) suicidal thoughts and/or behaviors.[13] These symptoms must be present for at least 2 weeks. Dysthymic disorder is a disorder in which there is a chronic depressed mood for most of the day, nearly every day, for at least a year (in children and adolescents).[13]

In adult burn survivors, the prevalence of major depressive disorder while in the acute phase has been noted to be about 4%.[23,52] Moderate depressive symptoms occurred in about 23% to 26% and severe depressive symptoms in 4% to 10% of adult patients within the first 10 days of hospitalization.[53,54] To our knowledge, the prevalence of depressive symptoms in pediatric burn patients while in the hospital has not been established.

Moderate to severe depressive symptoms in adults have been observed in 23% to 54% at 1 to 2 months,[23,53-55] 34% at 1 year,[23,52,55] and 45% at 2 years[55] postburn. A formal diagnosis of major depressive disorder has also been found in 7% to 10% and dysthymic disorder in 0% to 3% of adult burn survivors at 1 year following injury.[23,52] In addition, moderate to severe depressive symptoms were found in 18% to 30% of burn survivors in studies in which the average time since injury was at least 7 years.[56,57]

In terms of depressive symptoms in children postdischarge, Stoddard et al[14] conducted a study in which the average time since burn was nearly 9 years. Results revealed that the current (past month) and lifetime prevalence rates for major depressive disorder were 3% and 26%, respectively; the lifetime rate was higher than but not statistically different from the nonburned, matched control group. In addition, the incidences of current and lifetime dysthymic disorder in the sample were both 10%, which was also not statistically different from the control group.[14] However, Meyer et al[15] studied pediatric burn survivors who were young adults at follow-up, with an average time since injury of 14 years. Results indicated the current and

lifetime prevalence of major depressive disorder was 9% and 33%, respectively, with both rates higher than those in epidemiological samples.[15] The lifetime rate of dysthymic disorder was 6%.[15]

Predictors of depressive symptoms in adults while in the hospital include trait anxiety[53] and an ambivalent coping style,[58] and at 1 year postinjury include female gender and a burn to the head or neck.[55] At long-term follow-up, factors related to social comfort as well as body image and function were associated with depressive symptoms.[56,57] However, burn size was not predictive of depressive symptoms for adults at any of these time points.[53,55-57] In a similar manner, in 1 study, burn size did not appear to be related to depressive symptoms in children at a long-term follow-up.[59]

During the acute phase, a diagnosis of major depressive disorder can be difficult to make; some of the symptoms of this disorder are consistent with the patient's medical condition or may be due to other factors (eg, significant weight changes, low energy, sleep difficulties, or bereavement). Therefore, depressive symptoms may be identified by asking the patient about his or her mood, through behavioral observations, and/or via caregiver and health care staff reports. Depressive symptoms can be assessed with a clinical interview or with brief self-report assessments such as the child depression inventory.[60]

Concerning interventions, in a recent review of the literature on burn injuries and depression, Thombs et al[61] discovered there were no studies focusing on treatment and no recent investigations focusing on children. Nevertheless, the standard of care for treatment of depressive symptoms in adults[62-64] and children[65,66] is psychotherapy (eg, CBT) and/or medication.

## Grief and Loss

When children have been exposed to traumatic events, in addition to experiencing symptoms of anxiety and depression, they may be vulnerable to grief reactions.[67-70] The terms *bereavement*, *grief*, *traumatic grief*, and *mourning* can be confusing; however, they have distinct meanings.[68] *Bereavement* is defined as the experiences felt following the death of a loved one.[71] *Grief* is a more general term referring to the natural responses to loss, which include emotional, cognitive, behavioral, and physical reactions[68,72]; *traumatic grief* is characterized by the combination of post-traumatic stress and unresolved grief symptoms.[68,69] *Mourning*, on the other hand, is the process of responding to loss and is supported by cultural, family, and religious practices.[71,72]

Recently, research has focused on differentiating normal childhood grief responses to those of traumatic grief with children who experienced various types of trauma (eg, war, terrorism, natural disasters). Brown and Goodman[68] investigated the reactions of children who lost their fathers on the tragedy of September 11 and found that children who experienced normal grief responses retained a positive memory and an ongoing presence of their loved one. In contrast, children who suffered from traumatic grief had difficulty progressing through the normal grieving process, experienced post-traumatic stress disorder symptoms, and evidenced impairments in their general functioning.

Other studies have demonstrated the efficacy of treating childhood traumatic grief through cognitive-behavioral therapy or client-centered therapy.[69,73–75] However, few studies have examined the normal grief reactions of and interventions for children who sustained burns. Children who suffer burn injuries may face multiple changes and losses, such as separation from their home and loved ones, hospitalization, disfigurement, and, in some cases, death of a loved one or pet. These experiences can be confusing and frightening for the child.

In general, as children mature and age, their understanding of loss and death tends to change from perceiving death as temporary and reversible to viewing it as permanent, personal, and universal.[76,77] In addition, children tend to grieve more sporadically than adults, are more capable of putting grief aside, and may not have to deal with as many reminders of the loss.[77] However, grief reactions tend to vary from child to child and often depend on the type of loss experienced.[76–78] Some children experience immediate grief, while others have delayed responses.[77]

Three stages of grief children may experience include disorganization, transition, and reorganization. The disorganization stage encompasses the initial grief reaction and can be observed with behaviors ranging from regression, behavioral outburst, fears, and changes in mood. The transition stage is characterized by feelings of depression and despair, with some children withdrawing, becoming aggressive, and/or experiencing difficulty in school. In the final stage, reorganization, children move toward resolution and acceptance.[72,76]

### Disclosure Process

Talking with children about the traumatic event and resulting loss can be frightening for many caregivers, particularly as they may be uncertain about the appropriate time, delivery manner, and amount of information to provide to the child. Mental health professionals such as psychologists, counselors, child life specialists, and clergy are examples of persons who can facilitate the disclosure and healing process. Bronson and Price[78] from the Phoenix Society discuss important principles to keep in mind when working with pediatric burn survivors who are grieving. These principles include supportive and compassionate truth telling, accep-

tance, respect of differences and feelings, and nonjudgment. In addition, they recommend allowing the child an opportunity to say good-bye.

The process of helping a child work through his or her grief and loss can begin once the child arrives at the acute care unit of the hospital, is medically stable, and is able to verbally participate in conversations. The truth-telling process can be utilized to address various changes and losses such as the loss of body parts, family, friends, pets, material goods, and/or the home, as well as changes in appearance.

Robert et al[79] provided suggestions for the development and implementation of the truth-telling process. This process begins with an evaluation of the child's emotional and developmental readiness to hear the news. Important factors to consider during the evaluation process include factors related to the trauma, what the child knows and has asked, the wishes of the caregiver regarding the disclosure, and the cultural, religious, and spiritual needs of the child and family. It is important to obtain the full consent and participation of the caregiver when developing and implementing the truth-telling plan. Implementation of the plan can involve the caregiver alone or the caregiver in conjunction with the mental health professional. Additionally, other support systems may be asked to participate, including extended family, friends, or clergy. This process can take place in a single session or in multiple sessions, depending on the child's needs. Subsequent sessions can be beneficial to help the child and family work on coping strategies and to support the child's sense of safety.[79]

## SOCIAL ADJUSTMENT AND COMMUNITY REINTEGRATION

Social adjustment and community reintegration are important factors to consider with burn survivors. In adults, it has been noted that female gender, larger burns, and increased importance placed on appearance are related to body image dissatisfaction,[80] and in turn, body image dissatisfaction is predictive of psychosocial functioning at a 2-month[81] and 1-year[80] follow-up. In a study of adolescent burn survivors, it was noted that while they rated their appearance as less attractive than that of their peers, they ranked the importance of appearance as relatively low.[82] Moreover, in some studies, survivors of childhood burns reported that their body self-esteem was the same as or higher than the norm.[83–85]

In addition to body image, studies have focused on social competence. Results revealed that as a group, pediatric burn survivors evidence social competence levels within the normal range, even those with severe burns[86–90]; however, 20% to 30% of them demonstrate difficulties in this realm.[91] Research has also shown that healthy family relationships and environments,[92–94] as well as the presence of social support, are related to successful outcomes with these children.[84,95]

Despite the relatively positive outcomes reported, social anxiety may be present for some burn survivors, and school reentry interventions, social skills programs, and burn camps can help. Social anxiety can be described as distress related to social situations, which may or may not meet the threshold of a diagnosis of social phobia.

Symptoms of social phobia include (1) marked and persistent fear of 1 or more social or performance situations, (2) exposure to the feared social situation almost invariably provoking anxiety, (3) recognition that the fear is excessive or unreasonable (note: in children, this may be absent), and (4) avoidance of the feared social situations or performance, or an endurance of them with intense anxiety or distress.[13] In children, the anxiety must occur in peer settings (not just with adults), and symptoms may be expressed by crying, tantrums, or freezing.[13] This fear and avoidance must also interfere with normal functioning and, in children, must be present for at least 6 months.[13] The lifetime prevalence of social phobia in pediatric burn survivors who were young adults at follow-up has been noted to be nearly 9%.[15] Assessments for symptoms of social anxiety or social discomfort include a general clinical interview or self-report measures such as the social anxiety scales for children and adolescents (SAS)[96] or the social comfort questionnaire (SCQ),[97] for example.

## School Reentry and Social Skills Programs

Although results from one study indicated there was no difference between the preburn and postburn school functioning of children with relatively small burns and short hospital stays,[98] the academic performance of children, particularly those with larger burns, may be affected by frequent absences and diminished stamina. Moreover, changes in appearance (eg, scars, amputations), limited mobility, and the use of medical aids (a mask, splints, pressure garments, and prosthetics) can also make the process of returning to school uncomfortable initially, particularly due to the reactions of others.[99] Also, teachers and students in the traditional school system may be unfamiliar with the nature of burn injuries and with how these children can be reintegrated into the school setting.

The goal of school reintegration is to facilitate the successful transition from hospital to community and to lessen social discomfort. Hospital staff can educate teachers, school personnel, and other students about aspects of the child's injury, including changes in appearance and the use of medical devices as well as the child's current level of functioning. The hope is that this process will help dispel fears and myths as well as increase understanding of and empathy for the child with a burn. Communicating this information can be done via telephone, through the use of a video or DVD, or by way of a school visit from hospital staff (eg, child life and mental health professionals, nurses, and rehabilitation therapists). The type of intervention selected depends on the family's wishes, the child's developmental needs, and the available school resources.

Research on the efficacy of school reentry programs is limited. However, there is some evidence that teachers and parents are in favor of these types of interventions,[100] and in a study of a video reentry intervention, parents and children reported that the program was helpful and promoted socialization.[101]

New school reentry interventions have also been developed to meet the needs of burn survivors. The Phoenix Society for Burn Survivors developed a school reentry program called "The Journey Back," which is a comprehensive program to assist children with burns, the family, and the school community with the reentry process. This program consists of both print and video materials and can be used by anyone interested in assisting with the reentry process.

Different social skills programs have also been developed to facilitate community reintegration and improve the confidence of burn survivors. The programs provide effective strategies to handle difficult professional and social situations such as returning to school, attending job interviews, and responding to stares and questions from strangers. Examples of such programs include "Be Your Best," developed by a burn survivor, Barbara Kammerer Quayle of the Phoenix Society for Burn Survivors, and "Changing Faces," created by James Partridge, who is also a burn survivor.[102,103] "Changing Faces" has shown success with both adults with facial disfigurements[104] and adolescent burn survivors.[91]

## Burn Camps

Burn camps are another method of community reentry and were originally developed as a means of providing follow-up mental health and rehabilitation services to children once they left the hospital setting.[105] Currently, there are different types of camps. There are recreational camps that provide opportunities for socialization with peers through participation in different activities and rehabilitation camps that provide specialized services to promote independence.[105] Results from studies on the efficacy of camps in improving factors related to self-esteem and/or social competence have been mixed. Some reported improvements in self-esteem, even if not statistically significant,[106,107] whereas others did not.[108]

# SUMMARY

From the moment of initial injury, pediatric burn patients face a number of physical and psychosocial challenges. While great advances have been made in the physical aspects of burn care,[109] the most significant long-term problems for these individuals lie in the psychosocial domain.[15,110,111] The role of a mental health professional is to help alleviate discomfort during acute and outpatient phases of recovery as well as to assist the patient, family, friends, and community in the reintegration process.

# KEY POINTS

- The role of mental health professionals in pediatric burn units is ongoing.
- During the initial clinical interview, mental health professionals should gather information about the patient and family as well as assess the patient's current psychological functioning.
- If abuse and/or neglect are suspected, a risk assessment should be completed and a report to the appropriate state agency should be made.
- Mental health professionals should conduct ongoing assessments for symptoms of sleep difficulties, delirium and psychosis, anxiety, depression, and grief reactions.
- If the patient is experiencing psychological distress, appropriate treatments and interventions should be given, and the patient's medical team and family should be consulted.
- When the patient is ready to be discharged, mental health professionals should assist with the community reentry process.

# REFERENCES

1. Piazza-Waggoner C, Dotson C, Adams CD, Joseph K, Goldfarb IW, Slater H. Preinjury behavioral and emotional problems among pediatric burn patients. *J Burn Care Rehabil.* 2005; **26**(4): 371–378, discussion 369–370.

2. Rivlin E, Faragher EB. The psychological sequelae of thermal injury on children and adolescents: part 1. *Dev Neurorehabil.* 2007; **10**(2): 161–172.

3. Thomas CR, Ayoub M, Rosenberg L, Robert RS, Meyer WJ. Attention deficit hyperactivity disorder & pediatric burn injury: a preliminary retrospective study. *Burns.* 2004; **30**(3): 221–223.

4. Child Abuse Prevention and Treatment Act. Child Abuse Prevention and Treatment Act (CAPTA). Public Law: 93–247. 42 US.C. 5106g (2003).

5. Chester DL, Jose RM, Aldlyami E, King H, Moiemen NS. Non-accidental burns in children—are we neglecting neglect? *Burns.* 2006; **32**(2): 222–228.

6. Thombs BD. Patient and injury characteristics, mortality risk, and length of stay related to child abuse by burning: evidence from a national sample of 15,802 pediatric admissions. *Ann Surg.* 2008; **247**(3): 519–523.

7. Robert R, Blakeney P, Herndon D. Maltreatment by burning. In: Herndon DN, ed. *Total Burn Care.* Edinburgh, Scotland: Saunders Elsevier; 2007: 771–780.

8. Child Welfare Information Gateway. *Mandatory Reporters of Child Abuse and Neglect.* US Department of Health and Human Services (USDHHS); 2008: 1–5. State Statutes Series.

9. Lawrence JW, Fauerbach J, Eudell E, Ware L, and Munster A. The 1998 Clinical Research Award. Sleep disturbance after burn injury: a frequent yet understudied complication. *J Burn Care Rehabil.* 1998; **19**(6): 480–486.

10. Gottschlich MM, Jenkins ME, Mayes T, Khoury J, Kramer M, Warden GD, Kagan RJ. The 1994 Clinical Research Award. A prospective clinical study of the polysomnographic stages of sleep after burn injury. *J Burn Care Rehabil.* 1994; **15**(6): 486–492.

11. Armour A, Gottschlich MM, Khoury J, Warden GD, Kagan RJ. A randomized, controlled prospective trial of zolpidem and haloperidol for use as sleeping agents in pediatric burn patients. *J Burn Care Res.* 2008; **29**(1): 238–247.

12. Ratcliff Meyer WJ, Cuervo LJ, Villarreal C, Thomas CR, Herndon DN. The use of haloperidol and associated complications in the agitated, acutely ill pediatric burn patient. *J Burn Care Rehabil.* 2004; **25**(6): 472–478.

13. American Psychiatric Association. *Diagnostic and Statistical Manual of Mental Disorders.* 4th ed. Washington, DC: American Psychiatric Association; 2000.

14. Stoddard FJ, Norman DK, Murphy JM, Beardslee WR. Psychiatric outcome of burned children and adolescents. *J Am Acad Child Adolesc Psychiatry.* 1989; **28**(4): 589–595.

15. Meyer WJ, Blakeney P, Thomas CR, Russell W, Robert RS, and Holzer CE. Prevalence of major psychiatric illness in young adults who were burned as children. *Psychosom Med.* 2007; **69**(4): 377–382.

16. Harvey AG, Bryant RA. Acute stress disorder across trauma populations. *J Nerv Ment Dis.* 1999; **187**(7): 443–446.

17. Difede J, Ptacek JT, Roberts J, Barocas D, Rives W, Apfeldorf W, Yurt R. Acute stress disorder after burn injury: a predictor of posttraumatic stress disorder? *Psychosom Med.* 2002; **64**(5): 826–834.

18. McKibben JB, Bresnick MG, Wiechman Askay SA, Fauerbach JA. Acute stress disorder and posttraumatic stress disorder: a prospective study of prevalence, course, and predictors in a sample with major burn injuries. *J Burn Care Res.* 2008; **29**(1): 22–35.

19. Stoddard FJ, Saxe G, Ronfeldt H, Drake JE, Burns J, Edgren C, Sheridan R. Acute stress symptoms in young children with burns. *J Am Acad Child Adolesc Psychiatry.* 2006; **45**(1): 87–93.

20. Saxe G, Stoddard F, Chawla N, Lopez CG, Hall E, Sheridan R, King D, King L. Risk factors for acute stress disorder in children with burns. *J Trauma Dissociation.* 2005; **6**(2): 37–49.

21. Ratcliff SL, Brown A, Rosenberg L, Rosenberg M, Robert RS, Cuervo LJ, Villarreal C, Thomas CR, Meyer WJ. The effectiveness of a pain and anxiety protocol to treat the acute pediatric burn patient. *Burns.* 2006; **32**(5): 554–562.

22. Roca RP, Spence RJ, Munster AM. Posttraumatic adaptation and distress among adult burn survivors. *Am J Psychiatry.* 1992; **149**(9): 1234–1238.

23. Fauerbach JA, Lawrence J, Haythornthwaite J, Richter D, McGuire M, Schmidt C, Munster A. Preburn psychiatric history affects posttrauma morbidity. *Psychosomatics.* 1997; **38**(4): 374–385.

24. Perry S, Difede J, Musngi G, Frances AJ, Jacobsberg L. Predictors of posttraumatic stress disorder after burn injury. *Am J Psychiatry.* 1992; **149**(7): 931–935.

25. Van Loey NE, Maas CJ, Faber AW, Taal LA. Predictors of chronic posttraumatic stress symptoms following burn injury: results of a longitudinal study. *J Trauma Stress.* 2003; **16**(4): 361–369.

26. Difede J, Barocas D. Acute intrusive and avoidant PTSD symptoms as predictors of chronic PTSD following burn injury. *J Trauma Stress.* 1999; **12**(2): 363–369.

27. Ehde DM, Patterson DR, Wiechman SA, Wilson LG. Post-traumatic stress symptoms and distress 1 year after burn injury. *J Burn Care Rehabil.* 2000; **21**(2): 105–111.

28. Fauerbach JA, Lawrence JW, Schmidt CW, Munster AM, Costa PT. Personality predictors of injury-related posttraumatic stress disorder. *J Nerv Ment Dis.* 2000; **188**(8): 510–517.

29. Bryant RA. Predictors of post-traumatic stress disorder following burns injury. *Burns.* 1996; **22**(2): 89–92.

30. Drake JE, Stoddard FJ, Murphy JM, Ronfeldt H, Snidman N, Kagan J, Saxe G, Sheridan R. Trauma severity influences acute stress in young burned children. *J Burn Care Res.* 2006; **27**(2): 174–182.

31. Stoddard FJ, Ronfeldt H, Kagan J, Drake JE, Snidman N, Murphy JM, Saxe G, Burns J, Sheridan RL. Young burned children: the course of acute stress and physiological and behavioral responses. *Am J Psychiatry.* 2006; **163**(6): 1084–1090.

32. Saxe GN, Stoddard F, Hall E, Chawla N, Lopez C, Sheridan R, King D, King L, Yehuda R. Pathways to PTSD, part I: children with burns. *Am J Psychiatry.* 2005; **162**(7): 1299–1304.

33. Saxe G, Chawla N, Stoddard F, Kassam-Adams N, Courtney D, Cunningham K, Lopez C, Hall E, Sheridan R, King D, King, L. Child stress disorders checklist: a measure of ASD and PTSD in children. *J Am Acad Child Adolesc Psychiatry.* 2003; **42**(8): 972–978.

34. Robert R, Meyer WJ, Villarreal C, Blakeney PE, Desai M, Herndon D. An approach to the timely treatment of acute stress disorder. *J Burn Care Rehabil.* 1999; **20**(3): 250–258.

35. Cardena E, Koopman C, Classen C, Waelde LC, Spiegel D. Psychometric properties of the Stanford acute stress reaction questionnaire (SASRQ): a valid and reliable measure of acute stress. *J Trauma Stress.* 2000; **13**(4): 719–734.

36. Mindell JA, Owens JA. *A Clinical Guide to Pediatric Sleep: Diagnosis and Management of Sleep Problems.* Baltimore, MD: Lippincott Williams & Wilkins; 2003.

37. Tcheung WJ, Robert R, Rosenberg L, Rosenberg M, Villarreal C, Thomas C, Holzer CE, Meyer WJ. Early treatment of acute stress disorder in children with major burn injury. *Pediatr Crit Care Med.* 2005; **6**(6): 676–681.

38. Meighen KG, Hines LA, Lagges AM. Risperidone treatment of preschool children with thermal burns and acute stress disorder. *J Child Adolesc Psychopharmacol.* 2007; **17**(2): 223–232.

39. Todd RD, Joyner CA, Heath AC, Neuman RJ, Reich W. Reliability and stability of a semistructured *DSM-IV* interview designed for family studies. *J Am Acad Child Adolesc Psychiatry.* 2003; **42**(12): 1460–1468.

40. Roussos A, Goenjian AK, Steinberg AM, Sotiropoulou C, Kakaki M, Kabakos C, Karagianni S, Manouras V. Posttraumatic stress and depressive reactions among children and adolescents after the 1999 earthquake in Ano Liosia, Greece. *Am J Psychiatry.* 2005; **162**(3): 530–537.

41. Welner Z, Reich W, Herjanic B, Jung KG, Amado H. Reliability, validity, and parent-child agreement studies of the diagnostic interview for children and adolescents (DICA). *J Am Acad Child Adolesc Psychiatry.* 1987; **26**(5): 649–653.

42. Reich W, Cottler L, McCallum K, Corwin D, Van Eerdewegh M. Computerized interviews as a method of assessing psychopathology in children. *Compr Psychiatry.* 1995; **36**(1): 40–45.

43. Bradley R, Greene J, Russ E, Dutra L, Westen D. A multidimensional meta-analysis of psychotherapy for PTSD. *Am J Psychiatry.* 2005; **162**(2): 214–227.

44. Norton PJ, Price EC. A meta-analytic review of adult cognitive-behavioral treatment outcome across the anxiety disorders. *J Nerv Ment Dis.* 2007; **195**(6): 521–531.

45. Sherman JJ. Effects of psychotherapeutic treatments for PTSD: a meta-analysis of controlled clinical trials. *J Trauma Stress.* 1998; **11**(3): 413–435.

46. Adler-Nevo G, Manassis K. Psychosocial treatment of pediatric posttraumatic stress disorder: the neglected field of single-incident trauma. *Depress Anxiety.* 2005; **22**(4): 177–189.

47. Goenjian AK, Karayan I, Pynoos RS, Minassian D, Najarian LM, Steinberg AM, Fairbanks LA. Outcome of psychotherapy among early adolescents after trauma. *Am J Psychiatry.* 1997; **154**(4): 536–542.

48. March JS, Amaya-Jackson L, Murray MC, Schulte A. Cognitive-behavioral psychotherapy for children and adolescents with posttraumatic stress disorder after a single-incident stressor. *J Am Acad Child Adolesc Psychiatry.* 1998; **37**(6): 585–593.

49. Silverman W, Kurtines W. *Anxiety and Phobic Disorders: A Pragmatic Approach.* New York, NY: Plenum Press; 1996.

50. Borkovec TD, Ruscio AM. Psychotherapy for generalized anxiety disorder. *J Clin Psychiatry.* 2001; **62**(suppl 11): 37–42, discussion 43–45.

51. Cartwright-Hatton S, Roberts C, Chitsabesan P, Fothergill C, Harrington R. Systematic review of the efficacy of cognitive behaviour therapies for childhood and adolescent anxiety disorders. *Br J Clin Psychol.* 2004; **43**(pt 4): 421–436.

52. Madianos MG, Papaghelis M, Ioannovich J, Dafni R. Psychiatric disorders in burn patients: a follow-up study. *Psychother Psychosom.* 2001; **70**(1): 30–37.

53. Ptacek JT, Patterson DR, Heimbach DM. Inpatient depression in persons with burns. *J Burn Care Rehabil.* 2002; **23**(1): 1–9.

54. Thombs BD, Bresnick MG, Magyar-Russell G, Lawrence JW, McCann UD, Fauerbach JA. Symptoms of depression predict change in physical health after burn injury. *Burns.* 2007; **33**(3): 292–298.

55. Wiechman SA, Ptacek JT, Patterson DR, Gibran NS, Engrav LE, Heimbach DM. Rates, trends, and severity of depression after burn injuries. *J Burn Care Rehabil.* 2001; **22**(6): 417–424.

56. Thombs BD, Haines JM, Bresnick MG, Magyar-Russell G, Fauerbach JA, Spence RJ. Depression in burn reconstruction patients: symptom prevalence and association with body image dissatisfaction and physical function. *Gen Hosp Psychiatry.* 2007; **29**(1): 14–20.

57. Lawrence JW, Fauerbach JA, Thombs BD. Frequency and correlates of depression symptoms among long-term adult burn survivors. *Rehabil Psychol.* 2006; **51**(4): 306–313.

58. Fauerbach JA, Lawrence JW, Bryant AG, Smith JH. The relationship of ambivalent coping to depression symptoms and adjustment. *Rehabil Psychol.* 2002; **47**(4): 387–401.

59. Stoddard FJ, Stroud L, Murphy JM. Depression in children after recovery from severe burns. *J Burn Care Rehabil.* 1992; **13**(3): 340–347.

60. Kovacs M. *Children's Depression Inventory.* North Tonawanda, NY: Multi-Health Systems Inc; 1992.

61. Thombs BD, Bresnick MG, Magyar-Russell G. Depression in survivors of burn injury: a systematic review. *Gen Hosp Psychiatry.* 2006; **28**(6): 494–502.

62. DeRubeis RJ, Gelfand LA, Tang TZ, Simons AD. Medications versus cognitive behavior therapy for severely depressed outpatients: mega-analysis of four randomized comparisons. *Am J Psychiatry.* 1999; **156**(7): 1007–1013.

63. DeRubeis RJ, Hollon SD, Amsterdam JD, Shelton RC, Young PR, Salomon RM, O'Reardon JP, Lovett ML, Gladis MM, Brown LL, Gallop R. Cognitive therapy vs medications in the treatment of moderate to severe depression. *Arch Gen Psychiatry.* 2005; **62**(4): 409–416.

64. Gloaguen V, Cottraux J, Cucherat M, Blackburn IM. A meta-analysis of the effects of cognitive therapy in depressed patients. *J Affect Disord.* 1998; **49**(1): 59–72.

65. March J, Silva S, Petrycki S, Curry J, Wells K, Fairbank J, Burns B, Domino M, McNulty S, Vitiello B, Severe J. Fluoxetine, cognitive-behavioral therapy, and their combination for adolescents with depression: treatment for adolescents with depression study (TADS) randomized controlled trial. *JAMA.* 2004; **292**(7): 807–820.

66. Hetrick S, Merry S, McKenzie J, Sindahl P, Proctor M. Selective serotonin reuptake inhibitors (SSRIs) for depressive disorders in children and adolescents. *Cochrane Database Syst Rev.* 2007; (3): CD004851.

67. Kassam-Adams N, Winston FK. Predicting child PTSD: the relationship between acute stress disorder and PTSD in injured children. *J Am Acad Child Adolesc Psychiatry.* 2004; **43**(4): 403–411.

68. Brown EJ, Goodman RF. Childhood traumatic grief: an exploration of the construct in children bereaved on September 11. *J Clin Child Adolesc Psychol.* 2005; **34**(2): 248–259.

69. Cohen JA, Mannarino AP, Staron VR. A pilot study of modified cognitive-behavioral therapy for childhood traumatic grief (CBT-CTG). *J Am Acad Child Adolesc Psychiatry.* 2006; **45**(12): 1465–1473.

70. LaGreca AM, Silverman WK, Wasserstein SB. Children's predisaster functioning as a predictor of posttraumatic stress following hurricane Andrew. *J Consult Clin Psychol.* 1998; 66.

71. Stroebe MS, Hansson RO, Stroebe W, Schut H. *Handbook of Bereavement Research: Consequences, Coping, and Care.* Washington, DC: American Psychological Association; 2001.

72. Perry BD, Rosenfelt JL. The child's loss: death, grief and mourning. *Child Trauma Acad.* 1999; **3**(1): 1–12.

73. Cohen JA, Mannarino AP, Knudsen K. Treating childhood traumatic grief: a pilot study. *J Am Acad Child Adolesc Psychiatry.* 2004; **43**(10): 1225–1233.

74. Brown EJ, Pearlman MY, Goodman RF. Facing fears and sadness: cognitive-behavioral therapy for childhood traumatic grief. *Harv Rev Psychiatry.* 2004; **12**(4): 187–198.

75. Goodman RF, Morgan AV, Juriga S, Brown EJ. Letting a story unfold: a case study of client-centered therapy for childhood traumatic grief. *Harv Rev Psychiatry.* 2004; **12**(4): 199–212.

76. Keith K. Grief and children. http://childparenting.about.com/cs/emotionalhealth/a/childgrief.htm]. Published 2007. Accessed November 27, 2007.

77. Fitzgerald H. *The Grieving Child: A Parent's Guide.* New York, NY: Simon & Schuster; 1992.

78. Bronson MP, Price S. Grief, loss, and healing after burn trauma: helping children. *Burn Support News: Phoenix Society for Burn Survivors.* 2007; **4**: 13–15.

79. Robert R, Rosenberg L, Amrhein C, Blakeney P. Pediatric patients, their families, and truth telling. In: Association for the

Care of Children's Health, 34th Annual Conference; 1999; Long Beach, CA.

**80.** Thombs BD, Notes LD, Lawrence JW, Magyar-Russell G, Bresnick MG, Fauerbach JA. From survival to socialization: a longitudinal study of body image in survivors of severe burn injury. *J Psychosom Res.* 2008; **64**(2): 205–212.

**81.** Fauerbach JA, Heinberg LJ, Lawrence JW, Munster AM, Palombo DA, Richter D, Spence RJ, Stevens SS, Ware L, Muehlberger T. Effect of early body image dissatisfaction on subsequent psychological and physical adjustment after disfiguring injury. *Psychosom Med.* 2000; **62**(4): 576–582.

**82.** Robert R, Meyer W, Bishop S, Rosenberg L, Murphy L, Blakeney P. Disfiguring burn scars and adolescent self-esteem. *Burns.* 1999; **25**(7): 581–585.

**83.** Pope SJ, Solomons WR, Done DJ, Cohn N, Possamai AM. Body image, mood and quality of life in young burn survivors. *Burns.* 2007; **33**(6): 747–755.

**84.** Orr DA, Reznikoff M, Smith GM. Body image, self-esteem, and depression in burn-injured adolescents and young adults. *J Burn Care Rehabil.* 1989; **10**(5): 454–461.

**85.** Lawrence JW, Rosenberg LE, Fauerbach JA. Comparing the body esteem of pediatric survivors of burn injury with the body esteem of an age-matched comparing group without burns. *Rehabil Psychol.* 2007; **52**(4): 370–379.

**86.** Moore P, Moore M, Blakeney P, Meyer W, Murphy L, Herndon D. Competence and physical impairment of pediatric survivors of burns of more than 80% total body surface area. *J Burn Care Rehabil.* 1996; **17**(6, pt 1): 547–551.

**87.** Blakeney P, Meyer W, Moore P, Broemeling L, Hunt R, Robson M, Herndon D. Social competence and behavioral problems of pediatric survivors of burns. *J Burn Care Rehabil.* 1993; **14**(1): 65–72.

**88.** Blakeney P, Meyer W, Robert R, Desai M, Wolf S, Herndon D. Long-term psychosocial adaptation of children who survive burns involving 80% or greater total body surface area. *J Trauma.* 1998; **44**(4): 625–632, discussion 633–634.

**89.** Meyers-Paal R, Blakeney P, Robert R, Murphy L, Chinkes D, Meyer W, Desai M, Herndon D. Physical and psychologic rehabilitation outcomes for pediatric patients who suffer 80% or more TBSA, 70% or more third degree burns. *J Burn Care Rehabil.* 2000; **21**(1, pt 1): 43–49.

**90.** Piazza-Waggoner C, Butcher M, Adams CD, Goldfarb IW, Slater H. Assessing the relationship between locus of control and social competence in pediatric burn survivors attending summer camp. *J Burn Care Rehabil.* 2004; **25**(4): 349–356.

**91.** Blakeney P, Thomas C, Holzer C, Rose M, Berniger F, Meyer WJ. Efficacy of a short-term, intensive social skills training program for burned adolescents. *J Burn Care Rehabil.* 2005; **26**(6): 546–555.

**92.** Landolt MA, Grubenmann S, Meuli M. Family impact greatest: predictors of quality of life and psychological adjustment in pediatric burn survivors. *J Trauma.* 2002; **53**(6): 1146–1151.

**93.** LeDoux J, Meyer WJ, Blakeney PE, Herndon DN. Relationship between parental emotional states, family environment and the behavioural adjustment of pediatric burn survivors. *Burns.* 1998; **24**(5): 425–432.

**94.** Blakeney P, Portman S, Rutan R. Familial values as factors influencing long-term psychological adjustment of children after severe burn injury. *J Burn Care Rehabil.* 1990; **11**(5): 472–475.

**95.** Barnum DD, Snyder CR, Rapoff MA, Mani MM, Thompson R. Hope and social support in the psychological adjustment of children who have survived burn injuries and their matched controls. *Children's Health Care.* 1998; **27**(1): 15–30.

**96.** LaGreca AM. *Manual for the Social Anxiety Scales for Children and Adolescents.* Miami, FL: University of Miami; 1997.

**97.** Lawrence JW, Fauerbach JA, Heinberg LJ, Doctor M, Thombs BD. The reliability and validity of the perceived stigmatization questionnaire (PSQ) and the social comfort questionnaire (SCQ) among an adult burn survivor sample. *Psychol Assess.* 2006; **18**(1): 106–111.

**98.** Staley M, Anderson L, Greenhalgh D, Warden G. Return to school as an outcome measure after a burn injury. *J Burn Care Rehabil.* 1998; **20**(1): 91–94.

**99.** Blakeney P. School reintegration. *J Burn Care Rehabil.* 1995; **16**(2, pt 1): 180–187.

**100.** Blakeney P, Moore P, Meyer W, Bishop B, Murphy L, Robson M, Herndon D. Efficacy of school reentry programs. *J Burn Care Rehabil.* 1995; **16**(4): 469–472, discussion 466–468.

**101.** Rosenberg M, Bishop B, Amrhein C, Robert R, Chavirria A, Meyer W, Blakeney P. Assisting pediatric burn survivors from other countries returning to school. In: American Burn Association, 37th Annual Meeting; 2005; Chicago, IL.

**102.** Partridge J. About changing faces: promoting a good quality of life for people with visible disfigurements. *Burns.* 1997; **23**(2): 186–187.

**103.** Partridge J. Changing faces: taking up Macgregor's challenge. *J Burn Care Rehabil.* 1998; **19**(2): 174–180, discussion 169.

**104.** Robinson E, Rumsey N, Partridge J. An evaluation of the impact of social interaction skills training for facially disfigured people. *Br J Plast Surg.* 1996; **49**(5): 281–289.

**105.** Doctor ME. Burn camps and community aspects of burn care. *J Burn Care Rehabil.* 1992; **13**(1): 68–76.

**106.** Cox ER, Call SB, Williams NR, Reeves PM. Shedding the layers: exploring the impact of the burn camp experience on adolescent campers' body image. *J Burn Care Rehabil.* 2004; **25**(1): 141–147, discussion 140.

**107.** Rimmer RB, Fornaciari GM, Foster KN, Bay CR, Wadsworth MM, Wood M, Caruso DM. Impact of a pediatric residential burn camp experience on burn survivors' perceptions of self and attitudes regarding the camp community. *J Burn Care Res.* 2007; **28**(2): 334–341.

**108.** Arnoldo BD, Crump D, Burris AM, Hunt JL, Purdue GF. Self-esteem measurement before and after summer burn camp in pediatric burn patients. *J Burn Care Res*. 2006; **27**(6): 786–789.

**109.** Herndon DN. *Total Burn Care*. 3rd ed. Philadelphia: Saunders Elsevier; 2007.

**110.** Rosenberg M, Blakeney P, Robert R, Thomas C, Holzer C, Meyer W. Quality of life of young adults who survived pediatric burns. *J Burn Care Res*. 2006; **27**(6): 773–778.

**111.** Baker CP, Russell WJ, Meyer WJ, Blakeney P. Physical and psychologic rehabilitation outcomes for young adults burned as children. *Arch Phys Med Rehabil*. 2007; **88**(2): 57–64.

# CHAPTER TWENTY-EIGHT

# OUTPATIENT MANAGEMENT
# OF PEDIATRIC BURN PATIENTS

IBRAHIM SULTAN, MD

BRADLEY J. PHILLIPS, MD

## INTRODUCTION AND EPIDEMIOLOGY

Each year, more than a million people in the United States who have sustained thermal injury seek care at a medical center. Among this unique population, 250000 (>25%) are children,[1] of which approximately 15000 are hospitalized. Since the far majority of burned children are managed as outpatients, pediatricians, primary care physicians, and emergency room physicians must have a clear understanding of the assessment and management of such patients. It is imperative for the injured child to be closely followed in a controlled outpatient setting in order to minimize long-term disability and ensure optimal outcomes[2].

In general, traumatic injury is the most common cause of death in children who are younger than 18 years, accounting for 60% of deaths. This makes it a more common cause of death in children than all other causes combined. Nearly 16 million children are injured every year in the United States, and roughly a quarter of these pediatric patients require medical attention. Unfortunately, 55% of this population is left with a disability 1 year after injury. Studies have shown that children with severe blunt traumatic injuries have better outcomes when transferred to specialized pediatric centers once they are initially stabilized. Such centers have resources and personnel unique to helping children, beginning from initial management to rehabilitation and recovery. Understandably, the same principle applies to children who suffer from thermal injuries[3,4].

Pediatric burns, like traumatic injuries, can vary in severity with prognosis and treatment depending on the type of burn injury. Scald burns, typically due to spilled food, beverages, and hot tap water, still constitute the most common mode of thermal injury in children (approximately 80% incidence). Thermal burns incurred by contact with hot objects (stoves, clothing irons, curlers, and other heaters around the house) usually account for approximately 15% of all pediatric burn injuries; unfortunately, a number of children (2.5%) sustain burns secondary to fireworks, gasoline, and tobacco-related products. Other modes of injuries in children include chemical burns, typically due to mishandling of acid-based and alkali-based household cleaners. Electrical injuries also occur in children, commonly from a child reaching into an electrical outlet or chewing on a cord[5].

## INITIAL ASSESSMENT AND EVALUATION

Every burn patient, whether an adult or child, must be approached as a trauma patient until proven otherwise. As an example, a recent house fire brought 6 patients to our burn center: 4 adults and 2 children. The children were thrown from the second floor to escape the fire, and the mother jumped out the window after them; the children were caught by a neighbor, but the mom fractured her L2 spine and cervical disc. Despite the obvious and often dramatic presentation of a burn injury, *all* burn patients are trauma patients first.

When presented with trauma/burn patients, the ABCs (airway, breathing, circulation) must be addressed first. The airway should be secured with an endotracheal tube if any signs or symptoms of an inhalation injury are present. These include singed eyebrows, nares, and eyelashes, hoarseness, stridor, carbonaceous sputum, and perioral or nasal burns. If clinical signs of inhalation exist, a bronchoscopy should be done to document the level of injury to the trachea, carina, and primary and secondary bronchi. Although the pediatric population can be challenging, immediate intravenous access should be established. Any patient with burns > 20% total body surface area (TBSA) should begin resuscitation via the Parkland formula (4 ml × kg × % TBSA) in addition to receiving maintenance fluids. All clothing and any constricting garments must be promptly removed. The remainder of the history should be obtained in a timely manner, including past immunizations and congenital medical problems. Associated traumatic injuries, including fractures, should be ruled out during the secondary survey. Throughout the initial evaluation, it is key to keep patients warm and covered. Children dissipate heat quickly, and all efforts should be employed to minimize heat loss (warm fluids, sterile drapes over burned areas, warm blankets, increased ambient room temperatures, and so on).

During the secondary survey, particular attention should be paid to the presence of certain traumatic injuries known to significantly increase mortality, such as central nervous system (CNS) injuries. Unlike adults, where focal injuries are more common, children tend to develop diffuse cerebral edema, which contributes to such injuries being a leading cause of death in children who sustain trauma. For instance, a child who presents with a Glasgow Coma Scale (GCS) of <8 with a unilateral dilated pupil from a transcranial gunshot wound has an associated mortality of more than 80%. In children, neurologic exams are extremely helpful in detecting spinal cord injuries missed by imaging studies. Thoracic injuries are the second most common cause of death. In children, the unique compliance of their chest wall can lead to traumatic asphyxia after blunt chest injury. This causes sudden airway obstruction and the development of retrograde high pressure in the superior vena cava (SVC). As a result, these patients present with petechial hemorrhages over the neck and face and/or cyanosis because of vascular engorgement. Traumatic abdominal injuries also occur in children with splenic, hepatic, renal, and hollow viscus injuries most commonly. When one encounters a patient who has sustained traumatic injuries along with significant burns, it is not unreasonable to obtain detailed imaging studies as part of the secondary survey to rule out any traumatic injuries[6].

Once a patient's ABCs are secured and the primary survey is appropriately conducted, attention should be directed towards assessing the extent of the burn injuries. Anatomic location and depth of the injury as well as percentage of body area burned are critical factors in determining severity. Burns to the hand, face, or perineum or wounds that cross major joints should be paid particular attention because of their capacity to cause long-term disability. For partial-thickness and full-thickness burns, the % TBSA should be calculated to assess the extent of the injury. The rule of nines, typically used for adults, does not accurately apply to children and should not be used while calculating the % TBSA. Instead, the Lund Browder chart provides a more accurate approximation of % TBSA in children. When such charts are unavailable, the palm of the child, which is approximately 1% of body surface area, can be used to estimate the extent of injury[4,5].

It is also important to appreciate how a burn injury affects the skin. The most severely injured part of the burn wound, the zone of coagulation, is within the center of the wound and consists of dead tissue that is irreversibly destroyed. Just outside this is the zone of stasis, a tenuous layer that may continue to be devitalized or may be salvageable, depending on appropriate resuscitation and wound care. The outermost layer is the zone of hyperemia, named so because of increased blood flow secondary to inflammation.

Superficial burns (first-degree burns, eg, a sunburn) are injuries to the epidermal layer; the involved areas may appear red and painful but typically resolve without scarring when topical moisturizers are used (aloe, vitamin E, cocoa butter, etc). As such, epidermal burns are rarely referred to a burn center. Partial-thickness burns are divided into superficial or deep partial thickness. The former extend into the papillary dermis, whereas the latter progress into the reticular dermis. Superficial partial-thickness burns often blister and are erythematous and painful. These usually heal without scarring but require a moist environment for appropriate healing. It is advisable to observe superficial partial-thickness burns for roughly 10 to 14 days before surgical excision and grafting. Deeper burns can appear either red or even grey or white depending on the reticular layer involved. Deep partial-thickness burns may heal within 2 to 4 weeks but will likely leave a significant scar. Management of deep partial-thickness burns depends on location and 2 significant principles in burn surgical care: optimizing function and cosmesis. Full-thickness burns, on the other hand, appear leathery and white. Patients lose sensation over the region, and such areas do not bleed when stuck with a needle. Children with full-thickness burns should not be managed in an outpatient arena but rather promptly referred to a burn center for further evaluation and treatment[3,4,5].

It is important for providers to be able to detect signs and symptoms of abuse in children who present with thermal injuries. Sadly, up to 40% of burns in children are related to child abuse or neglect.[1] Specific patterns are suggestive of abuse, such as burns involving the buttocks, perineum, lower legs, and feet with sparing of the flexor surfaces in children who are dipped in scalding water. Cigarette burns are also common and cause "punched out" lesions, usually over the upper body. Another clue is a history which is inconsistent with the cause and pattern of injury; this should alert everyone to the possibility of abuse. When suspicious, it is recommended to have multiple-source documentation of the event and to secure objective photographic evidence of the injury pattern and depth; this can be as simple as the physician, nurse, and social worker each documenting his or her history and exam of the child while caregivers take digital pictures for the medical record. These few extra minutes can become quite valuable as the medical and possibly legal process evolves. Looking for and identifying associated or prior traumatic injuries is also important when considering abused children. Chronic subdural hematomas and multiple fractures (at different healing phases) are also commonly observed in children who are abused. One must maintain a low threshold to obtain skeletal surveys in children when abuse is suspected. Many children will hesitate to report if they were abused by someone at home because of fear of repercussions. Thus, one must be an astute observer in determining when such children can return home once medically cleared. Enlisting the assistance of social workers from the institution can further ensure appropriate support is available at home for children. The decision to treat a burned child as an outpatient is significant, involving multiple factors besides the medical aspects of care, and should not be taken lightly[8,9,10,11].

## MANAGEMENT

Although the topical management of burn wounds has been debated for decades, a definitive topical agent that can be used for any burn wound still does not exist. However, there are certain basic principles that apply to all burn wounds. Firstly, the wound should be kept clean and inspected periodically for signs of conversion to a deeper wound as well as for signs of infection such as erythema, discharge, odor, increased tenderness, or lympanginitis. If a topical agent is used, the wound should be rinsed twice a day with lukewarm water and a bland soap, followed by reapplication of the topical agent. Bacitracin is strongly preferred for wounds around mucus membranes. Ophthalmic ointments should be used for burns involving the eyes. After initial debridement is performed and it is determined that the child is safe to return home, the parent or guardian must be taught the basic steps in keeping the burn wound clean and healthy. The first dressing change should be done before discharge,

with the parent demonstrating proficiency in doing the same at home. As pain control may be a challenge, patients must be discharged with appropriate pain medications. An oral narcotic agent given an hour or half hour prior to a dressing change is typically sufficient to achieve adequate analgesia. Soaking dressings prior to removal may help in decreasing the amount of analgesia needed. Despite these measures, some children will need to be admitted to an acute care setting solely for pain control, anxiety, or the inability of the parent to adequately care for the child's burn wound. It may be useful to bring the child back to the emergency room for inspection of the wound before the patient presents to clinic in order to help avoid infections and detect conversion of superficial burns[13,14,17].

Superficial burns can be treated with nonalcoholic moisturizers for optimal healing, but are otherwise known to heal appropriately regardless of the kind of agent used. It is strongly recommended that patients use sunscreen with a sunscreen protection factor (SPF) of at least 15 to 30 following their initial injury. Partial-thickness burns, whether superficial or deep, must be initially debrided to determine the actual depth of injury since it is typically difficult and inaccurate to classify such burns without debridement. This can be done in the office, clinic, or emergency room. Blisters should be removed, particularly if they are around digits or cross over joints, in order to assess the underlying depth of injury and optimize the chances of maintaining full range of motion. Patients may need anxiolytics and/or pain medications to tolerate debridement. Debriding should be an active process, as there is no benefit to leaving nonviable, necrotic skin on the wound bed; this will only serve to increase colonization and subsequent infection of the burn wound. Areas within the burn which might be indeterminate should be considered deep until proven otherwise. Superficial partial-thickness burns may be treated with antitopicals to ensure a moist environment, and all dressings should be changed twice a day with active bathing. Gentle washing of wounds with soap and water is also encouraged and can be done twice a day with dressing changes. Deeper burns may require greater antibiosis with agents like silver sulfadiazine. Since it is a sulfa-based drug, it should not be used in patients with allergies to sulfa drugs, pregnant patients, newborns younger than 2 months, premature infants, or patients with *G6PD* deficiency. Deeper and full-thickness burns should be admitted for possible excision and grafting within 24 to 48 hours[17].

Pediatric electrical burns usually occur at home and are typically considered low voltage since these cables carry less than 1000 V. These patients can be treated as outpatients if their injuries are not extensive, a normal EKG is present on admission, and 4 hours of cardiac monitoring do not indicate any rhythm abnormalities. Urine myoglobin should be obtained, and aggressive treatment is indicated when the lab value is > 10,000. Most importantly, as with any other burns, before planning to discharge such patients, caregivers need to ensure parents are available to perform dressing changes as needed. The management of chemical burns should always begin with aggressive irrigation with water. Attempts to neutralize the offending agent with the opposing chemical are not advised. Patients with significant chemical burns should always be referred and evaluated at a burn center because such injuries are almost always underestimated and can cause significant long-term morbidity[8,12,14].

Wound membranes, by providing transient physiologic closure of the burn wound while the underlying dermis heals, have gained significant popularity over the past decades. They have been efficacious in preventing trauma and vapor transmission in addition to providing a barrier to bacteria. They also create a moist environment for the burn wound that leads to decreased bacterial counts. Wound membranes should only be used for superficial or partial-thickness wounds after they have been debrided with removal of devitalized tissue. While several types of wound membranes are available, the most common include allograft, Biobrane®, Acticoat®, Aquacel-Ag®, and AlloDerm®. Porcine xenograft was commonly used in the past, although its use has decreased in the past several years. Xenograft adheres to coagulum and improves pain control but inhibits range of motion when applied over joints. Biobrane®, discovered in the 1970s, consists of an outer silicone layer which acts as an epidermal barrier that is mainly protective in nature and an inner 3-D nylon layer that includes collagen peptides which bind to fibrin and endogenous collagen over the wound surface. Though it has a shelf life of 3 years, the disadvantages include high cost, decreased availability, and the possibility of creating a seal and trapping bacteria within the wound. Acticoat® is a nonadherent dressing that consistently delivers low concentrations of silver to the wound bed. It is advantageous over Biobrane® since it is nonadherent and requires less frequent dressing changes. It is helpful with large wounds, particularly dermatologic disorders. But, like Biobrane®, it is expensive. Integra®, which contains a porous collagen matrix overlaid with a thin silastic sheet, promotes the growth of neodermis through the collagen and rest of the matrix. However, it has not proven superior to Allograft in promoting wound regeneration. Aquacel-Ag® is also a synthetic wound membrane that delivers silver to the wound bed. The silver-impregnated dressings are theoretically superior because of the possible lower rates of infection. AlloDerm® consists of human dermal scaffold, but unfortunately requires immediate autografting for wound healing[17,18].

## CRITERIA FOR REFERRAL TO A BURN CENTER

The American Burn Association (ABA) and the American College of Surgeons have identified and established criteria for referral and admission of patients to a burn center. Below are some that apply specifically to the pediatric population:

- > 10% TBSA burns in children < 10 years
- > 20% TBSA in any other age group
- full-thickness burns
- partial-thickness or full-thickness burns to the face, ears, eyes, hands, genitalia, or perineum or over major joints
- circumferential burns
- significant electrical burns (will need cardiac monitoring depending on admission EKG)
- significant chemical burns
- inhalation injury
- any underlying medical conditions which may increase morbidity and mortality
- any suspicion of abuse, need for long-term rehabilitation, and emotional or social support for the child and/or family[19,20]

## FOLLOW-UP

Follow-up of pediatric patients with a burn surgeon is crucial, particularly in those patients with partial-thickness burns who were not admitted to the hospital. Follow-up in the clinic should typically occur in 3 to 7 days or earlier, depending on the actual thermal injury. During this visit, the surgeon will determine whether to continue conservative management or proceed with operative excision and grafting. In addition, patients should be assessed for the potential development of scars or contractures. Contractures, particularly over major joints, may cause severe functional deficits resulting in growth retardation and deformities. Earlier intervention may ensure cosmesis and functionality, and thus repeated visits are important to observe the progression of such injuries. Nonoperative approaches, such as silicon and pressure garments, can be employed for contractures. Along with the burn surgeon, a team of occupational and physical therapists can assist in identifying and treating such contractures before they interfere with functionality. Through the utilization of massage therapy, splints, and pressure therapy, contractures can be managed nonoperatively until scars mature. Although expensive, customized pressure garments are also available. They are typically worn throughout the day for 12 to 18 months until scar maturation occurs and should be refitted as the child grows. Several surgical options can be utilized for treatment of scars and contractures. Patients should be seen by a burn surgeon within 7 to 10 days if wounds do not appear to be healing adequately after the initial thermal injury. Excision with grafts, flaps, tissue expanders, and Z-plasties can be utilized depending on the location and size of scars.

An experienced multidisciplinary team is key to ensure successful treatment of the burned child. The outpatient setting should involve the entire spectrum of burn-trained providers: nurses, physicians, occupational therapists, physical therapists, child life specialists, and psychologists. Growth and nutritional assessments should be conducted on a regular basis (every 6 months), as should objective photographic documentation and formal assessment of significant scar patterns; past and present functional levels with range of motion should also be tracked and monitored over time. Social workers, counselors, and school teachers are all instrumental in ensuring the child's recovery and well-being.[21,22]

## PREVENTION OF BURN INJURIES

The saying "prevention is better than cure" cannot be overemphasized when considering thermal injuries in the pediatric population. As mentioned previously, scald burns are the most common type of burns in the pediatric population. Preventative measures include checking the temperature of bath water, which should never exceed 100°F. Moreover, a child should never be left alone in a bathtub. When heating hot beverages over a stove, the back burners should be used, with pot and pan handles turned away from the front of the stove. Any hot objects, including irons or curlers, should always be kept away from children. Because of the increased likelihood of burn injury from these items, parents need to be vigilant and focused when using such objects. Similarly, all chemicals should always be kept well out of reach of children. Childproof caps have been shown to decrease chemical injuries significantly. Flammable items, such as firecrackers, gasoline, and lighter fluid, should always be removed from a child's reach as well. More often, such injuries are noted in older children, and therefore education is the most efficacious way to prevent burn injuries[2].

## CONCLUSION

The majority of pediatric burn injuries are managed in outpatient environments. Emergency room physicians, pediatricians, and primary care physicians are usually the clinicians who will see such patients first. It is important to triage the pediatric burn patient appropriately. This includes treating the child as a trauma patient at all times during presentation. It also includes the important decision of whether or not to refer the patient to a burn center, and erring on the side of overreferral in the pediatric burn population is encouraged. It is crucial to look for signs and symptoms of abuse and involve appropriate personnel in order to ensure the child's safety. Children should be closely followed over time to ensure the best functional and cosmetic result. A multidisciplinary team should be employed for the full recovery of the burn child, while prevention of burn injuries should remain a focus.

# REFERENCES

**1.** The Burn Foundation Web site. http://www.burnfoundation. org/programs/resource.cfm?c=1&a=12. Accessed February 15, 2009.

**2.** O'Brien SP, Billmire DA. Prevention and management of outpatient pediatric burns. *J Craniofac Surg.* 2008; **19**(4): 1034–1039.

**3.** Passaretti D, Billmire DA. Management of pediatric burns. *Craniofac Surg.* 2003; **14**: 713–718.

**4.** Kassira W, Namias N. Outpatient management of pediatric burns. *Craniofac Surg.* 2008; **19**: 1007–1009.

**5.** Goodis J and Schraga DE. Thermal burns. eMedicine Web site. http://emedicine.medscape.com/article/926015-overview. Accessed February 16, 2009.

**6.** American Academy of Pediatrics. Management of pediatric trauma. *Pediatrics.* 2008. **121**(4): 849–854.

**7.** Zubair M, Besner G. Pediatric electric burns: management strategies. *Burns.* 1997; **23**: 413–420.

**8.** Cunningham PA. The need for cardiac monitoring after electric injury. *Med J Aust.* 1991; **155**: 301–303.

**9.** Rawlins JM, Khan AA, Shenton AF, Sharpe DT. Epidemiology and outcome analysis of 208 children with burns attending an emergency department. *Emerg Care.* 2007; **23**: 289–293.

**10.** Hall JR, Reyes HM, Meller JL, Loeff DS, Dembek R. The outcome for children with blunt trauma is best at a pediatric trauma center. *J Pediatr Surg.* 1996; **31**(1): 72–77.

**11.** Scheidt PC, Harel Y, Trumble AC, Jones DH, Overpeck MD, Bijur PE. The epidemiology of nonfatal injuries among US children and youth. *Am J Public Health.* 1995; **85**(7): 932–938.

**12.** Hu X, Wesson DE, Logsetty S, Spence LJ. Functional limitations and recovery in children with severe trauma: a one-year follow-up. *J Trauma.* 1994; **37**(2): 209–213.

**13.** Rimmer RB, Weigand S, Foster KN, Wadsworth MM, Jacober K, Matthews MR, Drachman D and Caruso DMScald burns in young children—a review of Arizona burn center pediatric patients and a proposal for prevention in the Hispanic community. *J Burn Care Res.* 2008; **29**(4): 595–605.

**14.** Brown RL, Greenhalgh DG, Warden GD, et al. Iron burns to the hand in the young pediatric patient: a problem in prevention. *J Burn Care Rehabil.* 1997; **18**(3): 279–282.

**15.** Peate WF. Outpatient management of burns. *Am Fam Physician.* 1992; **45**(3): 1321–1330.

**16.** Schonfeld N. Outpatient management of burns in children. *Pediatr Emerg Care.* 1990; **6**(3): 249–253.

**17.** Leon-Villapalos J, Jeschke MG, Herndon DN. Topical management of facial burns. *Burns.* 2008; **34**(7): 903–911.

**18.** Pham C, Greenwood J, Cleland H, Woodruff P, Maddern G. Bioengineered skin substitutes for the management of burns: a systematic review. *Burns.* 2007; **33**(8): 946–957.

**19.** Reed JL, Pomerantz WJ. Emergency management of pediatric burns. *Pediatr Emerg Care.* 2005; **21**(2): 118–129.

**20.** Johnson RM, Richard R. Partial-thickness burns: identification and management. *Adv Skin Wound Care.* 2003; **16**(4): 178–187.

**21.** Taylor K. The management of minor burns and scalds in children. *Nurs Stand.* 2001; **16**; 1145–1151.

**22.** Morgan ED, Bledsoe SC, Barker J. Ambulatory management of burns. *Am Fam Physician.* 2000: **62**(9) 2015–2026, 2029–2030.

**23.** Smith ML. Pediatric burns: management of thermal, electrical, and chemical burns and burn-like dermatologic conditions. *Pediatr Ann.* 2000; **29**(6): 367–378.

# CHAPTER TWENTY-NINE

# Pediatric Burn Care in Rural Environments

Felicia N. Williams, MD, Department of Surgery,
Brody School of Medicine, East Carolina University

Scott G. Sagraves, MD, FACS, Associate Professor and Chief,
Division of Trauma and Surgical Critical Care, Department of Surgery,
Brody School of Medicine, East Carolina University

Michael F. Rotondo, MD, FACS, Professor and Chairman,
Department of Surgery, Brody School of Medicine, East Carolina University

## Introduction

Major burn injury is a devastating and unfortunate reality to the burn victim and his or her family. Despite advances in resuscitation, nutrition, and wound care, the outcomes are all too often debilitating and moribund, if not fatal. While the advances in standards of care have been profound, there are a number of risk factors that have not changed the presentation of burn victims, such as age, location, demographics, and low socioeconomic status.[1,2] The people at risk for severe burn injury are those at the extremes of age—young children and the elderly[1]—due to impaired judgment and mobility. The latter population's risk is confounded by preexisting medical conditions, while the former is confounded by lack of proper supervision, access to hot liquids, and developmental limitations.[3] Although burn injuries occur more frequently in certain populations, there is not a single group unaffected by the public health debt caused by burns.

Location plays a major role in the risk, cost, and ease with which one seeks and receives medical attention for a burn. The available resources in a given community affect the delivery of appropriate and timely treatment, provision of education, and rehabilitation of burn victims. In fact, burn care requires the interdisciplinary collaboration of surgeons, anesthesiologists, occupational therapists and physiotherapists, nurses, nutritionists, rehabilitation therapists, and social workers just to accommodate the very basic needs of a major burn survivor.[4] While these resources are often very prevalent in metropolitan areas around the country, rural communities suffer from limited support systems, which can greatly affect morbidity and mortality. Furthermore, the isolated locations themselves can lead to a delay in resuscitation since the initial trauma care of an injured patient may occur at lengthy distances from the accident site. Prolonged discovery and transport times, a variety of different skill levels of prehospital providers, local or community protocols with selective access to trauma or burn centers, and a lack of resources all beleaguer the rural trauma system and often delay definitive trauma center patient care. The survival rate for all burns is 94.6%, but for at-risk populations or in communities lacking medical, legal, and public health resources, survival can be nearly impossible.[5,6]

## BURNS IN THE PEDIATRIC POPULATION

### Epidemiology

Fires and burn injuries account for the third most common cause of harm in young children.[7] Of the victims of residential fires, 40% are children.[8,9] In recent years, an estimated 1.1 million patients with burn injuries have sought medical attention; however, updated surveys from the American Burn Association (ABA) reported approximately 500000 burn injuries per year actually required medical attention, with only 10% warranting acute hospitalization.[10,11] Even though it appears that there has been a dramatic decline in the number of burn injuries per year, there is nonetheless a growing need for health care providers educated in basic trauma and burn care, particularly in rural communities and outpatient clinics, where the majority of these burn injuries present.

### Types of Burn Injury

Burn injuries to children commonly result from playing with fire, involvement in house fires, or scald injuries. Fires started by children occur when they play with matches, lighters, or fireworks. In fact, fires ignited by children are responsible for 40% of the childhood casualties of residential fires.[9] In 2002 the median age of children who started fires was 5 years, while the median age of a fatally burned child was 4 years. These fires account for nearly 14000 structure fires, hundreds of deaths, and over 300 million dollars' worth of damage.[12]

Four out of 5 fire deaths in the United States are from residential fires, with 5% to 10% due to children playing with fire.[1,8,9] In recent years, the mortality of very young children from residential fires has dramatically decreased, especially among minority groups.[13] However, there still remains a significant disparity among racial, ethnic, and socioeconomic groups.[14] Some estimates show a 3-fold-higher mortality rate for minority groups when compared to white children from residential fires.[13] As a whole, house fires account for greater than 2000 deaths annually and cost the nation billions of dollars.[1,9]

Scald injury, whether intentional or unintentional, is one of the most common mechanisms of burn injury among young children.[15,16] A scald injury occurs when a child has been immersed into extremely hot liquids or steam or has hot contents spilled or pulled onto him or her. Scald injuries are typically more prevalent among younger children, while flame or contact burns are more common among older children. In fact, among children hospitalized for burn-related injuries between the ages of 0 and 4 years, up to 65% of them are hospitalized for scald injury.[17,18] Factors leading to scald injuries include the thin skin of a child, lack of supervision, and environmental controls. Since children's skin is thinner, they are more vulnerable to significant burn injuries than adults are. Children have a decrease in their cognitive abilities to determine whether or not a situation or object is dangerous and rely on the abilities of their parents or guardians to control environmental factors that may be dangerous to their well-being. Any lapse in supervision or judgment in these regards may be harmful, not to mention deadly.[15,16] In terms of economic impact, scald injuries cost the United States up to 1 billion dollars annually.

### Abuse

Unfortunately, burns are frequently due to childhood abuse or neglect,[19] accounting for up to 25% of pediatric burns. Forms include flame or contact burns and pattern burns, in which various objects are used to inflict bodily harm (cigarettes or household appliances).[20] Scald burns are the most frequent type of abusive burn injuries, involving immersion or splash/spill injuries. The location and distribution of the injury often suggest whether the burn may have been intentional, with the face, hands, legs, feet, perineum, and buttocks being the most common sites of abuse. For example, when a child is forcibly immersed into hot liquid, there is usually uniform burn depth with clear lines of demarcation called tide marks, flexural sparing, a stocking and/or glove distribution, or donut-hole sparing. Stocking and glove burns result in circumferential, well-demarcated, symmetrical injuries from extremities being forcibly immersed into hot liquids. Sparing of flexural creases results from victims being in a flexed position when immersed, while donut-hole sparing occurs when the buttocks are pressed against a cool bathtub compared to the hot water already present in the bathtub.[20,21] Accidental immersions, in contrast, often demonstrate irregular markings, nonuniform depth, and are rarely full thickness due to a shorter contact time.[20]

Scalds by splashes and or spills are often accidental in nature, such as when a child reaches up to a counter or stove top and pulls pot handles or cords, allowing hot water to fall onto him or her. Abuse, however, occurs when hot liquids are poured on or thrown at children. Frequently, more splash marks are associated with this type of injury, which may make it more difficult to distinguish from accidental injury.[22] Characteristically, the burns are more superficial because the liquid disperses as it cools, causing less injury downstream from initial contact.[21,22]

Abusive burn injuries due to contact burns are often due to heating appliances, cigarettes, hair dryers, or irons [20,22] and are usually easier to distinguish from unintentional injuries. Unintentional contact burns are often superficial, singular, and irregular, whereas intentional burn injuries usually have more depth, are multiple, and are well demarcated.

## Evaluation

No matter the etiology of the burn injury, the victim must be immediately removed from the source. This includes removing all clothing, outerwear, and materials involved in the burning process since these items may prolong the contact time with the heating source. Patients should not be submerged or doused with cool water to alleviate the injury because this can lead to hypothermia. In general, it is advised not to immerse the affected body part in cool water if the injury exceeds 9% of the total body surface area (TBSA). The exception is with chemical burns, in which it may be necessary to copiously irrigate the wounds with room-temperature water in order to dilute the chemical substance. This is typically performed in a decontamination room warmed to 90°F.

A patient with burn injuries should be evaluated and managed as a trauma patient. Therefore, the algorithms for trauma evaluation should be diligently applied to the burn patient: ABCDE (airway, breathing, circulation, disability, and exposure).[23-25] Since the burn itself may be a distracting injury, care should be taken to avoid missing any simultaneously life-threatening injuries.

Due to the often limited resources and scarcity of specialized trauma and burn physicians in rural areas, it is important for communities with tertiary care facilities to be aware of the current guidelines and protocols regarding trauma care. This can be partially accomplished through participation in such courses as advanced cardiac life support (ACLS), advanced trauma life support (ATLS), or advanced burn life support (ABLS).

Assessment and management of the airway is the first step in evaluating a critically injured patient. Oxygen should be administered with frequent or continuous oxygen saturation monitoring. When an inhalation injury is suspected, it is important to obtain an arterial blood gas and carboxyhemoglobin level, as the saturation monitor may be falsely elevated due to carbon monoxide displacing oxygen off the hemoglobin molecule. Signs suggestive of inhalation injury

include tracheal tugging, carbonaceous sputum, soot around the airway passages, and singed facial or nasal hair. Signs of airway compromise entail the presence of wheezing, stridor, hoarseness, or tachypnea. If there are any concerns regarding patency of the airway, intubation and initiation of mechanical ventilatory support should be performed without delay. Children, in particular, with impending respiratory failure or substantial burn injuries should receive rapid, aggressive, and definitive airway management. Prior to proceeding with placement of an endotracheal tube, the patient should be preoxygenated with 100% oxygen administered via a non-rebreather or bag valve mask device. Basic airway maneuvers to open and maintain the airway should be employed (neutral, in-line position of the head, neck, and shoulders and anterior displacement of the chin and jaw to facilitate an open mouth[23]). In children, the appropriate size of the endotracheal tube is estimated by assessing the nares or fifth finger of the patient.[23] Typically, drug-assisted intubation (DAI) (formerly rapid-sequence intubation, RSI) is required for assisting with control of the airway. Pretreatment with atropine should be given in pediatric patients to limit secretions. Induction should then proceed with a sedative, such as etomidate, being given prior to administering a paralytic agent. Succinylcholine may be used for paralysis unless the burn is older than 12 to 24 hours (due to the risk of hyperkalemia). Once these medications have been given, proper positioning and cricoid pressure (Sellick's maneuver) should be applied to theoretically prevent gastric aspiration, particularly in the burn patient who is prone to developing an ileus. If an oral endotracheal tube cannot be placed, an early, standard cricothyroidotomy should be considered despite the presence of burned skin. Once a secure airway has been obtained with proof of placement, postintubation management should be initiated. This includes following arterial blood gases to ensure adequate oxygenation and ventilation, checking a chest X-ray, providing adequate sedation, and ensuring appropriate ventilatory strategies to limit tidal volumes and airway pressures.

Once the patient's airway is established, breathing should be carefully assessed. Examination involves inspection, palpation, and auscultation, with observation of air movement and chest expansion. Special attention should be given to a circumferential chest burn, as the eschar can serve as a restricting band that may limit adequate ventilation and require a shield escharotomy. The escharotomy can be easily completed with a scalpel or electocautery device at the bedside. Typically, additional sedation or analgesia is not required to perform this procedure as the eschar is insensate.

The respiratory rate and effort, breath sounds, and skin color reflect oxygenation and provide objective measurements of breathing.[23,24] A respiratory rate of less than 10 or greater than 60 may be a sign of impending respiratory failure[23] Signs of increased work of breathing include use of accessory muscles, manifested by supraclavicular, intercostal, subcostal, or sternal retractions, as well as the presence of grunting or nasal flaring.[23] Breath sounds may be altered due to inhalation of toxic material, but they are rarely abnormal from direct burn injury.

Cardiac assessment in the burn patient begins with assessment of peripheral and central pulses. The blood pressure in a child is typically 80 mm Hg plus 2 times their age. As a note of caution, a low blood pressure may be a late finding of hemodynamic instability in a pediatric patient due to increased vascular tone. Vital signs may be difficult to obtain in the burned victim, as burned extremities may impede the ability to obtain a blood pressure reading by a sphygmomanometer (blood pressure cuff). Often, arterial lines (particularly femoral lines) are necessary in order to continuously monitor blood pressure more accurately. While cardiac dysfunction after severe thermal injury is a well-documented complication, persistent tachycardia postinjury despite resuscitation should alert the medical staff to a missed injury.

The evaluation of disability involves recognizing a potentially lethal neurologic injury. A severe burn injury may distract the health care provider from the neurological status of the patient, particularly with regards to the presence of possible traumatic brain injuries. If feasible, prior to intubation, a rapid neurological survey should be completed in the burn patient suspected of having sustained a concomitant traumatic injury. The patient's level of consciousness should be assessed by the Glasgow Coma Score (GCS), which has 3 components: eye opening, verbal response, and motor response. A GCS of < 8 should warrant consideration of intubation for airway protection issues, regardless of the presence or absence of other injuries. Lack of extremity movement should suggest a spinal cord injury and prompt appropriate interventions to prevent significant complications.

Finally, the burn patient should be assessed for any other injuries by removing all clothing and exposing him or her to a full and thorough examination. While this is technically the last step in the trauma algorithm, exposure of the burned patient usually occurs earlier in the evaluation.

During the primary survey, these steps are often performed concurrently and diligently to begin the resuscitation and healing processes. Additional measures to consider include placement of a nasogastric or orogastric tube in the intubated patient in order to decompress the stomach.[26] Decompression is also imperative to assist with management of paralytic ileus, which is often seen postburn.[27] Furthermore, decompression is particularly important for patients transported at higher altitudes to a specialized burn center.[26]

## Resuscitation

Resuscitation is one of the most important steps in burn care. There is significant systemic capillary leak associated with severe burn injury that occurs up to 24 hours postburn.[28] This capillary leak, which is partially due to large losses in intravascular proteins, increases extravascular oncotic pressure, which then triggers intravascular hypovolemia.[28] The massive circulatory disturbances seen after burn injury are only partially caused by this large volume shift. Severe burn injury, typically considered to be a burn of greater than 30% TBSA, also causes a systemic decrease in cell transmembrane potential in both burned and unaffected cells.[29] This change in cell membrane potential results from depressed sodium ATPase activity causing increased intracellular sodium.[29] Findings revealed by Baxter in the 1970s showing resuscitative efforts to be only partially effective in restoring membrane potential and sodium concentrations would later help establish guidelines for fluid resuscitation.

In order to effectively resuscitate, treat, and minimize circulatory disturbances in the burn patient, intravenous (IV) access must be immediately obtained during the primary survey. Two large-bore peripheral IVs should be initially attempted, even if placed into burned skin. If this access is not possible, central or intraosseous access should be secured.

Resuscitation formula calculations should be based upon the time of the burn injury rather than the physical presentation of the patient to the care facility. The Parkland formula has served as a guideline for burn trauma resuscitation since its implementation in 1968.[30] It estimates the amount of fluid a burned patient requires in order to maintain adequate tissue perfusion.[30] As more evidence-based medicine has emerged, the Parkland formula has been reevaluated, particularly for pediatric patients.[31] In this population, postburn resuscitation remains a challenge as children generally require more fluid for burn shock resuscitation and may even require resuscitation for relatively small burns.[31] Fluid losses in children are proportionally much greater when compared to adults due to the differences in body weight and surface area. For example, total body water for neonates is approximately 75% to 80% of the total body composition compared to adults, whose total body water weight decreases to approximately 50% to 60%[32,33]. Thus, evaporative losses are more significant for a child than an adult, particularly with larger burns. In addition, children have a limited physiologic reserve. These factors underscore the importance of pediatric burn victims receiving prompt resuscitation. Research has shown that during the first 24 hours after a burn, a patient can lose up to 2000 mL of fluid/m[2] TBSA plus up to another 5000 mL of fluid/m[2] TBSA burned.[34,35] Thus, depending on the size of the patient and the burn, a patient can be substantially behind in fluid losses with as little as 1 hour delay in resuscitation.[35]

Any delays in resuscitation can lead to inadequate delivery of nutrients and oxygen as well as inadequate removal of waste products. Thus, the goals of resuscitation must be to restore and preserve perfusion in the tissues, prevent end organ damage, and replace the extracellular salt loss.[36–38] While replacing the fluid sequestered as a result of thermal injury, massive fluid shifts can occur even though the patient's total body water remains unchanged. Intracellular and interstitial volumes increase at the expense of plasma and blood volume, resulting in significant edema during the postburn period.[39]

Conventionally, crystalloid, specifically lactated Ringer's solution, is the resuscitative fluid of choice during the first 24 hours after thermal injury.[38] Those supporting the use of crystalloid solution alone for resuscitation report colloids to be more expensive while showing no advantages in maintaining intravascular volume.[40] Other crystalloids, such as hypertonic salt solutions, have also been shown to be effective in the resuscitation of burn patients.[41,42] Even though the infusion of hypertonic saline can produce elevated serum osmolarity and hypernatremia, the shift of intravascular water into the extracellular space[41,43] is reduced. By decreasing tissue edema, the need for escharotomies to alleviate vascular compromise due to edema or endotracheal intubations to protect edematous airways should be decreased.[38] In fact, Monafo[41] found that the use of hypertonic saline solutions with sodium concentrations of 240 to 300 mEq/L resulted in less edema because of smaller total fluid requirements when compared to lactated Ringer's solution. In 1991, Shimazaki et al[44] found that after resuscitating 46 patients with either lactated Ringer's solution or hypertonic saline, the sodium infusions were equivalent, but patients receiving lactated Ringer's required more interventions for airway edema.

Currently, a consensus regarding the optimal resuscitation fluid has yet to be reached. Studies have shown benefit of administering colloid with hypertonic solutions during the second 24 hours of resuscitation if the patient continues to exhibit signs of poor perfusion after large infusions of crystalloid.[38] Patients who were given colloid with crystalloid required less than 60% of the volume predicted by the Parkland formula, as compared to the 75% predicted volume for patients receiving hypertonic saline.[45] In another trial, patients in similar cohorts required fewer escharotomies, fewer days of mechanical ventilation, and less total fluid than patients resuscitated with crystalloid alone.[46]

Other institutions use modified solutions for resuscitation. Warden at the Shriners Hospital for Children has used a resuscitation fluid that contains 180 mEq of sodium (lactated Ringer's + 50 mEq sodium bicarbonate) for major

pediatric thermal injuries until any signs or indicators of metabolic acidosis have been reversed or up to 8 hours postinjury.[38] After the initial 8 hours, resuscitation is continued with lactated Ringer's to maintain adequate tissue perfusion.[38] According to Warden,[38] this hypertonic formula can be safely used in infants and the elderly without the accompanying risk of hypernatremia.[47,48]

The idea of using colloid solutions for resuscitation is based upon the goal of replacing plasma proteins into the circulation in order to generate an inward oncotic force to counteract the outward capillary hydrostatic force.[38] Massive edema results when there is a deficit of protein in the circulation due to the loss of plasma protein[38] after the burn. In a study by Goodwin et al[49] of 79 patients randomized to receive either crystalloid or colloid resuscitation, it was shown that there was no long-term benefit of colloids. Furthermore, in patients receiving colloids, there was significantly more accumulation of lung water when the edema was reabsorbed from the burn wound. Therefore, it was concluded that colloids are not recommended within the first 24 hours postburn since they appear to be no more effective than crystalloids to maintain intravascular volume and resulted in pulmonary edema. On the other hand, Demling[50] showed a benefit of colloid solutions given 8 to 12 hours after the burn injury, when they can then restore and maintain the concentration of plasma proteins. He recommends crystalloid only should be administered during the first 8 to 12 hours due to the massive fluid shifts. Recently, the Cochrane Central Register of Controlled Trials revealed that the use of albumin in the resuscitation of critically ill patients has no benefit over crystalloid in morbidity or mortality.[51,52] However, in patients with significant hypoalbuminemia or in children at increased risk for edema, albumin replacement to maintain serum albumin levels at more than 2.5 g/dL was helpful to maintain oncotic pressure.[53]

## Mortality

Traditional predictors of mortality from burns include the TBSA burned, presence of an inhalation injury, and extremes of age. Recent studies have also added delays in resuscitation efforts and initial responses to therapy to be predictors of poor outcomes.[35] However, studies from the last 3 decades have proven that advances in burn care, including early excision and grafting as well as improvements in nutrition and in treatments for burn wound infections, have increased the survival of severe burn victims.[54–56]

Despite these successes, patients with the highest mortality risk in the pediatric population remain those under 4 years of age, whose homes lack education and resources[57] and who suffer from delays in resuscitation. Additional risk factors include those from underserved communities and low socioeconomic backgrounds. Wolf et al[35] found that in pediatric patients with burns encompassing over 80% of TBSA, the best predictors of mortality were age, the size of the burn, presence of an inhalation injury, delays in resuscitation, and sepsis or multiorgan failure. Although the overall number of deaths has decreased nationally, these populations continue to experience the highest fatality rates. Rawlins et al[58] found that at-risk pediatric patients fit similar demographics in the United Kingdom and the United States.

## Endpoints

The endpoints of resuscitation are classically normalization of blood pressure, resolution of tachycardia, and acceptable urine output, which suggest adequate tissue perfusion. However, in children, these endpoints may be difficult to evaluate since tachycardia is often omnipresent and changes in urine output are often a late finding. Since burn shock is essentially a hypovolemic condition, it is characterized by profound hemodynamic changes, including decreased plasma volume and peripheral blood flow, diminished cardiac and urinary output, and elevated systemic vascular resistance.[59,60] Thus, resuscitation should be guided by a combination of basic laboratory values, invasive monitoring, and clinical findings.[29] Furthermore, the optimal guide to the endpoints of resuscitation should detect underresuscitation as well as overresuscitation in order to be predictive of patient mortality and outcome. Parker et al[61] recommend therapeutic endpoints for children as a capillary refill of less than 2 seconds, normal pulses, warm limbs, urine output of greater than 1 cc/kg body weight/h, normal mental status, decreased lactate, resolution of base deficit, and a superior vena cava or mixed venous oxygen saturation of greater than 70%. In addition, it is crucial to optimize preload in order to maintain adequate cardiac index (between 3.3 and 6.0 L/min/m²). For both adults and children, blood pressure by itself is not a reliable endpoint for assessing the adequacy of resuscitation. Children normally have a lower blood pressure than adults and can compensate for hypotension by increasing heart rate and vasoconstriction.[61]

Since children have a large cardiovascular reserve, they often do not exhibit signs of compromise until 25% of the circulating volume is lost.[53] Furthermore, their hearts are less compliant, and stroke volumes plateau at relatively low filling pressures, causing cardiac output to be almost completely dependent upon heart rate. Therefore, a transthoracic or transesophageal echocardiogram should be obtained early in the resuscitation to assess cardiac function in children who fail to respond to conventional therapy.[53] If additional information is necessary to optimize care, a low threshold for invasive monitoring, such as placement of a pulmonary artery catheter, should be considered.

## Hypermetabolism

A profound hypermetabolic response after a burn injury is directly proportional to the size of the burn injury. While immediately postburn the metabolic rate may be low (the ebb phase), the subsequent flow phase is associated with a hyperdynamic cardiovascular response, increased oxygen and glucose consumption,[62,63] and increased core temperature. Catecholamines and other catabolic agents, such as cortisol and glucagon, are upregulated, which causes increased oxygen consumption and energy expenditure as well as proteolysis, lipolysis, and glycogenolysis. In addition, delayed wound healing and immune depression have been noted.[64,65] Marked wasting of lean body and muscle mass occur within days of injury and can last up to 9 months after the initial insult.[66,67] Of burns encompassing greater than 40% TBSA, the metabolic rate can increase up to 200% of normal.[66,67] If prolonged, this metabolic dysfunction can lead to an increase in morbidity and mortality.

Interventions to curb this hypermetabolic response include early excision and grafting, prompt treatment of infection and sepsis, adequate nutrition and exercise, and implementation of pharmacologic modulators. Mlcak et al[68] showed that progressive resistance training and exercise during burn convalescence can maintain and possibly improve body mass while increasing muscle strength. Aili et al[69] showed that the administration of pharmacologic mediators such as recombinant human growth hormone prevented the often seen growth retardation in pediatric burn patients. Continuous small-dose insulin infusions have been shown to prevent muscle catabolism and conserve lean body mass.[70] Insulin also attenuates the inflammatory response postburn by decreasing proinflammatory proteins and increasing anti-inflammatory proteins.[71] More importantly, propranolol, a nonselective $\beta_1\beta_2$ antagonist, has been shown to successfully block the effects of endogenous catecholamines, the primary mediators of the hypermetabolic response,[72] and therefore reduce tachycardia and cardiac work.[73] Further, propranolol has been shown to reduce skeletal muscle wasting and resting energy expenditure while increasing lean body mass.[74]

## Nutrition

Nutritional support is critical in the recovery of burned pediatric patients. The importance of early initiation and maintenance of adequate nutrition is usually neglected for various reasons, such as frequent trips to the operating theatre, aggressive resuscitative efforts, and feeding intolerance caused by paralytic ileus and sepsis.[75]

Consequently, there is often an even more pronounced wasting in lean body mass. This is further complicated by a known hypermetabolic and hypercatabolic response.[76] Very aggressive nutritional support is therefore necessary to meet the increased energy requirements of these patients. Several studies have demonstrated the efficacy of early alimentation,[77,78] and most children will tolerate enteral feedings as early as 1 to 2 hours postburn. Enteral feedings can be administered through a flexible nasoduodenal feeding tube, bypassing the stomach and avoiding its decreased peristaltic action after the injury. In addition, early enteral feeding preserves gut mucosal integrity and improves intestinal blood flow and motility.[76] This is especially important postburn when the gastrointestinal response to burn is characterized by mucosal atrophy, increased intestinal permeability, and changes in digestive absorption.[27] These changes occur within 12 hours of injury and are directly proportional to the size of the burn insult.[79] The addition of antacids and early enteral nutrition can significantly decrease the incidence of such complications as mucosal ulceration and bleeding. Parenteral nutrition is usually contraindicated due to the increased risk of sepsis.[76]

The diet should consist of a substantial amount of carbohydrates, which are the major energy source for burn patients. Glucose is the preferred fuel for healing wounds, and accessory metabolic pathways to provide glucose are often very active in burn patients.[80] A small quantity of fat is an essential component of the diet since the hypermetabolic response postburn can lead to substantial lipolysis.[64,65] The inclusion of fat in the diet also limits the amount of carbohydrate calories needed and thus the glucose load. While the provision of carbohydrates and fat helps attenuate the hypermetabolic response, substantial amounts of protein must be supplied to reduce protein catabolism, curb the loss of lean body mass, and provide amino acids for wound healing and immune function.[81] Protein catabolism in burn patients can exceed 150 g/d,[80] with children requiring replacement of up to 3 g/kg body weight/d.[82,83] Feeding with high amounts of protein may not reduce the breakdown of endogenous protein stores, but it will facilitate protein synthesis while reducing the negative nitrogen balance.[84] In burned pediatric patients, a diet including increased protein (23% of total calories) was associated with improved immune function, decreased sepsis, and increased survival.[80,85]

## Rehabilitation

Rehabilitation is critical to the success of complete burn treatment and should be initiated as soon as possible after admission. Bedside therapy with passive and active range of motion is started early in the hospitalization. Early mobilization and ambulation after the grafts have taken are important to the success of the rehabilitation of burned children and are paramount to avoid contractures and other complications.

Splints should be utilized to minimize deformities and contractures. After patients are discharged from their acute care hospitalization, they should continue rigorous physical and occupational therapies, including stretching, range of motion, and strengthening exercises.

## Prevention

Prevention is the best way to manage pediatric burn injuries. Undoubtedly, national educational and preventive efforts have positively impacted the number of pediatric burns each year. For example, in 1994 the Consumer Product Safety Commission (CPSC) placed into effect a child-resistant lighter to protect children under 5 years of age, which decreased the number of fire fatalities by 58%[86] in subsequent years.[9] Educational programs to lower the temperature set on hot water heaters and provide resources to families in order to check bath water temperature before bathing a child have decreased scald injuries.[87] The risk of accidental explosions and fires has also significantly decreased after prevention groups provided education to hot water heater companies on the importance of raising gas water heaters 12 inches off the ground, away from infants and young children.[88] While these present positive steps towards protecting vulnerable children, more work still needs to be done.

Smoke alarms and detectors alone have been very effective in the prevention of residential fire-related deaths. Some estimates attribute a 40% to 50% risk reduction of residential fire fatalities.[8,89] Istre[14] found that families without smoke detectors in their homes were 8 times more likely to suffer fire-related injuries. CPSC safety standards are responsible for reductions of thousands of fires, hundreds of injuries and deaths, and millions of dollars in property loss. In societal savings, these programs have saved over hundreds of millions of dollars.[86] Prevention can be achieved by eliminating or reducing the risk of fire, removing agents that fuel the sites of potential fires, or altering the human behaviors that bring fuel and fire together.

## TEAM APPROACH TO BURN CARE

Major burns are physically, emotionally, and epidemiologically devastating and are often followed by significant pain, infirmity, and prolonged rehabilitation. Advances in burn care have led to increased survival and increased awareness in improving the quality of life of burn survivors.[35] Maintaining the relationship between research and clinical medicine is paramount in providing adequate and competent total burn care. A comprehensive approach to medicine and basic science by dedicated professionals with experience in burn injury is necessary to provide competent and compassionate care to this vulnerable patient population. Multidisciplinary representation in national and international organizations was established from pioneers in burn care.[90] The aforementioned advances in burn care underscore the value of such a system devoted to the concept of a group of clinicians, clinical researchers, and basic scientists seeking solutions to improve and practice total burn care.

## Members of a Burn Team

The burn team includes burn surgeons, nurses, dietitians, physical and occupational therapists, anesthesiologists, respiratory therapists, pharmacists, and social workers.[4] In addition, it may also involve input from epidemiologists, molecular biologists, microbiologists, physiologists, and other medical specialists.[4] In pediatric burn units, psychologists, school teachers, counselors, and child life specialists are significant members of the team as well.[4] It is essential that patients and their families be actively involved in the decisions about and rehabilitation of their injuries. Burn injury is a complex, systemic injury with potentially long-lasting effects that impact everyday life. Without the guidance and assistance of these health care members, the morbidity of these injuries would certainly overwhelm burn survivors.

The burn surgeon is the leader and key figure of the burn team, providing leadership and guidance while supervising management during the acute postburn period. A burn surgeon is usually a general or plastic surgeon with additional training in trauma and critical care as well as the techniques of acute care surgery, skin grafting, and amputations.[10] The surgeon must not only have a unique understanding of the physiological responses to the burn injury, but must also maintain current knowledge of evidence-based medicine.

The nurses of the burn team represent the largest single discipline involved in burn care. They are patient advocates who provide continuous coordinated care and are often the first to identify physical, emotional, and clinical changes in the patient. Nurses in the burn intensive care unit are usually trained in critical care, with further experience in burn injuries. Their expertise extends beyond basic patient management to providing compassion and empathy in complex and frequently emotional situations.

Respiratory therapists are essential in managing and coordinating care for patients with such pulmonary complications as inhalation injury and pneumonia.[91] They evaluate the pulmonary mechanics of burn patients, administer medications, and perform therapy to facilitate breathing. In addition, they are primarily responsible for recognizing and managing complex pulmonary issues as well as managing noninvasive or invasive mechanical ventilatory support.

Physiotherapy is essential in the management of burn patients. Both occupational therapists' and physical therapists' roles in the rehabilitation of burn patients begin on admission, when therapeutic interventions can maximize the potential of a functional recovery. Due to the burn injuries, skin grafting, and muscle wasting, burned patients require special positioning and splinting, pressure garments, strengthening exercises, early mobilization, and endurance activities to promote healing while controlling scar formation. In helping to prepare patients for activities of daily living, therapists must be knowledgeable and creative in designing and applying appropriate appliances. Clinically, they need to adapt to the evolving burn injury with its associated complications and prolonged, often painful recovery.

Early enteral nutrition is paramount in the management of burn patients.[77,78] The role of nutritionists or dietitians is essential in order to monitor daily caloric intake and weight and to provide optimal nutritional support to combat the hypermetabolic response of burn injury. Furthermore, nutritionists and dietitians provide expertise in the complex and controversial area of nutritional supplementation, such as administration of appropriate vitamins, minerals, and trace elements to promote wound healing and facilitate recovery.

Overall, the primary goal of the multidisciplinary burn care team is to provide comprehensive patient care while focusing on progression to a full, active, and productive life for the burn survivor. This requires extensive communication and collaboration among the team members, despite diverse professional backgrounds. In order to fully benefit from the expertise of the members, it is imperative that every voice be heard, acknowledged, and respected. As a whole, the burn care team must perform as one for the benefit of the patient.

## RURAL ACCESS TO BURN CARE

In order for the victim of a major burn to become a burn survivor, resources must be rapidly available. Burn centers were developed to provide multidisciplinary care in order to maximize healing potential and functional outcome. In order to benefit from the advantages of advances in resuscitation and burn wound care, burn victims must have access. When there is a paucity of available resources, the risks of complications and death significantly increase. Rural communities often lack specialized trauma and burn services. Between 1983 and 1985, the Federal Emergency Management Agency found that the death rate for fire-related deaths in rural populations was 35% higher than that of nonrural areas.[92,93]

Since rural areas are more isolated, less access to fire safety information programs and subsequent interventions is available. Rural households are also at greater risk of fire-related injuries and deaths due to greater use of alternative heating sources, wood or mobile homes, and a slower emergency response in extinguishing fires.[92,93] Fundamental differences between the rural and urban settings lie in the differences in fire characteristics with regards to etiology, causes of fires, and availability of preventive resources.

## Etiology

Annually, structural fires are responsible for more deaths and injuries in the United States than any other fire-related injuries. A higher proportion of these structural fires occur in the rural community compared to urban communities[92] and are usually caused by sources of heating. In fact, residential structure fires in rural areas are more than 2 times as likely to be caused by heating sources as fires in urban areas.[92] A study conducted by the US Fire Administration showed that the cause of such fires in rural communities is due to lack of maintenance of heating devices.[92] Up to 78% of homes in rural communities surveyed reported a lack of maintenance of their heating sources, attesting to a critical need for public awareness and education.[92] The lack of properly functioning smoke alarms and detectors in rural areas further complicates this issue, as evidenced by the fact that 73% of rural residential fires occurring between 1983 and 1995 were in homes without working smoke detectors.[92] Of this number, 58% of those rural homes did not have smoke detectors, and the other 15% actually had nonoperational devices. The higher incidence of rural residential fires in homes without smoke detectors may be directly related to the lack of public safety campaigns directed towards this population.

The devastation of fire is also profoundly affected by location. The actual extent of flame damage that residential structures sustain in rural areas is significantly worse than in metropolitan areas.[92] The US Fire Administration reported 29% of rural residential fires extended to the entire structure, compared to only 17% in metropolitan areas.[92] The US Fire Administration cites emergency response times and distance as factors for the prolonged length of time fires burn in rural areas.[92] Also, lower population densities may contribute to a longer burn time until fires are recognized.[92] Many rural fire companies are composed of volunteers and may be hampered by response time to the fire station, outdated equipment, and lack of an adequate water supply.

With the paucity of available resources for victims of burn injuries, burn care has become regionalized, with patients receiving appropriate initial care, then being readily transferred to specialized facilities. Warden and Heimbach[90] stressed that providing optimal burn care requires not only a physical place with the necessary monitoring and equipment for the burn patient, but a specialized team of caregivers as well. They recognized the dilemma of small burn centers: there is on average 1 burn center per 2 million people, with an average of 14 available beds per unit.[90] Since there are too few burn centers to accommodate all burn injuries, outpatient facilities and local trauma centers are required to assist with the burden of these complex patients.[94]

Of the 500000 burn injuries that require medical attention each year, only 10% require acute hospitalization.[10] The remainder are usually managed by primary care physicians, emergency departments, urgent care facilities, and outpatient facilities.[95] Upon initial evaluation, there are objective factors to estimate the probability of mortality and potentially assist tertiary care providers with difficult triage decisions. From the evaluation and treatment of 1665 patients, Ryan et al[96] identified 3 risk factors for death: age over 60 years, burns greater than 40% TBSA, and presence of inhalation injury. Patient mortality is 0.3% with no risk factors, 3% with 1 risk factor, 33% with 2 risk factors, and approximately 90% when all 3 risk factors are present.[96] Fortunately, most patients survive without receiving treatment at a burn center. Sagraves et al found that collaboration between burn centers and local trauma or tertiary care centers is beneficial on the basis of patient care, cost, travel time, patient satisfaction, and regional burn center capacity.[94] Their review of 311 patients from a rural population who were treated at a local trauma center found successful clinical outcomes with minimal complications in patients with burns less than 10% TBSA. Burn surgeons provided consultation via teleconference or e-mail to the trauma surgeons administering care to the burn patients. The local trauma center had dedicated occupational therapists and physical therapists to optimize functional outcomes as well as caseworkers, psychosocial experts, and rehabilitation facilities to assist with long-term rehabilitation.[94] Similar to this innovative idea, several burn centers have developed more comprehensive burn clinics and rehabilitation services with good results.[97,98] The previous evidence of successful collaboration provides a model for burn and trauma centers to develop burn clinics designed to unload minor burn care from regional burn centers and provide excellent and cost-effective clinical care to the local rural population while reserving complicated and more severe injuries for specialized burn centers.[94]

## SUMMARY

Burn victims encompass all ages, locations, demographics, and incomes. The population at increased risk for severe burn injury are those at the extremes of age—young children and the elderly.[1] The patients with the highest mortality risk in the pediatric population remain those under 4 years of age who receive delayed resuscitation and whose homes lack appropriate education and resources.[57] Burns in the pediatric population are particularly devastating regardless of size, depth, or etiology. Fires and burns are the third most common injury for young children,[7] who represent 40% of all residential fire victims[8,9]. The most common burn injuries to children arise from playing with fire, involvement in house fires, and scalds. Location plays a major role in the risk, cost, and feasibility with which one seeks and receives medical attention for a burn. The available resources in a given community greatly influence morbidity and mortality. A lack of adequate resources affects the education, rehabilitation, and survival rates for burn victims.[99] Despite advances in resuscitation, nutrition, burn wound care, and antimicrobial therapy, delays in reaching these resources result in an increased risk of morbidity and mortality. Total burn care requires a dedicated team of clinicians, therapists, psychosocial experts, and basic scientists to address the ever-changing needs of the burn patient. In the rural setting, burn care of the injured patient is often challenging due to the long distances from the site of injury[94] as well as long discovery and transport times. Collaboration between burn centers and local trauma or ambulatory care centers have revolutionized burn care by successfully outsourcing adequate burn care to resource-poor communities.[94]

## KEY POINTS

- Approximately 500000 burn injuries require medical attention per year; however, only 10% actually require acute hospitalization.
- Fires and burns are the third most common injury for young children.
- The most common burn injuries to children arise from playing with fire, involvement in house fires, and scalds.
- Unfortunately, a significant amount of burn injuries are due to childhood abuse or neglect; a high index of suspicion and diligent approach are warranted in such cases.
- Pediatric patients with the highest mortality risk are those under 4 years of age whose homes lack education and resources and who receive delays in resuscitation.
- Adequate and timely resuscitation is paramount in burn care, with delays leading to increased morbidity and mortality.
- Total burn care requires a multidisciplinary team of dedicated professionals to provide the extensive, complex, and challenging needs of burn patients.

- Because the death rate in rural populations is substantially higher than in metropolitan areas, collaboration between burn centers and tertiary care facilities is required to provide adequate care to all burn patients.
- Regionalization of burn care is often necessary due to the scarcity of burn centers to accommodate all burn injuries.

## REFERENCES

1. Fire Deaths and Injuries: Fact Sheet. 2007. (Accessed October 2, 2009, at http://www.cdc.gov/ncipc/factsheets/fire.htm.)

2. Hunt J AB, Purdue G. Prevention of burn injuries. In: Herndon D, ed. *Total Burn Care*. 3 ed. Philadelphia: Saunders Elsvier; 2007: 33–42.

3. Munro SA, van Niekerk A, Seedat M. Childhood unintentional injuries: the perceived impact of the environment, lack of supervision and child characteristics. *Child Care Health Dev.* 2006; **32:** 269–279.

4. Herndon D BP. Teamwork for total burn care: achievements, directions, and hopes. In: Herndon D, ed. *Total Burn Care*. 3 ed. Philadelphia: Saunders Elsvier; 2007: 9–13.

5. Gore DC, Hawkins HK, Chinkes DL, et al. Assessment of adverse events in the demise of pediatric burn patients. *J Trauma.* 2007; **63:** 814–818.

6. Miller S JJ, Bessey P, Caruso D, Gomez M, Kagan R, Latenser B, Lentz C, Purdue G et al. American Burn Association National Burn Repository 2005 Report. 2006.

7. 10 Leading Causes of Death, United States. 2005. (Accessed at http://webappa.cdc.gov/sasweb/ncipc/leadcaus10.html)

8. Barillo DJ, Goode R. Fire fatality study: demographics of fire victims. *Burns.* 1996; **22:** 85–88.

9. Istre GR, McCoy M, Carlin DK, McClain J. Residential fire related deaths and injuries among children: fireplay, smoke alarms, and prevention. *Inj Prev.* 2002; **8:** 128–132.

10. Guidelines for the operation of burn centers. *J Burn Care Res.* 2007; **28:** 134–141.

11. Fact Sheet: Trauma, Shock, Burn, and Injury: Facts and Figures. 2007. (Accessed October, 2009, at http://www.nigms.nih.gov/publications/factsheet_trauma.htm.)

12. National Fire Protection Association: Children Playing with Fire. National Fire Protection Association 2009. (Accessed 2009, at http://www.nfpa.org/assets/files/PDF/ChildrenPlayingExSummary.pdf.)

13. Pressley JC, Barlow B, Kendig T, Paneth-Pollak R. Twenty-year trends in fatal injuries to very young children: the persistence of racial disparities. *Pediatrics.* 2007; **119:** e875–884.

14. Istre GR, McCoy MA, Osborn L, Barnard JJ, Bolton A. Deaths and injuries from house fires. *N Engl J Med.* 2001; **344:** 1911–1916.

15. Cagle KM, Davis JW, Dominic W, Ebright S, Gonzales W. Developing a focused scald-prevention program. *J Burn Care Res.* 2006; **27**: 325–329.

16. Cagle KM, Davis JW, Dominic W, Gonzales W. Results of a focused scald-prevention program. *J Burn Care Res.* 2006; **27**: 859–863.

17. Morrow SE, Smith DL, Cairns BA, Howell PD, Nakayama DK, Peterson HD. Etiology and outcome of pediatric burns. *J Pediatr Surg.* 1996; **31**: 329–333.

18. Simon PA, Baron RC. Age as a risk factor for burn injury requiring hospitalization during early childhood. *Arch Pediatr Adolesc Med.* 1994; **148**: 394–397.

19. Andronicus M, Oates RK, Peat J, Spalding S, Martin H. Non-accidental burns in children. *Burns.* 1998; **24**: 552–558.

20. Kos L, Shwayder T. Cutaneous manifestations of child abuse. *Pediatr Dermatol.* 2006; **23**: 311–320.

21. Stratman E, Melski J. Scald abuse. *Arch Dermatol.* 2002; **138**: 318–320.

22. Purdue GF, Hunt JL, Prescott PR. Child abuse by burning—an index of suspicion. *J Trauma.* 1988; **28**: 221–224.

23. Bardella IJ. Pediatric advanced life support: a review of the AHA recommendations. American Heart Association. *Am Fam Physician.* 1999; **60**: 1743–1750.

24. Quan L, Seidel JS. Pediatric advanced life support: Instructor's Manual. Dallas: American Heart Association; 1997.

25. Trauma ACoSCo. Advanced Trauma Life Support for Doctors. 7th ed. Chicago: First Impression; 2004.

26. Mlcak R, Buffalo, M. Pre-hospital management, transportation, and emergency care. In: Herndon D, ed. *Total Burn Care.* Philadelphia: Saunders Elsvier; 2007: 81–92.

27. Wolf SE. Critical care in the severely burned: organ support and management of complications. In: Herndon D, ed. *Total Burn Care.* Philadelphia: Saunders Elsvier; 2007: 454–476.

28. Lehnhardt M, Jafari HJ, Druecke D, et al. A qualitative and quantitative analysis of protein loss in human burn wounds. *Burns.* 2005; **31**: 159–167.

29. Baxter CR. Fluid volume and electrolyte changes of the early postburn period. *Clin Plast Surg.* 1974; **1**: 693–703.

30. Baxter CR, Shires T. Physiological response to crystalloid resuscitation of severe burns. *Ann N Y Acad Sci.* 1968; **150**: 874–894.

31. Merrell SW, Saffle JR, Sullivan JJ, Navar PD, Kravitz M, Warden GD. Fluid resuscitation in thermally injured children. *Am J Surg.* 1986; **152**: 664–669.

32. Chumlea WC, Schubert CM, Sun SS, Demerath E, Towne B, Siervogel RM. A review of body water status and the effects of age and body fatness in children and adults. *J Nutr Health Aging.* 2007; **11**: 111–118.

33. D'Anci KE, Constant F, Rosenberg IH. Hydration and cognitive function in children. *Nutr Rev.* 2006; **64**: 457–464.

34. Carvajal HF. Fluid therapy for the acutely burned child. *Compr Ther.* 1977; **3**: 17–24.

35. Wolf SE, Rose JK, Desai MH, Mileski JP, Barrow RE, Herndon DN. Mortality determinants in massive pediatric burns. An analysis of 103 children with > or = 80% TBSA burns (> or = 70% full-thickness). *Ann Surg.* 1997; **225**: 554–565; discussion 65–69.

36. Moyer CA, Margraf HW, Monafo WW, Jr. Burn Shock and Extravascular Sodium Deficiency—Treatment with Ringer's Solution with Lactate. *Arch Surg.* 1965; **90**: 799–811.

37. Neely AN, Nathan P, Highsmith RF. Plasma proteolytic activity following burns. *J Trauma.* 1988; **28**: 362–367.

38. Warden GD. Fluid resuscitation and early management. In: Herndon DN, ed. *Total Burn Care.* 3 ed. Philadelphia: Saunders Elsvier; 2007: 107–118.

39. Hilton JG. Effects of fluid resuscitation on total fluid loss following thermal injury. *Surg Gynecol Obstet.* 1981; **152**: 441–447.

40. Pruitt BA, Jr., Mason AD, Jr., Moncrief JA. Hemodynamic changes in the early postburn patient: the influence of fluid administration and of a vasodilator (hydralazine). *J Trauma.* 1971; **11**: 36–46.

41. Monafo WW. The treatment of burn shock by the intravenous and oral administration of hypertonic lactated saline solution. *J Trauma.* 1970; **10**: 575–586.

42. Monafo WW, Halverson JD, Schechtman K. The role of concentrated sodium solutions in the resuscitation of patients with severe burns. *Surgery.* 1984; **95**: 129–135.

43. Caldwell FT, Bowser BH. Critical evaluation of hypertonic and hypotonic solutions to resuscitate severely burned children: a prospective study. *Ann Surg.* 1979; **189**: 546–552.

44. Shimazaki S, Yoshioka T, Tanaka N, Sugimoto T, Onji Y. Body fluid changes during hypertonic lactated saline solution therapy for burn shock. *J Trauma.* 1977; **17**: 38–43.

45. Griswold JA, Anglin BL, Love RT, Jr., Scott-Conner C. Hypertonic saline resuscitation: efficacy in a community-based burn unit. *South Med J.* 1991; **84**: 692–696.

46. Jelenko C, 3rd, Williams JB, Wheeler ML, et al. Studies in shock and resuscitation, I: use of a hypertonic, albumin-containing, fluid demand regimen (HALFD) in resuscitation. *Crit Care Med.* 1979; **7**: 157–167.

47. Baxter CR. Problems and complications of burn shock resuscitation. *Surg Clin North Am.* 1978; **58**: 1313–1322.

48. Du GB, Slater H, Goldfarb IW. Influences of different resuscitation regimens on acute early weight gain in extensively burned patients. *Burns.* 1991; **17**: 147–150.

49. Goodwin CW, Dorethy J, Lam V, Pruitt BA, Jr. Randomized trial of efficacy of crystalloid and colloid resuscitation on hemodynamic response and lung water following thermal injury. *Ann Surg.* 1983; **197**: 520–531.

50. Demling RH. Fluid resuscitation. In: Boswick JJ, ed. *The Art and Science of Burn Care.* Rockville, MD: Aspen; 1987: 189–202.

51. Alderson P, Bunn F, Lefebvre C, et al. Human albumin solution for resuscitation and volume expansion in critically ill patients. *Cochrane Database Syst Rev.* 2002: CD001208.

52. Alderson P, Bunn F, Lefebvre C, et al. Human albumin solution for resuscitation and volume expansion in critically ill patients. *Cochrane Database Syst Rev.* 2004: CD001208.

53. Lee J HD. The pediatric burned patient. In: Herndon D, ed. *Total Burn Care.* Philadelphia: Saunders Elsevier; 2007: 485–501.

54. Gallagher J W-BN, Villarreal C, Heggers J, Herndon D. Treatment of infection in burns. In: Herndon D, ed. *Total burn care.* 3 ed. Philadelphia: Saunders Elsevier; 2007: 136–176.

55. Herndon DN, Barrow RE, Stein M, et al. Increased mortality with intravenous supplemental feeding in severely burned patients. *J Burn Care Rehabil.* 1989; **10:** 309–313.

56. Herndon DN, Gore D, Cole M, et al. Determinants of mortality in pediatric patients with greater than 70% full-thickness total body surface area thermal injury treated by early total excision and grafting. *J Trauma.* 1987; **27:** 208–212.

57. Mallonee S, Istre GR, Rosenberg M, et al. Surveillance and prevention of residential-fire injuries. *N Engl J Med.* 1996; **335:** 27–31.

58. Rawlins JM, Khan AA, Shenton AF, Sharpe DT. Epidemiology and outcome analysis of 208 children with burns attending an emergency department. *Pediatr Emerg Care.* 2007; **23:** 289–293.

59. Andel D, Kamolz LP, Roka J, et al. Base deficit and lactate: Early predictors of morbidity and mortality in patients with burns. *Burns.* 2007; **33:** 973–978.

60. Germann G, Steinau HU. [Current aspects of burn treatment]. *Zentralbl Chir.* 1993; **118:** 290–302.

61. Parker MM, Hazelzet JA, Carcillo JA. Pediatric considerations. *Crit Care Med.* 2004; **32:** S591–594.

62. Reiss E, Pearson E, Artz CP. The metabolic response to burns. *J Clin Invest.* 1956; **35:** 62–77.

63. Turner WW, Jr., Ireton CS, Hunt JL, Baxter CR. Predicting energy expenditures in burned patients. *J Trauma.* 1985; **25:** 11–16.

64. Herndon DN. Mediators of metabolism. *Journal of Trauma.* 1981; **21:** 701–705.

65. Herndon DN, Tompkins RG. Support of the metabolic response to burn injury. *Lancet.* 2004; **363:** 1895–1902.

66. Hart DW, Wolf SE, Mlcak R, et al. Persistence of muscle catabolism after severe burn. *Surgery.* 2000; **128:** 312–319.

67. Pereira CT, Murphy KD, Herndon DN. Altering metabolism. *J Burn Care Rehabil.* 2005; **26:** 194–199.

68. Mlcak RP, Desai MH, Robinson E, McCauley RL, Robson MC, Herndon DN. Temperature changes during exercise stress testing in children with burns. *J Burn Care Rehabil.* 1993; **14:** 427–430.

69. Aili Low JF, Barrow RE, Mittendorfer B, Jeschke MG, Chinkes DL, Herndon DN. The effect of short-term growth hormone treatment on growth and energy expenditure in burned children. *Burns.* 2001; **27:** 447–452.

70. Aarsland A, Chinkes DL, Sakurai Y, Nguyen TT, Herndon DN, Wolfe RR. Insulin therapy in burn patients does not contribute to hepatic triglyceride production. *J Clin Invest.* 1998; **101:** 2233–2239.

71. Jeschke MG, Klein D, Herndon DN. Insulin treatment improves the systemic inflammatory reaction to severe trauma. *Ann Surg.* 2004; **239:** 553–560.

72. Wilmore DW, Long JM, Mason AD, Jr., Skreen RW, Pruitt BA, Jr. Catecholamines: mediator of the hypermetabolic response to thermal injury. *Ann Surg.* 1974; **180:** 653–669.

73. Minifee PK, Barrow RE, Abston S, Desai M, Herndon DN. Improved myocardial oxygen utilization following propranolol infusion in adolescents with postburn hypermetabolism. *J Pediatr Surg.* 1989; **24:** 806–810; discussion 10–1.

74. Wilmore DW. Nutrition and metabolism following thermal injury. *Clin Plast Surg.* 1974; **1:** 603–619.

75. Curreri PW. Supportive therapy in burn care. Nutritional replacement modalities. *J Trauma.* 1979; **19:** 906–908.

76. Mochizuki H, Trocki O, Dominioni L, Brackett KA, Joffe SN, Alexander JW. Mechanism of prevention of postburn hypermetabolism and catabolism by early enteral feeding. *Ann Surg.* 1984; **200:** 297–310.

77. Enzi G, Casadei A, Sergi G, Chiarelli A, Zurlo F, Mazzoleni F. Metabolic and hormonal effects of early nutritional supplementation after surgery in burn patients. *Crit Care Med.* 1990; **18:** 719–721.

78. McDonald WS, Sharp CW, Jr., Deitch EA. Immediate enteral feeding in burn patients is safe and effective. *Ann Surg.* 1991; **213:** 177–183.

79. Chung DH, Evers BM, Townsend CM, Jr., Huang KF, Herndon DN, Thompson JC. Role of polyamine biosynthesis during gut mucosal adaptation after burn injury. *Am J Surg.* 1993; **165:** 144–149.

80. Saffle JR, Graves C. Nutritional support of the burned patient. In: Herndon D, ed. *Total Burn Care.* 3 ed. Philadelphia: Saunders Elsevier; 2007: 398–419.

81. Gottschlich MM, Jenkins M, Warden GD, et al. Differential effects of three enteral dietary regimens on selected outcome variables in burn patients. *JPEN J Parenter Enteral Nutr.* 1990; **14:** 225–236.

82. Peck MD. Practice guidelines for burn care: Nutritional support. *J Burn Care Rehabil.* 2001; **22:** 59S–66S.

83. Waymack JP, Herndon DN. Nutritional support of the burned patient. *World J Surg.* 1992; **16:** 80–86.

84. Wolfe RR, Goodenough R, Burke J et al. Response of proteins and urea kinetics in burn patients to different levels of protein intake. *Ann Surg.* 1983; **197:** 163–171.

85. Alexander JW, MacMillan BG, Stinnett JD, et al. Beneficial effects of aggressive protein feeding in severely burned children. *Ann Surg.* 1980; **192:** 505–517.

86. Smith LE, Greene MA, Singh HA. Study of the effectiveness of the US safety standard for child resistant cigarette lighters. *Inj Prev.* 2002; **8:** 192–196.

87. Macarthur C. Evaluation of Safe Kids Week 2001: prevention of scald and burn injuries in young children. *Inj Prev.* 2003; **9:** 112–116.

88. Benjamin D HD. Successful prevention programs for gas hot water heater burn injuries. *J Burn Care Rehabil*. 2000; **21:** S152.

89. Hall JR, Jr. The U.S. experience with smoke detectors: who has them? How well do they work? When don't they work? *NFPA J*. 1994; **88:** 36–9, 41–46.

90. Warden GD, Heimbach D. Regionalization of burn care—a concept whose time has come. *J Burn Care Rehabil*. 2003; **24:** 173–174.

91. Mayhall CG. The epidemiology of burn wound infections: then and now. *Clin Infect Dis*. 2003; **37:** 543–550.

92. Administration UF. The rural fire problem in the United States. Federal Emergency Management Agency 1997.

93. Yang J, Peek-Asa C, Allareddy V, Zwerling C, Lundell J. Perceived risk of home fire and escape plans in rural households. *Am J Prev Med*. 2006; **30:** 7–12.

94. Sagraves SG, Phade SV, Spain T, et al. A collaborative systems approach to rural burn care. *J Burn Care Res*. 2007; **28:** 111–114.

95. Kagan RJ, Warden GD. Care of minor burn injuries: an analysis of burn clinic and emergency room charges. *J Burn Care Rehabil*. 2001; **22:** 337–340.

96. Ryan CM, Schoenfeld DA, Thorpe WP, Sheridan RL, Cassem EH, Tompkins RG. Objective estimates of the probability of death from burn injuries. *N Engl J Med*. 1998; **338:** 362–366.

97. Brandt CP, Yurko L, Coffee T, Fratianne R. Complete integration of inpatient and outpatient burn care: evolution of an outpatient burn clinic. *J Burn Care Rehabil*. 1998; **19:** 406–408.

98. Yurko LC, Coffee TL, Fusilero J, Yowler CJ, Brandt CP, Fratianne RB. Management of an inpatient-outpatient clinic an eight-year review. *J Burn Care Rehabil*. 2001; **22:** 250–254; discussion 49.

99. Thomas Wachtel MK. Burn management in disasters and humanitarian crises. In: Herndon D, ed. *Total Burn Care*. 3 ed. Philadelphia: Saunders Elsevier; 2007: 43–66.

# CHAPTER THIRTY

# PEDIATRIC BURNS IN DEVELOPING COUNTRIES

NELSON SARTO PICCOLO, MD,
CHIEF, PLASTIC SURGERY, PRONTO SOCORRO PARA QUEIMADURAS, GOIÂNIA, BRAZIL

MARIA THEREZA SARTO PICCOLO, MD, PhD,
DIRECTOR, SCIENTIFIC DEPARTMENT, PRONTO SOCORRO PARA QUEIMADURAS, GOIÂNIA, BRAZIL

CRISTINA LOPES AFONSO, PT,
DIRECTOR, PHYSIOTHERAPY DEPARTMENT, PRONTO SOCORRO PARA QUEIMADURAS, GOIÂNIA, BRAZIL

MÔNICA SARTO PICCOLO, MD,
DIRECTOR, PRONTO SOCORRO PARA QUEIMADURAS, GOIÂNIA, BRAZIL

## INTRODUCTION

Although burn patients who fulfill referral criteria for a burn center should be taken care of by a specialized team in an appropriate and dedicated environment, this is one of the greatest difficulties in developing countries. Reports from the developed world reveal the majority of burns (the vast majority of accidents result in injuries with burns less than 10% total body surface area [TBSA]) are treated in emergency rooms and clinics of major hospital centers. Even in these settings, care is not equal to that delivered by a specialized burn center. Ideally, the burn patient should receive treatment at a burn center from a multidisciplinary team of specialists with training and experience in the complexities of burn injuries.

Similarly to other third-world countries, Brazil has evolved slowly in relation to the creation and maintenance of tertiary burn centers. There are currently 51 burn services in our country, but only 32 are considered referral centers. Of these, the vast majority are owned and maintained by the city or state and financed with federal government funds. In an ideal world, such support should translate into centers of excellence for burn care; however, the centers which actually excel in this field owe their high level of quality to the local efforts of members of their burn teams. The unfortunate result is that burn patients in general receive inadequate care, often by personnel in crowded, nonspecialized institutions.[1,2,3]

When considering care for burned children, there are essentially 2 dedicated pediatric burn centers in our country, while other institutions care for pediatric patients on a pediatric ward or ICU within their facilities. Our hospital is an institution which is completely dedicated to adult and pediatric burn care. The institution also commonly receives patients with other skin disorders such as Stevens-Johnson syndrome and purpura fulminans.[4]

With this reality, in a country with an estimated population of 180+ million people, the patient who has suffered from a burn accident will most likely be seen by a nonspecialist on call in a city or state hospital, if the patient seeks medical care at all. In several inland cities with relatively larger populations (200000-300000), there remains a habit of pursuing expert opinions from the local pharmacist or even treating a burn wound with home remedies. This wide variation of burn practices often results in delayed and inappropriate care for the burn victim. Therefore, patients often present to burn centers underresuscitated, with unprotected or infected wounds, and with a poorly managed airway or lung damage.

Although these obstacles may also be encountered in developed countries, their occurrence in the third world can lead to devastating consequences, particularly in the pediatric patient population. Unfortunately, these patients are still often considered and treated as "small adults" by professionals who may not be acquainted with the specific characteristics children have, such as a relatively higher larynx and proportionally higher surface area compared to an adult.[5]

Burn care in general has greatly evolved over the past several decades and continues to do so. The developing world benefits from ongoing research which results in improvement of burn patient care. However, new and advanced technology remains out of reach for third-world countries, since governments are rarely willing to invest in the large financial expenses involved with burn care.[6] Regardless, where today's technology may not exist, older methods and techniques are employed to benefit patients. In addition, individual services and members in established burn centers often initiate several measures to improve and strive for better care of their patients.

Our institution analyzed 63532 patients seen over 5 years and noted that approximately 70% of small children are brought to the hospital within the first 24 hours after a burn, with over half in the first 3 hours after an accident (Table 1). This is probably due to the emotional impact of a burn injury to a small child, which causes a responsible parent or relative to act quickly and search for specialized care. In cities such as ours, where established services have been present for some time and are recognized by the population, patients can receive the benefits of specialized care immediately. Unfortunately, we have found that school-age children experience delays in initial treatment in a similar time frame as the working adult population. This most likely reflects the current widespread belief that burn accidents are not emergencies and therefore do not require immediate attention. A parallel activity of our institution provides education in public schools for children in elementary grades about burn prevention and timely care.

Unfortunately, there remains a great need for more widespread preventative campaigns as well as better education in primary schools regarding burn injuries. Since morbidity and mortality are mainly dependent on the size of a burn, there is still a stronger need for adequate initial care and more prompt referrals to burn centers.[7,8] Adequate burn care in the pediatric population requires involved members of the burn team having a thorough acquaintance of the epidemiology and natural history of the injury in these patients in order to offer the best possible treatment. The parents must also be closely involved with the treatment plan, which continuously evolves as the patient heals.

## EPIDEMIOLOGY

Characteristics of burn accidents in developing countries may vary from those commonly seen in the developed world. National burn societies in several countries, including our Brazilian Burn Society, have been able to institute and circulate better education and preventative campaigns about burn injuries. Although burn care has improved, such campaigns are unlikely to maintain a long-lasting effect since funds are limited and usually seasonally issued. Throughout the world there are several injuries, unique to each culture, which would require special messages for prevention. Examples include injuries from recently introduced electric water heaters in Taiwan, the use of steel chopsticks in Korea, and burns caused by high-temperature noodle soup.[9–15]

The major goal of any preventative campaign is to avert the most common injuries. As scalds are widely reported as the main cause of burn injury in the pediatric population, addressing bath-related and non-bath-related injuries separately may be of benefit. Reports from the third world usually show that scald-related deaths are similar in TBSA burned to nonscald burns, although inhalation injury is universally an indicator of higher morbidity and mortality. Lower socioeconomic groups, even those residing in first-world countries, appear to have a higher risk of burn accidents, particularly in young children. Fatal cases are largely due to infection, since several countries may lack appropriate facilities and/or medications to act in a timely manner to prevent such complications. In Latin America, the most frequent cause of pediatric burn injuries is hot liquids, followed by contact burns and flame burns. The typical injury is when a curious, unsupervised young child pulls a pan containing hot liquids from the stove. Since bathtubs are much rarer in developing countries, bath injuries are usually caused by inadequately cooled flame-heated water.[22–26]

Due to progressive socioeconomical changes in our country, a very significant shift in the epidemiology of burns in the pediatric and general population has been seen. Since the democracy assumed control 20 years ago, inflation has subsequently decreased, allowing thousands of families to now afford motorcycles for general transportation. As has been shown in the literature, any new device or appliance has the potential to be dangerous and cause accidents. This has been reflected in adults, with a major increase in friction burns (as one falls from a motorcycle) and contact burns (leg touching an exhaust tube). Children have also suffered contact burns from the hot exhaust tube of a recently parked motorcycle. Although similar accidents occur in the developed world, the incidence affects a much smaller percentage of the population. While the pattern of burn injuries has slowly changed over time in Brazil, hot liquids remain the primary cause of burns in preschool-age children. The main cause of death in children is attributed to flames from ethanol, responsible for 70% of deaths in the past 5 years. Tables 2 and 3 show the "evolution" of causative agents in our burn patient population.[27,28]

## INITIAL CARE AND RESUSCITATION

It is widely recognized that meticulous and extensive care must occur if adequate burn resuscitation is to benefit children, particularly infants. There are several reports in the literature which will corroborate the fact that infants and small children may need proportionally more fluids for resuscitation than adults or older children. The amount of fluid given is guided by a urinary output of 1 mL/kg/h, which usually indicates adequate renal perfusion and, most likely, adequate circulating volume. It is also known that the usual recommended resuscitation formulas may underestimate the needs of this patient population.[16–21] In addition to the calculated volume administered for a young child, basic maintenance fluid, which is calculated at 100 mL/kg for the first 10 kilograms of the child's weight + 50 mL/kg for the next 10 kilograms, is required as well.

Severe burns associated with inhalation injury significantly increase mortality. We favor the early use of noninvasive positive-pressure ventilation, but this modality is rarely possible in young children due to the lack of appropriately fitting masks. Bronchoscopy, when needed, is performed during the first operation. We use propanolol only after the resuscitation phase in stable patients to attenuate the hypermetabolic and catabolic responses seen in the severely burned victim. Also, special attention should be taken to avoid hyponatremia, which may result in very detrimental effects to the child.[22–26,29,30]

## NUTRITION

Adequate nutrition ensures a better chance of prompt recovery and possibly decreases morbidity and mortality. The formulas and formulations for nutritional support have evolved over recent years, with certain nutrient supplements not always available in a third-world burn center, although most are available in Brazil.

Patients with burns affecting ≤ 20% TBSA will usually obtain adequate caloric intake by mouth with the addition of specific nutrients. In those patients with TBSA ≥ 20% or previously nutritional deficiencies, tube feeding is started immediately after admission or with a diagnosis of major weight loss. Basic diets encompass 1000 to 1500 kcal/d, with a protein requirement of 3 to 4 gm/kg/d.

Nutritional support must be tailored to each patient and is offered regardless of timing. Variables to be considered are age, weight, metabolic stress, TBSA burned, burn depth, wound appearance, and, most importantly (in Brazil and third-world countries), previous nutritional status. Nutritional support usually involves commercially available industrial diets enriched with immunomodulators (hypercaloric and hyperproteic supplements with vitamins and minerals, dextrino-maltose modules, medium chain triglycerides, Ca+ caseinate, and glutamine). Although there is no consensus on the utilization of immunomodulators in children, they are widely used in our service as well as worldwide[31] (Figure 1).

The optimal goals of adequate nutritional support are to attain a positive nitrogen balance, replace losses, reverse catabolism, and maintain proper growth. These become difficult objectives since there are several severe alterations yielding very complex abnormalities on the overall homeostasis of these patients. The hypermetabolic response initiated by a major burn injury leads to a hyperdynamic state characterized by hyperthermia, increased lipolysis, glycogenolysis, proteolysis, increased oxygen and glucose consumption, increased $CO_2$ production, and greater futile substrate cycling. The body then turns for acquisition of energy through the consumption of protein and amino acids, with consequential degradation of muscle mass and progressive negative nitrogen balance.[32,33]

In our service, we favor enteral nutrition, either by mouth or via nasogastric tube. Usually tube feedings are administered via infusion pumps over 21 hours (6:00 am to 2:00 am, with 4 hours of rest). Nutrition is initiated immediately after admission with milk until calculations can be made for the proper formulation.

Although the gold standard for energy replacement measurements has been indirect calorimetry, it is rarely used in the third world due to its high cost. In actuality, equations are used to determine the nutritional needs of patients, although there is no consensus regarding which formula best approximates a patient's requirements, particularly in burn injuries.[29] Since children may need 50% to 100% more calories than adults, and since current equations may result in underestimation of a burned child's true metabolic expenditure, we favor the Grotte and O'Neil equations to calculate the daily needs for these young patients. Protein requirements are calculated with the Pennisi equation (3 gm/kg + 1 g x % TBSA burned). Calories are provided as follows: glucose (carbohydrates) 45% to 60%, proteins

15% to 20%, and lipids 30% to 45% (in infants younger than 6 months, 45% lipids are given, which is closer to human milk). A caloric density of 1 to 2 kcal/mL, with a ratio of 100:1 to 150:1 kcal/N is an optimum goal (Table 4).

Regardless of the equation used to calculate nutritional requirements for burned children, replacements should be individualized, the patient must be closely followed, and any necessary intervention must be promptly instituted.

In order to evaluate the efficiency of our enteral nutrition unit's material, methods, and manpower, we followed 200 sequential admissions in age groups ranging from 0 to 60 years during admission and ambulatory periods, until healing was achieved. The average TBSAs burned for these age groups were 21.2%, 22%, 23.8%, 18.6%, and 12.1%, respectively. Weight gain or loss was followed in every patient, who had nutritional replacements individually tailored for him or her.

Several interesting findings related to the nutritional status of these patients were discovered. Since our average admission period is relatively brief, there was very little variation in weight gain or loss during this period (Graph 1).

When analyzing the variation of weight during the admission period, ponderal gain or loss is more significant in the age groups of 0 to 4 years and 5 to 14 years. In the adult groups, at least 56% of patients gained weight during the admission period. On the contrary, approximately 70% of young and school age children did not gain weight during this period (Graphs 2 and 3).

During the treatment period, 36% of all patients returned to their original weight. There were more negative reversals (ie, weight loss) than positive reversals (ie, weight gain) during ambulatory care for the very young children. This probably reflects the inability of some parents to comply with the prescribed nutrition. There were no negative reversals for school-age children. Of the very young children who had lost weight during the admission period, 1 of 5 was able to reverse this situation during the ambulatory treatment period. No patient in the 5-to-14-year-old age group who had gained weight during the admission period lost weight during the ambulatory treatment period.

In this study, we were able to conclude that ponderal gain (or loss) is more significant in children ages 0 to 4 years and 5 to 14 years, with the most significant percentages of total weight loss in school-age children. Adults have an average greater weight loss, and as age increases, a less frequent positive reversal during ambulatory treatment was noted. This analysis suggests that more aggressive nutrition should be implemented, particularly in the 5-to-14-year-old age group, and continued during the entire treatment. After studying the results, we implemented actions to decrease the fasting period, place feeding tubes earlier, and provide diets until 4:00 am. In addition, more rigorous follow-up regarding ingestion of solid foods and augmenting the supply of liquids when necessary were enforced as well.

## WOUND CARE

Our routine of wound care begins when the patient presents to the emergency room. After a shower (or local wash in smaller wounds), the wound is cleansed with a solution of 2% chlorhexidine. Either zinc or silver sulphadiazine is then applied topically, after which a closed dressing is placed over the wound. The patient is then taken to the operating room, and in 98.7% of cases, the wound is debrided under anesthesia. Application of zinc or silver ointment with the addition of 10% sodium salicylate to act as a chemical debridant is the next step. Dressing changes are performed as needed—usually daily for inpatients and every 2 to 3 days for outpatients.

Excision of the burn wound became popular after Janzekovic revealed her clinical findings and experience in 1970.[35] This technique, however, requires a somewhat urgent need for immediate closure of the wound, since organic losses can be significant. Although autograft is the most desirable method to cover an excised wound, patients with extensive injury usually have very limited donor areas. The use of allograft (cadaver skin) suggested by Brown (1942) and Artz et al (1955) remains the gold standard, although several authors have suggested alternatives for coverage.[36,37]

Alternatives for coverage include inter vivo skin transplantation (allograft), xenografts, other biological tissues, and industrial or bioengineered products. Throughout the world, several alternatives are used to cover the burn wound, ranging from honey to potato peel to cultured keratinocytes, as well as a most diverse selection of biological tissues and bioengineered skin substitutes. Cuono (1987), Poulsen (1991), and Clugston (1991) all recommended cultured epithelial cells from the patient or other donors. Use of bioengineered tissue has been demonstrated as early as 1988 by Heimbach and in 1989 by Thompkins.[38-45] Allograft inter vivo skin transplantation has been practiced in our country for several decades, with the major difficulty being an availability of willing donors. The sudden news of a burn accident involving a loved one, along with the emotional impact accompanying the injury, may hinder clear decisions for relatives or close friends who would be the most logical donors. As a result, delays in performing this procedure in the recommended time frame (the first postburn week) are frequent.

In large burns with limited donor sites, cadaver skin (allograft) becomes the recommended way of covering an excised burn wound. In our country, the difficulty with this procedure is that with only 2 tissue banks providing skin for government-insured patients (about 2/3 of our burn patients), there is not enough skin for the 31 registered tertiary care burn centers in Brazil. The next feasible alternative is xenograft, since the industrial and/or bioengineered products are extremely expensive and not usually financially supported by most insurance plans.[46–50]

Pig skin has been used worldwide for several decades with good success by several clinicians, including Bondoc (1971), Yang (1980), Alexander (1981), and Heimbach (1987). The theory supporting its use is that the injured body does not recognize the foreign tissue for some time, while temporary adherence allows for healing of more superficial burns as well as good protection of deeper or excised wounds. Unfortunately, pig skin has been unavailable for some time due to government-imposed difficulties on the legal importation of this product. Consequently, it became extremely expensive, and over time, most companies lost interest in importation for commercial sales within Brazil.[51–55]

As a consequence of these difficulties, a search for alternatives was undertaken. Locally, the most logical choice was to attempt use of frog skin as a temporary biological cover for excised wounds. A practically unlimited supply of these animals was present in our region due to the large number of commercially raised frogs which are slaughtered for their meat. Although we originally and independently formulated this idea in 1989, a literature search subsequently discovered prior use by Fowler in 1899 and Ricketts in 1890. These surgeons used live frog skin placed directly over a burn wound.[57–59] Nevertheless, we proceeded to try frog skin from a species known as *Rana catesbeiana* (Shaw, or bullfrog)[56] on full-thickness burns on Wistar rats, and it was found to be a viable biological dressing since it possesses antibiotic properties and other active substances within its skin. Magainine, a dipetide with antibiotic properties which is present within the structure of the skin of the frog, was discovered by Zaziass.

Based on previous experiences with irradiated tissue by other authors, we have devised a study comparing "traditional" frog skin (prepared fresh and then kept frozen) with fresh prepared frog skin, which is irradiated, then stored at room temperature. If comparison shows similar results, its use would be more widespread, even to the most remote areas, where the maintenance of frozen products is a significant cost issue.[60]

Examination of fresh frog skin under the microscope demonstrates a relatively thick epidermis, similar to human or pig skin, and a thinner dermis. Biopsy of frozen frog skin reveals a thinner epidermis, with several dermal cell layers of vacuoles, apparently filled with water crystals. The basal lamina is very evident, with a cleft dividing the dermal stroma from the muscular plane. The stratum corneum

is apparently absent. An "older" specimen, removed from a wound at 12 days, will show a rather leathery appearance, with complete loss of cellular identity (Figures 2A–C).

Second-degree burns can greatly benefit from the use of this biological dressing since it provides a great deal of comfort and is practically painless for the patient (Figures 3A–D). Donor areas are also preferentially covered with frog skin (Figures 4A–F and 5), which can subsequently be removed at any time for definitive harvesting.

In deep burns, we favor the use of HeNe laser after excision or in patients with granulation tissue. This laser is generated in a chamber with a mixture of 90% helium and 10% neon. It has a wavelength of 632.8 nm, in the visible red light spectrum. Furthermore, its divergence is minimal and can be applied from a distance. Continuous power will yield 15 mW in tabletop sources and up to 30 mW in "cannon" sources. There is prompt absorption with superficial penetration (10-15 mm). Through biochemical, bioelectrical, and bioenergetical effects, a stimulus is generated to local microcirculation and cellular growth. This leads to an increase in intracellular ATP as well as analgesic and anti-inflammatory effects. Energy is applied proportionally to the desired effect, ranging from 2 to 4 J/cm$^2$ for analgesia to 3 to 6 J/cm$^2$ for regeneration of local tissue. The dose is progressively increased as evolution occurs. Contraindications include pregnancy, use in the eye and genital areas, and use in cancer patients[61–64] (Figure 6).

## PHYSIOTHERAPY/OCCUPATIONAL THERAPY

The physiotherapy and occupational therapy departments closely monitor patients from the time of their arrival to the hospital to long-term follow-up, even after the patient is healed. Therapists participate in daily rounds, constantly providing input in daily treatment and wound care. This aspect of a burned child's care can present a series of difficulties, since devices may be cumbersome and confusing as well as difficult to adapt to. Furthermore, pressure may be interpreted as pain in fearful situations, such as a postdressing changing or fitting. Also, specific areas of the body may prove frustrating to the entire team in relation to treatment, for example, hands and fingers in small children and full-thickness lesions of the neck, which may require repetitive surgery. Therapeutic resources employing ludic techniques are often applied during the acute and posthealing care as well and involve great participation of the therapists in this delicate aspect of burn care[65] (Figures 7–9). The use of techniques which involve playful behavior for children promotes happiness and comfort in a foreign and uncomfortable environment, surrounded by unfamiliar people. The stress and anxiety accompanying hospital surroundings may be significantly diminished through play.

Patients treated in this manner usually demonstrate more positive reactions not only in their daily activities, but also in relation to the prospect of returning home to their normal routines. Furthermore, playing can be a very important tool to deal with the various aspects of pediatric burn care, such as maintaining attention, adhering to treatment steps, and promoting independence while respecting a child's rights. Most importantly, the child will gain a fuller understanding of his or her injury and the associated consequences involved in the healing process. As a result, ease of communication between the child and burn care professional team may be facilitated. Following these principles, treatment objectives can be accomplished with much less suffering for the child and his or her family. Therapists apply such valuable resources in the form of stories for children (fairy tales and fables) and lullabies, as well as game activities which enforce use of the child's hands such as dominoes, jigsaw puzzles, drawings, and marionettes. These methods can be applied during dressing changes or after recovery from anesthesia. There are also separate daily motor physiotherapy sessions where the main activities are child dependent, involving active exercises to maintain or recover range of motion and physiological positions. Finally, ludic resources are used occasionally by gathering a small group of young patients with their siblings or relatives at the physiotherapy department in order to improve patient participation.[72–74]

## PAIN CONTROL

Although pain control methods are continuously evolving, there is still a need for frequent assessments to determine the level of acute and residual pain and provide appropriate pharmacological treatment. Several authors have reported alternative methods of controlling pain, even with virtual reality devices; of course, any method or device which can diminish the amount of pain perceived by the patient without increasing risk is welcome.[66]

Most children will benefit from a simple and honest explanation about the pain they may experience during their hospitalization. It is important to explain that the pain is transient, since small children may believe that their pain will not improve and may last forever. Physical restrains are not recommended during dressing changes since they can precipitate increased anticipation of fear and pain. Allowing patients to participate in dressing changes by removing bandages and applying the next dressing can assist with children's perceptions of pain as well. In Brazil, the primary medication used for pain control is metamizol or methylmelubrine, which is not available in the United States, Switzerland, Japan, Australia, or several other countries. It is a nonsteroidal anti-inflammatory agent with antipyretic and analgesic properties. In children, it is given at a dose of 30 to 50 mg/kg orally or intravenously. When more intense analgesia is required, tramadol at 1 mg/kg is usually administered intravenously. In instances where these medications are insufficient, the patient is taken into the operating room, where proper sedation, analgesia, and/ or anesthesia can be safely supervised by an anesthesiologist. Background pain is addressed by standing orders for appropriate medications, while procedural pain is treated as needed according to the expected amount of pain prior to initiation of a procedure.[67–71]

## RECONSTRUCTION

At our institution, we currently admit about 5.2% of all patients burned in Brazil per year, with approximately 42% being children. The average total burn surface area for admitted children under 4 years is 15.2% and for those 5 to 14 years is 16.46%. For these patients, the average length of stay is 9.6 days (5-39 days), with an average length of treatment of 28.4 days (6-120 days). Upon discharge, further clinical treatment is offered to approximately 60% of patients in order for them to continue treatment of their healed skin or scar tissue, striving towards a full recovery. For treatment of hypochromia, mechanical protection against the sun and ultraviolet light (computer monitors, fluorescent light bulbs, etc) and the use of protective garments during daylight hours are recommended. Pressure garments and the application of splints by the physiotherapy/occupational therapy department are often utilized.

Only 64% of treated patients remain compliant with ongoing therapy at 3 months and 56% at 6 months. Approximately 12% of all patients will be left with at least 1 permanent scar which he or she may want removed. Of all admitted children, 1.7% per year undergo an operation for removal or treatment of a scar. Other indications for surgical treatment include functional deficits such as lip or eyelid retraction, difficulties with flexion or extension of fingers or toes, and removal of mature scars. Our preferred method for scar removal is tissue expansion, which allows for acquisition of normal tissue while being a relatively safe technique with a short learning curve. Both esthetical and functional results can be obtained with this technique. Disadvantages to consider are the cost of the implants, the need for at least 2 procedures, and the presence of a deformity. In addition, complications are frequent and often higher in immediate reexpansions of the same site. One must also be aware of the possibility of skeletal deformities due to pressure from the growing implant, as well as the development of an infected pocket of bacteria which often originates from another source, such as otitis or pharyngitis. Furthermore, the possibility of several sequential expansions may be needed to remove an entire defect. Extra care must be taken in the pediatric population with the breast bud, which may delay procedures in children. As the scar is sequentially removed, additional procedures may also be necessary (ie, breast implants, liposuction, hair transplantation, and so on).[75-85]

The idea of tissue expansion was originated by Newman in 1957 when he unsuccessfully attempted to expand retroauricular skin with a latex balloon. In the late 1970s, Radovan devised round tissue expanders for use in breast reconstruction. This technique ushered in the modern era of tissue expansion, resulting in the manufacture of implants with several shapes and volumes. However, it was not until Austad and Rose in 1982 and Sasaki and Pang in 1984 understood the underlying mechanism that complications became known. In 1984 Manders, who had rapidly gained much experience in this area, advocated the need for meticulous surgical planning. It subsequently became obvious that this technique requires a very strict surgical design in order to augment success and minimize complication rates. In 1988 Nordstrom presented a series of cases of implant malfunction as an important cause of procedural failure and complications. Complication rates up to 48% are noted, including implant malfunctioning and widening of the original scar, which usually occurs in longer expansion periods (over 13 weeks) and should terminate expansion.[86-94]

Pitanguy, in 1985, recommended maintenance of the reactive capsule, mainly in cases of reexpansion. Most surgeons leave the reactive capsule which is formed around the implant while it is placed since it may allow better irrigation to the advanced flap. This is even more relevant in cases of reexpansion of the same site, where the capsule appears to lend some stability to the reexpanded flap.

We believe it is of utmost importance in order to prevent complications and gain the most from the expansion for the surgeon to follow precise preoperative and intraoperative steps. Planning must be very thorough, using precise "matching expanders" which resemble the shape of the defect, while employing a very meticulous operative technique which minimizes bleeding and trauma to the overlying flap. In addition, the surgeon must ensure that the tissue expander has the correct shape, is placed without folds or wrinkles, and lies flat within the cavity. This is particularly true in children whose normal peripheral skin may be proportionally smaller. Our technique involves initially marking the area to be undermined by placing the proposed tissue expander over the area where the pocket will be created. Then, a solution of 1:500000 epinephrine is injected subcutaneously and suprafascially in the proposed pocket area. A relatively small incision is placed parallel to the scar and at its border in order to create a suprafascial pocket according to the shape of the implant. When more than 1 implant is linearly placed in a single pocket, a "stepped up"

positioning to avoid "falls" or dislodgements is performed (Figures 10-12). A suction drain is then placed in the cavity, exiting through scarred tissue. The expander is then inserted and connected subcutaneously to the port cavity, which is usually created across (or under) the scar, through another incision. The pocket is closed with 2 to 3 layers of unabsorbable sutures. Injections are started within 2 weeks and then weekly, until the desired volume is obtained (Figures 13–15).

Some authors have recommended externally placed ports, particularly in children. However, we believe this is unnecessary, as children who are previously oriented to the procedure tolerate the subcutaneous port injections well and avoids the possibility of expander cavity infection.[97-99]

Although there have been reports in the published literature of the ability of some drugs, such as papaverine or verapamil, to enhance expansion, we have instead elected to gain a larger amount of expanded tissue through geometrically enhancing expansion.[100,101]

Our current approach in cases where there is a need for advancement in more than 1 plane tridimensionally, as with scars on the neck, shoulders, or breast, is to overlap 2 large expanders (following the croissant-shape principle) at their end, forming an L or a V, or as "fallen dominoes" (each end overlapping the next one and so on) around the defect. In this way, the extremities of the expanders grow to their "normal" nominal size, but at overlapping areas, there is exponential growth, and much more tissue can be advanced. Since this is a relatively new technique in our institution, we are still attempting to mathematically determine the exact proportion of growth in relation to single expanders. Thus far, the clinical results have been rather encouraging (Figures 16 and 17).

In patients for whom a distal lower extremity and/or foot expansion is planned, we prepare the area where the intended expanders are to be placed with 3 to 6 sessions of percutaneous saline injections with a 25-gauge butterfly needle. Progressive amounts of fluid are injected at 3-day intervals, aimed at creating the space where the folded expander will be placed. In general, the literature has warned surgeons about the extra care needed for expansion in the distal extremities and feet. However, our experience over the past 2 years has greatly decreased our concerns regarding potential complications of pressure of the expander upon the overlying flap (Figure 18).

## PREVENTION AND SOCIAL REINTEGRATION

Families of a burned child usually live with a completely different perspective of everyday life. After having a family member suffer from a burn injury, usually through a preventable accident, the entire family frequently commits to assist with circulation of preventative efforts regarding the risks of a burn injury and its consequences.

The road to full recovery is very long, and not always successful. Social reintegration involves several different measures, ranging from school and family activities to interpersonal relationships with other victims and nonburned children. For example, children who participate in a burn camp or regular vacation camp have been shown to achieve a significant improvement in self-esteem[102] (Figure 19).

As a means of supplying continuum of care for patients treated at our institution, we created the Nucleus for Protection of the Burn Victim (Núcleo de Proteção aos Queimados, NPQ) in 1999. Its mission includes prevention of burn accidents in the general population, supporting burn victims and their families, rehabilitating patients physically and psychologically, and promoting social and functional reintegration back into society. It also recognizes and promotes the necessity of a multidisciplinary approach in order to achieve proper care of the burn patient as well as the importance of adequate research facilities to advance the treatment of burn care. In addition, the nucleus promotes various actions amongst its members and the community to raise public awareness about burns, optimize and induce the habits of prevention, overcome the limitations imposed by sequelae, and promote research. The goal is to advocate and support the necessary measures for patients and their families to return to "normal life" as soon as possible after an accident.

## CONCLUSIONS

We believe that the successful care of burn patients in developing countries is primarily dependent on human resources rather than technology. The dedicated members of a burn team will employ their best efforts towards a patient's cure regardless of the lack of technological or financial support available in an institution. Of course, there is a constant struggle for the acquisition of new products, and these are progressively incorporated as proof of efficacy and cost benefit.

Another important issue is the surprising number of burn patients presenting to well-established burn centers. We believe this mainly occurs because of 2 very simple reasons: (1) despite the local efforts of burn centers as well as the Brazilian Burn Association to develop preventative campaigns, there is minimal assistance from the government, allowing many preventable accidents to continue; and (2) the population learns to trust the treatment provided by these centers, and the patient will therefore seek assistance at such places, mainly self-referred, despite the size of the burn. This also yields a realistic statistical profile of the population at risk, which in turn provides more data for us to present to politicians in order to convince them of the extreme need for primary prevention in burn care. Of course, society in general, due to the influence of burn centers, is much more aware of burn injuries overall. In general, people attempt to promote change and protect the unfortunate victims of such injuries. Unfortunately, adequate political and financial support is often lacking in many countries to achieve this goal. This is the reason why we and others around the world have created nongovernmental organizations to continue to fulfill the tremendous needs of these patients and hopefully assist them in the long and difficult journey towards living normal, productive, and happy lives.

## GRAPHS AND TABLES

### GRAPH 1
**Ponderal changes during the admission period.**

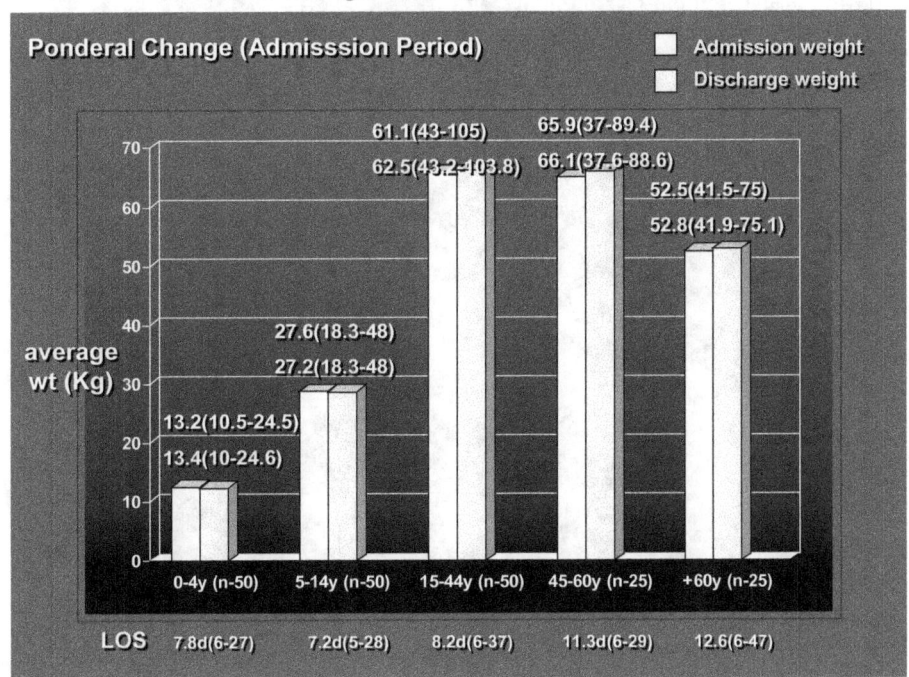

### GRAPH 2
**Percentage of ponderal changes during the admission period.**

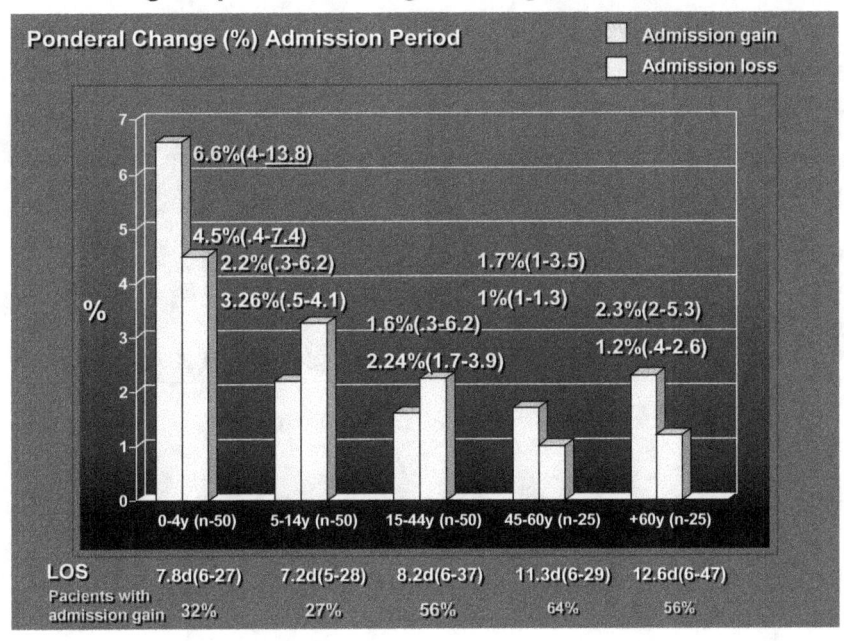

## GRAPH 3
### Percentages of ponderal changes during the treatment period.

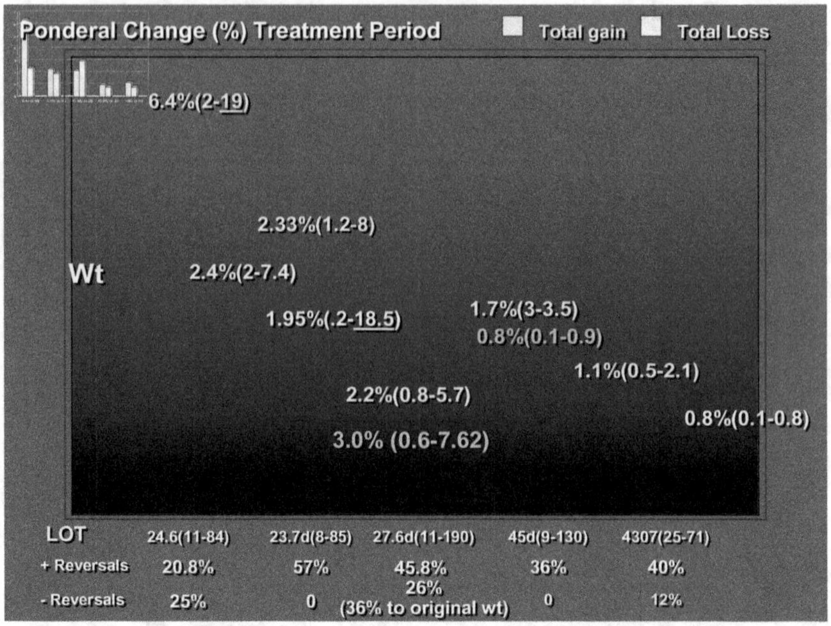

Ponderal Change (%) Treatment Period    ■ Total gain  ■ Total Loss

6.4%(2-19)

Wt    2.4%(2-7.4)    2.33%(1.2-8)

1.95%(.2-18.5)    1.7%(3-3.5)
0.8%(0.1-0.9)

1.1%(0.5-2.1)

2.2%(0.8-5.7)

0.8%(0.1-0.8)

3.0% (0.6-7.62)

| LOT | 24.6(11-84) | 23.7d(8-85) | 27.6d(11-190) | 45d(9-130) | 4307(25-71) |
|---|---|---|---|---|---|
| + Reversals | 20.8% | 57% | 45.8% | 36% | 40% |
| - Reversals | 25% | 0 | 26% (36% to original wt) | 0 | 12% |

## TABLE 1
### Delay for initial treatment.

|  | 0–4 yrs | 5–14 yrs | 15–44 yrs | 45–60 yrs | 60+ yrs |
|---|---|---|---|---|---|
| Up to 3 h | 42.5% | 28% | 27% | 24.4% | 22% |
| 3–6h | 12% | 12.8% | 12.6% | 8.8% | 8.5% |
| 6–12h | 4.6% | 5.4% | 6.4% | 5.2% | 4.2% |
| 12–24h | 11.7% | 14.2% | 13.3% | 11.4% | 10% |
| 24–48h | 11.2% | 14.1% | 13.9% | 13.7% | 11.3% |
| 48–72h | 6.7% | 8.3% | 8.6% | 9.2% | 8.5% |
| > 72h | 8.5% | 12.8% | 13.2% | 16.4% | 21% |
| > 7days | 2.4% | 3.8% | 1.7% | 3.2% | 6.8% |
| Total Patients N = 63532 | n = 7747 | n = 10156 | n = 38662 | n = 5287 | n = 1680 |

**TABLE 2**
**Causative agents of burns**
**according to age group in years (1988-1990).**

| Agent/Age Group | 0–4 | 5–14 | 15–44 | 45–60 | 60+ |
|---|---|---|---|---|---|
| Liquids | 44.2%* | 41.6%* | 33.7%* | 56.5%* | 54.8%* |
| Hot surface | 20.6% | 9.1% | 4.9% | 4.1% | 7.8% |
| Motorcycle | 15.5% | 12.0% | 21.9% | 6.3% | 10.0% |
| Flame | 12.4% | 19.5% | 13.6% | 19.1% | 20% |
| Electricity | 2.6% | 1.9% | 3.9% | 1.9% | 1.7% |
| Other | 5.7% | 15.9% | 21.3% | 11.3% | 12.2% |
| *N* = 12423 | | | | | |

* = Leading cause for age group; Motorcycle = falls and abrasions

**TABLE 3**
**Causative agents of burns**
**according to age group in years (2001-2005).**

| Agent/Age Group | 0–4 | 5–14 | 15–44 | 45–60 | 60+ |
|---|---|---|---|---|---|
| Liquids | 28.7% | 26.5% | 26.4% | 48.7%* | 53.3%* |
| Hot surface | 47.3%* | 27.7% | 20.8% | 19.9% | 13.7% |
| Motorcycle | 12.3% | 28.3%* | 39.6%* | 12% | 13.5% |
| Flame | 5% | 10.2% | 6.2% | 10.9% | 9.4% |
| Electricity | 3.5% | 2% | 1.7% | 2.6% | 1.8% |
| Other | 3.5% | 4.6% | 5.1% | 5.8% | 7.7% |
| # Patients | 7747 | 10156 | 38662 | 5287 | 1680 |
| *N* = 63532 patients | | | | | |

* = Leading cause for age group; Motorcycles = falls and abrasions

**TABLE 4**
**Calculating daily caloric needs.**

| Equation | Age | Less than 20% TBSA Burned | More than 20% TBSA Burned |
|---|---|---|---|
| Grotte | 0–1 y | 125 kcal/ kg | 150 kcal/kg |
| O'Neil | 1–3 y | 110 kcal/kg | 100 kcal/kg + 35 x burn % TBSA |
| O'Neil | 4–6 y | 85 kcal/kg | 70 kcal/kg + 35 x burn % TBSA |
| O'Neil | 7–10 y | 80 kcal/kg | 60 kcal/kg + 25 x burn % TBSA |
| O'Neil | 11–14 y | 55 kcal/kg | 25 kcal/kg + 40 x burn % TBSA |

## REFERENCES

1. Rawlins JM, Khan AA, Shenton AF, Sharpe DT. Epidemiology and outcome of children with burns attending an emergency department. *Pediatr Emerg Care*. 2007; **23**(5): 289–293.

2. Smith S, Duncan M, Mobley J, Kagan R. Emergency room management of minor burn injuries: a quality management situation. *J Burn Care Rehabil*. 1997; **18**: 76–80.

3. Schnitzler EJ. Pediatric intensive care in Argentina. *Crit Care Med*. 1993; **21**: S403–S404.

4. Brown DL, et al. Purpura fulminans: a disease best managed in a burn center. *J Burn Care Res*. 1998; **19**: 119–123.

5. Gore DC, et al. Assessment of adverse events in the demise of pediatric burn patients. *J Trauma*. 2007; **63**(4): 814–818.

6. Jeschke MG, et al. Sex differences in the long-term outcome after a severe thermal injury. *Shock*. 2007; **27**: 461–465.

7. Khojasteh VJ, Edwards-Jones V, Childs C, Foster HA. Prevalence of toxin producing strains of *Staphylococcus aureus* in a pediatric burns unit. *Burns*. 2007; **33**: 334–340.

8. Jeschke MG, et al. Burn size determines the inflammatory and hypermetabolic response. *Crit Care*. 2007; **11**: R90.

9. Enewi SD, et al. Mortality trends from burn injuries in Chile: 1954-1999. *Burns*. 2004; **30**: 348–356.

10. Spady DW, Saunders DL, Schopflocher DP, Svenson LW. Patterns of pediatric injury in children: a population-based approach. *Pediatrics*. 2004; **113**: 522–529.

11. Shalom A, et al. Noodles stay hotter longer. *J Burn Care Res*. 2007; **28**(3): 474–477.

12. Han T, et al. Pediatric hand injury induced by treadmill. *Burns*. 2005; **31**: 906–909.

13. Collier ML, et al. Home treadmill friction injuries: a five-year review. *J Burn Care Rehabil*. 2004; **25**: 441–444.

14. Maguina P, Palmieri T, Greenhalgh DG. Treadmills: a preventable source of pediatric friction burn injuries. *J Burn Care Rehabil*. 2004; **25**: 201–204.

15. Lee JW, Jang YC, Oh SJ. Pediatric electrical burn: outlet injury caused by steel chopstick misuse. *Burns*. 2004; **30**: 244–247.

16. Graves TA, et al. Fluid resuscitation of infants and children with massive thermal injury. *J Trauma*. 1988; **28**: 1656–1659.

17. Carvajal HF. Fluid resuscitation of pediatric burn victims: a critical appraisal. *Pediatr Nephrol*. 1994; **8**: 357–366.

18. Cocks AJ, O'Connell A, Martin H. Crystalloids, colloids and kids: a review of paediatric burns in intensive care. *Burns*. 1998; **24**: 717–724.

19. Okabayashi K, et al. The volume limit in fluid resuscitation to prevent respiratory failure in massively burned children without inhalation injury. *Hiroshima J Med Sci*. 2001; **50**: 41–45.

20. Cupera J, et al. Quality of prehospital management of patients with burn injuries—a retrospective study. *Acta Chir Plast*. 2002; **44**: 59–62.

21. Spies M, et al. Prediction of mortality from catastrophic burns in children. *Lancet*. 2003; **361**: 989–994.

22. Way C, Dhamrat R, Wade A, Walker I. Preioperative fluid therapy in children: a survey of current prescribing practice. *Br J Anaesth*. 2006; **97**: 371–379.

23. Holliday MA, Ray PE, Friedman AL. Fluid therapy for children: facts, fashions and questions. *Arch Dis Child*. 2007; **92**: 546–550.

24. Venter M. Rode H, Sive A, Visser M. Enteral resuscitation and early enteral feeding in children with major burns—effect McFarlane response to stress. *Burns*. 2007; **33**: 464–471.

25. Chong K, Bohn D. Maintenance parenteral fluids in the critically ill child. *J Pediatric (Rio J)*. 2007; **83**(2)(suppl): S3–S10.

26. Au AK, et al. Incidence of postoperative hyponatremia and complications in critically-ill children treated with hypotonic and normotonic solutions. *J Pediatr*. 2008; **152**: 33–38.

27. Chuang S, Yang Y, Tsai F. Electric water heaters: a new hazard for pediatric burns. *Burns*. 2003; **29**: 589–591.

28. Piccolo NP, Piccolo MTS, Piccolo MS. Two years in burn care—an analysis of 12,423 cases. *Burns*. 1991; **17**(6): 490–494.

29. Jeschke MG, et al. Propanolol does not increase inflammation, sepsis, or infectious episodes in severely burned children. *J Trauma*. 2007; **62**: 676–681.

30. Finnerty CC, Herndon DN, Jeschke MG. Inhalation injury in severely burned children does not augment the systemic inflammatory response. *Crit Care*. 2007; **11**: R22.

31. Saffle JR, et al. Randomized trial of immune-enhancing enteral nutrition in burn patients. *J Trauma*. 1997; **42**: 793–800.

32. Pereira C, Murphy K, Jeschke M, Herndon DN. Post burn muscle wasting and the effects of treatments. *Int J Biochem Cell Biol*. 2005, **37**: 1948–1961.

33. Herndon DN, Tompkins RG. Support of the metabolic response to burn injury. *Lancet*. 2004; **363**: 1895–1902.

34. Suman OE, MlCalk RP, Chinkes DL, Herndon DN. Resting energy expenditure in severely burned children: analysis of agreement between indirect calorimetry and predict equations using the Bland-Altman method. *Burns*. 2005; **32**: 335–342.

35. Janzekovic Z. A new concept in the early excision and immediate grafting. *J Trauma*. 1971; **10**: 1103–1108.

36. Brown JB, McDowell F. Massive repairs of burns with thick split skin grafts: emergency "dressings" with homografts. *Ann Surg*. 1942; **115**: 658–674.

37. Artz CP, Becker JM, Sako Y. Postmortem skin homografts in the treatment of extensive burns. *Arch Surg*. 1955; **71**: 682–687.

38. Cuono C, et al. Composite autologous-allogenic skin replacement: development and clinical application. *Plast Reconstr Surg*. 1987; **80**: 626–637.

39. Poulsen TD, et al. Polyurethane film (Opsite) versus impregnated gauze (Jelonet) in the treatment of burns: a prospective, randomized study. *Burns*. 1991; **17**: 59–61.

40. Clugston PA, et al. Cultured epithelial autografts: three years clinical experience with eighteen patients. *J Burn Care Rehabil.* 1991; **12**: 533–539.

41. Heimbach D, Luterman A, Burke J. Artificial dermis form major burns. *Ann Surg.* 1988; **208**: 313–320.

42. Thompkins RG, et al. Increased survival after massive thermal injuries in adults: a preliminary report using artificial skin. *Crit Care Med.* 1989; **17**: 734–740.

43. Subrahmanyam M. Honey dressing versus boiled potato peel in the treatment of burns: a prospective randomized study. *Burns.* 1996; **22**: 491–493.

44. Eldad A, et al. Cryopreserved cadaveric allografts for treatment of unexcised partial thickness flame burns: clinical experience with 12 patients. *Burns.* 1997; **23**: 608–614.

45. Noronha C, Almeida A. Local burn treatment—topical antimicrobial agents. *Ann Burns Fire Disasters.* 2000; **13**: 216–219.

46. Lakel A, et al. Substitutes cutanées. *Ann Dermatol Venereol.* 2002; **129**(10, pt 1): 1205–1210.

47. Ehrenreich M, Ruszczak Z. Update on tissue-engineered biological dressings. *Tissue Eng.* 2006; **12**(9): 2407–2424.

48. Gueugniaud PY, et al. Use of a biological film as cultured epidermal autograft support in the treatment of burns: preliminary report of a new technique. *Ann Burns Fire Disasters.* 1997; **10**: 33–39.

49. Dedovic Z, Koupilovia I, Suchanek I. Keratinocytes as biological dressing in treatment of partial thickness burns in children. *Ann Burns Fire Disasters.* 1998; **11**: 37–40.

50. Fernandes M, Sridhar MS, Sangwan VS, Rao GN. Amniotic membrane transplantation for ocular surface reconstruction. *Cornea.* 2005; **24**(6): 639–642.

51. Bondoc CC, Burke JF. Clinical experience with viable frozen human skin and a frozen skin bank. *Ann Surg.* 1971; **174**: 371–382.

52. Yang C, et al. The intermingled transplantation of autografts and homografts in severe burns. *Burns.* 1980; **6**: 141–145.

53. Alexander J, et al. Treatment of severe burns with widely meshed skin autograft and meshed allograft overlay. *J Trauma.* 1981; **21**: 433–438.

54. Heimbach DM. Early excision and grafting. *Surg Clin North Am.* 1987; **67**: 93–107.

55. Chiu T, Burd A. "Xenograft" dressing in the treatment of burns. *Clin Dermatol.* 2005; **23**(4): 419–423.

56. Turnbull AV, Rivier C. Corticotropin-releasing factor (CRF) and endocrine responses to stress: CRF receptors, binding protein and related peptides. *Proc Soc Exp Biol Med.* 1997; **215**(1): 1–10.

57. Fowler GR. On the transplantation of large strips of skin for covering extensive granulating surfaces, with report of a case in which human and frogskin were simultaneously used for this purpose. *Ann Surg.* 1889; **9**: 179–191.

58. Rickets BJ. Some observations on bone and skin grafting. *Trans N Y Med Assoc.* 1890: 362–370.

59. Piccolo NS, Piccolo MTS, Piccolo MS. Uso de pele de rã como curativo biológico com substituto temporário da pele em queimaduras. Experiência de doze anos. *Revista Brasileira de Queimaduras.* 2002; **2**: 18–23.

60. Gajiwala K, Gajiwala AL. Evaluation of lyophilised, gamma-irradiated amnion as a biological dressing. *Cell Tissue Bank.* 2004; **5**(2): 73–80.

61. Burr HS, Harvery SC, Taffel M. Bio-electric correlates of wound healing. *Yale J Biol Med.* 1938; **11**: 103–107.

62. Carvalho P, et al. Análise de fibras colágenas através da morfometria computadorizada em feridas cutâneas de ratos submetidos a irradiação do laser HeNe. *Ver Fisiot Brás.* 2003; **4**: 4–9.

63. Correa F, et al. O uso do laser HeNe. *Rev Fisiot Bras.* 2003; **4**: 335–340.

64. Medrado AR, Pugliese LS, Reis SR, Andrade ZA. Influence of low level laser therapy on wound healing and its biological action upon myofibroblasts. *Laser Surg Med.* 2003.

65. Sharp PA, Dougherty ME, Kagan RJ. The effect of positioning devices and pressure therapy on outcome after full-thickness burns of the neck. *J Burn Care Res.* 2007; **28**: 451–459.

66. Chan EA, et al. Application of a virtual reality prototype for pain relief of pediatric burn in Taiwan. *J Clin Nurs.* 2007; **16**: 786–793.

67. Kavanagh C. Psychological intervention with the severely burned child: report of an experimental comparison of two approaches and their effects on psychological sequelae. *J Am Acad Child Psychiatry.* 1983; **2**: 145–156.

68. Folwer PD. Aspirin, paracetamol and non-steroidal anti-inflammatory drugs—a comparative review of side-effects. *Med Toxicol.* 1987; **2**: 338–366.

69. Cederholm I, Bengtsson M. Long term high dose morphine, ketamine and midazolam infusion in a child with burns. *Br J Clin Pharmacol.* 1990; **30**: 901–905.

70. Garzone PD, Kroboth PD. Pharmacokinetics of the newer benzodiazepines. *Clin Pharmacokinet.* 1989; **16**: 337–364.

71. Serra MC, Chia CY. Analgesia em nível ambulatorial na criança queimada. *Arq Bras Pediatr.* 1996; **3**: 173–176.

72. Fujisawa DS. Formação academica do fisioterapeuta: utilização das atividades lúdicas nos atendimentos de crianças. *Ver Brás Educ Espec.* 2006; **12**: 1–47.

73. Machado MMP, et al. A criança hospitalizada: espaço potencial e o palhaço. *Boletim de Iniciação Científica em Psicologia.* 2002; **3**: 34–52.

74. Rossi LA, et al. A dor da queimadura—terrível para quem sente—estressante para quem cuida. *Ver Latin-Am Enf.* 2000; **8**: 18–26.

75. Borges Filho PT, et al. Soft tissue expansion in lower extremity reconstruction. *Clin Plast Surg.* 1991; **18**: 593–599.

76. Pandya AN, Vadodaria S, Coleman DJ. Tissue expansion on the limbs: a comparative analysis of limb and non-limb sites. *Br J Plast Surg.* 2002; **55**: 302–306.

77. Austad ED. Contraindications and complications in tissue expansion. *Facial Plast Surg.* 1988; **5**: 379–382.

78. Wyllie FJ, Gowar JP, Levick PL. Use of tissue expanders after burns and other injuries. *Burns Incl Therm Inj.* 1986; **12**: 277–282.

79. Buhrer DP, Hunag TT, Yee HW, Blackwell SJ. Treatment of burn alopecia with tissue expanders in children. *Plast Reconstr Surg.* 1988; **81**: 512–515.

80. Gibstein LA, et al. Tissue expansion in children: a retrospective study of complications. *Ann Plast Surg.* 1997; **38**: 358–364.

81. Mason AC, Davison SP, Manders EK. Tissue expander infections in children: look beyond the expander pocket. *Ann Plast Surg.* 1999; **43**: 539–541.

82. Youm T, et al. Complications of tissue expansion in a public hospital. *Ann Plast Surg.* 1999; **42**: 396–401.

83. Still JM, Law E, Craft-Coffman B. Skeletal deformities due to tissue expanders: report of two patients. *Ann Plast Surg.* 2000; **44**: 211–213.

84. Hudson DA, Lazarus D, Silfen R. The use of serial tissue expansion in pediatric plastic surgery. *Ann Plast Surg.* 2000; **45**: 589–593.

85. Cunha MS, et al. Tissue expander complications in plastic surgery: a 10-year experience. *Rev Hosp Clin Fac Med Sao Paulo.* 2002; **57**: 93–97.

86. Farzaneh FC, Kaldari S, Becker M, Wikstrom SO. Tissue expansion 1984-1999: a 15 year review. *Scand J Plast Reconstr Surg Hand Surg.* 2006; **40**: 89–92.

87. Fosutanos A, Zavrides H. Reconstruction of facial burn sequellae utilizing tissue expanders with embodiment injection site: case report. *Acta Chir Plast.* 2006; **48**: 103–107.

88. Tavares Filho JM, et al. Tissue expansion in burn sequellae repair. *Burns.* 2007; **33**: 246–251.

89. Stabellini G, et al. Tissue expander: histological and histochemical study 6 months after transplant—our experience. *J Long Term Eff Med Implants.* 2000; **10**: 279–290.

90. Manders EK, et al. Soft tissue expansion: concepts and complications. *Plast Reconstr Surg.* 1984; **74**: 493–507.

91. Pisasky BD. Tissue expander complications in the pediatric burn patient. *Plast Reconstr Surg.* 1998; **102**: 12.

92. Youm T, Margiotta M, Kasbian A, Karp N. Complications of tissue expansion in a public hospital. *Ann Plast Surg.* 1999; **42**: 396–401.

93. Iconomou TG, Michelou BG, Zucker RM. Tissue expansion in the pediatric patient. *Ann Plast Surg.* 1993; **31**: 134–140.

94. Friedman RM, et al. Risk factors for complications in pediatric tissue expansion. *Plast Reconstr Surg.* 1996; **98**: 1242–1246.

95. LoGiudice J, Gosain AK. Pediatric tissue expansion: indications and complications. *J Craniofac Surg.* 2003; **14**: 866–872.

96. Asian G, Tuncali D, Bingui F. Are new designs in expander technology possible in order to minimize complications? *Plast Reconstr Surg.* 2003; **112**: 1506–1507.

97. Dickson WA, Sharpe DT, Jackson IT. Experience with an external valve in small volume tissue expanders. *Br J Plast Surg.* 1988; **41**: 373–377.

98. Jackson IT, et al. Use of external reservoirs in tissue expansion. *Plast Reconstr Surg.* 1987; **80**: 266–273.

99. Lozano S, Drucker M. Use of tissue expanders with external ports. *Ann Plast Surg.* 2000; **44**: 14–17.

100. Copcu E, et al. Enhancement of tissue expansion by calcium channel blocker: a preliminary study. *World J Surg Oncol.* 2003; **9**: 1–19.

101. Tang Y, Luan J, Zhang X. Accelerating tissue expansion by application of topical papaverine cream. *Plast Reconstr Surg.* 2004; **114**: 1166–1169.

102. Rimmer RB, et al. Impact of a pediatric residential burn camp experience on burn survivors' perceptions of self and attitudes regarding the camp community. *J Burn Care Res.* 2007; **28**: 334–341.

# CARE OF THE HOSPITALISED PAEDIATRIC BURN PATIENT: A PERSPECTIVE FROM THE UNITED KINGDOM

KERRY DAVIES MSC, BSC (HONS), MBBS

## OUTLINE

## EPIDEMIOLOGY

Burn care in Britain has traditionally developed most rapidly at times of conflict and war. Very significant advances in the quality of burn surgery coincided with the Second World War, just prior to the introduction of the publicly funded National Health Service (NHS) in 1948. At that time, burn injuries of greater than 33% total body surface area (TBSA) were almost universally fatal.[1] In the 1950s and 1960s, the concept of the burn team was introduced in the NHS. Improved survival rates were augmented by vast improvements in the areas of fluid management and skin grafting techniques.[2] By the 1960s and 1970s, review of intensive care techniques facilitated the successful treatment of massive burns,[3] allowing support and treatment of individuals on dedicated intensive care burn units. Within the NHS, development of dedicated burns intensive care units (ICUs) was haphazard and uncoordinated, as it relied purely on the initiative of the local burn care teams to set up and implement. This has led to wide discrepancies in the working practices, staffing levels, and activities of the individual units.[4] As a result, it has been difficult to make direct comparisons between burn units globally due to the complexity and variability of burn injury and the lack of standardised and validated methodology and tools.

In the United Kingdom, it became apparent that there was a need for a national review of burn care services. The review of services was instigated by the British Burn Association (BBA), the association of professionals who specialise in burn care, in light of growing evidence that the current state of UK burn services was disorganised, fragmented, inadequate, and inequitable from the patients' perspective. Although historically British burn care was credited with being an innovative world leader, the quality of services had not developed in comparison with other world leading services over the last 2 decades. In September 1998, the Department of Health supported a national review of burn services. The committee of the National Burn Care Review (NBCR) was set up to consider burn care and its provision across the British Isles. The committee worked with clinical and nonclinical professionals and patients and their representatives to consider burn care from the time of injury through recovery, including the entire period of rehabilitation, reconstruction, and integration back in to society. The resultant publication, *Standards and Strategy for Burn Care*,[4] recommends standards for service organisations, stratification of burn care, and a process for implementing the recommendations with burn injury referral guidelines.

## UK DEMOGRAPHICS

In Britain there is no readily available way of identifying specialised burns activity from nonspecialised burns activity using current NHS information systems.[5] Diagnostic ICD-10 codes are of little use as there is no means of describing the severity of an injury. It is recommended that a new specialist code be created for use in the main speciality field of the Hospital Episode Statistics (HES) definition. The code would be used for any treatment required as a result of the individual having suffered a burn injury and should cover all clinical events, whether delivered by medical, nursing, or professions allied to medicine (PAMs).[5]

Burn injuries are experienced by around 250000 people in the United Kingdom annually due to contact with hot fluids and surfaces, flame, chemicals, and electrical sources. There are also rare skin disorders which cause massive burnlike wounds. Around 175000 people attend accident and emergency departments with burn injury each year, with 13000 admitted to hospitals. Not all are admitted to burns and plastic surgery units. Approximately 30% of children requiring admission are admitted to a nonspecialist unit. Approximately 1000 patients are admitted with

severe burns requiring fluid resuscitation per annum, about half of whom are children under 16 years of age.[4] Table 1 shows the incidence of burns admitted to tertiary hospitals throughout the United Kingdom with the data broken down into size of burn as indicated by TBSA.

The incidence of burn injuries is closely linked to social deprivation and exclusion, with large geographical variations throughout the United Kingdom. Qualitative research has shown that people from lower socioeconomic backgrounds may experience 50% more burn and scald injuries compared with people from higher socioeconomic backgrounds.[7] Deprivation factors include the use of poor quality products and facilities, overcrowding, lack of parental control of children, and increased use of deep-fat fryers and smoking materials.[6] Burn injury correlates with the population density. Burn injuries are largely accidental and reflect the vulnerability of groups to particular accidents, for example, children in the home and teenagers in cars.[8] Residential fires caused at least 67 deaths and 2500 nonfatal injuries to children aged 0 to 16 years in the United Kingdom in 1998. Very young children are disproportionally represented; 45% of those children suffering burns and scalds were under 5 years old, mostly as a result of domestic accidents. Teenage boys from deprived socioeconomic backgrounds are more likely to experience firework-related injuries than those from less deprived areas.[6]

There are around 155 burn injury admissions per million of the population per annum in the United Kingdom. This figure has been constant for at least 10 years.[8] However, admission rates vary enormously throughout Britain, with some health authorities with more than 2 standard deviations above the mean. For example, sustaining a burn in London, the patient would be close to burn care facilities where he or she could be treated as an outpatient. A similar injury in the north of Scotland is likely to result in an admission rather than referring to a distant burn unit in the south of the country. There are 300 deaths in hospital per annum in the United Kingdom. The risk of death remains largely unchanged in the over-60-year-old population but has decreased for those with similar injuries in the younger age groups, especially in children and young adults.[4]

## UK CLASSIFICATION OF BURNS

The NBCR[9] outlined its referral guidelines. Within these guidelines, it was necessary to classify the type and severity of burns to facilitate the correct referral patterns. It has been traditional to use the size of skin injury following a burn injury as the single criterion to guide referral. This approach has often been criticised as overly simplistic. Consideration of other important factors has proved difficult, as quantification of these is unclear or impossible. It has been recognised that practical clarification is needed, and the British Burn Association by way of the committee of the NBCR proposed the following guidance, outlined below. Such guidance is not to be viewed as rigid instruction but is used to help highlight some of the important features of burn injury that are known to predict a complex clinical course. It is proposed that burn injuries be referred to appropriate burn care hospitals based on the injury complexity for assessment and management.[9] In the opinion of the National Burn Care Review Committee (NBCRC) and the British Burn Association, there is no justification for injuries requiring hospital admission to be dealt with outside this system.

**TABLE 1**
**Complex: A burn is more likely to be complex if associated with the following criteria:**

| | |
|---|---|
| Age | Under 5 y or over 60 y |
| Site involvement (with dermal or full-thickness loss) | Face; hands; perineum; feet; any flexure, particularly the neck or axilla; or any circumferential dermal or full-thickness burn of the limbs, torso, or neck |
| Inhalation injury | Any significant such injury, excluding pure carbon monoxide poisoning |
| Mechanism of injury | Chemical injury (> 5% TBSA) Exposure to ionizing radiation injury High-pressure steam injury High-tension electrical injury Hydrofluoric acid injury (> 1% TBSA) Suspicion of nonaccidental burn injury, adult or paediatric |

**A complex burn injury is also suggested by one involving**

| | |
|---|---|
| Size of skin injury (with dermal or full-thickness loss) | Paediatric (under 16 y) > 5% TBSA or adult (16 y or over) > 10% TBSA |

**A burn injury may also be deemed complex if it occurs alongside**

| | |
|---|---|
| Existing conditions | Cardiac limitation &/or MI within 5 y, respiratory limitation of exercise, diabetes, pregnancy, immunosuppression for any reason, hepatic impairment, cirrhosis |
| Associated injuries | Crush injuries Fractures Head injury Penetrating injuries |

Associated injuries, such as those listed, complicate any burn injury and may make it complex. However, the range of presenting problems must be carefully considered and the most compelling injury dealt with first, according to clinical need. This may, in some circumstances, delay any referral for the burn injury to be dealt with. In such instances, advice as regards burn management should always be sought.

**TABLE 1 (continued)**

**A complex nonburn would include**

| | |
|---|---|
| Inhalation injury | Any significant such injury with no cutaneous burn, excluding pure carbon monoxide poisoning |
| Vesiculobullous disorders | Any over 5% TBSA Epidermolysis bullosa, staphylococcal scalded skin syndrome (Ritter's), Stevens-Johnson syndrome, toxic epidermal necrolysis (Lyell's) |

All injuries deemed to be complex need referral to the local burn centre or burn unit.

The criteria listed above put the patient at risk of a complex injury. While some are absolute, others, such as age < 5 years or > 60 years, coexisting medical problems, associated head injury, fractures, and burns to the face, hands, or feet, are open to interpretation if the burn is not more than 5% TBSA and has no area of deep burn. Under these circumstances, the burn may be treated locally in an accident and emergency (A&E) department, provided it is reviewed within 24 hours by an experienced A&E clinician and referred to the burns service if there is doubt about the extent or severity of the injury. A&E departments are advised to discuss these types of cases with their local burns service on initial presentation if there is any uncertainty about the nature, severity, or significance of each of the criteria.

TABLE 1 (*continued*)

**NONCOMPLEX:**
**All burn injuries felt not to be complex may be referred for assessment and admission according to the skin surface area involved.**

| | |
|---|---|
| Size of skin injury | Paediatric (under 16 y old) 2% to 5% TBSA if dermal or any smaller injury if full-thickness loss. Adult (16 y or over) 5% to 10% TBSA if dermal or any smaller injury if full-thickness loss. |

All noncomplex injuries referrals should be made to a local plastic surgery unit (burn facility). Other injuries not meeting the criteria laid out above are often suitable for care in an A&E department or in the community.

**NONACUTE REFERRALS:**
**Injuries that may require referral from A&E, general practitioner, practice nurse, or district nurse in the postacute phase include**

| | |
|---|---|
| Wound healing | Any wound unhealed at 14 days postinjury |
| Complications | Any significant infection, septic episode, or suggestion of a toxic shock–like illness |
| Rehabilitation | Any healed wound where the scarring suggests there will be a significant aesthetic impact &/or psychological disturbance<br>The need to consider skin camouflage<br>A significant functional limitation<br>The need to consider pressure therapy or other forms of scar modification<br>The need to consider surgical reconstruction |

## BURN FACILITIES

Key recommendations of the NBCR in 2003[4] were that all complex burns should be required to be referred to a local burn centre or burn unit and should not be managed by a plastic surgery unit or within a general hospital. A new structure of burn services is currently being developed nationally,[6] reflecting the complexity of the injury in an organised manner. Burn management will be organised in the following tier system:

- Burn centres for the most complex injuries as well as complex and noncomplex burn injuries
- Burn units for generally complex and noncomplex burn injuries
- Burn facilities for noncomplex burn injuries

In the document "The Case for Change,"[6] laid out by the Specialist Burn Care Commissioners' briefing, the structure of burn centres, burn units, and burn facilities was outlined as shown below.

## Burn Centre[6]

This level of inpatient burn care is for the highest level of injury complexity and offers a separately staffed, geographically discrete ward. The facilities are up to ICU level of critical care and have immediate operating theatre access.

- Purposely designed stand-alone ward for paediatric OR adult admissions (not both)
- Cubicle accommodation with environment control
- Designated burns nursing and other health professionals with training and experience
- Immediate access to a dedicated burn theatre (< 25 m)
- Dedicated burn anaesthetic input with nominated lead consultant
- Intensive care provided by intensivists either in the centre critical care beds or in a suitably equipped, adjacent (< 50 m) ICU or pediatric ICU
- Consultant burn surgeon on-call rota (24/7)
- Full range of support services and specialties

## Burn Unit[6]

This level of inpatient burn care is for the moderate level of injury complexity and offers a separately staffed, discrete ward. The facilities are up to HDU (High Dependency Unit) level for critical care and operating theatre access suitable for the case mix.

- Purposely designed stand-alone ward for paediatric OR adult admissions (not both)
- Cubicle accommodation of adequate size
- Designated burns nursing and other health professionals with training and experience
- Access to operating theatre (< 50 m) with fixed burn lists each week
- Intensive care access for any surgical patient, either paediatric or adult
- Plastic surgeon on-call rota (24/7)
- Single, named consultant lead for burn service
- District general hospital–level support services and specialties

## Burn Facility[6]

This level of inpatient burn care equates to a standard plastic surgical ward for the care of noncomplex burn injuries.

- An existing plastic surgery ward, paediatric OR adult (not both)
- Cubicle beds available
- Nursing and other health professionals with burn care training and experience
- Access to a trauma theatre
- Critical care access for any surgical patient, either paediatric or adult
- Plastic surgeon on-call rota (24/7)
- District general hospital–level support services and specialties
- Care provision for noncomplex injuries

Special attention needs to be paid to children requiring care for complex burns, including critical care. Each burn care service should be compliant with designation separately for paediatric and for adult care. In a limited number of hospitals, 2 burn services (1 paediatric, 1 adult) may coexist in an integrated burn care service which maintains paediatric care standards.

## BURN CARE NETWORKS

All children with burn injuries should receive specialist functional, aesthetic, and psychological rehabilitation, and this should be planned for on the day of admission. The NBCR[4] recommends that rehabilitation services are provided for throughout acute, subacute, early postdischarge, and community stages. They recommend that emphasis should be placed on

- Intensive (multispeciality) rehabilitation wards for patients with a range of traumatic injuries and burns
- Outreach teams linked to burn units and burn centres to ensure ongoing care for patients in their own homes via hospital outpatient departments and supportive educational health care professionals in the community, district general hospitals, or plastic surgery units
- Psychological rehabilitation of patient and family being coordinated by a named coordinator in each burn unit or centre

It is also the recommendation that locally based self-help groups and burn camps are actively developed with NHS supportive funding.

For noncomplex injuries, patients would be treated by their general (family) practitioner, practice nurse, or district (community) nurse. For the next level of severity, patients would receive treatment via emergency departments from which they can be referred to higher tiers if assessment indicates a more complex injury. Burn centres should admit all complex injuries with severe burns from a large geographical area, plus less complex injuries from a smaller area of the immediate population. This evens out peaks and troughs of workload and ensures that nursing staff in particular have a range of varying and interesting case loads to deal with. Collaboration is required between the small number of burn centres which operate within large geographical areas but have highly specialised services, and the burn units managing the moderate burn injury complexity providing a level of critical care (high dependency units) with operating theatre access at a more local level. These networks will be critical to the successful implementation of burn care management.[6]

Across the British Isles there are currently 49 plastic surgery services offering burn care of some kind, and in the United Kingdom mainland, 22 of these offer care to complex major injuries on a regular basis. There are currently 17 paediatric burn sites. All hospitals in the United Kingdom that have any form of defined burn care provision are clinically led by plastic surgeons. There is only 1 exception where a paediatric general surgeon is the clinical lead. Table 2 illustrates the proportion of children admitted to specialised burn units or to generalised hospitals with no specialist burn services.

**TABLE 1** (*continued*)
**Total Paediatric Burns Cases Admitted to Hospitals in England and Wales in 1997–1998.**

| Admitted burns patients 1997–1998 | Children < 16 y | Adults 16+ y |
|---|---|---|
| Burns units and plastic surgery units | 4600 | 5600 |
| Generalised hospitals with no defined burn service | 1800 | 4100 |

## STAFFING

In almost the whole British Isles, the surgical speciality that has clinical responsibility of severe burn injuries is plastic surgery. This subspeciality of burn surgery is part of the training for the FRCS(plast) examination, normally taken after year 4 of the Calman-style training. No other speciality in the United Kingdom has formal training and examination in the aspects of care for severe burn injury. It is the recommendation of the NBCRC[4] that services designated by purchasing health organisations to care for admissions with burn injury should ensure that the surgical service is provided by an accredited plastic surgeon working with at least 2 other plastic surgeons. Consideration must be given to the need to retain skills in dealing with children. The NBCRC recommends that burn unit or centre plastic surgeons should commit each week to at least 1 fixed session for a multidisciplinary ward round, 1 operative burn list, and 1 burns outpatient clinic. This commits at least approximately half the fixed sessions of the working week to the care of the burn injury. Most career surgeons will commit a greater proportion of the working week than this to the burn service. Plastic surgery and other specialist advisory committees should give urgent consideration to the establishment of burn fellowships as educational posts for trainees in years 5 and 6 of their training. The completion of a fellowship in the care of burn injury should be a necessity for any trainee wishing to take up a post in a burn centre in addition to the award of the certificate of completion of specialist training.[4]

Each burn unit or burn centre should admit at least 50 complex injuries per annum as a minimum and a total of 200 to 300 burn cases per annum. Within England and Wales, to manage the distribution of severe burns with reasonable geographical access for emergency transfer, it is anticipated that approximately 7 hospitals would act as burn centres. These centres would also be adult burns units for their immediate catchment areas. In addition, to ensure cross-country cover for the management of moderate burn injury, a further 1 or 2 additional adult burn units will be required. In 2002 to 2003, there were no hospitals in England and Wales dealing with children which had a paediatric ICU on the same site as the burns service.[4]

For the care of children with burns within England and Wales, a total of 3 paediatric burn networks are planned to include burn centres, with a possible 2 others acting as burn units. Burn centres and units would be responsible for the organisation and delivery of rehabilitation, including physical and psychosocial assessment for patients and their families, and for meeting the specific needs of children, including providing play therapists and teachers.[6]A programme of biannual visits to the services should be instigated for monitoring care services for their effectiveness and compliance with the recommendations.[10]

## NATIONAL BURN BED BUREAU

As medicine and surgery have developed, good intensive care services have developed in response. Specialised critical care services developed units for their own patients, but this was unplanned and haphazard.[11] The baseline for funded burn bed capacity in June 2007 was 393 across the British Isles. The total for each country are England 279, Scotland 49, Wales 32, Northern Ireland 19, and Ireland 14. On any given day, there are around 70 to 100 beds available across the United Kingdom for the treatment of burn injury. These are not necessarily in the right place, and most are only suitable for low-complexity care. Availability in ICUs is likely to be much lower (on some days it may be zero). It is necessary to have a detailed picture of bed types and the availability of specialist nursing staff.[8]

As part of the National Burn Care Group, the National Burn Bed Bureau (NBBB) was created in April 2003. The NBBB provides

- 24-hour coverage of availability in response to requests for patient transfers to specialist burn services across the British Isles
- Twice-daily establishment of bed capacity and availability
- A coordinated approach to bed availability
- Part of the nationwide response to a major incident involving burn injuries

The NBBB has kept details and records on the availability of, and transfers to, burn beds since 2003. If a patient who presents to an accident and emergency department requires admission to a burns unit or burns centre, the NBBB is contacted, and they will search for a suitably staffed, empty burn bed as geographically close as possible.[8] Figure 1 outlines the pathway for the allocation of burn beds in Britain using the NBBB.

Thirty burn care services across the British Isles have been asked by the Department of Health to complete a retrospective study into their admissions since January 2003 and have continued supplying information on a regular basis. This British Isles Burn Injury Database (BIBID) will be linked to the hospital episode statistics and the information from the NBBB to produce a national burn injury database providing a comprehensive report into burn admissions. This has been used for capacity planning and has for the first time provided a reliable method of identifying the complexity level of injuries and their treatment. Figure 2 outlines how accurate data on burns admissions will be collated for the national burn injury database.

## MAJOR INCIDENT PLANNING

A mass casualty incident is defined as a disastrous single event or simultaneous multiple events or other circumstances where the normal major incident response of several NHS organisations must be augmented by extraordinary measures in order to maintain an effective, suitable, and sustainable response. Such events have the potential to rapidly overwhelm or exceed the local capacity available to respond, even with the implementation of major incident plans.[14] The Health Services definition takes into account the severity of injury in its definition, as an incident resulting in a small number of casualties (10–20) may require a major incident response if all of the victims are severely injured.[15] It is the responsibility of all Category 1 (organisations core to the response, subject to the full set of civil protection duties, for example, NHS acute trusts and primary care trusts) and Category 2 responders (cooperating bodies affected by the response, for example, NHS strategic health authorities) under the Civil Contingencies Act 2004[16] to ensure an appropriate response to major incidents and to manage recovery whether incidents have effects locally, regionally, or nationally.[17] Central to a major incident is the integration of key health service organisations. This includes the ambulance strategic command which provides a coordinated response from the combined ambulance services; NHS and private (land and air); the NHS strategic command provides the responses of all NHS resources, including ambulances and the running of both emergency and routine clinical services; and public health advice.[18] The arrangements should enable a coordinated NHS response regardless of the nature or scale of the incident.

One area of concern highlighted by the NBCR was the absence of any coordinated plan to deal with a sudden surge in the number of complex burns, perhaps following a major transport accident like the Paddington rail crash in 1999 or an industrial fire like the Corus steelworks disaster in 2001. The possibility of terrorist attack has brought a further dimension to this concern. There is recognition that the majority of chemical and cutaneous radiation injuries as well as thermal injuries would ultimately receive care from burns services around the British Isles.[12] Major incidents, although not common, do occur, and when they do, they can involve large numbers of casualties affected by burns injury. Table 3 highlights some of the major incidents involving mass burn casualties in Europe in recent history.

The absence of a plan in itself reflected the lack of systematic knowledge of what specialist beds existed and where they might be available at any time. A best practice guidance was commissioned to create a general set of principles to NHS organisations in planning, preparing, and responding to all types of emergencies arising from any accident, natural disaster, failure of utilities or systems, or hostile act resulting in an abnormal casualty situation or posing any threat to the health of the community, or in the provision of services that involve significant numbers of burn-injured patients. The guidance covers adults and children and is intended to provide clinical guidance and to link with the NHS emergency planning guidance (2005),[12] which describes a set of principles to guide NHS organisations in their ability to respond to a major incident.

Burn services must ensure that they have a major incident plan that complements local major incident plans. If a major incident is declared or is put on standby, the burns unit must implement the plan and inform the NBBB of the implementation. Burn assessment teams (BATs) may be activated if there is a major incident to provide advice and support at the site of an incident or at the receiving hospitals. It is the responsibility of the burn care network in the area and the burn service to ensure that the individuals likely to form this team are aware of who they are and their role.[12] BATs will consist of 2 experienced burn surgeons, 1 of whom is a consultant. The BAT may also include a nurse if resources permit.[12] BATs will report back to a senior consultant in the burns service regarding the severity and number of casualties and in liaison with the hospital control team. Surgeons with extensive burns knowledge are required to assess patients whose burns are so extensive that the injury will inevitably be fatal. Accommodation with special treatment facilities is not necessary for this category.[20] Information from the NBBB will help to decide the destination of the patients.

Doctors without burns experience frequently overestimate the proportion of the body surface burnt. However, this task frequently falls to the less experienced because there are only 115 consultant plastic surgeons in Britain (1:487000 population). In addition, patients with burns may appear deceptively lucid in the first 4 to 6 hours postinjury.[21] Repatriation of patients to their local host services should be as soon as possible, and it is essential that following a major incident there is a formal debriefing process and analysis of the incident from which lessons may be learnt[12] from casualty profiles.[22]

## THE BRADFORD CITY FOOTBALL STADIUM FIRE, 1985[20]

On 11 May 1985, the main stand at the Bradford City football ground, which was mainly made of wood, caught fire. Out of a crowd of 10000 people, 3000 were in that stand. The fire is likely to have been due to rubbish that had accumulated in the corner of the stand catching fire. It spread so rapidly that within 4 minutes it was alight from end to end, and in addition, the bitumen coating of the roof was dripping down. Fifty-three people were burnt to death on the spot. These had been in direct contact with the flames and had tried to escape through the turnstiles but became trapped. A further 250 were injured; their burns were mainly due to radiant heat, not direct contact with the flames. This number would have been a lot higher, but as it was a cold day, spectators were dressed in many layers of clothing, protecting them from the thermal effects of the fire.

Casualties started to arrive at the local hospital, the Bradford Royal Infirmary, a few minutes after the fire started. Within 30 minutes, a total of 190 causalities had arrived. The casualty officer summoned the plastic surgeon on call, and a major accident emergency was declared. Nonurgent, nonburns patients were sent home and advised to see their own doctor or to come back the following day. Staff who were at home reported to the hospital. As many existing inpatient patients as possible were sent home to clear beds. The plastic surgery ward and 2 other wards were converted to burn wards.

Very few patients had any injuries other than burns. Patients with TBSA burns < 5% were considered fit for discharge. The physiotherapy gymnasium was converted into a dressing centre for the treatment of this group of patients. Patients with TBSA > 5% had dressings and were immediately admitted for further assessment. Those with TBSA > 10% were immediately fluid resuscitated and transferred to the ward. This was facilitated by the anaesthetic department. A total of 11 patients with the most severe burns were transferred to the local burns unit. The emergency department was empty 3 hours after the accident and was ready to resume normal service.

All nonemergency elective surgery was cancelled to free up 3 operating theatres. Nine plastic surgeons were transferred from 3 other hospitals—Leeds, Manchester, and Newcastle[21]—as well as extra surgical equipment. Teams of surgeons operated on a 24-hour basis in the 3 theatres simultaneously for the first 5 days. A total of 80 operating

hours, including 55 primary excisions with surgery ranging from 30 minutes to 3 hours, were performed.

## KING'S CROSS FIRE, LONDON UNDERGROUND STATION[23,24]

The King's Cross fire in November 1987 occurred when a wooden escalator caught fire. Superheated air rapidly rose up the escalator from the tunnels below, resulting in a "flash over" engulfing the central ticket area in a fireball, killing 58 people in the main ticket concourse at the top. Within 15 minutes, excess of 500 rescue workers were on the scene, including policemen, firemen, doctors, and religious personnel. Several hundred people were trapped underground but were successfully evacuated by stopping trains.

Casualties were distributed to 4 hospitals in the vicinity, and a major incident was declared. A total of 14 different ambulance services were coordinated at the scene. Fire fighters were on the scene for almost 24 hours. A total of 8 doctors were at the scene, including 5 from a volunteer agency. They played a vital role in triage and in certifying the dead. This enabled 13 casualties to be removed to a makeshift mortuary, freeing up ambulances and resources in the emergency department. Although many casualties were brought to the emergency department, many were certified dead on arrival. Only a relatively small number of patients required admission, and only 28 survivors were treated for thermal injuries, but the resources involved were considerable. Operating time approached 100 hours in total, and the bed occupancy involved 300 patient nights. Over 400 units of blood products were consumed from the National Blood Bank and 11 different medical and surgical specialities were involved in patient care.

## MANAGEMENT OF PAEDIATRIC CASES IN MAJOR INCIDENTS

Four to 5 major incidents occur in the United Kingdom each year, and many of them involve children.[15] In the United Kingdom, a 3-round Delphi process consisting of a multidisciplinary panel of 22 experts was performed to determine appropriate planning for the care of paediatric cases during major incidents. This is a structured process using a panel of experts to investigate complex or imprecise issues using a series of structured statements.[25] The number of children involved in major incidents has ranged from 10% to 100% of victims; however, at the time of the exercise, fewer than a third of hospitals in the United Kingdom had a plan for the care of children during major incidents.[25] Table 4 highlights major incidents involving children which have occurred in the United Kingdom since 1983.

The Delphi study highlighted 3 required aspects in preparation for a major incident: planning, equipment, and training. Regional planners should ensure that plans are in place for children at every receiving hospital and that a realistic assessment and statement of the paediatric resources available has been made at each hospital. Units should also make realistic estimates of seriously injured children that they are capable of receiving in 1 hour. Planning should assume that at least 15% to 20% of major incident patients require paediatric equipment. This should also be available for prehospital use in the form of snatch bags and should be available in the receiving areas of the emergency departments.[26] The recommended minimal amount of supplementary equipment required is outlined in Table 5.

All clinicians involved in the paediatric clinical response should be trained to at least the level of paediatric life support.[27] Tertiary services, especially intensive care and surgery, may be at a premium during a major incident. It is impractical to transfer all paediatric cases to specialist centres for assessment and treatment, as this would result merely in transferring a major incident from 1 hospital to another. It is proposed that paediatric assessment teams (PATs) triage casualties during major incidents. These teams would consist of senior, skilled staff experienced in travelling to and working in other hospitals (similar to those of intensive care retrieval teams). These teams could be supplemented with a paediatric surgeon when necessary. Membership will depend on local resources but should be made explicit in local and regional major incident plans.[25] PATs will travel to receiving hospitals to determine whether individual paediatric casualties warrant transfer to specialist services. Table 6 shows a proposed action card for PAT teams.[26]

It would be unlikely that there would be enough specialist paediatric staff to oversee treatment of every child admitted during a major accident. This is, however, unnecessary, as emergency staff are experienced in the treatment of paediatric cases. Severe paediatric cases should be seen by experienced paediatric staff. This can be achieved by forming paediatric treatment teams consisting of at least 1 paediatric doctor and 1 registered paediatric nurse. Their priorities would be to assess and treat seriously injured children and to provide advice and practical help to others involved in the care of paediatric cases. If the decision is made that a child needs to be transferred to a tertiary hospital, the child must be stabilised and transported by clinicians skilled in pediatric transfer.[26]

## CARE OF THE HOSPITALISED CHILD

Under the extension of the Patient's Charter Services for Children and Young People, issued in 1996, a list of minimal standards has been implemented in all NHS hospitals in Britain. Table 7 lists these standards.

The British government is currently developing a National Service Framework (NSF) for children, young people, and maternity services. NSFs set national standards, aiming to improve the quality of care and reduce unacceptable variations in health and social services. Children and young people should receive care that is integrated and coordinated around their particular needs and the needs of their family. They and their parents should be treated with respect and should be given support and information to enable them to understand and cope with the illness or injury and the treatment needed. They should be encouraged to be active partners in decisions about their health and care and, where possible, should be able to exercise choice. Children, young people, and their parents will participate in designing NHS and social care services that are readily accessible, respectful, and empowering, that follow best practice in obtaining consent, and that provide effective response to their needs.[28]

Child-centred hospital services are services that

- Consider the whole child, not simply the illness being treated
- Treat children as children and young people as young people
- Are concerned with the overall experience for the child and family
- Treat children, young people, and parents as partners in care
- Integrate and coordinate services around the child's and family's particular needs
- Graduate smoothly into adult services at the right time
- Work in partnership with children, young people, and parents to plan and shape services and to develop the workforce

The family unit has been recognised as a cohesive force, adding stability and continuity, and as a potentiator of recovery for a sick child. Experience does not allow parents to prepare themselves, their child, or their family. This may lead to high anxiety, interfere with communication, and add to stress. Information may have to be given frequently to family members, with further explanations, as their level of comprehension may be limited initially until they begin to cope with the situation. Parents have the right to truthful information, presented in a form they can understand.[29] Being in an age-appropriate environment that incorporates and addresses the different requirements that children and teenagers have with the opportunity to play indoors or outdoors, a family room, and age-related informational and play materials is considered vitally important. Additionally, a room where parents/

family members can retreat from the ward and talk to staff or other parents is deemed to be particularly important.[30]

## COORDINATION OF OTHER PROFESSIONALS

Burn care teams will include other professionals, for example, social workers, play specialists, occupational therapists, physiotherapists, and counsellors, all of whom can contribute to the psychosocial care of the burn-injured patients and their families. It is recommended that this input is overseen and led by a consultant lead clinical psychologist.[31]

## PSYCHOSOCIAL REHABILITATION

The National Burn Care Group, the purpose of which was 2-fold, convened a working party[31] to advise on the basis of the current evidence on the range of psychosocial interventions that might be required to meet the needs of children, young people, and adults who experience burn injuries and their families. It also produced detailed proposals for the staffing, roles, training, and costs of psychosocial rehabilitation at centre, unit, and facility levels and in the community that will meet the standards specified by the NBCG.

The report found that potential vulnerability markers for inpatient children included whether the child spent time on HDU and whether there was low parental extraversion. Injury indicators were not vulnerability markers. For children attending as outpatients, potential vulnerability markers included still being in the burn care system > 2 years postburn (not explained by TBSA/HDU), lower parental emotional stability, poorer family functioning, and younger age of mother. Injury indicators were again not found to be vulnerability markers.

It appeared that parental anxiety and depression reduced from the inpatient stage to the early postdischarge period, with residual anxiety evident for some parents. As time continued, and perhaps the permanence of the residual scar was realised, parental depression became more evident. Family dysfunction was also evident in the 2 to 3 months after returning home with the burned child and later on became a potential marker of psychosocial need. Social factors rather than injury variables were associated with parental adjustment, with younger mothers being more vulnerable to depression than their older counterparts. Injury variables may be markers for greater behavioural and emotional difficulties for the child as time continues. Burned children were also reported to have more problems with peers and with the reactions of other people to their appearance with increasing age. Time is not a healer in respect of those parents and children still in the burn care system at 2 to 3 years, especially as disfigurement from contractures

is associated with increased psychosocial problems.[32] Difficulties experienced may include relocation, finances, guilt, follow-up home care, daily trips to the hospital for many months, rehospitalisation for further surgery, reintegration into school, peer rejection, and depression.[33] Opportunity for support should be available for these "old hands" as well as for new burn patients, their parents, and their families.[31]

## RECOMMENDATIONS IN THE PROVISION OF PSYCHOSOCIAL SUPPORT IN BURNT CHILDREN[31]

Psychosocial support should encompass the needs of siblings, including normalising reactions, discussing responses, and explaining surgical intervention and outcome. Sibling involvement with their burned brother or sister's treatment should be encouraged where appropriate, and advice may be required about how to involve younger members of the family. Siblings can be advised on how to handle difficult or uncomfortable social situations which involve their burned brother or sister with explanations about the range of reactions that parents and burned children may exhibit following the accident. Advice and support for parents about sibling attention/"special time" and avoiding the sibling being overlooked.

Some children who present with minor burns may have witnessed a parent being burnt. Psychosocial support should encompass the needs of children of burned parents, including normalising reactions such as horror, fear, repulsion, or shock; in particular, facial burns and hand burns (which require "hand bags") seem to cause the most distress. There is a need for more information regarding burn injury aftereffects, scarring, time to heal, and outcome and an additional need for family support or child-specific support if there are changes in family dynamics. The child may require support and strategies for coping with situations in a way that does not have a negative impact, with advice on handling difficult or uncomfortable social situations which involve their burned parent and how to deal with situations where their parent can't do something (ie, when to step in and help and when not to).

The first indications that patients are in need of psychosocial intervention may occur later on in their care, when they may have moved from receiving inpatient care at a centre or unit to receiving follow-up care at the facility level. Consequently, it is recommended that psychosocial specialists should be an integral part of the staffing complement at all levels of burn care provision. Centralisation of psychological support may result in those who require such provision excluding themselves for pragmatic reasons (eg, unable to travel the distance, unable to arrange or afford child care cover, or unable to take the increased time off work). Adequate provision of psychological support necessarily requires a local option.[31]

## IMPLICATIONS FOR CARE

The evidence strongly indicates that psychosocial burn care should be developed within a managed clinical network of burn centres, units, and facilities as follows[31]:

- Routine care: the integration of psychological screening and support into the burn care process for patient and family should be routine from the start of a patient's journey for a period well beyond the completion of physical care.
- Promoting a patient-centred/family-centred approach: in light of the complexity and individuality of psychosocial needs, a whole-patient/whole-family approach should be adopted in order to more closely meet the range of needs (in contrast to existing care in which the focus is predominantly on excellence in the provision of surgical and medical interventions).

Realistically implementing these ideal guidelines may not be feasible, at least in the short term, as psychosocial rehabilitation has seriously been neglected in the UK burn arena. As a result, routine psychological care has not been carried out but has been reserved for those most severely affected. Routine screening normalises psychological issues after a burn and encourages a proactive and preventative approach rather than a reactive one. Some of the psychology required relates to basic skills that most allied health professionals already possess. Training these staff in the detection of psychological risk factors, the use of screening tools, and basic listening and support provide the first steps in a tiered approach where information is fed back to the psychologist in multidisciplinary meetings.[34]

## POST-TRAUMATIC STRESS DISORDER

Post-traumatic stress disorder (PTSD) develops following a stressful event or situation of an exceptionally threatening or catastrophic nature, which is likely to cause pervasive distress in almost anyone. The National Institute for Clinical Excellence (NICE)[35] has issued guidelines for the NHS on how to improve the recognition, screening, and treatment of PTSD in children and adults in primary and secondary care. PTSD can affect anyone and is common—around 5% of men and 10% of women will suffer from PTSD at some time in their life. Up to 30% of people exposed to a stressful event or situation of an exceptionally threatening or catastrophic nature (such as burns) will go on to develop

PTSD. Symptoms often develop immediately after the traumatic event, but the onset of symptoms may be delayed in some people. There is underrecognition of the condition in the NHS, particularly in children, yet PTSD is treatable even when problems present many years after the traumatic event. The guideline recommends that[35]

- Where symptoms are mild and have been present for less than 4 weeks after the trauma, watchful waiting, as a way of managing the difficulties presented by individual people with PTSD, should be considered.
- All others with PTSD should be offered a course of trauma-focused psychological treatment (trauma-focused cognitive behavioural therapy or eye movement desensitisation and reprocessing) on an individual outpatient basis.
- Children and young people with PTSD, including those who have been sexually abused, should be offered a course of trauma-focused cognitive behavioural therapy adapted as needed to suit their age, circumstances, and level of development.
- All disaster plans should contain provisions for a fully coordinated psychosocial response to the disaster, and health care workers involved in a disaster plan should have clear roles and responsibilities agreed in advance.
- For individuals who have experienced a traumatic event, the systematic provision to that individual alone of brief, single-session interventions that focus on the traumatic incident (often referred to as debriefing) should not be routine practice when delivering services.

## BURN CARE TEAM STAFF

The NBCG working party also recommends that the psychological advice/support from all members of the burn care team should be routine.[31] A distinction should be made between psychosocial care (which can be administered by the whole multidisciplinary burn care team) and the specialist task of psychological intervention (which should be the domain of properly trained psychological therapy staff and supervised by clinical psychologists). Psychologically trained staff should be fully integrated members of the core burn care team, ensuring that psychosocial support becomes collaborative, routine, and empowering rather than stigmatising, touchy-feely. or implying an inability to cope.[31]

Following the consensus achieved concerning the psychosocial standards of care, the next task was to map the way forward from the status quo and toward the adoption of these standards within each of the burns units in England and Wales. The British charity Changing Faces, together with the Centre for Appearance Research, performed semi-structured interviews with staff to determine perceptions of current psychosocial care provisions on burn units to determine the best way forward in the implementation of the recommended changes.[31]

The need for training was highlighted by participants as a crucial component in achieving the standards for several reasons. Training for staff at all levels would ensure that all members of the burn team have the same foundation of knowledge and would enable them to build an understanding of what their roles and responsibilities are in regards to facilitating psychosocial support. In addition to this, staff with considerable experience in burn care who perceived themselves as offering good levels of psychosocial support would also like to have their knowledge validated and extended by a programme of continuous professional development. This would increase their confidence in the care they are providing.

Psychosocial specialists identified the need of staff at all levels to have a working knowledge of psychosocial issues since the specialists rely on others to identify individuals that could benefit from seeing a psychosocial specialist. This is especially so as not all psychologists are located on the burn wards and many have limited presence, while staff such as nurses, physiotherapists, play specialists, and occupational therapists have a more continuous presence and more treatment interactions with the patients and their families. There was a consensus from all participants that all staff should become more integrated in facilitating basic psychosocial care than is currently the case. This would enable staff at higher levels to then address the more complex clinical issues and focus on other important components such as establishing and/or maintaining liaisons with other services and establishing collaborative networks between hospitals. These efforts will facilitate opportunities for research and enable psychosocial specialists to establish common approaches across burn centres/units.

Staff at all levels believe that an integrated, tiered approach would be beneficial for inpatient and outpatient care for patients of all age levels. It will optimise the chances that psychosocial support is fully accessible, appropriate, proactive, and preventive as well as reactive, and also that psychosocial advice and support is available to staff as well as to patients and their families. Another essential component of a comprehensive service is the provision of appropriate facilities that are conducive for psychological intervention, incorporating the specific needs of children and adolescents. Participants suggested that interventions should involve social skills training programmes and the opportunity to participate in burn camps.

## PLAY THERAPISTS

Children visiting or staying in hospital have a basic need for play and recreation that should be met routinely in all hospital departments providing a service to children. This applies equally to the siblings of patients and so is also a consideration for neonatal units. Play may also be used for therapeutic purposes, as part of the child's care plan and as a way of helping the child to assimilate new information, adjust to and gain control over a potentially frightening environment, and prepare to cope with procedures and interventions. There is evidence that play hastens recovery as well as reducing the need for interventions to be delivered under general anaesthesia. It has been recommended that all children staying in hospital have daily access to a play specialist.

The use of play techniques should be encouraged across the multidisciplinary team caring for children, including in accident and emergency departments, with play specialists taking a lead in modelling techniques that other staff can then adopt. The team should be able to offer a variety of play interventions to support the child at each stage in his or her journey through the hospital system.[28]

Play therapy is an effective therapy that helps children modify their behaviours, clarify their self-concept, and build up healthy relationships. In play therapy, children enter into a dynamic relationship with the therapist that enables them to express, explore, and make sense of their difficult and painful experiences. Play therapy helps children find healthier ways of communicating, develop fulfilling relationships, increase resiliency, and facilitate emotional literacy. Play therapists work closely with the child's parents throughout the play therapy intervention and occasionally undertake parent-child relationship interventions.[36] The child is granted confidentiality, with the exception of child protection protocols, so although the therapy contributes to reviews and shares general observations with the interprofessional team, details of the play are not divulged to protect the confidential nature of the work.[37]

Play therapy has long been criticized for a lack of an adequate research base to prove its efficacy. For 6 decades, while play therapists conducted small research studies, critics challenged the utility and efficacy of play therapy as a viable psychotherapy intervention. Ray et al (2001)[38] conducted a meta-analysis of 94 research studies focusing on the efficacy of play therapy. Play therapy appeared effective across modality, age, gender, clinical versus nonclinical populations, setting, and theoretical schools of thought.

Additionally, positive play therapy effects were found to be greatest when there was parent involvement in treatment and an optimal number of sessions provided.

With the migration of the early child psychotherapists to Britain in the 1930s, child psychotherapy has grown and developed as a strongly European tradition. Whilst play therapy has emerged from elements of child psychotherapy, the specific theoretical foundations emerged from the humanistic psychology tradition. In Britain, play therapy started to emerge as a new and differing tradition in the 1980s. Since then, the Children's Hour Trust has taught professionals the basic techniques of Axline's play therapy[39] that are used in a multitude of settings. In parallel, 2 drama therapists started using play therapy methods to inform their drama therapy practice with children. Elements of nondirective play therapy were integrated to formulate a British play therapy movement. In 1990, the Institute of Drama Therapy started to offer a certificate and diploma in play therapy.[40]

In 1992, the British Association of Play Therapists (BAPT) was started by a group of professionals studying at the Institute of Drama Therapy. Over the last 10 years, BAPT has developed the British play therapy movement and now validates training courses.[40] The BAPT has a duty to afford the highest possible standards of protection to the public and to promote the best standards of personal and professional conduct within the play therapy profession. The *Ethical Basis for Good Practice in Play Therapy* contains advice and guidance to all members of the BAPT on ethical principles, standards of competence, and good practice.[36]

## HOSPITAL PLAY STAFF

Play has a special function in the hospital environment, and NHS hospital play specialists lead playful activities and use play as therapeutic tool. They are neither play therapists nor play leaders. Play specialists work closely as part of the multidisciplinary team and

- organise daily play and art activities in the playroom or at the bedside
- provide play to achieve developmental goals
- help children master and cope with anxieties and feelings
- use play to prepare children for hospital procedures
- support families and siblings
- contribute to clinical judgements through their play-based observations
- teach the value of play for the sick child
- encourage peer group friendships to develop
- organise parties and special events

Play staff start work as play assistants and progress with further training and experience to work as basic grade hospital play specialists. With further experience and training, they may gain more responsibility as team leaders or team managers. New hospitals are designed with playrooms in place, and old ones are adapted to incorporate more play space. Children's hospitals in Britain have large play departments employing up to 40 hospital play specialists each. In general hospitals, small teams of play staff work in different areas of the hospital, such as outpatient clinics, children's units, and adolescent wards.[41]

## HOSPITAL PLAY THERAPISTS

Play therapy shares person-centred therapy's emphasis upon the client as trustworthy. Play therapy is based upon 3 critical theoretical principles[40]:

- Actualisation—Humans are motivated by an innate tendency to develop constructive and healthy capacities. This tendency is to actualise each person's inner potentials, including aspects of creativity, curiosity, and the desire to become more effective and autonomous.
- The need for positive regard—All people require warmth, respect, and acceptance from others, especially from significant others. As children grow and develop, this need for positive regard transforms into a secondary, learned need for positive self-regard.
- Play as communication—Children use play as their primary medium of communication. Play is a format for transmitting children's emotions, thoughts, values, and perceptions. It is a medium that is primarily creative.

Children/young people with burns, particularly large percentage burns, need to be able to have fun and feel motivated to participate in all areas of required therapy. The play therapist provides creative and expressive play activities which are not only developmentally appropriate, but which are chosen for their successful outcome given the medical circumstances. Other experiences offered include relaxation, medical play, and peer interaction groups.

Children are less articulate than adults in expressing their experience of pain. Children often revert to behaviour appropriate for younger children and may revert to a preverbal state and become introverted and silent. They may be reluctant to admit they are in pain for fear of being injected or subjected to other unpleasant treatment.[43] During painful and ongoing treatments, the play therapist provides procedural support. This is conducted in a team environment, with the play therapist offering support to the patient through speech and tactile contact and using imaginative and flexible techniques to provide distraction for children/ young people. Also, providing them with information to empower them helps to relieve their anxiety and increases their autonomy and ability to remain calm whilst undergoing these repetitive therapies.

The play therapist is also involved in maintaining confidence, optimism, and motivation in the patient despite long-term treatment prospects. This can be achieved by managing a positive rapport, providing the patient with absorbing activities, recognising interests and skills, and acknowledging the patient's value as a person whilst accessing a variety of resources.[44] Play therapy in paediatric burn patients has demonstrated reduced anxiety, mood elevation, and cooperation with staff.[45]

## Pain Relief

Play therapy can provide sufficient support so that medication is limited to pain relief rather than sedation of the patient. This aids their recovery from the procedure and therefore their continuation of the other required therapies. The child's environment may also reduce his or her distress and discomfort. Parental and sometimes sibling support, noise reduction, dimming lights at the child's normal bedtime, and distraction with music may all be appropriate.[46] Prior to venipuncture, topical local anaesthetics or, in infants, a sugar water (12% sucrose) solution given for 2 minutes can reduce pain and anxiety.[47]

Many physicians surveyed are dissatisfied with the levels of pain relief given to children during procedures.[48] Burns require frequent dressing changes and often painful debridement involving daily tankings, where the patient is placed in a hydrotherapy tub and devitalised surface tissues are removed.[33] If children are uncooperative despite attempts at distraction, procedural anaesthesia may be required to reduce suffering for the child and for parents who witness or participate in the restraint of their child.[49] Certain sedative agents such as the midazolam-fentanyl regime have been popular, but recovery is slow and monitoring with strict protocols is required due to the potential adverse reactions of such drugs.[50] Scoring systems[51,52] and anaesthesia monitors are commonly used to assess pain and sedation,[53] meaning that the child must be under constant supervision by at least 2 members of staff.

Children receiving care in specialised centres in the NHS can now expect to benefit from up-to-date techniques of pain management such as patient-controlled analgaesia, nurse-controlled analgaesia, and epidural infusions.[54] Patient-controlled anaesthesia (PCA) has gained popularity in the paediatric populations as an effective pain control.[55] It is usually appropriate for children aged 7 years and over, but this has been extended to the 5-to-7-year age group.[56] PCA patients administer more analgaesia in the first 24 hours postsurgery but less by 72 hours post-op, providing more effective drug management.[57] Doses of drugs such as morphine have been found in studies to be prescribed at subtherapeutic doses[58] and are associated with serious adverse effects.[59] Studies have shown that staff education can improve pain relief by increasing the accuracy of pain recognition by nurses.[60] PCA eliminates errors of underreporting of pain by staff, especially when children are afraid of receiving injections.[61]

## Inpatient Education

Staff, facilities, and equipment are required to meet the ongoing educational needs of children and young people staying in hospital, with reference to the Department for Education and Skills' guidelines on the education of sick children in hospital. This includes access to therapy input for children who need special equipment, such as seating and communication aids, in order to participate. Where a child's condition will affect schooling, hospital staff need to liaise with and involve the school from an early stage. This is particularly important if the child is likely to be away from school for some time or if the child's condition has long-term implications for education. Evidence suggests that this is not always handled effectively, which can have an impact on educational attainment. In addition, early education for 3-year-olds and 4-year-olds is an entitlement. If the hospital provision is included on the local education authority's (LEA's) directory of providers, then funding for this should be available from the LEA.[28]

## Rehabilitation

Disfigurement from scarring after burn injury is lifelong but can be improved by rehabilitation, reconstructive surgery, and other therapies. Children with severe burns receiving structured, supervised exercise programmes consisting of aerobic and progressive resistant exercises have been shown to have significantly less scar contractures requiring surgery.[62] A UK burn therapy standards audit[63] was conducted during 2003 to establish therapy compliance with these standards. Following analysis of the results and evaluation of the evidence base, burn therapists across the United Kingdom unanimously agreed that the standard should be further developed. The 6 standards cover all aspects of burn therapy assessment, treatment, and management, commencing with the acute phase, then progressing through the stages of intermediate rehabilitation and reintegration and finally onto later rehabilitation and reconstruction. It is acknowledged that not all of the standards are relevant to all patients; this is dependant upon the size, depth, and location of the burn injury as well as other physical and psychosocial factors. The burn therapist must therefore determine the relevant standards for each individual patient at a given time.[64]

## Standard One

The therapeutic management of the burn patient is determined by thorough assessment and formulation of a detailed list of problems, treatment goals, and a management plan. The patient is subject to regular, ongoing therapeutic reassessment and review with subsequent changes to the treatment goals and management plan.

## Standard Two

An individualised acute treatment management programme is implemented based on patient assessment. Wherever possible, this programme is developed in conjunction with the patient and/or his or her family and carers. This programme will typically include chest physiotherapy, limb elevation, correct positioning, splinting, active and passive exercises, functional/purposeful/play activities, and patient/family education and support.

## Standard Three

The transition from acute to intermediate rehabilitation is variable for each patient according to many factors, such as burn size, severity, and involvement of other body systems. Many patients (for example, those with a small % TBSA) will enter this phase almost immediately, whereas others may take several weeks or even months to become medically stable and thus appropriate for intermediate rehabilitation. This phase of therapy management may be delivered on an inpatient or outpatient basis and will vary in intensity according to patient need. During this stage, the main therapeutic focus is on function and purposeful activities. Where appropriate, the therapy sessions will often be based in the gymnasium, occupational therapy workshops, and activity areas. Significant wound healing will be taking place at this stage, and scar management will therefore usually commence at this stage of rehabilitation. Working as an integral part of the burns multidisciplinary team, the therapist assists, coordinates, and where appropriate leads the planning, implementation, and review of the patient's ongoing

care and management. For the burn patient, noncompliance with medical treatment is associated with very serious health consequences. Compliance with physiotherapy procedures is critical to prevent contractures and subsequent corrective surgeries.[33]

## Standard Four

Reintegration usually falls into the intermediate phase of rehabilitation, and the focus is on the patient's return to society and his or her gradual return to a maximal level of functioning and independence. Individuals with a major burn injury and/or complex psychosocial problems will often require a high level of MDT (multidisciplinary team) involvement in their integration back into society, whereas others (particularly those with less severe injuries) may require little or no assistance during this phase. Working as an integral part of the burns MDT, the therapist coordinates and facilitates the planning and implementation of the patient's return to society. Wherever possible (according to patient age, compliance, psychological state, etc), the patient is encouraged to take the lead in this reintegration process.

## Standard Five

In the later phase of rehabilitation, the burn wounds will usually be fully healed and the emphasis is on burn scar management, return to maximal function, independence, and continued psychosocial support. For individuals with significant scarring or complex psychosocial problems, the late phase of rehabilitation can continue for many months and often years (particularly for children). Individuals with minimal or nonproblematic scarring and minimal psychosocial problems will usually require very little input at this stage. The burn therapist provides ongoing assessment, treatment, advice, and psychosocial support to the patient and his or her family throughout the burn scar maturation period and, where necessary, post–scar maturation. The therapist implements a wide range of scar management modalities based on individualised assessment, including scar massage, pressure therapy, use of silicon products, splinting, and stretching.

## Standard Six

The reconstructive phase occurs during the later phase of rehabilitation. Burn patients with the following problems will usually be offered reconstructive surgery:

- cosmetically unacceptable scar
- unstable/hypersensitive/painful burn scar
- burn scar causing significant joint contracture
- burn scar causing significant functional limitation

Many children with major burn injuries will undergo reconstructive surgery at regular intervals throughout their childhood. There is no limitation on the timing of reconstruction. Indeed, some patients elect to undergo reconstruction many years after their initial burn injury. Following burn reconstruction, an individualised management programme is formulated and implemented by the burn therapist. This is based on thorough preoperative and postoperative assessment and formulation of a detailed list of problems, treatment goals, and a management plan. Wherever possible, this programme is developed in conjunction with the patient and/or his or her family.

## SOCIAL WORKERS

Relatives feel fear and shame when patients resume social living because they are imposing on others coexistence with people who no longer meet the accepted patterns. In view of this situation, the relatives think about the possibility of trying not to expose the sequelae, and change daily routines in an attempt to hide the patient.[65] The family's role in delivering care to a burned patient is very important, not only with respect to the technical aspects involved in caregiving, but particularly with respect to psychosocial aspects. Working with the family to promote cohesion reduces conflict and increases stability, but this can only be achieved effectively if the relatives are given sufficient support.[66]

A key component of psychosocial care is the incorporation of a social worker. The potential of having a knowledgeable person who knows how to access support and aid from social services, community services, and other institutions and how to support patients through the process of securing benefits is invaluable. This can improve the chances of those with complex problems to focus on their physical and psychological rehabilitation. It is crucial to provide high-quality psychosocial care at all facilities that deliver burn care. This is especially so since research indicates that the physical characteristics of the burn (eg, TBSA, depth, location) are not related to the degree of psychosocial distress and that psychosocial problems can persist for many years postburn. It is particularly important that a smooth transition from the inpatient to the outpatient settings is facilitated. The chances of achieving a positive outcome in the longer term could be increased through the provision of an outreach team that worked from outpatient clinics and/or through visits to patient's homes.

## DISCHARGE PLANNING

Discharge planning should commence as soon after admission as is practical and should be a process involving the multidisciplinary team in conjunction with the child and his or her relatives.[67] Clear instructions about pain control, wound care, mobilisation, and resumption of activities should be given to the family doctor. Arrangements for follow-up by a district nurse, health visitor, or family doctor and for review at the hospital outpatient department should be clearly documented.[68]

The two white papers "The NHS Plan: A Plan for Investment, a Plan for Reform" and "Modernising Social Services"[69,70] set out an agenda of intense reform, reinforcing the importance of health care and social care working together in the planning and delivering of care. Other policies that relate to and have an impact on avoiding unnecessary hospital admission, the effective use and coordination of health, social care, and housing resources, and hospital discharge planning are[71]

- The Health Act
- Building Capacity and Partnership in Care
- Patient and public partnership in the new NHS
- Carers (Recognition and Services) Act and the Carers and Disabled Children Act
- NHS-funded nursing care in nursing homes
- Fair Access to Care Services
- The National Service Framework for Mental Health
- Valuing people
- Supporting people
- Community Care (Delayed Discharge, etc) Bill (subject to Parliamentary approval)

The consistent and strong message within each of these is the need for statutory and independent agencies to work together with their local communities to plan, commission, and deliver services. Strong and positive engagement is therefore essential. An equally clear expectation is that those individuals who require services, and their carers, will be actively and fully informed participants in the planning and delivery of their care. Effective clinical governance arrangements are to underpin the delivery of health care, and for local authorities, best value reviews will ensure effective provision and use of social care services. The Health Act 1999 paved the way for the NHS and local authorities with social service responsibilities to work together.[72] The introduction of joint priorities for health care and social care adds further emphasis to the expectation that joint working will underpin the delivery of improved services and health gains in local communities.

## SUMMARY

Since the introduction of burn care services after the establishment of the NHS in 1948, burn care services have developed in a haphazard and uncoordinated manner, relying on individual burn units for planning and implementation. The NBCR has highlighted many areas for improvement, and this has sparked a nationwide review of all burn services, their roles, and their location in relation to their geographical need. Burn centres are merging into 7 adult and 3 major paediatric centres of excellence which will be required to meet national standards and coordinate care with other, smaller burn centres and with tertiary hospitals throughout the United Kingdom.

Central to these changes is the need to recognise the child as an individual with specialised needs and rights. The child and his or her parents should be involved at all stages in the multidisciplinary management of his or her injuries, and this management should include coordinated long-term goals for the postdischarge period, including reintegration into society.

## FIGURES AND TABLES

### FIGURE 1
### Protocol for referral to bed allocation of burn-injured patients.[13]

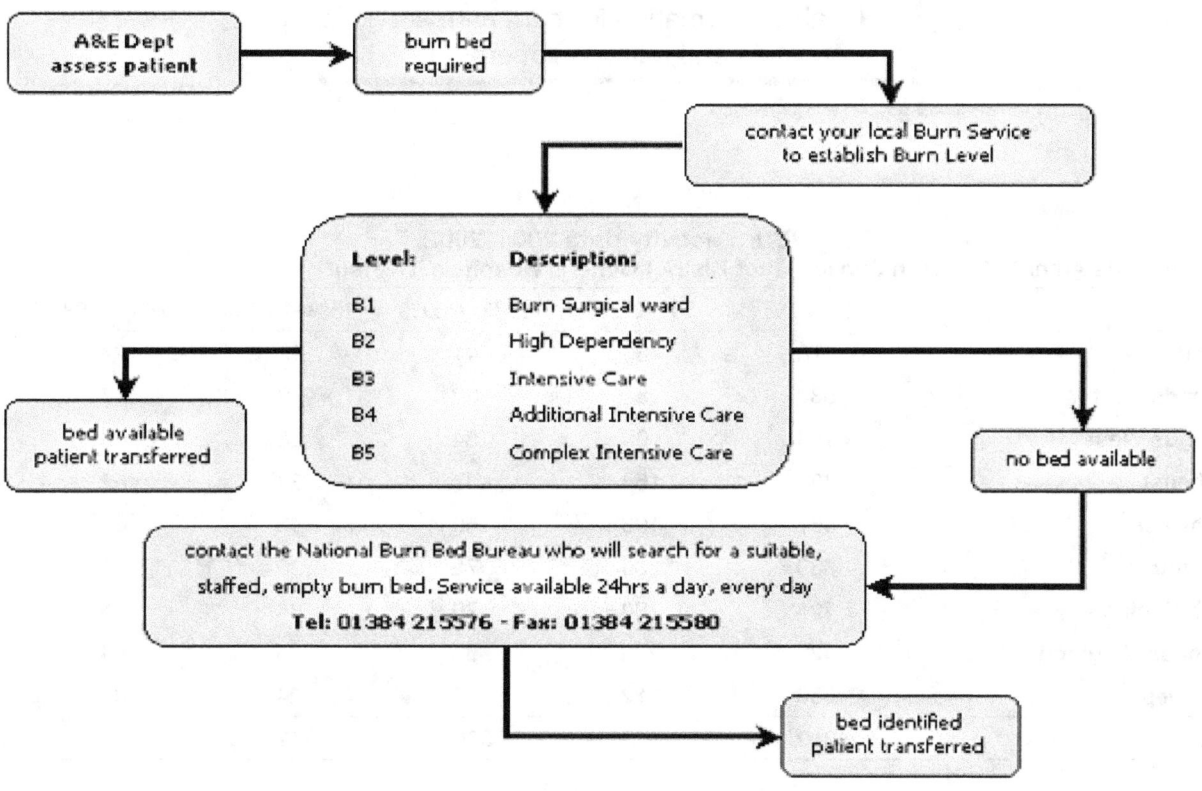

## Figure 2
### Input into the National Burn Injury Database.

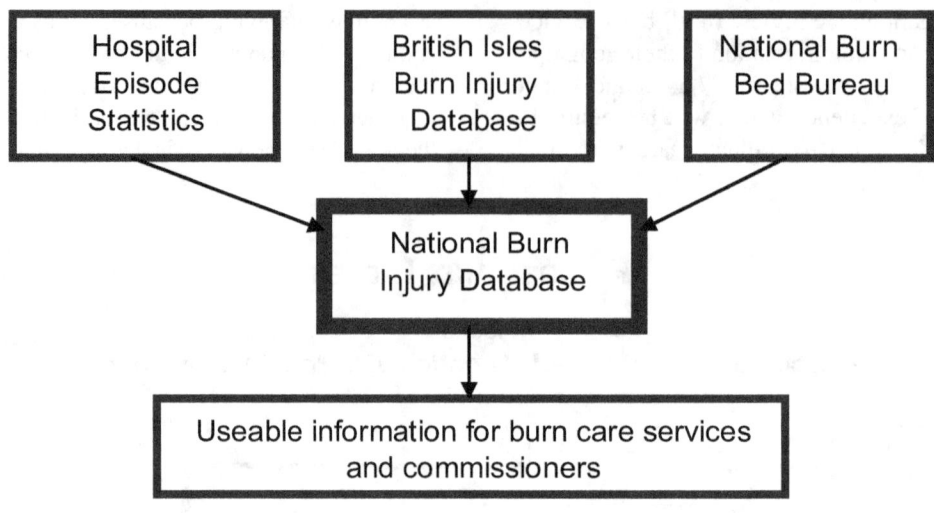

## Table 2
### Burn activity data 2001–2002.
#### a) Burn Injuries Admitted to Burn Services (not District General Hospitals [DGHs])[6]

|  | 0%–4.9% | 5%–9.9% | 10%–14.9% | 15%–19.9% | 20%–100% | Total |
|---|---|---|---|---|---|---|
| **Ireland** | 178 | 66 | 41 | 15 | 27 | 327 |
| **Midlands East** | 533 | 84 | 32 | 9 | 17 | 675 |
| **Midlands West** | 156 | 90 | 54 | 25 | 46 | 371 |
| **Northeast** | 437 | 154 | 67 | 34 | 62 | 754 |
| **Northwest** | 861 | 193 | 50 | 43 | 61 | 1208 |
| **Scotland** | 539 | 230 | 72 | 33 | 52 | 926 |
| **South England** | 424 | 180 | 70 | 34 | 86 | 794 |
| **Southeast England** | 429 | 236 | 65 | 25 | 54 | 809 |
| **Southwest** | 653 | 212 | 55 | 24 | 37 | 981 |
| **Total** | 4210 | 1445 | 506 | 242 | 442 | 6845 |

#### b) Burn Injuries in Children Admitted to Burn Services (Not DGHs)[6]

|  | 0%–4.9% | 5%–9.9% | 10%–14.9% | 15%–19.9% | 20%–100% | Total |
|---|---|---|---|---|---|---|
| **Ireland** | 60 | 26 | 13 | 5 | 9 | 113 |
| **Midlands East** | 254 | 44 | 12 | 5 | 5 | 320 |
| **Midlands West** | 76 | 48 | 28 | 14 | 19 | 185 |
| **Northeast** | 197 | 74 | 25 | 18 | 26 | 340 |
| **Northwest** | 476 | 114 | 11 | 24 | 23 | 648 |
| **Scotland** | 225 | 129 | 34 | 14 | 19 | 421 |

*(continued on next page)*

TABLE 2 (*continued*)

|  | 0%–4.9% | 5%–9.9% | 10%–14.9% | 15%–19.9% | 20%–100% | Total |
|---|---|---|---|---|---|---|
| South England | 111 | 73 | 22 | 15 | 26 | 247 |
| Southeast England | 209 | 139 | 26 | 8 | 17 | 399 |
| Southwest | 240 | 102 | 28 | 11 | 10 | 391 |
| Total | 1848 | 749 | 199 | 114 | 154 | 3064 |

c) Child Burn Deaths[6]

|  | 0%–4.9% | 5%–9.9% | 10%–14.9% | 15%–19.9% | 20%–100% | Total |
|---|---|---|---|---|---|---|
| Midlands West | 0 | 0 | 0 | 0 | 2 | 2 |
| Northeast | 0 | 0 | 0 | 0 | 1 | 1 |
| Northwest | 1 | 1 | 0 | 1 | 3 | 6 |
| Scotland | 0 | 0 | 0 | 0 | 1 | 1 |
| South England | 0 | 0 | 1 | 0 | 5 | 6 |
| Southeast England | 0 | 0 | 0 | 0 | 2 | 2 |
| Total | 1 | 1 | 1 | 1 | 14 | 18 |

TABLE 3
Major burn incidents in the European Union.[19]

| Date | Place | Type | Dead | Injured |
|---|---|---|---|---|
| 1973 | Summerland complex, Isle of Man | Building Fire | 48 | 70 |
| 1974 | Flixborough, Lancashire | Explosion | 28 | 89 |
| 1978 | Los Alfaques, Spain | Camping Fire | 216 | 200 |
| 1979 | Woolworth store, Manchester | Fire | 10 | 48 |
| 1981 | Stardust Club, Dublin | Disco Fire | 48 | 160 |
| 1982 | Cardowan mine, Glasgow | Mine Explosion | None | 40 |
| 1983 | Amoco refinery, Pembroke | Refinery Fire | 1 | 6 |
| 1984 | Abbeystead, Lancashire | Fire/Explosion | 16 | 36 |
| 1984 | Milford Haven, Pembs. | Ship explosion | 4 | 16 |
| 1984 | Oxford Circus, London | Station Fire | None | 15 |
| 1985 | Putney, London | Explosion | 8 | 10 |
| 1985 | Bradford, W. Yorkshire | Stadium Fire | 55 | 200 |
| 1985 | Manchester Airport | Plane Fire | 55 | 85 |
| 1987 | King's Cross, London | Station Fire | 32 | 60+ |
| 1988 | Ramstein, Germany | Plane Crash | 73 | 530 |
| 1988 | Piper Alpha, North Sea | Fire/Explosion | 165 | 25+ |
| 1992 | Amsterdam apartments | Plane crash | Unknown | Unknown |

(*continued on next page*)

TABLE 3 (*continued*)

| Date | Place | Type | Dead | Injured |
|------|-------|------|------|---------|
| 1992 | Faro Airport, Portugal | Plane crash | Unknown | 45 |
| 1994 | Smithfield, London | Cinema Fire | 11 | 12 |
| 1999 | Mont Blanc Tunnel, France | Lorry Fire | 42 | Unknown |
| 1999 | Ladbroke Grove, London | Train Crash | 31 | 415 |
| 2001 | Volendam, Netherlands | Fire | 14 | 207 |
| 2001 | Corus, Port Talbot, Wales | Explosion | 3 | 12 |
| 2004 | Belgium | Gas explosion | 15 | 120 |
| 2004 | Madrid, Spain | Multiple bombing | 191 | 1406 |

TABLE 4

**Incidents in the United Kingdom known to have involved large numbers of children.[25]**

| Major Incident | Year | Total Casualties | Child Casualties |
|----------------|------|------------------|------------------|
| M5 coach crash | 1983 | 31 | 27 |
| Enniskillin bombing | 1987 | 65 | 6 |
| Newton train crash | 1991 | 26 | 7 |
| Dimmocks train crash | 1992 | 45 | 12 |
| York coach crash | 1994 | 41 | 40 |
| West St. bus crash | 1994 | 33 | 33 |
| Abbeyhill junction, train crash | 1994 | 47 | 10 |
| Warrington coach crash | 1996 | 51 | 50 |
| Manchester bombing | 1996 | 217 | 30 |
| Dunblane mass shooting | 1996 | 30 | 28 |

TABLE 5

**Minimum supplementary paediatric equipment for 10 children.**

| | Item | Number |
|---|------|--------|
| Airway and cervical spine | Airways 00-2 | 5 each |
| | Endotracheal tubes 2.5-6.5 mm | 5 each |
| | Yankauer sucker (paediatric) | 10 |
| | Soft sucker 8-10 g | 10 each |
| | Semirigid cervical collars (paediatric) | 5 sets |
| Breathing | Child self-inflating bag | 2 |
| | Face masks 00-2 | 1 each |
| | Oxygen masks (with reservoir) (paediatric) | 10 |
| | Chest drains 24-28 F | 2 each |

(continued on next page)

TABLE 5 (*continued*)

| | Item | Number |
|---|---|---|
| Circulation | Venous cannulae 18-24 g | 20 each |
| | Intraosseous cannulae | 2 |
| | 50 mL syringes with luer lock | 2 |
| | Giving sets (paediatric) | 20 |
| | ECG electrodes (paediatric) | 25 |
| | Defibrillation pads (paediatric) | 2 pairs |
| Other | Urinary catheters 8-10 g | 2 each |
| | Nasogastric tubes 8-10 g | 2 each |
| | Weight-height or weight-age nomogram | 1 |
| | Spinal board (paediatric) | 1 |

TABLE 6
**Paediatric assessment team action card.**

**Responsibilities**

Estimate total number of children in receiving hospitals who may need paediatric tertiary services

Liaison with paediatric specialist services to ascertain the level of provision available

Identify individual children suitable for transfer to tertiary services

**Immediate action**

Proceed to lead paediatric hospital and report to the paediatric coordinator

Liaise with the paediatric coordinator to ascertain the number of children likely to be involved, the number of receiving hospitals, and the paediatric specialist services that may be required

Liaise with the relevant specialist paediatric services to ascertain preparedness and level of provision available

Proceed to the receiving units and liaise with the local paediatric coordinator to ascertain the number of children (if any) who need specialist provision

Estimate the relative need of each child for specialist provision

Match availability with need in each receiving unit

Arrange transfer of children who can be dealt with in the specialist units

Ensure that specialist units and receiving hospital staff have liaised regarding children who have not been transferred

**Priorities**

Estimation of the availability of specialist services

Estimation of the need for each specialist service within each receiving unit

Matching need with availability

## TABLE 7
### The Children's Charter.[27]

**The Children's Charter (1996)**

Care should be in a children's ward under the supervision of a consultant paediatrician.

Parents should be able to stay in the hospital with their child.

If the child is having surgery, the parents can expect to accompany him or her to the anaesthetic room and be present until he or she goes to sleep.

Parents should be informed about which pain relief will be given to their child.

The NHS should respect the privacy, dignity, and religious or cultural beliefs of the child.

The child should be offered a choice of children's menus.

There should be facilities for breastfeeding.

The child can wear his or her own clothes and have personal possessions.

The hospital should be clean, safe, and suitably furnished for children and young people.

There should be the opportunity for playing with and meeting other children.

The child has a right to receive suitable education.

Teenagers should have the choice of a children's ward, adult ward, or any specific accommodation for teenagers.

# REFERENCES

**1.** Colebrook L. *A New Approach to the Treatment of Burns and Scalds*. London: Fine Technical Publications; 1950.

**2.** MacMillan BG. Early excision of more than 25 percent of body surface in the extensively burned patient. *Arch Surg*. 1959; **77:** 369–376.

**3.** Jackson D, Tapley E, Cason JS, Lowbury EJL. Primary excision and grafting of large burns. *Ann Surg*. 1960; **152:** 167–169.

**4.** National Burn Care Review Committee. Standards and strategy for burn care. A review of burn care in the British Isles. National Burn Care Group, UK, www.nbcg.nhs.uk/EasySiteWeb/Gateway Link.aspx?alld=25770 (accessed June 2010).

**5.** Department of Health. Specialised services national definitions set. 2nd ed. Specialised burn care services (all ages)—definition no 9. 22 March 2004. Department of Health, The National Archives, http://webarchive.nationalarchives.gov.uk/+/www.dh.gov.uk/en/managingyourorganisation/commisioningspecialisedservices/specialised servicesdefinition/DH_4001838 (accessed June 2010).

**6.** Specialised Burn Care Commissioners briefing case for change. 18 January 2003. National Burn Care Group, UK, www.nbcg.nhs.uk/EasySiteWeb/GatewayLink.aspx?=25771 (accessed Oct 2009).

**7.** Consumer Affairs Directorate. Burns and scalds accidents in the home DTI. 1999. http: //webarchive.gov.uk/+/http: //www.dti.gov.uk/homesafetynetwork/bs_rhome.htm (accessed Oct 2009).

**8.** National Burn Care Group. Optimising burn care provision in England and Wales. www.nbcg.nhs.uk/EsySiteWeb/GatewayLink.aspx?alld=25772 (accessed Oct 2009).

**9.** National Burn Care Group. Referral guidelines. NBCR committee report: Standards and strategy for burn care. 2001. http://www.nbcg.uk/EsaySiteWeb/GatewayLink.aspx?alld=25770 (accessed Oct 2009).

**10.** National Burn Care Group. Burn care update. Issue 7, Feb 2006. www.nbcg.uk/EasySiteWeb/GatewayLink.aspx?alld=25755 (accessed Oct 2009).

**11.** Department of Health. Comprehensive critical care. A review of adult critical care services. 2000. www.dh.gov.uk/en/Publicationsandstatistics/Publications/PublicationsPolicyAndGuidance/DH_4006585 (accessed Oct 2009).

**12.** NHS emergency planning guidance 2005. Planning for the management of burn injured patients in the event of a major incident. Best practice guidance. 2007. http: //www.dh.gov.uk/publications (accessed Oct 2009).

**13.** National Burn Bed Bureau process. National Burn Care Group Web site. http: //www.nbcg.nhs.uk/national-burn-bed-bureau/process/ (accessed Oct 2009).

**14.** Department of Health, Emergency Preparedness Division. Mass casualties incidents—a framework for planning. 2007. http: //webarchive.nationalarchives.gov.uk/+/www.dh.gov.uk/en/consultations/Closedconsultations/DH_063395 (accessed Oct 2009).

**15.** Carley S, Mackway-Jones K, Donnan S. Major incidents in Britain over the past 28 years: the case for the centralised reporting of major incidents. *J Epidemiol Community Health*. 1998; **52:** 392–398.

**16.** Civil Contingencies Act 2004. http: //www.opsi.gov.uk/acts/acts2004/ukpga_20040036_en_1 (accessed Oct 2009).

17. Kemp V, Department of Health. NHS emergency planning guidance 2005: underpinning materials. Critical care contingency in the event of an emergency where the number of patients substantially exceeds normal critical care capacity. Best practice guidance. 2007. www.dh.gov.uk/en/Publicationsandstatistics/Publications/PublicationsPolicyAndGuidance/DH_081282 (accessed Oct 2009).

18. Storr P, Prepared by the Emergency Preparedness Division, Department of Health. Strategic command arrangements for the NHS during a major incident. 2007. www.dh.gov.uk/en/Publicationsandstatistics/Publications/PublicationsPolicyAndGuidance/DH_081507 (accessed Oct 2009).

19. National Burn Care Group; Burns Major Incident Planning Group. 2006. http://www.nationalburncaregroup.nhs.uk/burns-major-incident-plan/ (accessed Oct 2009).

20. Sharpe DT, Roberts AH, Barclay TL, et al. Treatment of burns casualties after fire at Bradford City football ground. *BMJ*. 1985; 291(5): 945–948.

21. Griffiths RW. Management of multiple casualties with burns. *BMJ*. 1985; **291**: 917–918.

22. Carley SD, Mackway-Jones K. The casualty profile from the Manchester bombing 1996; a proposal for the construction and dissemination of casualty profiles from major incidents. *J Accid Emerg Med*. 1997; **14**: 76–80.

23. Brough MD. The King's Cross fire. Part 1: the physical injuries. *Burns*. 1991; **17**(1): 6–9.

24. Sturgeon D, Rosser R, Shoenberg P. The King's Cross fire. Part 2: the psychological injuries. *Burns*. 1991; **17**(1): 10–13.

25. Carley SD, Mackway-Jones K, Donnan S. Delphi study into the planning for care of children in major incidents. *Arch Dis Child*. 1999; **80**: 406–409.

26. Mackway-Jones K, Carley SD, Robson J. Planning for major incidents involving children by implementing a Delphi study. *Arch Dis Child*. 1999; **80**: 410–413.

27. The Children's Charter. http://www.headlines.org.uk/charter.htm (accessed Oct 2009).

28. Department of Health. National Service framework for children, young people and maternity services. Part 1: standards for hospital services. 2004. http://www.dh.gov.uk/en/publicationandstatistics/publications/publicationspolicyandguidance/DH_4006182 (accessed Oct 2009).

29. Cunliffe PH. Communicating with children in the intensive care unit. *Intensive Care Nurs*. 1987; **3**: 71–77.

30. Persson M, Rumsey N, Spalding H, Partridge J. Bridging the gap between current care provision and the psychological standards of burn care. Changing Faces with the Centre for Appearance Research. 2007. www,nbcg.nhs.uk/EasySiteWeb/GatewayLink.aspx?alld=40002.

31. Psycho-social Working Party, National Burn Care Group. Psycho-social rehabilitation after burn injury. Report. 2006. www.nbcg.nhs.uk/EsaySiteWeb/Gateway Link.aspx?alld=25786 (accessed June 2010)

32. Madianos MG, Papaghelis M, Ioannovich J, Dafni R. Psychiatric disorders in burn patients: a follow-up study. *Psychother Psychosom*. 2001; **70**: 30–37.

33. Tarnowski KJ, Rasnake LK, Drabman RS. Behavioural assessment and treatment of pediatric burn injuries: a review. *Behav Ther*. 1987; **18**: 417–441.

34. Wisely JA, Hoyle E, Tarrier N, Edwards J. Where to start? Attempting to meet the psychological needs of burned patients. *Burns*. 2007; **33**: 736–746.

35. Post-traumatic stress disorder (PTSD). The management of PTSD in adults and children in primary and secondary care. NHS National Institute for Clinical Excellence. National Clinical Practice Number 26, National Collaborating Centre for Mental Health, Commissioned by the National Institute of Clinical Excellence, UK, http: //guideance.nice.org.uk/CG26/Guidance/pdf/English (accessed June 2010).

36. Ethical basis for good practice in play therapy. British Association of Play Therapists Web site. http: //www.bapt.info/ethicalbasis.htm (accessed Oct 2009).

37. Play therapy. The Children's Trust Web site. http: //www.thechildrenstrust.org.uk/ (accessed Oct 2009).

38. Ray D, Bratton S, Rhine T, Jones L. The effectiveness of play therapy: responding to the critics. *Int J Play Ther*. 2001; **10**(1): 85–108.

39. Play Therapy United Kingdom Web site. http: //www.playtherapy.org.uk/AboutPlayTherapy/PlayTherapyDefinition1.htm (accessed Oct 2009).

40. A history of play therapy. British Association of Play Therapists Web site. http: //www.bapt.info/historyofpt.thm (accessed Oct 2009).

41. Hospital play staff. NHS Careers Web site. http: //www.nhscareers.nhs.uk/details/Default.aspx?Id=911 (accessed Oct 2009).

42. Information for professionals. British Association of Play Therapists Web site. www.bapt.info/professionalinfo.htm (accessed Oct 2009).

43. Maurice SC, O'Donnell JJ, Beattie TF. Emergency analgesia in the paediatric population. Part 1: current practice and perspectives. *Emerg Med*. 2002; **19**: 4–7.

44. NSW Severe Burns Injury Service, Prepared by the Play Therapy Department, The Children's Hospital at Westmead 2003. Clinical practice guidelines. Play therapy for burn injured paediatric patients. 2003. www.health.nsw.gav.au/gmct/burninjury/index.asp (accessed June 2010).

45. Leinson P, Ousterhout DK. Art and play therapy with pediatric burn patients. *J Burn Care Rehabil*. 1980; **1**(1): 42–46.

46. Wolf AR, Jenkins IA. Sedation of the critically ill child. *Curr Paediatr*. 2005; **15**: 316–323.

47. Kharasch S. Pain treatment: opportunities and challenges. *Arch Pediatr Adolesc Med*. 2003; **157**: 1054–1056.

48. Juhl GA, Conners GP. Emergency physicians' practices and attitudes regarding procedural anaesthesia for nasogastric tube insertion. *Emerg Med*. 2005; **22**: 243–245.

**49.** Ellis DY, Hisain HM, Saetta JP, Walker T. Procedural sedation in paediatric minor procedures: a prospective audit on ketamine use in the emergency department. *Emerg Med J.* 2004; **21:** 286–289.

**50.** Gall O, Murat I. Sedation and analgesia for procedures outside the operating room in children. *Curr Opin Anaesthesiol.* 2001; **41:** 359–362.

**51.** Fumagali R, Ingelmo P, Sperti LR. Postoperative sedation and analgesia after pediatric liver transplantation. *Transplant Proc.* 2006; **38:** 841–843.

**52.** Suraseranivongse S, Kaosaard R, Intakong P, et al. A comparison of postoperative pain scales in neonates. *Br J Anaesth.* 2006; **97**(4): 540–544.

**53.** Fatovich DM, Gope M, Paech MJ. A pilot trail of BIS monitoring for procedural sedation in the emergency department. *Emerg Med Aust.* 2004; **16:** 103–107.

**54.** Lloyd-Thomas AR. Modern concepts of paediatric analgesia. *Pharmacol Ther.* 1999; **83:** 1–20.

**55.** Bozkurt P. The analgesic efficacy and neuroendocrine response in paediatric patients treated with two analgesic techniques: using morphine-epidural and patient-controlled analgesia. *Paediatr Anaesth.* 202; **12**(3): 248–254.

**56.** Schecter WP, Farmer D, Horn JK, Pietrocola DM, Wallace A. Special considerations in perioperative pain management: audio-visual distraction, geriatrics, paediatrics and pregnancy. *J Am Coll Surg.* 2005; **201**(4): 612–618.

**57.** Rodgers BM, Webb CJ, Stergios D, Newman BM. Patient-controlled analgesia in pediatric surgery. *J Pediatr Surg.* 1988; **23**(3): 259–262.

**58.** Jacob E, Puntillo KA. Variability of analgesic practices for hospitalised children on different pediatric speciality units. *J Pain Symptom Manage.* 2000; **20**(1): 59–67.

**59.** Zernikow B, Smale H, Michel E, Hasan C, Jorch N, Andler W. Paediatric cancer pain management using the WHO analgesic ladder—results of a prospective analysis from 2265 treatment days during a quality improvement study. *Eur J Pain.* 2006; **10:** 587–595.

**60.** Zernikow B, Hasan C, Hechler T, Huebner B, Gordon D, Michel E. Stop the pain! A nation-wide quality improvement programme in paediatric oncology pain control. *Eur J Pain.* 2008; **12:** 819–833.

**61.** Till H, Lochbuhler H, Lochbuhler HA, Kellnar ST, Bohm R, Joppich I. Patient controlled analgesia (PCA) in paediatric surgery: a prospective study following laparoscopic and open appendicectomy. *Paediatr Anaesth.* 1996; **6:** 29–32.

**62.** Young AE. The management of severe burns in children. *Curr Paediatr.* 2004; **14:** 202–207.

**63.** Evans L. Therapy standards in burn care: a multi-centre audit. Paper presented at: Burn Therapy Interest Group, Keele, UK. Unpublished.

**64.** Burn Therapy Standards Working Group. Standards of physiotherapy and occupational therapy practice in the management of burn injured adults and children. 2005. www.library.nhs.uk/guidelinesFinder/viewResource.aspx?resID=187932 (accessed June 2010).

**65.** Rossi LA, Vila V da SC, Zago MMF, Ferreira E. The stigma of burns: perceptions of burned patients' relatives when facing discharge from hospital. *Burns.* 2005; **31:** 37–44.

**66.** Davidson TN, Bowden ML, Tholen D, James MH, Feller I. Social support and post-burn adjustment. *Arch Phys Med Rehabil.* 1981; **62**(6): 274–278.

**67.** Intermediate Care and Integrated discharge planning. 2007. http://webarchive.nationalarchives.gov.uk/+/www.dh.gov.uk/en/Healthcare/IntegratedCare/Changeagentteam/DH_4049393 (accessed Oct 2009).

**68.** Lonnqvist P-A, Morton NS. Paediatric day-case anaesthesia and pain control. *Curr Opin Anaesthiol.* 2006; **19:** 617–621.

**69.** Audit Commission. Inpatient admissions and bed management in NHS acute hospital. London: The Stationery Office; 2000.

**70.** Preston C, Cheater F, Baker R, Hearnshaw H. Left in limbo: patients' views on care across the primary/secondary interface. *Qual Health Care.* 1999; **8:** 16–21.

**71.** Department of Health. Discharge from hospital pathway, process and practice. 2003. http: //www.dh.gov.uk/en/publicationsandstatistics/publications/publicationspolicyandguideance/DH_4003252 (accessed Oct 2009).

**72.** National Audit Office. The management and control of hospital acquired infection. London: The Stationery Office; 2000.

# CHAPTER THIRTY-TWO

# THE SURGICAL TREATMENT OF ACUTE BURNS: THE VIENNESE CONCEPT

L-P KAMOLZ, W HASLIK, DB LUMENTA, AND M FREY
VIENNA BURN CENTRE, DIVISION OF PLASTIC AND RECONSTRUCTIVE SURGERY,
DEPARTMENT OF SURGERY,
MEDICAL UNIVERSITY OF VIENNA, VIENNA, AUSTRIA

## INTRODUCTION

In the last few decades, burn care has improved to the extent that patients with severe burns frequently survive. The trend in current treatment extends beyond the preservation of life and function; the ultimate goal is the return of burn victims, as full participants, back to their families and communities. Hereby restoring function with an acceptable aesthetic appearance, including good pliability of the reconstructed tissue and minimal unstable scarring, are crucial in the difficult process of reintegration and a return to working life. In the past, great efforts were made to develop skin replacements to overcome the problem of poor skin quality and scar contraction in grafted areas.[1-5] Further important factors in burn care are early mobilisation, consequent hypertrophic scar prevention (eg, compression) management, and a tailored rehabilitation program in a specialized rehabilitation centre following discharge from the hospital.

This chapter was prepared to introduce the surgical treatment protocol of the Viennese Burn Centre.

## EPIDEMIOLOGICAL AND DEMOGRAPHIC CHARACTERISTICS

A review of our patient data (Vienna Burn Centre, Division of Plastic and Reconstructive Surgery, Department of Surgery, Medical University of Vienna) identified 365 cases with severe burn injuries over the last 3 years; 65% of patients were male and 35% female. The mean total body surface area (TBSA) burned was 32.6% +/− 23.3%. Hospital admission rates revealed 3 distinct age peaks: younger than 5 years, between 25 and 40 years of age, and older than 65 years. In general, the primary causes of burns were due to fire and flame sources resulting in scald and hot substance injuries. A relatively low but constant rate of admissions was due to self-inflicted burns, which contribute to yearly overall burn admission rates between 2% and 6%,[6,7] according to the literature and our data. Details on Austria and its health care system are presented in Table 1.

## Burn Wound Evaluation

One of the major problems facing any burn surgeon is the decision regarding the course of treatment, that is, conservative versus operative. In the case of an operative procedure, the decision involves determining the timing and planning on how to treat burn wounds, as well as accurately assessing the depth of the lesion and thereby the extent of tissue involvement.[8–12] Traditionally, the evaluation of burn depth has involved serial clinical examinations, which primarily involve subjective judgments. Various objective examination techniques supplementing the clinical diagnosis have been evaluated in our unit.[10–12] One of these techniques is ICG video angiography, which allows evaluation of dermal and subdermal vessel patency (evaluation of ICG uptake, steady state distribution, and clearance of dye-marked blood from the injured area) and thus estimates the extent of injury. Injured areas that demonstrate relatively bright and homogenous fluorescence, quick uptake, constant and high steady state distribution, and quick clearance all indicate patency of the small vessels of the subpapillary and dermal plexus and do not require operative intervention. Deep dermal injuries appear as darker areas yielding mottled fluorescence, slower uptake, and constant but less steady state distribution, thus indicating partial patency of the dermal plexus. Full-thickness skin lesions show only large and discrete vessels and little if any signs of fluorescence, indicating minimal or no remaining blood flow in the dermis. Scans in burns due to scalds, electrical injuries, and chemical injuries may initially suggest viable tissue, but during the next 24 to 48 hours, much more tissue will become necrotic as the injury progresses. Therefore, we would recommend an initial ICG video angiography on day 0 (after admission) and daily until no changes can be detected[10–12] (Figure 1). However, similar to other objective methods, there are limitations in the accuracy of this technique.[12] Moreover, although ICG video angiography is well studied for measuring flap and retinal perfusion, its use in burn and trauma surgery is still very limited. Therefore, in our daily routine, the serial clinical examination is still our gold standard to evaluate burn wound depth.

## Burn Wound Management

One of the most important functions of viable skin is to prevent infection. Nonviable and frequently necrotic burn wound eschar and granulating surfaces present a moist, protein-laden growth medium for microorganisms.[13] There is a general consensus that it is unrealistic to try to maintain a completely sterile burn wound. Therefore, our efforts are directed at controlling the microbial flora that colonize the local tissue environment through the use of silver products (eg, Flammazine®, Mepilex Ag,® and Acticoat® or Lavasorb® are the primary topical agents of choice on admission to our unit).

Biological dressings (eg, allografts, xenografts) applied to fully debrided, relatively uncontaminated wounds have been shown to adhere to the wound surface, thereby reducing wound colony counts, limiting fluid and protein loss, reducing pain, and increasing the rate of epithelialisation over that obtained with application of topical antimicrobial agents.[14]

Applications of special wound dressings (eg, Biobrane®, Suprathel®) are used to cover fresh deep dermal wounds because they provide a physiological environment for healing; however, the use of these dressings to granulating and deeply excised wounds is not recommended. Cadaver skin allografts are a more suitable alternative when the burn wound cannot be closed primarily with autografts. Our practice involves enzymatic debridement (using Varidase®) of untidy granulating wounds with serial application of biological dressings as a second choice in selective cases.

## Timing and Planning of Surgery

In the case of an operative procedure, the decision on when to excise burn wounds and how to accurately determine the depth of the lesion, and thereby the extent of tissue involvement, is needed. Controversies remain on how and when to proceed with excision, but it is widely accepted that if skin does not regenerate within a matter of a few weeks through healing of partial-thickness injury and closure of the wound, morbidity and scarring will be severe. Because the ultimate protection of the body from burn wound pathogens is obtained by healed and completely epithelialized skin,[15–17] the treatment of deep dermal partial-thickness and full-thickness burns leans toward very early excision and grafting in order to reduce the risk of infection, decrease scar formation, shorten hospital stay, and reduce costs. As opposed to deep dermal and full-thickness injuries, superficial burns generally heal without need for an operation within 2 to 3 weeks. Whenever a patient is hemodynamically stable and the risks of an operation are deemed acceptable (ie, no increase in mortality over that which would be expected from traditional treatment), then excision of as much of the burn wound as possible should be carried out. In patients with coinjuries such as an inhalation injury or comorbidities (eg, cardiac problems) and in the elderly, a carefully planned approach to surgical treatment is required in deciding when and how much to excise.[5]

We begin excision of all full-thickness burned areas within 72 hours of the time of injury (between 48 and 72 hours). Sequential layered tangential excision to viable bleeding points, even to fat, while minimizing loss of viable tissue, is the generally accepted technique in our unit. Excision of burn wounds to the fascia is reserved for large burns, where the risks of massive blood loss and the possibility of skin slough from less vascularized grafts on fat may lead to higher mortality.

In the case of full-thickness burns, we use expanded meshed autografts to cover wounds if sufficient donor sites are available. With facial or hand burns, we prefer using unmeshed skin grafts. The expansion rate of graft to wound area coverage ranges from 1:1.5 to 1:9.[18] As expansion rates higher than 1:3 heal in a suboptimal manner, we like to use larger meshed skin grafts (1:6 or 1:9) in combination with allografts or keratinocytes (sandwich technique in order to improve the aesthetic and functional outcome) (Figure 2). In very large burns, we like to use the Meek technique (Figure 3)[4] in ratios of 1:6 and 1:9. Donor sites for autografts in burns less than 40% TBSA are seldom a problem unless the patient is at risk of surgical complications resulting from age, cardiopulmonary problems, or coagulopathy. Since patients with more extensive burns have a paucity of available donor sites, we cover such areas with keratinocytes or Suprathel® (Figure 4).[4,19]

## LARGE BURNS > 60% TBSA

In massive burns, we organize body region topography according to the probability of skin take rate and functional importance in order to ultimately determine the need for surgical priority (Figures 5 and 6).[4] Surgical priority is generally given to areas of functional and aesthetic importance and superior take rate (Figures 5–7). Body regions with inferior take rate are preconditioned with silver nitrate or in fluidized microsphere bead beds and treated at a later phase,[4] as the patient's condition allows. Deep dermal and full-thickness burn wounds are initially treated with silver products. In addition, full-thickness burns that are not excised during the first operative sessions (days 3–9) are temporarily treated with silver products (Mepilex Ag®, Acticoat 7). Regions such as the dorsum, the dorsal aspect of the thighs, and the gluteal areas are treated by use of fluidized microsphere bead beds in order to keep the wounds dry.

## LOCATION-SPECIFIC TREATMENT

### Face

Superficial partial-thickness burns are treated conservatively by use of silver products (Figure 8). Deep partial-thickness (deep dermal) burns are dermabraded and covered with keratinocytes (Figure 9) or treated conservatively with Acticoat 7®. Full-thickness burns are excised and grafted with unmeshed skin grafts according to aesthetic units in the face.

### Hands

Superficial partial-thickness burns are treated conservatively by use of Flammazine®, Mepilex Ag®, or Acticoat 7®. Deep partial-thickness (deep dermal) burns are debrided tangentially and covered with keratinocytes or, when keratinocytes are lacking, with Suprathel®. Full-thickness burns are excised and grafted with Matriderm® and unmeshed skin grafts (Figure 10).[1–3,20,21]

## SKIN AND SKIN SUBSTITUTES

Over the past 3 decades, extraordinary advances have been made in our understanding of the pathobiology of wounds as well as the cellular and molecular processes involved in acute wound healing.[22,23] This knowledge has led to wound care innovations that have facilitated more rapid closure of chronic and acute wounds in addition to improved functional and aesthetic outcomes. Several products for wound treatment that germinated from our increased understanding of fundamental processes underlying wound healing have reached the market for therapy of recalcitrant wounds.[24]

The advent of tissue-engineered skin replacements revolutionized the therapeutic potential for recalcitrant wounds and injuries not amenable to primary closure. Two major approaches, in vitro and in vivo, have been utilized to develop engineered tissue. The in vitro method has received considerable attention since it attempts to create organs in tissue culture or bioreactors for implantation and replacement. In contrast, the in vivo approach attempts to create acellular biomaterial that contains matrices capable of stimulating tissue cell recruitment into the biomaterial and inducing cell differentiation to form the needed tissue. Ideally, tissue-engineered skin replacements should facilitate faster healing and promote the development of new tissue that bears a close structural and functional resemblance to the uninjured host tissue.[3]

Autologous and allogeneic epidermal replacement cultured autologous epidermal (CEA) sheets have been used to facilitate repair of both epidermal and partial-thickness wounds. Autologous epidermal sheets were first used to cover burn wounds, which have remained the major clinical target for both autologous and allogeneic epidermal replacement.[5,25–27]

Cultured epidermal sheet allografts were developed to overcome the necessity to obtain a biopsy from each patient for epidermal harvest, then await its associated 2-week cultivation until the final autograft product is ready. With the utilization of techniques for culturing epidermal sheets, epidermal cells from both cadavers and unrelated adult donors[27] have been used for the treatment of burns,[25] donor sites of skin grafts, and chronic leg ulcers. These allografts serve as biological active dressings in order to promote epithelialisation while also promoting accelerated healing and pain relief in a variety of wounds. To facilitate mass allograft production and wide availability, cryopreserved allografts, which gave comparable results to fresh allografts,[28] were developed.

Keratinocytes serve as permanent wound coverage since they yield adequate cosmetic results and the host does not reject them. However, graft take can vary widely due to wound preparation and its intrinsic status, a patient's underlying disease, and operator experience. Our experience with sheets of allogeneic keratinocytes for deep dermal burns in children appears to have allowed healing of wounds with better outcome in terms of scar formation compared to skin grafts (Figure 9).[25] Compared with other, previously reported methods, our modified technique of using keratinocytes on gels of fibrin containing living fibroblasts[26] offers the following advantages: (1) high expansion factor, (2) short culture time, (3) easy monitoring of keratinocyte growth, handling, and delivery for grafting, (4) elimination of enzymatic treatment, and (5) application of epithelial and mesenchymal cells in a single operative procedure. Overall, our culture system has improved the strategy for adequately closing burn wounds more quickly.

Suprathel® is a promising and fully synthetic copolymer with a porous membrane, mainly based on DL-lactidetrimethytencarbonate (>70%), trimethylenecarbonate, and e-caprolactone. Available with various pore and surface sizes, it can be employed after excision and haemostasis for second-degree burned areas (Figure 11) as well as for skin harvest regions (Figure 4). Proposed advantages of its utilization include a reduction in pain, accelerated epithelialisation, and the benefit for use in joint proximity and functionally stressed regions (eg, for early mobilization).[3,5,19]

While cultured epidermal sheets enhance healing, especially of burn wounds, they lack a dermal component that, if present, might prevent wound contraction and provide greater mechanical stability. Cadaver skin allografts containing both epidermis and dermis have been used for many years but provide only temporary coverage because of host rejection. Matriderm® is a very promising dermal substitute which is suitable for single-step repair of dermal tissue defects in combination with thin skin grafts.[1–5,20,21] Matriderm® is a thin, porous membrane consisting of native bovine collagen fibres coated with elastin hydrolysate (derived from bovine ligamentum nuchae) (Figure 12). The matrix, which is converted into native host collagen within weeks after application, can be stored at room temperature and is available as 1-mm- and 2-mm-thick sheets. Depending on local (intraoperative) conditions after debridement and meticulous haemostasis, it can either be applied after rehydration in 0.9% physiological saline solution or as it is onto the wound bed, from which rehydration can then proceed.

Sheets of 2-mm thickness and above are recommended for 2-step repairs, with a time interval of 7 days to allow for vascularisation of the matrix before the transplantation of split-thickness skin grafts. However, a 1-step procedure is feasible in the acute phase after burn trauma. Approximately a week after dressing removal, physiotherapy can be initiated. The take rate does not differ significantly as compared to "regular" split-thickness skin grafts. Moreover, the quality of the resulting scars is reported to be superior compared to skin grafting alone (Figure 10).

## TEMPORARY COVERAGE

If harvested split skin grafts are insufficient for coverage of full-thickness areas, we prefer to use allogeneic skin grafts as a temporary alternative. However, if allogeneic skin is not available, we are using Epigard® to temporarily wrap debrided full-thickness areas.

## NEGATIVE-PRESSURE WOUND THERAPY (VACUUM-ASSISTED CLOSURE)

A good take rate of the transplanted skin grafts is essential for fast wound healing and, thereby, for the patient's outcome. We prefer the vacuum-assisted closure (VAC®) for split-thickness skin fixation in moist and irregular wounds, for areas exposed to movement, and especially in older patients with comorbidities. This technique promotes good skin graft fixation in regions of inferior take,[4] while allowing for early mobilization in functionally important zones.[29] Our practice involves leaving the VAC in place for 3 to 5 days (Figure 13).

## FLUIDIZED MICROSPHERE BEAD BEDS

Fluidized microsphere bead beds are used for wound preconditioning as well as postoperative wound care. This method allows removal of moisture in order to keep wounds and dressings dry. The beds permit maintenance of constant levels of temperature in areas that are in direct contact with the bed's superficial fabric. Only thin, sterile covers are employed to shield dorsal burned areas while in these beds, and no extra ointments are applied. For wound coverage of freshly operated areas, we prefer fat gauze and dry sterile compresses.

## CONCLUSION

Our surgical strategy is primarily based on an exact evaluation of the burn wound (burn size and depth) and the precise planning and timing of surgery. Normally, we operate on full-thickness areas between days 3 and 5 depending on such factors as body region, age, and comorbidities. For deep dermal lesions, we prefer to use keratinocytes; when unavailable, Suprathel® is utilized. Split-thickness skin grafts (Meek, mesh) are used for permanent coverage of full-thickness skin defects. We employ fluidized microsphere bead beds for wound bed preparation. Other important aspects of our treatment strategy involve temporary coverage of wounds with allogeneic skin and skin substitutes (eg, Epigard®, Suprathel®, Matriderm®, allogeneic cultured keratinocyte sheets, and allogeneic split-thickness skin grafts) and negative-pressure wound therapy (vacuum-assisted closure) for skin graft fixation in selective cases. Other significant factors are early mobilisation, a consequent hypertrophic scar prevention (eg, compression) program, and a tailored rehabilitation program in a specialized rehabilitation centre following hospital discharge.

## KEY POINTS

- Exact determination of burn wound severity (burn depth and TBSA)
- Evaluation of the exact trauma mechanism
- Timing and planning of surgery
- Lesion-specific treatment (local therapy, debridement, and grafting)
- Early mobilisation and rehabilitation
- Close follow-up
- Surgical corrections (if indicated)

## REFERENCES

1. Haslik W, Kamolz LP, Nathschläger G, Andel H, Meissl G, Frey M. First experiences with the collagen-elastin matrix Matriderm as a dermal substitute in severe burn injuries of the hand. *Burns*. 2007; **33**: 364–368.

2. Haslik W, Kamolz LP, Manna F, Hladik M, Rath T, Frey M. Management of full-thickness skin defects in the hand and wrist region: first long-term experiences with the dermal matrix Matriderm®. *J Plast Reconstr Aesthet Surg*. 2008; **63**(2): 360–364.

3. Kamolz LP, Lumenta DB, Kitzinger HB, Frey M. Tissue engineering for cutaneous wounds: an overview of current standards and possibilities. *Eur Surg*. 2008; **40**: 19–26.

4. Lumenta DB, Kamolz LP, Frey M. Adult burn patients with more than 60% TBSA involved—Meek and other techniques to overcome restricted skin harvest availability—the Viennese concept. *J Burn Care Res*. 2009; **30**: 231–242.

5. Kamolz LP, Kitzinger HB, Andel H, Frey M. The surgical treatment of acute burns. *Eur Surg*. 2006; **38**: 417–423.

6. Titscher A, Lumenta DB, Belke V, Kamolz LP, Frey M. A new diagnostic tool for the classification of patients with self-inflicted burns (SIB): the SIB-typology and its implications for clinical practice. *Burns*. 2009; **35**: 733–737.

7. Kamolz LP, Andel H, Schmidtke A, Valentini D, Meissl G, Frey G. Treatment of patients with severe burn injuries: the impact of schizophrenia. *Burns*. 2003; **29**: 49–53.

8. Jackson DM. The diagnosis of the depth of burning. *Br J Surg*. 1953; **40**: 588.

9. Heimbach D, Engrav L, Grube B, Marvin J. Burn depth: a review. *World J Surg*. 1992; **16**(1): 10.

10. Kamolz LP, Andel H, Haslik W, et al. Indocyanine green video angiographics help to identify burns requiring operations. *Burns*. 2003; **29**(8): 785.

11. Kamolz LP, Andel H, Auer T, Meissl G, Frey M. Evaluation of skin perfusion by use of indocyanine green video angiographa: rational design and planning of trauma surgery. *J Trauma*. 2006; **61**: 635–641.

12. Haslik W, Kamolz LP, Andel H, Winter W, Meissl G, Frey M. The influence of dressings and ointments on the qualitative and quantitative evaluation of burn wounds by ICG video-angiography: an experimental setup. *Burns*. 2004; **30**(3): 232–235.

13. Herndon DN, Curreri PW, Abston S, Rutan TC, Barrow RE. Treatment of burns. *Curr Probl Surg*. 1987; **24**: 346.

14. Baxter CR. Topical use of 1, 0% silver sulfadiazine. In: *Contemporary Burn Management*. Boston, MA: Little Brown Co; 1971.

15. Engrav LH, Heimbach DM, Reus JL, Harnar TJ, Marvin JA. Early excision and grafting vs. nonoperative treatment of burns of indeterminant depth: a randomized prospective study. *J Trauma*. 1983; **23**(11): 1001.

16. Spurr ED, Shakespeare PG. Incidence of hypertrophic scarring in burned-children. *Burns*. 1990; **16**(3): 179.

17. Still JM, Law EJ, Belcher K, Thiruvaiyarv D. Decreased length of hospital stay by early excision and grafting of burns. *South Med J*. 1996; **89**: 578.

18. Snyder WH, Bowles, MacMillan BG. The use of expansion meshed grafts in the acute and reconstructive management of thermal injury: a clinical valuation. *J Trauma*. 1970; **10**: 740.

19. Schwarze H, Küntscher M, Uhlig C, et al. Suprathel, a new skin substitute, in the management of donor sites of split-thickness skin grafts: results of a clinical study. *Burns*. 2007; **33**: 850–854.

20. Ryssel H, Gazyakan E, Germann G, Ohlbauer M. The use of Matriderm in early excision and simultaneous autologous skin grafting in burns—a pilot study. *Burns*. 2008; **34**: 93–97.

21. Kamolz LP, Kitzinger HB, Karle B, Frey M. The treatment of hand burns. *Burns*. 2009; **35**: 327–337.

22. Singer AJ, Clark RA. Cutaneous wound healing. *N Engl J Med*. 1999; **341**: 738–746.

23. Clark RF, An JQ, Greiling D, Khan AJ, Schwarzbauer J. Fibroblast migration of fibronectin requires 3 distinct functional domains. *J Invest Dermatol*. 2003; **121**: 695–705.

24. Ehrenreich M, Ruszcak Z. Update on tissue-engineered biological dressings. *Tissue Eng.* 2006; **12:** 1–8.

25. Rab M, Koller R, Ruzicka M, et al. Should dermal scald burns in children be covered with autologous skin grafts or with allogeneic cultivated keratinocytes?—"The Viennese concept." *Burns.* 2005; **31:** 578–586.

26. Kamolz LP, Luegmair M, Wick N, et al. The Viennese culture method: cultured human epithelium obtained on a dermal matrix based on fibroblast containing fibrin glue gels. *Burns.* 2005; **31:** 25–29.

27. Koller R, Bierochs B, Meissl G, Rab M, Frey M. The use of allogeneic cultivated keratinozytes for the early coverage of deep burns—indications, results and problems. *Cell Tissue Bank.* 2002; **3:** 11–14.

28. Teepe RGC, Koebrugge EJ, Ponec M, Vermeer BJ. Fresh versus cryopreserved cultured allografts for the treatment of chronic skin ulcers. *Br J Dermatol.* 1990; **122:** 81–89.

29. Roka J, Karle B, Andel H, Kamolz L, Frey M. Use of V.A.C. therapy in the surgical treatment of severe burns: the Viennese concept. *Handchir Mikrochir Plast Chir.* 2007; **39:** 322–327.

# CHAPTER THIRTY-THREE

# PEDIATRIC BURNS: A GLOBAL PERSPECTIVE

MEHMET HABERAL, MD, FACS, FICS (HON),
PROFESSOR IN SURGERY, PRESIDENT OF BASKENT UNIVERSITY, PRESIDENT OF ISBI,
CHAIRMAN OF DEPARTMENT OF GENERAL SURGERY, TRANSPLANTATION AND BURNS, BASKENT UNIVERSITY
HOSPITALS, DIRECTOR OF BASKENT UNIVERSITY BURN AND FIRE DISASTER INSTITUTE

ÖZGÜR BAŞARAN, MD, ASSISTANT PROFESSOR IN SURGERY, DEPARTMENT OF GENERAL SURGERY,
BASKENT UNIVERSITY HOSPITALS

## INTRODUCTION

Burn injury is a serious worldwide health problem. A severe burn injury is not only a life-threatening matter for the injured patient, but it may also have serious physical, psychological, and financial effects on the patient, his or her family, and society. Burn injury in children represents a unique form of trauma that requires an experienced, multidisciplinary team for optimal outcomes. Burns remain common in children, particularly among lower socioeconomic groups, with major burns being more commonly associated with fatal outcomes in children than in adults.

Epidemiologic surveys provide objective information on hazardous agents and the settings in which burns are most likely to occur. There are an estimated 2.0 million burn injuries in the United States every year.[1] Although the number of burns has been decreasing in this country since the 1970s, accurate determination of its incidence is difficult owing to underreporting. Of the 30000 inpatient admissions yearly, approximately one-third of burn unit admissions are children under the age of 15 years. Nearly one-third of all burn deaths involve children, accounting for between 1000 and 5000 deaths per year. Burns are second only to motor vehicle accidents as the leading cause of death in children older than 1 year. Among burn injuries, accidents by children account for approximately 80%; in 20% there is some evidence or suspicion of neglect and abuse.[2] Along with the elderly, children have the highest rates of morbidity and mortality from thermal injuries.[3]

No one is truly aware of the prevalence of burn injuries affecting children throughout the world each year. The burn injury represents perhaps the widest spectrum of any form of trauma. Many injuries are often self-treated by the patient and/or parents, perhaps with advice from a pharmacist or health care practitioner other than a physician. Many more injuries will be treated by trained health care practitioners in a nonhospital setting such as a clinic. Some will be seen within a hospital setting only after suitable first aid and reassurance have been initially provided on an outpatient basis. The proportion of the pyramid of burn patients who are admitted to the hospital is relatively slight, with the smallest fraction represented by those with serious burn injuries. The numerical stratification of the burn pyramid is influenced by the local provision of services as well as the expectations of the population served.[4]

## EPIDEMIOLOGY

The global incidence of hospitalized pediatric burn patients is unknown.[4] One approach to determine a working estimate of the scope of the problem is to extrapolate information from relevant published studies. A literature search of the Medline database was performed to identify epidemiologic papers published since 1990 which addressed pediatric burn admissions.[4] Data from this search indicate the highest incidence of hospitalized pediatric burn patients in Africa and the lowest in the Americas. Europe, the Middle East, and Asia are similar in their incidences. Because of the considerably larger population of Asia, it bears over half of the world's pediatric burn population (Figure 1).

## ETIOLOGY

The leading causes of burns in children are scalds, flame burns, and electrical injuries. Scalds commonly result from inadequately cooled bath water which has not been checked by an adult. The contact time for a scald injury to occur drops significantly as water temperature rises above 120°F. For this reason, it is currently recommended that hot water heaters be set at or below this temperature.[5] Significant scalds to the face, hands, and shoulders occur because of children's inquisitive natures, which results in pulling electrical cords or containers located near the edge of a counter or table. Similarly, hot cooking grease from the stove may spill onto the curious child as well. Flame burns most commonly result from house fires but are also caused by trash fires, fireworks, and candles. House fires are the leading cause of mortality in pediatric burns, and one-third of these are linked to cigarette smoking. Death related to house fires is due to inhalation injury as well as direct thermal trauma.[3,6] It has been shown that smoke detectors and education can drastically decrease the risk of death in house fires.[7] Electrical burns result from a child biting an electrical cord or placing an object in an uncovered outlet. The resultant perioral injury and scarring can cause significant long-term morbidity. Contact burns can be caused by any number of common household items, including hair curlers, irons, space heaters, and ovens. Unrestricted access to household chemicals, including drain cleaners (lye), bleach, and acid cleansers, results in both contact burns and esophageal injury from ingestion. The risk of these injuries can be significantly limited with proper education and precautionary measures. Approximately 20% of pediatric burns are intentionally caused by a caregiver or parent. Because children are often too frightened or unable to report the exact cause of their injuries, the treating physician must remain vigilant to the possibility of abuse.[8,9] Intentional burns occur in predictable patterns, which can assist the physician in diagnosis. The "dipping" burn, in which a child is lowered into scalding water, involves the buttocks, perineum, and feet while sparing the flexion creases as a result of the child's defensive posturing.[10] Intentional cigarette burns cause a circular "punched out" injury that differs from the more random-appearing "dropped ash" burn.[10] Other signs of abuse include a repeated history of trauma, reports of the burn being caused by the child or a sibling, and accompaniment of the child by someone other than a parent.

## ETIOLOGY OF UNUSUAL SCALD BURNS

Scalding is the most common cause of burns in Turkish children.[11] In typical cases, the victim is scalded when hot fluid is splashed or spilled in the kitchen, often in the mother's presence. Tea, an extremely popular drink in Turkey, is traditionally brewed in 2 pots with narrow bottoms which are stacked on top of each other. Since the traditional pots are inherently unstable, this practice of tea-making is the main cause of burns in Turkish kitchens. Modern kettles have been advocated but are still not widely used.[12,13] Scalding is also relatively common in children who live in industrialized countries, where most accidents occur with electrical kettles.[14] Some anecdotal case reports from these regions describe burns caused by milk from baby bottles that have been inadvertently overheated in microwave ovens.[15,16] Preschool children are at especially high risk for burn accidents at home since they are very curious about their surroundings. At this age, even though they can stand, walk, and explore their environment, they do not fully understand the sometimes dangerous consequences of their actions. Furthermore, their size permits them to reach tabletops and surfaces and inadvertently grasp and spill a container with hot contents. Despite many prevention programs, scalding still causes significant morbidity and mortality in preschool children in all parts of the world.[3] This may be related to lack of a systematic preventive approach that targets major risk factors and risk groups.

Compared with water, cooking oil has a greater ability to hold heat (known as heat capacity) and adheres more strongly to skin because of its viscosity. The high boiling point, viscosity, and potential combustibility of oil equate to a greater potential for soft-tissue damage with oil accidents than with typical scald injuries from hot water.[17] Although oil is more viscous than water and becomes less so with heating, it still remains almost 20 times thicker than water at high temperatures.[17,18] Higher viscosity means longer contact time with skin and thus more extensive tissue destruction compared to other hot liquids that cool, become diluted, or evaporate more quickly.[19] Thus, oil causes deeper burns than similar volumes of water. Since hot milk contains fat, its effects on the skin can be similar to those of oil. In a previously reported study by our group, we demonstrated children scalded with hot milk tend to suffer from more extensive burns and thus have greater mortality than those scalded with hot water.[20]

Most people in the Anatolian region of Turkey live a customary lifestyle of making cheese and yoghurt in their own kitchens and backyards. The traditional method of producing cheese involves boiling milk in a very large tinned copper pot, cooling it, and then adding a special fermentation culture and storing it in optimal (relatively warm) conditions outdoors. The typical pot used for this process is large enough for a preschool-aged child to fit inside, is left open to the air with no lid or covering, and is heated over a wood fire at ground level. Adding to the hazardous situation, rural families in Turkey tend to have large numbers of children, with potentially less parental supervision per child. These factors conspire to produce severe scalding accidents when children fall into these vessels. Often, full-thickness burns result since children cannot readily escape from such a situation. Effective preventative measures would involve placing or building a physical barrier between the hot caldron and children's play areas, as well as use of smaller pots.

It has been shown in certain countries that various familial customs or characteristics related to families' ethnic backgrounds have a definite influence on the incidence and types of childhood injuries,[21] particularly to the degree with which children may be supervised. To design effective burn injury prevention programs in any given society, every detail regarding the lifestyles, traditions, and beliefs of families should be considered.

## TURKEY: BAŞKENT UNIVERSITY BURN AND FIRE DISASTERS INSTITUTE

In September 1980, Dr Mehmet Haberal and his team founded the Turkish Transplantation and Burn Foundation. The goals of this organization are as follows:

- to help burn patients manage financial difficulties
- to encourage research and training activities in burn medicine
- to support research projects
- to provide scholarships for research and treatment activities in transplant and burn medicine
- to establish institutes of higher education

Several years later, in 1986, Dr Haberal founded the Haberal Education Foundation, aimed at supporting and improving educational activities in Turkey. In September 1993, the Turkish Transplantation and Burn Foundation expanded its activities and facilities, leading to a merger with the Haberal Education Foundation and the establishment of Başkent University.

Başkent University then underwent another innovative step in 2003 to create Turkey's first Burn and Fire Disaster Institute, a nonprofit health agency under the umbrella of the university. In addition to its role in coordinating burn care activities at all facilities within the Başkent University Hospital Network, this institute became a collaboration center for all specialized burn units in Turkey.

The Başkent University Hospital Network involves 3 burn units located in the cities of Ankara, Adana, and Konya. The burn unit at Başkent University Ankara Hospital, established in 2003, is 1 of 5 burn units at different health care facilities in Ankara. These units serve a region of approximately 5 million people. Established in 1997, the burn unit at the Başkent University Adana Teaching and Medical Research Center is 1 of 4 burn units at different health care facilities in this city. Together with 3 other burn units, this unit provides services to a region with a population of approximately 3 million people. The only burn center in Konya, the Konya Teaching and Medical Research Center, was established in 2003 and provides burn care services to a region with a population of approximately 1.5 million people. The burn unit at Ankara hospital has acted as a referral center for the other burn units at the Adana and Konya hospitals since its establishment. Each unit is managed by a responsible general surgeon who leads a team of doctors from different specialties (eg, plastic surgery, pediatric surgery, and anesthesiology). Physicians at these units have 24-hour availability to the center in Ankara via the Internet or telephone, allowing consultation with patients, transfer of interactive images, discussion of possible treatments, and decisions regarding transfer of patients to the Ankara center if necessary. Although the different research teams at the university have been attempting to develop an effective telemedicine interface linking the electronic patient data systems of all the hospitals in the network, this is not currently available. Consequently, burn units utilize a standard Internet connection through which high-resolution pictures and webcam images can be transmitted, while patient details are described via e-mail or phone.[22]

## INSTITUTE'S 9-YEAR EXPERIENCE

Three hundred and sixty-two pediatric patients, including infants, toddlers, school-age children, and adolescents, were investigated retrospectively. To compare burn parameters,

4 groups were established according to activities and social behaviors which are predominant at different ages. The specifics of Turkish social life were incorporated using a modified version of a system described in previous reports.[23-24] The groups were as follows:

- 0–12 months: This group comprised infants who are dependent on their parents or caregivers, with limited ability of independent movements.
- 1–6 years: Children in this age group are capable of self-directed activity, are curious about their environment, and try to touch or grasp things within their reach. They require adult protection and supervision since they are unaware of potential dangers.
- 7–14 years: Children and adolescents in this age range are generally eager to engage in new events and activities. In Turkey, the mandatory age for starting primary education is 7 years, so children in this group are in school and more aware of possible dangers in their environment.
- 15–18 years: In Turkey, it is mandatory to complete 8 years of primary education. Consequently, this age group includes youths who have left school and taken jobs in industry and other sectors, as well as those continuing their education. The jobs noted here often involve exposure to substances or materials that can cause burns (ie, chemicals, electricity, steam, and hot liquids).

The findings in the above specified age groups were compared, as well as 2 pairs of subgroups: outpatients versus inpatients and urban versus rural children.

The 362 patients comprised 35.5% of all burn victims treated at 3 burn units. There were 183 boys and 179 girls (male to female ratio 1:0.98), with a mean total body surface area (TBSA) burned of 17.7% and 16.5%, respectively. The largest proportion of patients comprised the group of children aged 1 to 6 years. Figure 2 shows the distribution of patients among the 4 age categories.

The most frequent cause of burn injuries was scalding from spillage/splashing of hot water (referred to as nonbath scalding, 216 cases, 59.7%). The other causes, in order of descending frequency, were bath scalding (immersion in a large container of hot liquid such as milk or tomato paste, 94 cases, 26%), flame (32 cases, 8.8%), electrical (14 cases, 3.9%), and contact with hot surfaces/materials such as a stove or iron (6 cases, 1.7%). The most common environment where burns occurred was the home, whereas only 7 (1.9%) transpired in the workplace. The most frequently affected body site was the trunk (62.7% of cases), followed by the upper extremities (53%). Approximately 241 of the subjects (66.6%) lived in an urban environment, while 121 (33.4%) resided in rural areas

relatively near a burn unit. One hundred seventy-one patients (47.2%) received initial treatment directly at a burn unit, whereas the others (52.8%) were referred from other medical centers. Of these patients, 70.7% were referred to burn centers in the first 24 hours after burn injury, 86.5% were referred within 3 days of the injury, and 8.6% reached a burn unit at least 7 days after the injury. Around 124 (34.3%) of the 362 subjects were treated as outpatients, and 238 (65.7%) were hospitalized. The mortality rate was 8.9% (31 deaths).

## Outpatients Versus Inpatients

Approximately 238 of the patients (65.7%) were inpatients and 124 (34.3%) were outpatients. The majority of the inpatients (n = 172, 72.3%) and outpatients (n = 50, 40.3%) were between 1 and 6 years old. The mean TBSA burned in the inpatient subgroup was 16.1%; the corresponding finding in the outpatient group was 6.2%. A total of 178 inpatients (74.7%) were referred to burn units after treatment at other medical centers, and 145 (60.9%) were admitted within the first 24 hours after the burn injury. Only 13 outpatients (10.5%) were referred to the burn units after treatment at other centers, whereas 111 (89.5%) in this group were taken directly to our burn units within the first 24 hours. One hundred twenty children (97.6%) from urban areas and 3 patients (2.6%) from rural areas were treated as outpatients. Approximately 120 of the hospitalized patients (50.4%) were from urban areas and 118 (49.6%) were from rural areas. During the hospital stay, 92 inpatients (38.7%) were treated with daily dressings only, 128 (53.8%) required debridement only, and 75 (31.5%) required both debridement and grafting.

## Urban Versus Rural

As noted, 241 (66.6%) of the 362 patients lived in urban environments and 121 (33.4%) resided in rural areas. In both groups, the age group of 1-to-6-year-olds comprised the largest proportion of patients. Patients from rural areas had a significantly higher mean percentage of TBSA burned than did those from urban areas (27.1 [15%] vs 13.0 [2%]). Scalding from hot liquids other than water occurred significantly more often in patients in the rural group versus the urban group (36.4% vs 20.7%). Ninety-seven patients from rural areas (80.2%) were referred from other medical centers. A significantly higher proportion of patients from rural areas required hospitalization (rural vs urban: 97.5% vs 49.7%).

## Mortality

Thirty-one of the 362 patients in this series died (15 boys and 16 girls, male to female ratio 0.98:1, overall mortality rate 8.9%). The highest proportion of deaths (25 patients, 6.9%) occurred in the group of children aged 1 to 6 years; the second highest mortality was in those aged 0 to 12 months (3 patients, 0.8%). The range of TBSA burned for patients who died was 20.3% to 48.2%. The most common cause of burns among the nonsurvivors was bath scalds from hot liquids other than water (16 patients, 51.6%), followed by scalds from hot water (11 patients, 35.5%), then flame burns (12.9%). Twenty-one (67.7%) of the patients were from rural areas, and 10 (32.3%) lived in an urban environment. Nineteen patients (61.3%) died from multiple organ failure due to severe sepsis, while 12 (38.7%) expired from severe burn shock within 48 hours of hospitalization.

Over the past 9 years, our data reveal that the most common incidents in pediatric patients are scald burns in the home. The majority of our victims were children aged 1 to 6 years. Our research clearly shows that Turkish children and adolescents who live in rural areas are at higher risk for major burns than are those who reside in cities.[25]

## CURRENT STATUS OF BURN CARE IN TURKEY

While progress in burn care in Turkey is promising, the number and quality of burn units must be increased considerably (Figure 3). The Black Sea and southeast regions are currently the most underserved areas.[26] In addition to the need for national and international certification programs, courses, and continuing medical education programs aimed at training doctors and nurses in specialized burn care, burn centers should continue to improve their in-service training programs for nurses. There is a need to update Turkish laws related to the prevention of home and industrial burn accidents and to implement a strong program of continuing public education in the prevention of, and initial treatment for, burns. Strategies for cooperation and collaboration among countries in Europe and the Middle East during disaster situations also must be formulated and discussed.

Utilizing communication tools such as radio and television can be useful since they reach large populations. Başkent University is currently broadcasting education programs about burns and treatment on Channel-B television, a cable channel owned and operated by the university.

In addition, our institution founded a first aid training institute which conducts public education programs in first aid, including first aid for burns. We believe it is vital for these efforts to be extended to every region of Turkey. Publication and distribution of first aid brochures by local medical and educational personnel in rural areas may also help promote widespread education.

The wide variation in epidemiologic features for burn victims in Turkey to date suggests nationwide studies are required to obtain more reliable data regarding pediatric burns in our country.

## CONCLUSIONS

The majority of "epidemiologic" papers describing burn injury are not population-based studies. Although they can be useful in identifying patterns of injury aimed at developing possible preventive strategies, they do not, however, help to provide evidence to support resource allocation or redistribution at a national level. Nor can they truly assist in addressing the global scope of burn injuries. It is interesting that Asia, Europe, and the Middle East have comparable incidence rates of hospitalized pediatric burn patients. The reality of burn care in India is a disproportionate number of burn patients to available beds, while in China, access is restricted because patients must pay for treatment and many cannot afford hospital-based care. Such considerations are less likely to occur in Europe, where another aspect of burn care is a tendency to admit patients with smaller burns for hospital treatment. Thus, the population groups of hospitalized pediatric burn patients vary around the world. What is evident is that despite underreporting and varying indications for hospital admission, the magnitude of the problem in Asia eclipses the rest of the world by virtue of the size of the population involved.

In conclusion, the features of burns among children and adolescents differ from region to region. Every country must have a nationwide public education system aimed at preventing burns and ensuring that young burn victims receive first aid and burn care specific to their needs.

## KEY POINT

- Burns, children, adolescents, Turkey

# FIGURES

## FIGURE 1
## Epidemiology of pediatric burns worldwide.

| Continents | Pop in 2004 (million) | No of burns / year | Incidence rate |
|---|---|---|---|
| Asia | 3607 | 288,560 | 0.0080 |
| America | 867 | 38,148 | 0.0044 |
| Europe | 731 | 61,404 | 0.0084 |
| Middle East | 259 | 20,720 | 0.0080 |
| Africa | 893 | 96,444 | 0.0108 |
| Australasia | 24 | - | - |
| **Total** | **6357** | **505,276** | **0.0079** |

*Source.* Adapted from Burd A, Yuen C. A global study of hospitalized pediatric burn patients. *Burns.* 2005;31(4):432-438.

## FIGURE 2
## Distribution of patients among the 4 age categories analyzed in this study.

Distribution of Age groups

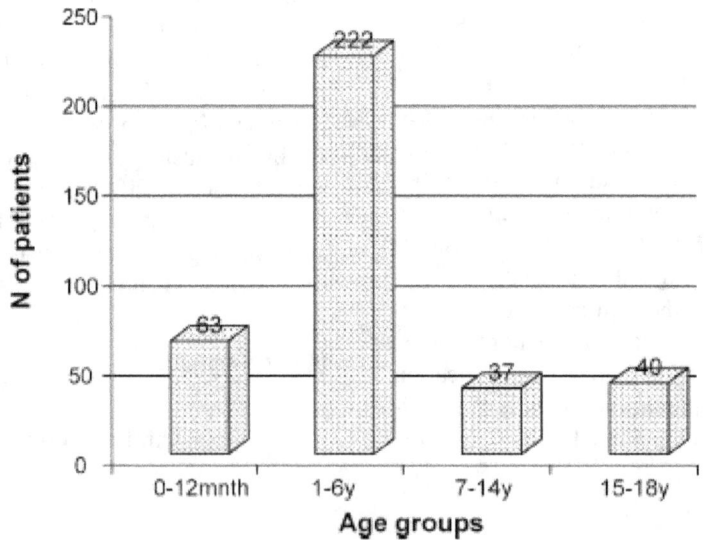

FIGURE 3
Distribution of burn centers (24 total) and hospitals with beds available (76 total) for burn patients among the 81 city/regions in Turkey. Every area outlined on the map represents a major city and its region. The numbers in the darkest fields indicate the number of burn centers in that city/region (ie, the Ankara region has 5 burn care centers).

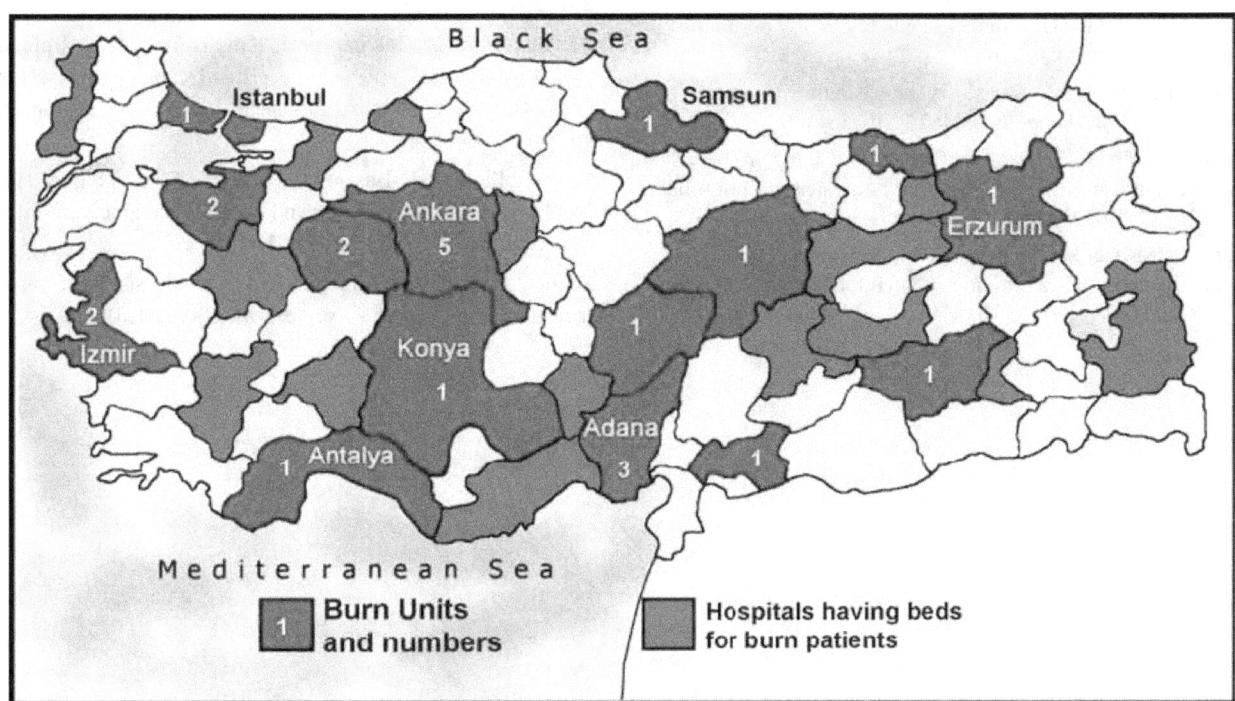

## REFERENCES

1. Brigham PA, McLoughlin E. Burn incidence and medical care use in the United States: estimates, trends, and data sources. *J Burn Care Rehabil.* 1996; **17**(2): 95–107.

2. Carvajal HF. Burns in children and adolescents: initial management as the first step in successful rehabilitation. *Pediatrician.* 1990; **17**(4): 237–243.

3. McLoughlin E, McGuire A. The causes, cost, and prevention of childhood burn injuries. *Am J Dis Child.* 1990; **144**(6): 677–683.

4. Burd A, Yuen C. A global study of hospitalized pediatric burn patients. *Burns.* 2005; **31**(4): 432–438.

5. Moritz A, Henriques F. Studies of thermal injury: II. The relative importance of time and surface temperature in the causation of cutaneous burns. *Am J Pathol.* 1947; **23**: 695–720.

6. Centers for Disease Control and Prevention, National Center for Injury Prevention and Control. Fire and burn injuries fact sheet. http://www.cdc.gov/ncipc/duip/burn.htm. Accessed November 29, 1999.

7. Marshall SW, Runyan CW, Bangdiwala SI, Linzer MA, Sacks JJ, Butts JD. Fatal residential fires: who dies and who survives? *JAMA.* 1998; **279**(20): 1633–1637.

8. McCauley RL, Stenberg BA, Rutan RL, Robson MC, Heggers JP, Herndon DN. Class C firework injuries in a pediatric population. *J Trauma.* 1991; **31**(3): 389–391.

9. Hight DW, Bakalar HR, Lloyd JR. Inflicted burns in children. Recognition and treatment. *JAMA.* 1979; **242**(6): 517–520.

10. Purdue GF, Hunt JL, Prescott PR. Child abuse by burning—an index of suspicion. *J Trauma.* 1988; **28**(2): 221–224.

11. Haberal M, Oner Z, Bayraktar U, Bilgin N. Epidemiology of adults' and childrens' burns in a Turkish burn center. *Burns Incl Therm Inj.* 1987; **13**(2): 136–140.

12. Nursal TZ, Yildirim S, Tarim A, Caliskan K, Ezer A, Noyan T. Burns in southern Turkey: electrical burns remain a major problem. *J Burn Care Rehabil.* 2003; **24**(5): 309–314.

13. Haberal M, Uçar N, Bilgin N. Epidemiological survey of burns treated in Ankara, Turkey and desirable burn-prevention strategies. *Burns.* 1995; **21**(8): 601–606.

14. Sheller JL, Thuesen B. Scalds in children caused by water from electrical kettles: effect of prevention through information. *Burns.* 1998; **24**(5): 420–424.

15. Dixon JJ, Burd DA, Roberts DG. Severe burns resulting from an exploding teat on a bottle of infant formula milk heated in a microwave oven. *Burns.* 1997; **23**(3): 268–269.

16. Möhrenschlager M, Weigl LB, Haug S, et al. Iatrogenic burns by warming bottles in the neonatal period: report of two cases and review of the literature. *J Burn Care Rehabil.* 2003; **24**(1): 52–55, discussion 49.

17. Schubert W, Ahrenholz DH, Solem LD. Burns from hot oil and grease: a public health hazard. *J Burn Care Rehabil.* 1990; **11**(6): 558–562.

18. Murphy JT, Purdue GF, Hunt JL. Pediatric grease burn injury. *Arch Surg.* 1995; **130**(5): 478–482.

19. Allen SR, Kagan RJ. Grease fryers: a significant danger to children. *J Burn Care Rehabil.* 2004; **25**(5): 456–460.

20. Tarim A, Nursal TZ, Basaran O, et al. Scalding in Turkish children: comparison of burns caused by hot water and hot milk. *Burns.* 2006; **32**(4): 473–476.

21. Türegün M, Celiköz B, Nişanci M, Selmanpakoğlu N. An extraordinary cause of scalding injury in childhood. *Burns.* 1997; **23**(2): 170–173.

22. Haberal M, Moray G, Kut A. The current status of burn centers and burn care in Turkey. In: Haberal M, Moray G, Kut A, eds. *Burn Care Facilities at Başkent University and Turkey.* Ankara, Turkey: Baskent University Publications; 2004: 1–7.

23. Kumar P, Chirayil PT, Chittoria R. Ten years' epidemiological study of pediatric burns in Manipal, India. *Burns.* 2000; **26**(3): 261–264.

24. Fukunishi K, Takahashi H, Kitagishi H, et al. Epidemiology of childhood burns in the critical care medical center of Kinki University Hospital in Osaka, Japan. *Burns.* 2000; **26**(5): 465–469.

25. Sakallioğlu AE, Başaran O, Tarim A, Türk E, Kut A, Haberal M. Burns in Turkish children and adolescents: nine years of experience. *Burns.* 2007; **33**(1): 46–51.

26. Kut A, Moray G, Haberal MA. Current status of burn care facilities: a nationwide survey. *Burns.* 2005; **31**(6): 679–686.

# CHAPTER THIRTY-FOUR

# PEDIATRIC BURNS IN WAR ENVIRONMENTS

DAVID J. BARILLO, MD, FACS, US ARMY INSTITUTE OF SURGICAL RESEARCH,
FT SAM HOUSTON, TEXAS

MOHAMMED BRISAM, MD, MBCHB, FICMS, AL-KINDY HOSPITAL BAGHDAD, IRAQ

The opinions or assertions contained herein are the private views of the authors and are not to be construed as official or as reflecting the views of the Department of the Army or Department of Defense. Brand names of commercial devices are provided for illustrative purposes and do not imply endorsement by the Department of the Army or Department of Defense. The authors have no financial interests in any commercial devices described.

## INTRODUCTION

When adults engage in armed conflict, children are often among the unintended victims. The mention of pediatric war injury conjures up mental images of badly burned children, injured as a result of aerial bombing, land mines, or mortar attacks. While the wartime delivery of pediatric burn care presents special challenges, in reality, most pediatric burn injuries have nothing to do with munitions or acts of war, but rather occur by common mechanisms resulting from the disruption of societal services or normal living arrangements. At the same time, the local medical system is frequently either significantly disrupted or overwhelmed, leaving few resources available to provide burn care. In such situations, military hospitals may find themselves tasked with the provision of burn care to the local populace. In this chapter, the recent experiences of civilian and military burn surgeons working in a war zone are reviewed.

## ETIOLOGY AND INCIDENCE

The key to an understanding of pediatric wartime burn injury is the appreciation of the extent that normal life becomes disrupted by war. Sectional fighting disrupts neighborhoods and causes families to leave and to move in with friends or relatives, resulting in severe overcrowding. The unavailability of electrical power leads to increased use of open flame sources for cooking, lighting, and heating. In Baghdad, Iraq, during the initial phases of Operation Iraqi Freedom, the deterioration of the economic status of the public along with disruption of distribution channels spawned a black market in gasoline for vehicles. Gasoline was bought, stored, and sold in whatever containers were available, and was frequently stored indoors within crowded living areas. In other conflicts, children have been pressed into service as laborers, where inexperience and lack of protective equipment expose them to the risk of occupational burn injury. Finally, in defiance of international norms, an estimated 300000 children are being inappropriately utilized as soldiers in over 30 countries.[1-5] Nevertheless, with this exception, it can be definitively stated that the majority of pediatric burns that occur during wartime are both unrelated to actual military operations and highly resistant to any type of burn prevention effort. These (mostly) domestic burn injuries are usually single, rarely associated with other serious injuries, and rarely result in mass casualties.[6]

Remarkably little information about war-related pediatric burn injury is in print. Coppola et al[7] reviewed civilian pediatric injuries treated at a US Air Force expeditionary hospital in Iraq between January 2004 and May 2005. Current US doctrine allows the use of deployed military medical facilities to treat civilians in instances of life-threatening, limb-threatening, or sight-threatening injury. There were 85 children treated with a mean age of 8 years, comprising 5.2% of all (military and civilian) patients and approximately 18% of all Iraqi civilians admitted during this time frame. Forty-eight children were treated for traumatic injury, including 25 fragmentation injuries, 11 gunshot or stab wounds, 3 blunt trauma cases, and 9 burn injuries.[7] Fragmentation injuries were most commonly caused by improvised explosive devices (IED). Two of the 5 reported deaths in the pediatric cohort resulted from burn injuries of 65% and 40% total body surface area (TBSA). Cancio et al[8] reported on 7920 patients seen at the 28th Combat Support Hospital over a 4-month period while deployed in Iraq in 2003. Of this group, there were 103 burn patients, including 86 requiring hospitalization (42 US or coalition forces and 44 Iraqi patients). Seven of the 44 Iraqi burn inpatients were children. The mean hospital length of stay was 2 days for US/coalition forces (range 1–4 days) and 10 days for Iraqi patients (range 1–53 days).[8] The length-of-stay disparity reflects the rapid evacuation of US and coalition forces out of country. A Czech Army field hospital deployed to Basra, Iraq, in 2003 treated a number of civilian burn patients of all ages.[9] Over a 3-month period, there were 442 outpatient burn dressings performed for first-degree and second-degree burns of 2% to 25% body surface area and 16 burn patients requiring admission, including 2 patients with burns > 75% TBSA. Age breakdown was not provided.

No study of war-related pediatric burn injury is complete without mention of land mine injuries. A related topic is unexploded ordnance (UXO). Land mines are small antipersonnel devices intentionally placed to cause injury or to deny access to a given area. UXO, on the other hand, comprises all types and sizes of munitions that pose a hazard because of partial or complete failure to detonate as intended. Both present a danger to civilian populations long after the conclusion of hostilities. Worldwide, land mines are present in at least 88 countries, including 23 countries in sub-Sahara Africa.[10] It is estimated that 35% of the land in Afghanistan and Cambodia remains unusable because of land mines remaining from prior conflicts.[10] Children are at particular risk for injury from land mines because of proximity to the ground and from UXO because of curiosity. In several large series, children comprised 25.6% of all land mine/UXO injuries or deaths in Chechnya[11]; 47.2% to 54% of land mine or UXO injuries in Afghanistan[12–14]; 20% of land mine injuries treated in Sri Lanka[15]; and 23.4% of

land mine or UXO injuries in Iran.[16] While these statistics are staggering, from the perspective of the burn care team it must be remembered that land mines and UXO usually cause fragmentation injuries and traumatic amputations rather than burns. An exception is injury caused by munitions containing white phosphorus[17] or situations where detonation of land mines or UXO causes ignition of adjacent flammable or combustible materials. As an example, during the Vietnam War, there were 143 US servicemembers evacuated to the United States and treated at the Institute of Surgical Research/US Army Burn Center for land mine–related burn injury. Of these, 135 patients were injured in a vehicle that struck a land mine. In most cases, burn injury occurred because mine detonation caused ignition of either the vehicle fuel tank or of other munitions carried within the vehicle.

## MANAGEMENT OF PEDIATRIC BURN PATIENTS IN DEPLOYED MEDICAL FACILITIES

Burn care is lengthy, resource intensive, and multidisciplinary, and the management of pediatric burn patients in deployed medical facilities is difficult. US Army combat support hospitals and US Air Force expeditionary hospitals are designed for the short-term resuscitative care of injured servicemembers, a group largely comprised of healthy, physically active young adults. Such facilities commonly do not stock pediatric-sized supplies, are not normally staffed with pediatricians or pediatric nurses, and cannot logistically support long-term care. US servicemembers do not remain in deployed hospitals for any length of time. Current doctrine emphasizes the long-range aeromedical transfer of the *stabilized*, rather than the *stable*,[18] and even the most massively injured normally arrive at military hospitals in the United States within a few days following injury. In the present conflict, US servicemembers burned in Iraq or Afghanistan arrive for definitive care at the US Army Institute of Surgical Research/US Army Burn Center (San Antonio, Texas) on an average of 3 to 4 days following injury. By comparison, during Operation Desert Storm, it took nearly 13 days to evacuate a burn patient back to San Antonio, and during the Vietnam conflict, burn patients arrived in San Antonio an average of 18 days after injury.

Deployed medical facilities are poorly equipped for definitive (long-term) burn management and even more poorly equipped or staffed for pediatric burn management. Cancio et al reported the difficulties encountered in a US Army combat support hospital tasked with civilian burn care early in Operation Iraqi Freedom.[8] After arrival in-country, emergency shipments of burn-specific medications, dressings, dermatomes, meshers, and other grafting supplies had to be arranged because these supplies were not stocked by the hospital.[8] Coppola et al noted a "short supply of the smallest endotracheal tubes sizes 3.5 to 5.0. Twenty-two and 24 gauge (vascular) catheters were quickly depleted."[7] Deployable hospitals are also poorly supplied with pediatricians. During operations Desert Shield, Desert Storm, and Provide Comfort, of 1460 deployed army, guard, and reserve physicians sent to southwest Asia, only 37 were (active duty) pediatricians and only 8 had completed pediatric subspecialty training.[19] There is a particular shortage of pediatric ICU nurses, pediatric intensivists, and pediatric anesthesiologists. Coppola reported that "the few individuals with this experience were often hard-pressed to cover prolonged periods when extremely ill children were present in the hospital."[7] Finally, it should be remembered that pediatric specialists are usually deployed to fill adult primary care or internal medicine positions and must cover their primary deployment responsibility in addition to the extra assigned task of civilian pediatric burn care.

Burned children presenting to deployed military facilities often travel long distances and are commonly accompanied by a relative other than a parent (who has other family responsibilities). In addition, the children frequently suffer from dehydration and malnutrition, which contribute to increased mortality.[7] Disruption of host-nation medical and transportation systems means that burned children will often arrive days or weeks after the acute burn injury, at a point where invasive burn wound sepsis is already evident, care is significantly complicated, and survival is unlikely. For the same reasons, long-term rehabilitation and follow-up is usually not possible. It is often necessary to keep burned children hospitalized until the point where they are well enough to travel long distances and to survive under the care of their families.[7]

For deployed burn team members, the provision of pediatric burn care in a forward medical facility requires flexibility, common sense, and an appreciation of imposed limitations. Probably the most important rule is to forget about how things are done back home, where patients arrive immediately after being burned, experienced personnel and burn supplies are readily accessible, physical and occupational therapy can be provided, and outpatient follow-up is easy to arrange. Instead, one must develop new burn care routines based upon available material, personnel, operating room time, and patient condition. For example, the technique of immediate excision and grafting would be inappropriate for a patient who presents a week or more after time of injury with no prior topical burn care treatment. In this case, invasive burn wound sepsis is likely, and the wounds will carry a significant bacterial burden.

Subeschar injection (clysis) of an antibiotic solution can be performed to decrease the bacterial load and lessen the expected postoperative hemodynamic instability. For invasive burn wound infection, clysis is performed immediately and 6 hours prior to surgery. If the patient is unstable and/or surgery must be delayed, this technique can be carried out twice a day for several days. One-half of the recommended daily dose of a semisynthetic penicillin (piperacillin or carbenicillin) is mixed in 1 L of normal saline and injected into the subeschar space using a spinal needle.[20-23]

Other modifications of practice include a change in surgical routine. When operating room availability is limited, it may be necessary to defer surgical excision and grafting to allow delineation of nonhealing full-thickness injury so that operative time can be minimized. Conversely, when bed space and nursing personnel are limited, it may be more practical to excise and graft as much as possible in 1 or 2 surgical procedures to get the wound rapidly closed.

Burn dressing changes present a particular problem. Local availability will dictate the topical agent of choice. Silver sulfadiazine and mafenide acetate cream are popular topical agents in the United States, but the far-forward stocking of such supplies in large quantity presents logistical difficulties in both shipment and storage. In austere circumstances, aqueous mafenide solution will also work well. In 1970, Mendelson developed a method of spraying 10% aqueous mafenide solution onto burn wounds while working in a civilian hospital in Saigon where burn creams, burn dressings, and sterile gloves where in short supply.[24] A 5% solution was utilized for facial burns. A bacteriostatic film formed over the burn wounds, which were treated without dressings to facilitate physical therapy, wound inspection, and conservation of scarce dressing supplies. A 5-pound drum of mafenide powder can be mixed with local water to provide sufficient 10% solution to cover 50% of the body surface area for 455 dressing changes. If mixed as a 5% solution, 910 dressing changes can be accomplished.[25] Aqueous 5% mafenide soaks are also an effective dressing for soft tissue blast wounds, complex open fractures, and large avulsion injuries; when these injuries are in proximity to thermal burns, aqueous 5% mafenide soaks provide ideal coverage.[26]

More recently, the use of silver-impregnated dressings for wartime burn care has become popular, with the advantage of being able to leave the dressing intact for several days to conserve nursing resources. The authors prefer the stretch-type of silver dressings, available in large sheets for the torso or in rolls for extremities (Silverlon® antibacterial silver burn wrap dressing, Argentum Medical LLC, Willowbrook, IL). The extremity rolls are applied similarly to Ace bandages and covered with loose gauze dressings which are then periodically moistened with water. In our experience, these dressings function best for short-term use and have become the dressing of choice for the long-range aeromedical transfer of burn patients, obviating the need for burn dressing changes in flight.

A final wound care consideration is that the intensive care unit of a deployed hospital will frequently be small, crowded, open bay, and located in a tent. This is not the ideal location for a lengthy burn dressing change. For this reason, we prefer to perform large burn dressing changes in the operating room under general anesthesia. When bedside dressing changes are attempted in the ICU, intravenous ketamine, sometimes augmented with small doses of intravenous fentanyl, provides safe and effective anesthesia for the duration of the procedure. The use of intravenous anesthesia is normally not possible on medical-surgical wards, and burn patients housed on the ward usually require a trip to the operating room for all but the most minimal dressing changes. An alternative is to take the patient to the ICU or postanesthesia recovery area for a planned dressing change under conscious sedation. This requires close coordination with both the anesthesiologist and the nursing staff. Finally, there are times when the initial wound debridement, escharotomy or even fasciotomy of a new burn patient must be performed in the emergency room because all of the operating rooms are busy with other trauma cases. Intravenous ketamine with or without IV fentanyl is an ideal anesthetic in this setting as well.

## WARTIME BURN CARE IN CIVILIAN FACILITIES

Civilian hospitals operating within the war zone share all of the limitations of deployed military medical facilities, and in addition, usually have greater difficulties in obtaining medical supplies and in providing hospital security. The hospital infrastructure may have been damaged during hostilities, and electrical, water, and sewer services frequently are unreliable or absent.

The civilian medical system in Iraq is a combination of public and private hospitals, with at least 1 public hospital in every municipality in and around Baghdad. Medical care is limited by the egress of physicians over the past several years. For example, it is estimated that half of the approximately 50 plastic surgeons previously in practice in Iraq have left the country. The Al Kindy Hospital is a public teaching hospital originally established in the 1970s as a facility of approximately 250 beds, and is known for the surgical specialties of otolaryngology, ophthalmology, and plastic surgery. Presently, Al Kindy has a very busy trauma practice and supports a wide zone of Baghdad with an overcrowded lower socioeconomic population. Mass

casualty incidents due to explosions and other accidents are common. The hospital is also the principal civilian burn hospital in Baghdad. In addition to shortages of medical and nursing staff, there are shortages of medical supplies and pharmaceuticals, particularly of antibiotics, antiseptics, and anesthesia equipment and drugs. The hospital buildings are in need of reconstruction. A continuous and reliable electrical supply is lacking.

The facility provides both pediatric and adult burn care. Since 2003, approximately 330 burned children have been managed at Al Kindy Hospital. The etiology of pediatric burn injury is presented in Table 1. The high incidence of flame and scald injuries reflects crowded living conditions and the use of alternative heating and cooking devices. Despite being located in a very active war zone, the number of pediatric burns directly attributable to war activities is low. A summary of war-related injuries is presented in Table 2.

## REHABILITATION AND RECONSTRUCTION

Rehabilitation and reconstruction of civilian pediatric burn patients in deployed medical facilities is challenging. Because the primary mission is emergency stabilization and rapid transfer, most deployed military medical facilities are neither equipped nor staffed for rehabilitation and reconstruction. As an example, during a recent deployment, 1 of the authors was assigned to a 400-person medical facility that included only 1 physical therapist. The physical therapist was wholly occupied in the outpatient orthopedic clinic, providing care to soldiers with sprains and knee injuries in order to rapidly return them to duty. The only available splinting material was a plaster cart in the operating room. Limited plastic surgery coverage was provided by the incidental assignment of 2 plastic surgeons who had previously completed general surgery training and thus were deployed as general surgeons. Despite these limitations, elective burn reconstruction can be accomplished if planned well enough in advance. As the active fighting slows down and hospital resources become more available, elective reconstructive surgery of burned children becomes both a strong "hearts and minds" mission and a morale boost for the surgical and nursing staff involved. In developing a reconstruction plan for a pediatric burn patient, it is important to remember that outpatient management is usually not feasible, rehabilitation services will not be available, and the patient will likely not be able to return for multiple surgical procedures over time due to the travel distances involved. Rather, multiple simultaneous procedures, such as Z-plasties of multiple body areas, should be performed at the same operative setting. Single-stage procedures are preferred over multistage procedures such as tissue expansion. The personnel and equipment necessary to perform free-tissue transfer will probably be unavailable. If possible, the burned child should remain hospitalized until wounds are closed, the flaps are healed, and the necessary procedures are completed. The family, if available, should become involved in dressing changes and should also be trained in stretching exercises with intent to prevent or minimize burn scar contractures after the patient has returned home.

## SUMMARY

The patient in photographs 5 through 9 summarizes the main points of this chapter. An 8-year-old boy received an electrical burn playing near a temporary electrical generator (burn resulting from disruption of delivery of utilities and services). He was treated at a local facility for several weeks while partial-thickness burns were allowed to heal nonoperatively (scarcity of surgical resources). He was referred for reconstruction of a nonhealing full-thickness chest wound that included exposed sternum. He travelled several hundred miles to the hospital accompanied by an uncle, as his parents were needed at home to care for the other children. He was electively admitted to a military medical facility at a point when casualty flow was slow. He underwent debridement, coverage of the exposed sternum with a pectoralis major pedicle muscle flap, and split-thickness skin grafting in a single procedure (conservation of surgical resources). He remained an inpatient on the surgical floor for several days (lack of outpatient surgery facility or outpatient housing), at which time he returned to the operating room for a dressing change under anesthesia (inability to perform conscious sedation on the ward). He remained in the hospital until the point where his wounds were completely healed and no further care was required. He subsequently made a several-hundred-mile journey back to his home and was unavailable for further follow-up.

## TABLES

### TABLE 1
### Mechanism of injury in pediatric burn patients treated at the Al Kindy Hospital.

| | |
|---|---|
| Flame injury | 65% |
| Hot liquids | 23% |
| War-related injuries | 10% |
| Electrical injuries | 2% |

### TABLE 2
### War-related injuries treated at Al Kindy Hospital.

| Case Number | Sex | Age (years) | Burn % | Mechanism of Burn | Fate |
|---|---|---|---|---|---|
| 1 | Male | 17 | 30% | Explosion | Survived |
| 2 | Male | 10 | 15% | Explosion | Survived |
| 3 | Male | 16 | 25% | Explosion | Survived |
| 4 | Male | 18 | 10% | Explosion | Survived |
| 5 | Female | 6 | 25% | Explosion | Survived |
| 6 | Male | 13 | 40% | Explosion | Died |
| 7 | Male | 16 | 25% | Explosion | Survived |
| 8 | Female | 10 | 30% | Bombarding | Survived |
| 9 | Female | 8 | 15% | Explosion | Survived |
| 10 | Male | 6 | 15% | Bombarding | Survived |

(continued on next page)

TABLE 2 (*continued*)

| Case Number | Sex | Age (years) | Burn % | Mechanism of Burn | Fate |
|---|---|---|---|---|---|
| 11 | Male | 8 | 60% | Explosion | Died |
| 12 | Male | 12 | 10% | Explosion | Survived |
| 13 | Male | 8 | 10% | Explosion | Survived |
| 14 | Male | 6 | 5% | Explosion | Survived |
| 15 | Male | 18 | 25% | Explosion | Survived |
| 16 | Male | 18 | 10% | Explosion | Survived |
| 17 | Male | 18 | 25% | Explosion | Survived |
| 18 | Male | 16 | 30% | Explosion | Survived |
| 19 | Male | 17 | 20% | Explosion | Survived |
| 20 | Female | 18 | 35% | Explosion | Survived |
| 21 | Male | 16 | 15% | Explosion | Survived |
| 22 | Male | 16 | 15% | Explosion | Survived |
| 23 | Male | 18 | 30% | Explosion | Survived |
| 24 | Male | 9 | 10% | Burning object from an airplane | Survived |
| 25 | Female | 10 | 3% | Bombarding | Survived |
| 26 | Male | 18 | 30% | Explosion | Survived |
| 27 | Male | 17 | 35% | Explosion | Survived |
| 28 | Male | 5 | 5% | Bombarding | Survived |
| 29 | Male | 18 | 20% | Explosion | Survived |
| 30 | Female | 15 | 10% | Explosion | Survived |
| 31 | Female | 16 | 10% | Bombarding | Survived |
| 32 | Male | 18 | 10% | Explosion | Survived |
| 33 | Female | 18 | 5% | Explosion | Survived |
| 34 | Female | 5 | 20% | Explosion | Survived |
| 35 | Male | 18 | 20% | Explosion | Survived |

## REFERENCES

1. Bosenberg AT. Pediatric anesthesia in developing countries. *Curr Opin Anaesthesiol*. 2007; **20**: 201–210.

2. Wexler ID, Branski D, Kerem E. War and children. *JAMA*. 2006; **296**: 579–581.

3. *Coalition to Stop the Use of Child Soldiers Global Report 2001*. London, England: Coalition to Stop the Use of Child Soldiers; 2001.

4. Albertyn R, Bickler SW, van As AB, et al. The effects of war on children in Africa. *Paediatr Surg Int*. 2003; **19**: 227–232.

5. Moss WJ, Ramakrishnan M, Storms D, et al. Child health in complex emergencies. *Bull World Health Organ*. 2006; **84**: 58–64.

6. Atiyeh BS, Gunn SWA, Hayek SN. Military and civilian burn injuries during armed conflicts. *Ann Burns Fire Disasters*. 2007; **10**: 203–215.

7. Coppola CP, Leininger BE, Rasmussen TE, Smith DL. Children treated at an expeditionary military hospital in Iraq. *Arch Pediatr Adolesc Med*. 2006; **160**: 972–976.

8. Cancio LC, Stout LR, Jezior JR, et al. Wartime burn care in Iraq: 28th Combat Support Hospital, 2003. *Mil Med*. 2007; **172**: 1148–1153.

9. Chmatal P, Bohonek M, Dobiasova M, Hasek R, Cernohous M. A humanitarian mission in southern Iraq: utilization of the 7th Field Hospital of the Army of the Czech Republic—a report on its medical activities and working conditions. *Mil Med*. 2005; **170**: 473–475.

10. Gosselin RA. War injuries, trauma and disaster relief. *Tech Orthop*. 2005; **20**: 97–108.

11. Bilukha OO, Tsitsaev Z, Ibragimov R, Anderson M, Brennanm M, Murtazaeva E. Epidemiology of injuries and deaths from landmines and unexploded ordnance in Chechnya, 1994 through 2005. *JAMA*. 2006; **296**: 516–518.

12. Bilukha OO, Brennan M. Injuries and deaths caused by unexploded ordnance in Afghanistan: review of surveillance data, 1997-2002. *BMJ*. 2005; **330**: 127–128.

13. Bilukha OO, Brennan M. Injuries and deaths from landmines and unexploded ordnance in Afghanistan, 2002-2006. *JAMA*. 2007; **298**: 526–528.

14. Centers for Disease Control and Prevention. Injuries associated with landmines and unexploded ordnance—Afghanistan 1997-2002. *MMWR*. 2003; **52**: 859–862.

15. Meade P, Mirocha J. Civilian landmine injuries in Sri Lanka. *J Trauma*. 2000; **48**: 735–739.

16. Zargar M, Khaji A, Soroush AR, et al. Injuries associated with landmines and unexploded ordnance in Iran. *Leading Abstracts of the Fourth European Congress on Emergency Medicine 2006*.

17. Barillo DJ, Cancio LC, Goodwin CW. Treatment of white phosphorus and other chemical burn injuries at one burn center over a 51 year period. *Burns*. 2004; **30**: 448–452.

18. Hurd WW, Jrtnigan JG, eds. *Aeromedical Evacuation, Management of Acute and Stabilized Patients*. New York, NY: Springer-Verlag: 2003.

19. Pierce JR. The role of the United States Army active component pediatricians in operations Desert Shield, Desert Storm and Provide Comfort. *Mil Med*. 1993; **158**: 105–108.

20. Barillo DJ, McManus AT. Infection in burn patients. In: Cohen J, Powderly WG, eds. *Infectious Diseases*. 2nd ed. Edinburgh, Scotland: Mosby Publishers; 2004.

21. Shirani KZ, Vaughn GM, Mason AD, Pruitt BA Jr. Update on current therapeutic approaches in burns. *Shock*. 1996; **5**: 4–16.

22. McManus WF, Mason AD, Pruitt BA Jr. Subeschar antibiotic infusion in the treatment of burn wound infection. *J Trauma*. 1980; **20**: 1021–1023.

23. McManus WF, Goodwin CW, Pruitt BA Jr. Subeschar treatment of burn wound infection. *Arch Surg*. 1983; **118**: 291–294.

24. Mendelson JA. The management of burns under conditions of limited resources using topical aqueous Sulfamylon (mafenide) hydrochloride spray. *J Burn Care Rehabil*. 1997; **18**: 238–244.

25. Mendelson JA. Topical mafenide hydrochloride aqueous spray in initial management of massive contaminated wounds with devitalized tissues. *Prehospital Disaster Med*. 2001; **16**: 172–174.

26. Barillo DJ. Using mafenide acetate in acute and chronic wounds. *Ostomy Wound Manage*. 2002; (suppl): 5–10.

# CHAPTER THIRTY-FIVE

# DISASTER MANAGEMENT: IMPLICATIONS FOR PEDIATRIC BURN PATIENTS

JOSE STERLING, MD, AND NICOLE GIBRAN, MD
UNIVERSITY OF WASHINGTON REGIONAL BURN CENTER

## INTRODUCTION

In spite of significant progress over the past 50 years, burn injuries continue to contribute significant morbidity, functional disability, and economic loss in the United States. Each year, greater than 500000 burn injuries require medical attention.[1] For pediatric populations, fire and burn injuries remain the fifth leading cause of child death[2]; children under 5 years old represent 12% of total burn cases (2007 National Burn Repository Report, http://www.ameriburn.org).[3] As a sharp contrast to the adult population, the majority of pediatric burn injuries are due to hot liquids.

With the wide adoption of transfer to burn centers, early excision and grafting, and improved critical care, survival for severely burned pediatric patients has improved over the past 30 years. Most burn centers incorporate a systematic multidisciplinary approach to provide comprehensive care. This comprehensive care includes coordinated surgical and critical care management, rehabilitation, and psychosocial intervention, all of which improve patient survival and aesthetic and functional outcomes.

The American Burn Association (ABA) has specific guidelines for transfer of a pediatric patient to a burn center (Table 1). Early burn center transfer has been associated with decreased complications, hospital length of stay, and rehabilitation days.[4] Exceptions to early transfer of burn patients to a burn center should be few (Table 2). The care of a pediatric burn patient requires the ability not only to achieve surgical excision and closure of the burn wound and critical care services, but also to provide patient and family psychosocial support and education, continuous long-term rehabilitation, mechanisms for reentry into society, and reconstructive surgical needs. Verified ABA and American College of Surgeons burn centers are often best suited to provide this care. These centers are required to care for at least 100 patients per year, guaranteeing that they have sufficient patients to justify a specialized multidisciplinary team. More importantly, verified centers must have stringent quality assurance programs to promote patient safety. Given the comprehensive standards of care provided by verified burn centers for burn patients, it makes sense that they would be best positioned to also care for burn patients in the event of a mass casualty disaster.

## Burn Mass Casualty Disaster Planning

In the aftermath of 9/11 and other national and international mass casualty burn disasters, the ABA has focused attention of optimal delivery of care during a burn disaster. Experience suggests that both manmade and natural disasters will likely result in large numbers of burn patients. The average burn size in a disaster will be 50% total body surface area (TBSA). Unlike trauma patients, who often require acute, high-intensity surgical and critical care for 24 hours to 7 days after an injury, burn patients are more likely to have longer hospital stays, averaging 1 day for every percent of TBSA burned. Hence, the resources required to care for burn patients can be enormous and could overwhelm a single burn center very quickly. Regardless, patients involved in a mass casualty burn disaster should receive gold standards of care whenever possible. In order to maintain these standards, the ABA drafted a national burn disaster plan that recommends that burn patients be triaged to a verified burn center within 24 hours of the disaster. Furthermore, if the closest regional burn center exceeds 150% of its normal capacity, the burn director should arrange secondary triage of patients to verified burn centers; if those resources become saturated, patients should be transferred to other, nonverified burn centers.[5] The report defines capacity to include not only bed vacancy but also staffing and ventilator, operating room, pharmaceutical, and blood availability. In this way, patients can be triaged away from the epicenter of the disaster and receive standard of care at a center that is not overwhelmed.

In spite of these recommendations, some events may prevent immediate transfer of survivors due to infrastructure damage, foul weather, or travel restrictions. For such events, staff at hospitals without a burn center and without pediatric specialization may benefit from a basic understanding of management of a critically injured child with a burn injury. In such situations, care during the first 24 to 72 hours should follow the defined guidelines detailed in the ABA-sponsored advanced burn life support course (http://www.ameriburn.org/ablsnow.php). As outlined in the ABA disaster management policy, every effort should be made to provide standard of care for patients with burn injuries.[5]

## Initial Assessment

It is important to remember that a burn patient, especially following a mass casualty disaster, is a trauma patient and requires the same primary and secondary trauma surveys.

Clearly, if the burn is an isolated injury with a known and documented history, a full trauma evaluation is not necessary. However, any question about the mechanism of injury justifies a workup as described by the Committee on Trauma, American College of Surgeons.[6] As with any type of trauma, first responders must control immediate life-threatening priorities: airway, breathing, circulation, disability, exposure, and fluid resuscitation.

Initial first aid for the burn patient must include stopping the burning process and removing clothing and jewelry to better assess the burn distribution and to anticipate swelling that occurs during the early response to injury and resuscitation.

During this process, an accurate assessment of burn size is essential for all subsequent management decisions. Several tools adequately estimate burn size. The rule of nines provides one easy assessment tool: each upper extremity equals 9% TBSA, each lower extremity is 18% TBSA, the anterior and posterior torso are each 18% TBSA, and the head is 9% TBSA. However, this method is best suited for patients older than 15 years due to surface area distribution in pediatric patients. Since children have larger heads than adults do, this formula may overestimate burns to the lower extremities and underestimate burns to the head. Alternatively, the patient hand size (including the fingers and palm) is 1% TBSA; estimating burn size by visualizing how many of the patient's hands would cover irregularly distributed burns (such as scald burns) can be convenient. The Lund-Browder diagram also accurately estimates burn size and has been modified for pediatric patients. Most burn centers use more sophisticated digital burn diagrams that calculate the burn size based on a drawing that is completed at the initial wound care.[7]

Cooling burns is not recommended; the burn patient must be kept warm and dry in clean blankets to prevent hypothermia, a major risk for pediatric burn patients that leads to complications in resuscitation, organ failure, and infection.[8–10] A chemical burn requires irrigation with copious tepid water, which should continue until the pH of the skin is neutral (as indicated by pH strips placed on the skin surface); depending on the exposure, this may involve 15 to 30 minutes of irrigation. With a hazardous material (hazmat) safety scenario, irrigation should occur at the scene prior to transport to a care facility. Emergency room treatment should include tetanus prophylaxis; every attempt should be made to determine the child's vaccination status since a child who is up to date should not need additional prophylaxis. Contrary to persistent erroneous beliefs among nonburn providers, systemic prophylactic antibiotics are contraindicated for burn patients because of the risk of multiresistant organism and fungus infections.

## AIRWAY MANAGEMENT

Not all patients with burns—even face burns—require intubation. Criteria for airway protection should include patient ability to protect the airway, presence of hoarseness or stridor, likelihood of massive upper airway swelling (as with large burns), and inhalation injury with thermal or chemical injury to the posterior pharynx or lower airway. A blood gas and a carboxyhemoglobin (carbon monoxide) level should be measured in any patient with a suspected inhalation injury. Patients with elevated carboxyhemoglobin levels should inhale 100% oxygen until the carbon monoxide level has normalized (< 5%); the half-life of carbon monoxide is approximately 40 minutes with 100% oxygen inspiration.

Several anatomical differences between pediatric and adult airways merit mention. The pediatric tongue is relatively larger and posterior. The epiglottis is short and the vocal cords are more cartilaginous, with a narrow opening. The airway is significantly smaller in diameter, with the narrowest point being the cricoid cartilage. Therefore, minimal airway edema can cause severe resistance, leading to airway obstruction. All of these factors complicate control of the pediatric airway and underscore the importance of choosing a proper size of endotracheal (ET) tube at the initial intubation; need for reintubation due to improper ET tube size can be life threatening in the presence of airway edema. There are multiple ways to estimate the proper size of the pediatric ET tube. Two quick observational approximations for ET tube size include the size of the child's nares or the diameter of the fifth digit. Also, several traditional age-based (AB) formulas determine ET tube size.[11]

$$ET \text{ tube size} = \frac{(Age + 16)}{4}$$

Perhaps the easiest and most reliable method during stressful situations is the body-length method, characterized by the Broselow pediatric resuscitation tape.[12] Based on body length, a wristband of a corresponding color is attached to the patient and used by all subsequent providers to guide catheter and instrument sizing.

## CIRCULATION

During the first 24 to 48 hours postinjury, the burn patient is in the resuscitative phase of the response to injury, when the injury triggers an overwhelming inflammatory response that causes the vasodilatation and capillary leak. Burn patients lose intravascular fluid proportionally to burn size and depth. If untreated, this capillary leak leads to hypovolemia, hypovolemic shock, and ultimately, multiorgan failure. Pediatric patients are susceptible to volume loss due to their small total blood volume. Delays in adequate fluid resuscitation are associated with increased mortality. Specific to the pediatric population, a delay in initiating fluid resuscitation of as short as 1 hour has been associated with poor outcomes and increased mortality.[13] Pediatric patients with burns larger than 15% TBSA require intravenous fluid resuscitation. Most pediatric burn patients with smaller burns (< 15% TBSA) can be adequately resuscitated by oral intake.

## FLUID RESUSCITATION

Whereas burn specialists debate potential benefits of one resuscitation formula over another, all resuscitation estimates provide starting points, and ongoing resuscitation should be continuously adjusted based on clinical responses. The most widely recommended formula is the Parkland or Baxter formula, which describes 3 to 4 mL lactated Ringer's solution/kg dry weight/% TBSA burn; half of this volume is administered over the first 8 hours and the other half over the next 16 hours. Children under 30 kg have inadequate glycogen stores to sustain the hormonal responses to injury and may develop severe hypoglycemia.[14,15] Therefore, in addition to the crystalloid resuscitation fluid, they also require weight-based maintenance intravenous fluid containing dextrose.

## ASSESSMENT OF RESUSCITATION ENDPOINTS

For children, successful resuscitation is observed by maintaining a mean arterial blood pressure over 60 mm Hg and a urine output of 1mL/kg/h. When the urine output decreases, the hourly volume of resuscitation fluid should be increased by 10% to 20%; if the mean arterial blood pressure drops below 60 mm Hg for a sustained time, a 10 to 20 mL/kg intravenous bolus and an accompanying increase in the hourly intravenous fluid rate should be administered.[16] In a similar fashion, if the urine output exceeds 1.5 kg/h, the hourly volume of resuscitation fluid should be decreased by 10% to 20%.

Patients may fail to maintain adequate clinical endpoints in spite of fluid resuscitation. Failure to resuscitate warrants reevaluation with a secondary survey. Reasons for failure to resuscitate include very deep burns, inhalation injury, associated trauma, delayed resuscitation, preinjury dehydration or intoxication, young age, or compartment syndrome (extremity, abdominal). No evidence supports the benefit of hypertonic saline for burn resuscitation at this time. Colloid may be indicated late in resuscitation (after 12 hours) when the capillary leak has closed.

## NUTRITION

Within the first 24 hours of thermal injury, enteral feeding should be initiated to decrease the incidence of ileus and subsequent stress ulcers.[17] Enteral nutrition decreases catabolic hormone secretion[18,19] and supports gut mucosal integrity, which may decrease enterogenic infection of the burn patient.[20] Whereas enteral burn resuscitation using the gastrointestinal tract is attractive, especially in times of disaster management when resources may be limited, this approach has never been definitively demonstrated to be feasible in patients with large burns over 20% TBSA.

## COMPARTMENT SYNDROMES

As resuscitation progresses, fluid extravasation leads to massive edema, swollen soft tissues, and compromised perfusion. In such situations, a circumferential extremity or torso burn may warrant an escharotomy to release an external band of restrictive eschar.[21] However, escharotomies are rarely indicated within the first few hours after a burn injury and should not be performed prophylactically. Elevation of limbs can often reduce swelling and prevent the need for these aesthetically distressing surgical interventions. Clinical indications for escharotomies include myoglobinuria, failure to resuscitate, and diminished distal pulses. An escharotomy incision should extend only through the eschar and should not violate underlying subcutaneous adipose tissue or the deep investing fascia. Escharotomies can be safely performed at the patient bedside with adequate analgesia and sedation. Fasciotomies are even less frequently indicated in patients with thermal injuries and usually only in patients with electrical injury leading to deep muscle damage. These procedures are better managed in the operating room to allow access to all compartments.

Burn patients can develop intra-abdominal hypertension leading to abdominal compartment syndrome due to massive resuscitation.[22] Decompressive laparotomy has been reported to be effective and may increase survival, especially in children.[23] Decompressive laparotomy can be performed at the bedside for patients who are too hemodynamically unstable to be transferred to the operating room. Like other decompressive procedures, this morbid intervention should not be performed prophylactically. Any patient requiring this level of care should be at a burn center.[24]

## PAIN CONTROL

Burn injuries cause tremendous pain and anxiety and should be treated accordingly. Pain and sedation assessments should be performed frequently. For critically injured patients, intravenous opioids can be used for pain management. Additional sedation with a benzodiazepine is crucial for the associated anxiety and should be included in all pain management plans. Because of the edema and impaired absorption, intramuscular, subcutaneous, or transdermal routes are not appropriate for patients with burn injuries.

## EARLY EXCISION AND GRAFTING

The most significant contribution to improved survival following a burn injury has been adoption of early excision of the burn with wound closure by grafting.[25,26] Given the decision tree for optimal wound coverage, including management of face and hand burns, children should be transferred to a verified burn center with experience caring for children before surgery is required. Since most burn specialists agree that excision of the burn wound should be started soon after resuscitation is complete, transfer to a burn center should occur within 72 hours of injury even in the face of a disaster.

## TRIAGE DECISIONS

Burn patient survival rates generally exceeded 96% in 2008; children especially enjoyed unprecedented survival rates. However, a mass casualty burn disaster involving large numbers of burn casualties in the United States will quickly exceed national capacity to care for patients. Resource utilization may necessitate triage decisions that are usually reserved for wars. Based on mortality and resource utilization in the National Burn Registry (http://www.ameriburn.org),[27] Saffle and colleagues created an algorithm to guide decisions about patient management in a mass casualty burn disaster.[28] The triage decision grid presents a benefit-to-resource ratio based on patient age and total burn size and suggests recommendations about levels of care for patients based on these factors. Patients with 20% burns who might be ordinarily admitted for daily wound care, education, pain management, and therapy could be managed as outpatients. Alternatively, patients at extremes of age and with very large burns may be treated with expectant care. End-of-life decisions are never easy, and inclusion of children who might survive under circumstances without constraints on the medical system increases emotional responses to such disaster plans. Whereas use of this evidence-based triage proposal would not be appropriate for most burn patients in 2008, disaster preparedness requires anticipating how to make hard and unpleasant decisions during a mass casualty.

## KEY POINTS

- The care of a pediatric burn patient requires the ability not only to achieve surgical excision and closure of the burn wound and critical care services, but also to provide psychosocial support and education, long-term rehabilitation, mechanisms for reentry into society, and reconstruction, all of which are provided by ABA-verified burn centers.

- Resources required to care for burn patients during a mass casualty burn disaster can be enormous and could overwhelm a single burn center very quickly.

- Patients involved in a mass casualty burn disaster should receive gold standards of care whenever possible and should be triaged to a verified burn center within 24 hours of the disaster.

- If the closest regional burn center to a disaster site exceeds 150% of its normal capacity, the burn director should arrange secondary triage of patients to verified burn centers; if those resources become saturated, patients should be transferred to other, nonverified burn centers.

- A mass casualty burn disaster involving large numbers of burn casualties may quickly exceed national capacity to care for burn patients. Resource utilization may necessitate triage decisions that require outpatient management of children who would otherwise be admitted to a hospital or expectant care for children with massive burns who would ordinarily be treated aggressively.

## TABLES

### TABLE 1
**American Burn Association transfer criteria (http://www.ameriburn.org/).**

| | |
|---|---|
| 1 | Second-degree burns (partial thickness) of greater than 10% of the body surface area |
| 2 | Third-degree burns (full thickness) in any age group |
| 3 | Inhalation injury |
| 4 | Burns involving the face, hands, feet, genitalia, major joints, or perineum |
| 5 | Electrical injury or burn (including lightning) |
| 6 | Burns associated with trauma or complicating medical conditions |
| 7 | Chemical burns |
| 8 | Burn injury in patients with preexisting medical disorders that could complicate management, prolong recovery, or affect mortality |
| 9 | Patients in hospitals without qualified personnel or equipment for the care of children |
| 10 | Burn injury in patients who will require special social, emotional, or rehabilitative intervention |

### TABLE 2
**Extenuating circumstances that may delay burn patient transfer to a regional burn center.**

| | |
|---|---|
| 1 | Natural or manmade disaster that overwhelms local and regional prehospital personnel |
| 2 | Severe weather that limits transport |
| 3 | Patient is remote such that multiple modes of transport must be coordinated |

# REFERENCES

1. Burn incidence and treatment in the US: 2007 fact sheet. 2007.

2. Report to the nation: trends in unintentional childhood injury mortality, 1987–2000. 2003.

3. *National Burn Repository—2007 Report.* American Burn Association, National Burn Repository, 2007.

4. Sheridan R. Early burn center transfer shortens the length of hospitalization and reduces complications in children with serious burn injuries. *J Burn Care Rehabil.* 1999; **20:** 347–350.

5. ABA Board of Trustees; Committee on Organization and Delivery of Burn Care. Disaster management and the ABA plan. *J Burn Care Rehabil.* 2005; **26**(2): 102–106.

6. American College of Surgeons. *Advance Trauma Life Support Program for Physicians.* 7th ed. Chicago: American College of Surgeons; 2004.

7. Neuwalder JM. A review of computer-aided body surface area determination: SAGE II and EPRI's 3D burn vision. *J Burn Care Rehabil.* 2002; **23**(1): 55–59.

8. Mozingo D. Acute resuscitation and transfer management of burned and electrically injured patients. *Trauma.* 1994; **11:** 94–113.

9. White C. Advances in surgical care: management of severe burn injury. *Crit Care Med.* 2008; **36**(7): S318–S324.

10. Ipaktchi K. Advances in burn critical care. *Crit Care Med.* 2006; **34**(9): S239–S244.

11. King B. Endotracheal tube selection in children: a comparison of four methods. *Ann Emerg Med.* 1993; **22**(3): 530–534.

12. Davis D. Pediatric endotracheal tube selection: a comparison of age-based and height-based criteria. *J Am Assoc Nurse Anesth.* 1998; **66**(3): 299–303.

13. Wolf SE. Mortality determinants in massive pediatric burns: an analysis of 103 children with >=80% TBSA burns (70% full-thickness). *Ann Surg.* 1997; **225**(5): 554–569.

14. Schulman CI. Pediatric fluid resuscitation after thermal injury. *J Craniofac Surg.* 2008; **19**(4): 910–912.

15. Parker MM. Pediatric considerations. *Crit Care Med.* 2004; **32:** 591–594.

16. Palmieri TL. Pediatric burn management. *Probl Gen Surg.* 2003; **20**(1): 27–36.

17. Hansbrough WB. Success of the immediate intragastric feeding of patients with burns. *J Burn Care Rehabil.* 1993; **14:** 512–516.

18. Mochizuki H. Mechanism of prevention of postburn hypermetabolism and catabolism by early enteral feeding. *Ann Surg.* 1984; **200:** 297–310.

19. Schulman CI. Nutritional and metabolic consequences in the pediatric burn patient. *J Craniofac Surg.* 2008; **19**(4): 891–894.

20. Peng Y. Effects of early enteral feeding on the prevention of enterogenic infection in severely burned patients. *Burns.* 2001; **27:** 145–149.

21. Harvey JS. Emergent burn care. *South Med J.* 1984; **77**(2): 204–214.

22. Oda J. Resuscitation fluid volume and abdominal compartment syndrome in patients with major burns. *Burns.* 2006; **32**(2): 151–154.

23. Tsoutsos D. Early escharotomy as a measure to reduce intraabdominal hypertension in full-thickness burns of the thoracic and abdominal area. *World J Surg.* 2003; **27**(12): 1323–1328.

24. Sheridan R. Early burn center transfer shortens the length of hospitalization and reduces complications in children with serious burn injuries. *J Burn Care Rehabil.* 1999; **20**(5): 347–350.

25. Pietsch J. Early excision of major burns in children: effect on morbidity and mortality. *J Pediatr Surg.* 1985; **20**(6): 754–757.

26. Engrav L. Early excision and grafting vs. nonoperative treatment of burns of indeterminant depth: a randomized prospective study. *Trauma.* 1983; **23:** 1001.

27. American Burn Association. NTRACS v5.0. 2008. Database available through ABA.

28. Saffle J. Defining the ratio of outcomes to resources for triage of burn patients in mass casualties. *J Burn Care Rehabil.* 2005; **26**(6): 478–482.

CHAPTER THIRTY-SIX

# BURNS RESEARCH AND THE FORGOTTEN TRAUMA OF CHILDHOOD

ANDREW J. A. HOLLAND, ASSOCIATE PROFESSOR OF PEDIATRIC SURGERY
DIRECTOR, THE CHILDREN'S HOSPITAL AT WESTMEAD BURNS RESEARCH INSTITUTE,
SYDNEY MEDICAL SCHOOL, THE UNIVERSITY OF SYDNEY, NEW SOUTH WALES, AUSTRALIA

## ABBREVIATIONS

| | |
|---|---|
| αSMA | α smooth muscle actin |
| BFAT | Burns first aid treatment |
| EMSB | Emergency management of severe burns |
| FDA | US Food and Drug Administration |
| HS | Hypertrophic scarring |
| LDF | Laser Doppler flowmetry |
| LDI | Laser Doppler imaging |
| NSW | New South Wales |
| PU | Perfusion unit |
| TBSA | Total body surface area |
| TGFβ1 | Transforming growth factor β1 |
| UK | United Kingdom |
| US | United States |

## INTRODUCTION

"Convictions are more dangerous enemies of truth than lies."—Nietzsche, *Human, All Too Human*, 1878–1886

Burns represent a unique form of that most complex of diseases, trauma. The most obvious effect of a burn injury remains a variable extent and level of skin necrosis.[1] The effects and treatment of burns have been recognized since antiquity: the Egyptian Papyrus Ebers dating from 1550 BC described the use of frogs boiled in oil as a burn remedy,[2] whereas Galen (AD 130–210) advocated vinegar and an open wound technique.[3] Richard Wiseman, a sergeant-surgeon to King Charles II, published an observational study of the healing of gunpowder burns in 1676 and was one of the first to establish the link between depth of burn and subsequent wound healing.[2]

As these early authors illustrate, understanding and managing burns requires that the injury be defined, an agreed classification system be established, and the extent of the problem be determined before treatments can be correctly evaluated and compared.[4] Such apparently simple steps have proven difficult, however, with consensus often difficult to achieve.[5] Whilst considerable advances have been made in the management of burn patients over the last century, many basic aspects of burn care, including analysis of epidemiological trends, lack scientific rigor or have been the subject of insufficient and sometimes conflicting data.[6]

How has this situation arisen? Why is it that in 2008 the American Burn Association practice guidelines on burn shock resuscitation commence with the statement that "[t]here are insufficient data to support a standard treatment at this time"?[7] The limited funding of trauma and burn research must represent a contributing factor: in 1998, Meyer estimated trauma received just 16% of the research funding allocated to cancer.[8] In Australia in 1997, research funding by the National Health and Medical Research Council for trauma, including burn injuries, was only 8% of that allocated to cardiovascular disease.[9] This, despite the fact that injury, in all its forms, had been identified as a national health priority since 1986.[9]

Burn clinicians, like their trauma colleagues, in addition to recognizing the special requirements of their pediatric patients, should appreciate the need for a blend of science and activism for research.[10] This does not necessarily require individual clinicians to conduct research themselves, although such involvement should always be encouraged under the guidance of an experienced mentor.[9] Rather, it requires that those involved in the care of these patients should approach new data with an open mind and accept that previously held convictions may need to be discarded and new models of care adopted.[11] With improved survival of burn patients now expected for even major burns, further advances to address the major morbidities of burn injury are likely to be more difficult to achieve and will require the participation of all those involved in the care of these patients.[12]

## EPIDEMIOLOGY AND ETIOLOGY

"Scalded at the table. Little children who can just reach the top of a table, often endeavor to drink from the spout of a tea-pot; and in consequence scald their mouths and throats; and die miserable deaths in a few hours."—*The Book of Accidents; Designed for Young Children.* New Haven, CT: S Babcock (Sidney's Press); 1830.[13] (Figure 1)

### Etiology

The most frequent burn injury seen in childhood is scald injury in a toddler. In addition to its frequency of well over 50% of all burn injuries in children, it illustrates many of the issues faced in addressing pediatric burns[14]: epidemiologically, in terms of the mechanism, age, gender, and location of the injury; prevention, particularly the demographic patterns of burn injury; anatomical and physiological differences, including the susceptibility and responses of children to burn injury, as well as the mixed-depth nature of the burn; and finally, the consequences of the burn, in terms of functional, cosmetic, and psychological issues for the life of a child.[15]

The scald-at-table scenario also highlights 2 other important issues: how we define and categorize burn injury and what constitutes the pediatric population.[16] A burn may be defined as a thermal injury caused by extremes of temperature or a physical or chemical agent producing a similar effect to heat. Typically, burns in childhood have been classified based on the mechanism of injury, such as scald, flame, contact, electrical, chemical, and sunburn.[17] Do these categories adequately reflect our patient population? How should a flash or spark burn be classified? Is a splash from hot oil a contact or scald burn? In the course manual for the emergency management of severe burns (EMSB), the classification of burns etiology implies that oil burns be classified as scalds for adults and contact for children.[17] The increasing use of home exercise equipment, particularly treadmills, has led to a dramatic rise in the number of friction burns in children.[18] Friction burns have also been seen as part of the injury complex found in those children run over in their own driveway.[19] Finally, perhaps in association with the increased survival of premature and low-birth-weight infants, our center has seen a corresponding rise in the frequency of burns from inappropriate use of hot packs and skin loss from malposition of an intravenous cannula containing hypertonic fluids.

The issue of classification remains vexed, with guidelines unclear even in standard texts.[12] Such confusion does not assist clinicians and researchers, and for this reason a categorization system with definitions has been proposed (Table 1). Further, such collected data should be reviewed by institutions and burn centers regularly, as traditional patterns of disease may change over time. In our unit, a rise in the frequency of contact burns between 2003 and 2007 was seen, which replaced flame as the second most frequent type of burn injury seen in childhood.[17,20] This changing pattern has also been seen in other centers and serves as a reminder of the need to constantly review patterns of disease to identify new risks and guide preventative initiatives.[21,22]

### Epidemiology

The literature remains unclear regarding the true frequency of burn injury and how this is reflected in numbers of patients treated in burn units.[23] Several North American studies have suggested a steady decline in the frequency of burn-related deaths and admissions. Brigham and McLoughlin, after allowing for the expected population increase, suggested that burns in adults and children had decreased by 50% in the United States between 1971 and 1991.[24] Spinks et al reviewed pediatric (defined as 19 years of age and under) burns in Canada between 1994 and 2003; they identified a nearly 5% reduction per annum in the frequency of burn deaths and admissions.[22] These data would suggest a positive impact from various burn prevention initiatives, coupled with increased treatment of patients in ambulatory care settings.[25]

Other data, however, have suggested a true increase in patient numbers and certainly in burn unit workload. In Adelaide, South Australia, adult burn unit admissions increased by approximately 20% per annum between 1996 and 2004, with an overall increase in patient numbers of 107%.[26] In part, this increase seemed to reflect significant changes in local referral patterns, with many patients previously treated by local medical centers and hospitals now routinely referred irrespective of burn injury severity. The incidence of pediatric burns, particularly from scalds, was found to increase in Iceland between 1982 and 1995 when compared to similar data from the 1950s and 1960s.[27] Another center in the United Kingdom suggested that patient numbers have remained relatively static between 1956 and 1991.[28] In Bangladesh, a developing country, the incidence of nonfatal burn injury in children (defined as under 18 years of age) was estimated from a household survey to be 288 per 100000 children-years, with a peak between 1 and 4 years of age.[29]

These apparently conflicting data highlight the importance of accurate definitions and data collection: admissions versus presentations, adults and children, children and adolescents, or only children under 16 years of age. Accuracy of these data would seem crucial in persuading politicians and health care managers of the need for appropriate funding and resources for those centers charged with the care of these patients, correctly classified or otherwise.

Age remains crucially important to all surgeons involved in the care of children as a result of its intimate link with likely pathology and outcome. Thus, in neonates and immobile infants, nonaccidental burns and non-burn-related skin loss remain a frequent reason for referral to a burn unit.[22,27] As infants become mobile, scald and contact burns become more common and predominate in toddlers and preschool-age children.[22,27,30] Although flame burns remain in third place, they become more common in older, school-age children.[22,27] Gender and trauma appear closely linked, with males consistently overrepresented in all forms of traumatic injury, including burns, from birth.[31]

Such data are of more than academic interest to the burn clinician. Whilst burns in general remain more common in children from families of low socioeconomic status, a careful history should always be sought to ensure this is consistent with the developmental status of the child and the clinical findings.[32] Poulos et al reviewed New South Wales (NSW) hospital injury admission data between 1999 and 2005 for children under 15 years of age and correlated this with socioeconomic status.[33] Children suffering from fire-related or burn-related injury were strongly associated with low socioeconomic status, with a relative risk of 1.37 to 2.00. Australia, as with many other Western countries, has a large migrant population. At least initially, this group typically is non-English speaking, of low socioeconomic status, and, like those from a remote and rural background, greatly overrepresented in trauma statistics.[34,35] Thus, the increased relative risk of burn injury seen in these children was similar to the increased risk of pedestrian and motor vehicle passenger injuries seen in the same group of patients.[33,36] This highlights the scope for greater cooperation and communication between trauma and burn services, based not only on similar patient populations, prevention, and management challenges, but also on the potential for the burn patient to suffer additional injuries or for the trauma patient to suffer burns.[16,23]

The definition of childhood, paradoxically, would seem more controversial than classification of burn injury, with upper limits for age ranging from 14 years to even 21 years.[37,38] The importance of such limits should not be underestimated by well-meaning clinicians, with considerable impact on resources and the likely outcomes of treatment depending on the exact population studied. A review by Klein et al determined that hospital costs alone associated with the care of a typical pediatric burn patient at a US burn center with a median total body surface area (TBSA) burn of 9.3% between 1994 to 2004 averaged $9026.[39] For those patients with a burn of greater than 20% TBSA, this average cost rose to $63806.

Yet these costs represent just the tip of the total burns pyre of expenditure. A review of 898 patients treated at a burn center in Valencia, Spain, between 1997 and 2001 identified an average total patient cost to the community of $95551. What is sobering to reflect is that a typical patient at this center was not a geriatric patient with a 70% flame burn, but a 10-year-old boy with a scald burn. In Australia, all but minor burns in children are typically treated by a multidisciplinary team led by a pediatric or plastic surgeon with a commitment to burn care. Such arrangements are not uniform between states, however, and will clearly vary significantly between countries. Whilst accepting that the location of patient treatment will likely be decided based largely on local resources and patterns of referral, clear definitions and corresponding funding arrangements need to be in place for optimal outcomes.

That these resources remain difficult to access in many parts of the world would perhaps not surprise many burn clinicians. What should perhaps worry these same clinicians is the failure of many non-activity-based health care models in more established countries to acknowledge, adapt to, and resource current models of burn care.[22,39,40] Multiple factors involved in funding implications not always recognized by health care coding systems include the importance of such units in leading burn prevention programs, the mounting reluctance of nonspecialists to direct management of children with burn injuries, burn centers' increased involvement in the care of patients from remote and rural areas, and adolescent patients and children with non-burn-related skin loss.[40] Coupled with the trend for increased subspecialization in all areas of patient care, the scene would seem to be set for a dramatic increase in referrals to burn units, placing an additional burden upon already overstretched staff.[41]

## FIRST AID

Burns first aid treatment (BFAT) is the initial treatment of a patient's burn wound. Despite the obvious importance of this topic, traditional recommendations have largely been based on anecdotal observations with limited supporting data.[42,43] This has been reflected in poor compliance with recommendations in both community and health care settings, with at best only half of all children receiving adequate BFAT within 3 hours of their burn injury despite its clear analgesic benefit.[44-46] A significant contributing factor has been lack of knowledge of the correct recommendations, with as few as 19% of health care workers able to correctly select appropriate BFAT when completing a questionnaire study with 4 common burn scenarios.[47]

Yet this topic has special relevance to the pediatric population since their generally thinner skin renders them more susceptible to deeper thermal injury than the majority of adults with injury in an equivalent location.[48] This same physical characteristic of skin, however, should also potentially enhance the effectiveness of BFAT. In addition, children's normal developmental immaturity compared to adults predisposes them to injury in general and its adverse consequences as a result of an inappropriate response to thermal trauma.[49,50] These characteristics, whilst well recognized, often appear poorly understood by parents and caregivers, leading to an overrepresentation of children with readily preventable burn injuries.[51]

Whilst it remains clear that the first step should always involve stopping the burning process, scientific observations to support the EMSB course recommendations to cool the burn with cold running water for 20 minutes have generally been lacking.[17] In part this has reflected the apparent ethical and experimental difficulties associated with developing and investigating an appropriate burn wound model.[52-54] In this context, ethics committees need to accept that they also have an important duty to the community to act as facilitators for clinically important research in light of rigid journal guidelines on scientific protocols and standards.[54]

## Epidemiological Evidence Supporting Efficacy of BFAT

Prior to the development of contemporary models to investigate the physical efficacy of BFAT and its influence on subsequent burn wound healing, epidemiological evidence of its positive impact has been slowly accumulating.

Nguyen et al reviewed the importance of BFAT in 695 children under 15 years of age with burns between 10% and 60% TBSA admitted to the National Burn Institute in Hanoi, Vietnam, between 1997 and 1999.[55] They identified an inverse relationship between early cooling and the subsequent requirement for skin grafting, with cooling reducing the need for skin grafting by 32%. Although a retrospective review with limited information concerning the definition of immediate cooling, these data nevertheless support the concept of BFAT.

Skinner et al prospectively reviewed the impact of a multimedia burns prevention and first aid educational campaign in Auckland, New Zealand, over two 4-month study intervals between 1997 and 2002.[56] In addition to demonstrating improved use of BFAT following the campaign, a statistically significant reduction in the requirement for admission (64% to 36%) and surgical procedures (26% to 11%), including skin grafting, was documented. Similar findings following a campaign targeting families with a non-English-speaking background (NESB) were made in Sydney, Australia, in 1999, with surgical procedures for this high-risk group falling from 88% prior to the campaign to 37% in the subsequent year.[34,57]

## Scientific Evidence Supporting Efficacy of BFAT

Empirical and epidemiological findings support the efficacy of BFAT in reducing the pain associated with burn wound injury and the requirement for subsequent surgical intervention. It is only recently, however, with the development of appropriate animal burn wound models analogous to the acute paediatric scald burn, that experimental evidence to support BFAT has been found.[52,53,58]

Jandera et al reported the outcome of burn wound cooling in a porcine partial-thickness scald burn wound model, with evaluation of the wounds by an independent clinician and pathologist at 7, 14, and 21 days postinjury.[58] The authors compared immediate application of packs soaked in cold water and changed every 3 minutes for 1 hour with *Melaleuca* hydrogel applied immediately or after 30 minutes for the same period. Statistically significant improvement in burn wound healing, which correlated with the fall in skin temperature with BFAT, was observed in both treatment groups.

Yuan et al modified this model to more closely reflect the situation seen in paediatric clinical practice.[53] A piglet model of an acute scald contact burn injury was used, with a control group receiving no first aid compared with 20 minutes of 3 treatment modalities applied immediately: cold running tap water, wet towels replaced every 3 minutes, and a cold water spray every 30 seconds. Analysis of intradermal skin temperature (Figure 2), clinical assessment of burn wound healing, and histological analysis of burn depth by independent clinicians provided compelling, statistically significant experimental evidence of the efficacy of cold running tap water over other treatment modalities whilst avoiding hypothermia.

Subsequent work with the same model has shown the optimal duration of cooling with cold running water does indeed appear to be 20 minutes.[59] Based on the experience of our center with typical durations of first aid in clinical practice, the EMSB-recommended duration of 20 minutes was compared with a control wound and cold running water for 5, 10, and 30 minutes.[44] In addition to confirming the effectiveness of cold running water in cooling the acute burn wound, this study revealed that it was only statistically significantly associated with improved burn wound healing with a duration of 20 minutes. Importantly, cold running water for shorter or longer durations was less effective, which suggests, at least in this model, a potential dose response curve.

More recent studies have suggested that delayed cooling with cold running water for up to 1 hour was as effective as immediate BFAT.[60] Clearly, further work is needed in this area to investigate longer durations of delayed cooling to confirm the EMSB recommendation of the efficacy of delayed cooling of up to 3 hours postburn. Further, the relative impact of delayed compared to prompt cooling in terms of burn wound healing, development of scarring, and the subsequent requirement for surgical intervention warrants further study. The development of a similar porcine model with evidence of subsequent hypertrophic scarring (HS) by Cuttle et al should facilitate this process.[52]

## Barriers to the Use of Optimal First Aid

Evidence from several audits of burns in children has consistently highlighted the frequency of scald injury and the inadequacy of optimal BFAT.[14,22,44] A component of this reflects lack of knowledge, both within the community and amongst health care professionals, which would be amenable to educational intervention.[47,57,61]

There remain other barriers, however, to effective BFAT. In the home environment, the most common location of burn wounds in children, the caregiver may panic, or, as a result of cultural beliefs or inexperience, utilize inappropriate treatment modalities.[62] Even when telephone advice is sought or medical assistance arrives in the form of ambulance or paramedical personnel, BFAT may be less than ideal.[63] Whilst confusion of what represents optimal BFAT may exacerbate this situation, a lack of consensus and standardization will undoubtedly represent significant contributing factors.[63]

Practical and safety issues are also relevant: clearly, cold running water cannot be utilized effectively and safely whilst the patient is being transported to a health care facility. Considerable interest has been expressed by ambulance services, primary health care providers, and the military in the use of commercial burn wound first aid products.[64] In Australia, these include Burnaid® and WaterJel®, both products consisting largely of sterile water with *Melaleuca* oil and emulsifiers impregnated into a foam dressing. Clear data on the efficacy of these products compared with cold running water appears lacking. Whilst Jandera et al demonstrated equivalence with the use of cold water packs, this was shown by Yuan et al to be much less effective than cold running water in a similar scald burn wound.[53,58] Further, Cuttle et al found Burnaid® to be ineffective when compared with cold running water, as were saliva and aloe vera.[65]

Finally, a real concern in children relates to the development of hypothermia from cooling an acute burn wound.[17,66] Whilst cooling is clearly of benefit, this needs to be conducted in a safe fashion to reduce the risk of hypothermia and the major adverse impact this may have on the child as well as the burn injury.[44]

Clearly, further studies, which should be encouraged and supported by the burn research community, ethics committees, and granting bodies, are required before any of these practical issues can be addressed.

## PREDICTION OF BURN WOUND OUTCOME

Assessment of burn depth has long been known to correlate with burn wound healing.[67-69] In general, the deeper the burn, the greater the risk of infection, the longer the healing time, and the worse the final cosmetic and functional outcome.[23,69,70] Thus, the ability to correctly diagnose burn depth or to predict burn wound healing has been considered important, as the diagnosis of those burns likely to heal within a defined time period facilitates patient management and planning of surgical intervention for those unlikely to heal.[68,71,72] Equally if not more important would be the development of an objective measurement of burn depth to facilitate comparison of burn wounds and allow fair and balanced review of different treatment approaches and novel interventions.[23,73,74]

## Classification of Burn Wound Depth

Whilst burns have been recognized since antiquity, Jean de Vigo in 1483 was one of the first to suggest the link between burn wound treatment and underlying severity of the burn.[2,75] Although Peter Lowe used the terms *superficial, average,* and *great* to categorize burns in 1597, it was Fabricius who classified burns into first, second, and third degree in 1610.[68,75] Whilst early clinicians suggested more complex systems of categorization of burn injury, including Dupuytren's 6 degrees, it is perhaps William Clowes (1540–1604) who first clearly articulated a recognizable, contemporary description of burn depth classification in 1943.[2,75]

Jackson made a major contribution when he published the results of his clinical and histopathological study of burns in 1953.[1] He described the relationship between burn wound appearance, burn depth progression, and cutaneous microvascular blood flow. Based on these observations, 3 zones of burn injury were defined: a peripheral zone of reactive hyperemia, a central zone of coagulative necrosis, and an intermediate zone of stasis (Figure 3). Whilst Forage's historical review of the classification of burns is clear, his statement that "without doubt, a fairly accurate estimate can be made of the relative depths of an exposed burn by observation of the varying superficial appearances over it" would be challenged by the majority of burn clinicians caring for children.[68,75] Jackson believed the zone of stasis would inevitably become necrotic and concluded that at the end of the first week after burn injury, "[a]lthough one knows that the tissue of the two inner zones will be cast off, it is not possible by surface inspection alone to tell whether those zones include the whole thickness of the skin or not."[1]

These conclusions should be evaluated in the context of the 1950s standard of burn care; subsequent experimental and clinical work has indicated that with optimal management, particularly in terms of fluid resuscitation and treatment of the burn wound, the zone of stasis may yet be salvaged.[17,76,77]

## Assessment of Burn Depth and Prediction of Burn Wound Outcome

Having determined the importance of burn depth in terms of prediction of burn wound outcome and its healing potential, the question arises as to how this is best assessed. Traditionally, partly through the influence of historical observational studies with later clinical work by Jackson and others, this has been made by serial clinical examination of the burn wound by an experienced burn clinician.[67,68,75] Whilst there have been numerous evaluations in both adults and children, clinician assessment alone has not proven reliable, with accuracy rates of 50% to 75% typically reported despite the enthusiasm of the clinician.[67,78,79]

Children represent a particularly problematic group to judge due to their thin skin rendering them more susceptible to thermal injury and due to the difficulties associated with examination of a potentially uncooperative, nonverbal patient. Preschool-age children with scald burns are the most difficult group in which to make an early diagnosis of burn depth, particularly given their heterogeneous nature.[80] Unfortunately, they also comprise the most prevalent population; teenagers with flame burns are much more easily assessed.[80,81]

The results of inaccurate case selection were well illustrated by Desai et al's study in 1991.[81] The authors randomized 24 children of similar age and % TBSA burn with indeterminate-depth scald injuries at presentation to either early or late excision. Those in the early group were grafted within 72 hours, whereas a nonoperative approach was adopted for the first 2 weeks postburn in the late group. They found that those patients in the late excision group had significantly ($P < .05$) smaller areas grafted, required fewer blood transfusions, and spent less time in the operating theater. As with all studies, there were limitations: length of stay was not compared statistically between the 2 groups, nor was long-term wound outcome assessed. Rather than validating the superiority of the delayed approach to surgery in this setting, arguably the most important message of this study was the importance of accurate diagnosis, a fact recognized by the authors.

Diagnostic tools to assist in determining the healing potential of burn wounds have been used for over 50 years, with early descriptions in the literature describing histological analysis, the use of fluorescein dyes, and radioactive isotopes.[1,82,83] Subsequently, new modalities such as thermography, ultrasound, and differential reflectance photometry have all been advocated. Unfortunately, despite a plethora of techniques, none have proven either practical or useful long-term for the pediatric patient population.[71,84–86]

## Laser Doppler Imaging

Laser Doppler imaging (LDI) was first reported in the biomedical engineering literature by Essex and Byrne in 1991 to assess skin blood flow.[87] The device was based on the

Doppler effect, named after the Austrian mathematician and physicist who first described the change in frequency when a sound source and observer are in relative motion away from or toward each other.[87] The same phenomenon occurs when a coherent, monochromatic laser light is used to illuminate a moving object: the light reflected by the object undergoes a frequency shift that correlates with the speed of movement.[88]

Initially, the technique, termed *laser Doppler flowmetry* (LDF), required a probe be placed in contact with the skin. It was first reported in the assessment of burn wounds by Alsbjorn et al, based on the principle that superficial burns would be expected to show dramatically increased blood flow, whereas a deep burn would show low or comparatively normal blood flow.[1,68,89] This technique had several disadvantages, especially in relation to the pediatric patient. First, the probe required warming prior to application to the skin surface. Secondly, the pressure used to apply the probe was operator dependent, which might affect skin blood flow. Thirdly, and perhaps most importantly, only skin in direct contact with the probe could be assessed, with the technique subject therefore to both selection bias and an increased risk of wound infection.[71,85,90]

In contrast, the development of LDI offered the ability to assess the whole burn without requiring direct patient contact. The initial device (Figure 4) consisted of a Class IIIa visible-red helium neon laser operating at a wavelength of 632.8 nm with a power of 2 mW (moorLDI, Moor Instruments Ltd, Axminster, Devon, UK). The laser beam was directed onto the skin surface with reflected laser light collected by a mirror and directed to photodiodes. Subsequent analysis by a Doppler signal processor produced a detailed color perfusion map in relative perfusion units (PUs) of skin blood flow in the area scanned (Figure 5). Mounted on a mobile stand with a panel PC, the device could be brought to the patient with relative ease.

The first report of the clinical application of LDI for the assessment of burn depth was by Niazi et al in 1993.[84] Data were presented on 13 adult patients who presented within 24 hours with burns of less than 12% TBSA. Patients were scanned in a room at 25°C using the LDI at 24, 48, and 72 hours at a fixed distance of 1.6 m from the scanner. Punch wound biopsies for histological analysis were taken at 72 hours "based on clinical assessment or scan trend."[84] The perfusion scan was then compared with burn wound healing at 21 days, with LDI not allowed to influence clinical management. This study documented absolute correlation between LDI scanning and histological diagnosis of burn wound depth. Optimal accuracy appeared to occur between 48 and 72 hours postburn. Overall, LDI correlated with clinical assessment of burn wound depth in 10 patients and correctly diagnosed 2 patients with superficial burns

that were clinically evaluated as deep and 1 patient with a deep burn that was initially considered superficial. This early report has now been followed by subsequent studies with similar findings from several centers.[91–94]

The first evaluation of this technique in the pediatric population occurred in 2002.[71] Fifty-seven patients between 5 months and 15 years of age were scanned between 36 and 72 hours postburn, with the operator blinded to the treating clinician's assessment and the treating clinician blinded to the results of the LDI scan. Patients were scanned immediately following their dressing change and burn wound debridement, with the majority of scans performed on a high-resolution setting and requiring between 3 and 7 minutes to perform. Comparison of the sensitivity of LDI in this study was 90%, compared to 60% for an experienced burn surgeon, with the sensitivity scores 96% and 71%, respectively.

Subsequent reports in the literature have confirmed the accuracy of LDI in predicting burn wound outcome in both adult and pediatric patients.[85,92,93,95–97] A study by La Hei et al has demonstrated consistent accuracy in the pediatric age group, even when the reporter was not the operator of the LDI and did not examine either the patient or the burn wound.[98] This investigation used a refined version of the Moor LDI2, featuring a 2.5 mW Class IIIR near-infrared helium neon laser operating at a frequency of 780 nm, together with low-resolution color images produced with an integrated CCD camera. This version of the LDI, based on the near-infrared spectrum, also raised the possibility that imaging could be performed through wound dressings that were opaque to visible light. This would potentially reduce the number of dressing changes, with significant benefits in reducing patient discomfort and economic advantages through reduced nursing time. A recent study with the Moor LDI2-BI on a standardized cutaneous injury model has confirmed the potential applicability of LDI in this setting, but further studies will be required to confirm its validity in clinical practice.[99]

Despite such encouraging results, LDI is not without its disadvantages. It may be inaccurate in the presence of tattoos, silver-based dressings such as Acticoat®, wound infections, and excessive movement.[71,92,98,100] Whilst tattoos remain an infrequent confounding factor in the pediatric population, excessive movement represents a challenge. The use of various forms of distraction therapy has been shown to be of considerable benefit in this setting.[71,98,101] Further development of the device, including the use of a multichannel laser, should greatly reduce scanning times from several minutes to under 1 minute. Safety concerns in relation to use of a laser appear unfounded, with no issues reported despite many years in clinical practice.[71,85] There remains room for further research to validate the accuracy of LDI performed within the first 24 hours of burn injury, particularly with the advent of newer dressings allowing earlier discharge and the increasing use of ambulatory care.[102]

LDI has been approved by the US Food and Drug Administration (FDA) for use in burn wound assessment, the only device with such approval.[85] Despite a body of evidence and FDA approval, there remains considerable skepticism of this investigative modality amongst burn clinicians, with continual searching for alternative modalities.[72,85,103] Clinicians should understand that LDI is utilized in conjunction with clinical examination and judgment and does not represent loss of direct involvement in patients' care.[71,98] Given the significant costs associated with purchase and maintenance, perhaps further evidence of the economic benefits of LDI regarding earlier treatment decisions and facilitation of increased use of ambulatory care in burn patients is required.[92,99,104,105] Burn clinicians should consider the significant advantages of an objective measure of burn wound depth and healing potential, not only in clinical practice, but also as a research tool for facilitating accurate comparative trials.[23,85]

## BURN WOUND SCARRING

One of the major challenges facing burn clinicians who treat children is scarring (Figure 6).[70] Despite considerable advances in other areas of burn care, with significant reductions in length of stay, cost, and mortality, HS remains a major cause of morbidity.[23,25,39,106,107] The problem is compounded in children due to their higher incidence of HS complicating burn injury compared with adults.[69,70,81,108] Further, as a result of continuing growth and development, scarring and contracture may evolve with the patient and remain a lifelong issue.[109,110] Careful review of the present literature and several recent developments have provided insight into how improvements might be made in this area.

### Early Surgical Intervention and Hypertrophic Scarring

In 1947, Cope et al were one of the first groups of surgeons to report the benefits of early excision in 38 adult and pediatric patients with 52 full-thickness burns.[111] Although no control group was described, time to healing and discharge dramatically improved, with a 95% graft take and a "minimum of scarring, keloids, contractures, and disability."[111]

Subsequently, there have been several clinical audit studies focusing on the benefits of early debridement of both adult and pediatric burns in terms of optimal wound outcome and a reduction in HS.[4,112,113] Deitch et al sought to determine the risk factors associated with HS by studying

59 children and 41 adults admitted to the Shreveport Burn Unit in Louisiana between 1980 and 1981.[69] They prospectively assessed the outcome of 245 burn wounds clinically thought to be superficial or moderate partial-thickness depth. The influence of anatomic site, racial origin, age, and depth on the subsequent development of HS were compared. Patients were followed for a minimum of 9 months, with HS defined as an elevated area at least 2 cm in diameter independent of the use of pressure therapy. The highest risk of HS in children was 70% in those with burn wounds that healed within 21 to 30 days. This risk, however, increased from just 6% of those healing within 10 days, through 14% for those healing within 10 to 14 days, to 42% of those healing within 14 to 21 days.

Engrav et al conducted a prospective, randomized controlled trial of early excision and wound closure versus nonoperative treatment of indeterminate depth burns of less than 20% TBSA in both children and adults.[114] Between 1979 and 1980, 47 patients were treated at the Washington Burn Center in Seattle. A comparison of age, extent of burn, cost, length of treatment, cosmetic outcome, and functional outcome was made. Age and extent of burn were not significantly different between the 2 groups. Early excision was associated with significantly shorter length of inpatient care ($P < .01$), reduced medical costs ($P < .05$), and more rapid return to work or school ($P < .05$). Long-term review, however, showed no statistically significant difference between the 2 groups, although those treated by early excision required fewer late grafts for closure and had a lower incidence of hypertrophic scarring (14% vs 28%).

Unfortunately, these studies have typically included mixed populations of patients with both adults and children, and perhaps even more importantly, have either focused on those patients with major, deep burns or relied on clinical assessment of burn depth only. A 2006 meta-analysis concluded that the only clear evidence regarding early excision of burns was a significant reduction in mortality and increased use of blood products, with "no conclusive evidence…in terms of duration of sepsis, wound healing time and skin graft take."[73]

The reality of those responsible for the treatment of children with acute burn injuries is that the majority will be relatively minor, mixed, or intermediate-depth scald burns that may well heal within 14 to 21 days. The optimal treatment in terms of subsequent HS remains less clear for this important group, with some recent data suggesting early surgical intervention might even increase the risk of subsequent HS. Cubison et al sought to establish the link between healing time and HS in a nonrandomized study of 337 children with scald burns treated between 1997 and 2003 at East Grinstead and Newcastle, United Kingdom.[115] This retrospective review was conducted over different time periods at the 2 centers. A third subgroup of patients with hot tea scalds from East Grinstead previously examined was also included but analyzed separately because of tea's reported anti-inflammatory properties. Standard practice for intermediate depth burns, as assessed clinically, was to excise and graft at the Newcastle center but to treat nonoperatively at East Grinstead. Healing time and HS were determined by the recording of these facts in the patient's notes or assumed by the use of silicone gel, steroid injections, and pressure garments. Of the 106 children treated surgically, HS was highest in those requiring more than 30 days to heal, at 88%, then fell to 59% and 19% in those healing between 22 to 30 days and 15 to 21 days, respectively. Surprisingly, those healing between 10 to 14 days developed HS in 33% of cases, more than those grafted between 15 and 21 days.

Whilst this study has a number of methodological limitations, it would seem to suggest caution in recommending a single optimal approach to the child with an indeterminate-depth scald burn that has not healed within 14 days, but might heal within 21 days. Whether early or late surgical intervention in this group is subsequently found to be optimal, what is clear remains the need for accurate and objective prediction of burn wound outcome, which is perhaps the real message of this and similar studies.[1,23,67,81,93]

## How Can We Reduce Scarring?

With the advent of early, tangential excision using a variety of sharp dissection techniques, the focus has been on debridement of all necrotic material until tissue viability can be assured.[4,73,116] This forms an adequate basis for subsequent surgical wound closure, typically with meshed split-thickness autograft.[116,117]

This concept, as well as questions in relation to the optimal timing of surgical intervention, has been challenged by several recent developments in the burn care literature.[115] The first relates to the use of Acticoat® as a primary burn wound dressing and its impact on burn wound healing, including the need for subsequent grafting. The second has been the introduction of the Versajet® hydrosurgery system, facilitating preservation of a greater proportion of the dermis. Thirdly, a novel subpopulation of circulating leucocytes, whose appearance may be associated with HS, has now been identified in acute burn wounds.

## Scarring and Dressings

Acticoat® was developed by Burrell in the 1990s and consists of an absorbent rayon/polyester core which is bonded on either side with a layer of high-density polyethylene impregnated with silver in a nanocrystalline form

(Figure 7).[118] When exposed to moisture, silver clusters and ions are released over several days with antibacterial, antifungal, and anti-inflammatory effects.[119] Since its introduction, Acticoat® has been shown to be effective in reducing the rate of burn wound infection.[120] Of perhaps equal importance has been a consequent reduction in the need for daily dressing changes, associated pain, and nursing costs, as Acticoat® retains its antibacterial properties for up to 3 days.[120,121] This benefit has been further extended with the introduction of Acticoat7®, with its 3 layers of nanocrystalline silver enabling its antimicrobial activity to be extended for up to 7 days.

Cuttle et al conducted a nonrandomized, retrospective cohort study in children of Acticoat® compared with their historical control dressing, Silvazine® (silver sulphadiazine with 0.2% chlorhexidine digluconate).[102] Between January 2000 and July 2003, 328 patients were treated with Silvazine®, followed by 241 patients treated with Acticoat®. The authors found that 26% of those treated with Silvazine® required grafting compared with 15% in the Acticoat® group ($P = .001$). Once those patients that required grafting were excluded, there was also a significant reduction in overall wound healing time in the Acticoat® group, with a trend for reduced incidence of subsequent HS. Although this study was limited by its use of historical controls and a comparative dressing that many clinicians would consider of historical interest only, these findings have been supported by similar studies.[122,123]

Additional studies have confirmed the anti-inflammatory properties of Acticoat®, suggesting a possible mechanism for its apparent association with reduced healing times and requirement for subsequent grafting.[123,124] In the absence of randomized controlled trials, however, these data need to be viewed with caution, with a clear need for further studies, as suggested by Fong and Wood.[123]

## Scarring and Debridement

The Versajet® hydrosurgery system consists of a disposable handpiece with an 8-mm or 14-mm window or blade, which is connected to a foot-activated power console with variable settings that supplies saline under high pressure. This fluid, together with any debris, is then evacuated as a result of the Venturi effect created by the high-pressure jet into a sealed waste container (Figure 8). Its first reported use in burn debridement was by Klein et al from Seattle, Washington, in 2005.[125] They commented on the value of the device for small, difficult-to-access areas such as the web spaces between digits. Subsequently, the device has been applied for larger burns in both adults and children in other centers.[126,127] Cubison et al utilized the device in children and suggested that the more accurate debridement allowed by the Versajet® might reduce subsequent HS as a result of an increase in the ability of the surgeon to preserve viable dermis.[126] Although not documented in their study, others have also made this observation.[127,128]

In addition to allowing preservation of viable dermis, it is interesting to speculate that an additional benefit of the Versajet® system in burn wound debridement may perhaps be related to its unique mechanical action promoting survival of the zone of stasis and reduced blood loss. Once again, further evaluation of this technique in both adults and children is required to better define its clinical role and potential benefits in practice in relation to its initial purchase and maintenance costs.

## Role of the Fibrocyte

Fibrocytes represent a specific subpopulation of leucocytes first described by Bucala et al in 1994.[129] These cells account for less than 0.5% of all circulating leucocytes and are thought to be derived from bone marrow.[130] They appear to have an active role in inflammation and wound healing in addition to producing connective tissue proteins such as collagen I and α-smooth muscle actin (αSMA).[131,132] This raises the possibility that fibrocytes may be involved in both acute burn wound healing and the development of subsequent HS.[133] Fibrocytes have been identified in postburn HS in adults and adolescents, with their number and differentiation toward a fibroblast-type appearance positively correlated with the serum level of the regulatory cytokine transforming growth factor β1 (TGFβ1).[134] Interestingly, TGFβ1 has been shown to be elevated in adult patients with burn injury, with peak values typically found between 15 and 21 days.[135,136]

Fibrocytes remain difficult to identify, however, and although expressing specific cell surface markers, some may only be expressed at specific points in the life cycle of a cell.[134,137,138] Despite these challenges, fibrocytes have now been identified in pediatric burn wounds.[139] A total of 53 burn wounds were examined in 33 children between 7 months and 15 years of age presenting to the pediatric burns unit in NSW, Australia. Fibrocytes were identified in 18 patients (55%) (Figure 9). Perhaps of more interest, however, was the finding that in those children that subsequently developed HS, fibrocytes were present in 88%.

These studies suggest a role for fibrocytes in pediatric burn wound healing and subsequent HS. Perhaps modulation of their activity might alter the wound healing process, either through changes in the level of TGFβ1 or as part of a generalized direct anti-inflammatory process. It has been speculated that the antiproliferative action of fetuin, a glycoprotein present in fetal serum, on TGFβ1 in cell culture may represent a possible treatment.[139,140] It is also possible that 1 component of the anti-inflammatory effect of nano-crystalline silver might be a direct effect on the proliferation or development of fibrocytes. To further determine the role of fibrocytes and assess the impact of potential treatments in burn would healing will require their identification in an appropriate animal model.[133]

## CONCLUSION

"It was the best of times, it was the worst of times."
—Charles Dickens, *A Tale of Two Cities* (1859)

The great advances in pediatric burn care made over the last 50 years have brought new challenges. Patients that would not previously have survived now represent considerable reconstructive and rehabilitation challenges to the burn care team. Issues of funding and increased patient numbers with limited resources persist, as does the challenge of reinventing effective burn prevention strategies. Many basic questions in burn treatment remain unanswered and require further research, such as the optimal time for surgical intervention of the intermediate-depth burn. There appears considerable scope for collaborative research between centers to facilitate these studies. Existing developments in our understanding of the biology of burn wound healing may offer greatly enhanced scar management in the future.

## KEY POINTS

- Contact burns are more common than flame burns.
- Friction burns from treadmill injuries are increasingly common.
- Apparent increased frequency of burns may reflect a greater number of transfers from remote and rural, adult-orientated, and nonspecialized centers.
- Optimal BFAT consists of cold running water for 20 minutes, while avoiding hypothermia.
- If not able to be used immediately, optimal BFAT is still effective if utilized at least up to 1 hour postburn.
- The efficacy of commercial burn first aid products is unproven.
- LDI has high sensitivity and specificity in predicting the healing potential of burn wounds in children.
- LDI represents the only technology approved by the FDA for assessment of burn wounds.
- LDI facilitates objective assessment of burn wounds for comparative research and clinical trial purposes.

# REFERENCES

**1.** Jackson DM. The diagnosis of the depth of burning. *Br J Surg.* 1953; **40:** 588–596.

**2.** Haeger K. *The Illustrated History of Surgery.* London, England: Harold Starke; 1988.

**3.** Thomas S, Barrow RE, Herndon DN. History of the treatment of burns. In: Herndon D, ed. *Total Burn Care.* London, England: Saunders; **2002:** 1–10.

**4.** Herndon DN, Barrow RE, Rutan RL, et al. A comparison of conservative versus early excision. *Ann Surg.* 1989; **209:** 547–553.

**5.** Greenhalgh DG, Saffle JR, Holmes JH, et al. American Burn Association consensus conference to define sepsis and infection in burns. *J Burn Care Res.* 2007; **28:** 776–790.

**6.** Mann R, Heimbach D. Prognosis and treatment of burns. *West J Med.* 1996; **165:** 215–220.

**7.** Pham TN, Cancio LC, Gibran NS. American Burn Association practice guidelines burn shock resuscitation. *J Burn Care Res.* 2008; **29:** 257–266.

**8.** Meyer AA. Death and disability from injury: a global challenge. *J Trauma: Inj, Infect Crit Care.* 1998; **44:** 1–12.

**9.** Strategic Research Development Committee of the National Health and Medical Research Council. Injury: from problem to solution. Canberra, Australia: NHMRC; 1999.

**10.** Roberts I, Diguiseppi C. Injury prevention. *Arch Dis Child.* 1999; **81:** 200–201.

**11.** Montgomery BJ. Consensus for treatment of 'the sickest patients you'll ever see.' *JAMA.* 1979; **241:** 345–346.

**12.** Pruitt BA Jr, Goodwin CW, Mason AD Jr. Epidemiological, demographic, and outcome characteristics of burn injury. In: Herndon D, ed. *Total Burn Care.* London, England: Saunders; **2002:** 16–30.

**13.** Cone TE Jr. Burns. *Pediatrics.* 1970; **46:** 636.

**14.** Dewar DJ, Magson CL, Fraser JF, et al. Hot beverage scalds in Australian children. *J Burn Care Rehabil.* 2004; **25:** 224–227.

**15.** Griffiths HR, Thornton KL, Clements CM, Burge TS, Kay AR, Young AER. The cost of a hot drink scald. *Burns.* 2006; **32:** 372–374.

**16.** O'Neill JA. Advances in the management of pediatric trauma. *Am J Surg.* 2000; **180:** 365–369.

**17.** Australian and New Zealand Burn Association: Education Committee. *Emergency Manual of Severe Burns Course Manual.* Australian and New Zealand Burn Association Limited; 2006.

**18.** Wong A, Maze D, La Hei E, et al. Pediatric treadmill injuries: a public health issue. *J Pediatr Surg.* 2007; **42:** 2086–2089.

**19.** Holland AJA, Cass DT. Driveway motor vehicle injuries in children. *Med J Aust.* 2000; **173:** 503.

**20.** Abeyasundara SL, Rajan V, Holland AJA, Harvey JG. The changing trend of paediatric burns in NSW. *ANZ J Surg.* 2008; 78(suppl 1): A13–A14.

**21.** Spallek M, Nixon J, Bain C, et al. Scald prevention campaigns: do they work? *J Burn Care Res.* 2007; **28**(2): 328–333.

**22.** Spinks A, Wasiak J, Cleland H, et al. Ten-year epidemiological study of pediatric burns in Canada. *J Burn Care Res.* 2008; **29**(3): 482–488.

**23.** Holland AJ. Pediatric burns: the forgotten trauma of childhood. *Can J Surg.* 2006; **49:** 272–277.

**24.** Brigham PA, McLoughlin E. Burn incidence and medical care use in the United States: estimates, trends, and data sources. *J Burn Care Rehabil.* 1996; **17:** 95–107.

**25.** Foglia RP, Moushey R, Meadows L, et al. Evolving treatment in a decade of pediatric burn care. *J Pediatr Surg.* 2004; **39:** 957–960.

**26.** Greenwood JE, Tee R, Jackson WL. Increasing numbers of admissions to the adult burns service at the Royal Adelaide Hospital 2001–2004. *ANZ J Surg.* 2007; **77:** 358–363.

**27.** Elisdottir R, Ludvigsson P, Einarsson O, et al. Paediatric burns in Iceland. Hospital admissions 1982–1995, a populations-based study. *Burns.* 1999; **25:** 149–151.

**28.** Eadie PA, Williams R, Dickson WA. Thirty-five years of paediatric scalds: are lessons being learned? *Br J Plast Surg.* 1995; **48:** 103–105.

**29.** Mashreky SR, Rahman A, Chowdhury SM, et al. Epidemiology of childhood burn: yield of largest community based injury survey in Bangladesh. *Burns.* 2007; **34**(6): 856–862.

**30.** Nguyen DQ, Tobin S, Dickson WA, et al. Infants under 1 year of age have a significant risk of burn injury. *Burns.* 2008; **34**(6): 863–867.

**31.** Udry JR. Why are males injured more frequently than females? *Inj Prev.* 1998; **4:** 94–95.

**32.** Chester DL, Jose RM, Aldlyami E, et al. Non-accidental burns in children—are we neglecting neglect? *Burns.* 2006; **32:** 222–228.

**33.** Poulos R, Hayen A, Finch C, et al. Area socioeconomic status and childhood injury morbidity in New South Wales, Australia. *Inj Prev.* 2007; **13:** 322–327.

**34.** Livingston A, Holland AJA, Dickson D. Language barriers and paediatric burns: does education make a difference? *Burns.* 2006; **32:** 482–486.

**35.** Carey V, Vimpani G, Taylor R. Childhood injury mortality in New South Wales: geographical and socio-economic variations. *J Paediatr Child Health.* 1993; **29:** 136–140.

**36.** Ng DK, Cherk SW, Yu WL, et al. Review of children with severe trauma or thermal injury requiring intensive care in a Hong Kong hospital: retrospective study. *Hong Kong Med J.* 2002; **8:** 82–86.

**37.** Benjamin D, Herndon DN. Special considerations of age: the pediatric burned patient. In: Herndon DN, ed. *Total Burn Care.* London, England: Saunders; **2002:** 427–438.

**38.** Rivara FP. Pediatric injury control in **1999:** where do we go from here? *Pediatrics.* 1999; **103:** 883–888.

**39.** Klein MB, Hollingworth W, Rivara FP, et al. Hospital costs associated with pediatric burn injury. *J Burn Care Res.* 2008; **29**(4): 632–637.

**40.** Casemix Technical Development Section. *Australian Refined Diagnosis Related Groups.* Canberra: Australian Government Department of Health and Ageing; 2006.

**41.** Sanchez JL, Pereperez SB, Bastida JL, et al. Cost-utility analysis applied to the treatment of burn patients in a specialized center. *Arch Surg.* 2007; **142:** 50–57.

**42.** Wallace AB. Early and first-aid treatment of burns. *Proc R Soc Med.* 1955; **48:** 440–442.

**43.** Barnett JS. Immediate surface cooling in treatment of burns. *Med J Aust.* 1968; **1:** 240–241.

**44.** McCormack RA, La Hei ER, Martin HC. First-aid management of minor burns in children: a prospective study of children presenting to the Children's Hospital at Westmead, Sydney. *Med J Aust.* 2003; **178:** 31–33.

**45.** Rea S, Wood F. Minor burn injuries in adults presenting to the regional burns unit in Western Australia: a prospective descriptive study. *Burns.* 2005; **31:** 1035–1040.

**46.** Lam NN, Dung NT. First aid and initial management for childhood burns in Vietnam—an appeal for public and continuing medical education. *Burns.* 2008; **34:** 67–70.

**47.** Rea S, Kuthubutheen J, Fowler B, et al. Burns first aid in Western Australia—do healthcare workers have the knowledge? *Burns.* 2005; **31:** 1029–1034.

**48.** Agache P, Makki S, Blanc D, et al. Skin care in childhood. *Curr Med Res Opin.* 1982; **7:** 15–22.

**49.** Dougherty J, Pucci P, Hemmila MR, et al. Survey of primary school educators regarding burn-risk behaviours and fire-safety education. *J Int Soc Burn Inj.* 2007; **33:** 472–476.

**50.** Rivara FP. Developmental and behavioral issues in childhood injury prevention. *J Dev Behav Pediatr.* 1995; **16:** 362–370.

**51.** Peleg K, Goldman S, Sikron F. Burns prevention programs for children: do they reduce burn-related hospitalizations? *Burns.* 2005; **31:** 347–350.

**52.** Cuttle L, Kempf M, Phillips GE, et al. A porcine deep dermal partial thickness burn model with hypertrophic scarring. *Burns.* 2006; **32:** 806–820.

**53.** Yuan J, Wu C, Holland AJA, et al. Assessment of cooling on an acute burn wound in a porcine model. *J Burn Care Res.* 2007; **28:** 514–520.

**54.** Savulescu J, Chalmers I, Blunt J. Are research ethics committees behaving unethically? Some suggestions for improving performance and accountability. *BMJ.* 1996; **313:** 1390–1393.

**55.** Nguyen NL, Gun RT, Sparnon AL, et al. The importance of immediate cooling—a case series of childhood burns in Vietnam. *Burns.* 2002; **28:** 173–176.

**56.** Skinner AM, Brown TL, Peat BG, et al. Reduced hospitalisation of burns patients following a multi-media campaign that increased adequacy of first aid treatment. *Burns.* 2004; **30:** 82–85.

**57.** King L, Thomas M, Gatenby K, et al. "First aid for scalds" campaign: reaching Sydney's Chinese, Vietnamese, and Arabic speaking communities. *Inj Prev.* 1999; **5:** 104–108.

**58.** Jandera V, Hudson DA, de Wet PM, et al. Cooling the burn wound: evaluation of different modalities. *Burns.* 2000; **26:** 265–270.

**59.** Bartlett N, Yuan J, Holland AJ, et al. Optimal duration of cooling for an acute scald contact burn injury in a porcine model. *J Burn Care Res.* 2008; **29**(5): 828–834.

**60.** Bartlett N, Tahtouh E, Holland AJA, Martin HCO, La Hei ER, Harvey JG. Delayed cooling of an acute burn injury in a porcine model: is it worthwhile? *J Burn Care Res.* 2009; **30**(4): 729–734.

**61.** Rivara FP, Aitken M. Prevention of injuries to children and adolescents. *Adv Pediatr.* 1998; **45:** 37–72.

**62.** Nguyen T. Cultural influences in the initial care of paediatric burn wounds administered by parents. *Aust N Z Burns Assoc Bull.* 1997; **20:** 11–13.

**63.** Allison K. The UK pre-hospital management of burn patients: current practice and the need for a standard approach. *Burns.* 2002; **28:** 135–142.

**64.** Price J. Burnaid. *Burns.* 1998; **24:** 80–82.

**65.** Cuttle L, Kempf M, Kravchuk O, et al. The efficacy of aloe vera, tea tree oil and saliva as first aid treatment for partial thickness burn injuries. *Burns.* 2008; **34**(8): 1176–1182.

**66.** Hudspith J, Rayatt S. First aid and treatment of minor burns. *Br Med J.* 2004; **328:** 1487–1489.

**67.** Heimbach DM, Engrav L, Grube B, et al. Burn depth: a review. *World J Surg.* 1992; **16:** 10.

**68.** Shakespeare PG. Looking at burn wounds: the A. B. Wallace Memorial Lecture 1991. *Burns.* 1992; **18:** 287–295.

**69.** Deitch EA, Wheelahan TM, Rose MP, Clothier J, Cotter J. Hypertrophic burn scars: analysis of variables. *J Trauma.* 1983; **23**(10): 895–898.

**70.** Spurr ED, Shakespeare PG. Incidence of hypertrophic scarring in burn-injured children. *Burns.* 1990; **16**(3): 179–181.

**71.** Holland AJ, Martin HC, Cass DT. Laser Doppler imaging prediction of burn wound outcome in children. *Burns.* 2002; **28:** 11–17.

**72.** Shakespeare PG. Prognostic indicators of burns. *Burns.* 2003; **29:** 105–106.

**73.** Ong YS, Samuel M, Song C. Meta-analysis of early excision of burns. *Burns.* 2006; **32:** 145–150.

**74.** Wood FM, Kolybab ML, Allen P. The use of cultured epithelial autograft in the treatment of major burn injuries: a critical review of the literature. *Burns.* 2006; **32:** 395–401.

**75.** Forage AV. The history of the classification of burns (diagnosis of depth). *Br J Plast Surg.* 1963; **16:** 239–242.

76. Zawacki BE. The natural history of reversible burn injury. *Surg Gynecol Obstet*. 1974; **139**: 867–872.

77. Isik S, Sahin U, Ilgan S, et al. Saving the zone of stasis in burns with recombinant tissue-type plasminogen activator (r-tPA): an experimental study in rats. *Burns*. 1998; **24**: 217–223.

78. Godina M, Derganc M, Bircic A. The reliability of clinical assessment of the depth of burns. *Burns*. 1977; **4**: 92–96.

79. Heimbach DM, Afromowitz MA, Engrav LH, et al. Burn depth estimation—man or machine. *J Trauma*. 1984; **24**: 373–378.

80. Phillips W, Mahairas E, Hunt D, et al. The epidemiology of childhood scalds in Brisbane. *Burns*. 1986; **12**: 343–350.

81. Desai MH, Rutan RL, Herndon DN. Conservative treatment of scald burns is superior to early excision. *J Burn Care Rehabil*. 1991; **12**: 482–484.

82. Bennett JE, Dingman RO. Evaluation of burn depth by the use of radioactive isotopes. *Plast Reconstr Surg*. 1957; **20**: 261.

83. Dingwall JA. A clinical test for differentiating second from third degree burns. *Ann Surg*. 1943; **118**: 427–429.

84. Niazi ZB, Essex TJ, Papini R, et al. New laser Doppler scanner, a valuable adjunct in burn depth assessment. *Burns*. 1993; **19**: 485–489.

85. Monstrey S, Hoeksema H, Verbelen J, et al. Assessment of burn depth and burn wound healing potential. *Burns*. 2008; **34**: 761–769.

86. Pham TN, Gibran NS, Heimbach DM. Evaluation of the burn wound: management decisions. In: Herndon DN, ed. *Total Burn Care*. Philadelphia, PA: Saunders Elsevier; 2007: 119–126.

87. Essex TJH, Byrne PO. A laser Doppler scanner for imaging blood flow in skin. *J Biomed Eng*. 1991; **13**: 189–194.

88. Watkins D, Holloway GA. An instrument to measure cutaneous blood flow using the Doppler shift of laser light. *IEEE Trans Biomed Eng*. 1978; **25**: 28–33.

89. Alsbjorn B, Micheels J, Sorensen B. Laser Doppler flowmetry measurements of superficial dermal, deep dermal and subdermal burns. *Scand J Plast Reconstr Surg*. 1984; **18**: 75–79.

90. Atiles L, Mileski W, Spann K, et al. Early assessment of pediatric burn wounds by laser Doppler flowmetry. *J Burn Care Rehabil*. 1995; **16**: 596–601.

91. Droog EJ, Steenbergen W, Sjoberg F. Measurement of depth of burns by laser Doppler perfusion imaging. *Burns*. 2001; **27**: 561–568.

92. Jeng JC, Bridgeman A, Shivnan L, et al. Laser Doppler imaging determines need for excision and grafting in advance of clinical judgment: a prospective blinded trial. *Burns*. 2003; **29**: 665–670.

93. Pape SA, Skouras CA, Byrne PO. An audit of the use of laser Doppler imaging (LDI) in the assessment of burns of intermediate depth. *Burns*. 2001; **27**: 233–239.

94. Yeong EK, Mann R, Goldberg M, et al. Improved accuracy of burn wound assessment using laser Doppler. *J Trauma*. 1996; **40**: 956–961.

95. Hemington-Gorse SJ. A comparison of laser Doppler imaging with other measurement techniques to assess burn depth. *J Wound Care*. 2005; **14**: 151–153.

96. Mileski WJ, Atiles L, Purdue G, et al. Serial measurements increase the accuracy of laser Doppler assessment of burn wounds. *J Burn Care Rehabil*. 2003; **24**: 187–191.

97. Renshaw A, Childs C. Assessment of burn depth in children using laser Doppler imaging. British Burns Association Annual Scientific Meeting; April 25–27, 2001; Essex, England.

98. La Hei ER, Holland AJA, Martin HCO. Laser Doppler imaging of paediatric burns: can burn wound outcome be predicted independent of clinical examination? *Burns*. 2006; **32**: 550–553.

99. Holland AJA, Ward D, Farrell B. The influence of burn wound dressings on laser Doppler imaging assessment of a standardized cutaneous injury model. *J Burn Care Res*. 2007; **28**: 871–878.

100. McGill DJ, Taggart I. Tattoos: a confounding issue in laser Doppler imaging of burn depth. *Burns*. 2005; **31**: 657–659.

101. Miller K, Bucolo S, Patterson E, et al. The emergence of multi-modal distraction as a paediatric pain management tool. *Stud Health Technol Inform*. 2008; **132**: 287–292.

102. Cuttle L, Naidu S, Mill J, et al. A retrospective cohort study of Acticoat versus Silvazine in a paediatric population. *Burns*. 2007; **33**: 701–707.

103. McGill DJ, Sorensen K, MacKay IR, et al. Assessment of burn depth: a prospective, blinded comparison of laser Doppler imaging and videomicroscopy. *Burns*. 2007; **33**: 833–842.

104. Pape SA, Byrne PO. Burn depth measurement by laser Doppler imaging (LDI) reduces the surgical workload of a burn unit. 9th Congress of the European Burns Association; September 12–15, 2001; Lyon, France.

105. Kim LHC, Ward D, Lam L, Holland AJA. The impact of Laser Doppler imaging on time to grafting decisions in pediatric burns. *J Burn Care Res*. 2010; **31**(2): 328–332.

106. Pereira C, Murphy K, Herndon D. Outcome measures in burn care. Is mortality dead? *Burns*. 2004; **30**: 761–771.

107. Sheridan RL. Burns. *Crit Care Med*. 2002; **30**: S500–S514.

108. Bombaro KM, Engrav LH, Carrougher GJ, et al. What is the prevalence of hypertrophic scarring following burns? *Burns*. 2003; **29**: 299–302.

109. Rosenberg M, Blakeney P, Robert R, Thomas C, Holz C, Meyer W. Quality of life of young adults who survived pediatric burns. *J Burn Care Rehabil*. 2006; **27**(6): 773–778.

110. Lee JO, Herndon DN. The pediatric burned patient. In: Herndon DN, ed. *Total Burn Care*. Philadelphia, PA: Saunders Elsevier; 2007: 485–495.

111. Cope O, Langohr JL, Moore FD, et al. Expeditious care of full-thickness burn wounds by surgical excision and grafting. *Ann Surg*. 1947; **125**: 1–22.

112. Sjoberg F, Danielsson P, Andersson L, et al. Utility of an intervention scoring system in documenting effects of changes in burn treatment. *Burns*. 2000; **26**: 553–559.

113. Tompkins RG, Remensnyder JP, Burke JF, et al. Significant reductions in mortality for children with burn injuries through the use of prompt eschar excision. *Ann Surg.* 1988; **208**: 577–585.

114. Engrav LH, Heimbach DM, Reus JL, et al. Early excision and grafting vs. nonoperative treatment of burns of indeterminant depth: a randomized prospective study. *J Trauma.* 1983; **23**: 1001–1004.

115. Cubison TC, Pape SA, Parkhouse N. Evidence for the link between healing time and the development of hypertrophic scars (HTS) in paediatric burns due to scald injury. *Burns.* 2006; **32**: 992–999.

116. Janzekovic Z. A new concept in the early excision and immediate grafting of burns. *J Trauma.* 1970; **10**: 1103–1108.

117. Muller M, Gahankari D, Herndon DN. Operative wound management. In: Herndon DN, ed. *Total Burn Care.* Philadelphia, PA: Saunders Elsevier; **2007**: 177–195.

118. Wright JB, Lam K, Burrell RE. Wound management in an era of increasing bacterial antibiotic resistance: a role for topical silver treatment. *Am J Infect Control.* 1998; **26**: 572–577.

119. Burrell RE. A scientific perspective on the use of topical silver preparations. *Ostomy Wound Manage.* 2003; **49**: 19–24.

120. Tredget EE, Shankowsky HA, Groeneveld A, et al. A matched-pair, randomized study evaluating the efficacy and safety of Acticoat silver-coated dressing for the treatment of burn wounds. *J Burn Care Rehabil.* 1998; **19**: 531–537.

121. Varas RP, O'Keeffe T, Namias N, et al. A prospective, randomized trial of Acticoat versus silver sulfadiazine in the treatment of partial-thickness burns: which method is less painful? *J Burn Care Rehabil.* 2005; **26**: 344–347.

122. Peters DA, Verchere C. Healing at home: comparing cohorts of children with medium-sized burns treated as outpatients with in-hospital applied Acticoat to those children treated as inpatients with silver sulfadiazine. *J Burn Care Res.* 2006; **27**: 198–201.

123. Fong J, Wood F. Nanocrystalline silver dressings in wound management: a review. *Int J Nanomedicine.* 2006; **1**: 441–449.

124. Nadworny PL, Wang J, Tredget EE, et al. Anti-inflammatory activity of nanocrystalline silver in a porcine contact dermatitis model. *Nanomedicine.* 2008; **4**: 241–251.

125. Klein MB, Hunter S, Heimbach DM, et al. The Versajet water dissector: a new tool for tangential excision. *J Burn Care Rehabil.* 2005; **26**: 483–487.

126. Cubison TCS, Pape SA, Jeffery SLA. Dermal preservation using the Versajet hydrosurgery system for debridement of paediatric burns. *Burns.* 2006; **32**: 714–720.

127. Gravante G, Delogu D, Esposito G, et al. Versajet hydrosurgery versus classic escharectomy for burn debridement: a prospective randomized trial. *J Burn Care Res.* 2007; **28**: 720–724.

128. Kimble RM, Mott J, Joethy J. Versajet hydrosurgery system for the debridement of paediatric burns. *Burns.* 2008; **34**: 297–298.

129. Bucala R, Spiegel LA, Chesney J, et al. Circulating fibrocytes define a new leukocyte subpopulation that mediates tissue repair. *Mol Med.* 1994; **1**: 71–81.

130. La Rue AC, Ogawa M. Hematopoietic origin of fibrocytes. In: Bucala R, ed. *Fibrocytes: New Insights Into Tissue Repair and Systemic Fibroses.* Hackensack, NJ: World Scientific; **2006**: 61–74.

131. Abe R, Donnelly SC, Peng T, et al. Peripheral blood fibrocytes: differentiation pathway and migration to wound sites. *J Immunol.* 2001; **166**: 7556–7562.

132. Quan TE, Cowper S, Wu SP, et al. Circulating fibrocytes: collagen-secreting cells of the peripheral blood. *Int J Biochem Cell Biol.* 2004; **36**: 598–606.

133. Wang JF, Wu Y, Medina A, et al. The role of fibrocytes in post-burn hypertrophic scarring. In: Bucala R, ed. *Fibrocytes: New Insights into Tissue Repair and Systemic Fibroses.* Hackensack, New Jersey: World Scientific Publishing Co Pte Ltd; **2007**: 75–104.

134. Yang L, Scott PG, Dodd C, et al. Identification of fibrocytes in postburn hypertrophic scar. *Wound Repair Regen.* 2005; **13**: 398–404.

135. Yang L, Scott PG, Giuffre J, et al. Peripheral blood fibrocytes from burn patients: identification and quantification of fibrocytes in adherent cells cultured from peripheral blood mononuclear cells. *Lab Invest.* 2002; **82**: 1183–1192.

136. Ghahary A, Shen YJ, Scott PG, et al. Enhanced expression of mRNA for transforming growth factor-ß, type I and type III procollagen in human post-burn hypertrophic scar tissues. *J Lab Clin Med.* 1993; **122**: 465–473.

137. Quan TE, Cowper SE, Bucala R. The role of circulating fibrocytes in fibrosis. *Curr Rheumatol Rep.* 2006; **8**: 145–150.

138. Werner S, Grose R. Regulation of wound healing by growth factors and cytokines. *Physiol Rev.* 2003; **83**: 835–870.

139. Holland AJ, Tarran SL, Medbury HJ, et al. Are fibrocytes present in pediatric burn wounds? *J Burn Care Res.* 2008; **29**: 619–626.

140. Demetriou M, Binkert C, Sukhu B, et al. Fetuin/$\alpha_2$-HS glycoprotein is a transforming growth factor-$\alpha$ type II receptor mimic and cytokine antagonist. *J Biol Chem.* 1996; **271**: 12755–12761.

# Long-Term Outcomes After Burn Injury in Children

Kathryn Butler, MD

Robert Sheridan, MD

## Introduction

An estimated 1 million American children suffer burns annually. Of this number, 3% of patients sustain injuries to greater than 70% of their total body surface area (TBSA).[1] Fifty years ago, only half of children who suffered burns greater than 50% TBSA survived the acute hospitalization period. With the innovation of early excision and grafting, topical antibiotics, and resuscitation algorithms, now half of children with > 85% TBSA burns survive.[2] As advances in burn care over the past 20 years have prolonged patient survival, the quality of life of these patients and the long-term sequelae of their injuries and the therapies they receive have fallen under scrutiny.

## Physical Disability

Research on the long-term outcomes of pediatric burn patients focus on 2 endpoints: functional disability and psychosocial development. With regard to the first category, the current data suggest that with appropriate rehabilitation therapy, the majority of severely burned children return to an age-appropriate level of activity. This finding was first suggested by Herndon et al in 1986, in one of the earliest reports in the literature.[3] In this retrospective study of 12 children surviving > 80% TBSA burns, whom the group examined at a mean of 1.5 years after discharge (range 0.8

to 2.8 years), patients demonstrated deficiencies in fine motor skills as well as growth retardation, heat intolerance, hyperesthesias, and joint pain. Despite these deficits, 50% of the patients studied were completely independent in their activities of daily living. The majority attended all-day age-appropriate school programs and participated in most physical education activities.

Recent studies have echoed these findings from the 1980s. In 2007, Baker et al found that in young adult survivors of severe burns seen in long-term follow-up, 26% had deficiencies in wrist strength, particularly with flexion.[2] Despite these impairments, 99% of patients were independent in areas of hygiene and home management skills. Feeding skills were more varied, but even for this category, 88% of patients demonstrated complete independence.

In 1998, Sheridan et al at the Shriners Hospital in Boston closely examined upper extremity fine motor skills in long-term survivors of burns.[4] They reported results of a 10-year retrospective review of 495 children sustaining 698 hand burns. The patients underwent ranging and splinting throughout their hospital stay as well as prompt sheet autograft closure and axial pin fixation and flaps when indicated. They received long-term follow-up, hand therapy, and reconstructive surgery and were evaluated for at least 1 year and for an average of > 5 years at an outpatient burns clinic. Data revealed that with appropriate splinting and rehabilitation methods, the majority of patients had excellent functional results. Ninety-seven percent of patients who required no surgery and 85% who underwent autografting alone maintained completely normal function on follow-up. Of the patients in these categories with functional deficits, only 1.5% and 6%, respectively, could not perform activities of daily living (ADLs). Patients who underwent bone reconstruction—15% of the total population studied—were an exception to this trend, with significantly worse impairments and only 20% with normal function. However, even 50% of these patients could perform ADLs.

A second study by the same research group evaluated 83 patients admitted with > 70% TBSA burns between the years of 1969 to 1992 and used the SF-36 quality of life assessment tool to measure 8 domains: general health, physical functioning, social functioning, physical role, emotional role, mental health, energy/vitality, and bodily pain. The study revealed that patients who followed up consistently in a multidisciplinary burn clinic for 2 years had higher physical functioning.[1] While length of stay and age at injury were not statistically significant, early reintegration into age-appropriate activities as well as consistent clinic visits had positive correlations with domain scores. Most children had a quality of life comparable with age-matched controls in the general population. Such data highlight the impact of rehabilitation and long-term multidisciplinary care on patients' motor skills and functioning.

## PSYCHOLOGICAL IMPAIRMENT

Difficulties in psychosocial adjustment despite independence in age-appropriate activities recurs as a theme in the literature. In their study in 1986, Herndon et al reported that one-third of patients they evaluated demonstrated excessive fear, regression, and neurotic and somatic complaints.[3] The parents of these patients confirmed these findings, observing in their children moderate to severe problems with body image, self-esteem, anxiety level, fears, and interpersonal relationships.

Baker et al noted similar pathology in 2007. In their evaluation of 83 patients aged 18 to 28 years who were burned > 30% TBSA at least 2 years before the time of their assessment, 45% of patients had at least 1 Axis I diagnosis on follow-up.[2] Anxiety disorders demonstrated the highest prevalence, at 31%, and overall the prevalence of current and lifetime psychiatric diagnoses in these patients were twice those seen nationally. One year later, this same group evaluated 80 young adult survivors of pediatric burns at least 2 years postburn. Thirty percent of the survivors experienced moderate to severe psychological and social difficulties during the recovery process.[6]

Interestingly, the extant data demonstrate little correlation between these psychosocial difficulties and the physical challenges that patients face. For example, in 2008 Baker et al found that mobility, stability, strength, and ADL scores had no correlation with psychological findings in the 80 patients whom they studied.[6] SF-36 scores in this study suggested that patients considered their physical function comparable to that of the general population. Scores on a different survey, the QLQ (a composite quality of life measure), indicated that patients rated their quality of life lower than the reference group to a degree that was statistically significant. Such data reveal the importance of long-term psychological counseling in pediatric burn patients and suggest rehabilitation should include routine assessment for emotional disturbances and anxiety disorders.

## THE ROLE OF THE FAMILY

In addition to active and early rehabilitation, a supportive family environment critically influences patients' long-term recovery. In their research from 2000, Sheridan et al reported that the functional status of the family predicted a higher physical role in the studied patients. "Because a child's outcome is so significantly affected by the degree of family function," they concluded, "it is important that family services be an integral part of acute management and aftercare."[1] Blakeney et al mirrored this conclusion in 1988 when they examined 38 young adults who had suffered > 40% TBSA burns.[5] Most subjects in the study were in school or employed and were within normative limits on measures of their psychological adjustment. However, those who did have psychological disturbances differed from their peers in their perceptions of family cohesiveness and independence. Similarly, 20 years later, Baker et al also noted that parent factors, such as depression, anxiety, and coping processes, had a significant impact in the functional outcomes of children 6 months following burn injury.[6] Psychological and physical recovery thus appear directly linked to a patient's family environment, and the functional status of the family should be assessed on an outpatient basis to ensure optimal recovery and development for pediatric burn patients.

## HYPOXIC BRAIN INJURY

Patients who suffer hypoxic injury represent a unique population at risk for long-term cognitive impairment. In 2005, Rosenberg et al published a 20-year case-control study that compared 39 children with hypoxic brain injury (defined as $PaO_2 < 80$ or $CO > 10\%$) to 21 controls matched for age, % TBSA, and time of injury. Patients were evaluated for a mean period of 4.5 years postburn, with a range of 1 to 18 years. One-third of patients in this study who survived from the hypoxic group had cognitive difficulties on follow-up.[7]

The degree of deficit correlated directly with the severity of the event and the area of the brain injured. In the patients who suffered burns without hypoxic injury, only 1 had cognitive impairments, although several had emotional and behavioral problems. Explicit testing of the hypoxic-injury patients unveiled deficits in attention, memory, language, and speech. Patients in this group also demonstrated anxiety disorders and emotional disturbances, but when paired with the control group, the difference was not statistically significant. In light of their findings, Rosenberg et al recommended that in addition to the rehabilitation and counseling critical for all severely burned pediatric patients, patients who suffer hypoxic brain injury should undergo routine neuropsychological assessment to assist them in their cognitive development.

## SEX-SPECIFIC SEQUELAE

With regard to burn rehabilitation, data imply discrepancies between the sexes. From a physiologic standpoint, in the acute period, girls demonstrate decreased hypermetabolism and increased anabolic hormones compared to boys, with shorter average ICU stays. A study in 2007 by Jeschke et al, however, revealed that this benefit does not persist long-term. In their examination of patients evaluated months after discharge, boys and girls demonstrated similar growth curves, suggesting equal normalization of metabolism for both sexes.[8] Psychosocial development, meanwhile, maintains disparate patterns. In 2007, Baker et al reported that male young adult burn survivors reported more somatic complaints than females on long-term follow-up, and the studied female patients reported more externalizing and total problems than their male counterparts.[2] Sheridan et al also suggested differences in their study of 2000; females scored higher than males in the domains of general health, physical functioning, and physical role, while males scored higher in the domain of emotional role.[1] The significance of these findings is uncertain, and further study is required to elucidate whether or not rehabilitation should target goals specific to male and female patients.

## THE NEXT PHASE

As survival from massive burns is only a recent phenomenon, outcomes research in such patients is in its infancy. The information is of great potential value as focused efforts to enhance these outcomes may make the difference between many decades of dependency and depression or many decades of productivity and contentment. Knowledge of the expected outcomes, and of the factors impacting those outcomes, might allow for directed interventions to improve long-term function, appearance, and emotional health of children suffering severe burns.

## REFERENCES

**1.** Sheridan RL, Hinson MI, Liang MH, et al. Long-term outcome of children surviving massive burns. *JAMA*. 2000; **283**(1): 69–73.

**2.** Baker CP, Russell WJ, Meyer W, Blakeney P. Physical and psychological rehabilitation outcomes for young adults burned as children. *Arch Phys Med Rehabil*. 2007; **88**(2): S57–S64.

**3.** Herndon DN, LeMaster J, Beard, S, et al. The quality of life after major thermal injury in children: an analysis of 12 survivors with > = 80% TBSA, 70% 3rd degree burns. *J Trauma*. 1986; **26**(7): 609–619.

**4.** Sheridan RL, Baryza MJ, Pessina MA, et al. Acute hand burns in children: management and long-term outcome based on a 10-year experience with 698 injured hands. *Ann Surg*. 1998; **229**(4): 558–564.

**5.** Blakeney P, Herndon DN, Desai MH, Beard S, Wales-Seale P. Long-term psychosocial adjustment following burn injury. *J Burn Care Rehabil*. 1988; **9**: 661–665.

**6.** Baker CP, Rosenberg M, Mossberg KA, et al. Relationships between the quality of life questionnaire and the SF-36 among young adults burned as children. *Burns*. 2008; **34**: 1163–1168.

**7.** Rosenberg M, Robertson C, Murphy KD, et al. Neuropsychological outcomes of pediatric burn patients who sustain hypoxic episodes. *Burns*. 2005; **31**: 883–889.

**8.** Jeschke MG, Przkora R, Suman OE, et al. Sex differences in the long-term outcome after a severe thermal injury. *Shock*. 2007; **27**(5): 461–465.

# INDEX